Lippincott's

Nursing Procedures

SIXTH EDITION

Lippincott's

Nursing Procedures

SIXTH EDITION

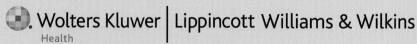

Wolters Kluwer | Lippincott Williams & Wilkins
Health

Philadelphia • Baltimore • New York • London
Buenos Aires • Hong Kong • Sydney • Tokyo

Staff

Publisher
Jay Abramovitz

Chief Nurse
Judith A. Schilling McCann, RN, MSN

Clinical Director
Joan M. Robinson, RN, MSN

Clinical Project Manager
Melissa Morris, RN, MBE, JD

Clinical Editors
Kate Stout, RN, MSN, CCRN
Mary Ann Foley, RN, BSN

Product Director
David Moreau

Senior Product Manager
Diane Labus

Editor
Margaret Eckman

Copy Editor
Debra Share

Editorial Assistants
Megan L. Aldinger, Karen J. Kirk, Jeri O'Shea, Linda K. Ruhf

Art Director
Elaine Kasmer

Design
Joseph John Clark, MW Design (Cover)

Design Assistant
Karen Kappe Nugent

Vendor Manager
Cynthia Rudy

Senior Manufacturing Coordinator
Beth J. Welsh

Production Services
Aptara, Inc.

Library of Congress Cataloging-in-Publication Data

Lippincott's nursing procedures.—6th ed.
   p. ; cm.
   Nursing procedures
   Includes bibliographical references and index.
   ISBN 978-1-4511-4633-2 (alk. paper)
   I. Lippincott Williams & Wilkins.   II. Title: Nursing procedures.
   [DNLM: 1. Nursing Care. WY 100.1]

   610.73–dc23   2012021642

Contents

D

 E

 F

G

H

Contributors and consultants

Deborah Hutchinson Allen, RN, MSN, AOCNP, APRN-BC, FNP
Clinical Nurse Specialist and Nurse Practitioner
Duke University Health System
Durham, N.C.

Anna Alvarez, RN, MSN, ANCC
Program Manager
Cardinal Hill Rehabilitation Hospital
Lexington, Ky.

Catherine Amero, RN, MSN/Ed, CRNI
Infusion Therapy
Milford Regional Medical Center
Milford, Mass.

Lisa M. Anderson, RN, MSN, APRN, CCNS, CCRN
Nurse Manager—MSN
Franklin Woods Community Hospital
Johnson City, Tenn.

Peggy D. Baikie, RN, DNP, NNP-BC, PNP-BC
Nurse Practitioner/Program Manager
Denver Health
Denver, Col.

Lynda K. Ball, RN, MSN, CNN
Quality Improvement Director
Northwest Renal Network
Seattle, Wash.

Robin Bankhead, CRNP, MS, CS
Nurse Practitioner, Department of Surgery
Temple University Hospital
Philadelphia, Pa.

M. Brucene Bechtel, RN, MSN, NCI, PMHCNS
Psychiatric Clinical Nurse Specialist
Gaston Memorial Hospital—CaroMont Health
Gastonia, N.C.

Lisa Ann Behrend, RN, MSN, AC-CNS, CCRN-CSC
Critical Care Nurse
Fountain Valley Regional Medical Center
Fountain Valley, Calif.

Dina Salvatore BenDavid, RN, MSN, APRN, NP-C
Surgical Services Nurse
Martha's Vineyard Hospital
Oak Bluffs, Mass.

Lorraine Bigony, RN, BSN, CNOR, ONC
Nurse Manager, Perioperative Services
Aria Health, Bucks County Campus
Langhorne, Pa.

Michele Blacksberg, RN, BSN, MS
Independent Contractor, Freelance Health Writer
Scottsdale, Ariz.

Donna Bond, RN-BC, DNP, AE-C, CCNS
Pulmonary Clinical Nurse Specialist
Carilion Clinic
Roanoke, Va.

Julie Calvery Carman, RN, MS, APN, FNP-BC
Nurse Practitioner
Van Buren Family Medical Clinic
Van Buren, Ariz.

Jennifer Chaikin, RN-BC, MSN/MHA, CCRN
Director, Educational Initiatives
Gannet Healthcare Group
Falls Church, Va.

Hannah Chatillon, RN, MSN, CRNI
Education Specialist
Yale New Haven Hospital
New Haven, Conn.

Martha D. Cobb, RN, MS, MEd, ACNS-BC, CWOCN
Nurse Consultant
Tucson, Ariz.

Laura A. Conklin, RN, MSN, MSA, CNE, CWS, Dip. AAWM, FCCWS, LNCE, ONC
Professor
Wayne County Community College District—Northwest Campus
Detroit, Mich.

Kathleen Conn, RN, MSN
Nurse Educator
Stevens-Henager College
Murray, Utah
Medical-Surgical and Psychiatric Nurse
Duke University Health System
Durham Regional Hospital
Durham, N.C.

Laura M. Criddle, RN, PhD, CNRN, FAEN
Clinical Nurse Specialist
The Laurelwood Group
Scappoose, Ore.

Evelyn Dean, RN, MSN, ACNS-BC, CCRN
Clinical Nurse Specialist
Heart Failure Department
Saint Luke's Hospital of Kansas City
Kansas City, Mo.

Scott DeBoer, RN, MSN, CCRN, CEN, CFRN, CPEN
Flight Nurse
University of Chicago Hospitals
Chicago, Ill.

Sylvia Dlugokinski-Plenz, RN, MSN, ANP-BC, CNRN
Nurse Practitioner
Family Choice
Depew, N.Y.

Kate Douglass, RN, MS, APN,C, CRNI
President
Performance Strategies, LLC
Ridgewood, N.J.

Shelba Durston, RN, MSN, CCRN
Nursing Instructor
San Joaquin Delta College
Stockton, Calif.

Fran Feltovich, RN, MBA, CIC, CPHQ
Project Director, Business
    Practices/Regulatory Compliance
The Methodist Hospital
Houston, Tex.

Valerie Gail Fisher, BA, RRT
Respiratory Therapist
Lehigh Valley Health Network
Allentown, Pa.

Jan Foecke, RN, MS, ONC
Director of Programs
National Association of Orthopaedic
    Nurses
Chicago, Ill.

Ellie Z. Franges, CRNP, MSN, CNRN, CRNP
Nurse Practitioner Neurosurgery
Main Line Health
Paoli, Pa.

Debra L. Furtado, RN-BC, BSN, MA, MSN(C)
Facility Administrator, CEO
DaVita Dialysis
Brookline, Mass.

Gayle K. Gilmore, RN, MA, MIS, CIC
Consultant
Duluth, Minn.

Sheryl Gilson, RN, MSN
Clinical Specialist
Memorial Regional Hospital
Hollywood, Fla.

Molly Groban, RN, MS, MAEd, CCRN, CEN
Director of Education
JFK Memorial Hospital
Indio, Calif.

Sandy Hamilton, RN, BSN, MEd, CHPN
Triage Nurse, Case Manager II
Nathan Adelson Hospice
Pahrump, Nev.

Carey Heck, RN, MSN, ACNP-CS, CCRN, CNRN
Clinical Specialist
Thomas Jefferson University Hospital
Philadelphia, Pa.

Kathleen M. Hill, RN, MSN, CCNS-CSC
Clinical Nurse Specialist, Surgical
    Intensive Care Unit
Cleveland Clinic
Cleveland, Ohio

Christine Hoener, RN, ADN
Lead Charge Nurse
Cape Fear Valley Behavioral Health Care
Fayetteville, N.C.

Karin Hoffmann, RN, ADN, TNCC
Staff Nurse
CHRISTUS Hospital–St. Elizabeth
Beaumont, Tex.

Timothy L. Hudson, RN, PhD,
CCRN, FACHE
Battalion Commander
264th Medical Battalion
Fort Sam Houston, Tex.

Priscilla Huggins, RN, PhD(C)
Adjunct Faculty
Miller-Motte Community College
Fayetteville, N.C.

Gretchen Hunt, RN, MSN, CNS-BC
Director ICU/PCU/MS
Texas Health Resources Harris
    Hospital—Southwest
Ft. Worth, Tex.

Julia Isen, RN, MS, FNP-C
Assistant Clinical Professor/Family Nurse
    Practitioner
University of California, San Francisco
San Francisco, Calif.

Lois Jackson, RN, MSN, CEN
Intensive Care Director
University Physicians Hospital
Tucson, Ariz.

Jennifer L. Jennings, RN, MS, FNP-BC
Clinical Assistant Professor
University at Buffalo
Buffalo, N.Y.

Fiona S. Johnson, RN, MSN, CCRN
Clinical Education Consultant
Memorial Health University Medical
    Center
Savannah, Ga.

Nancy Banfield Johnson, RN, MSN
Nurse Manager
Kendal at Ithaca
Ithaca, N.Y.

Christine Kennedy, RN, MSN
Hospital Clinical Instructor
VA Connecticut Healthcare Systems
West Haven, Conn.

Daphne Lee Knill, RN, BS, MAEd
Hospital Staff Educator
Sentara Obici Hospital
Suffolk, Va.

Merita Konstantacos, RN, MSN, CCNS
Staff Nurse CVSICU
Aultman Hospital
Canton, Ohio

Charles Kunkle III, RN, MSN, BC-NA,
CCRN, CEN
Director of Emergency/Pediatric
    Services
St. Mary Medical Center
Langhorne, Pa.

Veronica W. Lacambra, RN, MSN
Staff Nurse
Christus Schumpert Health System
Shreveport, La.

Patricia Lemelle-Wright, RN, MS
Staff Nurse
University of Chicago Hospitals
Chicago, Ill.
Associate Director of Nursing
Dabney University School of Nursing
Hammond, Ind.

Sandra S. Lucas, RN, MS, CCRN, NE-BC
Director of Education
Kent Hospital
Warwick, R.I.

Margaret Malone, RN, MN, CCRN
Clinical Nurse Specialist
St. John Medical Center
Longview, Wash.

Fran McAdams, RN, MSN, AOCNS
Clinical Director, Infusion Services
Fox Chase Cancer Center
Philadelphia, Pa.

Julia McAvoy, RN, MSN, CCRN
Director, Quality Management and Staff
    RN in the Critical Care Unit
The Washington Hospital
Washington, Pa.

Lorraine Micheletti, RN, BSN, MA, CCRN
Nurse Manager, ICU and CCU
Lower Bucks Hospital
Bristol, Pa.

Deanna R. Miller, RN, MSN/Ed, HCE
Manager, Critical Care and Staff
  Development
UH Geneva Medical Center
Geneva, Ohio

Pamela Moody, RN, DNP, PhD, CRNP
Nurse Administrator
Alabama Department of Public Health
Tuscaloosa, Ala.

Robin Nelson, RN, MSN/Ed, CRNI, NE-BC
Director of Education and Clinical Practice
Morgan Hospital and Medical Center
Martinsville, Ind.

Patricia A. Normandin, RN, DNP, CEN,
CPEN, CPN
Emergency Department Staff Nurse
Tufts Medical Center
Nursing Instructor
Northeastern University
Boston, Mass.

Jennifer M. Pedretti, RN, MSN
Assistant Clinical Manager, RN
Advocate Christ Medical Center
Oak Lawn, Ill.

Cathy Peterson, RN, CNOR
Clinical Nurse Educator
St. James Hospital and Medical Centers
Chicago Heights, Ill.

Rexann G. Pickering, RN, MSN, PhD, CIM, CIP
Administrator, Human Protection
Methodist Healthcare
Memphis, Tenn.

Susan Poole, RN, BSN, MS, CIC,
CNSN, CRNI
Infection Prevention Coordinator
Haven Behavioral Health Care
Remuda Ranch
Wickenburg, Ariz.

Michelle C. Quigel, RN, BSN, CWOCN
Certified Wound, Ostomy, Continence
  Nurse Specialist
Holy Redeemer Hospital
Meadowbrook, Pa.

Anabel Quintanar, RN, MSN, PHN, CEN
Nurse Care Manager
VA Greater Los Angeles Healthcare
  System, Santa Maria CBOS
Santa Maria, Calif.
Nursing Supervisor
Lompoc Valley Medical Center
Lompoc, Calif.

Cheryl L. Rader, RN, BSN, CCRN-CSC
Registered Nurse IV
Saint Luke's Hospital
Kansas City, Mo.

Teofila U. Rafael, RN, MSN
Clinical Practitioner/Educator
Northshore University Health
  System–Glenbrook Hospital
Glenview, Ill.

Susan M. Raymond, RN, MSN, CCRN
Deputy Commander for Nursing
  (Chief Nursing Officer)
Weed Army Hospital
Fort Irwin, Calif.

Charles W. Reick, MS, RRT
Consultant
Greater Baltimore Medical Center
Towson, Md.

Stephen Risch, RN, MSN, CCNS, CCRN
Clinical Educator
Georgetown University Hospital
Washington, D.C.

Noraliza Salazar, RN, MSN, CCNS
Critical Care Nurse Educator
UCSF Medical Center
San Francisco, Calif.

Laura S. Savage, RN, MSN, PCCN
Cardiothoracic Clinical Nurse
  Specialist
Virginia Commonwealth University
  Health System
Richmond, Va.

Donna Scemons, RN, PhD, CNS,
CWOCN, FNP-BC
President
Healthcare Systems, Inc.
Castaic, Calif.

Mary Clare A. Schafer, RN, MS, CRRN, ONC
Clinical Nurse Educator, Orthopaedics
Kennedy Health System
Turnersville, N.J.

Louise Schwabenbauer, RN, MSN, MEd
Nursing Instructor
University of Pittsburgh
Titusville, Pa.

S. Kay Sedlak, RN, MS, CEN, FAEN
Faculty/Laboratory Manager
Western Nevada College
Carson City, Nev.

Alexander John Siomko, RN, MSN,
APRN-BC, CRNP
Lead Nurse Practitioner
Primary Home Care
Elkins Park, Pa.

Jody K. Smith, RN, MSN, CNE, FNP-C
Family Nurse Practitioner
Greystone Medical Clinic
Cabot, Ark.

Jennifer A. Smoltz, RN, MSN, ACNP-BC,
CWOCN
Nurse Practitioner
University of Virginia Health System
Charlottesville, Va.

Dawn M. Specht, RN, PhD, CCNS,
CCRN, CEN, PCCN
Advanced Practice Nurse/Clinical Nurse
  Specialist, Emergency
AtlantiCare Regional Medical Center—
  City Campus
Atlantic City, N.J.

Gretta M. Tarter, RN, MSN, FNP-C
Medical-Surgical Clinical Educator
Lake Cumberland Regional Hospital
Somerset, Ky.

Allison J. Terry, RN, PhD
Assistant Professor
Auburn University at Montgomery School
  of Nursing
Mongtomery, Ala.

Genevieve M. Thul, RN, MSN, PhD(C)
Student
Medical University of South Carolina
Charleston, S.C.

Peggy Thweatt, RN, MSN
Nursing Instructor
Medical Careers Institute, LPN Program
Newport News, Va.

Leigh Ann Trujillo, BSN, RN
Nurse Educator
St. James Hospital and Health Centers
Olympia Fields, Ill.

Laura J. Tucco, RN, MSN, APN (CNS/NP), CEN
Family Nurse Practitioner
Minute Clinic
Minneapolis, Minn.

Rebecca Unruh, RN, MSN
Manager, Nursing Education
North Kansas City Hospital
North Kansas City, Mo.

Linda A. Valdiri, RN, MSN, CCNS
Assistant Deputy Commander for
  Nursing
Weed Army Community Hospital
Fort Irwin, Calif.

Barbara Wyand Walker, RN, BSN, CIC
Infection Control and Employee Health
  Coordinator
Greenbrier Valley Medical Center
Ronceverte, W. Va.

Patricia Weiskittel, RN, MSN, ACNP, CNN
Renal/Hypertension Nurse Practitioner
Cincinnati VA Medical Center
Cincinnati, Ohio

Nancy A. Welch, RN, BSN, MSEd
Staff Development Coordinator
The Ohio State University Medical Center
Columbus, Ohio

Karen Wilkinson, RN, MN, ARNP
Pediatric Nurse Practitioner
Seattle Children's Hospital
Seattle, Wash.

Cynthia A. Worley, RN, BSN, CWOCN
Wound, Ostomy and Continence Nurse
The University of Texas MD Anderson
  Cancer Center
Houston, Tex.

Janice Zagari, RN, MSN
Unit Director
University of Pittsburgh Medical Center
Pittsburgh, Pa.

Dawn M. Zwick, RN, CRNP
Assistant Professor/Adult Nurse
  Practitioner
Kent State University
North Canton, Ohio

How to use this book

As a nurse, you're expected to know how to perform or assist with literally hundreds of procedures. From the most basic patient care, to complex treatments, to assisting with the most intricate surgical procedures, you need to be able to carry out nursing procedures with skill and confidence. But mastering so many procedures is a tall order.

Newly updated with the latest evidence-based research, this sixth edition of *Lippincott's Nursing Procedures* provides step-by-step guidance on the most commonly performed nursing procedures you need to know, making it the ideal resource for providing the professional hands-on care your patients deserve.

The A to Zs of organization

With over 400 procedures covered in detail, the current edition of *Lippincott's Nursing Procedures* seeks to present this wealth of information in the most efficient way possible, resulting in a new way to organize the book. Previous editions organized procedures into such categories as fundamental procedures, body systems, and other types of procedures (such as psychiatric care). But with the proliferation in the number and types of procedures you need to understand, such an organization can become difficult to manage.

To address this, the sixth edition has organized all procedures into an easy-to-use A-to-Z listing, making the book faster and easier to use than ever. Now when you need to find a particular procedure quickly, you simply look it up by name. No need to scan through the table of contents. No time lost turning to the index, looking for the name of the procedure you want, and then finding the right page in the book.

Once you've found the entry for a particular procedure in the alphabetical listing, you'll find that each entry uses the same clear, straightforward structure. An introductory section appears first. After that, most or all of the following sections appear, depending on the particular procedure:

■ The *Equipment* section lists all the equipment you'll need, including all the variations in equipment that might be needed. For instance, in the "endotracheal intubation" entry, you'll see a general equipment list, which is followed by separate lists of the additional equipment you'll need

for direct visualization intubation and blind nasotracheal intubation.

■ As the name implies, the *Preparation of equipment* section guides you through preparing the equipment for the procedure.

■ In the *Implementation* section—the heart of each entry—you'll find the step-by-step guide to performing the particular procedure.

■ *Special considerations* alerts you to factors to keep in mind that can affect the procedure.

■ *Patient teaching* covers procedure-related and home care information you need to teach to the patient and his family.

■ *Complications* details procedure-related complications to watch for.

■ The *Documentation* section helps you keep track of everything you need to document related to the procedure.

■ The expanded *References* section includes numbered citations keyed to the main text of each entry. These numbered citations serve as the clinical evidence that underpins the information and step-by-step procedures presented in the entry. (There'll be more on this in the next section of this "how to" guide.)

■ The *Additional references*—the final section in each entry—presents even more clinical background research for the reader who wants to delve deeper.

The overall A-to-Z organization of the sixth edition and the clear structure of each entry make this book a powerful tool for finding and understanding the procedures you need to know.

Evidently speaking...

Now here in *Lippincott's Nursing Procedures* is the shift to a more evidenced-based approach to nursing care clearer than in the extensive numbered *References* section that appears in each entry. As mentioned earlier, the numbered citations are keyed to information that appears throughout each procedure.

As you read through an entry and come across a bullet describing a particular step in a procedure, you'll notice one or more red superscript numbers following the bullet. These numbers, in turn, refer to citations in the *References* section;

the studies in these citations supply clinical evidence or detail best practices related to that bulleted step in the procedure. This is what is meant by *evidence-based practice*: A particular practice—say, performing hand hygiene—is supported by the clinical evidence. This evidence-based approach means the procedures you'll read about in *Lippincott's Nursing Procedures* are best-practice procedures that rely on solid, authoritative evidence.

As you look at the numbered references in each entry, you may notice that many of them are followed by a level number. This level number appears in parentheses after the reference as the word "Level" followed by a Roman numeral that ranges from I to VII. These level numbers give you an indication of the strength of the particular reference, with Level I being the strongest and Level VII, the weakest.

Here's how the rating system for this hierarchy of evidence works:

- *Level I*: Evidence comes from a systematic review or meta-analysis of all relevant randomized, controlled trials.
- *Level II*: Evidence comes from at least one well-designed randomized, controlled trial.
- *Level III*: Evidence comes from well-designed, controlled trials without randomization.
- *Level IV*: Evidence comes from well-designed case-control and cohort studies.
- *Level V*: Evidence comes from systematic reviews of descriptive and qualitative studies.
- *Level VI*: Evidence comes from a single descriptive or qualitative study.
- *Level VII*: Evidence comes from the opinion of authorities, reports of expert committees, or both.

In this book, the majority of cited references followed by a level are rated "Level I." These Level I references provide the strongest level of evidence to support a particular practice. You can use these levels to gauge the strength of supporting evidence for any particular practice or procedure.

Another important way *Lippincott's Nursing Procedures* provides a more evidence-based approach is by offering rationales for many procedures steps. These rationales are set off from the main text in italics. For instance, you may see a bullet like this:

"Answer all the patient's questions *to decrease anxiety and improve cooperation*." The second part of that bullet—the italicized-portion—is the rationale, or reason, for performing the first part. The practice of answering the patient's questions is supported by the clinical evidence of the patient's decreased anxiety and increased cooperation.

Just the highlights, please

Lippincott's Nursing Procedures, Sixth Edition, also benefits from other features that make it easy to use. Throughout, you'll find highlighting that greatly enhances the main text.

Some examples:

- As mentioned earlier, footnotes appear in red for easier spotting.
- Colored letter tabs at the top of each page make finding a particular entry quick and easy.
- Full-color photos highlight the main text, illustrating many of the step-by-step procedures in the *Implementation* section of each entry.
- Special alerts—with eye-catching graphic icons—appear in many entries. Pediatric alerts and Elder alerts warn you of particular precautions to take for these patients, and general Nursing alerts let you know about potentially dangerous actions or clinically significant findings related to a procedure.
- Short, boxed-off articles appear through the book. Several are set off with their own eye-catching logos—including Equipment, Troubleshooting, and Patient teaching logos—and many are enhanced with illustrations or full-color photos. These short pieces run the gamut, from explaining procedures in more detail, to highlighting equipment, to offering tips for clearer documentation, to name just a few.

Your go-to guide

Now that you know what the sixth edition of *Lippincott's Nursing Procedures* has to offer—and have learned how to use it quickly and adeptly—you're ready to take on the task of preforming a variety of nursing procedures. Whether you're a nursing student, a recent graduate, or an experienced practitioner, you're ready to provide all your patients with expert nursing care, with your go-to guide at your fingertips.

ABDOMINAL PARACENTESIS, ASSISTING

As a bedside procedure, abdominal paracentesis involves the aspiration of fluid from the peritoneal space through a needle or trocar and cannula inserted in the abdominal wall. Used to diagnose and treat massive ascites resistant to other therapies, the procedure helps to determine the cause of ascites while relieving the pressure it creates.

Abdominal paracentesis may also precede other procedures, including radiography, peritoneal dialysis, and surgery; detect intra-abdominal bleeding after a traumatic injury; and be used to obtain a peritoneal fluid specimen for laboratory analysis. The procedure must be performed cautiously in pregnant patients as well as in patients with bleeding tendencies, a severely distended bowel, or an infection at the intended insertion site.

Equipment

Tape measure ■ sterile gloves ■ mask ■ gloves ■ gown ■ goggles ■ linen-saver pads ■ Vacutainer tubes ■ two large Vacutainer bottles (1,000 mL or larger) ■ sterile pressure dressing ■ laboratory request forms ■ antiseptic cleaning solution ■ local anesthetic (multidose vial of 1% or 2% lidocaine with epinephrine) ■ 4″ × 4″ sterile gauze pads ■ sterile paracentesis tray ■ sterile drapes ■ marking pen ■ 5-mL syringe with 21G or 25G needle ■ Optional: alcohol sponge, 50-mL syringe, suture materials, salt-poor albumin.

If a preassembled tray isn't available, you will need to gather the following sterile supplies: trocar with stylet, 16G to 20G needle, 25G or 27G 1½″ needle, 20G or 22G spinal needle, scalpel, no. 11 knife blade, three-way stopcock.

Implementation

■ Perform hand hygiene and put on gloves.[1,2,3]

■ Confirm the patient's identity using at least two patient identifiers according to your facility's policy.[4]

■ Explain the procedure to the patient *to ease his anxiety and promote cooperation*. Reassure him that he should feel no pain, but that he may feel a stinging sensation from the local anesthetic injection and pressure from the needle or trocar and cannula insertion.

■ Make sure that an informed consent has been obtained and is documented in the patient's medical record.[5]

■ Instruct the patient to void before the procedure. Or, insert an indwelling urinary catheter, if ordered, *to minimize the risk of accidental bladder injury from the needle or trocar and cannula insertion.*

■ Conduct a preprocedure verification process *to make sure that all relevant documentation, related information, and equipment are available and correctly identified to the patient's identifiers.*[6]

■ Obtain and record baseline values: vital signs, weight, and abdominal girth. (Use the tape measure to measure the patient's abdominal girth at the umbilical level.) Indicate the abdominal area measured with a felt-tipped marking pen. *Baseline data will be used to monitor the patient's status.*

■ Position the patient supine or on his side *to allow the fluid to pool in dependent areas.*[7]

■ Expose the patient's abdomen from diaphragm to pubis. Keep the rest of the patient covered *to avoid chilling him.*

■ Make the patient as comfortable as possible, and place a linen-saver pad under him *for protection from drainage.*

■ Remind the patient to stay as still as possible during the procedure *to prevent injury from the needle or trocar and cannula.*

■ Remove and discard your gloves. Perform hand hygiene. Put on sterile gloves, a gown, and goggles *to prevent cross-contamination.*[1,2,3,8]

■ Open the paracentesis tray using sterile technique *to ensure a sterile field.*[8]

■ Label all medications, medication containers, and other solutions on and off the sterile field.[9]

■ Conduct a time-out immediately before starting the procedure *to identify the correct patient, site, positioning, and procedure and to ensure that, as applicable, all relevant information and necessary equipment are available during and after the procedure.*[10]

■ Assist the doctor as he prepares the patient's abdomen with antiseptic cleaning solution, drapes the operative site with sterile drapes, and administers the local anesthetic.

■ If the paracentesis tray doesn't contain a sterile ampule of anesthetic, wipe the top of a multidose vial of anesthetic solution with an alcohol sponge, and invert the vial at a 45-degree angle. *This step allows the doctor to insert the sterile 5-mL syringe with the 21G or 25G needle and withdraw the anesthetic without touching the nonsterile vial.*

■ Using the scalpel, the doctor may make a small incision before inserting the needle or trocar and cannula (usually 1″ to 2″ [2.5 to 5 cm] below the umbilicus). Listen for a popping sound, *which signifies that the needle or trocar has pierced the peritoneum.*

■ Assist the doctor with collecting specimens in the proper containers. If the doctor orders substantial drainage, aseptically connect the three-way stopcock and tubing to the cannula. Run the other end of the tubing to a large, sterile Vacutainer. Or, aspirate the fluid with a three-way stopcock and 50-mL syringe.

■ Gently turn the patient from side to side *to enhance drainage*, if necessary.

■ As the fluid drains, monitor the patient's vital signs according to the doctor's orders. Observe the patient closely for vertigo, faintness, diaphoresis, pallor, heightened anxiety, tachycardia, dyspnea, and hypotension—especially if more than 1,500 mL of peritoneal fluid was aspirated at one time. *This loss may induce a fluid shift and hypovolemic shock.*[7]

■ Immediately report signs of shock to the doctor; he may order you to administer salt-poor albumin IV *to prevent hypovolemia and a decline in renal function.*

■ When the procedure ends and the doctor removes the needle or trocar and cannula, he may suture the incision.

■ Remove and discard your gloves. Perform hand hygiene and put on sterile gloves.[1,2,3,8]

■ Apply the sterile pressure dressing to the site.

■ Help the patient assume a comfortable position.

■ Monitor the patient's vital signs and check the dressing for drainage according to your facility's policy *to detect delayed reactions to the procedure.* Be sure to note drainage color, amount, and character.

■ Label the Vacutainer specimen tubes in the presence of the patient *to prevent mislabeling*, and send them to the laboratory with the appropriate laboratory request forms. If the patient is receiving antibiotics, note this information on the request form *for consideration during the fluid analysis.*

■ Dispose of all equipment and supplies in the appropriate receptacles.

■ Remove and discard your gloves. Perform hand hygiene.[1,2,3,8]

■ Document the procedure.[11]

Special considerations

■ Throughout this procedure, try to help the patient remain still *to prevent accidental perforation of abdominal organs.*

■ If the patient shows any signs of hypovolemic shock, reduce the vertical distance between the needle or the trocar and cannula and the drainage collection container *to slow the drainage rate.* If necessary, stop the drainage.

■ *To prevent fluid shifts and hypovolemia*, limit aspirated fluid to between 1,500 and 2,000 mL. If peritoneal fluid doesn't flow easily, try repositioning the patient *to facilitate drainage.*

■ After the procedure, observe for peritoneal fluid leakage. If this develops, notify the doctor.

■ Always maintain daily patient weights and abdominal girth records. Compare these values with the baseline figures *to detect recurrent ascites.*

Complications

Removing large amounts of fluid may cause hypotension, oliguria, and hyponatremia. If an excessive amount of fluid (more than 2 L) is removed, ascitic fluid tends to form again, drawing fluid from extracellular tissue throughout the body. Other complications include perforation of abdominal organs, wound infection, bleeding, and peritonitis.

Documentation

Record the date and time of the procedure, the puncture site location, and whether the wound was sutured. Document the amount, color, viscosity, and odor of aspirated fluid. Record all assessments, vital signs, weight, and abdominal girth measurements before and after the procedure. Also note the patient's tolerance of the procedure and any complications during the procedure. Note all specimens sent to the laboratory.

REFERENCES

1 Centers for Disease Control and Prevention. (October 2002). Guideline for hand hygiene in health-care settings. *Morbidity and Mortality Weekly Report, 51* (RR-16), 1–45. (Level I)

2 World Health Organization. (2009). *WHO guidelines on hand hygiene in health care: First global patient safety challenge. Clean care is safer care.* Geneva, Switzerland: World Health Organization. (Level I)

3 The Joint Commission. (2012). Standard NPSG.07.01.01. *Comprehensive accreditation manual for hospitals: The official handbook.* Oakbrook Terrace, IL: The Joint Commission. (Level I)

4 The Joint Commission. (2012). Standard NPSG.01.01.01. *Comprehensive accreditation manual for hospitals: The official handbook.* Oakbrook Terrace, IL: The Joint Commission. (Level I)

5 The Joint Commission. (2012). Standard RI.01.03.01. *Comprehensive accreditation manual for hospitals: The official handbook.* Oakbrook Terrace, IL: The Joint Commission. (Level I)

6 The Joint Commission. (2012). Standard UP.01.01.01 *Comprehensive accreditation manual for hospitals: The official handbook.* Oakbrook Terrace, IL: The Joint Commission. (Level I)

7 Lynn-McHale Wiegand, D. (Ed.). (2011). *AACN procedure manual for critical care* (6th ed.). Philadelphia, PA: Saunders.

8 The Joint Commission. (2012). Standard NPSG.07.05.01. *Comprehensive accreditation manual for hospitals: The official handbook.* Oakbrook Terrace, IL: The Joint Commission. (Level I)

9 The Joint Commission. (2012). Standard NPSG.03.04.01. *Comprehensive accreditation manual for hospitals: The official handbook.* Oakbrook Terrace, IL: The Joint Commission. (Level I)

10 The Joint Commission. (2012). Standard UP.01.03.01. *Comprehensive accreditation manual for hospitals: The official handbook.* Oakbrook Terrace, IL: The Joint Commission. (Level I)

11 The Joint Commission. (2012). Standard RC.01.03.01. *Comprehensive accreditation manual for hospitals: The official handbook.* Oakbrook Terrace, IL: The Joint Commission. (Level I)

ADDITIONAL REFERENCE

Hou, W., & Sanyal, A.J. (2009). Ascites: Diagnosis and management. *Medical Clinics of North America, 93*(4), 801–817.

ADMISSION

Admission to the nursing unit prepares the patient for his stay in the health care facility. Whether the admission is scheduled or follows emergency treatment, effective admission procedures should include certain steps to accomplish important goals. These steps include verifying the patient's identity using at least two patient identifiers according to your facility's policy,[1] assessing his clinical status, making him as comfortable as possible, introducing him to roommates and staff members, orienting him to the environment and routines, and providing any supplies and special equipment needed for daily care.

During your assessment, prioritize the patient's needs, and always be conscious of the patient's levels of fatigue and comfort. Maintain the patient's privacy while obtaining his health history; he also has the right to expect that his examinations, consultations, and treatment will be conducted in a manner that protects his privacy.

Effective admission routines that show appropriate concern for the patient can ease his anxiety and promote cooperation and receptivity to treatment. Conversely, admission routines that the patient perceives as careless or excessively impersonal can heighten the patient's anxiety, reduce cooperation, impair his response to treatment, and possibly aggravate symptoms.

Equipment

Gown ■ personal property form ■ valuables envelope ■ admission form ■ nursing assessment form ■ sphygmomanometer ■ stethoscope ■ thermometer ■ Optional: emesis basin, bedpan, urinal, bath basin, urine specimen container, towel, washcloth.

Preparation of equipment

Obtain a gown. Position the bed as the patient's condition requires. If the patient is ambulatory, place the bed in the low position; if he's arriving on a stretcher, place the bed in the high position. Fold down the top linens. Prepare any emergency or special equipment, such as oxygen or suction, as needed.

Implementation

■ Adjust the lights, temperature, and ventilation in the room.
■ Quickly review the admission form and the doctor's orders. Note the reason for admission, any restrictions on activity or diet, and any orders for diagnostic tests requiring specimen collection.
■ Perform hand hygiene.[2,3,4]
■ Speaking slowly and clearly, greet the patient by his proper name and introduce yourself and any other staff members present.
■ Confirm the patient's identity using at least two patient identifiers according to your facility's policy.[1] Verify the name and spelling with the patient. Notify the admission office of any corrections.
■ Escort the patient to his room and, if he isn't in great distress, introduce him to his roommate.
■ Help the patient change into a gown or pajamas; if the patient is sharing a room, provide privacy.
■ Itemize all valuables, clothing, and prostheses on the nursing assessment form (or in your notes if your facility doesn't use such a form). Encourage the patient to store valuables or money in the safe or, preferably, to send them home along with any medications he may have brought.
■ Show the ambulatory patient where the bathroom and closets are located.
■ Take and record the patient's vital signs, and collect specimens, if ordered. Measure his height and weight if possible. If he can't stand, use a chair or bed scale and ask him his height. *Knowing the patient's height and weight is important for planning treatment and diet and for calculating medication and anesthetic dosages.*
■ Show the patient how to use the equipment in his room. Include the call system, bed controls, television controls, telephone, and lights.
■ Explain the routine at your health care facility. Mention when to expect meals, vital sign checks, and medications. Review visiting hours and any restrictions.
■ Obtain a complete patient history. Include all previous hospitalizations, illnesses, surgeries, and food or drug allergies.
■ Make sure that a complete list of the medications the patient was taking at home (including doses, routes, and frequency) has been obtained and documented in the patient's medical record. This list should be compared with the patient's current medications, and any discrepancies (omissions, duplications, adjustments, deletions or additions) should be reconciled and documented in the patient's medical record *to reduce the risk of transition-related adverse drug events.*[5]

Using patient care reminders

When placed at the head of the patient's bed, care reminders call attention to the patient's special needs and help ensure consistent care by communicating these needs to the health care facility's staff members, the patient's family, and other visitors.

You can use a specially designed card or a plain piece of paper to post important information about the patient, such as:
■ allergies
■ dietary restrictions
■ fluid restrictions
■ needed specimen collection
■ infection-control or isolation procedures
■ whether a patient is deaf or hearing impaired and if so, in which ear
■ whether a foreign language is spoken.

You can also use care reminders to post special instructions, such as:
■ complete bed rest
■ no blood pressure on right arm
■ turn every hour
■ nothing by mouth.

Never violate the patient's privacy by posting his diagnosis, details about surgery, or any information he might find embarrassing.

■ Determine whether the patient has an advance directive and ask for a copy to be placed in the medical record. If the patient doesn't have an advance directive, provide information about such directives to the patient.[6] (See "Advance directives," page 6.)
■ Ask the patient to tell you why he came to the facility. Record the answers (in the patient's own words) as the chief complaint. Follow up with a physical assessment, emphasizing complaints. Record any marks, bruises, discolorations or wounds on the nursing assessment form.
■ Perform a comprehensive pain assessment using techniques that are appropriate for the patient's age, condition, and ability to understand.[7]
■ If the patient has a drug allergy, attach an allergy-alert bracelet to his arm according to your facility's policy.
■ After assessing the patient, inform him of any tests that have been ordered and when they're scheduled. Describe what he should expect.
■ Before leaving the patient's room, make sure he's comfortable and safe. Adjust his bed, and place the call button and other personal items within easy reach.
■ Post patient care reminders (concerning such topics as allergies or special needs) at the patient's bedside *to notify coworkers.* (See *Using patient care reminders.*)
■ Perform hand hygiene.[2,3,4]
■ Document the procedure.[8]

Managing emergency admissions

For the patient admitted through the emergency department (ED), immediate treatment takes priority over routine admission procedures. After ED treatment, the patient arrives on the nursing unit with a temporary identification bracelet, a doctor's order sheet, and a record of treatment. Read this record and talk to the nurse who cared for the patient in the ED *to ensure continuity of care and to gain insight into the patient's condition and behavior.*

Next, record any ongoing treatment such as an IV infusion in your notes. Trace catheters or tubing from the patient to their point of origin *to make sure that they're attached to the proper connection ports.* If the patient has more than one connection to a port of entry into the body (for example, if an IV catheter has more than one infusion infusing through it), label each tube near the insertion site. If the patient is receiving infusions by different administration routes, place the infusion pumps on opposite sides of the bed *to prevent administration errors.*

Obtain and record the patient's vital signs, and follow the doctor's orders for treatment. If the patient is conscious and not in great distress, explain any treatment orders. If family members accompany the patient, ask them to wait in the lounge while you assess the patient and begin treatment. Permit them to visit the patient after he's settled in his room. When the patient's condition allows, proceed with routine admission procedures.

Special considerations

■ Keep in mind that the patient admitted from the emergency department requires special procedures. (See *Managing emergency admissions.*)
■ If the patient brings medication from home, take an inventory and record this information on the nursing assessment form. Instruct the patient not to take any medication unless authorized by the doctor. Send authorized medication to the pharmacy for identification and relabeling. Send other medication home with a responsible family member, or store it in the designated area outside the patient's room until he's discharged. *Use of unauthorized medication may interfere with treatment or cause an overdose.*
■ Find out the patient's normal routine, and ask him if he would like to make any adjustments to the facility regimen; for instance, he may prefer to shower at night instead of in the morning. *By accommodating the patient with such adjustments whenever possible, you can ease his anxiety and help him feel more in control of his potentially threatening situation.*
■ Patients requiring isolation precautions should be placed in an isolation room *to reduce the risk of transmission.*[9]
■ Teach the patient and his family about the importance of proper hand hygiene in preventing the spread of infection. Encourage them to speak up if a health care worker fails to per-

form hand hygiene before having contact with the patient or the patient's environment.

Documentation

After leaving the patient's room, complete the nursing assessment form or your notes, as required. The completed form should include the patient's vital signs, height, weight, allergies, and drug and health history; a list of his belongings and those sent home with family members; the results of your physical assessment; and a record of specimens collected for laboratory tests.

REFERENCES

1 The Joint Commission. (2012). Standard NPSG.01.01.01. *Comprehensive accreditation manual for hospitals: The official handbook.* Oakbrook Terrace, IL: The Joint Commission. (Level I)
2 The Joint Commission. (2012). Standard NPSG.07.01.01. *Comprehensive accreditation manual for hospitals: The official handbook.* Oakbrook Terrace, IL: The Joint Commission. (Level I)
3 Centers for Disease Control and Prevention. (October 2002). Guideline for hand hygiene in health-care settings. *Morbidity and Mortality Weekly Report, 51* (RR-16), 1–45. (Level I)
4 World Health Organization. (2009). *WHO guidelines on hand hygiene in health care: First global patient safety challenge. Clean care is safer care.* Geneva, Switzerland: World Health Organization. (Level I)
5 The Joint Commission. (2012). Standard MM.03.01.05. *Comprehensive accreditation manual for hospitals: The official handbook.* Oakbrook Terrace, IL: The Joint Commission. (Level I)
6 The Joint Commission. (2012). Standard RI.01.05.01. *Comprehensive accreditation manual for hospitals: The official handbook.* Oakbrook Terrace, IL: The Joint Commission. (Level I)
7 The Joint Commission. (2012). Standard PC.01.02.07. *Comprehensive accreditation manual for hospitals: The official handbook.* Oakbrook Terrace, IL: The Joint Commission. (Level I)
8 The Joint Commission. (2012). Standard RC.01.03.01. *Comprehensive accreditation manual for hospitals: The official handbook.* Oakbrook Terrace, IL: The Joint Commission. (Level I)
9 Siegel, J.D., et al. "2007 guideline for isolation precautions: Preventing transmission of infectious agents in healthcare settings" [Online]. Accessed June 2011 via the Web at http://www.cdc.gov/hicpac/2007ip/2007isolationprecautions.html (Level I)

ADDITIONAL REFERENCES

American Hospital Association. (2003). *The patient care partnership: Understanding expectation, rights, and responsibilities.* Chicago, IL: American Hospital Association.
Bickey, L. (2010). *Bates' guide to physical examination and health history taking* (10th ed.). Philadelphia, PA: Lippincott Williams & Wilkins.
Institute of Safe Medication Practices. (2010). Preventing catheter/tubing misconnections: Much needed help is on the way. ISMP medication safety alert! *Nurse Advise-ERR, 8*(12).

ADMIXTURE OF DRUGS IN A SYRINGE

Combining two drugs in one syringe avoids the discomfort of two injections. Usually, drugs can be mixed in a syringe in one of four ways: They may be combined from two multidose vials (for example, regular and long-acting insulin), from one multidose vial and one ampule, from two ampules, or from a cartridge-injection system combined with either a multidose vial or an ampule. Such combinations are contraindicated when the drugs aren't compatible and when combined doses exceed the amount of solution that can be absorbed from a single injection site.

Equipment

Prescribed medications ■ patient's medication record and chart ■ alcohol pads ■ sterile syringe and needle ■ Optional: cartridge-injection system, safety needle, filter needle.

The type and size of the syringe and needle depend on the prescribed medications, the patient's body build, and the route of administration. Medications that come in prefilled cartridges require a cartridge-injection system. (See *Cartridge-injection system.*)

Implementation

■ Verify that the drugs to be administered agree with the patient's medication record and the doctor's orders.[1]
■ Calculate the dose to be given.
■ Perform hand hygiene.[2,3,4]

Mixing drugs from two multidose vials

■ Using an alcohol pad, wipe the rubber stopper on the first vial *to decrease the risk of contaminating the medication as you insert the needle into the vial.*
■ Pull back the syringe plunger until the volume of air drawn into the syringe equals the volume to be withdrawn from the drug vial.
■ Without inverting the vial, insert the needle into the top of the vial, making sure that the needle's bevel tip doesn't touch the solution. Inject the air into the vial and withdraw the needle. *This step replaces air in the vial, thus preventing the creation of a partial vacuum on withdrawal of the drug.*
■ With a new needle, repeat the steps above for the second vial. Then, after injecting the air into the second vial, invert the vial, withdraw the prescribed dose, and then withdraw the needle (as shown below).

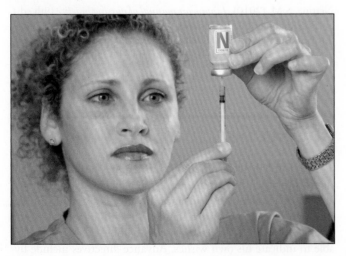

Cartridge-injection system

A cartridge-injection system, such as Tubex or Carpuject, is a convenient, easy-to-use method of injection that facilitates accuracy and sterility. The device consists of a plastic cartridge-holder syringe and a prefilled medication cartridge with needle attached.

The medication in the cartridge is premixed and premeasured, which saves time and helps ensure an exact dose. The medication remains sealed in the cartridge and sterile until the injection is administered to the patient.

The disadvantage of this system is that not all drugs are available in cartridge form. However, compatible drugs can be added to partially filled cartridges.

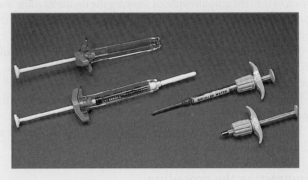

■ Wipe the rubber stopper of the first vial again and insert the needle, taking care not to depress the plunger. Invert the vial, withdraw the prescribed dose, and then withdraw the needle.
■ Change the needle on the syringe, if indicated.

Mixing drugs from a multidose vial and an ampule

■ Using an alcohol pad, wipe the rubber stopper on the vial *to decrease the risk of contaminating the medication as you insert the needle into the vial.*
■ Pull back the syringe plunger until the volume of air drawn into the syringe equals the volume to be withdrawn from the drug vial.
■ Insert the needle into the top of the vial and inject the air. Then invert the vial and keep the needle's bevel tip below the level of the solution as you withdraw the prescribed dose. Put the sterile needle cover over the needle.
■ Tap the stem of the ampule *to move any medication from the stem into the body of the ampule.*
■ Wrap a sterile gauze pad or an alcohol pad around the ampule's neck *to protect yourself from injury in case the glass splinters.* Break open the ampule, directing the force away from you.
■ Change to a filter needle *to filter out any glass splinters.*[5]

■ Insert the needle into the ampule. Be careful not to touch the outside of the ampule with the needle. Draw the correct dose into the syringe.

■ Change the filter needle back to a regular needle to administer the injection.

Mixing drugs from two ampules

■ An opened ampule doesn't contain a vacuum; therefore, you don't need to inject air before withdrawing the medication.

■ Tap the stem of the ampule *to move any medication from the stem into the body of the ampule.*

■ Open each ampule by wrapping a small gauze pad or alcohol pad around the neck of the ampule and quickly snapping off the top along the scored line at the neck. Snap the neck in the direction away from your body.

■ Insert a syringe (with a filter needle attached *to filter out any glass splinters*) into the ampule without allowing the needle to come into contact with the rim of the ampule. Be sure the needle is in the solution.[5]

■ Withdraw the amount ordered from the first ampule and remove the needle from the solution. Check to ensure that the dose is accurate.

■ Repeat the above steps with the second ampule, changing the needles as necessary.

■ When the syringe is prepared, change to a regular needle to administer the medication.

Completing the procedure

■ Discard all equipment in appropriate receptacles.

■ Perform hand hygiene.[2,3,4]

■ Document the procedure.[6]

Special considerations

■ Insert a needle through the vial's rubber stopper at a slight angle, bevel up, and exert slight lateral pressure. *This way you won't cut a piece of rubber out of the stopper, which can then be pushed into the vial.*

■ When mixing drugs from multidose vials, be careful not to contaminate one drug with the other. Change the needle after drawing the first medication into the syringe.

■ Never combine drugs if you're unsure of their compatibility, and never combine more than two drugs. *Although drug incompatibility usually causes a visible reaction, such as clouding, bubbling, or precipitation, some incompatible combinations produce no visible reaction, even though they alter the chemical nature and action of the drugs.* Check appropriate references and consult a pharmacist when you're unsure about specific compatibility. When in doubt, administer two separate injections.

■ Some medications are compatible for only a brief time after being combined and should be administered within 10 minutes after mixing. After this time, environmental factors, such as temperature, exposure to light, and humidity, may alter compatibility.

■ *To reduce the risk of contamination,* most facilities dispense parenteral medications in single-dose vials. Insulin is one of the few drugs still packaged in multidose vials. Be careful when mixing regular and long-acting insulin. Draw up the regular insulin first

to avoid contamination by the long-acting suspension. (If a minute amount of the regular insulin is accidentally mixed with the long-acting insulin, it won't appreciably change the effect of the long-acting insulin.) Check your facility's policy before mixing insulins.

■ When you combine a cartridge-injection system and a multidose vial, use a separate needle and syringe to inject air into the multidose vial. *This prevents contamination of the multidose vial by the cartridge-injection system.*

Complications

Complications, such as adverse drug reactions, may occur if an incorrect dose of medication is prepared or incompatible medications are mixed and administered.

Documentation

Record the drugs administered, injection site, and time of administration. Document any adverse drug reactions or other pertinent information.

REFERENCES

1　The Joint Commission. (2012). Standard MM.06.01.01. *Comprehensive accreditation manual for hospitals: The official handbook.* Oakbrook Terrace, IL: The Joint Commission. (Level I)

2　The Joint Commission. (2012). Standard NPSG.07.01.01. *Comprehensive accreditation manual for hospitals: The official handbook.* Oakbrook Terrace, IL: The Joint Commission. (Level I)

3　Centers for Disease Control and Prevention. (October 2002). Guideline for hand hygiene in health-care settings. *Morbidity and Mortality Weekly Report, 51* (RR-16), 1–45. (Level I)

4　World Health Organization. (2009). *WHO guidelines on hand hygiene in health care: First global patient safety challenge. Clean care is safer care.* Geneva, Switzerland: World Health Organization. (Level I)

5　Standard 28. Filters. Infusion nursing standards of practice. (2011). *Journal of Infusion Nursing 29*(1S), S33. (Level I)

6　The Joint Commission. (2012). Standard RC.01.03.01. *Comprehensive accreditation manual for hospitals: The official handbook.* Oakbrook Terrace, IL: The Joint Commission. (Level I)

ADDITIONAL REFERENCES

Nettina, S.M. (2010). *Lippincott manual of nursing practice* (9th ed.). Philadelphia, PA: Lippincott Williams & Wilkins.

Taylor, C., et al. (2011). *Fundamentals of nursing: The art and science of nursing care* (7th ed.). Philadelphia, PA: Lippincott Williams & Wilkins.

ADVANCE DIRECTIVES

The Patient Self-Determination Act[1] requires health care facilities to provide information about the patient's right to choose and refuse treatment. An advance directive is a legal document used as a guideline for providing life-sustaining medical care to a patient with an advanced disease or disability who is no longer able to indicate his own wishes. Advance directives include living wills and health care proxies.

All patients should be encouraged to have an advance directive as part of any admission, before any routine medical treatment, or at their primary doctor's office on annual physical examinations. All adults, regardless of their current health status, should make their preferences about medical treatment known before any serious injury or unplanned illness occurs. The advance directive should be discussed with the patient's doctor, family, and health care proxy.

If a person is terminally ill or in a persistent vegetative state or coma, a living will instructs health care providers about the patient's preferences about life-sustaining treatment. In making a living will, a legally competent patient states which procedures he does or doesn't want carried out, such as endotracheal intubation and mechanical ventilation, feeding tubes, artificial nutrition and hydration, antibiotics, dialysis, and cardiopulmonary resuscitation. The living will goes into effect when a person can no longer communicate his choices on medical care. (See *The living will,* page 8.)

In the health care proxy (also called *durable power of attorney for health care*), the patient designates another person to make decisions about medical care if the patient can't make his own decisions. (See *Health care proxy,* page 9.)

Equipment

Advance directive forms ■ medical record ■ Optional: witness or notary public (as required by the state).

Implementation

■ Confirm the patient's identity using at least two patient identifiers according to your facility's policy.[2]
■ Ask the patient if he has an advance directive as set forth in the Patient Self-Determination Act.

If the patient has an advance directive

■ Review the advance directive with the patient and confirm that it still reflects his wishes.
■ Place a copy of the advance directive in the medical record *so that it's easily accessible to all health care providers.*[3]
■ Notify the doctor that the patient has an advance directive *so that it can be used to guide care.*[4]
■ Determine whether the health care proxy has a copy of the advance directive.
■ Encourage the patient to discuss his advance directive with his family and health care proxy *so that they understand the patient's wishes and can ask questions while the patient is competent and can explain his decisions.*
■ Document the procedure and that the patient has an advance directive.[4,5]

If the patient doesn't have an advance directive

■ Provide the patient with verbal and written information about advance directives *so that he can make an informed decision about developing one.*[4]

■ Answer the patient's questions about advance directives or have a social worker or patient representative discuss advance directives with him *to provide accurate information.*[4]
■ Assist in the assessment of the patient's level of competency *to assure he can make decisions.* This process may include the patient's ability to understand information, consider the alternatives, evaluate the alternatives in relation to his own situation, make a decision, and communicate his choice. According to facility policy, the patient's capacity for making decisions may be determined by a doctor or advanced practice nurse.
■ Document the procedure and note that the patient doesn't have an advance directive at this time.[4,5]

Special considerations

■ If family members express opposition to the patient's advance directive, notify the patient's doctor, the nursing supervisor, and the risk manager. Encourage family members to discuss their feelings with the patient and these individuals. A consult to the facility ethics committee may be made, as indicated.
■ The patient may revoke or change his advance directive at any time.[1,4] For example, the patient may revoke his directive if he changes his mind about his previous decision or if his condition mandates that he revise his directive. The patient can revoke an advance directive either orally or in writing.

Documentation

Document the presence of an advance directive[4] and that the doctor was notified of its presence. Include the name of the doctor and the time of notification. Include the name, address, and telephone number of the health care proxy. If the patient's wishes differ from those of his doctor or family, note the discrepancies.

If the patient doesn't have an advance directive, document that he was given written information concerning his rights under state law to make decisions regarding health care. If the patient refuses information on an advance directive, document this refusal using the patient's own words, in quotes, if possible. Record any conversations with the patient regarding his decision making. Document that proof of competence was obtained.

REFERENCES

1 Patient Self-Determination Act of 1990, §§ 4206 and 4751 of the Omnibus Reconciliation Act of 1990, Pub. L. No. 101–508 (November 5, 1990).
2 The Joint Commission. (2012). Standard NPSG.01.01.01. *Comprehensive accreditation manual for hospitals: The official handbook.* Oakbrook Terrace, IL: The Joint Commission. (Level I)
3 The Joint Commission. (2012). Standard RC.02.01.01. *Comprehensive accreditation manual for hospitals: The official handbook.* Oakbrook Terrace, IL: The Joint Commission. (Level I)
4 The Joint Commission. (2012). Standard RI.01.05.01. *Comprehensive accreditation manual for hospitals: The official handbook.* Oakbrook Terrace, IL: The Joint Commission. (Level I)
5 The Joint Commission. (2012). Standard RC.01.03.01. *Comprehensive accreditation manual for hospitals: The official handbook.* Oakbrook Terrace, IL: The Joint Commission. (Level I)

The living will

The living will is an advance care document that specifies a person's wishes with regard to medical care, should he become terminally ill, incompetent, or unable to communicate. This will is commonly used in combination with the patient's health care proxy.

All states and the District of Columbia have living will laws that outline the documentation requirements for living wills. The sample document below is from Ohio.

Living will

If my attending doctor and one other doctor who examines me determine, to a reasonable degree of medical certainty and in accordance with reasonable medical standards, that I am in a terminal condition or in a permanently unconscious state, and if my attending doctor determines that at that time I no longer am able to make informed decisions regarding the administration of life-sustaining treatment, and that, to a reasonable degree of medical certainty and in accordance with reasonable medical standards, there is no reasonable possibility that I will regain the capacity to make informed decisions regarding the administration of life-sustaining treatment, then I direct my attending doctor to withhold or withdraw medical procedures, treatment, interventions, or other measures that serve principally to prolong the process of my dying, rather than diminish my pain or discomfort.

I have used the term "terminal condition" in this declaration to mean an irreversible, incurable, and untreatable condition caused by disease, illness, or injury from which, to a reasonable degree of medical certainty as determined in accordance with reasonable medical standards of my attending doctor and one other doctor who has examined me, both of the following apply:

1. There can be no recovery.
2. Death is likely to occur within a relatively short time if life-sustaining treatment is not administered.

I have used the term "permanently unconscious state" in this declaration to mean a state of permanent unconsciousness that, to a reasonable degree of medical certainty, is determined in accordance with reasonable medical standards by my attending doctor and one other doctor who has examined me, as characterized by both of the following:

1. I am irreversibly unaware of myself and my environment.
2. There is a total loss of cerebral cortical functioning, resulting in my having no capacity to experience pain or suffering.

Nutrition and hydration

I hereby authorize my attending doctor to withhold or withdraw nutrition and hydration from me when I am in a permanent unconscious state if my attending doctor and at least one other doctor who has examined me determine, to a reasonable degree of medical certainty and in accordance with reasonable medical standards, that nutrition or hydration will not or no longer will serve to provide comfort to me or alleviate my pain.

[Sign here for withdrawal of nutrition or hydration] _____

I hereby designate [Print name of person to decide] as the person who I wish my attending doctor to notify at any time that life-sustaining treatment is to be withdrawn or withheld pursuant to this Declaration.

_____   _____
          [Sign your name here]   [Today's date]

Witnessed by: _____

[Living will person's name] voluntarily signed or directed another individual to sign this Living Will in the presence of the following who each attests that the Declarant appears to be of sound mind and not under or subject to duress, fraud, or undue influence.

_____   _____
          [First witness signs here]   [Second witness signs here]

Health care proxy

The sample document below is an example of a health care proxy, which allows a competent patient to delegate to another person the authority to consent to or refuse health care treatment for him. This document helps the patient ensure that his wishes will be carried out if he should become incompetent.

Each state with a health care proxy law has specific requirements for executing the document. The sample form below is from Nebraska.

Power of attorney for health care

I appoint ——————————————————————————————

whose address is ——————————————————————————

and whose telephone number is ————————————————

as my attorney-in-fact for health care. ———————————————

I appoint ——————————————————————————————

whose address is ——————————————————————————

and whose telephone number is ————————————————

as my successor attorney-in-fact for health care. ——————————

I authorize my attorney-in-fact appointed by this document to make health care decisions for me when I am determined to be incapable of making my own health care decisions. I have read the warning that accompanies this document and understand the consequences of executing a power of attorney for health care.

I direct that my attorney-in-fact comply with the following instructions or limitations (optional):

I direct that my attorney-in-fact comply with the following instructions on life-sustaining treatment (optional):

I direct that my attorney-in-fact comply with the following instructions on artificially administered nutrition and hydration (optional):

I have read this power of attorney for health care. I understand that it allows another person to make life and death decisions for me if I am incapable of making such decisions. I also understand that I can revoke this power of attorney for health care at any time by notifying my attorney-in-fact, my physician, or the facility in which I am a patient or resident. I also understand that I can require in this power of attorney for health care that the fact of my incapacity in the future be confirmed by a second physician.

———————————————————   ———————————————————

[Signature of person making designation]   [Date]

ADDITIONAL REFERENCES

Bacon D., et al. (2007). Position statement on laws and regulations concerning life-sustaining treatment, including artificial nutrition and hydration, for patients lacking decision-making capacity. *Neurology* 68(14), 1097–1100.

Duke, G., et al. (2007). Factors influencing completion of advance directives in hospitalized patients. *International Journal of Palliative Nursing* 13(1), 39–43.

Nishimura, A., et al. (2007). Patients who complete advance directives and what they prefer. *Mayo Clinic Proceedings* 82(12), 1480–1486.

EQUIPMENT

Respirator seal check

After you properly put on your respirator, perform a seal check. To do so, place your hands over the face piece, as shown below, and then exhale gently. The seal is considered satisfactory if a slight positive pressure builds up inside the face piece without air leaking from the seal. Evidence of air leaking from the seal includes fogging of your glasses, a feeling of air trickling down your uncovered face, and lack of pressure buildup under the face piece.

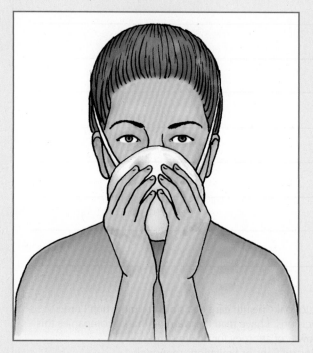

If the respirator has an exhalation valve, cover the filter surface with your hands as much as possible and then inhale. The seal is considered satisfactory if the face piece collapses on your face and you don't feel air passing between your face and the face piece.

AIRBORNE PRECAUTIONS

Airborne precautions, used in addition to standard precautions, prevent the spread of infectious droplet nuclei (small particles that become suspended in the air and disperse over long distances by air currents). Because the infectious particles can become suspended in the air, they may be inhaled by susceptible individuals who haven't had face-to-face contact with their source (the infected individual).[1] (See *Conditions requiring airborne precautions.*)

Effective airborne precautions require an airborne infection isolation room—a single-patient room that's equipped with monitored negative pressure (in relation to the surrounding area). An airborne infection isolation room should have 12 air exchanges/hour if the room has been newly constructed or renovated, or 6 air exchanges/hour in existing rooms. The air is either vented directly to the outside of the building or filtered through high-efficiency particulate air (HEPA) filtration before recirculation.[1,2] According to the Centers for Disease Control and Prevention (CDC), air pressure should be monitored daily, using visual indicators, while the room is in use. The door to the room should be kept closed to maintain the proper air pressure balance between the isolation room and the adjoining hallway or corridor. An anteroom is preferred.

Respiratory protection must be worn by everyone who enters an airborne infection isolation room. Such protection is provided by a disposable respirator (such as an N95 respirator or a HEPA respirator) or a reusable respirator (such as a HEPA respirator or a powered air-purifying respirator [PAPR]).[1,2] Regardless of the type of respirator used, the health care worker must ensure proper fit to the face each time the worker wears one by performing a user seal check.[1,2] When using a PAPR, the health care worker must ensure proper functioning of the unit.

NURSING ALERT *When a patient comes to your facility complaining of respiratory symptoms and an airborne infection is suspected, put a surgical mask on him (if tolerated) and immediately place him in a private room with the door closed until an airborne infection isolation room is available. If the patient is unable to tolerate a mask, place him in a private room with the door closed and wear a respirator to care for him.*

Equipment

Respirators (either disposable N95 or HEPA respirators or reusable HEPA respirators or PAPRs) ▪ surgical masks ▪ isolation sign ▪ other personal protective equipment, as needed, for standard precautions.

Preparation of equipment

Gather any additional supplies for patient care, such as a thermometer, stethoscope, and blood pressure cuff. Keep all airborne precaution supplies outside the patient's room in a wall- or door-mounted cabinet, a cart, or an anteroom.

Implementation

▪ Perform hand hygiene.[4,5,6]
▪ Situate the patient in a single-patient airborne infection isolation room with the door closed.[1] Preferably, the room will have an anteroom. If a private bathroom is available, make sure the bathroom is also under negative air pressure. Monitor negative pressure according to regulations and your facility's policy.
▪ Explain isolation precautions to the patient and his family *to ease patient anxiety and promote cooperation.*
▪ Keep the patient's door (and the anteroom door) closed at all times *to maintain negative pressure and contain the airborne pathogens.*[1] Put the airborne precautions sign on the door *to alert anyone entering the room to don a respirator.*
▪ Pick up your respirator and put it on according to the manufacturer's directions. Adjust the straps for a firm but comfortable fit. Check the fit. (See *Respirator seal check.*)

Conditions requiring airborne precautions[2]

If a patient is known to have a condition requiring airborne precautions, the facility should follow the Centers for Disease Control and Prevention (CDC) isolation precautions to prevent the spread of organisms spread by the airborne route.[3]

CONDITION	PRECAUTIONARY PERIOD	SPECIAL CONSIDERATIONS (AS APPLICABLE)
Avian influenza	■ For 14 days after onset of symptoms or until alternate diagnosis is confirmed	
Chickenpox (varicella)	■ Until lesions are crusted and no new lesions appear	
Herpes zoster (disseminated disease in any patient or localized disease in immunocompromised patient until disseminated disease is ruled out)	■ For duration of illness	■ Susceptible health care workers shouldn't enter the room if immune caregivers are available. ■ Contact precautions should be instituted.
Measles (rubeola)	■ For 4 days after onset of rash; for duration of illness in immunocompromised patients	■ Susceptible health care workers shouldn't enter the room if immune caregivers are available.
Monkeypox	■ Until disease is confirmed and smallpox is excluded	■ Contact precautions should be instituted until lesions have crusted.
Severe acute respiratory syndrome	■ For duration of illness plus 10 days after resolution of fever	■ Eye protection (goggles or face shield) should be worn. ■ Contact precautions should be instituted. ■ Vigilant environmental disinfection should be performed.
Smallpox	■ For duration of illness until all scabs have crusted and separated (typically 3 to 4 weeks)	■ Contact precautions should be instituted. ■ Unvaccinated health care workers shouldn't provide care when immune health care workers are available.
Tuberculosis, extrapulmonary, draining lesion	■ Until patient improves clinically and drainage has ceased or until three consecutive negative cultures of continued drainage are obtained	■ Contact precautions should be instituted.
Tuberculosis, pulmonary or laryngeal disease, confirmed	■ Until patient improves clinically while on effective therapy (decreased cough and fever, improved chest X-ray) and has three consecutive sputum smears negative for acid-fast bacillus, collected on separate days	
Tuberculosis, pulmonary or laryngeal disease, suspected	■ Until active tuberculosis is deemed highly unlikely and either there is another diagnosis that explains the clinical findings or the results of three consecutive sputum smears for acid-fast bacillus, collected 8 to 24 hours apart, are negative	■ At least one of the three sputum specimens should be collected in the morning.

- If using a PAPR, check for proper function, battery life, and air flow.
- Remove the patient's mask, if he has one on.
- Instruct the patient to cover his nose and mouth with a facial tissue while coughing or sneezing. Place a sign in the patient's room as a reminder.
- Tape an impervious bag to the patient's bedside *so the patient can dispose of facial tissues correctly.*
- Remove and discard your gloves; remove other personal protective equipment, if applicable; and perform hand hygiene.[4,5,6]
- Remove your respirator after leaving the patient's room and closing the door. To remove your respirator, grasp the bottom and then the top elastic; avoid touching the front of the respirator *because the front is considered contaminated.* Discard the respirator in the appropriate receptacle, or follow your facility's policy if you're permitted to reuse it.[1]
- Perform hand hygiene.[4,5,6]
- Document the procedure.[7]

Special considerations

- Teach visitors how to properly wear respiratory protection and make sure that they wear respiratory protection while in the patient's room.[2]
- Limit the patient's movement from the room. If he must leave for essential procedures, make sure he wears a surgical mask, covering his nose and mouth.[1,2] Notify the receiving staff of the patient's isolation precautions *so that the precautions will be maintained and the patient can be returned to his room promptly.*
- Depending on the type of respirator and recommendations from the manufacturer, follow your facility's policy and either discard your respirator or store it until the next use.[1] If your respirator is to be stored until the next use, store it in a dry, well-ventilated place (not a plastic bag) *to prevent microbial growth.* Nondisposable respirators must be cleaned according to the manufacturer's recommendations.
- If the patient on airborne precautions requires surgery, try to schedule the procedure when a minimal number of health care workers and other patients are present. If possible, schedule the procedure as the last case of the day so more time is available to clean and disinfect the operating room. Use an operating room with an anteroom, if possible. All staff members involved in the surgery should wear respiratory protection.[2]
- If possible, the airborne infection isolation room should be left vacant according to your facility's policy after a patient is discharged *to allow for a full air exchange.*

Complications

Social isolation is a complication of airborne precautions.

Documentation

Record the need for airborne precautions on the nursing care plan and as otherwise indicated by your facility. Document initiation and maintenance of the precautions, the patient's tolerance of the procedure, and any patient or family teaching and their understanding of your teaching. Also document the date airborne precautions were discontinued.

REFERENCES

1 Siegel, J.D., et al. "2007 guideline for isolation precautions: Preventing transmission of infectious agents in healthcare settings" [Online]. Accessed June 2011 via the Web at http://www.cdc.gov/hicpac/2007ip/2007isolationprecautions.html (Level I)
2 Centers for Disease Control and Prevention. (December 2005). Guidelines for preventing the transmission of *Mycobacterium tuberculosis* in health care settings. *Morbidity and Mortality Weekly Report* 54(RR-17), 1–141. (Level I)
3 The Joint Commission. (2012). Standard IC.01.05.01. *Comprehensive accreditation manual for hospitals: The official handbook.* Oakbrook Terrace, IL: The Joint Commission. (Level I)
4 Centers for Disease Control and Prevention. (October 2002). Guideline for hand hygiene in health-care settings. *Morbidity and Mortality Weekly Report, 51* (RR-16), 1–45. (Level I)
5 The Joint Commission. (2012). Standard NPSG.07.01.01. *Comprehensive accreditation manual for hospitals: The official handbook.* Oakbrook Terrace, IL: The Joint Commission. (Level I)
6 World Health Organization. (2009). *WHO guidelines on hand hygiene in health care: First global patient safety challenge. Clean care is safer care.* Geneva, Switzerland: World Health Organization. (Level I)
7 The Joint Commission. (2012). Standard RC.01.03.01. *Comprehensive accreditation manual for hospitals: The official handbook.* Oakbrook Terrace, IL: The Joint Commission. (Level I)

ADDITIONAL REFERENCES

Centers for Disease Control and Prevention. (June 2003). Guidelines for environmental infection control in health-care facilities: Recommendations of CDC and the health care infection control practices advisory committee (HICPAC). *Morbidity and Mortality Weekly Report 52*(RR-10), 1–42.
Siegel, J.D., et al. (2006). "Management of multidrug-resistant organisms in healthcare settings, 2006" [Online]. Accessed June 2011 via the Web at www.cdc.gov/ncidod/dhqp/pdf/ar/MDRO Guideline2006.pdf

AIR-FLUIDIZED THERAPY BED USE

Originally designed for managing burns, the air-fluidized therapy bed is now used for patients with various debilities. By allowing harmless contact between the bed's surface and grafted sites, the bed promotes comfort and healing.

The traditional air-fluidized therapy bed is actually a large tub that supports the patient on a thick layer of silicone-coated microspheres of lime glass. Another version combines the air-fluidized section with a low-air-loss or cushioned section. (See *The air-fluidized therapy bed.*) A monofilament polyester filter sheet covers the microsphere-filled tub. Warmed air, propelled by a blower beneath the bed, passes through it. The resulting fluid-like surface reduces pressure on the skin to avoid obstructing capillary blood flow, thereby helping to prevent pressure ulcers and to promote wound healing.[1] The bed's air temperature can be adjusted

EQUIPMENT

The air-fluidized therapy bed

The air-fluidized therapy bed is a large tub filled with microspheres that are suspended by air pressure and give the patient fluidlike support. The bed provides the advantages of flotation without the disadvantages of instability, patient positioning difficulties, and immobility.

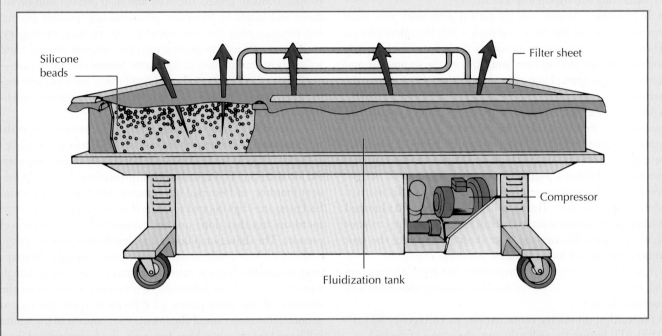

Silicone beads

Filter sheet

Compressor

Fluidization tank

to help control hypothermia and hyperthermia. The microprocessor technology also allows manipulation of various sections of the unit for optimum adjustment. Some models come with adjustable back and leg supports to promote positioning.

The air-fluidized therapy bed may be contraindicated for a patient with an unstable spine. It may also be contraindicated for a patient who can't mobilize and expel pulmonary secretions because the lack of back support impairs productive coughing. Operation of the air-fluidized therapy bed is complex and requires special training.

Equipment

Air-fluidized therapy bed with microspheres (about 1,650 lb [750 kg]) ▪ filter sheet ▪ flat sheet ▪ elastic cord ▪ Optional: gloves.

Preparation of equipment

Normally, a manufacturer's representative or a trained staff member prepares the bed for use. If you must help with the preparation, make sure the microspheres reach to within ½″ (1.3 cm) of the top of the tank. Then position the filter sheet on the bed with its printed side facing up. Match the holes in the sheet to the holes in the edge of the bed's frame. If the bed has detachable aluminum rails, place them on the frame, with the studs in the proper holes. Depress the rails firmly, and secure them by tightening the knurled knobs to seal the filter sheet. Place a flat sheet over the filter sheet or use the specialized sheet provided by the bed company, and secure it with the elastic cord. Turn on the air current *to activate the microspheres and to ensure that the bed is working properly;* then turn it off.

Implementation

▪ Perform hand hygiene and put on gloves.[2,3,4]
▪ Confirm the patient's identity using at least two patient identifiers according to your facility's policy.[5]
▪ Explain and, if possible, demonstrate the operation of the air-fluidized therapy bed. Tell the patient the reason for its use and that he'll feel as though he's floating.
▪ With the help of three or more coworkers, transfer the patient to the bed using a lift sheet.
▪ Use the foam wedge to elevate the head of the bed if the patient has a feeding tube *to prevent aspiration.*
▪ Turn on the air pressure to activate the bed, and remove the lift sheet.
▪ Adjust the air temperature as necessary. *Because the bed usually operates within 10° to 12° F (5.6° to 6.7° C) of ambient air temperature,* set the room temperature to 75° F (23.9° C). If microsphere temperature reaches 105° F (40.6° C), the bed automatically shuts off. It restarts automatically after 30 minutes.
▪ Remove and discard your gloves and perform hand hygiene.[3,4]
▪ Document the procedure.[6]

Special considerations

■ Monitor fluid and electrolyte status *because the air-fluidized therapy bed increases evaporative water loss.* Because of this drying effect, always cover a mesh graft for the first 2 to 8 days, as ordered. If the patient has excessive upper respiratory tract dryness, use a humidifier and mask, as ordered. Encourage coughing and deep breathing. After prolonged use of an air-fluidized bed, watch for hypocalcemia and hypophosphoremia.

■ To position a bedpan, roll the patient away from you, place the bedpan on the flat sheet, and push it into the microspheres. Then reposition the patient. To remove the bedpan, hold it steady and roll the patient away from you. Turn off the air pressure and remove the bedpan. Then turn the air on and reposition the patient.

■ Don't secure the filter sheet with pins or clamps, *which may puncture the sheet and release microspheres.* Take care to avoid puncturing the bed when giving injections. Holes or tears may be repaired with iron-on patching tape. Sieve the microspheres monthly or between patients *to remove any clumped microspheres.* Handle them carefully to avoid spills; *spilled microspheres may cause falls.* Treat a soiled filter sheet and clumped microspheres as contaminated items; handle according to your facility's policy. Change the filter sheet and operate the unit unoccupied for 24 hours between patients.

■ Assess the patient's skin and reposition him every 2 hours; specialty beds don't eliminate the need for frequent assessment and position changes.

■ For cardiopulmonary resuscitation, an emergency STOP/ DEFLATE button immediately stops the action of the bed.

Documentation

Record the duration of therapy and the patient's response to it. Document the condition of the patient's skin, pressure ulcers, and other wounds.

REFERENCES

1 VanGilder, C. et al. (2010). Air-fluidized therapy: Physical properties and clinical uses. *Annals of Plastic Surgery, 65*(3), 364–370.

2 Centers for Disease Control and Prevention. (October 2002). Guideline for hand hygiene in health-care settings. *Morbidity and Mortality Weekly Report, 51* (RR-16), 1–45. (Level I)

3 The Joint Commission. (2012). Standard NPSG. 07.01. *Comprehensive accreditation manual for hospitals: The official handbook.* Oakbrook Terrace, IL: The Joint Commission. (Level I)

4 World Health Organization. (2009). *WHO guidelines on hand hygiene in health care: First global patient safety challenge. Clean care is safer care.* Geneva, Switzerland: World Health Organization. (Level I)

5 The Joint Commission. (2012). Standard NPSG.01.01.01. *Comprehensive accreditation manual for hospitals: The official handbook.* Oakbrook Terrace, IL: The Joint Commission. (Level I)

6 The Joint Commission. (2012). Standard RC.01.03.01. *Comprehensive accreditation manual for hospitals: The official handbook.* Oakbrook Terrace, IL: The Joint Commission. (Level I)

ALIGNMENT AND PRESSURE-REDUCING DEVICES

Various assistive devices can be used to maintain correct body positioning and to help prevent complications that commonly arise when a patient must be on prolonged bed rest. Alignment and pressure-reducing devices, or pressure-redistribution devices, include boots to protect the heels and help prevent skin breakdown and footdrop; abduction pillows to help prevent internal hip rotation after femoral fracture, hip fracture, or surgery; trochanter rolls to help prevent external hip rotation; and hand rolls to help prevent hand contractures. Several of these devices—cradle boots, trochanter rolls, and hand rolls—are especially useful when caring for patients who have a loss of sensation, mobility, or consciousness.

Cradle boots, made of sponge rubber with heel cutouts, cushion the ankle and foot without completely enclosing it. Other commercial boots are available, but not all help to prevent external hip rotation. Footboards with anti-rotation blocks help prevent footdrop and external hip rotation, but they don't prevent heel pressure. High-topped sneakers may be used to help prevent footdrop, but they don't prevent external hip rotation or heel pressure. The abduction pillow is a wedge-shaped piece of sponge rubber with lateral indentations for the patient's thighs. Its straps wrap around the thighs to maintain correct positioning. Although a properly shaped bed pillow may temporarily substitute for the commercial abduction pillow, it's difficult to apply and fails to maintain the correct lateral alignment. The commercial trochanter roll is made of sponge rubber, but it can also be improvised from a rolled blanket or towel. The hand roll, available in hard and soft materials, is held in place by fixed or adjustable straps. It can be improvised from a rolled washcloth secured with roller gauze and adhesive tape. (See *Common preventive devices.*)

Equipment

Cradle boots ■ abduction pillow ■ trochanter rolls ■ hand rolls.

Preparation of equipment

If you're using a device that's available in different sizes, select the appropriate size for the patient.

Implementation

■ Perform hand hygiene.[1,2,3]

■ Confirm the patient's identity using at least two patient identifiers according to your facility's policy.[4]

■ Explain the purpose and steps of the procedure to the patient.

Applying a cradle boot

■ Open the slit on the superior surface of the boot. Then place the patient's heel in the circular cutout area. If the patient is positioned laterally, you may apply the boot only to the bottom foot and support the flexed top foot with a pillow.

■ If appropriate, insert the other foot in the second boot.

■ Position the patient's legs properly in alignment *to prevent strain on hip ligaments and pressure on bony prominences.*

EQUIPMENT

Common preventive devices

Equipment is available to reduce pressure or help maintain positioning, depending upon the patient's needs.

Cradle boot
Prevents footdrop, skin breakdown, and external hip rotation

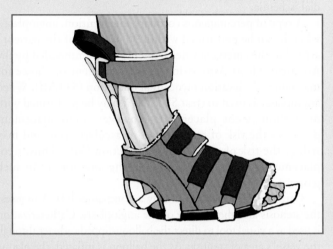

Trochanter roll
Prevents external hip rotation

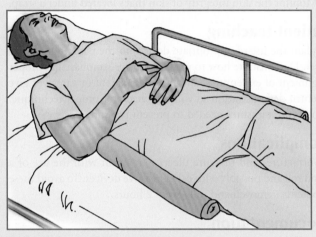

Abduction pillow
Prevents internal hip rotation and hip abduction

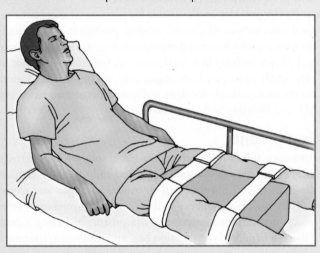

Hand roll
Prevents hand contractures

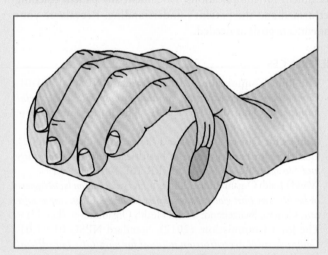

Applying an abduction pillow
■ Position the patient supine and place the pillow between the patient's legs. Slide it toward the groin so that it touches the legs all along its length.
■ Place the upper part of both legs in the pillow's lateral indentations and secure the straps *to prevent the pillow from slipping.*

Applying trochanter rolls
■ Position one roll along the outside of the thigh, from the iliac crest to midthigh. Then place another roll along the other thigh. Make sure neither roll extends as far as the knee *to avoid peroneal nerve compression and palsy, which can lead to footdrop.*

■ If you've fashioned trochanter rolls from a towel or rolled-up sheet, leave several inches unrolled and tuck this under the patient's thigh *to hold the device in place and maintain the patient's position.*

Applying a hand roll
■ Place one roll in the patient's hand to maintain the neutral position.
■ Secure the strap, if present, or apply roller gauze and secure with nonallergenic or adhesive tape.
■ Place another roll in the other hand.

Completing the procedure
- Perform hand hygiene.[1,2,3]
- Document the procedure.[5]

Special considerations
- Remember that the use of assistive devices doesn't preclude regularly scheduled patient positioning, range-of-motion exercises, and skin care.
- Monitor the skin integrity of skin that's located under a strap.

Patient teaching
Explain the use of appropriate devices to the patient and caregiver. Demonstrate how to use each device, emphasizing proper alignment of extremities, and have the patient or caregiver give a return demonstration so you can check for proper technique. Emphasize measures needed to prevent pressure ulcers.

Complications
Contractures and pressure ulcers may occur with the use of a hand roll and possibly with other assistive devices. To avoid these problems, remove hand rolls every 2 hours.

Documentation
Record the use of these devices in the patient's chart and the nursing care plan, include the reason for the device, and indicate assessment for complications. Document any patient teaching performed and the patient's understanding. Reevaluate your patient care goals as needed.

REFERENCES

1 The Joint Commission. (2012). Standard NPSG.07.01.01. *Comprehensive accreditation manual for hospitals: The official handbook.* Oakbrook Terrace, IL: The Joint Commission. (Level I)
2 Centers for Disease Control and Prevention. (October 2002). Guideline for hand hygiene in health-care settings. *Morbidity and Mortality Weekly Report, 51* (RR-16), 1–45. (Level I)
3 World Health Organization. (2009). *WHO guidelines on hand hygiene in health care: First global patient safety challenge. Clean care is safer care.* Geneva, Switzerland: World Health Organization. (Level I)
4 The Joint Commission. (2012). Standard NPSG.01.01.01. *Comprehensive accreditation manual for hospitals: The official handbook.* Oakbrook Terrace, IL: The Joint Commission. (Level I)
5 The Joint Commission. (2012). Standard RC.01.03.01. *Comprehensive accreditation manual for hospitals: The official handbook.* Oakbrook Terrace, IL: The Joint Commission. (Level I)

ADDITIONAL REFERENCES

Baranoski, S., & Ayello, E. (2008). *Wound care essentials practice and principles* (2nd ed.). Philadelphia, PA: Lippincott Williams & Wilkins.
National Pressure Ulcer Advisory Panel. (2007). "Pressure Ulcer Prevention Points" [Online]. Accessed June 2011 via the Web at http://www.npuap.org/PU_Prev_Points.pdf

ANGIOPLASTY CARE

A nonsurgical approach to opening coronary vessels narrowed by arteriosclerosis, percutaneous transluminal coronary angioplasty (PTCA) uses a balloon-tipped catheter that's inserted into a narrowed coronary artery. This procedure, performed in the cardiac catheterization laboratory under local anesthesia, helps restore circulation to the heart, relieving pain caused by angina and myocardial ischemia.

A type of percutaneous coronary intervention, angioplasty, when it can be performed within 90 minutes of the patient's arrival to the emergency department, is recommended by the American Heart Association as the treatment of choice for managing ST-elevation myocardial infarction (STEMI). When angioplasty is used to treat STEMI, it may be performed with or without stent placement. However, stent placement decreases the risk of target vessel revascularization and may reduce the risk of myocardial reinfarction (MI). Thus, stent placement has become routine during angioplasty in such patients.[1,2]

Cardiac catheterization usually accompanies PTCA to assess the stenosis and the efficacy of the angioplasty. Catheterization is used as a visual tool to direct the balloon-tipped catheter through the vessel's area of stenosis. As the balloon is inflated, the plaque is compressed against the vessel wall, allowing coronary blood to flow more freely. (See *Performing PTCA.*)

PTCA provides an alternative for patients who are poor surgical risks because of chronic medical problems. It's also useful for patients who have total coronary occlusion, unstable angina, and plaque buildup in several areas and for those with poor left ventricular function. After angioplasty, it's important to monitor the patient closely for signs and symptoms of coronary spasm, MI, and bleeding at the insertion site.

Equipment
Antiseptic solution (chlorhexidine-based solution is preferred) ■ local anesthetic ■ IV solution as ordered and tubing ■ electrocardiogram (ECG) monitor and electrodes ■ oxygen and oxygen delivery system ■ clippers ■ sedative ■ contrast medium ■ emergency medications ■ emergency equipment, including a defibrillator, a handheld resuscitation bag, and intubation equipment ■ heparin for injection ■ introducer kit for PTCA catheter ■ eye protection ■ gloves ■ sterile gown, gloves, and drapes ■ surgical cap, mask, and eye protection ■ Optional: nitroglycerin, pulmonary artery (PA) catheter, transparent dressing.

Implementation
Preprocedure care
- Confirm the patient's identity using at least two patient identifiers according to your facility's policy.[3]
- Explain the procedure to the patient and his family *to reduce the patient's fear and promote cooperation.*
- Inform the patient that the procedure lasts from 1 to 4 hours and that he may feel some discomfort from lying on a hard table for that long.

Performing PTCA

Percutaneous transluminal coronary angioplasty (PTCA) is a procedure that opens an occluded coronary artery without opening the chest. It's performed in the cardiac catheterization laboratory after coronary angiography confirms the presence and location of the occlusion. When the occlusion is located, the doctor threads a guide catheter through the patient's femoral artery and into the coronary artery under fluoroscopic guidance.

When the guide catheter's position at the occlusion site is confirmed by angiography, the doctor carefully introduces into the catheter a double-lumen balloon that's smaller than the catheter lumen. He then directs the balloon through the lesion, where a marked pressure gradient will be obvious. The doctor alternately inflates and deflates the balloon until an angiogram verifies successful arterial dilation and the pressure gradient has decreased.

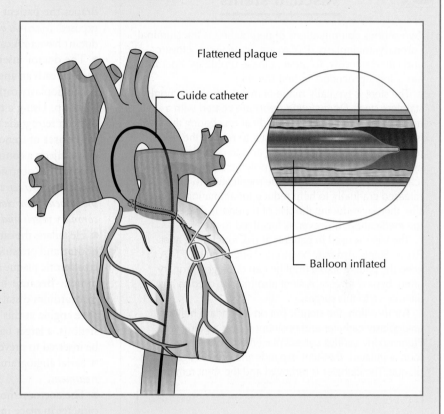

Flattened plaque

Guide catheter

Balloon inflated

Tell him that a catheter will be inserted into an artery or a vein in his groin and that he may feel pressure as the catheter moves along the vessel.

■ Reassure him that although he'll be awake during the procedure, he'll be given a sedative. Explain that the doctor or nurse will ask him how he's feeling and that he should tell them if he experiences any chest pain.

■ Explain that the doctor will inject a contrast medium *to outline the lesion's location.* Warn the patient that he may feel a hot, flushing sensation or transient nausea during the injection.

■ Conduct a preprocedure verification process *to make sure that all relevant documentation, related information, and equipment are available and correctly identified to the patient's identifiers.*[4]

■ Check the patient's history for allergies; if he has had allergic reactions to shellfish, iodine, or contrast media, notify the doctor.

■ Make sure that informed consent has been obtained and is documented in the patient's medical record.[5]

■ Restrict food and fluids for at least 6 hours before the procedure, or as ordered.

■ Ensure that the results of coagulation studies, complete blood count, serum electrolyte studies, and blood typing and cross-matching are available.

■ Perform hand hygiene and put on gloves.[6,7,8]

■ Administer antiplatelet drugs and antithrombotic drugs as ordered, following safe medication administration practices.[2,9]

■ Insert an IV catheter *in case emergency medications are required.* (See "IV catheter insertion and removal," page 421.)

■ Clip hair from the insertion site (groin or brachial area).[10]

■ Clean the area of skin at the insertion site with antiseptic solution.

■ Give the patient a sedative as ordered, following safe medication administration practices.

■ Obtain baseline vital signs and assess peripheral pulses in all extremities.

■ Remove and discard your gloves and perform hand hygiene.[6,7,8]

■ Communicate information about the patient's history, condition, and care to the nurse who will care for the patient during PTCA and then give her the opportunity to ask questions. *Hand-off communication between caregivers promotes patient safety and prevents errors.*

■ Document your preparation of the patient.[11]

Intraprocedure care

■ Perform hand hygiene and put on gloves.[6,7,8]

■ When the patient arrives at the cardiac catheterization laboratory, confirm the patient's identity using at least two patient identifiers according to your facility's policy.[3]

■ Conduct a preprocedure verification process *to make sure that all relevant documentation, related information, and equipment are available and correctly identified to the patient's identifiers.*[4]

EQUIPMENT

Vascular stents

Two serious complications of percutaneous transluminal coronary angioplasty (PTCA) are acute vessel closure and late restenosis. To prevent these problems, doctors are using a procedure called *stenting*.

The stent is typically made of metal, most commonly stainless steel. *Drug-eluting stents* are coated with a medication or polymer. The medication coating the stent is released at the implantation site to reduce the risk of restenosis. The polymer coating acts to decrease platelet aggregation. In addition, some polymers contain medication. The polymer allows the medication to be released gradually to help reduce inflammation at the site, thereby reducing the risk of restenosis. The effect of the medication, however, is localized to the area.

The stent is used in patients at risk for clotting after PTCA. Stents also may be inserted after a failed PTCA to keep the patient stable until he can undergo coronary artery bypass surgery. A stent also may be used as an alternative to this surgery.

For insertion, the stent is put on a standard balloon angioplasty catheter and positioned over a guide wire. Fluoroscopy verifies correct placement. When the balloon is inflated, the stent expands and presses against the plaque. The catheter is removed and the stent remains.

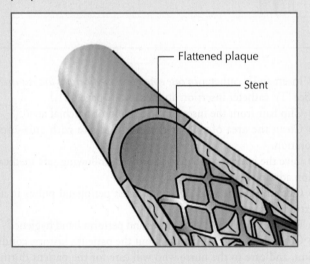

Flattened plaque

Stent

■ Confirm that the correct procedure has been identified for the correct patient at the correct site.[4]
■ Apply ECG electrodes and ensure IV catheter patency.
■ Administer oxygen through an appropriate oxygen delivery device.
■ Conduct a time-out immediately before starting the procedure *to determine that the correct patient, site, positioning, and procedure are identified and confirmed, as applicable, and that relevant information and necessary equipment are available.*[12]
■ The doctor will put on a surgical cap, a mask, a sterile gown, and gloves. Put on the same personal protective equipment.

■ Open the sterile supplies and label all medications, medication containers, and other solutions on and off the sterile field.[13]
■ The doctor prepares the site, injects a local anesthetic, and then drapes the patient from head to toe, leaving the insertion site exposed. *Maximal barrier precautions prevent infection.* If the patient doesn't have a PA catheter in place, the doctor may insert one now.
■ The doctor inserts a large guide catheter into the artery and then threads an angioplasty catheter through the guide catheter. An angioplasty catheter is thinner and longer and has a balloon at its tip. Using a thin, flexible guide wire, he then threads the catheter retrograde through the aorta and into the coronary artery to the area of stenosis.
■ He injects a contrast medium through the angioplasty catheter and into the obstructed coronary artery *to outline the lesion's location and help assess the blockage.* He also injects heparin *to prevent the catheter from clotting,* and intracoronary nitroglycerin *to dilate coronary vessels and prevent spasm, if needed.*
■ He inflates the catheter's balloon, gradually increasing the amount of time and pressure. The expanding balloon compresses the atherosclerotic plaque against the arterial wall, expanding the arterial lumen. Because balloon inflation blocks blood flow to the myocardium distal to the inflation area, the patient may experience angina at this time. If balloon inflation fails to decrease the stenosis, a larger balloon may be used. A vascular stent may also be inserted to prevent vessel closure. (See *Vascular stents.*)
■ Serial angiograms are done *to help determine the effectiveness of treatment.*
■ The doctor removes the angioplasty catheter, leaving the guide catheter in place *in case the procedure needs to be repeated because of vessel occlusion.* The guide catheter is usually sutured at this time and is generally removed 2 to 24 hours after the procedure.
■ Remove and dispose of equipment in appropriate receptacles. Perform hand hygiene.[6] Document the procedure.[11]

Postprocedure care
■ When the patient returns to the unit, perform hand hygiene and put on gloves.[6,7,8]
■ Confirm his identity using at least two patient identifiers according to your facility's policy.[3]
■ When the patient returns to the unit, he may be receiving anticoagulants. If he's bleeding at the catheter insertion site, he may also have a compression device on it *to prevent a hematoma.* Alternatively, manual pressure may be applied. If bleeding at the site occurs, apply pressure approximately 2 to 3 cm above the puncture site.
■ Assess the patient's vital signs every 15 minutes for the first hour, then every 30 minutes for 4 hours, or according to your facility's policy.
■ Assess peripheral pulses distal to the catheter insertion site as well as the color, sensation, temperature, and capillary refill of the affected extremity every 15 minutes for the first hour, then every 30 minutes for 4 hours, or according to your facility's policy.
■ Monitor and record ECG rhythm and arterial pressures.
NURSING ALERT *Because coronary spasm may occur during or after PTCA, monitor the patient's ECG for ST- and T-wave changes, and obtain vital signs frequently. Be alert for signs*

and symptoms of ischemia, which requires emergency coronary revascularization.

■ Instruct the patient to remain in bed for the amount of time specified by the doctor and to keep the affected extremity straight and immobilized while he's on bed rest. Elevate the head of the bed 15 to 30 degrees. *Bed rest times vary depending on the technique used for closure during PTCA, the size of the sheath used, whether the patient receives antiplatelet therapy after the procedure, and facility policy.*

■ Assess the catheter site for hematoma, ecchymosis, and hemorrhage. If an area of expanding hematoma appears, mark the site and alert the doctor. If bleeding occurs, locate the artery and apply manual pressure; then notify the doctor.

■ Administer IV fluids, as ordered (usually 100 mL/hour) *to promote excretion of the contrast medium.* Be sure to assess for signs of fluid overload (distended jugular veins, atrial and ventricular gallops, dyspnea, pulmonary congestion, tachycardia, hypertension, and hypoxemia).

■ Perform hand hygiene and then put on gloves.[6,7,8] After the catheter is removed, apply direct pressure for at least 10 minutes and monitor the site often. Place a dressing over the site, preferably a transparent film dressing.[14]

■ Remove and discard your gloves and perform hand hygiene.[6,7,8]

■ Document the procedure.[11]

Special considerations

■ Devices to prevent lower extremity embolism are recommended for use during PTCA.

■ The current recommendation is to administer 75 mg of clopidogrel daily or 10 mg of prasugrel daily after the procedure for a period of 1 to 12 months, depending on the exact procedure completed. If the patient isn't already receiving long-term aspirin therapy, 300 to 325 mg/day of aspirin may also be prescribed for 1 to 6 months, depending on the patient's condition and status. This is typically followed by a regimen of 75 to 162 mg/day.[2]

■ If the patient exhibits signs and symptoms of an MI after the procedure, a 12-lead ECG and CK-MB and troponin levels should be obtained.

■ If the patient is restless, moving his extremities, and at risk for self-injury, apply soft restraints, if necessary.

Complications

The most common complication of PTCA is restenosis. Others include prolonged angina, coronary artery perforation, balloon rupture, reocclusion (necessitating a coronary artery bypass graft), MI, pericardial tamponade, hematoma, hemorrhage, reperfusion arrhythmias, and closure of the vessel.

Documentation

Note the patient's status before the procedure and response during the procedure. Include vital signs and the condition of the extremity distal to the insertion site. Document any complications and interventions performed before, during, or after the procedure.

REFERENCES

1 American Heart Association. (2010). American Heart Association guidelines for cardiopulmonary resuscitation and emergency cardiovascular care. *Circulation, 122*(Suppl. 3), S787–S817. (Level I)

2 Kushner, F., et al. (2009). 2009 focused updates: ACC/AHA guidelines for the management of patients with ST-elevation myocardial infarction (updating the 2004 Guideline and 2007 focused Update) and ACC/AHA/SCAI guidelines on percutaneous coronary intervention (updating the 2005 guideline and 2007 focused update): A Report of the American College of Cardiology Foundation/American Heart Association Task Force on Practice Guidelines. *Circulation, 120*(22), 2271–306. (Level I)

3 The Joint Commission. (2012). Standard NPSG.01.01.01. *Comprehensive accreditation manual for hospitals: The official handbook.* Oakbrook Terrace, IL: The Joint Commission. (Level I)

4 The Joint Commission. (2012). Standard UP.01.01.01. *Comprehensive accreditation manual for hospitals: The official handbook.* Oakbrook Terrace, IL: The Joint Commission. (Level I)

5 The Joint Commission. (2012). Standard RI.01.03.01. *Comprehensive accreditation manual for hospitals: The official handbook.* Oakbrook Terrace, IL: The Joint Commission. (Level I)

6 The Joint Commission. (2012). Standard NPSG.07.01.01. *Comprehensive accreditation manual for hospitals: The official handbook.* Oakbrook Terrace, IL: The Joint Commission. (Level I)

7 Centers for Disease Control and Prevention. (October 2002). Guideline for hand hygiene in health-care settings. *Morbidity and Mortality Weekly Report, 51* (RR-16), 1–45. (Level I)

8 World Health Organization. (2009). *WHO guidelines on hand hygiene in health care: First global patient safety challenge. Clean care is safer care.* Geneva, Switzerland: World Health Organization. (Level I)

9 King, S., et al. (2007). 2007 focused update of the ACC/AHA/SCAI 2005 guideline update for percutaneous coronary intervention: A report of the American College of Cardiology/American Heart Association Task Force on Practice Guidelines (2007 writing group to review new evidence and update the ACC/AHA/SCAI 2005 guidelines for percutaneous coronary intervention). *Circulation, 117*(1), 261–295. (Level I)

10 The Joint Commission. (2012). Standard NPSG.07.05. *Comprehensive accreditation manual for hospitals: The official handbook.* Oakbrook Terrace, IL: The Joint Commission. (Level I)

11 The Joint Commission. (2012). Standard RC.01.03.01. *Comprehensive accreditation manual for hospitals: The official handbook.* Oakbrook Terrace, IL: The Joint Commission. (Level I)

12 The Joint Commission. (2012). Standard UP.01.03.01. *Comprehensive accreditation manual for hospitals: The official handbook.* Oakbrook Terrace, IL: The Joint Commission. (Level I)

13 The Joint Commission. (2012). Standard NPSG.03.04. *Comprehensive accreditation manual for hospitals: The official handbook.* Oakbrook Terrace, IL: The Joint Commission. (Level I)

14 Mcle, S., et al. Transparent film dressing vs pressure dressing after percutaneous transluminal coronary angiography. *American Journal of Critical Care, 18*(1), 14–19. (Level IV)

ADDITIONAL REFERENCES

Hirsch, J., et al. (2008). Antithrombotic and thrombolytic therapy: American College of Chest Physicians Evidence-Based Clinical Practice Guidelines (8th edition). *Chest, 133*(6 Suppl.), 110S–112S.

Maluenda, G., et al. (2009). The clinical significance of hematocrit values before and after percutaneous coronary intervention. *American Heart Journal, 158*(6), 1024–1030.

Manoukian, S.V. (2009). Predictors and impact of bleeding complications in percutaneous coronary intervention, acute coronary syndromes, and ST-segment elevation myocardial infarction. *American Journal of Cardiology, 104*(5 Suppl.), 9C–15C.

Rolley, J.X., et al. (2009). Review of nursing care for patients undergoing percutaneous coronary intervention: A patient journey approach. *Journal of Clinical Nursing, 18*(17), 2394–2405.

Ruiz-Nodar, J.M., et al. (2008). Anticoagulant and antiplatelet therapy use in 426 patients with atrial fibrillation undergoing percutaneous coronary intervention and stent implantation: Implications for bleeding risk and prognosis. *Journal of the American College of Cardiology, 51*(8), 818–825.

Zibaeenezhad, M.J., & Mazloum, Y. (2009). Heparin infusion after successful percutaneous coronary intervention: A prospective, randomized trial. *Acta Cardiologica, 64*(1), 65–70.

ANTIEMBOLISM STOCKING APPLICATION

Elastic antiembolism stockings help prevent deep vein thrombosis (DVT) and pulmonary embolism by compressing superficial leg veins. This compression increases venous return by forcing blood into the deep venous system rather than allowing it to pool in the legs and form clots. Antiembolism stockings can provide equal pressure over the entire leg or a graded pressure that's greatest at the ankle and decreases over the length of the leg. Usually indicated for postoperative, bedridden, elderly, or other patients at risk for DVT, these stockings shouldn't be used on patients with dermatoses or open skin lesions, gangrene, severe arteriosclerosis or other ischemic vascular diseases, pulmonary or any massive edema, recent vein ligation, or vascular or skin grafts. For patients with chronic venous problems, intermittent pneumatic compression stockings may be ordered during surgery and postoperatively. (See "Sequential compression therapy," page 645.)

Equipment

Tape measure ▪ antiembolism stockings of correct size and length ▪ talcum powder.

Preparation of equipment
Before applying a knee-length stocking
Measure the circumference of the patient's calf at its widest point and leg length from the bottom of the heel to the back of the knee. (See *Measuring for antiembolism stockings.*)

Before applying a thigh-length stocking
Measure the circumference of the calf and thigh at their widest points and the leg length from the bottom of the heel to the gluteal fold.

Before applying a waist-length stocking
Measure the circumference of the calf and thigh at their widest points and the leg length from the bottom of the heel along the side to the waist.

Obtain the correct size stocking according to the manufacturer's specifications. If the patient's measurements are outside the range indicated by the manufacturer or if his legs are deformed or edematous, ask the doctor if he wants to order custom-made stockings.

Implementation
- Check the doctor's order.
- Confirm the patient's identity using at least two patient identifiers according to your facility's policy.[1]
- Provide privacy and explain the procedure to the patient.
- Perform hand hygiene.[2,3,4]
- Assess the patient's condition. If his legs are cold or cyanotic, notify the doctor before proceeding.
- Have the patient lie down. Then dust his ankle with talcum powder *to ease application.*

Applying a knee-length stocking
- Insert your hand into the stocking from the top and grasp the heel pocket from the inside. Holding the heel, turn the stocking inside out so that the foot is inside the stocking leg. *This method allows easier application than gathering the entire stocking and working it up over the foot and ankle.*
- With the heel pocket down, hook the index and middle fingers of both your hands into the foot section. Facing the patient, ease the stocking over the toes, stretching it sideways as you move it up the foot.
- Support the patient's ankle with one hand and use the other hand to pull the heel pocket under the heel. Then center the heel in the pocket.
- Gather the loose portion of the stocking at the toe and pull only this section over the heel (as shown below).

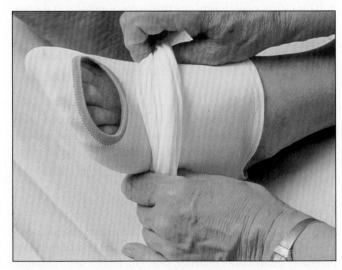

Measuring for antiembolism stockings

Measure the patient carefully to ensure that his antiembolism stockings provide enough compression for adequate venous return.

To choose the correct knee-length stocking, measure the circumference of the calf at its widest point (top left) and the leg length from the bottom of the heel to the back of the knee (bottom left).

To choose a thigh-length stocking, measure the calf as for a knee-length stocking and the thigh at its widest point (top right). Then measure leg length from the bottom of the heel to the gluteal fold (bottom right).

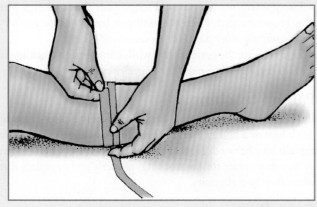 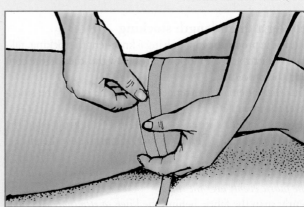

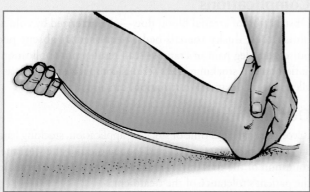 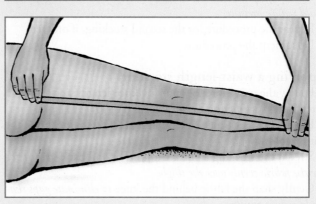

■ Gather the loose material at the ankle and slide the rest of the stocking up over the heel with short pulls, alternating front and back (as shown below).

■ Insert your index and middle fingers into the gathered stocking at the ankle and ease the fabric up the leg to the knee (as shown below).

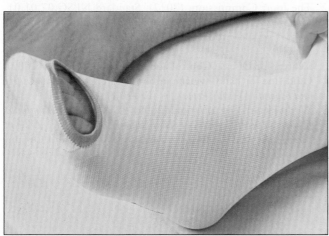 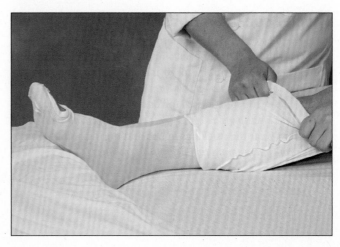

■ Supporting the patient's ankle with one hand, use your other hand to stretch the stocking toward the knee, front and back, *to distribute the material evenly.* The stocking top should be 1″ to 2″ (2.5 to 5 cm) below the bottom of the patella.

■ Gently snap the fabric around the ankle *to ensure a tight fit and eliminate gaps that could reduce pressure.*

■ Adjust the foot section *for fabric smoothness and toe comfort* by tugging on the toe section. Properly position the toe window, if any.

■ Repeat the procedure for the second stocking, if ordered.

■ Document the procedure.[5]

Applying a thigh-length stocking

■ Follow the procedure for applying a knee-length stocking, taking care to distribute the fabric evenly below the knee before continuing the procedure.

■ With the patient's leg extended, stretch the rest of the stocking over the knee.

■ Flex the patient's knee, and pull the stocking over the thigh until the top is 1″ to 3″ (2.5 to 7.5 cm) below the gluteal fold.

■ Stretch the stocking from the top, front and back, *to distribute the fabric evenly over the thigh.*

■ Gently snap the fabric behind the knee *to eliminate gaps that could reduce pressure.*

■ Repeat the procedure for the second stocking, if ordered.

■ Document the procedure.[5]

Applying a waist-length stocking

■ Follow the procedure for applying knee-length stockings and extend the stocking top to the gluteal fold.

■ Flex the patient's knee, and pull the stocking to the top of the gluteal fold.

■ Stretch the stocking from the top, front and back, *to distribute the fabric evenly over the thigh.*

■ Gently snap the fabric behind the knee *to eliminate gaps that could reduce pressure.*

■ Fit the patient with the adjustable belt that accompanies the stockings. Make sure that the waistband and the fabric don't interfere with any incision, drainage tube, catheter, or other device.

■ Document the procedure.[5]

Special considerations

■ Apply the stockings in the morning, if possible, *before edema develops.* If the patient has been ambulating, ask him to lie down and elevate his legs for 15 to 30 minutes before applying the stockings *to facilitate venous return.*

■ Don't allow the stockings to roll or turn down at the top or toe *because the excess pressure could cause venous strangulation.* Have the patient wear the stockings in bed and during ambulation *to provide continuous protection against thrombosis.*

■ Check the patient's toes at least every 4 hours—more often in the patient with a faint pulse or edema. Note skin color and temperature, sensation, swelling, and ability to move. If complications occur, remove the stockings and notify the doctor immediately.

■ Be alert for an allergic reaction *because some patients can't tolerate the sizing in new stockings.* Laundering the stockings before applying them reduces the risk of an allergic reaction to sizing. Remove the stockings at least once daily *to bathe the skin and observe for irritation and breakdown.*

■ Using warm water and mild soap, wash the stockings when they become soiled. Keep a second pair handy *for the patient to wear while the other pair is being laundered.*

■ Don't elevate the patient's legs while compression stockings are on him *because of the risk of decreased circulation.*

Patient teaching

If the patient will require antiembolism stockings after discharge, teach him or a family member how to apply them correctly and explain why he needs to wear them.[6] Instruct the patient or family member to care for the stockings properly and to replace them when they lose elasticity.

Complications

Obstruction of arterial blood flow—characterized by cold and bluish toes, dusky toenail beds, decreased or absent pedal pulses, and leg pain or cramps—can result from application of antiembolism stockings. Less serious complications, such as an allergic reaction and skin irritation, can also occur.

Documentation

Record the date and time of stocking application, stocking length and size, condition of the leg and foot before and after treatment, condition of the toes during treatment, any complications, and the patient's tolerance of the treatment.

REFERENCES

1 The Joint Commission. (2012). Standard NPSG.01.01.01. *Comprehensive accreditation manual for hospitals: The official handbook.* Oakbrook Terrace, IL: The Joint Commission. (Level I)

2 The Joint Commission. (2012). Standard NPSG.07.01.01. *Comprehensive accreditation manual for hospitals: The official handbook.* Oakbrook Terrace, IL: The Joint Commission. (Level I)

3 Centers for Disease Control and Prevention. (October 2002). Guideline for hand hygiene in health-care settings. *Morbidity and Mortality Weekly Report, 51* (RR-16), 1–45. (Level I)

4 World Health Organization. (2009). *WHO guidelines on hand hygiene in health care: First global patient safety challenge. Clean care is safer care.* Geneva, Switzerland: World Health Organization. (Level I)

5 The Joint Commission. (2012). Standard RC.01.03.01. *Comprehensive accreditation manual for hospitals: The official handbook.* Oakbrook Terrace, IL: The Joint Commission. (Level I)

6 Court, A., et al. (2008). The Joanna Briggs Institute: Graduated compression stockings for the prevention of post-operative venous thrombosis. *International Journal of Evidence-Based Healthcare, 4*(4):43–50. (Level I)

ADDITIONAL REFERENCES

ACOG Committee on Practice Bulletins. (2001, reaffirmed 2008). ACOG practice bulletin 19. Thromboembolism in pregnancy. *International Journal of Gynecology and Obstetrics, 75* (2), 203–212.

Brady, D., et al. (2007). The use of knee-length versus thigh-length compression stockings and sequential compression devices. *Critical Care Nursing Quarterly, 30*(3), 255–262.

Craven, R.F., & Hirnle, C.J. (2009). *Fundamentals of nursing: Human health and function* (6th ed.). Philadelphia, PA: Lippincott Williams & Wilkins.

Hilleren-Listerud, A.E. (2009). Graduated compression stocking and intermittent pneumatic compression device length selection. *Clinical Nurse Specialist, 23*(1), 21–24.

Hirsch, J., et al. (2008). American College of Chest physicians evidence-based clinical practice guidelines (8th Edition). *Chest, 133*(6), 71s–109s.

Nettina, S.M. (2010). *Lippincott manual of nursing practice* (9th ed.). Philadelphia, PA: Lippincott Williams & Wilkins.

Snow, V., et al. (2007). Management of venous thromboembolism: A clinical practice guideline from the American College of Physicians and the American Academy of Family Physicians. *Annals of Internal Medicine, 146*(3), 204–210.

Taylor, C., et al. (2011). *Fundamentals of nursing: The art and science of nursing care* (7th ed.). Philadelphia, PA: Lippincott Williams & Wilkins.

Winslow, E.H., and Brosz, D.L. (2008). Graduated compression stockings in hospitalized postoperative patients: Correctness of usage and size. *AJN, 108*(9), 40–50.

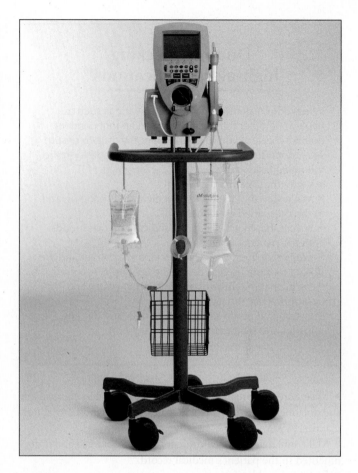

AQUAPHERESIS

Aquapheresis is a therapy that uses ultrafiltration to remove fluid from the blood. It provides an alternative method for relieving congestion caused by fluid overload in patients with decompensated heart failure who are resistant to diuretics.[1]

Aquapheresis is provided using venovenous access and a device known as the Aquadex FlexFlow ultrafiltration system (as shown at right on top). This device mechanically withdraws blood through a catheter and passes it through a hemofilter, which removes excess sodium and water, restoring fluid balance. After the patient's blood is filtered, it's returned to the patient through the infusion port of the catheter.

NURSING ALERT *Only individuals who have received specialized training in administering aquapheresis therapy are permitted to administer the therapy.[2]*

Equipment

Aquadex FlexFlow pump ▪ sterile, disposable, single-use extracorporeal blood circuit set ▪ IV heparin bolus ▪ heparin infusion ▪ 500-mL IV bag of normal saline solution ▪ 10-mL syringes ▪ graduated liquid waste receptacle ▪ gloves ▪ sterile end caps ▪ alcohol pads ▪ venovenous access device (a 6 French dual-lumen extended-length peripheral catheter, a 5 French single-lumen extended-length peripheral catheter, and an 18G IV catheter, or a 7 or 8 French dual-lumen central venous access catheter).

Preparation of equipment

Before therapy is initiated, the doctor or specially trained nurse will insert a venovenous access device. The catheter must be able to accommodate a blood flow of 10 to 40 mL/minute.

Gather all the equipment in the patient's room. Inspect the sterile packages *to make sure they're intact.* Don't use a blood circuit system that's damaged or that has kinks in the tubing. Follow sterile technique throughout the therapy.[3,4]

Implementation

▪ Verify the doctor's order for aquapheresis in the patient's medical record, and make sure that diuretic and electrolyte replacement therapy has been discontinued before initiating therapy.

- Make sure that preprocedure laboratory test results are available and documented in the patient's medical record; report any abnormalities.
- Make sure that informed consent has been obtained and is documented in the patient's medical record.[5]
- Perform hand hygiene.[4,6,7]
- Confirm the patient's identity using at least two patient identifiers, according to your facility's policy.[8]
- Explain the procedure to the patient *to allay his fears and promote cooperation.*
- Obtain the patient's weight.
- Begin anticoagulant therapy at least 30 minutes before the procedure, as ordered, following safe medication administration practices. *Typically an IV bolus dose of heparin is given, followed by a continuous heparin infusion.*

NURSING ALERT *When administered IV, heparin is considered a high-alert medication* because it can cause significant patient harm when used in error. *Another nurse must double-check certain preparation steps* to ensure safe medication administration.[9]

- Before starting the heparin infusion, have another nurse perform an independent double-check according to your facility's policy. (See *Double-checking high-alert medications.*)
- After comparing results of the independent double-check with the other nurse, begin infusing the heparin (through the withdrawal port of the access device) if there are no discrepancies. If discrepancies exist, rectify them before beginning the infusion.[10]
- Perform hand hygiene and put on gloves.[4,6,7]
- Verify patency of the access catheter.

Priming the blood circuit
- Plug the power cord into a grounded electrical outlet.

- Press the ON/OFF key on the front panel. (See *A look at the aquapheresis circuit.*)
- Place the blood pump cartridge into the blood pump on the machine console and snap it into place. Turn the knob clockwise until you hear a beep.
- Insert the ultrafiltrate cartridge in the side of the console and snap it into place. Turn the knob clockwise until you hear a beep.
- Insert the tubing into the blood leak and air sensors.
- Put the pressure sensor cables into their proper connectors, located on the console.
- Insert the data key provided with the blood circuit system into the reader on the front of the console; *this data key facilitates many of the system's functions.*[3]
- Hang the empty ultrafiltrate collection bag on the machine's weight scale hook and close the drain valve located at the bottom of the bag.
- Remove the end caps from the infusion tubing of the circuit and the priming adapter on the ultrafiltrate drainage bag, and then attach the circuit infusion tubing to the priming adaptor on the ultrafiltrate drainage bag.
- Remove the end caps from the withdrawal tubing and the priming spike adapter, and then attach the withdrawal tubing to the withdrawal priming spike adapter.
- Spike the 500-mL priming bag of normal saline solution with the priming spike, and then hang the bag on the priming hook, making sure that the ultrafiltrate bag hangs freely.
- Open the clamps on the withdrawal tubing, infusion tubing, and ultrafiltrate bag priming adapter.
- Press the PRIME key and follow the onscreen instructions; priming should be completed and the system should be free from air in about 4 minutes.
- Empty the priming solution from the fluid collection bag before starting therapy. *Priming solution drains into the collection bag; emptying the collection bag ensures the accuracy of the patient's output measurement.*
- Close the clamps on the blood circuit set, remove the end cap on the withdrawal catheter lumen, disconnect the withdrawal line from the IV spike, and connect the withdrawal line to the withdrawal catheter lumen.
- Remove the end cap from the infusion catheter lumen, disconnect the infusion line from the ultrafiltrate priming adapter, and connect the infusion line to the infusion catheter lumen.
- Trace the tubings from the patient to their points of origin to make sure that you've attached them to the proper catheter lumens.[10]
- Put sterile end caps on the saline priming spike and the ultrafiltrate priming adaptor.

Beginning therapy
- Open the withdrawal and infusion tubing clamps.
- Press the RUN key to begin therapy.[3]
- If your unit has a hematocrit (HCT) monitor, make sure that the sensor clip is attached to the blood chamber on the blood circuit. Allow 5 to 10 minutes to elapse in the RUN mode to complete the initial baseline measurement of the patient's HCT. The text "Baselining" will appear; after "Baselining" is complete, press the HCT key to set the HCT limit, using the up and down arrows.

EQUIPMENT

A look at the aquapheresis circuit

Aquapheresis requires a circuit like the one below to filter fluid and sodium from patients with fluid overload.

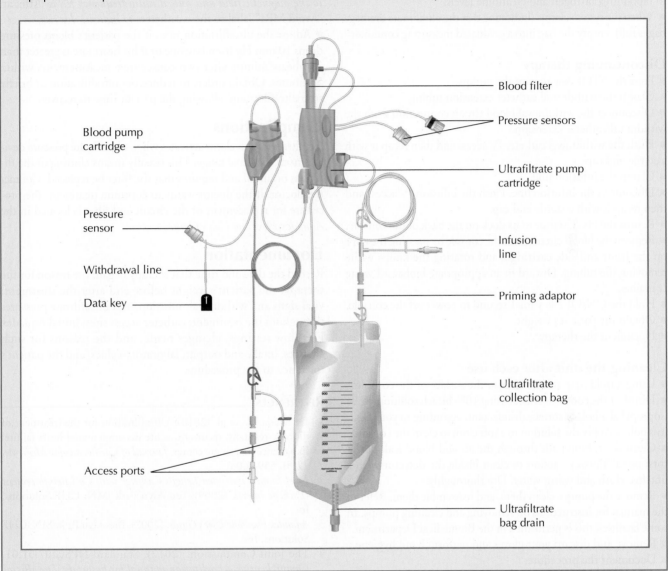

- Blood filter
- Pressure sensors
- Ultrafiltrate pump cartridge
- Infusion line
- Priming adaptor
- Ultrafiltrate collection bag
- Ultrafiltrate bag drain
- Blood pump cartridge
- Pressure sensor
- Withdrawal line
- Data key
- Access ports

The HCT limit automatically restricts the fluid removal rate *to help prevent excessive volume depletion.*[3]

■ Set the blood flow rate by pressing the BLOOD FLOW key. Use the arrow keys to adjust the value. For a central venous catheter, begin the flow rate at 40 mL/minute. For a peripheral dual-lumen extended-length catheter, begin the flow rate at 25 mL/minute.

■ After the blood flow rate is stable, increase the rate in increments of 10 mL/hour until an adequate rate is determined. Use the arrow keys to adjust the rate. The average removal rate is 250 mL/hour. Patients in volume-sensitive states, such as those with right-sided heart failure, hepatic disease, or cardiogenic shock, usually require lower rates (50 to 100 mL/hr).[12]

■ Monitor the patient and the system for 10 minutes after beginning therapy. If after 10 minutes the system functions without alarming, secure the catheter.

■ Monitor vital signs every 15 minutes during the first hour of treatment, then every hour or more frequently, as indicated by the patient's condition.[13]

■ Record intake and output hourly; include the ultrafiltrate in the patient's output volume.[3,12]

■ Monitor the system and respond to any alarms according to the manufacturer's guidelines. *The system has sensors to detect air bubbles in the blood circuit line, blood leaks in the ultrafiltrate line, and pressure in both lines.*[3,13]

- Monitor the system for signs of clotting, such as frequent and unexpected infusion or withdrawal occlusions.[3,13]
- Maintain the patient's fluid restriction.
- Monitor the patient for signs of hypovolemia, such as tachycardia, hypotension, diminished urinary output, and elevations in blood urea nitrogen and creatinine levels.[11]
- When the system alarms (indicating that the ultrafiltrate drainage bag is full), empty the bag into a graduated measuring container.[3]

Discontinuing therapy

- Press the STOP key to stop the pumps.[3]
- Clamp the withdrawal catheter extension tubing.
- Disconnect the withdrawal blood circuit connection from the withdrawal catheter extension.
- Flush the withdrawal catheter IV access and then recap it with a sterile end cap.
- Clamp the infusion line.
- Disconnect the infusion line. Flush the infusion IV access and then recap it with a sterile end cap.
- Return the HCT sensor to its dock on the back of the console.
- Remove the blood circuit from the console by pressing the clips on the front and side cartridges and rotating the knobs while removing the tubing. Discard in an appropriate biohazard waste container.[3,14]
- Hold the ON/OFF key for 1 second to power off the console.
- Obtain the patient's weight.
- Document the therapy.[15]

Cleaning the unit after each use

- Using a mild soap solution, clean the surface of the console.
- Disinfect the console surfaces using 10% bleach solution, 95% isopropyl alcohol, or surface disinfectant, according to your facility's policy. Apply the solution to a soft cloth to clean the console.[3]
- Clean the tubing path through the air and blood leak detectors; use a "flossing" action to clean inside the detector with a lint-free cloth and warm water. Dry thoroughly.[3]
- Remove the pumps, clean them, and reassemble them. Refer to the manual for instructions on removing and cleaning pumps. In some facilities, this is performed in the Biomedical Department.[3]
- Remove and discard your gloves and perform hand hygiene.[3]
- Document the procedure.[15]

Special considerations

- Monitor partial thromboplastin time (PTT) at intervals during therapy, as ordered or according to your facility's policy. The recommended therapeutic range for therapy is 80 to 100 seconds.
- Patients receiving warfarin (Coumadin) who have an International Normalized Ratio greater than 2 typically start on a continuous heparin infusion and aren't given an initial bolus of the drug. If heparin is contraindicated, argatroban may be prescribed.
- You can safely remove up to 500 mL or 1.1 lb of fluid per hour. The average treatment is 24 hours, with 6 L or 13.2 lb of fluid removed.[3]
- Although a patient can sit up in a chair and walk to the bathroom using the unit's battery backup, blood is pumped more efficiently through the filter with less patient movement, decreasing the length of the procedure.
- Magnetic resonance imaging (MRI) is contraindicated with the dual-lumen catheter *because the reinforcement coil may experience rotational or translational forces or temperature increases due to the magnetic field and pulsed radio frequency fields.* Affix an "Avoid MRI" label to these catheters *to indicate this risk.*
- Adjust the ultrafiltration rates if the patient's blood pressure drops 10 mm Hg from baseline or if his heart rate is greater than 130 beats/minute after two consecutive measurements within 5 minutes. Obtain orders to reduce the ultrafiltration or briefly stop ultrafiltration, allowing the patient time to recover.

Complications

An ultrafiltration alarm activates when ultrafiltrate pressure deviates from the usual range. This usually means clotting of the filter has occurred and requires that the filter be replaced. Contact the doctor. If the doctor wants to continue treatment, the procedure for replacement of the circuit and filter is located in the *Aquadex FlexFlow User's Guide.*[3]

Documentation

Record the date and time that therapy began; the reason for the therapy; the patient's weight before and after the treatment; vital signs and withdrawal, infusion, and ultrafiltrate pressures throughout the treatment; catheter access sites; initial Aquadex FlexFlow settings, changes made, and the reasons for such changes; intake and output; laboratory values, and the patient's tolerance to the procedure.

REFERENCES

1 De Maria, E., et al. (2010). Ultrafiltration for the treatment of diuretic-resistant, recurrent, acute decompensated heart failure: Experience in a single center. *Journal of Cardiovascular Medicine, 11*(8), 559–604.

2 *Duel Lumen Extended Length Catheter with Coil Reinforcement (Package Insert).* (2009). Brooklyn Park, MN: CHF Solutions, Inc.

3 *Aquadex FlexFlow User's Guide.* (2007). Brooklyn Park, MN: CHF Solutions, Inc.

4 The Joint Commission. (2012). Standard NPSG.07.01.01. *Comprehensive accreditation manual for hospitals: The official handbook.* Oakbrook Terrace, IL: The Joint Commission. (Level I)

5 The Joint Commission. (2012). Standard RI.01.03.01. *Comprehensive accreditation manual for hospitals: The official handbook.* Oakbrook Terrace, IL: The Joint Commission. (Level I)

6 Centers for Disease Control and Prevention. (October 2002). Guideline for hand hygiene in health-care settings. *Morbidity and Mortality Weekly Report, 51* (RR-16), 1–45. (Level I)

7 World Health Organization. (2009). *WHO guidelines on hand hygiene in health care: First global patient safety challenge. Clean care is safer care.* Geveva, Switzerland: World Health Organization. (Level I)

8 The Joint Commission. Standard NPSG.01.01.01. *Comprehensive accreditation manual for hospitals: The official handbook.* Oakbrook Terrace, IL: The Joint Commission. (Level I)

9 Institute for Safe Medication Practices. "ISMP's List of High-Alert Medications" [Online]. Accessed July 2011 via the Web at http://www.ismp.org/tools/highalertmedications.pdf

10 Institute for Safe Medication Practices. (2008). "Conducting an Independent Double-check." *ISMP Medication Safety Alert! Nurse Advise-ERR, 6*(12), 1 [Online]. Accessed July 2011 via the Web at http://www.ismp.org/newsletters/nursing/Issues/NurseAdviseERR200812.pdf

11 U.S. Food and Drug Administration (2009). "Look. Check. Connect.: Safe Medical Device Connections Save Lives" [Online]. Accessed July 2011 via the Web at www.fda.gov/downloads/MedicalDevices/Safety/AlertsandNotices/UCM134873.pdf

12 Mielniczuk, L. et al. (2010). Ultrafiltration in the management of acute decompensated heart failure. *Current Opinions in Cardiology, 25*(2), 155–160.

13 The Joint Commission. (2012). Standard RC.02.01.01. *Comprehensive accreditation manual for hospitals: The official handbook.* Oakbrook Terrace, IL: The Joint Commission. (Level I)

14 National Health Service. (2008). Evaluation report: CHF solutions Aquadex FlexFlow Ultrafiltration System. CEP 07017.

15 The Joint Commission. (2012). Standard RC.01.03.01. *Comprehensive accreditation manual for hospitals: The official handbook.* Oakbrook Terrace, IL: The Joint Commission. (Level I)

ADDITIONAL REFERENCES

Costanzo, M. (2008). Ultrafiltration in the management of heart failure. *U.S. Cardiology: Touch Briefings, 5*(1), 66–69.

Costanzo, M., et al. (2007). Ultrafiltration versus intravenous diuretics for patients hospitalized for acute decompensated heart failure. *Journal of the American College of Cardiology, 49*(6), 675–684.

Kale, P., et al. (2008). Devices in acute heart failure. *Critical Care Medicine, 36*(Suppl. 1), 121–28.

Mielniczuk, L. et al. (2010). Ultrafiltration in the management of acute decompensated heart failure. *Current Opinions in Cardiology, 25*(2), 155–160.

Occupational Safety and Health Administration. "Bloodborne Pathogens, Standard Number 1910.1030" [Online]. Accessed July 2011 via the Web at http://www.osha.gov/pls/oshaweb/owadisp.show_document?p_table=STANDARDS&p_id=10051 (Level I)

Peterangelo, M. (2008). Incorporating aquapheresis into the hospital setting: A practical approach. *Progress in Cardiovascular Nursing, 23*(4), 168–172.

Peterangelo, M. (2009). Incorporating aquapheresis into therapy options for the treatment of volume overload: A CNS driven project. *Heart & Lung: The Journal of Acute and Critical Care. 38*(3), 269–70.

Walsh, C., et al. (2007). Peripheral ultrafiltration for patients with volume overload. *Critical Care Nursing Quarterly, 30*(4), 329–336.

ARTERIAL AND VENOUS SHEATH REMOVAL

The number of endovascular procedures performed by cardiologists and vascular surgeons has dramatically increased in the past decade. Following these procedures, arterial sheaths, venous sheaths, or both may be left in place. Removing the sheath may improve patient comfort and shorten the amount of bed rest required, which can lead to positive patient outcomes. However, sheath removal isn't without risk, and nurses need appropriate training for the procedure.

Various methods help control bleeding following sheath removal, including manual compression (used alone or with a hemostasis pad), mechanical compression devices, collagen plug devices, or percutaneous suture-mediated closure devices. Manual compression can cause fatigue and injury, possibly leading to carpal tunnel problems for the health care worker applying the compression. Mechanical compression techniques help prevent such problems and effectively prevent hematoma formation.

Equipment

Gloves ▪ gown ▪ goggles or face shield with mask ▪ electrocardiogram (ECG) monitor ▪ blood pressure monitor ▪ permanent marker ▪ antiseptic solution (chlorhexidine-based skin preparation) ▪ sterile gauze ▪ sterile gloves ▪ suture removal kit (if the sheath is sutured in place) ▪ hypoallergenic tape ▪ linen-saver pad ▪ sterile saline solution (if using noninvasive hemostasis pad) ▪ transparent dressing (if using noninvasive hemostasis pad) ▪ Optional: mechanical compression device, noninvasive hemostasis pad.

Preparation of equipment

Perform hand hygiene[1,2,3] and bring the equipment to the patient's bedside. Using sterile technique, open the suture removal kit and gauze packages and place them within reach. If a hemostasis pad is being used, open it using sterile technique and open the normal saline solution. (See "Sterile technique, basic," page 671.)

Implementation

▪ Perform hand hygiene.[1,2,3]
▪ Verify the doctor's order for sheath removal.
▪ Confirm the patient's identity using at least two patient identifiers according to your facility's policy.[4]

Preparing for sheath removal

▪ Explain the procedure to the patient *to reduce anxiety and enhance cooperation.* Include activity restrictions, discomfort caused by pressure to the site, and signs and symptoms to report following the procedure.
▪ Before sheath removal, assess for bleeding disorders and check the patient's platelet count, prothrombin time, International Normalized Ratio, partial thromboplastin time, complete blood count, and activated clotting time *to assure that hemostasis can be achieved.*
▪ Obtain vital signs, and check the ECG *to establish a baseline.* Check that systolic blood pressure is less than 150 mm Hg *to facilitate hemostasis.*
▪ Assess neurovascular status in the extremity distal to the sheath insertion site *to establish a baseline.*
▪ Mark the pulses distal to the sheath insertion site using a permanent marker *to facilitate finding the pulses.*
▪ Administer an analgesic 20 to 30 minutes before the procedure *to promote patient comfort.*

■ Confirm that the patient has a patent IV catheter *in case emergency fluids or medications are required.*

■ Position the patient with the head of the bed flat *to promote hemostasis.*

■ Place the linen-saver pad underneath the affected extremity *to keep the bed linen clean and to provide a place to set the sheath after removal.*

■ If a mechanical compression device is being used, place it under the patient before sheath removal *to reduce patient movement and the risk of bleeding after the sheath is removed.*

■ If the sheath is sutured in place, open the suture removal kit using sterile technique.

■ Perform hand hygiene[1,2,3] and put on goggles, a mask, gloves, and a gown.

■ Carefully remove the dressing covering the sheath insertion site.

■ Clean the insertion site with antiseptic solution.

■ Remove and discard your gloves, and perform hand hygiene *to reduce the risk of transmission of microorganisms.*[1,2,3]

■ Put on sterile gloves.

■ Remove sutures, if present. (See "Suture removal," page 688.)

Sheath removal using manual or mechanical compression

■ Locate the femoral pulse proximal to the insertion site *so that compression (manual or mechanical) can be properly positioned 1 to 2 cm above the insertion site.*

■ Hold the sheath with one hand while applying manual or mechanical pressure over the femoral artery with the other hand *to reduce bleeding.*

■ Remove the sheath slowly while the patient exhales, *to prevent Valsalva's maneuver,* while continuing to apply pressure manually or with the mechanical device.

■ Apply continuous pressure to the artery for approximately 20 minutes.[5] Ensure that the pressure is strong enough to stop the bleeding but not so strong that it obscures the pedal pulse.

Sheath removal using a noninvasive hemostasis pad with manual compression

■ Moisten the pad with sterile saline *to activate the hemostatic system.*

■ Apply pressure 1 to 2 cm proximal to the insertion site.

■ Apply a sterile gauze pad over the insertion site, and then place the moistened pad over the gauze and apply pressure.

■ Gently remove the sheath as described above.

■ Reduce proximal pressure to let a small amount of blood from the insertion site moisten the noninvasive hemostasis pad, and then reapply proximal pressure.

■ Slowly let up on applying pressure proximal to the insertion site after 3 to 4 minutes while continuing to apply pressure to the insertion site for no less than 10 minutes.

■ Remove manual pressure once hemostasis is achieved.

■ Apply another sterile gauze pad over the hemostasis pad and cover the site with a transparent dressing.

■ Leave the hemostasis pad in place for 24 hours.

Venous sheath removal

■ Remove the venous sheath, if present, 5 to 10 minutes after removal of the arterial sheath *because pressure at the arterial site needs to be maintained for a longer time.*[5]

■ Apply pressure over the venous and arterial sites for 10 more minutes or until bleeding has stopped.

■ If a hemostasis pad is used, follow the previous directions for its use.

Follow-up care

■ Apply a sterile dressing to the arterial and venous insertion sites to *keep the area clean and reduce the risk of infection.*

■ Assess neurovascular status, vital signs, and the insertion site in the affected limb every 15 minutes for 1 hour, then every 30 minutes for 1 hour, then every hour for 4 hours, or according to your facility's policy, *to ensure adequate circulation and neurologic function.*

■ Tell the patient not to elevate the head of the bed more than 30 degrees *to reduce the risk of disrupting hemostasis and to relieve back discomfort.*

■ Instruct the patient to report any bleeding from the site, if the dressing becomes saturated, or if he feels wetness and warmth on his groin or leg.

■ Tell the patient to report coolness, numbness, tingling, or pain in the affected extremity.

■ Keep the patient on bed rest for 2 to 6 hours, or according to your facility's policy, when applying mechanical or manual pressure after arterial sheath removal *to reduce the complications of bed rest and back discomfort.* Clinical studies have shown that bed rest doesn't increase the risk of vascular complications.[6]

■ Keep the patient on bed rest for 1 to 4 hours, or according to your facility's policy, when achieving hemostasis through percutaneous suture–mediated closure and hemostasis pads.

■ Keep the patient on bed rest for no more than 4 hours, or according to your facility's policy, following venous sheath removal.

■ Remove and discard your gloves. Perform hand hygiene.[1,2,3]

■ Assess for pain and medicate as prescribed.

■ Document the procedure.[7]

Special considerations

■ If the patient is obese, a second person may be required to help hold back skin and abdominal folds.

■ The patient with hypertension may need pressure applied for a longer period of time *to ensure hemostasis.*

■ Read the manufacturer's instructions and check your facility's policy for correct use of mechanical compression devices. *Tissue damage can occur if the device is used incorrectly.*

■ Keep in mind that the compression time required to control bleeding depends on several factors, including the size of the sheath, whether the patient received heparin and antiplatelet drugs, and blood coagulation levels.

Patient teaching

Provide the patient and his family with written and oral discharge instructions. Tell the patient that he shouldn't lift anything heavier than 10 lb (4.5 kg) for 3 days and that he shouldn't drive or operate machinery for 24 hours. Tell him that he may remove the dressing and shower after 24 hours but that he shouldn't take a tub bath or swim until the skin is healed. After the initial 24 hours, the patient may clean the site with soap and water and apply a small adhesive bandage. Tell the patient to inspect the site daily and to notify his doctor as soon as possible of any bleeding, redness, or discharge or if he develops a fever.

Complications

The most common complication following sheath removal is bleeding, which occurs most frequently at the femoral artery access site. Retroperitoneal bleeding may also occur. Vascular complications include hematoma, pseudoaneurysm, arteriovenous fistula formation, embolus, and thrombus. Sensory or motor impairment may occur in the affected limb. Vasovagal complications may also occur.

Documentation

Record the date and time of sheath removal. Note whether an arterial sheath, a venous sheath, or both were removed and their locations. Record any patient and family teaching about the removal procedure and activity restrictions following sheath removal. Include the patient's level of discomfort, using a 0 to 10 scale as well as the name, dose, route, and time of any analgesics given. Document that laboratory values were checked before the sheath was removed and that they were within normal limits. Record vital signs, neurovascular status, and heart rhythm before sheath removal. State whether pulses distal to the sheath insertion sites were marked.

Note that the patient has a patent IV. Include that the patient was placed in a flat position for sheath removal. Describe the condition of the sheath insertion sites, noting any redness, skin breakdown, drainage, bleeding, or hematoma formation. Note how many sutures were removed. Explain any difficulties encountered during sheath removal. Record the type of pressure or hemostasis used and how long until hemostasis was achieved. Document the frequent neurovascular, vital signs, and sheath removal site checks. Note the patient's tolerance of the procedure.

Record any complications, the time and name of the person notified, orders given, nursing actions taken, and the patient's response. Include the patient's position following sheath removal and how long bed rest was maintained.

REFERENCES

1 Centers for Disease Control and Prevention. (October 2002). Guideline for hand hygiene in health-care settings. *Morbidity and Mortality Weekly Report, 51* (RR-16), 1–45. (Level I)
2 The Joint Commission. (2012). Standard NPSG.07.01.01. *Comprehensive accreditation manual for hospitals: The official handbook.* Oakbrook Terrace, IL: The Joint Commission. (Level I)
3 World Health Organization. (2009). *WHO guidelines on hand hygiene in health care: First global patient safety challenge. Clean care is safer care.* Geneva, Switzerland: World Health Organization. (Level I)
4 The Joint Commission. (2012). Standard NPSG.01.01.01. *Comprehensive accreditation manual for hospitals: The official handbook.* Oakbrook Terrace, IL: The Joint Commission. (Level I)
5 Lynn-McHale Wiegand, D. (Ed.). (2011). *AACN procedure manual for critical care* (6th ed.). Philadelphia, PA: Saunders.
6 Walker, S., et al. (2008). Comparison of complications in percutaneous coronary intervention patients mobilized at 3, 4, and 6 hours after femoral arterial sheath removal. *Journal of Cardiovascular Nursing, 23*(5), 407–413. (Level II)
7 The Joint Commission. (2012). Standard RC.01.03.01. *Comprehensive accreditation manual for hospitals: The official handbook.* Oakbrook Terrace, IL: The Joint Commission. (Level I)

ADDITIONAL REFERENCES

Juergens, C.P., et al. (2009). Vaso-vagal reactions during femoral arterial sheath removal after percutaneous coronary intervention and impact on cardiac events. *International Journal of Cardiology, 127*(2), 252–254.

Mego, D., et al. (2010). A poly-*n*-acetyl glucosamine hemostatic dressing for femoral artery access site hemostasis after percutaneous coronary intervention: A pilot study. *Journal of Invasive Cardiology, 22*(1), 35–39.

Narins, C.R., et al. (2008). A prospective, randomized trial of topical hemostasis patch use following percutaneous coronary and peripheral intervention. *Journal of Invasive Cardiology, 20*(11), 579–584.

Rastan, A., et al. (2008). VIPER-2: A prospective, randomized single-center comparison of 2 different closure devices with a hemostatic wound dressing for closure of femoral artery access sites. *Journal of Endovascular Therapy, 15*(1), 83–90.

Shoulders-Odom, B. (2008). Management of patients after percutaneous coronary interventions. *Critical Care Nurse, 28*(5), 26–41.

ARTERIAL PRESSURE MONITORING

Direct arterial pressure monitoring permits continuous measurement of systolic, diastolic, and mean arterial pressures and allows for arterial blood sampling. Because direct measurement reflects systemic vascular resistance as well as blood flow, it's generally more accurate than indirect methods (such as palpation and auscultation of Korotkoff, or audible pulse, sounds), which are based on blood flow.

Direct monitoring is indicated when highly accurate or frequent blood pressure measurements are required, such as for patients with low cardiac output and high systemic vascular resistance. It may also be used for hospitalized patients who are obese or have severe edema—conditions that may make indirect measurement difficult to perform. It's also useful for patients receiving titrated doses of vasoactive drugs and for those requiring frequent blood sampling.

Arterial pressure monitoring is used in critical care settings. To carry out monitoring, the doctor inserts an arterial catheter, which allows for direct arterial pressure monitoring. The procedure can be performed at the bedside under surgically sterile conditions.

Arterial monitoring equipment permits waveform evaluation and allows the nurse to make clinical decisions about changes in the patient's therapy. (See *Understanding the arterial waveform,* page 30.)

Understanding the arterial waveform

Normal arterial blood pressure produces a characteristic waveform, representing ventricular systole and diastole. The waveform has five distinct components: the anacrotic limb, systolic peak, dicrotic limb, dicrotic notch, and end diastole.

The *anacrotic limb* marks the waveform's initial upstroke, which results as blood is rapidly ejected from the ventricle through the open aortic valve into the aorta. The rapid ejection causes a sharp rise in arterial pressure, which appears as the waveform's highest point. This is called the *systolic peak*.

As blood continues into the peripheral vessels, arterial pressure falls, and the waveform begins a downward trend. This part is called the *dicrotic limb*. Arterial pressure usually will continue to fall until pressure in the ventricle is less than pressure in the aortic root. When this occurs, the

aortic valve closes. This event appears as a small notch on the waveform's downside, called the *dicrotic notch*. When the aortic valve closes, diastole begins, progressing until the aortic root pressure gradually descends to its lowest point. On the waveform, this is known as *end diastole*.

Normal arterial waveform

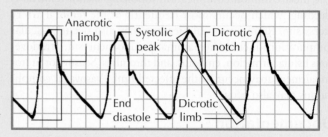

A patient being monitored with an arterial pressure monitoring system can have blood samples for laboratory testing withdrawn from the arterial catheter. The arterial pressure monitoring system can be open or closed. An *open system* is one in which a Vacutainer is attached to the stopcock, withdrawing 5 to 10 mL of blood for waste, which is then discarded. A *closed system* has an attached reservoir that withdraws the waste; when all appropriate blood samples have been obtained, the blood in the reservoir can be returned to the patient.

According to the Centers for Disease Control and Prevention and the Infusion Nurses Society, the tubing and flush solution for an arterial line is considered a closed system and should be changed every 96 hours, immediately if contamination is suspected, or when the integrity of the product is compromised.[1,2] In some cases, however, you may need to change the flush solution more frequently due to use.

Removal of an arterial catheter should occur as soon as possible to decrease the risk of complications, such as thrombosis and infection.[1]

Equipment

For catheter insertion

Disposable pressure transducer system ▪ 250-mL bag of normal saline solution ▪ arterial catheter ▪ unvented or dead-end caps ▪ pressure tubing ▪ pressure bag or IV pump ▪ transducer holder on an IV pole ▪ monitoring system and equipment (module, bedside monitor, cable, and hookup) ▪ suture material ▪ sterile transparent dressing ▪ sterile hypoallergenic tape ▪ carpenter's level ▪ Optional: arm board or limb-immobilization device, chlorhexidine-impregnated sponge.

For blood sampling

Gloves ▪ gown ▪ mask ▪ protective eyewear ▪ linen-saver pad ▪ laboratory request forms and labels ▪ appropriate blood sample collection tubes ▪ laboratory biohazard transport bag ▪ antisep-

tic wipes (alcohol, tincture of iodine, or chlorhexidine-based) ▪ sterile nonvented cap ▪ vacutainer ▪ needleless Vacutainer luer adapter.

For tubing change

Gloves ▪ gown ▪ mask ▪ protective eyewear ▪ linen-saver pad ▪ preassembled arterial pressure tubing with flush device and disposable pressure transducer ▪ sterile gloves ▪ 500-mL bag of IV flush solution (typically normal saline solution) ▪ antiseptic solution swabs ▪ sterile dressing ▪ medication label ▪ pressure bag ▪ site care kit ▪ tubing labels.

For catheter removal

Gloves ▪ mask ▪ gown ▪ protective eyewear ▪ two sterile 4″ × 4″ gauze pads ▪ linen-saver pad ▪ 3- or 5-mL syringe ▪ sterile suture removal set ▪ dressing ▪ hypoallergenic tape ▪ Optional: sterile scissors, laboratory biohazard transport bag, sterile container, hemostatic pad, patch, or powder.

Preparation of equipment

Before setting up and priming the monitoring system, perform hand hygiene.[3,4,5,6] Set up and prime the monitoring system. (See "Transducer system setup," page 739.) Make sure you keep all parts of the pressure monitoring system sterile. Label all medications, medication containers, and other solutions on and off the sterile field.[7] When you've completed equipment preparation, turn on the bedside monitor alarms according to your facility's policy.

Implementation

▪ Confirm the patient's identity using at least two patient identifiers according to your facility's policy.[8]
▪ Maintain asepsis by wearing personal protective equipment throughout all procedures described.
▪ Position the patient for easy access to the catheter insertion site. Place a linen-saver pad under the site.

Inserting an arterial catheter

■ Explain the procedure to the patient and his family, including the purpose of arterial pressure monitoring and the anticipated duration of catheter placement.

■ Make sure that informed consent has been obtained and is documented in the patient's medical record.[9]

■ Check the patient's history for any allergy or hypersensitivity to iodine, heparin, or the ordered anesthetic.

■ If the catheter will be inserted in the radial artery, perform Allen's test *to assess collateral circulation in the hand.*

■ Obtain baseline data, including vital signs, level of consciousness, and hemodynamic stability, *to help identify acute changes in the patient.*

■ Assist the doctor as needed during catheter placement. After insertion and while the doctor holds the catheter in place, activate the fast-flush release *to flush blood from the catheter.* After each fast-flush operation, observe the drip chamber *to verify that the continuous flush rate is as desired.* A waveform should appear on the bedside monitor.

■ The doctor may suture the catheter in place, or you may secure it with sterile tape. Cover the insertion site with a chlorhexidine-impregnated sponge (according to your facility's policy) and then a sterile occlusive dressing (as specified by your facility's policy), and label the dressing with the date and time.[10]

■ Immobilize the insertion site. With a radial or brachial site, use an arm board. With a femoral site, maintain the patient on bed rest, with the head of the bed raised no more than 30 degrees *to prevent the catheter from kinking.*

■ Level the zeroing stopcock of the transducer with the phlebostatic axis. Then zero the system to atmospheric pressure.

NURSING ALERT *Keep the catheter site visible at all times. Don't allow linens to cover the site; intra-arterial catheter dislodgment requires prompt recognition and intervention to reduce the risk for exsanguination.*

■ Make sure that the monitor alarms are activated and set appropriately according to your facility's policy.

■ Continuously observe the arterial waveform quality on the monitor and record variances *to ensure the accuracy of the waveform and to detect changes in the patient's hemodynamic status.* A normal waveform has a peak systole, clear dicrotic notch, and end diastole. Compare the intra-arterial pressure with blood pressure readings obtained by a cuff at least once per shift.

■ Monitor for potential complications of the arterial catheter, and notify the doctor immediately if any occur.

■ Troubleshoot the arterial waveform, as needed. Notify the doctor, as appropriate. If the waveform suddenly becomes dampened, check the patient before attempting to determine its cause or fix the problem *because a sudden hypotensive episode can look like a dampened waveform on the monitor and can be potentially life-threatening if not treated properly.* (See *Recognizing abnormal waveforms,* page 32.)

■ Remove and discard your gloves. Perform hand hygiene.[3,4,5,6]

■ Document the procedure.[11]

Obtaining a blood sample

■ Perform hand hygiene. Put on gloves and other personal protective equipment, as needed.[3,4,5,6]

■ Explain the procedure to the patient.

■ Position the patient for easy access to the catheter insertion site. Place a linen-saver pad under the site.

■ Assemble the equipment following sterile technique, taking care not to contaminate the nonvented cap and stopcock.

■ Label the discard blood sample collection tube *to prevent accidentally confusing it with a true specimen.*

For an open monitoring system

■ Attach the needleless luer adapter to the Vacutainer.

■ Temporarily silence the monitor alarms.

■ Locate the blood sampling port of the stopcock nearest the patient. Remove the nonvented cap from the stopcock.

■ Thoroughly disinfect the stopcock port with an antiseptic pad, using friction.[1,12]

■ Connect the needleless adapter of the Vacutainer into the sampling port of the stopcock and turn off the stopcock to the flush solution.

■ Insert the labeled blood sample collection tube for the discard sample into the Vacutainer. (This sample is discarded *because it's diluted with flush solution.*) Follow your facility's policy on how much discard blood to collect. In most cases, you'll withdraw 5 to 10 mL.

■ Insert each blood sample collection tube into the Vacutainer, keeping the stopcock turned off to the flush solution. *Because the Vacutainer is a nonvented system,* there won't be any backflow of blood from the patient. If the doctor has ordered coagulation tests, obtain blood for this sample last *to prevent dilution from the flush device.*

■ After you've obtained blood for the final sample, turn off the stopcock to the Vacutainer. Activate the fast-flush release *to clear the tubing.*

■ Turn off the stopcock to the patient, attach a labeled discard blood sample collection tube to the Vacutainer, and repeat the fast flush *to clear the stopcock port.*

■ Turn off the stopcock to the stopcock port, and remove the Vacutainer. Place a new sterile, nonvented cap on the blood sampling port; *blood or debris left in the existing cap increases the risk for infection.*[12,13,14,15]

For a closed monitoring system

■ Holding the reservoir upright, grasp the flexures and slowly fill the reservoir with blood over a 3- to 5-second period. *(This blood serves as discard blood.)* If you feel resistance, reposition the affected extremity and check the catheter site for obvious problems (such as kinking). Then resume blood withdrawal.

■ Turn the one-way valve off to the reservoir by turning the handle perpendicular to the tubing. Thoroughly disinfect the sampling port with antiseptic solution, using friction.[1,12,13,14] Using a syringe with attached cannula, insert the cannula into the sampling port. (Make sure the plunger is depressed to the bottom of the syringe barrel.) Slowly fill the syringe. Repeat the procedure as needed to fill the required number of syringes. Then grasp the cannula near the sampling site and remove the syringe and cannula as one unit. If the doctor has ordered coagulation tests, obtain

Recognizing abnormal waveforms

Understanding a normal arterial waveform is relatively straightforward. However, an abnormal waveform is more difficult to decipher. Abnormal patterns and markings may provide important diagnostic clues to the patient's cardiovascular status, or they may simply signal trouble in the monitor. Use this chart to help you recognize and resolve waveform abnormalities.

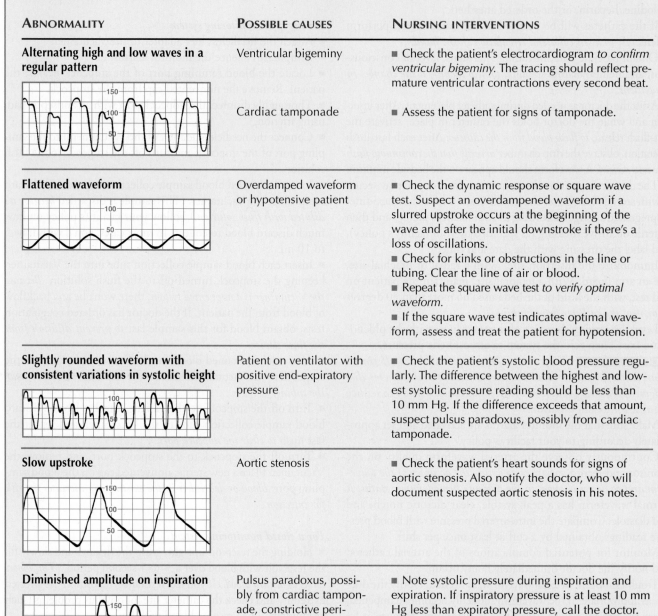

ABNORMALITY	POSSIBLE CAUSES	NURSING INTERVENTIONS
Alternating high and low waves in a regular pattern	Ventricular bigeminy	▪ Check the patient's electrocardiogram *to confirm ventricular bigeminy*. The tracing should reflect premature ventricular contractions every second beat.
	Cardiac tamponade	▪ Assess the patient for signs of tamponade.
Flattened waveform	Overdamped waveform or hypotensive patient	▪ Check the dynamic response or square wave test. Suspect an overdampened waveform if a slurred upstroke occurs at the beginning of the wave and after the initial downstroke if there's a loss of oscillations. ▪ Check for kinks or obstructions in the line or tubing. Clear the line of air or blood. ▪ Repeat the square wave test *to verify optimal waveform*. ▪ If the square wave test indicates optimal waveform, assess and treat the patient for hypotension.
Slightly rounded waveform with consistent variations in systolic height	Patient on ventilator with positive end-expiratory pressure	▪ Check the patient's systolic blood pressure regularly. The difference between the highest and lowest systolic pressure reading should be less than 10 mm Hg. If the difference exceeds that amount, suspect pulsus paradoxus, possibly from cardiac tamponade.
Slow upstroke	Aortic stenosis	▪ Check the patient's heart sounds for signs of aortic stenosis. Also notify the doctor, who will document suspected aortic stenosis in his notes.
Diminished amplitude on inspiration	Pulsus paradoxus, possibly from cardiac tamponade, constrictive pericarditis, or lung disease	▪ Note systolic pressure during inspiration and expiration. If inspiratory pressure is at least 10 mm Hg less than expiratory pressure, call the doctor. ▪ If you're also monitoring pulmonary artery pressure, observe for a diastolic plateau. This occurs when the mean central venous pressure (right atrial pressure), mean pulmonary artery pressure, and mean pulmonary artery wedge pressure (pulmonary artery obstructive pressure) are within 5 mm Hg of one another.

blood for those tests from the final syringe to prevent dilution from the flush solution.

■ After filling the syringes, turn the one-way valve to its original position, parallel to the tubing.

■ Smoothly and evenly push down on the plunger until the flexures lock in place in the fully closed position and all fluid has been reinfused. The fluid should be reinfused over a 3- to 5-second period.

■ Activate the fast-flush release *to clear blood from the tubing and reservoir.*

■ Thoroughly disinfect the sampling port with an antiseptic pad, using friction.[1,12] Place a new sterile, nonvented cap on the sampling port; *blood or debris left in the existing cap increases the risk for infection.*[12]

Completing a blood-sampling procedure
■ Reactivate the monitor alarms.

■ Check the monitor for return of the arterial waveform and pressure reading. (See *Understanding the arterial waveform,* page 30.)

■ Label all blood sample collection tubes in the presence of the patient *to prevent mislabeling.*

■ Send all samples to the laboratory in a laboratory biohazard transport bag with the appropriate documentation.

■ Remove and discard your personal protective equipment and perform hand hygiene.[3,4,5,6,15,16]

■ Document the procedure.[11]

Changing the arterial line tubing
■ Explain the procedure to the patient.

■ Position the patient for easy access to the catheter site. Place a linen-saver pad under the site.

■ Perform hand hygiene and put on personal protective equipment.[3,4,5,6]

■ Assemble the new pressure transducer system. (See "Transducer system setup," page 739.)

■ Inflate the pressure bag to 300 mm Hg and check it for air leaks. Then release the pressure.

■ Prepare the IV flush solution according to your facility's policy, and prime the pressure tubing and transducer system. Apply the appropriate medication labels. Place the IV flush solution in the pressure bag. Apply 300 mm Hg of pressure to the system. Then hang the IV bag on a pole.

■ Label all tubing *to prevent an unintentional injection of drugs or other substances into the artery.*[7]

■ Remove the dressing from the catheter insertion site, taking care not to dislodge the catheter or cause vessel trauma. Temporarily silence the monitor alarms.[17]

■ Turn off the flow clamp of the tubing segment that you'll change. Disconnect the tubing from the catheter hub, taking care not to dislodge the catheter.[18] Immediately insert new tubing into the catheter hub. Trace the tubing from the patient to its point of origin *to make sure you've connected it to the proper port.*[19] Secure the tubing *to prevent misconnections* and then activate the transducer's fast-flush release to clear the catheter of blood.

■ Reactivate the monitor alarms.

■ Remove and discard your gloves, perform hand hygiene, and then put on sterile gloves.[3,4,5,6,16]

■ Clean the insertion site with an antiseptic swab (preferably a chlorhexidine-based antiseptic) and then allow it to dry.

■ Apply an appropriate sterile occlusive dressing (gauze, which is preferred if the patient is diaphoretic or the site is oozing or bleeding, or transparent semipermeable dressing) and label it with the date, time, and your initials.[7]

■ Level the zeroing stopcock of the transducer with the phlebostatic axis, and zero the system to atmospheric pressure.

■ Remove and discard your gloves and perform hand hygiene.[3,4,5,6]

■ Document the procedure.[11]

Removing an arterial line
■ Consult your facility's policy *to determine whether you're permitted to perform this procedure.*

■ Check the patient's coagulation studies before catheter removal *to determine if you will need to hold pressure for a longer time in order to achieve hemostasis.*

■ Gather all equipment.

■ Perform hand hygiene.[3,4,5,6]

■ Confirm the patient's identity using at least two patient identifiers according to your facility's policy.[8]

■ Explain the procedure to the patient.

■ Observe standard precautions, including wearing personal protective equipment as needed for this procedure.

■ Record the patient's systolic, diastolic, and mean blood pressures. If a manual, indirect blood pressure hasn't been assessed recently, obtain one now *to establish a new baseline.*

■ Turn off the monitor alarms. Then turn off the flow clamp to the flush solution.

■ Position the patient for easy access to the insertion site.

■ Carefully remove the dressing over the insertion site. Remove any sutures, using the suture removal kit, and then carefully check that all sutures have been removed.[17]

■ Assess the site for signs of infection, such as redness, swelling, and drainage from the insertion site. Notify the doctor immediately if you note any such signs.

■ Turn the stopcock off to flush the solution.

■ Apply pressure directly above the insertion site.

■ Withdraw the catheter using a gentle, steady motion. Keep the catheter parallel to the artery during withdrawal *to reduce the risk of traumatic injury.*

■ Immediately after withdrawing the catheter, apply pressure to the site with a sterile 4″ × 4″ gauze pad.[20] Maintain pressure until hemostasis is achieved; you may need to apply a hemostatic pad, patch, or powder to encourage clot formation. Apply additional pressure to a femoral site or if the patient has coagulopathy or is receiving anticoagulants.[20] Some facility policies allow you to use a compression device to apply pressure to the femoral site. (See "Femoral compression," page 309.)

■ Apply a pressure dressing to the site *to help prevent rebleeding.*[20]

■ If the doctor has ordered a culture of the catheter tip (to diagnose a suspected infection), gently place the catheter tip on a 4″ × 4″ sterile gauze pad. When the bleeding is under control, hold the catheter over the sterile container. Using sterile scissors, cut the tip so it falls into the sterile container. Label the specimen in the presence of the patient *to prevent mislabeling* and send it to the laboratory in a biohazard transport bag.

■ Dispose of supplies appropriately, remove personal protective equipment, and perform hand hygiene.[3,4,5,6]

■ Observe the site for bleeding. Assess circulation in the extremity distal to the site by evaluating color, pulses, and sensation.[20] Repeat this assessment as ordered by the doctor or according to your facility's policy.

■ Document the procedure.[11]

Special considerations
Catheter insertion
■ Be aware that several factors can lead to incorrect pressure readings, including a clotted catheter; positional, loose connections; the addition of extra stopcocks or extension tubing; inadvertent entry of air into the system; and improper calibrating, leveling, or zeroing of the monitoring system. If the catheter lumen clots, the flush system may be improperly pressurized. Regularly assess the amount of flush solution in the IV bag, and maintain 300 mm Hg of pressure in the pressure bag.

■ Observe the pressure waveform on the monitor to help assess arterial pressure. An abnormal waveform may reflect an arrhythmia (such as atrial fibrillation) or other cardiovascular problems, such as aortic stenosis, aortic insufficiency, pulsus alternans, or pulsus paradoxus.

■ Perform hand hygiene before changing a dressing, and use sterile technique and sterile gloves when redressing the site. When removing the current dressing, observe for signs of infection, such as redness, warmth, swelling, and purulent drainage, and note any complaints of tenderness.

■ Change the pressure tubing every 96 hours or if the integrity of the system is compromised.

■ Change the dressing at the catheter site at intervals specified by your facility's policy.

■ Regularly assess the site for signs of infection, such as redness and swelling. Notify the doctor immediately if you note any such signs.

Blood sampling
■ Limit the number of times you enter the arterial pressure monitoring system by grouping blood draws, if possible, *to minimize the risk of infection.*

■ Always assess the arterial waveform before and after blood withdrawal *to ensure the system is operating properly.*

■ Use the minimal amount of blood for discard *to prevent anemia.*

■ Monitor hemoglobin and hematocrit levels and report decreasing levels to the doctor *to detect nosocomial anemia.*

■ Assess the need for the catheter daily during multidisciplinary rounds, and discontinue the catheter as soon as it's no longer needed *to reduce the risk for infection.*

Tubing change
■ Some facilities may add 500 to 1,000 units of heparin to the flush bag *to help ensure a patent arterial line.*

■ Observing the pressure waveform on the monitor can enhance assessment of arterial pressure. An abnormal waveform may reflect an arrhythmia (such as atrial fibrillation) or other cardiovascular problems, such as aortic stenosis, aortic insufficiency, pulsus alternans, or pulsus paradoxus.

■ Assess the site for signs of infection, such as redness and swelling. Notify the doctor immediately if you note such signs.

■ Be aware that erroneous pressure readings may result from a catheter that is clotted or positional, loose connections, the addition of extra stopcocks or extension tubing, inadvertent entry of air into the system, or improper calibrating, leveling, or zeroing of the monitoring system. If the catheter lumen clots, the flush system may be improperly pressurized. Regularly assess the amount of flush solution in the IV bag, and maintain 300 mm Hg of pressure in the pressure bag.

Catheter removal
■ Teach the patient about reporting signs and symptoms of bleeding, infection, and phlebitis after catheter removal.

Complications
Arterial catheter insertion and pressure monitoring can cause such complications as arterial bleeding; infection at the insertion site, which can spread into the bloodstream; clot formation within the catheter, which can then be carried into the general circulation; catheter perforation of the vessel wall, which can be associated with excessive bleeding and extravasation of flush solution into the surrounding tissue; air embolism; arterial spasm; and impaired circulation to the extremity distal to the catheter insertion site which, if not treated promptly, can lead to loss of tissue or, ultimately, the limb.

Other complications can occur as well. If the radial artery is used, prolonged hyperextension of the wrist can cause transient median nerve conduction deficits. Blood sampling from an arterial catheter can cause such complications as arterial bleeding, infection, air embolism, or arterial spasm; an arterial line tubing change may also result in arterial bleeding, infection, or air embolism. Removal of an arterial catheter can cause arterial bleeding and hematoma formation, infection, air embolism, arterial spasm, or thrombosis.

Documentation
If you assisted with insertion, record the date and time of insertion, assessment findings, the insertion site used, catheter size used, type of flush solution used, and the patient's response to the procedure. Document the color, warmth, sensation, and pulse strength of the extremity distal to the catheter insertion site before insertion, immediately after insertion, and at regular intervals, according to your facility's policy. Document alarm settings.

Record the patient's position for zeroing the transducer *so that other health care team members can replicate the placement.* Record the patient's manual blood pressure in comparison with the blood pressure obtained through the arterial catheter. Document dressing, tubing, and flush solution changes, when appropriate.

Document the date, time, and type of blood samples drawn, along with any laboratory test results (when available). Document the quality of the arterial waveform before specimen collection as well as any unexpected outcomes and interventions after specimen collection.

Record the date and time of a tubing change, the type of flush solution used, your assessment findings, and the patient's response to the procedure. Carefully document the amount of flush solution infused.

Document any patient teaching and the patient's understanding of your teaching.

REFERENCES

1 O'Grady, N.P., et al. (2011). "Guidelines for the prevention of intravascular catheter-related infections, 2011" [Online]. Accessed July 2011 via the Web at http://www.cdc.gov/hicpac/pdf/guidelines/bsi-guidelines-2011.pdf (Level I)

2 Standard 43. Administration set change. Infusion nursing standards of practice. (2011). *Journal of Infusion Nursing, 34*(1S), S55–57. (Level I)

3 Centers for Disease Control and Prevention. (October 2002). Guideline for hand hygiene in health-care settings. *Morbidity and Mortality Weekly Report, 51* (RR-16), 1–45. (Level I)

4 Centers for Disease Control and Prevention. (August 2002). Guidelines for the prevention of intravascular catheter-related infections. *Morbidity and Mortality Weekly Report, 51*(RR-10), 1–26. (Level I)

5 The Joint Commission. (2012). Standard NPSG.07.01.01. *Comprehensive accreditation manual for hospitals: The official handbook.* Oakbrook Terrace, IL: The Joint Commission. (Level I)

6 World Health Organization. (2009). *WHO guidelines on hand hygiene in health care: First global patient safety challenge. Clean care is safer care.* Geneva, Switzerland: World Health Organization. (Level I)

7 The Joint Commission. (2012). Standard NPSG.03.04.01. *Comprehensive accreditation manual for hospitals: The official handbook.* Oakbrook Terrace, IL: The Joint Commission. (Level I)

8 The Joint Commission. (2012). Standard NPSG.01.01.01. *Comprehensive accreditation manual for hospitals: The official handbook.* Oakbrook Terrace, IL: The Joint Commission. (Level I)

9 The Joint Commission. (2012). Standard RI.01.03.01. *Comprehensive accreditation manual for hospitals: The official handbook.* Oakbrook Terrace, IL: The Joint Commission. (Level I)

10 Marschall, J., et al. (2008). SHEA/IDSA practice recommendation: Strategies to prevent central line-associated bloodstream infections in acute care hospitals, *Infection Control and Hospital Epidemiology, 29*(S1), S22–S30. (Level I)

11 The Joint Commission. (2012). Standard RC.01.03.01. *Comprehensive accreditation manual for hospitals: The official handbook.* Oakbrook Terrace, IL: The Joint Commission. (Level I)

12 Standard 27. Needleless connectors. Infusion nursing standards of practice. (2011). *Journal of Infusion Nursing, 34*(1S), S32–33. (Level I)

13 The Joint Commission. (2012). Standard NPSG.07.04.01. *Comprehensive accreditation manual for hospitals: The official handbook.* Oakbrook Terrace, IL: The Joint Commission. (Level I)

14 Standard 18. Infection prevention. Infusion nursing standards of practice. (2011). *Journal of Infusion Nursing, 34*(1S), S25–26. (Level I)

15 Siegel, J.D., et al. "2007 guideline for isolation precautions: Preventing transmission of infectious agents in healthcare settings" [Online]. Accessed June 2011 via the Web at http://www.cdc.gov/hicpac/2007ip/2007isolationprecautions.html

16 Standard 19. Hand hygiene. Infusion nursing standards of practice. (2011). *Journal of Infusion Nursing, 34*(1S), S26–27. (Level I)

17 Standard 46. Vascular access device site care and dressing changes. Infusion nursing standards of practice (2011). *Journal of Infusion Nursing, 34*(1S), S63–64. (Level I)

18 Standard 27. Needless connectors. Infusion nursing standards of practice. (2011). *Journal of Infusion Nursing, 34* (1S), S32–33. (Level I)

19 U.S. Food and Drug Administration (2009). "Look. Check. Connect.: Safe Medical Device Connections Save Lives" [Online]. Accessed July 2011 via the Web at www.fda.gov/downloads/MedicalDevices/Safety/AlertsandNotices/UCM134873.pdf

20 Standard 44. Vascular access device removal: Infusion nursing standards of practice. (2011). *Journal of Infusion Nursing, 34*(1S), S57–63. (Level I)

ADDITIONAL REFERENCES

Lynn-McHale Wiegand, D. (Ed.). (2011). *AACN procedure manual for critical care* (6th ed.). Philadelphia, PA: Saunders.

Occupational Safety and Health Administration. "Bloodborne Pathogens, Standard Number 1910.1030" [Online]. Accessed July 2011 via the Web at http://www.osha.gov/pls/oshaweb/owadisp.show_document?p_table=STANDARDS&p_id=10051

Standard 11. Patient education: Infusion nursing standards of practice. (2011). *Journal of Infusion Nursing, 34*(1S), S16.

ARTERIAL PUNCTURE FOR BLOOD GAS ANALYSIS

Obtaining an arterial blood sample requires percutaneous puncture of the brachial, radial, or femoral artery or withdrawal of a sample from an arterial line. Once collected, the sample can be analyzed to determine arterial blood gas (ABG) values.

ABG analysis evaluates ventilation by measuring blood pH and the partial pressures of arterial oxygen (PaO_2) and carbon dioxide ($PaCO_2$). Blood pH measurement reveals the blood's acid-base balance, PaO_2 indicates the amount of oxygen that the lungs deliver to the blood, and $PaCO_2$ indicates the lungs' capacity to eliminate carbon dioxide. ABG samples can also be analyzed for oxygen content and saturation and for bicarbonate values.[1]

Typically, ABG analysis is ordered for patients who have chronic obstructive pulmonary disease, pulmonary edema, acute respiratory distress syndrome, myocardial infarction, or pneumonia. It's also performed during episodes of shock and after coronary artery bypass surgery, resuscitation from cardiac arrest, changes in respiratory therapy or status, and prolonged anesthesia.

Most ABG samples can be drawn by a respiratory technician or specially trained nurse. Collection from the femoral artery, however, is usually performed by a doctor. Before attempting a radial puncture, you should perform Allen's test. (See *Performing Allen's test,* page 36.)

Equipment

Preheparinized ABG plastic luer-lock syringe specially made for drawing blood for ABG analysis ▪ 1-mL ampule of aqueous heparin (1:1,000), if a preheparinized syringe isn't available ▪ 0G to 25G 1″ to 1½″ needle ▪ 22G 1″ needle ▪ gloves ▪ goggles ▪ chlorhexidine solution ▪ two 2″ × 2″ gauze pads ▪ rubber cap for syringe hub ▪ ice-filled plastic bag ▪ label ▪ laboratory request form ▪ small

Performing Allen's test

To perform Allen's test, rest the patient's arm on the mattress or bedside stand and support his wrist with a rolled towel. Then tell him to clench his fist. Using your index and middle fingers, press on the radial and ulnar arteries. Hold this position for a few seconds.

Without removing your fingers from the patient's arteries, ask him to unclench his fist and hold his hand in a relaxed position. The palm will be blanched *because pressure from your fingers has impaired the normal blood flow.*

Blanched palm

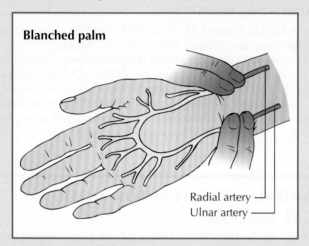

Radial artery
Ulnar artery

Release pressure on the patient's ulnar artery. If the hand becomes flushed, *which indicates blood filling the vessels,* you can safely proceed with the radial artery puncture. If the hand doesn't flush, select another site for the puncture.[1]

Flushed palm

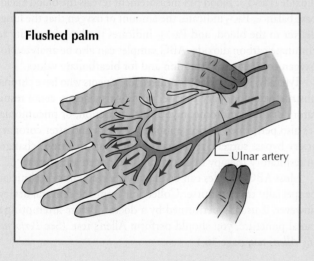

Ulnar artery

towel ■ adhesive bandage ■ Optional: 1% lidocaine solution without epinephrine or lidocaine and prilocaine cream, 1-mL syringe with 25G needle.

Many health care facilities use a commercial ABG kit that contains most of the equipment listed above.

Preparation of equipment

Verify the doctor's order and then prepare the collection equipment before entering the patient's room. Perform hand hygiene.[2,3,4] Open the ABG kit and remove the sample label and the plastic bag. Record on the label the patient's name and room number, the date and collection time, and the doctor's name. Fill the plastic bag with ice and set it aside. Label the syringe in the presence of the patient.[5]

If the syringe isn't heparinized, you will have to do so. To heparinize the syringe, first attach the 22G needle to the syringe. Then open the ampule of heparin. Draw all the heparin into the syringe *to prevent the sample from clotting.* Hold the syringe upright, and pull the plunger back slowly to about the 7-mL mark. Rotate the barrel while pulling the plunger back *to allow the heparin to coat the inside surface of the syringe.* Then slowly force the heparin toward the hub of the syringe, and expel all of the heparin.

Implementation

■ Confirm the patient's identity using at least two patient identifiers according to your facility's policy.[5]

■ Review the patient's current anticoagulation therapy, known blood dyscrasias, and pertinent laboratory values *to determine the patient's risk of prolonged bleeding after the procedure.*

■ Tell the patient you need to collect an arterial blood sample, and explain the procedure *to help ease anxiety and promote cooperation.* Tell him that the needle stick will cause some discomfort but that he must remain still during the procedure.

■ Perform hand hygiene and put on gloves and goggles.[2,3,4]

■ Place a rolled towel under the patient's wrist *for support.* Locate the artery, palpate it for a strong pulse, and perform Allen's test.

■ Clean the puncture site with chlorhexidine using a back-and-forth motion while applying friction for 30 seconds.

■ Allow the skin to dry.

■ If indicated, administer a local anesthetic to the puncture site. However, consider use of lidocaine carefully *because it delays the procedure, the patient may be allergic to the drug, or the resulting vasoconstriction may prevent successful puncture.*

■ Palpate the artery with the index and middle fingers of one hand while holding the syringe over the puncture site with the other hand. The puncture site should be between your index and middle fingers as they palpate the pulse.

■ Hold the needle bevel up at a 30- to 60-degree angle. (See *Arterial puncture technique.*)

■ Puncture the skin and the arterial wall in one motion, following the path of the artery.

■ Watch for blood backflow in the syringe. Don't pull back on the plunger *because arterial blood should enter the syringe automatically.* Obtain 1 mL of blood. Withdraw the needle.

■ After collecting the sample, press a gauze pad firmly over the puncture site until the bleeding stops, at least 5 minutes. If the patient is receiving anticoagulant therapy or has a blood dyscrasia, apply pressure for 10 to 15 minutes; if necessary, ask a coworker to hold the gauze pad in place while you prepare the sample for transport to the laboratory. Don't ask the patient to hold the pad. *If he fails to apply sufficient pressure, a large, painful hematoma may form, hindering future arterial punctures at that site.*

- Check the syringe for air bubbles. If any appear, remove them by holding the syringe upright and slowly ejecting some of the blood onto a 2″ × 2″ gauze pad.[2]
- Remove the needle and place a rubber cap directly on the syringe tip *to prevent the sample from leaking and to keep air out of the syringe.*
- Gently roll the syringe in your hands for 30 seconds.
- Put the labeled sample in the ice-filled plastic bag. Attach a properly completed laboratory request form, and send the sample to the laboratory immediately.[6]
- When bleeding stops, apply a small adhesive bandage to the site.
- Monitor the patient's vital signs, and observe for signs of circulatory impairment, such as swelling, discoloration, pain, numbness, or tingling in the arm or leg. Watch for bleeding at the puncture site.
- Dispose of used equipment in the appropriate receptacles.
- Remove and discard your gloves and perform hand hygiene.[2,3,4]
- Document the procedure.[7]

Special considerations

- If the patient is receiving oxygen, make sure that his therapy has been underway for 20 to 30 minutes before collecting an arterial blood sample. If the patient is receiving mechanical ventilation, wait at least 10 minutes after a change before collecting a blood sample.
- Unless ordered, don't turn off existing oxygen therapy before collecting arterial blood samples. Be sure to indicate on the laboratory request slip the amount and type of oxygen therapy the patient is receiving.
- If the patient isn't receiving oxygen, indicate that he's breathing room air. If the patient has received a nebulizer treatment, wait about 20 minutes before collecting the sample.
- If necessary, you can anesthetize the puncture site with 1% lidocaine solution or 0.9% benzyl alcohol.
- When filling out a laboratory request form for ABG analysis, be sure to include the following information *to help the laboratory staff calibrate the equipment and evaluate results correctly:* the patient's current temperature, most recent hemoglobin level, current respiratory rate and, if the patient is on a ventilator, fraction of inspired oxygen, tidal volume, and ventilatory frequency.

Complications

If you use too much force when attempting to puncture the artery, the needle may touch the periosteum of the bone, causing the patient considerable pain, or you may advance the needle through the opposite wall of the artery. If this happens, slowly pull the needle back a short distance and check to see if you obtain a blood return. If blood still fails to enter the syringe, withdraw the needle completely and attempt the puncture with a new needle and syringe. Don't make more than two attempts to withdraw blood from the same site. *Probing the artery may injure it and the radial nerve. Also, hemolysis will alter test results.*

If arterial spasm occurs, blood won't flow into the syringe and you won't be able to collect the sample. If this happens, replace the needle with a smaller one and try the puncture again. *A smaller-bore needle is less likely to cause arterial spasm.*

Arterial puncture technique

The angle of needle penetration in arterial blood gas sampling depends on which artery will be sampled. For the radial artery, which is used most often, the needle should enter bevel up at a 30- to 60-degree angle over the radial artery.

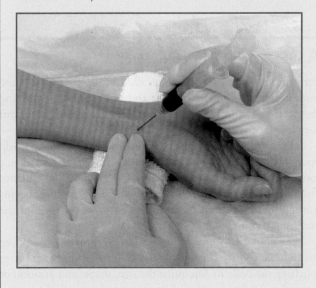

Documentation

Record the results of Allen's test, the time the sample was drawn, the patient's temperature, the site of the arterial puncture, the amount of time that pressure was applied to the site to control bleeding, and the type and amount of oxygen therapy the patient was receiving.

REFERENCES

1 American Association for Respiratory Care. (1992). Clinical practice guidelines. Sampling for arterial blood gas analysis. *Respiratory Care, 37*(8), 891–897. (Level I)
2 Centers for Disease Control and Prevention. (October 2002). Guideline for hand hygiene in health-care settings. *Morbidity and Mortality Weekly Report, 51* (RR-16), 1–45. (Level I)
3 The Joint Commission. (2012). Standard NPSG.07.01.01. *Comprehensive accreditation manual for hospitals: The official handbook.* Oakbrook Terrace, IL: The Joint Commission. (Level I)
4 World Health Organization. (2009). *WHO guidelines on hand hygiene in health care: First global patient safety challenge. Clean care is safer care.* Geneva, Switzerland: World Health Organization. (Level I)
5 The Joint Commission. (2012). Standard NPSG.01.01.01. *Comprehensive accreditation manual for hospitals: The official handbook.* Oakbrook Terrace, IL: The Joint Commission. (Level I)
6 The Joint Commission. (2012). Standard NPSG.03.04.01. *Comprehensive accreditation manual for hospitals: The official handbook.* Oakbrook Terrace, IL: The Joint Commission. (Level I)
7 The Joint Commission. (2012). Standard RC.01.03.01. *Comprehensive accreditation manual for hospitals: The official handbook.* Oakbrook Terrace, IL: The Joint Commission. (Level I)

ADDITIONAL REFERENCES

Lynn-McHale Wiegand, D. (Ed.). (2011). *AACN procedure manual for critical care* (6th ed.). Philadelphia, PA: Saunders.

National Committee for Clinical Laboratory Standards. (2004). "Procedures for the Collection of Arterial Blood Specimens, 4th ed. Approved standard H11-A4" [Online]. Accessed July 2011 via the Web at http://www.clsi.org/source/orders/free/H11-a4.pdf

Nettina, S.M. (2010). *Lippincott manual of nursing practice* (9th ed.). Philadelphia, PA: Lippincott Williams & Wilkins.

ASSESSMENT TECHNIQUES

Performing a physical assessment calls for four basic techniques: inspection, palpation, percussion, and auscultation. Performing these techniques correctly helps elicit valuable information about the patient's condition.

Inspection requires the use of vision, hearing, touch, and smell. Special lighting and various equipment—such as an otoscope, a tongue blade, or an ophthalmoscope—may be used to enhance vision or examine an otherwise hidden area. Inspection begins during the first patient contact and continues throughout the assessment.

Palpation usually follows inspection, except when examining the abdomen or assessing infants and children. Palpation involves touching the body to determine the size, shape, and position of structures; to detect and evaluate temperature, pulsations, and other movement; and to elicit tenderness. The four palpation techniques include light palpation, deep palpation, light ballottement, and deep ballottement. Ballottement is the technique used to evaluate a flowing or movable structure. The nurse gently bounces the structure by applying pressure against it and then waits to feel it rebound. This technique may be used, for example, to check the position of an organ or a fetus.

Percussion uses quick, sharp tapping of the fingers or hands against body surfaces to produce sounds, detect tenderness, or assess reflexes. Percussing for sound helps locate organ borders, identify organ shape and position, and determine whether an organ is solid or filled with fluid or gas. Organs and tissues produce sounds of varying loudness, pitch, and duration, depending on their density. For example, air-filled cavities, such as the lungs, produce markedly different sounds from those produced by the liver and other dense organs and tissues. Percussion techniques include indirect percussion, direct percussion, and blunt percussion.

Auscultation involves listening to various sounds of the body—particularly those produced by the heart, lungs, vessels, stomach, and intestines. Most auscultated sounds result from the movement of air or fluid through these structures.

Typically, auscultation comes last after the other assessment techniques. When examining the abdomen, however, auscultation takes place after inspection but before percussion and palpation so that bowel sounds can be heard before palpation disrupts them. Auscultation is also best performed first on infants and young children, who may start to cry when palpated or percussed. Auscultation is most successful when performed in a quiet environment with a properly fitted stethoscope.

Equipment

Flashlight or gooseneck lamp, as appropriate ▪ patient drape ▪ stethoscope ▪ alcohol pad.

Implementation

- Gather all equipment.
- Perform hand hygiene.[1,2,3]
- Confirm the patient's identity using at least two patient identifiers according to your facility's policy.[4]
- Explain all aspects of the procedure to the patient, have him undress, and drape him appropriately.
- Make sure the room is warm and adequately lit *to make the patient comfortable and aid visual inspection.*
- Warm your hands and the stethoscope.

Inspection

- Focus on areas related to the patient's chief complaint. Use your eyes, ears, and sense of smell to observe the patient.
- To inspect a specific body area, first make sure the area is sufficiently exposed and adequately lit. Then survey the entire area, noting key landmarks and checking its overall condition. Next, focus on specifics—color, shape, texture, size, and movement. Note unusual findings as well as predictable ones.

Palpation

- Tell the patient what to expect such as occasional discomfort as pressure is applied. Encourage him to relax *because muscle tension or guarding can interfere with performance and results of palpation.*
- Provide just enough pressure to assess the tissue beneath one or both hands. Then release pressure and gently move to the next area, systematically covering the entire surface to be assessed. (See *Performing palpation*, page 39.
- To perform light palpation, depress the skin, indenting ½" to ¾" (1 to 2 cm). Use the lightest touch possible *because excessive pressure blunts your sensitivity.*
- If the patient tolerates light palpation and you need to assess deeper structures, palpate deeply by increasing your fingertip pressure, indenting the skin about 1½" to 2½" (4 to 6 cm). Place your other hand on top of the palpating hand *to control and guide your movements.*
- To perform light ballottement, apply light, rapid pressure from quadrant to quadrant on the patient's abdomen. Keep your hand on the skin *to detect tissue rebound.*
- To perform deeper ballottement, apply abrupt, deep pressure and then release it. Maintain fingertip contact.
- Use both hands (bimanual palpation) to trap a deep, underlying, hard-to-palpate organ (such as the kidney or spleen) or to fix or stabilize an organ (such as the uterus) with one hand while you palpate it with the other.

Percussion

- First, decide which of the percussion techniques best suits your assessment needs. Indirect percussion helps reveal the size and density of underlying thoracic and abdominal organs and tissues. Direct percussion helps assess an adult's sinuses for tenderness and elicits

Performing palpation

You should be familiar with four palpation techniques: light palpation, deep palpation, light ballottement, and deep ballottement. Remember to use the flattened finger pads for palpating tender tissues, feeling for crepitus (crackling) at the joints, and lightly probing the abdomen. Use the thumb and index finger for assessing hair texture, grasping tissues, and feeling for lymph node enlargement. Use the back, or dorsal, surface of the hand when feeling for warmth.

Light palpation

With the tips of two or three fingers held close together, press gently on the skin to a depth of ½″ to ¾″ (1 to 2 cm).[5] Use the lightest touch possible; too much pressure blunts your sensitivity.

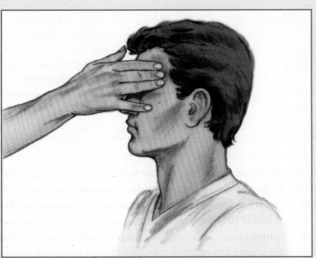

Light ballottement

Apply light, rapid pressure to the abdomen, moving from one quadrant to another. Keep your hand on the skin surface *to detect tissue rebound*.

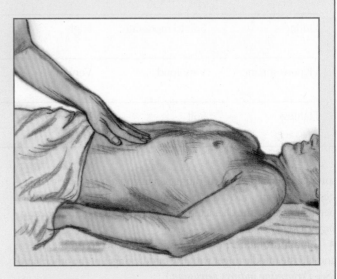

Deep palpation (bimanual palpation)

Place one hand on top of the other. Then press down about 1½″ to 2½″ (4 to 6 cm) with the fingertips of both hands.[5]

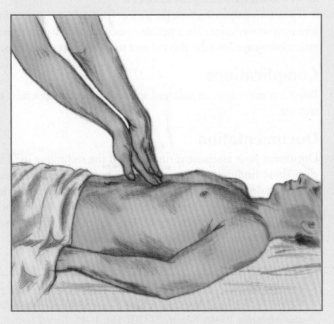

Deep ballottement

Apply abrupt, deep pressure on the patient's abdomen. Release the pressure completely, but maintain fingertip contact with the skin.

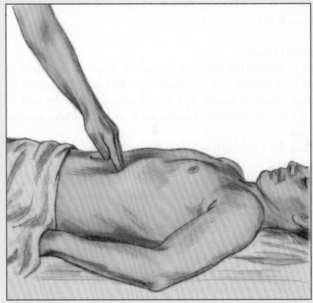

Identifying percussion sounds

Percussion produces sounds that vary according to the tissue being percussed. This chart lists important percussion sounds along with their characteristics and typical sources.

SOUND	INTENSITY	PITCH	DURATION	QUALITY	SOURCE
Resonance	Moderate to loud	Low	Long	Hollow	Normal lung
Tympany	Loud	High	Moderate	Drumlike	Gastric air bubble, intestinal air
Dullness	Soft to moderate	High	Moderate	Thudlike	Liver, full bladder, pregnant uterus
Hyperresonance	Very loud	Very low	Long	Booming	Hyperinflated lung (as in emphysema)
Flatness	Soft	High	Short	Flat	Muscle

sounds in a child's thorax. Blunt percussion aims to elicit tenderness over organs, such as the kidneys, gallbladder, or liver. When percussing, note the characteristic sounds produced. (See *Identifying percussion sounds*.)

■ To perform indirect percussion, place one hand on the patient and tap the middle finger with the middle finger of the other hand. (See *Performing indirect percussion*.)

■ To perform direct percussion, tap your hand or fingertip directly against the body surface.

■ To perform blunt percussion, strike the ulnar surface of your fist against the body surface. Or place the palm of one hand against the body, make a fist with the other hand, and strike the back of the first hand.

Auscultation

■ First, determine whether to use the diaphragm or bell of your stethoscope. Use the diaphragm to detect high-pitched sounds, such as breath and bowel sounds. Use the bell to detect lower-pitched sounds, such as heart and vascular sounds.

■ Place the diaphragm or bell of the stethoscope over the appropriate area of the patient's body and place the earpieces in your ears.

■ Listen intently to individual sounds, and try to identify their characteristics. Determine the intensity, pitch, and duration of each sound, and check the frequency of recurring sounds.

■ Disinfect your stethoscope with an alcohol pad.[6]

■ Perform hand hygiene.[1,2,3]

■ Document the procedure.[7]

Special considerations

■ Avoid palpating or percussing an area of the body known to be tender at the start of your examination. Instead, work around the area; then gently palpate or percuss it at the end of the examination. *This progression minimizes the patient's discomfort and apprehension.*

■ To assess the abdomen, inspect visually first. Then auscultate bowel sounds before palpation and percussion, *which alter these sounds.*

■ To pinpoint an inflamed area deep within the patient's body, perform a variation on deep palpation: Press firmly with one hand over the area you suspect is involved, and then lift your hand away quickly. If the patient reports that pain increases when you release the pressure, then you've identified rebound tenderness.

NURSING ALERT *Suspect peritonitis if you elicit rebound tenderness when examining the abdomen.*

■ If you can't palpate because the patient fears pain, try distracting him with conversation. Then perform auscultation and gently press your stethoscope into the affected area to try to elicit tenderness.

Complications

Palpation may cause an enlarged spleen or infected appendix to rupture.

Documentation

Document your assessment findings and the technique used to elicit those findings—for example, "Right lower quadrant tenderness on deep palpation, no rebound tenderness." Indicate who you notified of any abnormal findings and the time of the notification. Document interventions required to treat those findings as well as the patient's response to them.

REFERENCES

1 Centers for Disease Control and Prevention. (October 2002). Guideline for hand hygiene in health-care settings. *Morbidity and Mortality Weekly Report, 51* (RR-16), 1–45. (Level I)

Performing indirect percussion

To perform indirect percussion, use the middle finger of your nondominant hand as the pleximeter (the mediating device used to receive the taps) and the middle finger of your dominant hand as the plexor (the device used to tap the pleximeter). Place the pleximeter finger firmly against a body surface such as the upper back. With your wrist flexed loosely, use the tip of your plexor finger to deliver a crisp blow just beneath the distal joint of the pleximeter. Be sure to hold the plexor perpendicular to the pleximeter. Tap lightly and quickly, removing the plexor as soon as you have delivered each blow. Move your nondominant hand to cover the entire area to be percussed.

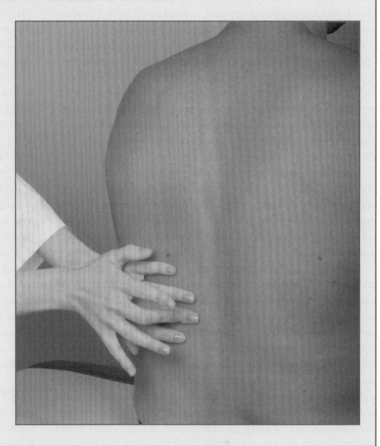

2   The Joint Commission. (2012). Standard NPSG.07.01.01. *Comprehensive accreditation manual for hospitals: The official handbook.* Oakbrook Terrace, IL: The Joint Commission. (Level I)

3   World Health Organization. (2009). *WHO guidelines on hand hygiene in health care: First global patient safety challenge. Clean care is safer care.* Geneva, Switzerland: World Health Organization. (Level I)

4   The Joint Commission. (2012). Standard NPSG.01.01.01. *Comprehensive accreditation manual for hospitals: The official handbook.* Oakbrook Terrace, IL: The Joint Commission. (Level I)

5   Jensen, S. (2011). *Nursing health assessment: A best practice approach.* Philadelphia, PA: Lippincott Williams & Wilkins.

6   Rutala, W.A., et al. (2008). "Guideline for disinfection and sterilization in healthcare facilities, 2008" [Online]. Accessed July 2011 via the Web at http://www.cdc.gov/ncidod/dhqp/pdf/guidelines/Disinfection_Nov_2008.pdf (Level I)

7   The Joint Commission. (2012). Standard RC.01.03.01. *Comprehensive accreditation manual for hospitals: The official handbook.* Oakbrook Terrace, IL: The Joint Commission. (Level I)

ADDITIONAL REFERENCES

Bickley, L.S., & Szilaqyi, P.G. (2009). *Bate's guide to physical examination and history taking* (10th ed.). Philadelphia, PA: Lippincott Williams & Wilkins.

Craven, R.F., & Hirnle, C.J. (2009). *Fundamentals of nursing: Human health and function* (6th ed.). Philadelphia, PA: Lippincott Williams & Wilkins.

Nettina, S.M. (2010). *Lippincott manual of nursing practice* (9th ed.). Philadelphia, PA: Lippincott Williams & Wilkins.

AUTOLOGOUS BLOOD COLLECTION, PREOPERATIVE

Also called *autotransfusion,* autologous blood transfusion is the collection, filtration, and reinfusion of the patient's own blood. Autologous transfusion is becoming increasingly common because of the declining rate of blood donation, the concerns related to the risks involved with allogenic blood transfusions, and the costs associated with blood transfusions.

Indications for autologous transfusion include elective surgery (blood is donated over time); perioperative and emergency blood salvage during and after thoracic or cardiovascular surgery and hip, knee, or liver resection and during surgery for ruptured ectopic pregnancy and hemothorax; and perioperative and emergency blood salvage for traumatic injury of the lungs, liver, chest wall, heart, pulmonary vessels, spleen, kidneys, inferior vena cava, and iliac, portal, or subclavian veins.

Autologous transfusion has several advantages over transfusion of bank blood. Transfusion reactions don't occur, diseases aren't transmitted, anticoagulants aren't added (except in post-operative autologous transfusion, when acid citrate dextrose is added), and the blood supply isn't depleted. Also, unlike bank blood, autologous blood contains normal levels of 2 3-diphos-phoglycerate, which is helpful in tissue oxygenation.

There are three techniques for autologous transfusion: pre-operative blood donation, perioperative blood donation, and acute normovolemic hemodilution.[1] Preoperative collection is used when a patient is donating his own blood before a planned procedure. Perioperative blood donation (sometimes called *intra-operative* or *postoperative*), in which blood is collected during or after surgery, is used in vascular and orthopedic surgery and in the treatment of traumatic injury.

The third option, acute normovolemic hemodilution, is used mainly in open-heart surgery. It's performed the same way as pre-operative blood donation. One or two units of blood are collected immediately before or just after anesthesia induction. The blood volume is replaced with crystalloid or colloid solution to produce normovolemic anemia. The blood is then reinfused after surgery.

Autologous blood transfusion does have its drawbacks. With preoperative donation, one must consider that collected blood has an expiration date. If the procedure must be rescheduled, the patient may have to donate again. The donation process may also involve additional fees for the patient. Finally, not all patients may be candidates to donate the amount of blood that is needed. Contraindications include existing infections or known inflam-matory disease, antibiotic use, long-term corticosteroids or non-steroidal anti-inflammatory medication use, malignant neoplasms, coagulopathies, cardiovascular disease with compromised hemo-dynamic reserves, anemia, contamination of blood with bowel contents, malnutrition or excessive weight loss due to illness, use of antiplatelet agents in the weeks prior to surgery, and severe preexisting lung or renal dysfunction.

Equipment

Gloves ▪ face shield ▪ gown ▪ tourniquet ▪ rubber ball ▪ 14G to 24G catheter ▪ equipment for venipuncture ▪ blood collection bags ▪ IV line ▪ inline filter for reinfusion ▪ IV fluids (if ordered).

Implementation

▪ Review the doctor's order for autologous blood collection.[2]
▪ Confirm the patient's identity using at least two patient iden-tifiers according to your facility's policy.[3]
▪ Explain the procedure to the patient. Explain that he can donate one unit of blood every 7 days until surgery, as ordered by his doctor.[2]
▪ *To prevent hypovolemia,* encourage the patient to drink plenty of fluids before the donations. Explain that he may feel light-headed during the donation but the problem can be treated.
▪ Verify that the patient's hemoglobin level is 11 g/dL or higher.
▪ Perform hand hygiene and put on gloves.[4,5,6]
▪ Obtain and record vital signs before starting the donation.
▪ Help the patient into a supine position.
▪ Put on a face shield and gown. Follow standard precautions.
▪ Prepare the collection bags according to the manufacturer's instructions.

▪ Prepare replacement IV fluids, if ordered.
▪ Select an appropriate IV catheter insertion site.
▪ Prepare the patient's arm and IV catheter insertion site. Insert a large-bore catheter (14G to 24 G). (See "IV catheter insertion and removal," page 421.)
▪ Connect the collecting system according to the manufacturer's instructions. Have the patient squeeze the rubber ball *to promote the blood flow into the collecting bag.*
▪ Monitor the patient for adverse reactions.
NURSING ALERT *Monitor the patient's vital signs closely for signs of hypotension during this process.*[7]
▪ Administer replacement IV fluids, if ordered.
▪ When blood collection is complete, remove the IV catheter and perform site care according to your facility's policy.
▪ Recheck the patient's vital signs.
▪ Send a blood sample obtained from the patient to the labora-tory to be checked for the patient's coagulation profile, hemo-globin and hematocrit, and calcium levels.
▪ Clearly label the collection bag with the patient's name, iden-tifying numbers, and an AUTOLOGOUS BLOOD label. *This labeling ensures that the blood isn't subjected to rigorous blood bank testing or given to another patient.*
▪ Send the blood to the blood bank according to your facility's policy.
▪ Remove and discard your personal protective equipment and perform hand hygiene.[4,5,6]
▪ Document the procedure.[8]

Special considerations

▪ In the 4 to 6 weeks before surgery, the patient may be pre-scribed iron supplements *to prevent depletion of his iron stores.*
▪ Monitor the patient closely during and after the donation. Although vasovagal reactions are usually mild and easy to treat, they can quickly progress to severe reactions, such as loss of con-sciousness and seizures.
▪ Have the patient remain supine for 10 minutes after the dona-tion. If he feels light-headed or dizzy, advise him to sit down immediately and to lower his head between his knees. He may also lie down with his head lower than his body until his symp-toms resolve.
▪ Instruct the patient to drink more fluids than usual for a few hours after the donation and to eat heartily at his next meal.
▪ Instruct the patient to monitor his IV site for a few hours after the donation. If some bleeding occurs, he should apply firm pres-sure for 5 to 10 minutes. If the bleeding continues, instruct him to notify his doctor.

Complications

Preoperative donation may cause vasovagal reactions and hypo-volemia. (See *Managing problems of autologous transfusion.*)

Documentation

Document the time the donation began and ended, the amount of blood the patient donated, and his tolerance of the procedure. Note the condition of the IV site. Note that the blood sample was sent to the laboratory and that the blood was sent to the blood bank.

Managing problems of autologous transfusion

PROBLEM	POSSIBLE CAUSES	NURSING INTERVENTIONS
Citrate toxicity (rare, unpredictable)	■ Citrate in citrate phosphate dextrose (CPD) combines with calcium and magnesium ■ Predisposing factors, including hyperkalemia, hypocalcemia, acidosis, hypothermia, myocardial dysfunction, and liver or kidney problems	■ Watch for hypotension, arrhythmias, and myocardial contractility. ■ Prophylactic calcium chloride may be administered if more than 2,000 mL of CPD-anticoagulated blood is given over 20 minutes. ■ Stop infusing CPD and correct acidosis. Measure arterial blood gas values and serum calcium levels frequently to assess for toxicity.
Coagulation	■ Not enough anticoagulant ■ Blood not defibrinated in mediastinum	■ Add CPD or another regional anticoagulant at a ratio of 7 parts blood to 1 part anticoagulant. Keep blood and CPD mixed by shaking collection bottle regularly. ■ Check for anticoagulant reversal. Strip chest tubes as needed.
Coagulopathies	■ Reduced platelet and fibrinogen levels ■ Platelets caught in filters ■ Enhanced levels of fibrin split products	■ Patients receiving autologous transfusions of more than 4,000 mL of blood may also need transfusion of fresh frozen plasma or platelet concentrate.
Emboli	■ Microaggregate debris ■ Air	■ Don't use equipment with roller pumps or pressure infusion systems. Before reinfusion, remove air from blood bags. ■ Reinfuse with a 20- to 40-unit microaggregate filter.
Hemolysis	■ Trauma to blood caused by turbulence or roller pumps	■ Don't skim operative field or use equipment with roller pumps. When collecting blood from chest tubes, keep vacuum below 30 mm Hg; when aspirating from a surgical site, keep vacuum below 60 mm Hg.
Sepsis	■ Lack of sterile technique ■ Contaminated blood	■ Give broad-spectrum antibiotics. Use strict sterile technique. Reinfuse patient within 4 hours. ■ Don't infuse blood from infected areas or blood that contains feces, urine, or other contaminants.

REFERENCES

1 Cardone, D., & Klein, A.A. (2009). Perioperative blood conservation. *European Journal of Anesthesiology, 26*(9), 722–729.
2 American Association of Blood Banks. (2009). Process controls. In *Standards for blood banks and transfusion services* (26th ed.). Bethesda, MD: American Association of Blood Banks. (Level I)
3 The Joint Commission. (2012). Standard NPSG.01.01.01. *Comprehensive accreditation manual for hospitals: The official handbook.* Oakbrook Terrace, IL: The Joint Commission. (Level I)
4 Centers for Disease Control and Prevention. (October 2002). Guideline for hand hygiene in health-care settings. *Morbidity and Mortality Weekly Report, 51* (RR-16), 1–45. (Level I)
5 The Joint Commission. (2012). Standard NPSG.07.01.01. *Comprehensive accreditation manual for hospitals: The official handbook.* Oakbrook Terrace, IL: The Joint Commission. (Level I)

6 World Health Organization. (2009). *WHO guidelines on hand hygiene in health care: First global patient safety challenge. Clean care is safer care.* Geneva, Switzerland: World Health Organization. (Level I)
7 John, T., et al. (2008). Blood conservation in a congential cardiac surgery program. *AORN Journal, 87*(6), 1180–1190.
8 The Joint Commission. (2012). Standard RC.01.03.01. *Comprehensive accreditation manual for hospitals: The official handbook.* Oakbrook Terrace, IL: The Joint Commission. (Level I)

ADDITIONAL REFERENCES

Bouchard, D., et al. (2008). Preoperative autologous blood donation reduces the need for allogeneic blood products: A prospective randomized study. *Canadian Journal of Surgery, 51*(6), 422–427.
World Health Organization. (2002). *The clinical use of blood handbook.* Geneva, Switzerland: World Health Organization.

Autologous blood recovery systems

Autologous blood recovery systems are used in surgical procedures to salvage red blood cells (RBCs) when there is rapid bleeding or high-volume blood loss. Shed blood is collected and stored in a reservoir, where waste is separated from the healthy RBCs. The waste collects into a separate bag; healthy RBCs are then returned to the patient. This process can be performed in 3 to 7 minutes. In emergent situations, the autologous blood recovery system can process up to 800 mL of blood each minute. Advantages to autologous blood recovery systems, such as the Cell Saver® 5+ shown, include:

- up-to-date microprocessor and sensor technologies
- automated operation and manual operation options
- platelet sequestration
- RBC bags with integrated microaggregate filters
- features to ensure consistent processing and a high-quality blood product
- fast processing
- built-in safety features.

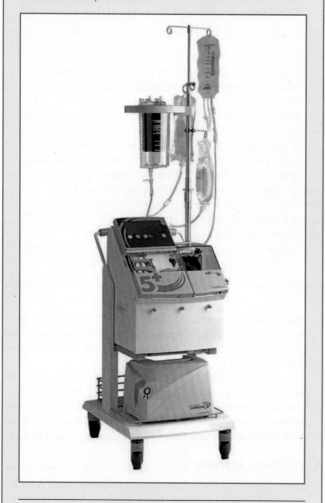

The photograph of the Cell Saver® 5+ autologous blood recovery system is used by permission of Haemonetics Corporation. Haemonetics® and Cell Saver® are registered trademarks of Haemonetics Corporation in the United States, other countries, or both.

AUTOLOGOUS BLOOD TRANSFUSION, PERIOPERATIVE

Both preoperative blood donation and acute normovolemic hemodilution involve collecting the patient's own blood preoperatively. (See "Autologous blood collection, preoperative," page 41.) In contrast, in perioperative autologous blood transfusion, blood is collected during or after surgery.[1] This perioperative blood donation (sometimes called *intraoperative* or *postoperative*) is used in the treatment of traumatic injury as well as during vascular and orthopedic surgery because considerable bleeding may follow these surgeries. Blood may be collected during surgery or up to 12 hours afterward in a process called *red blood cell (RBC) salvage*.

Blood collected during surgery undergoes a process in which RBCs are washed and packed and then transfused immediately. (See *Autologous blood recovery systems.*) Blood obtained postoperatively may be collected from chest tubes, mediastinal drains, or wound drains that are placed in the surgical wound during surgery with devices such as the Solcotrans autotransfusion system or Pleur-evac drains for blood recovery. Blood recovered postoperatively from wound drains is typically filtered, and the total volume is infused into the patient with an approximate hematocrit of 30%. Blood collected postoperatively must be reinfused within 6 hours of being collected because of the increased risk of infection.[2] Blood collected intraoperatively may be used for 6 to 8 hours. Check you facility's policy for specifics.

Contraindications for perioperative autologous transfusion are the same as for preoperative autologous transfusions. Intraoperative collection devices may also cause problems if they're used improperly. The blood units returned to the patient may be overdiluted during the washing process, or the units may not be washed well, exposing the patient to the anticoagulant medications that were used to keep the blood from clotting in the collection container as well as to other debris that may have been suctioned from the surgical wound.

Equipment

Gloves ▪ face shield ▪ gown ▪ data recording form ▪ 250-mL bag of normal saline IV solution ▪ standard blood administration IV tubing set with gravity drip and microaggregate filter ▪ wall suction with pressure gauge, as needed ▪ autotransfusion device with necessary supplies; for a Cell Saver® 5+ unit, suction tubing and collection kit; an autotransfusion drain usually has stand-alone functioning.

Implementation

- Confirm the patient's identity using at least two patient identifiers according to your facility's policy.[3]
- Verify the doctor's order for the rate of reinfusion and the amount of blood to be reinfused.
- Verify the presence of consent for blood and blood product transfusion according to your facility's policy.
- Call the perfusionist to set up the autotransfusion device and connect the tubing to the setup according to your facility's policy and the autotransfusion manufacturer's instructions. (Note that the person responsible for this step may vary by facility. The

perioperative nurse or anesthesia care provider may set up the device in some facilities.)

- Perform hand hygiene.[4,5,6]
- Put on a gown, gloves, and a face shield. Follow standard precautions.[7]
- Make sure the collection chamber and the blood transfer bag are clearly marked with the patient's name, identifying numbers, and an AUTOLOGOUS BLOOD label.
- Obtain and record the patient's vital signs according to your facility's policy.
- Check that the patient has a patent, acceptable venous access site available for blood administration according to your facility's policy. The access may be peripheral or central and should be 24G or larger.[8] (See "Transfusion of blood and blood products," page 742.) To assess patency, aspirate the catheter for blood return using a 10-mL syringe, and then flush with preservative-free normal saline solution.[9]
- Insert one spike of the standard Y-type blood administration set into the 250-mL bag of normal saline solution. Close all clamps and hang the set on an IV pole.
- The anesthesia care provider, perioperative nurse, or perfusionist will start the collection of shed blood according to your facility's policy and the autotransfusion manufacturer's instructions. (Some devices process and centrifuge the blood automatically.)

NURSING ALERT *Monitor the patient's vital signs closely for signs of hypotension during this process.* Hypotension may occur as the result of hypovolemia.

- Monitor the status of the blood collection.
- When enough blood has been collected to reinfuse, spike the blood transfer bag with the open port of the standard blood administration IV set. Remove all air from the blood transfer bag. Hang it on the IV pole.
- Open the clamp from the normal saline solution and prime the filter and tubing. Close the clamp from the normal saline solution. Remove all air from the tubing.
- Open the clamp from the blood transfer bag to the drip chamber of the blood administration set and prime the filter and tubing with blood.
- If using a postprocedure transfusion device, follow the manufacturer's instructions to properly connect the device to the patient. (Staff members should receive training on all transfusion devices before use.)
- Thoroughly disinfect the IV catheter hub with a disinfectant pad using friction.[10]
- Attach the blood tubing to the venous access device and then trace the tubing from the patient to its point of origin *to make sure it's connected to the proper port.*[11]
- Begin the reinfusion according to your facility's policy.
- Monitor the patient for transfusion reactions.
- Make sure the reinfusion is completed within your facility's recommended time frame.
- Record the patient's vital signs after the reinfusion is complete.
- Depending on facility policy, disconnect the blood collection setup from the patient's drains or have the anesthesia care provider, perioperative nurse, or perfusionist do so according to your facility's policy.

- Recheck the laboratory data for coagulation profile, hemoglobin and hematocrit, and calcium levels after the reinfusion is complete, or as ordered by the doctor.
- Remove and discard your personal protective equipment and perform hand hygiene.[4,5,6]
- Document the procedure.[12]

Special considerations

- If multiple units are to be reinfused, change the blood administration setup and filter, as needed, according to your facility's policy.
- Clotting factors may need to be replaced if large volumes of blood are reinfused.
- Certain religious groups refuse blood transfusions because of the belief that blood is sacred. However, many of these groups permit autologous blood transfusion if it's kept in a continuous closed circuit.[13]
- Frozen blood units usually expire after about 30 days. Once thawed, they are good for 24 hours.[14]

Complications

There are more complications associated with the reinfusion of filtered, unwashed blood than with the transfusion of filtered, washed blood. These complications include fever, hypotension, myocardial infarction, infections, particulate and air embolism, and thrombocytopenia. Complications are more pronounced when the time from salvage to transfusion is greater than 6 hours. (See *Managing problems of autologous transfusion*, page 43.)

Documentation

Document the time the collection was initiated, the time the reinfusion started and ended, and the venous access site used for the reinfusion. Include the patient's vital signs before and after reinfusion per your facility's policy. Note the amount of blood that was collected, processed, and reinfused and the method used. Also document any post-reinfusion laboratory studies that were obtained. Document the patient's tolerance of the procedure.

REFERENCES

1 Cardone, D., & Klein, A.A. (2009). Perioperative blood conservation. *European Journal of Anesthesiology, 26*(9), 722–729.
2 Recommended practices for hand hygiene in the perioperative setting. (2010). In R. Conner, et al. (Eds.). *Perioperative standards and recommended practices.* Denver, CO: AORN. (Level I)
3 The Joint Commission. (2012). Standard NPSG.01.01.01. *Comprehensive accreditation manual for hospitals: The official handbook.* Oakbrook Terrace, IL: The Joint Commission. (Level I)
4 Centers for Disease Control and Prevention. (October 2002). Guideline for hand hygiene in health-care settings. *Morbidity and Mortality Weekly Report, 51* (RR-16), 1–45. (Level I)
5 The Joint Commission. (2012). Standard NPSG.07.01.01. *Comprehensive accreditation manual for hospitals: The official handbook.* Oakbrook Terrace, IL: The Joint Commission. (Level I)
6 World Health Organization. (2002). *The clinical use of blood handbook.* Geneva, Switzerland: World Health Organization. (Level I)

Understanding the AED

The AED interprets the victim's cardiac rhythm and gives the operator step-by-step directions on how to proceed if defibrillation is indicated.

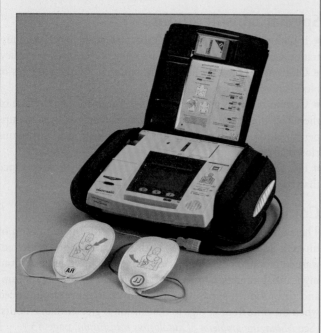

7 Siegel, J.D., et al. "2007 guideline for isolation precautions: Preventing transmission of infectious agents in healthcare settings" [Online]. Accessed June 2011 via the Web at http://www.cdc.gov/hicpac/2007ip/2007isolationprecautions.html

8 Standard 66. Transfusion therapy. Infusion nursing standards of practice. (2011). *Journal of Infusion Nursing, 34*(1S), S93–95. (Level I)

9 Standard 45. Flushing and locking. Infusion nursing standards of practice. (2011). *Journal of Infusion Nursing, 34*(1S), S59–63. (Level I)

10 Standard 27. Needleless connectors. Infusion nursing standards of practice. (2011). *Journal of Infusion Nursing, 34*(1S), S32–33. (Level I)

11 U.S. Food and Drug Administration. (2009). "Look. Check. Connect.: Safe medical device connections save lives" [Online]. Accessed July 2011 via the Web at www.fda.gov/downloads/MedicalDevices/Safety/AlertsandNotices/UCM134873.pdf

12 The Joint Commission. (2012). Standard RC.01.03.01. *Comprehensive accreditation manual for hospitals: The official handbook.* Oakbrook Terrace, IL: The Joint Commission. (Level I)

13 John, T., et al. (2008). Blood conservation in a congential cardiac surgery program. *AORN Journal, 87*(6), 1180–1190.

14 American Association of Blood Banks. (2009). Process controls. In *Standards for blood banks and transfusion services* (26th ed.). Bethesda, MD: American Association of Blood Banks. (Level I)

ADDITIONAL REFERENCE

Bouchard, D., et al. (2008). Preoperative autologous blood donation reduces the need for allogeneic blood products: A prospective randomized study. *Canadian Journal of Surgery, 51*(6), 422–427.

AUTOMATED EXTERNAL DEFIBRILLATION

Automated external defibrillators (AEDs) are commonly used to meet the need for early defibrillation, which is currently considered the most effective treatment for ventricular fibrillation (VF) and pulseless ventricular tachycardia. Some facilities now require an AED on every noncritical care unit. Their use is common in such public places as shopping malls, sports stadiums, and airplanes. Instruction in using the AED is required as part of both basic life support (BLS) and advanced cardiac life support (ACLS) training, pediatric advanced life support (PALS), and heartsaver AED courses. Studies have shown that attempts to resuscitate victims of sudden cardiac arrest resulting from VF using public defibrillation equipment and administered by laypeople trained to use an AED have a survival rate of 41% to 74% when cardiopulmonary resuscitation (CPR) is initiated immediately and defibrillation occurs within 3 to 5 minutes.[1]

The 2010 American Heart Association (AHA) guidelines for CPR and emergency cardiovascular care (ECC) recommend rapid integration of CPR with the use of an AED. These guidelines include the following:

■ Initiate CPR immediately, and then use the AED as soon as it's available.

■ When two rescuers are available, one rescuer should begin CPR immediately while the second rescuer activates the emergency response system and prepares the defibrillator.

■ Coordinate CPR and defibrillation to minimize the time between stopping compressions and administering the shock.

■ First-responding personnel should receive AED training with the goal of delivering the first shock for any spontaneous cardiac arrest within 3 minutes of collapse.

■ An AED can be used for children ages 1 to 8; however, for this age group, an AED with a pediatric dose attenuator system should be used, if available. If one isn't available, a standard AED can be used.

■ If pediatric pads aren't available, adult pads can be used on a child. Place the pads at least 1 inch apart or use an anterior-posterior pad position.[2]

■ An AED shouldn't be used for infants; instead, a manual defibrillator is preferred. However, if a manual defibrillator isn't available, an AED with a pediatric dose attenuator system may be used. If neither defibrillator is available, an AED without a dose attenuator may be used as a last resort.[1]

AEDs provide early defibrillation, even when no health care provider is present. (See *Understanding the AED.*) The AED is equipped with a microcomputer that senses and analyzes a patient's heart rhythm at the push of a button. Then it audibly or visually prompts the operator to deliver a shock. AED models all have the same basic function but offer different operating options. For example, all AEDs communicate display directions on a screen, give voice commands, or both. Some AEDs simultaneously display a patient's heart rhythm.

All devices record the operator's interactions with the patient during defibrillation, either on a cassette tape or in a solid-state memory module. Some AEDs have an integral printer for immediate event documentation. Facility policy determines who is responsible for reviewing all AED interactions; the patient's doctor always has that option. Local and state regulations govern who is responsible for collecting AED case data for reporting purposes.

Equipment

AED ■ two prepackaged, unopened AED electrodes ■ gloves ■ Optional: clippers.

Implementation

■ Perform hand hygiene.[3,4,5]

■ Put on gloves and follow standard precautions throughout the procedure.[6]

■ After discovering that your patient is unresponsive to your questions and apneic or only gasping, start CPR and follow BLS and ACLS protocols.[1] Ask a colleague to activate the emergency response system, bring the AED into the patient's room, and set it up as described below before the code team arrives.

■ Turn on the AED and follow the visual or audible prompts.

■ Open the foil packets containing the two electrode pads.

■ Expose the patient's chest. Remove the plastic backing film from the pads, and place one electrode pad on the right side of the patient's bare, dry chest just below the clavicle. Place the second electrode pad on the left side of the patient's bare, dry chest to the left of the heart's apex.[1] Depending on the manufacturer, images showing proper placement are located on the anterior surface of the pads. Avoid placing the pads over any implanted devices or medication patches.[1]

■ Attach one electrode pad to each electrode cable (if not already attached), and then connect the cable to the AED.

■ Ask everyone to stand clear, and press the ANALYZE button when the machine prompts you to. Be careful not to touch or move the patient while the AED is in analysis mode. (If you get the message "Check electrodes," make sure the electrodes are correctly placed and the patient cable is securely attached; then press the ANALYZE button again.)

■ In 15 to 30 seconds, the AED will analyze the patient's rhythm. If the patient needs a shock, the AED will prompt a "Stand clear" message and emit a beep that changes into a steady tone as it's charging.

■ When the AED is fully charged, it will prompt you to press the SHOCK button. (Some fully automatic AED models automatically deliver a shock within 15 seconds after analyzing the patient's rhythm. If a shock isn't needed, the AED will prompt "No shock indicated" and advise you to "Check patient.")

■ Make sure no one is touching the patient or his bed, and call out "Stand clear." Then press the shock button on the AED.

■ After the shock is delivered, resume CPR for 2 minutes. Don't delay compressions to recheck rhythm or pulse. After five cycles of CPR, the AED should analyze the rhythm again and deliver another shock, if indicated.[1]

■ If a nonshockable rhythm is detected, the AED will instruct you to check the patient. If unable to defect a pulse, resume CPR.

■ After the code, remove and transcribe the AED's computer memory module or tape, or prompt the AED to print a rhythm strip with code data. Follow facility policy for analyzing and storing code data.

■ Remove and discard your gloves and perform hand hygiene.[3,4,5]

■ Document the procedure.[7]

Special considerations

■ AEDs vary from one manufacturer to the next, so familiarize yourself with your facility's equipment.

■ AED operation should be checked according to your facility's policy.

■ Acceptable alternative electrode placement includes biaxillary positioning, with pads placed on the right and left lateral chest walls, or placement of one pad in the standard apical position, with the other pad on the right or left upper back.[1]

■ Excessive chest hair can interfere with optimal pad adhesion and may need to be removed. Use clippers to remove the hair or rapidly remove an adhesive AED pad and apply a new one.[1]

Complications

Defibrillation can cause accidental electric shock to those providing care.

Documentation

Document the following: the patient's name, age, medical history, and chief complaint; the time you found the patient in cardiac arrest; when you started CPR; when you applied the AED; how many shocks the patient received; if the patient regained a pulse at any point; what postarrest care was provided; and physical assessments findings.

REFERENCES

1 American Heart Association. (2010). 2010 American Heart Association guidelines for cardiopulmonary resuscitation and emergency cardiovascular care, *Circulation, 122*(3 Suppl.), S706–719. (Level I)

2 Lynn-McHale Wiegand, D. (Ed.). (2011). *AACN procedure manual for critical care* (6th ed.). Philadelphia, PA: Saunders.

3 World Health Organization. (2009). *WHO guidelines on hand hygiene in health care: First global patient safety challenge. Clean care is safer care.* Geneva, Switzerland: World Health Organization. (Level I)

4 The Joint Commission. (2012). Standard NPSG.07.01.01. *Comprehensive accreditation manual for hospitals: The official handbook.* Oakbrook Terrace, IL: The Joint Commission. (Level I)

5 Centers for Disease Control and Prevention. (October 2002). Guideline for hand hygiene in health-care settings. *Morbidity and Mortality Weekly Report, 51* (RR-16), 1–45. (Level I)

6 Siegel, J.D., et al. "2007 Guideline for isolation precautions: Preventing transmission of infectious agents in healthcare settings" [Online]. Accessed June 2011 via the Web at http://www.cdc.gov/hicpac/2007ip/2007isolationprecautions.html

7 The Joint Commission. (2012). Standard RC.01.03.01. *Comprehensive accreditation manual for hospitals: The official handbook.* Oakbrook Terrace, IL: The Joint Commission. (Level I)

ADDITIONAL REFERENCES

Nettina, S.M. (2010). *Lippincott manual of nursing practice* (9th ed.). Philadelphia, PA: Lippincott Williams & Wilkins.

Rhee, J.E., et al. (2009). Is there any room for shortening hands-off time further when using an AED? *Resuscitation, 80*(2), 231–237.

Yamamoto, T., et al. (2008). Inappropriate analyses of automated external defibrillators used during in-hospital ventricular fibrillation. *Circulation Journal, 72*(4), 679–681.

BACK CARE

Regular bathing and massage of the neck, back, buttocks, and upper arms promotes patient relaxation and allows assessment of the patient's skin condition. Particularly important for the bedridden patient, massage causes cutaneous vasodilation, helping to prevent pressure ulcers from prolonged pressure on bony prominences or perspiration. Gentle back massage can be performed after myocardial infarction but may be contraindicated in patients with rib fractures, surgical incisions, or other recent traumatic injury to the back.

Equipment

Basin ▪ skin cleaner ▪ bath blanket ▪ bath towel ▪ washcloth ▪ back lotion with lanolin base ▪ gloves, if the patient has open lesions or has been incontinent.

Preparation of equipment

Fill the basin two-thirds full with warm water.

Implementation

▪ Gather the equipment at the patient's bedside.
▪ Perform hand hygiene and put on gloves, as needed.[1,2,3]
▪ Confirm the patient's identity using at least two patient identifiers according to your facility's policy.[4]
▪ Explain the procedure to the patient and provide privacy.[5] Ask him to tell you if you're applying too much or too little pressure.
▪ Adjust the bed to a comfortable working height and lower the head of the bed, if allowed.
▪ Place the patient in the prone position, if possible, or on his side. Position him along the edge of the bed nearest you *to prevent back strain*.
▪ Untie the patient's gown, and expose his back, shoulders, and buttocks. Then drape the patient with a bath blanket *to prevent chills and minimize exposure.* Place a bath towel next to or under the patient's side *to protect bed linens from moisture*.
▪ Fold the washcloth around your hand to form a mitt *to prevent the loose ends of the cloth from dripping water onto the patient and to keep the cloth warm longer.* (See *Making a washcloth mitt*.) Then apply skin cleaner.
▪ Using long, firm strokes, bathe the patient's back, beginning at the neck and shoulders and moving downward to the buttocks. Rinse and dry well *because moisture trapped between the buttocks can cause chafing and predispose the patient to formation of pressure ulcers.* While giving back care, closely examine the patient's skin, especially the bony prominences of the shoulders, the scapulae, and the coccyx, for redness or abrasions.
▪ Pour a small amount of lotion into your palm. Rub your hands together *to warm and distribute the lotion.* Then apply the lotion

to the patient's back, using long, firm strokes. *The lotion reduces friction, making back massage easier.*
▪ Massage the patient's back, beginning at the base of the spine and moving upward to the shoulders. For a relaxing effect, massage slowly; for a stimulating effect, massage quickly. Alternate the three basic strokes: effleurage, friction, and petrissage, (See *How to give a back massage*, page 50.) Add lotion, as needed, keeping one hand on the patient's back *to avoid interrupting the massage*.
▪ Compress, squeeze, and lift the trapezius muscle *to help relax the patient*.
▪ Finish the massage by using long, firm strokes, and blot any excess lotion from the patient's back with a towel. Then, retie the patient's gown and straighten or change the bed linens as necessary.
▪ Return the bed to its original position, and make the patient comfortable. Empty and clean the basin. Dispose of gloves, if used, and return equipment to the appropriate storage area.
▪ Perform hand hygiene.[1,2,3]
▪ Document the procedure.[6]

Special considerations

▪ Before giving back care, assess the patient's body structure and skin condition, and tailor the duration and intensity of the massage accordingly. If you're giving back care at bedtime, have the patient ready for bed beforehand, *so the massage can help him fall asleep*.
▪ Use separate lotion for each patient *to prevent cross-contamination.* If the patient has oily skin, substitute a lotion of the patient's choice.
▪ When massaging the patient's back, stand with one foot slightly forward and your knees slightly bent *to allow effective use of your arm and shoulder muscles*.
▪ Don't massage the patient's legs unless ordered *because reddened legs can signal clot formation, and massage can dislodge the clot, causing an embolus.* Develop a turning schedule and give back care at each position change.

Documentation

Document back care in the patient's medical record. Record redness, abrasion, or change in skin condition in your notes.

REFERENCES

1 Centers for Disease Control and Prevention. (October 2002). Guideline for hand hygiene in health-care settings. *Morbidity and Mortality Weekly Report, 51* (RR-16), 1–45. (Level I)
2 The Joint Commission. (2012). Standard NPSG.07.01.01. *Comprehensive accreditation manual for hospitals: The official handbook.* Oakbrook Terrace, IL: The Joint Commission. (Level I)
3 World Health Organization. (2009). *WHO guidelines on hand hygiene in health care: First global patient safety challenge. Clean care is safer care.* Geneva, Switzerland: World Health Organization. (Level I)
4 The Joint Commission. (2012). Standard NPSG.01.01.01. *Comprehensive accreditation manual for hospitals: The official handbook.* Oakbrook Terrace, IL: The Joint Commission. (Level I)

Making a washcloth mitt

To make a washcloth mitt, take a clean, dry washcloth and fold it in thirds lengthwise around your hand. Fold the top of the washcloth down and tuck it into the bottom of the mitt.

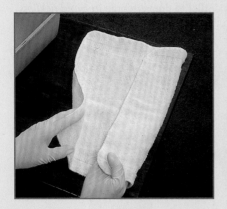 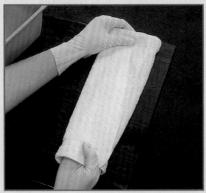 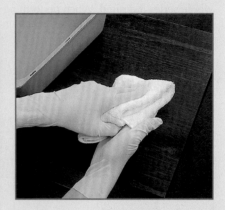

5   The American Hospital Association. (2003). *The patient care partnership: Understanding expectation, rights, and responsibilities.* Chicago, IL: American Hospital Association.
6   The Joint Commission. (2012). Standard RC.01.03.01. *Comprehensive accreditation manual for hospitals: The official handbook.* Oakbrook Terrace, IL: The Joint Commission. (Level I)

ADDITIONAL REFERENCES

Billhult, A., et al. (2007). Massage relieves nausea in women with breast cancer who are undergoing chemotherapy. *Journal of Alternative and Complementary Medicine, 13*(1), 53–57.
Garner, B., et al. (2008). Pilot study evaluating the effect of massage therapy on stress, anxiety and aggression in a young adult psychiatric inpatient unit. *Australian and New Zealand Journal of Psychiatry, 42*(5), 414–422.

BALLOON VALVULOPLASTY CARE

Although the treatment of choice for valvular heart disease is surgery, balloon valvuloplasty is an alternative to valve replacement in patients with critical stenoses. This technique enlarges the orifice of a heart valve that has been narrowed by a congenital defect, calcification, rheumatic fever, or aging. It evolved from percutaneous transluminal coronary angioplasty and uses the same balloon-tipped catheters for dilatation.

Balloon valvuloplasty was first performed successfully on pediatric patients, then on elderly patients who had stenotic valves complicated by other medical problems such as chronic obstructive pulmonary disease. It's indicated for patients who face a high risk from surgery and for those who refuse surgery. In addition, balloon valvuloplasty has proved to be more tolerable than surgery for older patients.

This procedure is performed in the cardiac catheterization laboratory under local anesthesia. The doctor inserts a balloon-tipped catheter through the patient's femoral vein or artery, threads it into the heart, and repeatedly inflates it against the leaflets of the diseased valve. This process increases the size of the orifice, improving valvular function and helping prevent complications from decreased cardiac output. (See *How balloon valvuloplasty works,* page 51.) Studies have shown that balloon valvuloplasty can provide excellent results for many years.[1,2]

Equipment
Before and during balloon valvuloplasty
Antiseptic solution ▪ local anesthetic ▪ valvuloplasty or balloon-tipped catheter ▪ IV solution and tubing ▪ electrocardiogram (ECG) monitor and electrodes ▪ oxygen and oxygen delivery device ▪ sterile label ▪ sterile marker ▪ sedative ▪ emergency medications ▪ scissors ▪ heparin for injection ▪ introducer kit for balloon catheter ▪ sterile gown, gloves, mask, cap, and drapes ▪ Optional: nitroglycerin, pulmonary artery (PA) catheter.

Postprocedure balloon valvuloplasty
IV solution and tubing ▪ ECG monitor and electrodes ▪ pulmonary artery monitor, if necessary ▪ oxygen and oxygen delivery device ▪ emergency medications ▪ Doppler stethoscope ▪ programmable pumps with dosing limits.

Implementation
▪ Perform hand hygiene.[3,4,5]
▪ Confirm the patient's identity using at least two patient identifiers according to your facility's policy.[6]
▪ Reinforce the doctor's explanation of balloon valvuloplasty, including its risks and alternatives, to the patient and his family.
▪ Reassure the patient that although he'll be awake during the procedure, he'll receive a sedative and a local anesthetic beforehand.

How to give a back massage

Three strokes commonly used when giving a back massage are effleurage, friction, and petrissage. Start with effleurage, go on to friction, and then to petrissage. Perform each stroke at least six times before moving on to the next; then repeat the whole series if desired. When performing effleurage and friction, keep your hands parallel to the vertebrae *to avoid tickling the patient*. For all three strokes, maintain a regular rhythm and steady contact with the patient's back *to help him relax*.

Effleurage
Using your palm, stroke from the buttocks up to the shoulders, over the upper arms, and back to the buttocks. Use slightly less pressure on the downward strokes.

Friction
Use circular thumb strokes to move from buttocks to shoulders; then, using a smooth stroke, return to the buttocks, as shown below.

Petrissage
Using your thumb to oppose your fingers, knead and stroke half the back and upper arms, starting at the buttocks and moving toward the shoulder. Then knead and stroke the other half of the back, rhythmically alternating your hands.

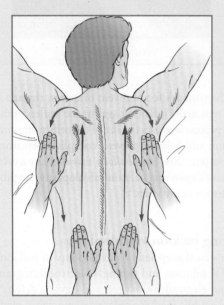
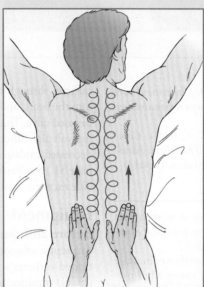
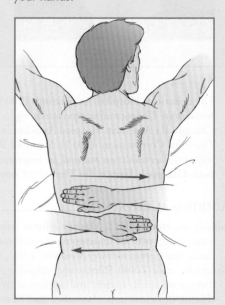

■ Teach the patient what to expect. For example, inform him that the hair in his groin area will be clipped and the skin cleaned with an antiseptic; he'll feel a brief, stinging sensation when the local anesthetic is injected; and he may feel pressure as the catheter moves along the vessel. Describe the warm, flushed feeling he's likely to experience from injection of the contrast medium.

■ Tell the patient that the procedure may last up to 4 hours and that he may feel discomfort from lying on a hard table for that long.

Before balloon valvuloplasty

■ Make sure that the patient isn't allergic to shellfish, iodine, or contrast media.

■ Perform a preprocedure verification *to make sure that all relevant documentation, related information, and equipment are available and correctly identified to the patient's identifiers.*[7]

■ Verify that laboratory and imaging studies have been completed, as ordered, and that the results are in the patient's medical record;

notify the doctor of any unexpected results. Make sure that the results of blood typing and crossmatching are available.[7]

■ Make sure that informed consent has been obtained and is documented in the patient's medical record.[8]

■ Hold food and fluids (except for medications) for at least 6 hours before balloon valvuloplasty, or as ordered (usually after midnight the night before the procedure).

■ Perform hand hygiene and put on gloves.[3,4,5]

■ Insert an IV catheter *to provide access for medications.* (See "IV catheter insertion and removal," page 421.)

■ Obtain baseline vital signs and peripheral pulses in all extremities.

■ Clip hair from insertion sites; then clean the sites with antiseptic solution.

■ Have the patient void.

■ Administer a sedative, as ordered, following safe medication administration practices.

■ Upon arrival at the cardiac catheterization laboratory, apply ECG electrodes and ensure IV catheter patency.

How balloon valvuloplasty works

In balloon valvuloplasty, the doctor inserts a balloon-tipped catheter through the femoral vein or artery and threads it into the heart. After locating the stenotic valve, he inflates the balloon, increasing the size of the valve opening.

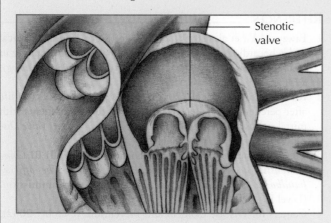

Stenotic valve

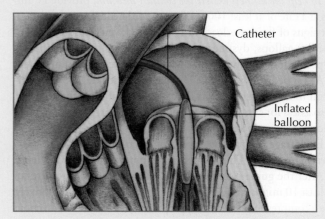

Catheter

Inflated balloon

■ Remove and discard your gloves and perform hand hygiene.[3,4,5]
■ Document the procedure.[9]

During balloon valvuloplasty

■ Administer oxygen via nasal cannula.
■ The doctor will put on a sterile gown, gloves, a mask, and a cap and open the sterile supplies.[10] A member of the team labels all medications, medication containers, and other solutions on and off the sterile field.[11] Assist as necessary.
■ The team conducts a time-out before starting the procedure *to perform a final assessment that the correct patient, site, positioning, and procedure are identified and, as applicable, that all relevant information and equipment are available.*[12]
■ The doctor uses maximal barrier precautions and prepares and anesthetizes the catheter insertion site (usually at the femoral artery). He may insert a PA catheter if one isn't already in place.
■ The doctor then inserts a large guide catheter into the site and threads a valvuloplasty or balloon-tipped catheter up into the heart.
■ The doctor injects a contrast medium *to visualize the heart valves and assess the stenosis.* He also injects heparin *to prevent the catheter from clotting.*
■ Using low pressure, the doctor inflates the balloon on the valvuloplasty catheter for a short time, usually 15 to 30 seconds, gradually increasing the time and pressure. If the stenosis isn't reduced, a larger balloon may be used.
■ After completion of valvuloplasty, a series of angiograms is taken *to evaluate the effectiveness of the treatment.* Assist as necessary.
■ The doctor then sutures the guide catheter in place. He'll typically remove it within 4 hours.
■ Remove and discard personal protective equipment and perform hand hygiene.[3,4,5]
■ Document the procedure.[9]

After balloon valvuloplasty

■ Perform hand hygiene and put on gloves.[3,4,5]
■ Upon receiving the patient on the unit, confirm his identity using at least two patient identifiers according to your facility's policy.[6]
■ When the patient returns to the unit, he may be receiving IV heparin or nitroglycerin; administer them using programmable pumps with dosing limits *to prevent life-threatening dosing errors.* Perform an independent double-check of the medications *to make sure that the medications correspond to the patient's diagnosis, the correct formulations are hanging, dosage calculations are correct, the pumps are set to the proper settings, and the tubings are attached to the proper ports.* The patient may also have a compression device at the insertion site *to prevent hematoma formation.*
■ Monitor ECG rhythm, arterial pressure, and pulmonary artery pressure as appropriate.
■ Assess the insertion site frequently for signs of hemorrhage *because exsanguination can occur rapidly.*
■ *To prevent excessive hip flexion and migration of the catheter,* keep the affected leg straight and elevate the head of the bed no more than 15 degrees. If necessary, place a sheet both over and under the unaffected extremity, then tuck in on both sides to serve as a reminder to keep the leg straight.
■ Monitor vital signs every 15 minutes for the first hour, every 30 minutes for the next 2 hours, and then hourly for the next 4 hours, or according to your facility's policy. If vital signs are unstable, notify the doctor and continue to monitor them every 5 minutes.
■ When you obtain vital signs, assess peripheral pulses distal to the catheter insertion site as well as the color, sensation, temperature, and capillary refill time of the affected extremity. Compare findings bilaterally.
■ Assess the catheter site for hematoma, ecchymosis, and hemorrhage. If hematoma expands, mark the site and alert the doctor.

■ Assess the patient's respiratory status; *changes in rate and pattern can be the first sign of a complication, such as embolism.*

■ Auscultate regularly for murmurs, which may indicate worsening valvular insufficiency. Notify the doctor if you detect a new or worsening murmur.

■ *To help the kidneys excrete the contrast medium,* provide IV fluids at a rate of at least 100 mL/hour as ordered. Assess the patient for signs of fluid overload: distended neck veins, atrial and ventricular gallops, dyspnea, pulmonary congestion, tachycardia, hypertension, and hypoxemia. Monitor intake and output closely.

■ Assess pedal pulses with a Doppler stethoscope. They'll be difficult to detect, especially if the catheter sheath remains in place. Also assess for complications: embolism, hemorrhage, chest pain, and cardiac tamponade.

■ Encourage the patient to perform deep-breathing exercises *to prevent atelectasis.* This is especially important in elderly patients.

■ After the guide catheter is removed, apply direct pressure for at least 10 minutes and monitor the site frequently. Alternatively, use a compression device, as appropriate. (See "Arterial and venous sheath removal," page 27.)

■ Remove and discard your gloves and perform hand hygiene.[3,4,5]

■ Document the procedure.[9]

Special considerations

■ Assess the patient's vital signs continually during the procedure, especially if it's an aortic valvuloplasty. During balloon inflation, the aortic outflow tract is completely obstructed, causing blood pressure to fall dangerously low. Ventricular ectopy is also common during balloon positioning and inflation. Start treatment for ectopy when signs and symptoms develop or when ventricular tachycardia is sustained.

■ Carefully assess the patient's respiratory status; *changes in rate and pattern can be the first sign of a complication such as embolism.*

■ Using heparin and a large-bore catheter can lead to arterial hemorrhage. This complication can be reversed with protamine sulfate when the sheath is removed, or the sheath can be left in place and removed 6 to 8 hours after the heparin is discontinued.

■ If the patient is receiving heparin, maintain the infusion according to your facility's policy. Monitor partial thromboplastin time according to your facility's policy.

■ Chest pain can result from obstruction of blood flow during aortic valvuloplasty; assess for signs and symptoms of myocardial ischemia. Also be alert for signs of cardiac tamponade (decreased or absent peripheral pulses, pale or cyanotic skin, hypotension, and paradoxical pulse), which requires emergency surgery.

Complications

Severe complications, such as myocardial infarction or calcium emboli (embolization of debris released from the calcified valve), are rare. Other complications include bleeding or hematoma at the insertion site, arrhythmias, circulatory disorders distal to the insertion site, guide wire perforation of the ventricle leading to tamponade, disruption of the valve ring, restenosis of the valve, and valvular insufficiency, which can contribute to heart failure and reduced cardiac output. Infection and an allergic reaction to the contrast medium can also occur.

Documentation

Document vital signs, your assessments, diagnostic test results, any complications and interventions, and the patient's tolerance of the procedure. Document patient teaching and the patient's understanding of your teaching.

REFERENCES

1 Fawzy, M.E., et al. (2009). Long-term (up to 18 years) clinical and echocardiographic results of mitral balloon valvuloplasty in 531 consecutive patients and predictors of outcome. *Cardiology, 113*(3), 213–221. (Level VI)

2 Krittayaphong, R., et al. (2007). Improvement in quality of life after percutaneous balloon mitral valvulotomy in patients with mitral stenosis: Does rhythm matter? *Journal of Heart Valve Disease, 16*(1), 13–18. (Level VI)

3 The Joint Commission. (2012). Standard NPSG.07.01.01 *Comprehensive accreditation manual for hospitals: The official handbook.* Oakbrook Terrace, IL: The Joint Commission. (Level I)

4 Centers for Disease Control and Prevention. (October 2002). Guideline for hand hygiene in health-care settings. *Morbidity and Mortality Weekly Report, 51* (RR-16), 1–45. (Level I)

5 World Health Organization. (2009). *WHO guidelines on hand hygiene in health care: First global patient safety challenge. Clean care is safer care.* Geneva, Switzerland: World Health Organization. (Level I)

6 The Joint Commission. (2012). Standard NPSG.01.01.01. *Comprehensive accreditation manual for hospitals: The official handbook.* Oakbrook Terrace, IL: The Joint Commission. (Level I)

7 The Joint Commission. (2012). Standard UP.01.01.01. *Comprehensive accreditation manual for hospitals: The official handbook.* Oakbrook Terrace, IL: The Joint Commission. (Level I)

8 The Joint Commission. (2012). Standard RI.01.03.01. *Comprehensive accreditation manual for hospitals: The official handbook.* Oakbrook Terrace, IL: The Joint Commission. (Level I)

9 The Joint Commission. (2012). Standard RC.01.03.01. *Comprehensive accreditation manual for hospitals: The official handbook.* Oakbrook Terrace, IL: The Joint Commission. (Level I)

10 The Joint Commission. (2012). Standard NPSG.07.05.01. *Comprehensive accreditation manual for hospitals: The official handbook.* Oakbrook Terrace, IL: The Joint Commission. (Level I)

11 The Joint Commission. (2012). Standard NPSG.03.04.01. *Comprehensive accreditation manual for hospitals: The official handbook.* Oakbrook Terrace, IL: The Joint Commission. (Level I)

12 The Joint Commission. (2012). Standard UP.01.03.01. *Comprehensive accreditation manual for hospitals: The official handbook.* Oakbrook Terrace, IL: The Joint Commission. (Level I)

ADDITIONAL REFERENCES

Bonow, R.O., et al. (2008). 2008 focused update incorporated into the ACC/AHA 2006 guidelines for the management of patients with valvular heart disease: A report of the American College of Cardiology/American Heart Association Task Force on practice guidelines (writing committee to revise the 1998 guidelines for the management of patients with valvular heart disease): Endorsed by the Society of Cardiovascular Anesthesiologists, Society for Cardiovascular Angiography and Interventions, and Society of Thoracic Surgeons. *Circulation, 118*(15), e523–e661.

Centers for Medicare & Medicaid Services, Department of Health and Human Services. (2006). "Conditions of Participation: Patients' Rights" 42 CFR part 482.13 [Online]. Accessed November 2011 via the Web at https://www.cms.gov/CFCsAndCoPs/downloads/finalpatientrightsrule.pdf

Maluenda, G., et al. (2009). The clinical significance of hematocrit values before and after percutaneous coronary intervention. *American Heart Journal, 158*(6).

Rolley, J.X., et al. (2009). Review of nursing care for patients undergoing percutaneous coronary intervention: A patient journey approach. *Journal of Clinical Nursing, 18*(17), 2, 394–405.

Siegel, J.D., et al. "2007 guideline for isolation precautions: Preventing transmission of infectious agents in healthcare settings" [Online]. Accessed June 2011 via the Web at http://www.cdc.gov/hicpac/2007ip/2007isolationprecautions.html

Zibaeenezhad, M.J., & Mazloum, Y. (2009). Heparin infusion after successful percutaneous coronary intervention: A prospective, randomized trial. *Acta Cardiologica, 64*(1):65–70.

BARIATRIC BED USE

Obesity affects nearly one-third of all Americans. A patient is considered obese if his body mass index (BMI) is 30 kg/m² or greater. Typical hospital beds are designed to hold patients weighing up to 450 lb and who don't have a wide abdominal girth. Bariatric beds are a recent addition to hospital equipment that are designed to accommodate these larger patients. Various bariatric beds are available, ranging from those that are simply a larger version of a standard bed to low-air-loss mattresses that provides pressure relief (as shown below).

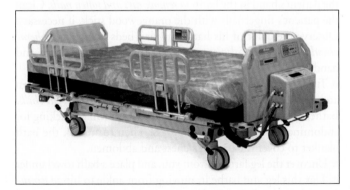

Bariatric beds provide more comfort for obese patients than standard-size beds. They help preserve self-esteem by providing these patients with a bed that easily fits their larger body size as well as special side rails that help them turn and reposition themselves. Bariatric beds allow caregivers to perform such routine care as boosting, turning, and transferring in and out of bed with greater ease and less risk of injury. Most bariatric beds have a built-in scale that allows the nurse to more easily weigh the patient. Some bariatric beds also convert to a cardiac chair.

Equipment

Bariatric bed ▪ Optional: overhead trapeze, special sheets.

Preparation of equipment

Obtain the bariatric bed from central supply or contact the company representative to have the bed delivered, according to facility protocol. Prepare the bed according to the manufacturer's guidelines. A company representative may be involved in the patient assessment to ensure that the appropriate type and size of bed are provided. Choose the appropriate type of mattress to meet your patient's needs. Specialized sheets may be necessary. Attach an overhead trapeze, if indicated.

Implementation

▪ Verify the doctor's order for a bariatric bed.
▪ Perform hand hygiene.[1,2,3]
▪ Confirm the patient's identity using at least two patient identifiers according to your facility's policy.[4]
▪ Discuss the need for a specialized bed with the patient *so that he understands its benefits and therapeutic effects.*
▪ Consult with other health care team members, such as the doctor, surgical team, physical therapy, occupational therapy, wound care specialist, and respiratory therapy, *to choose the appropriate type of bed for the patient's needs.*
▪ If the bed is rented, ask the company representative for an in-service appointment so that all health care team members understand the bed's use and provide safe care.
▪ Ensure that written instructions come with the bed, and keep them at the bedside.
▪ Provide the patient with product information, and orient him to the bed functions and controls *so that the he understands its many features and safe use.*
▪ Perform hand hygiene.[1,2,3]
▪ Document the procedure.[5]

Special considerations

▪ Provide for other bariatric equipment, such as hospital gowns, commodes, wheelchairs, lifts, scales, and stretchers *for patient comfort and safety.*
▪ When sending the patient to other departments, call first to be sure they can accommodate a larger bed and are familiar with its use.

Documentation

Document the type of bed and indicate that the patient was oriented to the safe use of the bed and that he gave a return demonstration. Note if written information was given to the patient or left at the bedside. Record other equipment provided, such as an overhead trapeze or special sheets. Note the type of mattress on the bed. Document the patient's skin condition when placed on the bed. Record the patient's response to the bed.

REFERENCES

1 Centers for Disease Control and Prevention. (October 2002). Guideline for hand hygiene in health-care settings. *Morbidity and Mortality Weekly Report, 51* (RR-16), 1–45. (Level I)
2 The Joint Commission. (2012). Standard NPSG.07.01.01. *Comprehensive accreditation manual for hospitals: The official handbook.* Oakbrook Terrace, IL: The Joint Commission. (Level I)

3 World Health Organization. (2009). *WHO guidelines on hand hygiene in health care: First global patient safety challenge. Clean care is safer care.* Geneva, Switzerland: World Health Organization. (Level I)

4 The Joint Commission. (2012). Standard NPSG.01.01.01. *Comprehensive accreditation manual for hospitals: The official handbook.* Oakbrook Terrace, IL: The Joint Commission. (Level I)

5 The Joint Commission. (2012). Standard RC.01.03.01. *Comprehensive accreditation manual for hospitals: The official handbook.* Oakbrook Terrace, IL: The Joint Commission. (Level I)

ADDITIONAL REFERENCE

National Institutes of Health; National Heart, Lung, and Blood Institute. (1998). *Clinical guidelines of the identification, evaluation, and treatment of overweight and obesity in adults: The evidence report.* Bethesda, MD: U.S. Department of Health and Human Services.

BED BATH

A complete bed bath cleans the skin, stimulates circulation, provides mild exercise, and promotes comfort. Bathing also allows assessment of skin condition, joint mobility, and muscle strength. Depending on the patient's overall condition and duration of hospitalization, he may have a complete or partial bath daily. A partial bath, including hands, face, axillae, back, genitalia, and anal region, can replace the complete bath for the patient with dry, fragile skin or extreme weakness and can supplement the complete bath for the diaphoretic or incontinent patient.

Equipment

Bath basin ▪ bath blanket ▪ skin cleaner ▪ towel ▪ washcloth ▪ skin lotion ▪ orangewood stick ▪ gloves ▪ deodorant ▪ hospital-grade disinfectant ▪ Optional: chlorhexidine-impregnated cloth, bath oil, perineal pad, abdominal (ABD) pad, and linen-saver pad.

Preparation of equipment

Adjust the temperature of the patient's room, and close any doors or windows *to prevent drafts and provide privacy.* Determine the patient's preference for skin cleaner or other hygiene aids *because some patients are allergic to soap or prefer bath oil or lotions.* Gather the equipment on an overbed table or bedside stand.

Implementation

▪ Confirm the patient's identity using at least two patient identifiers according to your facility's policy.[1]
▪ Perform hand hygiene.[2,3,4]
▪ Tell the patient you'll be giving him a bath, and provide privacy. Offer him a bedpan or urinal. Position the patient supine if possible. If the patient's condition permits, encourage him to assist with bathing *to provide exercise and promote independence.*
▪ Fill the bath basin two-thirds full of warm water (about 115° F [46° C]), and bring it to the patient's bedside. If a bath thermometer isn't available, test the water temperature carefully *to avoid scalding or chilling the patient;* the water should feel comfortably warm.
▪ Raise the patient's bed to a comfortable working height *to avoid back strain.*
▪ If the bed will be changed after the bath, remove the top linen. If not, fanfold it to the foot of the bed.
▪ Cover the patient with a bath blanket *to provide warmth and privacy.*
▪ Put on gloves.
▪ Remove the patient's gown and other articles, such as elastic stockings, elastic bandages, and restraints (as ordered).
▪ Place a towel under the patient's chin. To wash his face, begin with the eyes, working from the inner to the outer canthus without soap. Use a separate section of the washcloth for each eye *to avoid spreading ocular infection.*
▪ If the patient tolerates skin cleaner, apply it to the cloth and wash the rest of his face, ears, and neck, using firm, gentle strokes. Rinse thoroughly *because residual soap can cause itching and dryness.* Then dry the area thoroughly, taking special care in skin folds and creases. Observe the skin for irritation, scaling, or other abnormalities.
▪ Turn down the bath blanket, and drape the patient's chest with a bath towel. While washing, rinsing, and drying the chest and axillae, observe the patient's respirations. Wash skin folds under the female patient's breasts by lifting each breast. Use firm strokes *to avoid tickling the patient.* If the patient tolerates deodorant, apply it.
▪ Place a bath towel beneath the patient's arm farthest from you. Then bathe his arm, using long, smooth strokes and moving from wrist to shoulder *to stimulate venous circulation.* If possible, soak the patient's hand in the basin *to remove dirt and soften nails.* Clean the patient's fingernails with the orangewood stick, if necessary. Observe the color of his hand and nail beds *to assess peripheral circulation.* Follow the same procedure for the other arm and hand.
▪ Turn down the bath blanket to expose the patient's abdomen and groin, keeping a bath towel across his chest *to prevent chills.* Bathe, rinse, and dry the abdomen and groin while checking for abdominal distention or tenderness. Then turn back the bath blanket to cover the patient's chest and abdomen.
▪ Uncover the leg farthest from you, and place a bath towel under it. Flex this leg and bathe it, moving from ankle to hip *to stimulate venous circulation.* Don't massage the leg, however, *to avoid dislodging any existing thrombus, possibly causing a pulmonary embolus.* Rinse and dry the leg.
▪ If possible, place a basin on the patient's bed, flex the leg at the knee, and place the foot in the basin. Soak the foot, and then wash and rinse it thoroughly. Remove the foot from the basin, dry it, and clean the toenails. Observe skin condition and color during cleaning *to assess peripheral circulation.* Repeat the procedure for the other leg and foot.
▪ Cover the patient with the bath blanket *to prevent chilling.* Then lower the bed and raise the side rails *to ensure patient safety while you change the bath water.*
▪ Remove your gloves and perform hand hygiene, and put on new gloves.[2,3,4]

■ When you return, roll the patient on his side or stomach, place a towel beneath him, and cover him *to prevent chilling.* Bathe, rinse, and dry his back and buttocks.

■ Massage the patient's back with lotion. Check for redness, abrasions, and pressure ulcers. Avoid massaging over red areas.

■ Bathe the anal area from front to back *to avoid contaminating the perineum.* Rinse and dry the area well.

■ After lowering the bed and raising the side rails *to ensure the patient's safety,* change the bath water again. Remove your gloves, perform hand hygiene, and put on new gloves.[2,3,4] Then turn the patient on his back and bathe the genital area thoroughly but gently, using a different section of the washcloth for each downward stroke. Bathe from front to back, avoiding the anal area. Rinse thoroughly and pat dry.

■ If applicable, perform indwelling urinary catheter care. Apply perineal pads or scrotal supports as needed.

■ Dress the patient in a clean gown, and reapply any elastic bandages, elastic stockings, or restraints removed before the bath.

■ Empty, clean, and disinfect the basin.

■ Remake the bed or change the linens, and remove the bath blanket.

■ Place a bath towel beneath the patient's head *to catch loose hair,* and then brush and comb his hair.

■ Return the bed to its original position and make the patient comfortable.

■ Carry soiled linens to the hamper with outstretched arms. *To avoid spreading microorganisms,* don't let soiled linens touch your clothing.

■ Remove and discard your gloves.

■ Perform hand hygiene.[2,3,4]

■ Document the procedure.[5]

Special considerations

■ In areas in your facility where central line–associated bloodstream infection rates are higher than desired, bathe patients daily who are older than 2 months of age with a chlorhexidine-impregnated cloth according to the manufacturer's guidelines *to reduce the risk of central line–associated bloodstream infections.*[6,7,8,9]

■ Fold the washcloth around your hand to form a mitt while bathing the patient. *This technique keeps the cloth warm longer and avoids dribbling water on the patient from the cloth's loose ends.* Change the water as often as necessary *to keep it warm and clean.*

■ Carefully dry creased skin-fold areas—for example, under breasts, in the groin area, and between fingers, toes, and buttocks. Dust these areas lightly with powder after drying *to reduce friction.* Use powder sparingly *to avoid caking and irritation and to avoid provoking coughing in patients with respiratory disorders.*

■ If the patient has very dry skin, use bath oil instead of skin cleaner. No rinsing is necessary. Warm the lotion before using it for back massage *because cold lotion can startle the patient and induce muscle tension and vasoconstriction.* (See "Back care," page 48.)

■ A bag bath involves the use of 8 to 10 premoistened, warmed, disposable cloths contained in a plastic bag or prepackaged pouch.

The cloths contain a no-rinse surfactant. Before use, the cloths are warmed in a microwave or a special warming unit supplied by the manufacturer. A separate cloth is used to wash each part of the body. *A bag bath saves time compared with the conventional bed bath because no rinsing is required.*

■ *To improve circulation, maintain joint mobility, and preserve muscle tone,* move the body joints through their full range of motion during the bath.

■ If the patient is incontinent, loosely tuck an ABD pad between his buttocks and place a linen-saver pad under him *to absorb fecal drainage.* Together, these pads help prevent skin irritation and reduce the number of linen changes.

Documentation

Record the date and time of the bed bath in the flowchart. Note the patient's tolerance for the bath, his range of motion, and his self-care abilities, and report any unusual findings.

REFERENCES

1 The Joint Commission. (2012). Standard NPSG.01.01.01. *Comprehensive accreditation manual for hospitals: The official handbook.* Oakbrook Terrace, IL: The Joint Commission. (Level I)

2 The Joint Commission. (2012). Standard NPSG.07.01.01. *Comprehensive accreditation manual for hospitals: The official handbook.* Oakbrook Terrace, IL: The Joint Commission. (Level I)

3 World Health Organization. (2009). *WHO guidelines on hand hygiene in health care: First global patient safety challenge. Clean care is safer care.* Geneva, Switzerland: World Health Organization. (Level I)

4 Centers for Disease Control and Prevention. (October 2002). Guideline for hand hygiene in health-care settings. *Morbidity and Mortality Weekly Report, 51* (RR-16), 1–45. (Level I)

5 The Joint Commission. (2012). Standard RC. 01.03.01. *Comprehensive accreditation manual for hospitals: The official handbook.* Oakbrook Terrace, IL: The Joint Commission. (Level I)

6 Dixon, J., & Carver, R. (2010). Daily chlorhexidine gluconate bathing with impregnated cloths results in statistically significant reduction in central line–associated bloodstream infections. *American Journal of Infection Control, 38*(10), 817–821.

7 Evans, H., et al. (2010). Effect of chlorhexidine whole-body bathing on hospital-acquired infections among trauma patients. *Archives of Surgery, 145*(3), 240–246.

8 Marschall, J., et al. (2008). Strategies to prevent central line-associated bloodstream infections in acute care hospitals. *Infection Control and Hospital Epidemiology, 29*(S1), S22–S30. (Level I)

9 Bleasdale, S. C., et al. (2007). Effectiveness of chlorhexidine bathing to reduce catheter-associated bloodstream infections in medical intensive care unit patients. *Archives of Internal Medicine, 167*(19). 2073–2079.

ADDITIONAL REFERENCE

Craven, R.F., & Hirnle, C.J. (2009). *Fundamentals of nursing: Human health and function* (6th ed.). Philadelphia, PA: Lippincott Williams & Wilkins.

BED EQUIPMENT, SUPPLEMENTAL

Certain equipment can promote the bedridden patient's comfort and help prevent pressure ulcers and other complications of immobility. A wood or hard plastic footboard helps prevent foot-drop by maintaining proper alignment. It also raises bed linens off of the patient's feet. The foot cradle, a horizontal or arched bar over the end of the bed, keeps bed linens off of the patient's feet, preventing skin irritation and breakdown, especially in patients with peripheral vascular disease or neuropathy. A bed board, made of wood or wood covered with canvas, firms the mattress and is especially useful for the patient with spinal injuries. The metal basic frame and the metal trapeze (a triangular piece attached to this frame) allow the patient with arm mobility and strength to lift himself off the bed, facilitating bed making and bedpan positioning. The metal overbed cradle, a cagelike frame positioned on top of the mattress, keeps bed linens off of the patient with burns, open wounds, or a wet cast.

A vinyl water mattress used to prevent or treat pressure ulcers exerts less pressure on the skin than the standard hospital mattress. An alternating pressure pad (a vinyl pad divided into chambers filled with air or water and attached to an electric pump) serves the same purpose, but it also stimulates circulation by alternately inflating and deflating its chambers.

The reusable water mattress replaces the standard hospital mattress and rests on a sheet of heavy cardboard placed over the bedsprings; the smaller, less bulky disposable mattress rests on top of the standard hospital mattress. All supplemental bed equipment is optional, depending on the patient's needs. Reusable and disposable water mattresses are also available. (See *Types of supplemental bed equipment.*)

Equipment

Footboard and cover ▪ drawsheet ▪ bath blanket ▪ foot cradle ▪ bed board ▪ basic frame with trapeze ▪ overbed cradle ▪ roller gauze ▪ water mattress ▪ stretcher ▪ alternating pressure pad ▪ pump and tubing ▪ footstool ▪ linen-saver pad ▪ safety pins ▪ sandbag, bath blanket, or pillow, if necessary.

The exact equipment needed depends on what supplemental bed equipment is being added to the patient's bed.

Preparation of equipment

If you're preparing a footboard for use, place a cover over it *to provide padding.* Or pad it with a folded drawsheet or bath blanket: Bring the top and side edges of the sheet or blanket to the back of the footboard, miter the corners, and secure them at the center with safety pins. *Padding cushions the patient's feet against pressure from the hard footboard, helping to prevent skin irritation and breakdown.* Avoid wrinkles *to prevent skin irritation.* For a portable water mattress, check with the maintenance department before transferring the mattress *because its weight may rule out use on some electric beds.*

Implementation

▪ Perform hand hygiene.[1,2,3]

▪ Confirm the patient's identity using at least two patient identifiers according to your facility's policy.[4]
▪ Tell the patient what you're going to do and describe the equipment.

Using a footboard

▪ Move the patient up in bed *to allow room for the footboard.* Loosen the top linens at the foot of the bed, and then fold them back over the patient *to expose his feet.*
▪ Lift the mattress at the foot of the bed and place the lip of the footboard between the mattress and the bedsprings. Or secure the footboard under both sides of the mattress.
▪ Adjust the footboard so that the patient's feet rest comfortably against it. If the footboard isn't adjustable, tuck a folded bath blanket between the board and the patient's feet.
▪ Unless the footboard has side supports, place a sandbag, a folded bath blanket, or a pillow alongside each foot *to maintain 90-degree foot alignment.*
▪ Fold the top linens over the footboard, tuck them under the mattress, and miter the corners.

Using a foot cradle

▪ Move the patient up in bed *to allow room for the foot cradle.* Loosen the top linens at the foot of the bed and fold them over the patient or to one side.
▪ When using a one-piece cradle, place one side arm under the mattress, carefully extend the arch over the bed, and place the other side arm under the mattress on the opposite side.
▪ Adjust the tension rods *so that they rest securely over the edge of the mattress.*
▪ When using a sectional cradle with two side arms, first place the side arms under the mattress. Secure the tension rods over the edge of the mattress. Then carefully place the arch over the bed and connect it to the side arms. When using a sectional cradle with one side arm, connect the side arm and horizontal cradle bar before placement. Then place the side arm under the mattress on one side of the bed.
▪ Cover the cradle with the top linens, tuck them under the mattress at the foot of the bed, and miter the corners.

Using a bed board

▪ Transfer the patient from his bed to a stretcher or a chair. Obtain assistance if necessary.
▪ Strip the linens from the bed. If you plan to reuse them, fold each piece neatly and hang it over the back of a chair. Otherwise, place soiled linens in a laundry bag.
▪ If the bed board consists of wooden slats encased in canvas, lift the mattress at the head of the bed and center the board over the bedsprings *to prevent it from jutting out and causing accidental injury.* Unroll the slats to cover the bedsprings at the head of the bed. Then lift the mattress at the foot of the bed and unroll the remaining slats.
▪ If the bed board consists of one solid or two hinged pieces of wood, lift the mattress on one side of the bed and center the board over the bedsprings.
▪ After positioning the bed board, replace the linens. Then return the patient to bed.

EQUIPMENT

Types of supplemental bed equipment

Adjustable footboard

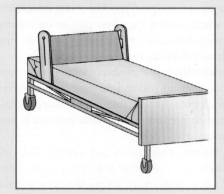

Sectional cradle with one side arm

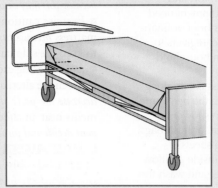

Overbed cradle

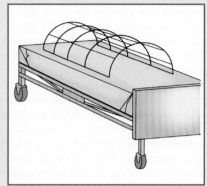

Alternating pressure mattress

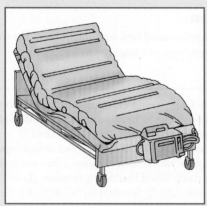

Trapeze and basic frame

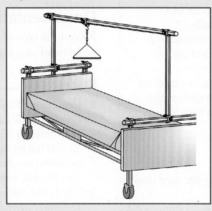

Alternating pressure pad

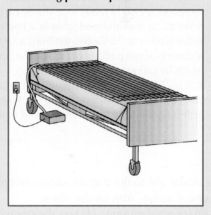

Using a basic frame with trapeze
■ If an orthopedic technician isn't available to secure the frame and trapeze to the patient's bed, get assistance to attach these devices to the bed, as necessary. Be sure to hang the trapeze within the patient's easy reach *so he won't need to strain to reach it.*

Using an overbed cradle
■ Loosen and remove the top linens.
■ Carefully lower the cradle onto the patient's bed and secure it in place.
■ Wrap roller gauze around both sides of the cradle. Then pull the gauze taut and attach it to the bedsprings.
■ Cover the cradle with the top linens, tuck them under the mattress at the foot of the bed, and miter the corners.

Using a portable water mattress
■ Ensure that the patient isn't prone to motion sickness *because the movement of the water in the mattress may cause nausea.*
■ Obtain several coworkers to help transfer the mattress from the stretcher to the patient's bed *because the mattress is heavy and bulky.*

■ Position the mattress on the bed and place the protective cover over it. Then place a bottom sheet over the cover and tuck it in loosely.
■ Place a sheepskin, linen-saver pad, or drawsheet over the bottom sheet, as needed. Adding these items doesn't decrease the effectiveness of this mattress.
■ Position the patient comfortably on the mattress. Then cover him with the top linens and tuck them in loosely.
■ Check the water mattress daily *to ensure adequate flotation.* To do so, place your hand under the patient's thighs. If you can feel the bottom of the mattress, arrange to have water added.

Using an alternating pressure pad
■ If possible, transfer the patient from his bed to a chair or stretcher. Get help, if necessary.
■ Strip the linens from the bed.
■ Inspect the plug and electrical cord of the alternating pressure pad for defects. Don't use the unit if it appears damaged.
■ Unfold the pad on top of the mattress with the appropriate side facing up.
■ Place the motor on a linen-saver pad on the floor or on a footstool near the mattress outlets. Connect the tubing securely to

PATIENT TEACHING

Helping patients improvise assistive devices at home

Assistive devices can increase patient comfort and improve care given in the home. This equipment need not be expensive. If the patient's illness is brief or financial constraints exist, teach patients and caregivers to improvise assistive devices with common household items. For example:

■ Side rails can be made by placing kitchen chairs along the sides of a bed and securing their legs to the bed frame.

■ Linen-saver pads can be fashioned from shower curtains, plastic tablecloths, a plastic raincoat, or trash bags.

■ Absorbent pads can be made by placing sheets of newspaper and a bottom layer of plastic inside a pillowcase. When damp, discard the newspaper and wash the pillowcase.

■ An ironing board, a wooden crate with two sides removed, a child's table, or a sturdy cardboard box can serve as an over-the-bed table or a bed cradle.

■ Backrests can be fashioned from a large item such as a cutting board padded on top and supported underneath by pillows.

■ A pull rope to assist the patient in turning or sitting up can be made by braiding nylon stockings together and fastening the rope to the side or end of the bed.

the motor and to the mattress outlets and plug the cord into an electrical outlet. Turn on the motor.

■ After several minutes, observe the emptying and filling of the pad's chambers, and check the tubing for kinks *because they could interfere with the pad's function.*

■ Place a bottom sheet over the pad and tuck it in loosely. *To avoid tube constriction,* don't miter the corner where the tubing is attached.

■ Position the patient comfortably on the pad, cover him with the top linens, and tuck them in loosely.

■ If the pad becomes soiled, clean it with a damp cloth and mild soap, and then dry it well. *To avoid damaging the pad's surface,* don't use alcohol.

■ When the patient no longer needs the pad or is discharged, turn off the motor, disconnect the tubing, and unplug the cord from the wall outlet. Remove the pad from the patient's bed, and fold and discard it. Or, if applicable, give the pad to the patient to take home. Inform him that the motor needed to power the pad can usually be rented from a surgical supply store. Explain to the patient or a caregiver how to operate the pad at home. (See *Helping patients improvise assistive devices at home.*)

■ Coil the tubing and electrical cord, and then strap them to the motor. Return the motor unit to the central supply department.

Completing the procedure

■ Perform hand hygiene.[1,2,3]

■ Document the procedure.[5]

Special considerations

■ Place the patient in bed before positioning and securing an overbed or foot cradle *to ensure its proper placement and to prevent patient injury.* Similarly, remove the cradle before the patient gets out of bed. When turning or positioning the patient on his side, make sure the foot cradle's tension rod doesn't rest against his skin *because this may cause pressure and predispose him to skin breakdown.*

■ Exercise caution when turning the obese patient on a water mattress *because turning displaces a large volume of water.* Be sure to keep the side rails raised during turning *to prevent falls.*

■ Avoid placing excessive layers of drawsheets or linen-saver pads between the alternating pressure pad and the patient *because these decrease the pad's effectiveness.* Avoid using pins or sharp instruments near an alternating pressure pad or water mattress *to prevent accidental puncture.*

NURSING ALERT Because a plastic-covered mattress slides off a bed board easily, *make sure a coworker is standing on the opposite side of the bed when you're transferring the patient from stretcher to bed.*

Documentation

Record the type of supplemental bed equipment used, the time and date of use, and the patient's response to treatment.

REFERENCES

1 Centers for Disease Control and Prevention. (October 2002). Guideline for hand hygiene in health-care settings. *Morbidity and Mortality Weekly Report, 51* (RR-16), 1–45. (Level I)

2 World Health Organization. (2009). *WHO guidelines on hand hygiene in health care: First global patient safety challenge. Clean care is safer care.* Geneva, Switzerland: World Health Organization. (Level I)

3 The Joint Commission. (2012). Standard NPSG.07.01.01. *Comprehensive accreditation manual for hospitals: The official handbook.* Oakbrook Terrace, IL: The Joint Commission. (Level I)

4 The Joint Commission. (2012). Standard NPSG.01.01.01. *Comprehensive accreditation manual for hospitals: The official handbook.* Oakbrook Terrace, IL: The Joint Commission. (Level I)

5 The Joint Commission. (2012). Standard RC.01.03.01. *Comprehensive accreditation manual for hospitals: The official handbook.* Oakbrook Terrace, IL: The Joint Commission. (Level I)

ADDITIONAL REFERENCES

Craven, R.F., & Hirnle, C.J. (2009). *Fundamentals of nursing: Human health and function* (6th ed.). Philadelphia, PA: Lippincott Williams & Wilkins.

Taylor, C., et al. (2011). *Fundamentals of nursing: The art and science of nursing care* (7th ed.). Philadelphia, PA: Lippincott Williams & Wilkins.

BEDMAKING, OCCUPIED

For a bedridden patient, linen changes promote comfort and help prevent skin breakdown and health care–acquired infection. Such changes require the use of side rails to prevent the patient from rolling out of bed and, depending on the patient's condition, the use of a turning sheet to move him from side to side.

Making a traction bed

For a patient in traction, obtain help from a coworker to make the bed. Work from head to toe *to minimize the risk for traction misalignment.*

Preparation
■ Perform hand hygiene.[1,2,3] Put on gloves, if necessary. Bring clean linens and arrange them in the order of use on the bedside stand or a chair.
■ Explain the procedure, provide privacy, and remove unnecessary furniture.

Changing the linens
■ Lower both side rails. Stand near the headboard, opposite your coworker.
■ Gently pull the mattress to the head of the bed. Avoid sudden movements; *they can misalign traction and cause patient discomfort.*
■ Remove the pillow from the bed. Loosen the bottom linens and roll them from the headboard toward the patient's head. Then remove the soiled pillowcase and replace it with a clean one.
■ Fold a clean bottom sheet crosswise and place the sheet across the head of the bed. Tell the patient to raise her head and upper shoulders by grasping the trapeze above the bed (as shown below). With your coworker, quickly fanfold the bottom sheet from the head of the bed under the patient's shoulders so that it meets the soiled linen. Tuck at least 12" (30.5 cm) of the bottom sheet under the head of the mattress. Miter the corners and tuck in the sides.
■ Tell the patient to raise her buttocks by grasping the trapeze. As a team, move toward the foot of the bed and, in one movement, quickly and carefully roll soiled linens and clean linens under the patient.
■ Instruct the patient to release the trapeze and to rest. Place a pillow under her head for comfort.
■ If allowed, remove any pillows from under the patient's extremity. If pillow removal is contraindicated, continue to move linens toward the foot of the bed and under the patient's legs and traction while your coworker lifts the pillows and supports the patient's extremity.
■ Put soiled linens in a laundry bag or pillowcase.
■ Tuck the remaining loose linens securely under the mattress. *To ensure a tight-fitting bottom sheet,* have the patient

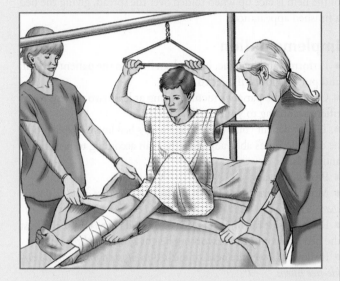

raise herself off the bed by simultaneously grasping the trapeze and raising her buttocks while you pull the sheet tight. As needed, place a drawsheet or linen-saver pad under her. Complete the bed making alone.
■ If the bottom sheet doesn't cover the foot of the mattress, cover it with a drawsheet. Miter its corners and tuck in the sides.
■ Replace the pillows under the patient's extremity, and then cover her with a clean top sheet. Fold over the top hem of the sheet approximately 8" (20.5 cm). If one or both legs are in traction, fit the lower end of the sheet loosely over the traction apparatus; don't press on the traction ropes. To secure the sheet, tuck in the corner opposite the traction under the foot of the bed and miter the corner. Neatly tuck in the lower corner of the sheet on the traction side *to expose the leg and foot.*
■ If the traction equipment exposes the patient's sides, cover her with a drawsheet—not a full sheet or spread.
■ Lower the bed, but don't allow the traction weights to touch the floor. Raise the side rails *to prevent falls.* If allowed, leave one side rail down *so the patient can reach the bedside stand.*
■ Remove and discard your gloves, if applicable, and perform hand hygiene.[1,2,3]

Making an occupied bed may require more than one person. It also entails loosening the bottom sheet on one side and fanfolding it to the center of the mattress instead of loosening the bottom sheet on both sides and removing it, as in an unoccupied bed. Also, the foundation of the bed must be made before the top sheet is applied instead of both the foundation and top being made on one side before being completed on the other side. (See *Making a traction bed.*)

Equipment

Two sheets (one fitted, if available) ■ pillowcase ■ one or two drawsheets ■ spread ■ one or two bath blankets ■ gloves ■ comfort-enhancing device, as needed ■ Optional: laundry bag, linen-saver pad.

Preparation of equipment

Obtain clean linen, which should be folded in half lengthwise and then folded again. If the linen is folded incorrectly, refold it. The bottom sheet should be folded so the rough side of the hem is facedown when placed on the bed; *this helps prevent skin irritation caused by the rough hem edge rubbing against the patient's heels.* The top sheet should be folded similarly, so that the smooth side of the hem is face up when folded over the spread, giving the bed a finished appearance.

Implementation

■ Perform hand hygiene, bring clean linen to the patient's room, and put on gloves, if needed.[1,2,3]

■ Confirm the patient's identity using at least two patient identifiers according to your facility's policy.[4]

■ Tell the patient you will be changing his bed linens. Explain how he can help if he's able, adjusting the plan according to his abilities and needs.

■ Provide privacy.

■ Move any furniture away from the bed *to ensure ample working space.*

■ Raise the side rail on the far side of the bed *to prevent falls.* Adjust the bed to a comfortable working height *to prevent back strain.*

■ If allowed, lower the head of the bed *to ensure tight-fitting, wrinkle-free linens.*

■ When stripping the bed, watch for belongings among the linens.

■ Cover the patient with a bath blanket *to avoid exposure and provide warmth and privacy.*

■ Fanfold the top sheet and spread from beneath the bath blanket, and bring them back over the blanket.

■ Loosen the top linens at the foot of the bed and remove them separately. If reusing the top linens, fold each piece and hang each piece over the back of the chair. Otherwise, place each piece in the laundry bag. *To avoid dispersing microorganisms,* don't fan the linens, hold them against your clothing, or place them on the floor.

■ If the mattress slid down when the head of the bed was raised, pull it up again. *Adjusting the mattress after the bed is made loosens the linens.* If the patient is able, ask him to grasp the head of the bed and pull with you; otherwise, ask a coworker to help you.

■ Roll the patient to the far side of the bed, and turn the pillow lengthwise under his head *to support his neck.* Ask him to help (if he can) by grasping the far side rail as he turns *so that he's positioned at the far side of the bed.*

■ Loosen the soiled bottom linens on the side of the bed nearest you. Then roll the linens toward the patient's back in the middle of the bed (as shown below).

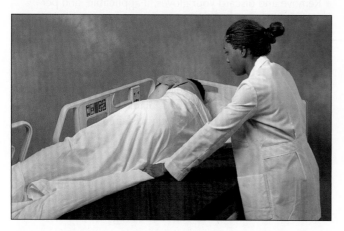

■ Place a clean bottom sheet on the bed, with its center fold in the middle of the mattress. For a fitted sheet, secure the top and bottom corners over the side of the mattress nearest you. For a flat sheet, place its end even with the foot of the mattress. Miter the top corner as you would for an unoccupied bed *to keep linens firmly tucked under the mattress, preventing wrinkling.*

■ Fanfold the remaining clean bottom sheet toward the patient, and place the drawsheet, if needed, about 15″ (38 cm) from the top of the bed, with its center fold in the middle of the mattress. Tuck in the entire edge of the drawsheet on the side nearest you. Fanfold the remaining drawsheet toward the patient (as shown below).

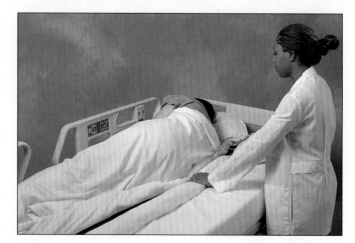

■ If necessary, position a linen-saver pad on the drawsheet *to absorb excretions or surgical drainage,* and fanfold it toward the patient.

■ Raise the other side rail, and roll the patient to the clean side of the bed.

■ Move to the unfinished side of the bed and lower the side rail nearest you. Then loosen and remove the soiled bottom linens separately and place them in the laundry bag.

■ Pull the clean bottom sheet taut. Secure the fitted sheet or place the end of a flat sheet even with the foot of the bed, and miter the top corner. Pull the drawsheet taut and tuck it in. Unfold and smooth the linen-saver pad, if used.

■ Assist the patient to the supine position if his condition permits.

■ Remove the soiled pillowcase, and place it in the laundry bag. Then slip the pillow into a clean pillowcase, tucking its corners well into the case *to ensure a smooth fit.* Place the pillow beneath the patient's head, with its seam toward the top of the bed *to prevent it from rubbing against the patient's neck, causing irritation.* Place the pillow's open edge away from the door *to give the bed a finished appearance.*

■ Unfold the clean top sheet over the patient with the rough side of the hem facing away from the bed *to avoid irritating the patient's skin.* Allow enough sheet to form a cuff over the spread.

■ Remove the bath blanket from beneath the sheet, and center the spread over the top sheet.

■ Tuck the top sheet and spread under the foot of the bed, and miter the bottom corners. Fold the top sheet over the spread *to give the bed a finished appearance.*

■ Make a 3″ (7.6-cm) toe pleat, or vertical tuck, in the top linens *to allow room for the patient's feet and prevent pressure that can cause discomfort, skin breakdown, and footdrop.*

■ Raise the head of the bed to a comfortable position, make sure both side rails are raised, and then lower the bed and lock its wheels *to ensure the patient's safety.* Assess the patient's body alignment.

■ Place the call button within the patient's easy reach. Remove the laundry bag from the room.

■ Remove and discard your gloves, if applicable, and perform hand hygiene *to prevent the spread of health care–acquired infections.*[1,2,3]

Special considerations

■ Use a fitted sheet, when available, *because a flat sheet slips out from under the mattress easily, especially if the mattress is plastic-coated.*

■ Prevent the patient from sliding down in bed by tucking a tightly rolled pillow under the top linens at the foot of the bed.

■ For the diaphoretic or bedridden patient, fold a bath blanket in half lengthwise and place it between the bottom sheet and the plastic mattress cover; *the blanket acts as a cushion and helps absorb moisture. To help prevent sheet burns on the heels and bony prominences,* center a bath blanket or sheepskin over the bottom sheet and tuck the blanket under the mattress.

■ If the patient can't help you move or turn him, devise a turning sheet *to facilitate bed making and repositioning.* To do this, first fold a drawsheet or bath blanket and place it under the patient's buttocks. Make sure the sheet extends from the shoulders to the knees *so that it supports most of the patient's weight.* Roll the sides of the sheet to form handles. Next, ask a coworker to help you lift and move the patient. With one person holding each side of the sheet, you can move the patient without wrinkling the bottom linens. If you can't get help and must turn the patient yourself, stand at the side of the bed. Turn the patient toward the rail and, if he's able, ask him to grasp the opposite rolled edge of the turning sheet. Pull the rolled edge carefully toward you and turn the patient.

Documentation

Although linen changes aren't usually documented, record their dates and times in your notes for patients with incontinence, excessive wound drainage, pressure ulcers, or diaphoresis.

REFERENCES

1 World Health Organization. (2009). *WHO guidelines on hand hygiene in health care: First global patient safety challenge. Clean care is safer care.* Geneva, Switzerland: World Health Organization. (Level I)

2 Centers for Disease Control and Prevention. (October 2002). Guideline for hand hygiene in health-care settings. *Morbidity and Mortality Weekly Report, 51* (RR-16), 1–45. (Level I)

3 The Joint Commission. (2012). Standard NPSG.07.01.01. *Comprehensive accreditation manual for hospitals: The official handbook.* Oakbrook Terrace, IL: The Joint Commission. (Level I)

4 The Joint Commission. (2012). Standard NPSG. 01.01.01. *Comprehensive accreditation manual for hospitals: The official handbook.* Oakbrook Terrace, IL: The Joint Commission. (Level I)

ADDITIONAL REFERENCES

Craven, R.F., & Hirnle, C.J. (2009). *Fundamentals of nursing: Human health and function* (6th ed.). Philadelphia, PA: Lippincott Williams & Wilkins.

Taylor, C., et al. (2011). *Fundamentals of nursing: The art and science of nursing care* (7th ed.). Philadelphia, PA: Lippincott Williams & Wilkins.

BEDMAKING, UNOCCUPIED

Although considered routine, daily changing and periodic straightening of bed linens promotes patient comfort and prevents skin breakdown. When preceded by hand hygiene, performed using clean technique, and followed by proper handling and disposal of soiled linens, this procedure helps control health care–acquired infections.

Equipment

Two sheets (one fitted, if available) ■ pillowcase ■ bedspread ■ gloves ■ Optional: bath blanket, laundry bag, linen-saver pads, drawsheet.

Preparation of equipment

Obtain clean linen, which should be folded in half lengthwise and then folded again. If the linen is folded incorrectly, refold it. The bottom sheet should be folded so the rough side of the hem is facedown when placed on the bed; *this helps prevent skin irritation caused by the rough hem edge rubbing against the patient's heels.* The top sheet should be folded similarly, so that the smooth side of the hem is face up when folded over the spread, giving the bed a finished appearance.

Implementation

■ Perform hand hygiene, bring clean linen to the bedside, and put on gloves, if needed.[1,2,3]

■ Confirm the patient's identity using at least two patient identifiers according to your facility's policy.[4]

■ Tell the patient that you're going to change his bed. Help him to a chair if necessary.

■ Move any furniture away from the bed *to provide ample working space.*

■ Lower the head of the bed and side rails *to make the mattress level and ensure tight-fitting, wrinkle-free linens.* Then, raise the bed to a comfortable working height *to prevent back strain.*

■ When stripping the bed, watch for any belongings that may have fallen among the linens.

■ Remove the pillowcase and place it in the laundry bag or in the middle of the bed. Set the pillow aside.

■ Lift the mattress edge slightly and work around the bed, untucking the linens. If you plan to reuse the top linens, fold the top hem of the spread down to the bottom hem. Then pick up the hemmed corners, fold the spread into quarters, and hang it over the back of the chair. Do the same for the top sheet. Otherwise, carefully remove and place the top linens in the laundry bag or pillowcase. *To avoid spreading microorganisms,* don't fan the linens; hold them against your clothing, or place them on the floor.

■ Remove the soiled bottom linens and place them in the laundry bag.

■ If the mattress has slid downward, push it to the head of the bed. *Adjusting it after bed making loosens the linens.*

■ Place the bottom sheet with its center fold in the middle of the mattress.

■ For a fitted sheet, secure the top and bottom corners over the mattress corners on the side of the bed nearest you. For a flat sheet, align the end of the sheet with the foot of the mattress and miter the top corner *to keep the sheet firmly tucked under the mattress.* To miter the corner, first tuck the top end of the sheet evenly under the mattress at the head of the bed. Then lift the side edge of the sheet about 12″ (30.5 cm) from the mattress corner and hold it at a right angle to the mattress. Tuck in the bottom edge of the sheet hanging below the mattress. Finally, drop the top edge and tuck it under the mattress. (See *Making a mitered corner.*)

■ After tucking under one side of the bottom sheet, place the drawsheet or linen-saver pad (if either are needed) about 15″ (38 cm) from the top of the bed, with its center fold in the middle of the bed. Then tuck in the entire edge of the drawsheet on that side of the bed.

■ Place the top sheet with its center fold in the middle of the bed and its wide hem even with the top of the bed. Position the rough side of the hem face up *so that the smooth side shows after folding.* Allow enough sheet at the top of the bed to form a cuff over the spread.

■ Place the spread over the top sheet, with its center fold in the middle of the bed. (If the patient will be returning from surgery, use the alternative technique. [See *Making a surgical bed,* page 64.])

■ Make a 3″ (7.6-cm) toe pleat, or vertical tuck, in the top linens *to allow room for the patient's feet and to prevent pressure that can cause discomfort, skin breakdown, and footdrop.*

■ Tuck the top sheet and spread under the foot of the mattress. Then miter the bottom corners.

■ Move to the opposite side of the bed and repeat the procedure.

■ After fitting all corners of the bottom sheet or tucking them under the mattress, pull the sheet at an angle from the head toward the foot of the bed. *Doing so tightens the linens, making the bottom sheet taut and wrinkle-free and promoting patient comfort.*

■ Fold the top sheet over the spread at the head of the bed *to form a cuff and to give the bed a finished appearance.* When making an open bed, fanfold the top linens to the foot of the bed. If a linen-saver pad is needed, place it on top of the bottom sheets.

■ Slip the pillow into a clean case, tucking in the corners. Then place the pillow with its seam toward the top of the bed *to prevent it from rubbing against the patient's neck, causing irritation,*

and its open edge facing away from the door *to give the bed a finished appearance.*

■ Lower the bed and lock its wheels *to ensure the patient's safety.*

■ Return furniture to its proper place, and place the call button within the patient's easy reach. Carry away soiled linens in outstretched arms *to avoid contaminating your uniform.*

■ After disposing of the linens, remove your gloves (if used) and perform hand hygiene *to prevent the spread of microorganisms.*[1,2,3]

Special considerations

■ Because a hospital mattress is usually covered with plastic *to protect it and to facilitate cleaning between patients,* a flat-bottom sheet tends to loosen and become untucked. Use a fitted sheet, if available, to prevent this.

■ If a fitted sheet isn't available, the top corners of a flat sheet may be tied together under the top of the mattress *to prevent the sheet from becoming dislodged.*

■ A bath blanket placed on top of the mattress, under the bottom sheet, helps to absorb moisture and prevent dislodgment of the bottom sheet.

Documentation

Although linen changes aren't usually documented, record their dates and times in your notes for patients with incontinence, excessive wound drainage, or diaphoresis.

REFERENCES

1 World Health Organization. (2009). *WHO guidelines on hand hygiene in health care: First global patient safety challenge. Clean care is safer care.* Geneva, Switzerland: World Health Organization. (Level I)

2 Centers for Disease Control and Prevention. (October 2002). Guideline for hand hygiene in health-care settings. *Morbidity and Mortality Weekly Report, 51* (RR-16), 1–45. (Level I)

3 The Joint Commission. (2012). Standard NPSG.07.01.01. *Comprehensive accreditation manual for hospitals: The official handbook.* Oakbrook Terrace, IL: The Joint Commission. (Level I)

4 The Joint Commission. (2012). Standard NPSG.01.01.01. *Comprehensive accreditation manual for hospitals: The official handbook.* Oakbrook Terrace, IL: The Joint Commission. (Level I)

ADDITIONAL REFERENCES

Craven, R.F., & Hirnle, C.J. (2009). *Fundamentals of nursing: Human health and function* (6th ed.). Philadelphia, PA: Lippincott Williams & Wilkins.

Taylor, C., et al. (2011). *Fundamentals of nursing: The art and science of nursing care* (7th ed.). Philadelphia, PA: Lippincott Williams & Wilkins.

BEDPAN AND URINAL USE

Bedpans and urinals permit elimination by a bedridden patient and accurate observation and measurement of urine and stool by the nurse. A bedpan is used by a female patient for defecation and urination and by a male patient for defecation; a urinal is used by a male patient for urination. Either device should be offered frequently, before meals, visiting hours, morning and

Making a mitered corner

■ To make a mitered corner, after placing the sheet on the bed, grasp the side edge of the sheet and lift it up to form a triangle.

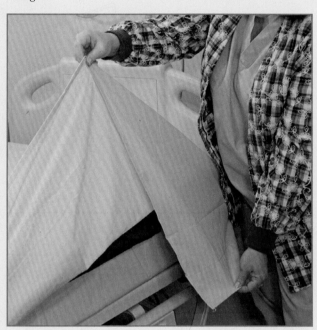

■ Then, place the sheet on the top of the bed, making a flat triangular fold.

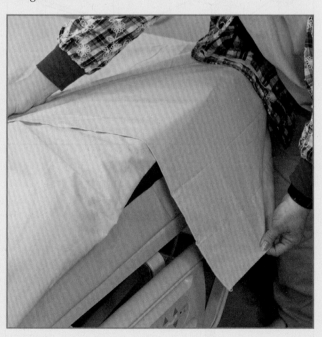

■ While holding the point of the triangle on the bed, tuck the sheet under the mattress.

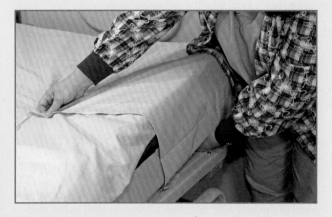

■ Take the triangular fold from the mattress and place it over the side of the mattress.

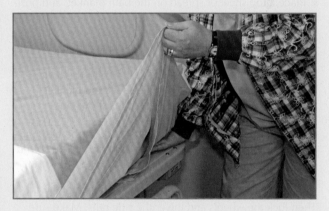

■ Tuck the remaining end of the triangular linen fold under the mattress.

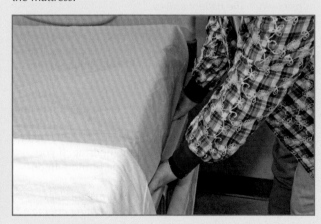

Making a surgical bed

Preparation of a surgical bed permits easy patient transfer from surgery and promotes cleanliness and comfort. To make such a bed, take the following steps:

■ Perform hand hygiene, bring clean linen to the bedside, and put on gloves, if needed. [1,2,3]

■ Assemble linens as you would for making an unoccupied bed, including two clean sheets (one fitted, if available), a drawsheet, a bath blanket, a spread or sheet, a pillowcase, facial tissues, a trash bag, and linen-saver pads. Raise the bed to a comfortable working height *to prevent back strain.*

■ Slip the pillow into a clean pillowcase and place it on a nearby table or chair.

■ Make the foundation of the bed using the bottom sheet and drawsheet.

■ Place an open bath blanket about 15″ (38 cm) from the head of the bed with its center fold positioned in the middle of the bed. *The blanket warms the patient and counteracts the decreased body temperature caused by anesthesia.*

■ Place a top sheet or spread on the bath blanket, and position it as you did the blanket. Then fold the blanket and sheet back from the top so that the blanket shows over the sheet. Similarly, fold the sheet and blanket up from the bottom (as shown in illustration 1).

■ On the side of the bed where you'll receive the patient, fold up the two outer corners of the sheet and blanket so they meet in the middle of the bed (as shown in illustration 2).

■ Pick up the point hanging over this side of the bed and fanfold the linens back to the other side of the bed *so the linens won't interfere with patient transfer* (as shown in illustration 3).

■ Raise the bed to the high position if you haven't already. Then lock the wheels and lower the side rails. Make sure the side rails work properly. Move the bedside stand and other objects out of the stretcher's path *to facilitate easy transfer when the patient arrives.*

■ After the patient is transferred to the bed, position the pillow for his comfort and safety. Cover him by pulling the top point of the sheet and blanket over him and opening the folds. After covering the patient, tuck in the linens at the foot of the bed and miter the corners.

■ *To make the patient comfortable and to prevent unnecessary movement and linen changes,* try to anticipate and be ready for his special needs. For nausea, keep an emesis basin, facial tissues, and linen-saver pads at the bedside. Also, remove all liquids from the bedside. If you expect bleeding or discharge, place one or more linen-saver pads on the bed.

■ Keep extra pillows handy *to elevate arms and legs and to promote circulation, thereby preventing edema.* If necessary, have IV equipment, suction apparatus, a roller for patient transfer, or other special equipment ready.

1.

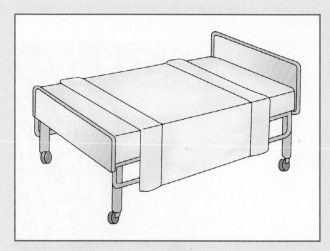

2.

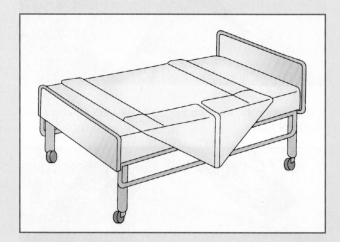

3.

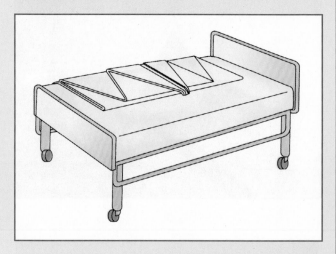

evening care, and any treatments or procedures. Whenever possible, allow the patient privacy.

Equipment

Bedpan, fracture pan, or urinal with cover ▪ toilet tissue ▪ two washcloths ▪ soap ▪ gloves ▪ towel ▪ linen-saver pad ▪ bath blanket ▪ pillow ▪ Optional: air freshener.

Available in adult and pediatric sizes, a bedpan may be disposable or reusable (the latter can be sterilized). The fracture pan, a type of bedpan, is used when spinal injuries, body or leg casts, or other conditions prohibit or restrict turning the patient. Like the bedpan, the urinal may be disposable or reusable.

Preparation of equipment

Obtain the appropriate bedpan or urinal. For a thin patient, place a linen-saver pad at the edge of the bedpan or use a fracture pan *to minimize pressure on the coccyx.*

Implementation

▪ Perform hand hygiene and put on gloves *to prevent contact with body fluids and comply with standard precautions.*[1,2,3]
▪ Confirm the patient's identity using at least two patient identifiers according to your facility's policy.[4]
▪ Provide privacy.
▪ Explain the procedure to the patient.

Placing a bedpan

▪ If allowed, elevate the head of the bed slightly *to prevent hyperextension of the spine when the patient raises the buttocks.*
▪ Rest the bedpan on the edge of the bed. Then, turn down the corner of the top linens and draw up the patient's gown. Ask him to raise his buttocks by flexing his knees and pushing down on his heels. While supporting the patient's lower back with one hand, center the curved, smooth edge of the bedpan beneath his buttocks.
▪ If the patient can't raise his buttocks, lower the head of the bed to horizontal and help the patient roll onto one side, with his buttocks toward you. Position the bedpan properly against his buttocks, and then help the patient roll back onto the bedpan. Once the patient is positioned comfortably, raise the head of the bed as indicated.
▪ After positioning the bedpan, elevate the head of the bed further to 30 degrees or higher, if allowed, until the patient is sitting erect. *This position, like the normal elimination posture, aids in defecation and urination.* (For information on another device that permits normal elimination posture, see *Using a commode.*)
▪ If elevation of the head of the bed is contraindicated, tuck a small pillow or folded bath blanket under the patient's back *to cushion his sacrum against the edge of the bedpan and support his lumbar region.*
▪ If the patient can be left alone, place the bed in a low position and raise the side rails *to ensure his safety.* Place toilet tissue and the call button within the patient's reach, and instruct him to push the button after elimination. If the patient is weak or disoriented, remain with him.

Using a commode

An alternative to a bedpan, a commode is a portable chair made of plastic or metal with a large opening in the center of the seat. It may have a bedpan or bucket that slides underneath the opening, or it may slide directly over the toilet, adding height to the standard toilet seat. Unlike a bedpan, a commode allows the patient to assume his normal elimination posture, which aids in defecation.

Before the patient uses it, inspect the commode's condition and make sure it is clean. Roll or carry the commode to the patient's room. Place it parallel and as close as possible to the patient's bed, and secure its brakes or wheel locks. If necessary, block its wheels with sandbags. Assist the patient onto the commode, provide toilet tissue, and place the call button within his reach. Instruct the patient to push the call button when he has finished.

If necessary, assist the patient with cleaning. Help him into bed and make him comfortable. Offer the patient soap, water, and a towel to wash his hands. Then close the lid of the commode or cover the bucket. Roll the commode or carry the bucket to the bathroom. If ordered, observe and measure the contents before disposal. Rinse and clean the bucket, and then spray or wipe the bucket and commode seat with disinfectant. Use an air freshener, if appropriate.

▪ Before removing the bedpan, lower the head of the bed slightly. Then ask the patient to raise his buttocks off the bed. Support his lower back with one hand, and gently remove the bedpan with the other *to avoid skin injury caused by friction.* If the patient can't raise his buttocks, ask him to roll to the opposite side so that his buttocks are toward you while you assist with one hand. Hold the pan firmly with the other hand to avoid spills. Cover the bedpan and place it on the chair.
▪ Help clean the anal and perineal area, as necessary, *to prevent irritation and infection.* Turn the patient on his side, wipe carefully with toilet tissue, clean the area with a damp washcloth and soap, and dry well with a towel. Clean a female patient from front to back *to avoid introducing rectal contaminants into the vaginal or urethral openings.*

Placing a urinal

▪ Lift the corner of the top linens, hand the urinal to the patient, and allow him to position it.
▪ If the patient can't position the urinal himself, spread his legs slightly and hold the urinal in place *to prevent spills.*
▪ After the patient voids, carefully withdraw the urinal and close the lid or cover it.

After use of a bedpan or urinal

■ Give the patient a clean, damp, warm washcloth for his hands. Check the bed linens for wetness or soiling, and straighten or change them, if needed. Make the patient comfortable. Place the bed in the low position and raise the side rails if appropriate.

■ Take the bedpan or urinal to the bathroom or utility room. Observe the color, odor, amount, and consistency of its contents. If ordered, measure urine output or liquid stool, or obtain a specimen for laboratory analysis.

■ Empty the bedpan or urinal into the toilet or designated waste area. Rinse with water and clean it thoroughly, using a disinfectant solution. Dry, cover, and return it to the patient's bedside stand.

■ Use an air freshener, if necessary, *to eliminate offensive odors and minimize embarrassment.*

■ Remove and discard your gloves and perform hand hygiene.[1,2,3]

■ Document the procedure.[5]

Special considerations

■ Explain to the patient that drug treatment and changes in his environment, diet, and activities may disrupt his usual elimination schedule. Try to anticipate elimination needs, and offer the bedpan or urinal frequently *to help reduce embarrassment and minimize the risk for incontinence.*

■ Avoid placing a bedpan or urinal on top of the bedside stand or overbed table *to avoid contamination of clean equipment and food trays.* Similarly, avoid placing it on the floor *to prevent the spread of microorganisms from the floor to the patient's bed linens when the device is used.*

■ If the patient feels pain during turning or feels uncomfortable on a standard bedpan, use a fracture pan. Unlike the standard bedpan, the fracture pan is slipped under the buttocks from the front rather than the side. Because it's shallower than the standard bedpan, you need only lift the patient slightly to position it. If the patient is obese or otherwise difficult to lift, ask a coworker to help you.

■ If the patient has an indwelling urinary catheter in place, carefully position and remove the bedpan *to avoid tension on the catheter, which could dislodge it or irritate the urethra.* After the patient defecates, wipe, clean, and dry the anal region, taking care to avoid catheter contamination. If necessary, clean the urinary meatus according to your facility's policy.

■ Avoid leaving the urinal, fracture pan, or bedpan in place for extended periods *to prevent skin breakdown.*

Documentation

Record the time, date, and type of elimination in the flowchart and the amount of urine output or liquid stool on the intake and output record, as needed. In your notes, document the amount, color, clarity, and odor of the urine or stool and the presence of blood, pus, or other abnormal characteristics in urine or stool. Document the condition of the perineum.

REFERENCES

1 World Health Organization. (2009). *WHO guidelines on hand hygiene in health care: First global patient safety challenge. Clean care is safer care.* Geneva, Switzerland: World Health Organization. (Level I)

2 Centers for Disease Control and Prevention. (October 2002). Guideline for hand hygiene in health-care settings. *Morbidity and Mortality Weekly Report, 51* (RR-16), 1–45. (Level I)

3 The Joint Commission. (2012). Standard NPSG.07.01.01. *Comprehensive accreditation manual for hospitals: The official handbook.* Oakbrook Terrace, IL: The Joint Commission. (Level I)

4 The Joint Commission. (2012). Standard NPSG.01.01.01. *Comprehensive accreditation manual for hospitals: The official handbook.* Oakbrook Terrace, IL: The Joint Commission. (Level I)

5 The Joint Commission. (2012). Standard RC.01.03.01. *Comprehensive accreditation manual for hospitals: The official handbook.* Oakbrook Terrace, IL: The Joint Commission. (Level I)

ADDITIONAL REFERENCE

Siegel, J.D., et al. "2007 guideline for isolation precautions: Preventing transmission of infectious agents in healthcare settings" [Online]. Accessed June 2011 via the Web at http://www.cdc.gov/hicpac/2007ip/2007isolationprecautions.html

BEDSIDE SPIROMETRY

Bedside spirometry measures forced vital capacity (FVC) and forced expiratory volume (FEV), allowing calculation of other pulmonary function indices, such as timed forced expiratory flow rate. Depending on the type of spirometer used, bedside spirometry can also allow direct measurement of vital capacity and tidal volume.

Bedside spirometry aids in diagnosing obstructive or restrictive pulmonary dysfunction, evaluating its severity, and determining the patient's response to therapy. It's also useful for evaluating preoperative anesthesia risk. Because the required breathing patterns can aggravate conditions such as bronchospasm, use of the bedside spirometer requires a review of the patient's history and close observation during testing.

Equipment

Spirometer ■ disposable mouthpiece ■ breathing tube, if required ■ spirographic chart and recording pen, if required ■ gloves ■ Optional: vital capacity predicted-values table, noseclips, bacteria filter if required by your facility's infection control policy.

Preparation of equipment

Review the manufacturer's instructions for assembly and use of the spirometer. If necessary, firmly insert the breathing tube *to ensure a tight connection.* If the tube comes preconnected, check the seals for tightness and the tubing for leaks. Check the operation of the recording mechanism, and insert a chart and pen, if necessary. Insert the disposable mouthpiece and make sure it's tightly sealed. Make sure that the unit has been calibrated according to the manufacturer's guidelines.

Implementation

■ Confirm the patient's identity using at least two patient identifiers according to your facility's policy.[1]

■ Explain the procedure to the patient. Emphasize that his cooperation is essential *to ensure accurate results.*

- Instruct the patient to remove or loosen bras, belts, and other constricting clothing *to prevent alteration of test results from restricted thoracic expansion and abdominal mobility.*
- Instruct the patient to void *to prevent abdominal discomfort.*
- Obtain the patient's weight and height without shoes. *These measurements are needed to calculate predicted lung volumes.*
- If the patient wears dentures that fit well, leave them in place *to promote a tight seal around the mouthpiece.* However, if the dentures fit poorly, have the patient remove them *to prevent incomplete closure of his mouth around the mouthpiece, which could allow air to leak around the mouthpiece.*
- Plug in the spirometer, and set the baseline time.
- Perform hand hygiene and put on gloves.[2,3,4]
- Make sure the patient is sitting straight in a chair or standing with his head slightly elevated.
- If desired, allow the patient to practice the required breathing technique with the breathing tube unhooked. After practice, replace the tube and check the seal.
- Tell the patient not to breathe through his nose. If the patient has difficulty complying, apply noseclips.[5]
- To measure vital capacity, instruct the patient to inhale as deeply as possible, and then insert the mouthpiece so that his lips are sealed tightly around it *to prevent air leakage and ensure an accurate digital readout or spirogram recording.*
- Tell him to exhale normally but completely and then remove the mouthpiece *to prevent recording his next inspiration.*
- Allow the patient to rest. Then repeat the procedure twice.
- To measure FEV and FVC, repeat this procedure with the chart or timer on, but instruct the patient to exhale as forcefully and completely as possible in one exhalation. Tell him when to start, and turn on the recorder or timer at the same time. Coach the patient throughout inspiration and exhalation.
- Allow the patient to rest. Then repeat the procedure twice.
- Monitor the patient for increased shortness of breath, light-headedness, paroxysmal coughing, and chest pain.
- Compare vital capacity values between each maneuver.

NURSING ALERT *If any subsequent vital capacity is 20% lower than the original value and you're confident there is no leak in the system, terminate the study.* Potentially dangerous air trapping may be resulting from the forced exhalation.

- After completing the procedure, discard the mouthpiece, remove the spirographic chart, and follow the manufacturer's instructions for cleaning and sterilizing the spirometer.[5]
- Remove and discard your gloves and perform hand hygiene.[2,3,4]
- Document the procedure.[6]

Special considerations

- Don't perform pulmonary function tests immediately after a large meal *because the patient may experience abdominal discomfort.*
- Encourage the patient to perform maximally during the test; *doing so may help him to exhale more forcefully.* If the patient coughs during expiration, wait until coughing subsides before repeating the measurement.
- Read the vital capacity directly from the readout or spirogram chart. The vital capacity is the greatest measurement volume on

complete exhalation after the deepest inhalation without forced or rapid effort. It's usually recorded in liters or milliliters. Of the three trials, accept the highest recorded exhalation volume as the vital capacity result.

- To determine the percentage of predicted vital capacity, first determine the patient's predicted value from the vital capacity predicted-values table; then calculate the percentage by using the following formula:

$$\frac{\text{observed vital capacity}}{\text{predicted vital capacity}} \times 100 = \% \text{ predicted vital capacity}$$

- Read the FVC directly from the readout or spirogram chart. Although the FVC is normally approximately equal to the vital capacity, it may be reduced in obstructive disease, whereas the vital capacity remains normal. In restrictive disease, both the vital capacity and FVC may be reduced.
- To determine the FEV for a specified time, mark the point on the spirogram where it crosses the desired time, and draw a straight line from this point to the side of the chart, which indicates volume in liters. This measurement is usually calculated for 1, 2, and 3 seconds and reported as a percentage of FVC. A healthy patient will have exhaled 75%, 85%, and 95%, respectively, of his FVC. Calculate this percentage by using the following formula:

$$\frac{\text{observed FEV}}{\text{observed FVC}} \times 100 = \% \text{ FVC}$$

Complications

Forced exhalation can cause dizziness or light-headedness, precipitate or worsen bronchospasm, rapidly increase exhaustion (possibly to where the patient will require mechanical support), and increase air trapping in the emphysemic patient.

Documentation

Record the date and time of the procedure; the patient's sex, age, height, and weight at the time of the study; the measured and calculated values, including FEV at 1, 2, and 3 seconds; any complications and the nursing action taken; and the patient's tolerance of the procedure.

REFERENCES

1. The Joint Commission. (2012). Standard NPSG.01.01.01. *Comprehensive accreditation manual for hospitals: The official handbook.* Oakbrook Terrace, IL: The Joint Commission. (Level I)
2. The Joint Commission. (2012). Standard NPSG.07.01.01. *Comprehensive accreditation manual for hospitals: The official handbook.* Oakbrook Terrace, IL: The Joint Commission. (Level I)
3. World Health Organization. (2009). *WHO guidelines on hand hygiene in health care: First global patient safety challenge. Clean care is safer care.* Geneva, Switzerland: World Health Organization. (Level I)
4. Centers for Disease Control and Prevention. (October 2002). Guideline for hand hygiene in health-care settings. *Morbidity and Mortality Weekly Report, 51* (RR-16), 1–45. (Level I)

5 American Association for Respiratory Care. (1996). "AARC Clinical Practice Guideline. Incentive Spirometry, 1996 Update" [Online]. Accessed July 2011 via the Web at http://www.aarc.org/daz/rcjournal/rcjournal/x.RCJOURNAL.COM%2002.21.07/online_resources/cpgs/spirupdatecpg.html (Level I)

6 The Joint Commission. (2012). Standard RC.01.01.03. *Comprehensive accreditation manual for hospitals: The official handbook.* Oakbrook Terrace, IL: The Joint Commission. (Level I)

BINDER APPLICATION

Also known as *self-closures,* binders are lengths of cloth or elasticized material that encircle the chest, abdomen, or groin to provide support, keep dressings in place (especially for patients allergic to tape), and reduce edema, tension on wounds and suture lines, and breast engorgement in mothers who aren't breast-feeding. Binders also promote patient comfort and the healing process. Typically, cloth binders are fastened with safety pins, and elasticized binders are fastened with Velcro.

Equipment

Tape measure ▪ binder of appropriate size and type ▪ safety pins ▪ gloves, if necessary ▪ dressing materials.

Commercial elastic binders are now commonly used instead of standard cotton straight and Scultetus binders that require pins. Disposable T-binders are available, and scrotal supports typically replace binders for male patients, except after abdominal-perineal resection.

Preparation of equipment

Measure the area that the binder must fit, and obtain the proper size and type of binder from the central supply department.

Implementation

▪ Check the doctor's order.
▪ Perform hand hygiene and put on gloves, as needed.[1,2,3]
▪ Confirm the patient's identity using at least two patient identifiers according to your facility's policy.[4]
▪ Provide privacy and explain the procedure to the patient.
▪ Raise the patient's bed to a comfortable working height *to avoid muscle strain when applying the binder.*
▪ Position the patient in a supine position, with his head slightly elevated and his knees slightly flexed *to decrease tension on the abdomen.*
▪ Assess the patient's condition.
▪ Remove the dressing and inspect the wound or suture line, if appropriate.
▪ Redress the wound and then remove and discard your gloves.

Applying a straight abdominal binder

▪ Accordion-fold half of the binder, slip it under the patient, and pull it through from the other side. Make sure the binder is straight, free of wrinkles, and evenly distributed under the patient. Its lower edge should extend well below the hips.

▪ Overlap one side snugly onto the other.
▪ Starting at the lower edge, close the Velcro closure.
▪ Make darts in the binder, as needed. Avoid making the binder too tight around the diaphragm *because it may interfere with breathing.* Then insert one finger under the binder's edge *to ensure a snug fit that's still loose enough to avoid impaired circulation and patient discomfort.*
▪ *For maximum support,* wrap the binder so that it applies even pressure across the body section. Eliminate all wrinkles, and avoid placing pressure over bony prominences (as shown below).

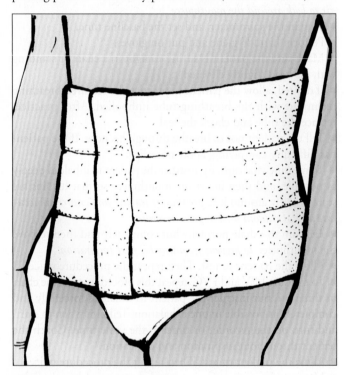

Applying a breast binder

▪ Wash and thoroughly dry under pendulous breasts. Place 4″ × 4″ gauze pads under breasts, as necessary, *to prevent skin irritation.*
▪ Slip the binder under the patient's chest so that its lower edge aligns with the waist.
▪ Straighten the binder to distribute it evenly on either side.
▪ Place the binder so that the patient's nipples are centered in the breast tissue. *This position ensures proper breast alignment and support and produces faster tissue involution.*
▪ *For maximum support,* wrap the binder so that it applies even pressure across the body section. Eliminate all wrinkles, and avoid placing pressure over bony prominences.
▪ Pull the binder's edges snugly together and begin closing the Velcro closures upward from the waist.

■ Adjust the shoulder straps to fit properly and secure them with the Velcro fasteners (as shown below).

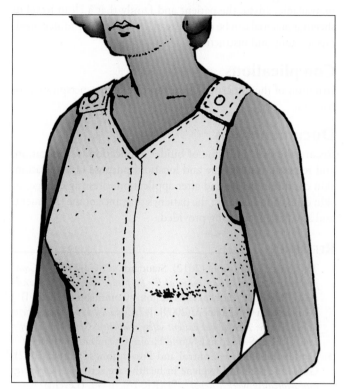

Applying a Scultetus binder

■ Slide the binder under the patient's hips and buttocks so that its top aligns with the waist and its lowest tail crosses the extreme lower abdomen.

■ Adjust the binder so that its solid part is centered under the patient and its tails are evenly distributed on either side. Spread the tails out flat *so you can pick them up easily.*

■ Beginning at the lower edge of the binder, bring one tail straight across the patient's abdomen. If the tail is too long, fold it over flat at the end. Hold this tail snugly in place as you bring the opposite tail across on top of it, overlapping the first tail's upper half and continuing with succeeding tail pieces. (See *Applying a Scultetus binder,* page 70.)

■ Secure the top strap with the Velcro.

Applying a T-binder

■ Slip the T-binder under the patient's waist, with its tails extending below the buttocks. Smooth the waistband and tails *to remove twists, which can chafe the patient's skin.*

■ Pull the waistband snugly into position at the patient's waistline or lower across the abdomen. Then fasten the Velcro closure. Next, bring the free tail up between the patient's legs over the dressing or perineal pad.

■ For a female patient, bring the single tail up to the center of the waist, loop it behind and over the waistband, and secure it to the waistband with the Velcro closures. For a male patient, bring the two tails up on either side of the penis *to provide even support for the testes.* Loop the ends behind and over the waistband on either

side of the midline, and fasten them to the waistband by closing the Velcro closures.

■ *For maximum support,* wrap the binder so that it applies even pressure across the body section. Eliminate all wrinkles and avoid placing pressure over bony prominences (as shown below).

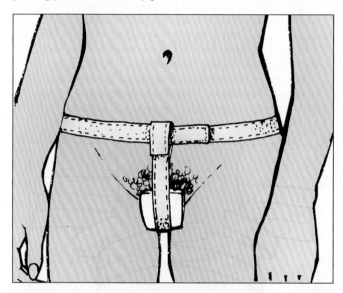

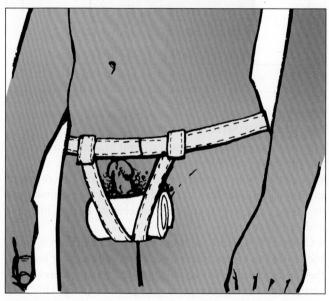

■ Tell the patient to call for assistance when he needs to void or defecate *to unfasten and reapply the binder.*

Completing the application of any binder

■ Ask the patient if the binder feels comfortable. Tell him that it may feel tight initially but should feel comfortable shortly. Instruct the patient to notify you immediately if the binder feels too tight or too loose or comes apart.

■ Return the bed to its lowest position *for patient safety.*

■ If the patient can ambulate, ask him to do so *to evaluate the fit of the binder.*

■ Perform hand hygiene.[1,2,3]

■ Document the procedure.[5]

Applying a Scultetus binder

After centering the binder's solid portion under the patient, with tails distributed evenly on each side, bring the lowest tail straight across the patient's abdomen, hold it snugly, and bring the next higher tail across to overlap it. Alternate tails in this manner, with the next higher tail overlapping the one below it by about half its width. *For maximum support,* wrap the binder so that it applies even pressure across the body section. Eliminate all wrinkles, and avoid placing pressure over bony prominences.

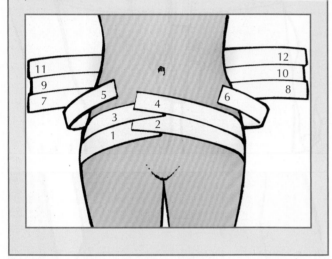

Special considerations

■ In surgical applications, fasten straight binders from the bottom upward *to relieve gravitational pull on the wound.*

■ Be careful not to compress any tubes, drains, or catheters and not to position them so that they are working against gravity. Also, make sure that binder placement doesn't interfere with elimination.

■ Observe the patient and check binder placement every 4 hours, and as needed. Check the skin for color, palpate it for warmth, check pulses, and assess for tingling or numbness. Check respiratory status, and encourage coughing and deep breathing.

■ Check the patient's lower extremities for color, pulses, and edema. Encourage movement of the patient's feet and legs *to prevent deep vein thrombosis.*

■ Reapply the binder when a dressing needs changing, when the binder becomes loose or too tight, and at other times according to the doctor's orders. When changing the binder, observe the skin for signs of irritation. Provide appropriate skin care before reapplying the binder.

Patient teaching

If the patient will need a binder after discharge, teach him and a family member how to remove it, inspect the skin, bathe the area, and reapply the binder. Tell the patient and family member where binders can be purchased and how to care for them. For a patient with cancer, the American Cancer Society may provide assistance in obtaining binders. If commercially manufactured binders are unavailable, advise the patient and family that a clean towel or sheeting material can be used instead. Periodically reinforce previous teaching and instructions.

Complications

Irritation of the underlying skin can result from perspiration or friction.

Documentation

Record the date and time of binder application, reapplication, and removal; binder type and location; purpose of application; skin condition before and after application; dressing changes or skin care; complications; the patient's tolerance of the treatment; and any patient teaching provided.

REFERENCES

1 The Joint Commission. (2012). Standard NPSG.07.01.01. *Comprehensive accreditation manual for hospitals: The official handbook.* Oakbrook Terrace, IL: The Joint Commission. (Level I)
2 World Health Organization. (2009). *WHO guidelines on hand hygiene in health care: First global patient safety challenge. Clean care is safer care.* Geneva, Switzerland: World Health Organization. (Level I)
3 Centers for Disease Control and Prevention. (October 2002). Guideline for hand hygiene in health-care settings. *Morbidity and Mortality Weekly Report, 51* (RR-16), 1–45. (Level I)
4 The Joint Commission. (2012). Standard NPSG.01.01.01. *Comprehensive accreditation manual for hospitals: The official handbook.* Oakbrook Terrace, IL: The Joint Commission. (Level I)
5 The Joint Commission. (2012). Standard RC.01.03.01. *Comprehensive accreditation manual for hospitals: The official handbook.* Oakbrook Terrace, IL: The Joint Commission. (Level I)

ADDITIONAL REFERENCES

Craven, R.F., & Hirnle, C.J. (2009). *Fundamentals of nursing: Human health and function* (6th ed.). Philadelphia, PA: Lippincott Williams & Wilkins.
Larson, C.M., et al. (2009). The effect of abdominal binders on postoperative pulmonary function. *The American Surgeon, 75*(2), 169–71.
Taylor, C., et al. (2011). *Fundamentals of nursing: The art and science of nursing care* (7th ed.). Philadelphia, PA: Lippincott Williams & Wilkins.
Toft, M.H., et al. (2008). Haemodynamic and respiratory effects of an abdominal compression binder. *Clinical Physiology and Functional Imaging, 28*(6), 398–402.

BISPECTRAL INDEX MONITORING

Bispectral index monitoring involves the use of an electronic device that converts EEG waves into a number. This number, statistically derived from raw EEG data, indicates the depth or level of a patient's sedation and provides a direct measure of the effects of sedatives and anesthetics on the brain. Rather than relying on subjective assessments and vital signs, bispectral index monitoring

EQUIPMENT

Bispectral index monitoring

Bispectral index monitoring consists of a monitor and cable connected to a sensor applied to the patient's forehead (as shown below).

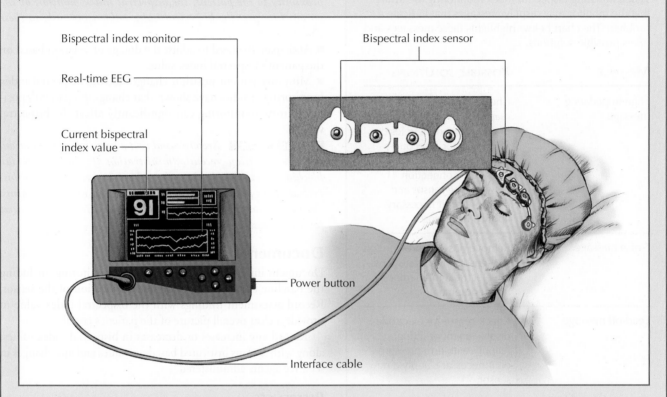

Bispectral index monitor

Bispectral index sensor

Real-time EEG

Current bispectral
index value

Power button

Interface cable

provides objective, reliable data on which to base care, thus minimizing the risks of oversedation and undersedation. When used appropriately, bispectral index monitoring can decrease the total amount of sedation needed to keep a patient adequately sedated.

The bispectral index monitor is attached to a sensor applied to the patient's forehead. The sensor obtains information about the patient's electrical brain activity and then translates this information into a number from 0 (indicating no brain activity) to 100 (indicating a patient who's awake and alert). In the critical care unit, bispectral index monitoring is used to assess sedation when the patient is receiving mechanical ventilation or neuromuscular blockers or during barbiturate coma or bedside procedures.

Equipment
Bispectral index monitor and cable ▪ bispectral index sensor ▪ alcohol pads ▪ gauze pad ▪ soap and water.

Implementation
▪ Gather the necessary equipment.
▪ Place the bispectral index monitor close to the patient's bed, and plug the power cord into the wall outlet.
▪ Turn on the monitor to allow it to initiate a self-test *to make sure the equipment is functioning properly.*

▪ Confirm the patient's identity using at least two patient identifiers according to your facility's policy.[1]
▪ Explain the procedure and rationale to the patient and his family. (See *Bispectral index monitoring.*)
▪ Provide privacy.
▪ Perform hand hygiene and follow standard precautions.[2,3,4]
▪ Clean the patient's forehead with soap and water and allow it to dry. If necessary, wipe the forehead with an alcohol pad and then dry it with a gauze pad *to ensure that the skin is oil-free.*
▪ Open the sensor package and apply the sensor to the patient's forehead. Position the circle labeled "1" midline approximately 1½″ (about 4 cm) above the bridge of the nose.
▪ Position the circle labeled "3" vertically on the right or left temple area, at the level of the outer canthus of the eye, between the corner of the eye and the patient's hairline.
▪ Ensure that the circle labeled "4" and the line below it are parallel to the eye on the appropriate side.
▪ Position the circle labeled "2" between the circles labeled "1" and "4."
▪ Apply gentle but firm pressure around the edges of the sensor, including the areas in between the numbered circles, *to ensure proper adhesion.*

TROUBLESHOOTING

Troubleshooting sensor problems

When initiating bispectral index monitoring, be aware that the monitor may display messages that indicate a problem. The chart below highlights these messages and offers possible solutions.

MESSAGE	POSSIBLE SOLUTIONS
High impedance message	Check sensor adhesion; reapply firm pressure to each of the numbered circles on the sensor for 5 seconds; if the message continues, check the connection between the sensor and the monitor; if necessary, apply a new sensor.
Noise message	Remove possible pressure on the sensor; investigate possible electrical interference from equipment.
Lead-off message	Check sensor for electrode displacement or lifting; reapply with firm pressure or, if necessary, apply a new sensor.

■ Press firmly on each of the numbered circles for about 5 seconds *to ensure that the electrodes adhere to the skin.*
■ Connect the sensor to the interface cable and monitor.
■ Watch the monitor for information related to impedance (electrical resistance) testing.
NURSING ALERT *Be aware that for the monitor to display a reading, impedance values must be below a specified threshold. If they aren't, be prepared to troubleshoot sensor problems. (See* Troubleshooting sensor problems.*)*
■ Select a smoothing rate (the time during which data is analyzed for calculation of the bispectral index; usually 15 or 30 seconds) using the "advance setup" button based on your facility's policy.
■ Read and record the bispectral index value.
■ Check the sensor site according to facility policy. Change the sensor every 24 hours.
■ Perform hand hygiene.[2,3,4]
■ Document the procedure.[5]

Special considerations

■ Always evaluate the bispectral index value in light of other patient assessment findings. Don't rely on the bispectral index value alone. (See *Interpreting bispectral index values.*)

■ Keep in mind that movement may occur with low bispectral index values. Be alert for artifacts that could falsely elevate bispectral index values.
NURSING ALERT *Bispectral index values may be elevated because of muscle shivering, tightening, or twitching, or with the use of mechanical devices either with the patient or in close proximity to the patient, the bispectral index monitor, or the sensor. Interpret the bispectral index value cautiously in these situations.*
■ Anticipate the need to adjust the dosage of sedation based on the patient's bispectral index value.
■ Minimize patient position changes during bispectral index monitoring. Studies have shown that changing a patient's position during monitoring can significantly affect the bispectral values.
NURSING ALERT *Keep in mind that a decrease in stimulation, increased sedation, recent administration of a neuromuscular blocking agent or analgesia, or hypothermia may decrease the bispectral index, indicating the need for a decrease in sedative agents. Pain may cause an elevated bispectral index, indicating a need for an increase in sedation.*

Documentation

Document initiation of bispectral index monitoring, including the baseline bispectral index value and location of the sensor. Record assessment findings with the bispectral index value to provide a clear overall picture of the patient's condition.

Record any increases or decreases in bispectral index values, along with actions instituted based on values and any changes in sedative agents administered.

REFERENCES

1 The Joint Commission. (2012). Standard NPSG.01.01.01. *Comprehensive accreditation manual for hospitals: The official handbook.* Oakbrook Terrace, IL: The Joint Commission. (Level I)
2 The Joint Commission. (2012). Standard NPSG.07.01.01. *Comprehensive accreditation manual for hospitals: The official handbook.* Oakbrook Terrace, IL: The Joint Commission. (Level I)
3 Centers for Disease Control and Prevention. (October 2002). Guideline for hand hygiene in health-care settings. *Morbidity and Mortality Weekly Report, 51* (RR-16), 1–45. (Level I)
4 The Joint Commission. (2012). Standard NPSG.01.01.01. *Comprehensive accreditation manual for hospitals: The official handbook.* Oakbrook Terrace, IL: The Joint Commission. (Level I)
5 The Joint Commission. (2012). Standard RC.01.03.01. *Comprehensive accreditation manual for hospitals: The official handbook.* Oakbrook Terrace, IL: The Joint Commission. (Level I)

ADDITIONAL REFERENCES

Kaki, A.M., & Almarakbi, W.A. (2009). Does patient position influence the reading of the bispectral index monitor? *Anesthesia and Analgesia, 109*(6), 1843–1846.
Lynn-McHale Wiegand, D.J. (Ed.). (2011). *AACN procedure manual for critical care* (6th ed.). Philadelphia, PA: Saunders.
Myles, P.S., et al. (2009). Prediction of neurological outcome using bispectral index monitoring in patients with severe ischemic-hypoxic brain injury undergoing emergency surgery. *Anesthesiology, 110*(5), 1106–1115.

Olson, D.M., et al. (2009). A randomized evaluation of bispectral index-augmented sedation assessment in neurological patients. *Neurocritical Care, 11*(1), 20–27.

Punjasawadwong, Y., et al. (2007). Bispectral index for improving anaesthetic delivery and postoperative recovery. *Cochrane Database of Systematic Reviews,* (4), CD003843.

BLADDER ULTRASONOGRAPHY

Urine retention, a potentially life-threatening condition, may result from neurologic or psychological disorders or obstruction of urine flow. Medications such as anticholinergics, antihistamines, and antidepressants may also cause urine retention. Traditionally, the amount of urine retained in the bladder was measured by urinary catheterization, placing the patient at risk for infection. Noninvasive bladder ultrasonography provides an assessment of bladder volume while lowering the risk of urinary tract infection.

Equipment

Bladder ultrasonography unit with scanhead ▪ ultrasonic transmission gel ▪ antiseptic pads ▪ washcloth ▪ gloves.

Implementation

▪ Check the doctor's order.
▪ Confirm the patient's identity using at least two patient identifiers according to your facility's policy.[1]
▪ Bring the bladder ultrasonography unit to the bedside. Explain the procedure to the patient *to help reduce his anxiety.*
▪ Perform hand hygiene.[2,3,4]
▪ Provide privacy.
▪ If this is a postvoiding scan, ask the patient to void; assist as necessary.
▪ Place the patient in a supine position.
▪ Put on gloves and clean the rounded end of the scanhead with an antiseptic pad.
▪ Expose the patient's suprapubic area.
▪ Turn on the ultrasonography unit by pressing the button (designated by a dot within a circle) on the far left and then press SCAN.
▪ Place ultrasonic gel on the scanhead *to promote an airtight seal for optimal sound wave transmission.*
▪ Tell the patient that the gel will feel cold when placed on the abdomen.
▪ Locate the symphysis pubis, and place the scanhead about 1″ (2.5 cm) superior to the symphysis pubis.
▪ Locate the icon (a rough figure of a patient) on the probe and make sure the head of the icon points toward the head of the patient.
▪ Press the scanhead button marked with a sound wave pattern to activate the scan. Hold the scanhead steady until you hear the beep.
▪ Look at the aiming icon and screen, which displays the bladder position and volume. Reposition the probe and scan until the bladder is centered in the aiming screen. The largest measurement will be saved.

Interpreting bispectral index values

Use the following guidelines to interpret your patient's bispectral index value:

BISPECTRAL INDEX	
100	Awake
80	Light to moderate sedation
70	Deep sedation (low probability of explicit recall)
60	General anesthesia (low probability of consciousness)
40	Deep hypnotic state
0	Flat-line EEG

Light hypnotic state

Moderate hypnotic state

▪ Press DONE when finished.
▪ The bladder ultrasonography unit will display the measured urine volume and the longitudinal and horizontal axis scans.
▪ Press PRINT to obtain a hard copy of your results.
▪ Turn off the unit. Use an antiseptic pad to clean the gel off the scanhead.
▪ Using a washcloth, remove the gel from the patient's skin.
▪ Remove and discard your gloves and perform hand hygiene.[2,3,4]
▪ Document the procedure.[3,4]

Special considerations

▪ Some scanners require you to choose a sex. If the patient has had a hysterectomy, select the male category.

Documentation

Write the patient's name, the date, and the time on the printout and attach it to the patient's medical record. Also document the procedure and urine volume as well as any treatment in the patient's medical record.

REFERENCES

1 The Joint Commission. (2012). Standard NPSG.01.01.01. *Comprehensive accreditation manual for hospitals: The official handbook.* Oakbrook Terrace, IL: The Joint Commission. (Level I)

2 The Joint Commission. (2012). Standard NPSG.07.01.01. *Comprehensive accreditation manual for hospitals: The official handbook.* Oakbrook Terrace, IL: The Joint Commission. (Level I)

3 Centers for Disease Control and Prevention. (October 2002). Guideline for hand hygiene in health-care settings. *Morbidity and Mortality Weekly Report, 51* (RR-16), 1–45. (Level I)

4 The Joint Commission. (2012). Standard RC.01.03.01. *Comprehensive accreditation manual for hospitals: The official handbook.* Oakbrook Terrace, IL: The Joint Commission. (Level I)

BLOOD CULTURE SAMPLE COLLECTION

Normally bacteria-free, blood is susceptible to infection through infusion lines as well as from thrombophlebitis, infected shunts, or bacterial endocarditis resulting from prosthetic heart valve replacements. Bacteria may also invade the vascular system from local tissue infections through the lymphatic system and the thoracic duct.

Blood cultures are performed to detect bacterial invasion (bacteremia) and the systemic spread of such an infection (septicemia) through the bloodstream. In this procedure, a venous blood sample is collected by venipuncture at the patient's bedside and then transferred into two bottles, one containing an anaerobic medium and the other, an aerobic medium. The bottles are incubated, encouraging any organisms present in the sample to grow in the media. Blood cultures allow identification of about 67% of pathogens within 24 hours and up to 90% within 72 hours. Two or three sets of blood culture samples should be drawn over a period of 24 hours.

Equipment

Tourniquet ▪ gloves ▪ alcohol pad ▪ chlorhexidine swabs ▪ 20-mL syringe for an adult; 10-mL syringe for a child (1 syringe for each set of cultures) ▪ three or four 20G 1½″ needles ▪ two or three blood culture bottles (50-mL bottles for adults; 20-mL bottles for infants and children) with sodium polyethanol sulfonate added (one aerobic bottle containing a suitable medium, such as Trypticase Soy Broth with 10% carbon dioxide atmosphere; one anaerobic bottle with prereduced medium; and, possibly, one hyperosmotic bottle with 10% sucrose medium) ▪ laboratory request form ▪ laboratory biohazard transport bag ▪ 2″ × 2″ sterile gauze pads ▪ small adhesive bandages ▪ labels.

Preparation of equipment

Check the expiration dates on the culture bottles and replace outdated bottles.

Implementation

▪ Verify the doctor's order.
▪ Gather the appropriate equipment.
▪ Perform hand hygiene and put on gloves.[1,2,3]
▪ Confirm the patient's identity using at least two patient identifiers according to your facility's policy.[4]
▪ Tell the patient that you need to collect a series of blood samples to check for infection. Explain the procedure *to ease his anx-*

iety and promote cooperation. Explain that the procedure usually requires two blood samples collected from two different sites.
▪ Tie a tourniquet 2″ (5 cm) proximal to the area chosen. (See "Venipuncture," page 781.)
▪ Clean the venipuncture site with an alcohol pad, starting in the center and moving outward in a circular motion.
▪ Next, clean the area with a chlorhexidine swab. Scrub the site for at least 30 seconds. Wait 30 seconds for the skin to dry.
▪ Perform a venipuncture, drawing 20 mL of blood from an adult.

PEDIATRIC ALERT *Draw 2 to 6 mL of blood from a child.*

▪ Remove the tourniquet. Apply pressure to the venipuncture site using a sterile 2″ × 2″ gauze dressing. Then cover the site with a small adhesive bandage.
▪ Wipe the diaphragm tops of the culture bottles with an alcohol pad.
▪ Inject 10 to 20 mL of blood into each bottle or 1 to 2 mL into a 20-mL pediatric culture bottle, using a needleless transfer device if available. *Doing so ensures the most accurate culture results.*
▪ Label the culture bottles in the presence of the patient *to prevent mislabeling.*[5] Label the bottles and the laboratory request form according to your facility's policy.
▪ Discard syringes, needles, and gloves in the appropriate receptacles.[6]
▪ Send the samples in a laboratory transport bag to the laboratory immediately.
▪ Perform hand hygiene.[1,2,3]
▪ Document the procedure.[7]

Special considerations

▪ Obtain each set of cultures from a different site.
▪ Avoid using existing blood lines for cultures unless there is no peripheral access available.

Complications

The most common complication of venipuncture is formation of a hematoma.

Documentation

Record the date and time of blood sample collection, name of the test, amount of blood collected, number of bottles used, the patient's temperature, and adverse reactions to the procedure.

REFERENCES

1 The Joint Commission. (2012). Standard NPSG.07.01.01. *Comprehensive accreditation manual for hospitals: The official handbook.* Oakbrook Terrace, IL: The Joint Commission. (Level I)

2 World Health Organization. (2009). *WHO guidelines on hand hygiene in health care: First global patient safety challenge. Clean care is safer care.* Geneva, Switzerland: World Health Organization. (Level I)

3 Centers for Disease Control and Prevention. (October 2002). Guideline for hand hygiene in health-care settings. *Morbidity and Mortality Weekly Report, 51* (RR-16), 1–45. (Level I)

4 The Joint Commission. (2012). Standard NPSG.01.01.01. *Comprehensive accreditation manual for hospitals: The official handbook.* Oakbrook Terrace, IL: The Joint Commission. (Level I)

5 The Joint Commission. (2012). Standard NPSG.03.04.01. *Comprehensive accreditation manual for hospitals: The official handbook.* Oakbrook Terrace, IL: The Joint Commission. (Level I)

6 Occupational Safety and Health Administration. "Bloodborne Pathogens, Standard Number 1910.1030" [Online]. Accessed July 2011 via the Web at http://www.osha.gov/pls/oshaweb/owadisp.show_document?p_table=STANDARDS&p_id=10051 (Level I)

7 The Joint Commission. (2012). Standard RC.01.03.01. *Comprehensive accreditation manual for hospitals: The official handbook.* Oakbrook Terrace, IL: The Joint Commission. (Level I)

ADDITIONAL REFERENCES

Craven, R.F., & Hirnle, C.J. (2009). *Fundamentals of nursing: Human health and function* (6th ed.). Philadelphia, PA: Lippincott Williams & Wilkins.

Fischbach, F.T., & Dunning, M.B. (2009). *A manual of laboratory and diagnostic tests* (8th ed.). Philadelphia, PA: Lippincott Williams & Wilkins.

BLOOD GLUCOSE MONITORING

Blood glucose monitors measure blood glucose concentrations. A drop of blood is placed on a blood glucose test strip before or after the strip is inserted into the monitor. A portable blood glucose monitor provides quantitative measurements that compare in accuracy with other laboratory tests. Most monitors store successive test results electronically to help determine glucose patterns.

Equipment

Gloves ▪ portable blood glucose monitor ▪ alcohol pads ▪ gauze pads ▪ disposable lancets or mechanical blood-letting devices ▪ blood glucose test strips ▪ Optional: small adhesive bandage.

Preparation of equipment

When using a blood glucose monitor, calibrate it and run it with a quality control test *to ensure accurate test results.* Most hospital-based glucose monitors must have quality control tests performed every 24 hours. Follow the manufacturer's instructions for calibration. If appropriate, ensure that the code strip number on the test strip matches the code number on the monitor.

Implementation

▪ Verify the doctor's order.
▪ Perform hand hygiene and put on gloves.[1,2,3]
▪ Confirm the patient's identity using at least two patient identifiers according to your facility's policy.[4]
▪ Explain the procedure to the patient.
▪ Next, select the puncture site—usually the fingertip or earlobe.
▪ If necessary, dilate the capillaries by applying warm, moist compresses to the area for about 10 minutes.

▪ Wipe the intended puncture site with an alcohol pad and allow it to dry completely (as shown below).

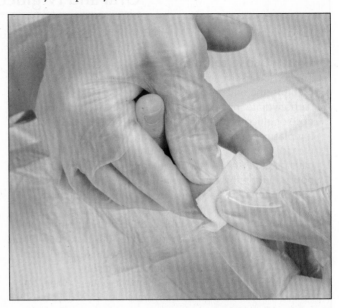

▪ To collect a sample from the fingertip with a disposable lancet (smaller than 2 mm), position the lancet on the side of the patient's fingertip perpendicular to the lines of the fingerprints. Pierce the skin sharply and quickly *to minimize the patient's anxiety and pain and to increase blood flow.* Alternatively, you can use a mechanical blood-letting device, such as an Autolet, which uses a spring-loaded lancet (as shown below).

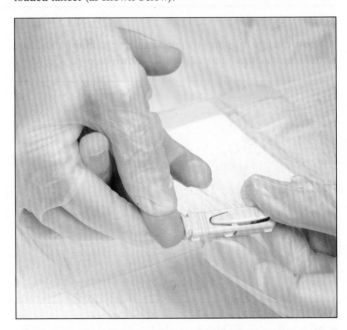

▪ After puncturing the finger, gently massage the base of the finger, stroking toward the puncture site but not squeezing the puncture site *to avoid diluting the sample with tissue fluid.*
▪ Turn on the monitor.
▪ Touch a drop of blood to the test area of the test strip; make sure the entire test area is covered.

Oral and IV glucose tolerance tests

For monitoring trends in glucose metabolism, two tests may offer benefits over testing blood with reagent strips.

Oral glucose tolerance test

The most sensitive test for detecting borderline diabetes mellitus, the oral glucose tolerance test (OGTT) measures carbohydrate metabolism after ingestion of a challenge dose of glucose. The body absorbs this dose rapidly, causing plasma glucose levels to rise and peak within 30 minutes to 1 hour. The pancreas responds by secreting insulin, causing glucose levels to return to normal within 2 to 3 hours. During this period, plasma and urine glucose levels are monitored to assess insulin secretion and the body's ability to metabolize glucose.

Although you may not collect the blood and urine specimens (usually five of each) required for this test, you will be responsible for preparing the patient for the test and monitoring his physical condition during the test.

Begin by explaining the OGTT to the patient. Then, tell him to maintain a high-carbohydrate diet for 3 days and to fast for 10 to 16 hours before the test, as ordered. The patient must not smoke, drink coffee or alcohol, or exercise strenuously for 8 hours before or during the test. Inform him that he'll then receive a challenge dose of 100 g of carbohydrate (usually a sweetened carbonated beverage or gelatin).

Tell the patient who will perform the venipunctures and when and that he may feel slight discomfort from the needle punctures and the pressure of the tourniquet. Reassure him that collecting each blood sample usually takes less than 3 minutes. As ordered, withhold drugs that may affect test results. Remind him not to discard the first urine specimen voided after waking.

During the test period, watch for signs and symptoms of hypoglycemia—weakness, restlessness, nervousness, hunger, and sweating—and report these to the doctor immediately. Encourage the patient to drink plenty of water to promote adequate urine excretion. Provide a bedpan, urinal, or specimen container when necessary.

IV glucose tolerance test

This test may be chosen for patients who are unable to absorb an oral dose of glucose—for example, those with malabsorption disorders or short-bowel syndrome or those who have had a gastrectomy. This test measures blood glucose after an IV infusion of 50% glucose over 3 or 4 minutes. Blood samples are then drawn after 30 minutes, 1 hour, 2 hours, and 3 hours. After an immediate glucose peak of 300 to 400 mg/dL (accompanied by glycosuria), the normal glucose curve falls steadily, reaching fasting levels within 1 to 1¼ hours. Failure to achieve fasting glucose levels within 2 to 3 hours typically confirms diabetes.

■ Insert the test strip into the blood glucose monitor according to the manufacturer's instructions (as shown below).

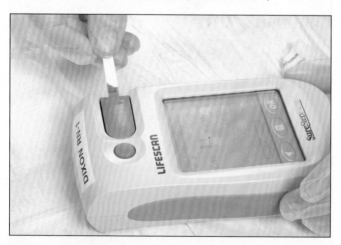

■ After collecting the blood sample, briefly apply pressure to the puncture site *to prevent painful extravasation of blood into subcutaneous tissues.* Ask the patient to hold a gauze pad firmly over the puncture site until bleeding stops.
■ Read the digital display when the alarm sounds.
■ Remove the test strip and dispose of it according to your facility's policy.

■ After bleeding has stopped, you may apply a small adhesive bandage to the puncture site.
NURSING ALERT *If you obtain an extremely low or high blood glucose monitor result, obtain a serum blood glucose level immediately* to confirm the result.
■ Clean and disinfect the blood glucose monitor between each patient contact, according to your facility's policy.
■ Remove your gloves and perform hand hygiene.[1,2,3]
■ Document the procedure.[5]

Special considerations

■ Follow your facility's policy and procedure for bedside point-of-care testing.
■ Avoid selecting cold, cyanotic, or swollen puncture sites *to ensure an adequate blood sample.* If you can't obtain a capillary sample, perform venipuncture and place a large drop of venous blood on the test strip. If you want to test blood from a refrigerated sample, allow the blood to return to room temperature before testing it.
■ *To help detect abnormal glucose metabolism and diagnose diabetes mellitus,* the doctor may order other blood glucose tests. (See *Oral and IV glucose tolerance tests.*)
■ Some blood glucose monitors require smaller amounts of blood, and the puncture may also be done on the patient's arm.

■ Store the test strips away from heat and humidity *because these can affect the accuracy of the results.*

Patient teaching

If the patient will perform blood glucose monitoring at home, teach him the proper use of the lancet or Autolet and portable blood glucose monitor, as necessary. Also provide written guidelines.

Documentation

Record the reading in your notes or in a special flowchart, if available. Also record the time and date of the test.

REFERENCES

1 The Joint Commission. (2012). Standard NPSG.07.01.01. *Comprehensive accreditation manual for hospitals: The official handbook.* Oakbrook Terrace, IL: The Joint Commission. (Level I)

2 World Health Organization. (2009). *WHO guidelines on hand hygiene in health care: First global patient safety challenge. Clean care is safer care.* Geneva, Switzerland: World Health Organization. (Level I)

3 Centers for Disease Control and Prevention. (October 2002). Guideline for hand hygiene in health-care settings. *Morbidity and Mortality Weekly Report, 51* (RR-16), 1–45. (Level I)

4 The Joint Commission. (2012). Standard NPSG.01.01.01. *Comprehensive accreditation manual for hospitals: The official handbook.* Oakbrook Terrace, IL: The Joint Commission. (Level I)

5 The Joint Commission. (2012). Standard RC.01.03.01. *Comprehensive accreditation manual for hospitals: The official handbook.* Oakbrook Terrace, IL: The Joint Commission. (Level I)

ADDITIONAL REFERENCES

American Diabetes Association. (2009). Standards of medical care in diabetes—2010. *Diabetes Care, 32*(Suppl. 1), S13–S61.

Occupational Safety and Health Administration. "Bloodborne Pathogens, Standard Number 1910.1030" [Online]. Accessed July 2011 via the Web at http://www.osha.gov/pls/oshaweb/owadisp.show_document&p_table=standards&p_id=10051.

Rutala, W.A., et al. (2008). "Guideline for disinfection and sterilization in healthcare facilities, 2008" [Online]. Accessed July 2011 via the Web at http://www.cdc.gov/ncidod/dhqp/pdf/guidelines/Disinfection_Nov_2008.pdf

BLOOD PRESSURE ASSESSMENT

Defined as the lateral force exerted by blood on the arterial walls, blood pressure depends on the force of ventricular contractions, arterial wall elasticity, peripheral vascular resistance, and blood volume and viscosity. Systolic, or maximum, pressure occurs during left ventricular contraction and reflects the integrity of the heart, arteries, and arterioles. Diastolic, or minimum, pressure occurs during left ventricular relaxation and directly indicates blood vessel resistance.

Pulse pressure, the difference between systolic and diastolic pressures, varies inversely with arterial elasticity. Rigid vessels, incapable of distention and recoil, produce high systolic pressure and low diastolic pressure. Normally, systolic pressure exceeds dias-

tolic pressure by about 40 mm Hg. Narrowed pulse pressure—a difference of less than 30 mm Hg—occurs when systolic pressure falls and diastolic pressure rises. These changes reflect reduced stroke volume, increased peripheral resistance, or both. Widened pulse pressure—a difference of more than 50 mm Hg between systolic and diastolic pressures—occurs when systolic pressure rises and diastolic pressure remains constant, or when systolic pressure rises and diastolic pressure falls. These changes reflect increased stroke volume, decreased peripheral resistance, or both.

Frequent blood pressure measurement is critical after serious injury, surgery, or anesthesia and during any illness or condition that threatens cardiovascular stability. (Frequent measurement may be performed with an automated vital signs monitor.) Regular measurement is indicated for patients with a history of hypertension or hypotension, and annual screening is recommended for all adults.

Blood pressure should be measured using the recommendations set by the Seventh Report of the Joint National Committee on Prevention, Detection, Evaluation, and Treatment of High Blood Pressure (JNC VII). Until recently, patients with hypertension were stratified based on blood pressure readings alone. However, the JNC VII also considers the patient's individual risk factors, meaning that those with more risk factors are treated more aggressively. (See *Classification of blood pressure,* page 78.)

Equipment

Aneroid sphygmomanometer ■ stethoscope ■ alcohol pad ■ automated vital signs monitor (if available).

The sphygmomanometer consists of an inflatable compression cuff linked to a manual air pump and an aneroid gauge. A recently calibrated aneroid gauge should be used. To obtain an accurate reading, rest the gauge in any position but view it directly from the front. Cuffs come in sizes ranging from newborn to extra-large adult. Disposable cuffs and thigh cuffs are available.

The automated vital signs monitor is a noninvasive device that measures pulse rate, systolic and diastolic pressures, and mean arterial pressure at preset intervals. (See *Using an electronic vital signs monitor,* page 79.)

Preparation of equipment

Carefully choose a cuff of appropriate size for the patient; the bladder should encircle at least 80% of the upper arm. *An excessively narrow cuff may cause a falsely high pressure reading; an excessively wide one, a falsely low reading.* (For information on other situations that can cause false-high or false-low readings, see *Correcting problems of blood pressure measurement,* page 80.) If you aren't using your own stethoscope, disinfect the earpieces with an alcohol pad before placing them in your ears *to avoid cross-contamination.*

To use an automated vital signs monitor, collect the monitor, dual air hose, and pressure cuff. Then make sure the monitor unit is firmly positioned near the patient's bed.

Implementation

■ Perform hand hygiene.[1,2,3]
■ Confirm the patient's identity using at least two patient identifiers according to your facility's policy.[4]

Classification of blood pressure

The Seventh Report of the Joint National Committee on Prevention, Detection, Evaluation, and Treatment of High Blood Pressure recommends that a person's risk factors be considered in the treatment of hypertension. The patient with more risk factors should be treated more aggressively.

CATEGORY	SBP MM HG		DBP MM HG
Normal	less than 120	and	less than 80
Prehypertension	120 to 139	or	80 to 89
Hypertension, stage 1	140 to 159	or	90 to 99
Hypertension, stage 2	160 or higher	or	100 or higher

Key: SBP = systolic blood pressure; DBP = diastolic blood pressure.

Adapted from the Seventh Report of the Joint National Committee on Prevention, Detection, Evaluation, and Treatment of High Blood Pressure. (2003). NIH Publication No. 03-5231. Bethesda, Md: National Institutes of Health; National Heart, Lung, and Blood Institute; National High Blood Pressure Education Program.

■ Have the patient rest for at least 5 minutes before measuring his blood pressure. Make sure he hasn't smoked or had caffeine for at least 30 minutes.

■ Tell the patient that you're going to take his blood pressure.

■ The patient can lie supine or sit erect during blood pressure measurement. If the patient is sitting erect, make sure he has both feet on the floor *because crossing the legs may increase blood pressure.* His arm should be extended at heart level and be well supported. *If the artery is below heart level, you may get a false-high reading.* Make sure the patient is relaxed and comfortable when you take his blood pressure *so it stays at its normal level.*

■ Wrap the deflated cuff snugly around the upper arm. (See *Positioning the blood pressure cuff,* page 81.)

■ If the arm is very large or misshapen and the conventional cuff won't fit properly, take a leg or forearm measurement.

■ To obtain a thigh blood pressure, apply the appropriate-size cuff to the thigh and auscultate the pulsations over the popliteal artery (as shown below). To obtain a forearm blood pressure, apply the appropriate-size cuff to the forearm 5″ (13 cm) below the elbow.

■ If necessary, connect the appropriate tube to the rubber bulb of the air pump and the other tube to the gauge.

■ To determine how high to pump the blood pressure cuff, first estimate the systolic blood pressure by palpation. As you feel the radial artery with your fingers of one hand, inflate the cuff until the radial pulse disappears. Read this pressure on the gauge and add 30 mm Hg to it. Use this sum as the target inflation *to prevent discomfort from overinflation.* Deflate the cuff.

■ Locate the brachial artery by palpation. Center the bell of the stethoscope over the part of the artery where you detect the strongest beats, and hold it in place with one hand. *The bell of the stethoscope transmits low-pitched arterial blood sounds more effectively than does the diaphragm.*

■ Using the thumb and index finger of your other hand, turn the thumbscrew on the rubber bulb of the air pump clockwise to close the valve.

■ Pump up the cuff to the predetermined level. Then insert the stethoscope earpieces into your ears.

■ Carefully open the valve of the air pump, and then slowly deflate the cuff—no faster than 2 to 3 mm Hg/second. While releasing air, watch the mercury column or aneroid gauge and auscultate for the sound over the artery.

■ When you hear the first beat or clear tapping sound, note the pressure on the column or gauge. This is the systolic pressure. (The beat or tapping sound is the first of five Korotkoff sounds. The second sound resembles a murmur or swish; the third sound, crisp tapping; the fourth sound, a soft, muffled tone; and the fifth, the last sound heard.)

■ Continue to release air gradually while auscultating for the sound over the artery.

■ Note the pressure where the sound disappears. This is the diastolic pressure—the fifth Korotkoff sound.

Using an electronic vital signs monitor

An electronic vital signs monitor allows you to track a patient's vital signs continually, without having to reapply a blood pressure cuff each time. In addition, the patient won't need an invasive arterial line to gather similar data.

Some automated vital signs monitors are lightweight and battery-operated and can be attached to an IV pole for continual monitoring, even during patient transfers. Make sure you know the capacity of the monitor's battery and plug the machine in whenever possible *to keep it charged.* Regularly calibrate the monitor to ensure accurate readings.

Before using any monitor, check its accuracy. Determine the patient's pulse rate and blood pressure manually, using the same arm you'll use for the monitor cuff. Compare your results when you get initial readings from the monitor. If the results differ, call your supply department or the manufacturer's representative.

Check the manufacturer's guidelines *because most automated monitoring devices are intended for serial monitoring only and may be inaccurate for a one-time measurement.*

Preparing the device
■ Explain the procedure to the patient. Describe the alarm system *so he won't be frightened if it's triggered.*
■ Make sure the power switch is off. Then plug the monitor into a properly grounded wall outlet. Secure the dual air hose to the front of the monitor.
■ Connect the pressure cuff's tubing into the other ends of the dual air hose, and tighten connections *to prevent air leaks.* Keep the air hose away from the patient *to avoid accidental dislodgment.*
■ Squeeze all air from the cuff and wrap it loosely around the patient's arm about 1" (2.5 cm) above the antecubital fossa. Never apply the cuff to a limb that has an IV catheter in place. Position the cuff's "artery" arrow over the palpated brachial artery. Then secure the cuff for a snug fit.

Selecting parameters
■ When you turn on the monitor, it will default to a manual mode. (In this mode, you can obtain vital signs yourself before switching to the automatic mode.) Press the AUTO/MANUAL button to select the automatic mode. The monitor will give you baseline data for the pulse rate, systolic and diastolic pressures, and mean arterial pressure.
■ Compare your previous manual results with these baseline data. If they match, you're ready to set the alarm parameters. Press the SELECT button to blank out all displays except systolic pressure.
■ Use the HIGH and LOW limit buttons to set the specific parameters for systolic pressure. (These limits range from a high of 240 to a low of 0.) You'll also do this three more times for mean arterial pressure, pulse rate, and diastolic

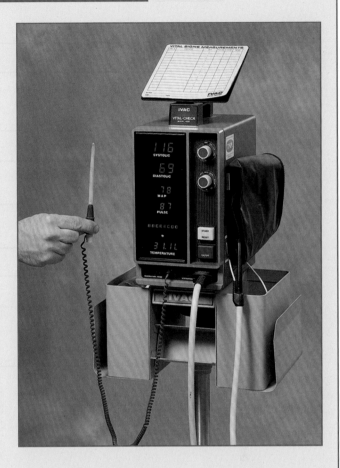

pressure. After you've set the parameters for diastolic pressure, press the SELECT button again to display all current data. Even if you forget to do this last step, the monitor will automatically display current data 10 seconds after you set the last parameters.

Collecting data
■ You also need to program the monitor according to the desired frequency. Press the SET button until you reach the desired time interval in minutes. If you've chosen the automatic mode, the monitor will display a default cycle time of 3 minutes. You can override the default cycle time to set the interval you prefer.
■ You can obtain a set of vital signs at any time by pressing the START button. Also, pressing the CANCEL button will stop the interval and deflate the cuff. You can retrieve stored data by pressing the PRIOR DATA button. The monitor will display the last data obtained along with the time elapsed since then. Scrolling backward, you can retrieve data from the previous 99 minutes.
■ Make sure that the patient's vital signs are documented frequently on a vital sign assessment sheet.

Correcting problems of blood pressure measurement

REACTION AND CAUSES	NURSING ACTIONS
FALSE-HIGH READING	
Cuff too small	Make sure the cuff bladder length is 80% of the arm circumference and the width is at least 40% of arm circumference (a length-to-width ratio of 2:1).
Cuff wrapped too loosely, reducing its effective width	Tighten the cuff.
Slow cuff deflation, causing venous congestion in the arm or leg	Never deflate the cuff more slowly than 2 mm Hg/heartbeat.
Poorly timed measurement (after patient has eaten, ambulated, appeared anxious, or flexed arm muscles)	Postpone blood pressure measurement or help the patient relax before taking pressures.
FALSE-LOW READING	
Incorrect position of arm or leg	Make sure the arm or leg is level with the patient's heart.
Failure to notice auscultatory gap (sound fades out for 10 to 15 mm Hg, then returns)	Estimate systolic pressure by palpation before actually measuring it. Then check this pressure against the measured pressure.
Inaudible low-volume sounds	Before reinflating the cuff, instruct the patient to raise the arm or leg to decrease venous pressure and amplify low-volume sounds. After inflating the cuff, tell the patient to lower the arm or leg. Then deflate the cuff and listen. If you still fail to detect low-volume sounds, chart the palpated systolic pressure.

■ After you hear the last Korotkoff sound, deflate the cuff slowly for at least another 10 mm Hg *to ensure that no further sounds are audible.*

■ Rapidly deflate the cuff. Record the pressure, wait 2 minutes, and then repeat the procedure. If the average of the readings is greater than 5 mm Hg, take the average of two or more readings. Remove and fold the cuff and return it to storage or, if using a blood pressure cuff that isn't dedicated for single patient use, clean and disinfect it before returning it to storage according to your facility's policy.

■ Clean and disinfect your stethoscope using an alcohol pad.

■ Perform hand hygiene.[1,2,3]

■ Document your measurements.[5]

Special considerations

■ Frequent blood pressure readings may be taken for unstable patients as well as for those receiving a blood transfusion or oral or IV medication to stabilize blood pressure.

■ If you can't auscultate blood pressure, you may estimate systolic pressure. To do this, first palpate the brachial or radial pulse. Then inflate the cuff until you no longer detect the pulse. Slowly deflate the cuff and, when you detect the pulse again, record the pressure as the palpated systolic pressure.

■ Palpation of systolic blood pressure also may be important *to avoid underestimating blood pressure in patients with an auscultatory gap.* This gap is a loss of sound between the first and second Korotkoff sounds that may be as great as 40 mm Hg. You may find an auscultatory gap in patients with venous congestion or hypotension.

■ If your patient is crying or anxious, delay blood pressure measurement, if possible, until the patient becomes calm *to avoid falsely elevated readings.*

■ Occasionally, blood pressure must be measured in both arms or with the patient in two different positions (such as lying and standing or sitting and standing). In such cases, observe and record any significant difference between the two readings and record the blood pressure as well as the extremity and position used.

■ Measure the blood pressure of patients taking antihypertensive medications while they're in a sitting position *to ensure accurate measurements.*

Complications

Don't take a blood pressure reading in the arm on the affected side of a patient who has had a mastectomy *because taking the reading may decrease already compromised lymphatic circulation, worsen edema, and damage the arm*. Likewise, don't take a blood pressure reading on the affected arm of a patient with an arteriovenous fistula or a hemodialysis shunt *because blood flow through the vascular device may be compromised*.

Documentation

In the patient's medical record, record blood pressure as systolic over diastolic pressures, such as 120/78 mm Hg. Document an auscultatory gap, if present. If required by your facility, document blood pressures on a graph, using dots or checkmarks. Also, document the extremity used and the patient's position. Include patient teaching about lifestyle modifications, drug therapy, and follow-up care. Record the name of any doctor notified about blood pressure results and any orders given.

REFERENCES

1 The Joint Commission. (2012). Standard NPSG.07.01.01. *Comprehensive accreditation manual for hospitals: The official handbook.* Oakbrook Terrace, IL: The Joint Commission. (Level I)
2 World Health Organization. (2009). *WHO guidelines on hand hygiene in health care: First global patient safety challenge. Clean care is safer care.* Geneva, Switzerland: World Health Organization. (Level I)
3 Centers for Disease Control and Prevention. (October 2002). Guideline for hand hygiene in health-care settings. *Morbidity and Mortality Weekly Report, 51* (RR-16), 1–45. (Level I)
4 The Joint Commission. (2012). Standard NPSG.01.01.01. *Comprehensive accreditation manual for hospitals: The official handbook.* Oakbrook Terrace, IL: The Joint Commission. (Level I)
5 The Joint Commission. (2012). Standard RC.01.03.01 *Comprehensive accreditation manual for hospitals: The official handbook.* Oakbrook Terrace, IL: The Joint Commission. (Level I)

ADDITIONAL REFERENCES

Craven, R.F., & Hirnle, C.J. (2009). *Fundamentals of nursing: Human health and function* (6th ed.). Philadelphia, PA: Lippincott Williams & Wilkins.
National Institutes of Health; National Heart, Lung, and Blood Institute. (2004). *The seventh report of the Joint National Committee on Prevention, Detection, and Treatment of High Blood Pressure.* NIH Publication No. 03-5233. Bethesda, MD: U.S. Department of Health and Human Services.
Rutala, W.A., et al. (2008). "Guideline for disinfection and sterilization in healthcare facilities, 2008" [Online]. Accessed July 2011 via the Web at http://www.cdc.gov/ncidod/dhqp/pdf/guidelines/Disinfection_Nov_2008.pdf

BODY JEWELRY REMOVAL

Piercings and body jewelry may be present on virtually any body part. The most common sites are the ears, nose, tongue, eyebrows, lips, and umbilicus. Less common sites include the nipples and genitals.

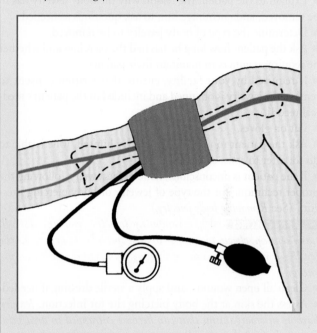

Positioning the blood pressure cuff

Palpate the brachial artery. Position the cuff 1" (2.5 cm) above the site of pulsation, center the bladder above the artery with the cuff fully deflated, and wrap the cuff evenly and snugly around the upper arm.

Depending on the risk to the patient, the medical interventions to be performed, and your facility's policy, the doctor may order for body jewelry to be removed to reduce the risk for such complications as electrical burns, aspiration, pressure injuries, or tissue injures. However, urgent medical care should never be delayed while attempting to remove body jewelry.

If you're helping a patient to remove body jewelry or removing it from an unconscious patient, you must make sure that the patient isn't harmed during the process and that the patient's dignity is preserved. You must also take steps to avoid damaging the jewelry during the removal process and retain the jewelry for reinsertion later.

Equipment

Gloves ■ ring-opening tool or ring-spreading pliers ■ tongue stabilizer or ring forceps ■ ball-grabber tool or bead tweezers ■ lubricating gel ■ antiseptic solution ■ personal belongings envelope ■ Optional: inert plastic radiolucent retainer that's approved by the Food and Drug Administration (FDA), microbore extension tubing, thick suture material, epidural catheter.

Implementation

■ Perform hand hygiene.[1,2,3]
■ Confirm the patient's identity using at least two patient identifiers according to your facility's policy.[4]

■ Ask the patient whether he's wearing body jewelry, especially jewelry that isn't readily visible. If the patient is unconscious, ask the patient's family about known body jewelry and note the presence of body jewelry during the physical examination.

■ Verify the doctor's orders for body jewelry removal and review the patient's medical record for scheduled diagnostic tests or surgical procedures.

■ Explain to the patient the reason why the body jewelry has to be removed, and encourage him to ask questions as needed.

■ Determine the type of body jewelry to be removed.

■ Ask the patient how long he has had the piercings and whether he requires retainers to maintain their patency.

■ If required by your facility, ensure that written consent to remove the jewelry is obtained and included in the patient's medical record.

■ Put on gloves.

■ Ask the patient to remove the jewelry himself, if he is able to do so; offer to assist as needed.

■ If the patient is unconscious, remove the jewelry, following the proper technique for the type of jewelry or body piercing present.[5] (See *Removing body jewelry.*)

NURSING ALERT *When removing jewelry from the nostril, nasal septum, cheek, tongue, or lip, use special care to prevent the jewelry from slipping into the airway, which may result in aspiration.*

■ Clean all open wounds, and apply a sterile dressing if needed.

■ Assess the skin at the body piercing site for infection. *Jewelry harbors microorganisms that can become entrapped in area skin. Removal of jewelry provides an opportunity to effectively remove microorganisms from the piercing site.*

■ Assist the patient with inserting a retainer (or insert one on an unconscious patient), if needed, *to maintain patency of the piercing.*

■ Clean soiled jewelry with antiseptic solution. *Consider all piercings contaminated with body fluids.*

■ Place the jewelry in a personal belongings envelope that's labeled with the patient's name and identification number, and give it to a family member or secure it according to facility policy.

■ Remove your gloves and perform hand hygiene.[1,2,3]

■ Document the procedure.[6]

Special considerations

■ If the patient refuses to remove the jewelry, notify the doctor *so that the risks of proceeding with any scheduled procedures can be reevaluated.*

■ Gloves can provide additional traction and grip when removing body jewelry.

■ Jewelry located on the face, eyebrows, nose, or mouth should be removed while the patient is sitting upright *to minimize the risk of aspiration.*

■ For procedures requiring electrocautery, metal jewelry that's between the active and dispersive electrodes should be removed *to minimize the risk of burns in the operating room.*

■ *Because jewelry harbors microorganisms,* body jewelry that's near the surgical site should be removed preoperatively and before the skin is prepped.

■ Removing jewelry from a piercing that isn't completely healed or well established (which can take 6 to 12 months for some piercings) can result in rapid closure of the piercing, making reinsertion difficult or impossible. Inert plastic, FDA-approved retainers are commercially available and can be inserted through a piercing to replace metal jewelry. Alternatively, if such a retainer isn't available, microbore extension tubing, thick suture material, or an epidural catheter can be threaded through the piercing and secured so that the hole doesn't close.

Complications

Jewelry cut from a piercing site may have rough, burred edges that can damage tissue when removed, creating a source for possible infection. Infection can also occur through a piercing that hasn't completely healed. Tissue trauma can occur when removing a tongue piercing; it can also create airway management problems. Aspiration can occur during intubation if jewelry located in and around the mouth loosens and dislodges.

NURSING ALERT *Don't delay emergency intubation to remove body jewelry.*

Burns can result if metal jewelry heats up as a result of exposure to electrical currents during cauterization in the operating room. Pressure injuries may result if an unconscious patient is positioned on a body part with jewelry in place. Traumatic injury may occur if body jewelry accidentally becomes entangled in bedding or caught on equipment.

Documentation

Record the patient teaching provided as well as any questions asked by the patient and your responses. Document whether the patient or nurse removed the jewelry, the type of jewelry removed and its location on the body, the condition of the skin at the piercing site, any drainage noted at the piercing site, the disposition of the jewelry, and measures applied to the site to prevent closure and infection.

REFERENCES

1 The Joint Commission. (2012). Standard NPSG.07.01.01. *Comprehensive accreditation manual for hospitals: The official handbook.* Oakbrook Terrace, IL: The Joint Commission. (Level I)

2 World Health Organization. (2009). *WHO guidelines on hand hygiene in health care: First global patient safety challenge. Clean care is safer care.* Geneva, Switzerland: World Health Organization. (Level I)

3 Centers for Disease Control and Prevention. (October 2002). Guideline for hand hygiene in health-care settings. *Morbidity and Mortality Weekly Report, 51* (RR-16), 1–45. (Level I)

4 The Joint Commission. (2012). Standard NPSG.01.01.01. *Comprehensive accreditation manual for hospitals: The official handbook.* Oakbrook Terrace, IL: The Joint Commission. (Level I)

Removing body jewelry

JEWELRY TYPE	JEWELRY DESCRIPTION	REMOVAL TECHNIQUE	REMOVAL TOOLS
Barbell, straight, curved, or circular 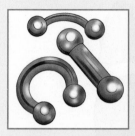	Straight, curved, or circular post with balls on the ends; one or both of the balls unscrew from the rod	■ Grasp the removable ball with the tweezers or forceps while holding the opposite end still, and turn it counterclockwise to loosen it. ■ After loosening the ball, fully unscrew it by hand and pull the open end of the post toward the side of the stationary ball to remove it. ■ Use caution when pulling the post through the body part *to prevent injury from any screw threads on the end of the post.*	■ Gloves ■ Ball grabber ■ Bead tweezers ■ Tongue stabilizer or ring forceps
Beaded closure, capture ball ring, or captive bead ring 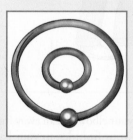	Sphere (or other shape) held in place by the tension of the ring	■ Insert ring-opening pliers into the middle of the ring, and slowly pry the ring open. ■ Remove the ball and then the ring. ■ Use care when removing the ball, *which can fall when separated from the ring.*	■ Gloves ■ Ring-opening or ring-spreading pliers ■ Ring forceps
Labret or Monroe 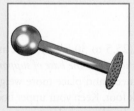	Straight barbell with one flat end resembling the head of a nail; the ball may be attached to the post with either internal or external threading	■ Stabilize the stud with the bead tweezers, and rotate the ball counterclockwise. ■ Use caution when pulling the post through the body part *to prevent injury from any screw threads on the end of the post.*	■ Gloves ■ Ball grabber ■ Bead tweezers ■ Tongue stabilizer or ring forceps
Tunnel, plug, or eyelet 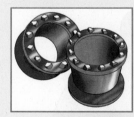	Large, round tube usually held in place with an O-ring; the tunnel may be flared on one end	■ If the tunnel has an O-ring, slide it off and remove the tube. ■ If the tunnel has a flared outer edge held in place by the surface tension of the skin, use gentle traction and lubricating gel during removal. ■ If the metal tunnel consists of two separate pieces screwed together, grasp each half (front and back) and rotate counterclockwise to separate.	■ Gloves ■ Ring forceps ■ Lubricating gel

5 Perioperative Patient Safety Subcommittee of the Committee on Clinical, Administrative, Professional and Emergency Services. (2006). *Guidelines for caring for patients with body jewelry/piercings in the operating room and procedure areas.* Chicago, IL: Metropolitan Chicago Healthcare Council.

6 The Joint Commission. (2012). Standard RC.03.01.01. *Comprehensive accreditation manual for hospitals: The official handbook.* Oakbrook Terrace, IL: The Joint Commission. (Level I)

ADDITIONAL REFERENCES

Conner, R., et al. (Eds.). (2010). *Perioperative standards and recommended practice.* Denver, CO: Association of periOperative Registered Nurses.

DeBoer, S., et al. (2008). Body piercing and airway management: Photo guide to tongue jewelry removal techniques. *AANA Journal, 76*(1), 19–23.

DeBoer, S., et al. (2008). Puncturing myths about body piercing and tattooing. *Nursing, 38*(11), 50–54.

Diccini, S., et al. (2009). Body piercing among Brazilian surgical patients. *AORN Journal, 89*(1), 161–165.

BODY MECHANICS

Many patient care activities require the nurse to push, pull, lift, and carry. By using proper body mechanics, you can avoid musculoskeletal injury and fatigue and reduce the risk for injuring patients.

Correct body mechanics can be summed up in three principles: First, keep a low center of gravity by flexing the hips and knees instead of bending at the waist. This position distributes weight evenly between the upper and lower body and helps maintain balance. Second, create a wide base of support by spreading the feet apart. This tactic provides lateral stability and lowers the body's center of gravity. Third, maintain proper body alignment and keep the body's center of gravity directly over the base of support by moving the feet rather than twisting and bending at the waist. Keep the back, neck, pelvis, and feet aligned.

Implementation

Follow the directions below to push, pull, stoop, lift, and carry correctly.

Pushing and pulling correctly

■ Stand close to the object, and place one foot slightly ahead of the other, as in a walking position. Tighten your leg muscles and set your pelvis by simultaneously contracting the abdominal and gluteal muscles.

■ To push, place your hands on a stable part of the object and flex your elbows. Lean into the object by shifting weight from your back leg to your front leg, and apply smooth, continuous pressure (as shown below).

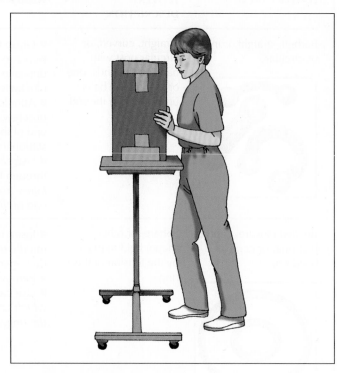

■ To pull, grasp the object and flex your elbows. Lean away from the object by shifting weight from your front leg to your back leg. Pull smoothly, avoiding sudden, jerky movements.

■ After you've started to move the object, keep it in motion; *stopping and starting uses more energy.*

Stooping correctly

■ Stand with your feet 10″ to 12″ (25.5 to 30.5 cm) apart and one foot slightly ahead of the other *to widen the base of support.*

■ Lower yourself by flexing your knees, and place more weight on your front foot than on your back foot. Keep your upper body straight by not bending at the waist (as shown below).

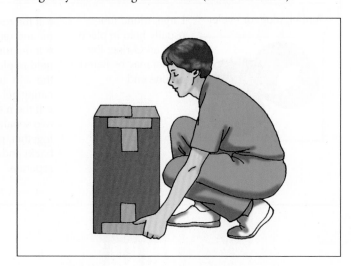

■ To stand up again, straighten your knees and keep your back straight.

Lifting and carrying correctly

■ Assume the stooping position directly in front of the object *to minimize back flexion and avoid spinal rotation when lifting.*
■ Grasp the object, and tighten your abdominal muscles.
■ Stand up by straightening your knees, using your leg and hip muscles. Always keep your back straight *to maintain a fixed center of gravity.* Keep the weight of the object as close to your body as possible (as shown below).

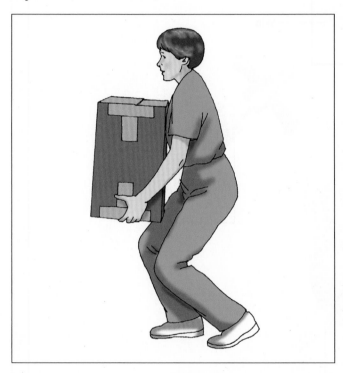

■ Carry the object close to your body at waist height—near the body's center of gravity—*to avoid straining your back muscles.*

Special considerations

■ Wear shoes with low heels, flexible nonslip soles, and closed backs *to promote correct body alignment, promote proper body mechanics, and prevent accidents.*
■ When possible, pull rather than push an object *because the elbow flexors are stronger than the extensors.* Pulling an object allows the use of hip and leg muscles and avoids the use of lower back muscles.
■ When doing heavy lifting or moving, remember to use assistive or mechanical devices, if available, or obtain assistance from coworkers; know your limitations and use sound judgment.
■ Mechanical and other assistive devices have been shown to significantly decrease the incidences of low back injury in nursing personnel.[1]

REFERENCE

1 Taylor, C., et al. (2011). *Fundamentals of nursing: The art and science of nursing care* (7th ed.). Philadelphia, PA: Lippincott Williams & Wilkins.

ADDITIONAL REFERENCES

Craven, R.F., & Hirnle, C.J. (2009). *Fundamentals of nursing: Human health and function* (6th ed.). Philadelphia, PA: Lippincott Williams & Wilkins.
Nelson, A., & Baptiste, A.S. (2006). Evidence-based practices for safe patient handling and movement. *Online Journal of Issues in Nursing, 25*(6), 366–379.
Viera, E. R., et al. (2006). Low back problems and possible improvements in nursing jobs. *Journal for Advanced Nursing, 55*(1), 79–89.

BONE MARROW ASPIRATION AND BIOPSY

Bone marrow is the major site of blood cell formation. A bone marrow specimen may be obtained by aspiration or needle biopsy. Obtaining a specimen allows for evaluation of overall blood composition, blood elements, precursor cells, and abnormal or malignant cells. (See *Obtaining a bone marrow specimen,* page 86.)

Aspiration helps diagnose various disorders and cancers, such as oat cell carcinoma and leukemia as well as such lymphomas as Hodgkin's disease. Cells are removed through a needle inserted into the marrow cavity of the bone. A biopsy removes a small, solid core of marrow tissue through the needle.

Both procedures are usually performed by a doctor, but some facilities authorize specially trained chemotherapy nurses or nurse clinicians to perform them with an assistant. The procedures are usually performed at the same time to stage the disease and monitor the patient's response to treatment. Note, however, that bone marrow biopsy is contraindicated in patients with severe bleeding disorders.

Equipment
For aspiration

Sterile gloves, masks, gowns, and goggles for the doctor and assistant ■ antiseptic solution pads ■ two sterile fenestrated drapes ■ ten 4″ × 4″ gauze pads ■ ten 2″ × 2″ gauze pads ■ two 10-mL syringes ■ 22G 1″ or 2″ needle ■ scalpel ■ sedative, as ordered ■ specimen containers ■ bone marrow needle ■ 70% isopropyl alcohol ■ 1% lidocaine (unopened bottle) ■ 26G or 27G ½″ to ⅝″ needle ■ adhesive tape ■ glass slides and cover glass ■ labels ■ sterile marker ■ sterile labels.

Most of the equipment above is available in a sterile, prepackaged tray. Familiarize yourself with your facility's tray and obtain any additional equipment needed.

For biopsy

All equipment listed above ■ Vim-Silverman, Jamshidi, Illinois sternal, or Westerman-Jensen needle ■ Zenker's fixative.

Implementation

■ Gather the appropriate equipment.
■ Perform hand hygiene and put on gloves.[1,2,3]
■ Confirm the patient's identity using at least two patient identifiers according to your facility's policy.[4]

Obtaining a bone marrow specimen

Aspiration removes cells through a needle inserted into the marrow cavity of the bone; a biopsy removes a small, solid core of marrow tissue through the needle. The illustration below shows the removal of bone marrow from the posterior iliac crest.

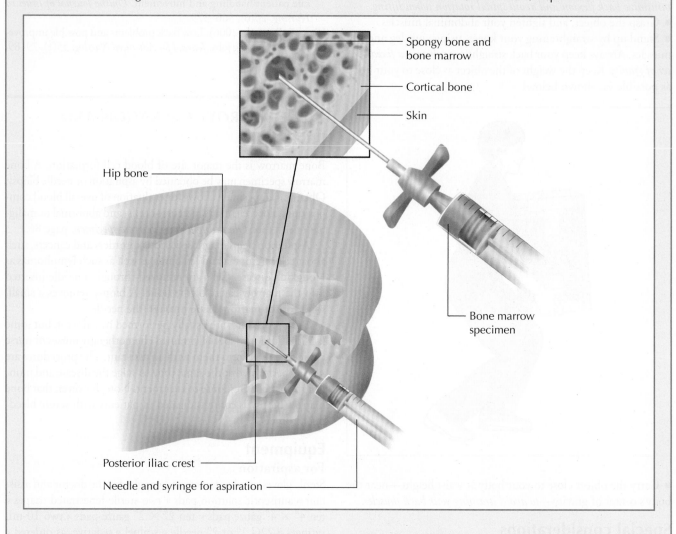

Spongy bone and bone marrow

Cortical bone

Skin

Hip bone

Bone marrow specimen

Posterior iliac crest

Needle and syringe for aspiration

■ Tell the patient that the doctor will collect a bone marrow specimen, and explain the procedure *to ease his anxiety and ensure cooperation.* Tell him which bone will be aspirated. Inform him that he'll receive a local anesthetic and feel heavy pressure from insertion of the biopsy or aspiration needle, as well as a brief pulling sensation. Tell him the doctor may make a small incision *to avoid tearing the skin.*

■ If the patient has osteoporosis, tell him that the needle pressure may be minimal; if he has osteopetrosis, inform him that a drill may be needed.

■ Make sure the patient or a responsible family member understands the procedure and signs a consent form obtained by the doctor.[5]

■ Inform the patient that the procedure normally takes about 20 minutes and that more than one marrow specimen may be required.

■ Check the patient's history for hypersensitivity to the local anesthetic.

■ Conduct a preprocedure verification process *to make sure that all relevant documentation, information, and equipment are available and correctly identified to the patient's identifiers.*[6,7,8]

■ Provide a sedative, as ordered, following safe medication administration practices.

■ Label all medications, medication containers, and other solutions on and off the sterile field.[9]

■ Verify that the doctor has marked the aspiration site with his initials or another unambiguous mark as determined by your facility's policy. Confirm that the correct procedure has been identified for the correct patient at the correct site.[6,7,8]

■ Position the patient according to the selected puncture site and instruct him to remain as still as possible. (See *Common sites for bone marrow aspiration and biopsy.*)

Common sites for bone marrow aspiration and biopsy

The posterior superior iliac crest is the preferred site for aspiration *because the risk of pain is decreased, accessibility is increased, and no vital organs or vessels are nearby.* The patient is placed in the lateral position with one leg flexed or in the prone position. The anterior iliac crest may be used with patients who can't lie prone or when the posterior iliac crest is unapproachable or not available because of infection, injury, or morbid obesity, although this location is generally not preferred *because of its dense cortical layer,* which makes obtaining specimens more difficult, necessitates smaller specimens, and increases the risk of pain.

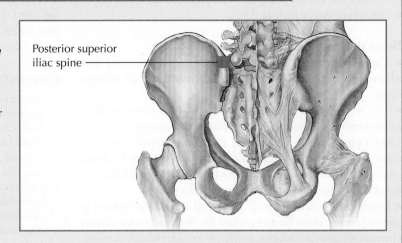

Posterior superior iliac spine

The spinous process of the third or fourth lumbar vertebra is the preferred site if multiple punctures are necessary or marrow is absent at other sites. The patient sits on the edge of the bed, leaning over the bedside stand.

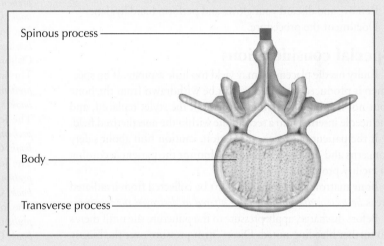

Spinous process

Body

Transverse process

■ Conduct a time-out immediately before starting the procedure *to ensure that the correct patient, site, positioning, and procedure are identified and that, as applicable, all relevant information and necessary equipment are available during and after the procedure.*[6,7,8]

■ Using sterile technique, the puncture site is cleaned with antiseptic solution and allowed to dry; then the area is draped.

■ To anesthetize the site, the doctor infiltrates it with 1% lidocaine, using a 26G or 27G ½" to ⅝" needle to inject a small amount intradermally and then a larger 22G 1" to 2" needle to anesthetize the tissue down to the bone.

■ When the needle tip reaches the bone, the doctor anesthetizes the periosteum by injecting a small amount of lidocaine in a circular area about ¾" (2 cm) in diameter. The needle should be withdrawn from the periosteum after each injection.

■ After allowing about 1 minute for the lidocaine to take effect, a scalpel may be used to make a small stab incision in the patient's skin to accommodate the bone marrow needle. *This technique avoids pushing skin into the bone marrow and also helps avoid unnecessary skin tearing to help reduce the risk of infection.*

Bone marrow aspiration

■ The doctor inserts the bone marrow needle and lodges it firmly in the bone cortex. If the patient feels sharp pain instead of pressure when the needle first touches bone, the needle was probably inserted outside the anesthetized area. If this happens, the needle should be withdrawn slightly and moved to the anesthetized area.

■ The needle is advanced by applying an even, downward force with the heel of the hand or the palm, while twisting it back and forth slightly. A crackling sensation means that the needle has entered the marrow cavity.

■ Next, the doctor removes the inner cannula, attaches the syringe to the needle, aspirates the required specimen (usually 3 to 5 mL), and withdraws the needle. The specimen is placed on glass slides and covered with the coverglass.

■ Label the specimen in the presence of the patient with the patient's name and the date.[9]

■ Remove your gloves, perform hand hygiene, put on clean gloves.[1,2,3]

■ Apply pressure to the aspiration site with a gauze pad for 5 minutes to control bleeding while an assistant prepares the marrow slides. Then clean the area with alcohol to remove the antiseptic solution, dry the skin thoroughly with a 4″ × 4″ gauze pad, and apply a sterile pressure dressing.

■ Remove and discard your gloves and perform hand hygiene.[1,2,3]
■ Document the procedure.[10]

Bone marrow biopsy

■ The doctor inserts the biopsy needle into the periosteum and advances it steadily until the outer needle passes into the marrow cavity.

■ The biopsy needle is directed into the marrow cavity by alternately rotating the inner needle clockwise and counterclockwise. Then a plug of tissue is removed, the needle assembly is withdrawn, and the marrow specimen is expelled into a properly labeled specimen bottle containing Zenker's fixative or formaldehyde.

■ Label the specimen in the presence of the patient.[9]

■ Firmly press a sterile 2″ × 2″ gauze pad against the incision *to control bleeding,* clean the area around the biopsy site with alcohol *to remove the antiseptic solution,* and apply a sterile pressure dressing.

■ Remove and discard your gloves and perform hand hygiene.[1,2,3]
■ Document the procedure.[10]

Special considerations

■ Faulty needle placement may yield too little aspirate. If no specimen is produced, the needle must be withdrawn from the bone (but not from the overlying soft tissue), the stylet replaced, and the needle inserted into a second site within the anesthetized field.

■ If the patient has received sedation, caution him about safety concerns and driving restrictions. Monitor the patient according to facility protocol.

■ Bone marrow specimens shouldn't be collected from irradiated areas *because radiation may have altered or destroyed the marrow.*

■ Before discharge, apply pressure to the puncture site until there's no further bleeding noted. Direct, firm pressure over the biopsy site can be supplemented by having the patient lie supine.

Patient teaching

Instruct the patient to leave the sterile dressing in place for 24 to 48 hours, depending on your facility's guidelines. Advise the patient to avoid tub baths, hot tubs, swimming pools, and whirlpool baths for 48 hours after the procedure *to allow the biopsy site adequate time to heal.* Tell the patient that he may experience mild to moderate discomfort at the site for 24 to 48 hours. He may take analgesics as needed; however he should avoid aspirin and nonsteroidal anti-inflammatory drugs for 24 to 48 hours *to minimize the risk of bleeding from the site.* Instruct the patient to call the doctor if he experiences bleeding or fever after discharge.

Complications

Bleeding and infection are potentially life-threatening complications of aspiration or biopsy at any site. Complications of sternal needle puncture are uncommon but include puncture of the heart and major vessels, causing severe hemorrhage; puncture of the mediastinum, causing mediastinitis or pneumomediastinum; and puncture of the lung, causing pneumothorax.

If a hematoma occurs around the puncture site, apply warm soaks. Give analgesics for site pain or tenderness.

Documentation

Chart the time, date, and location as well as the patient's tolerance of the procedure. Note the amount and color of marrow aspirated, laboratory tests ordered, and time the specimen was sent. Chart the patient's vital signs, pain level, complications, and type of dressing applied. Also document patient teaching.

REFERENCES

1 The Joint Commission. (2012). Standard NPSG.07.01.01. *Comprehensive accreditation manual for hospitals: The official handbook.* Oakbrook Terrace, IL: The Joint Commission. (Level I)

2 World Health Organization. (2009). *WHO guidelines on hand hygiene in health care: First global patient safety challenge. Clean care is safer care.* Geneva, Switzerland: World Health Organization. (Level I)

3 Centers for Disease Control and Prevention. (October 2002). Guideline for hand hygiene in health-care settings. *Morbidity and Mortality Weekly Report, 51* (RR-16), 1–45. (Level I)

4 The Joint Commission. (2012). Standard NPSG.01.01.01. *Comprehensive accreditation manual for hospitals: The official handbook.* Oakbrook Terrace, IL: The Joint Commission. (Level I)

5 The Joint Commission. (2012). Standard RI.01.03.01. *Comprehensive accreditation manual for hospitals: The official handbook.* Oakbrook Terrace, IL: The Joint Commission. (Level I)

6 The Joint Commission. (2012). Standard UP.01.01.01. *Comprehensive accreditation manual for hospitals: The official handbook.* Oakbrook Terrace, IL: The Joint Commission. (Level I)

7 The Joint Commission. (2012). Standard UP.01.02.01. *Comprehensive accreditation manual for hospitals: The official handbook.* Oakbrook Terrace, IL: The Joint Commission. (Level I)

8 The Joint Commission. (2012). Standard UP.01.03.01. *Comprehensive accreditation manual for hospitals: The official handbook.* Oakbrook Terrace, IL: The Joint Commission. (Level I)

9 The Joint Commission. (2012). Standard NPSG.03.04.01. *Comprehensive accreditation manual for hospitals: The official handbook.* Oakbrook Terrace, IL: The Joint Commission. (Level I)

10 The Joint Commission. (2012). Standard RC.01.03.01. *Comprehensive accreditation manual for hospitals: The official handbook.* Oakbrook Terrace, IL: The Joint Commission. (Level I)

ADDITIONAL REFERENCES

Lynn-McHale Wiegand, D.J. (Ed.). (2011). *AACN procedure manual for critical care* (6th ed.). Philadelphia, PA: Saunders.

Nettina, S.M. (2010). *Lippincott manual of nursing practice* (9th ed.). Philadelphia, PA: Lippincott Williams & Wilkins.

Talamo, G., et al. (2010). Oral administration of analgesia and anxiolysis for pain associated with bone marrow biopsy. *Supportive Care in Cancer, 18*(3), 301–305.

BRAIN TISSUE OXYGEN MONITORING AND CARE

Brain tissue oxygen ($P_{bt}O_2$) monitoring is used to measure oxygen delivery to the cerebral tissue and to identify cerebral ischemia and hypoxia in patients with traumatic brain injury, stroke, or aneurysm or traumatic subarachnoid hemorrhage. It's also used to monitor other patients at risk for secondary brain injury. Secondary brain injury typically results when complications, such as elevated intracranial pressure (ICP), shivering, agitation, seizures, fever, hypotension, hypovolemia, anemia, and hypoxia, cause cerebral hypoxia. Cerebral hypoxia, in turn, can lead to cerebral ischemia.

$P_{bt}O_2$ monitoring is achieved using a $P_{bt}O_2$ probe that's inserted through an intracranial bolt or tunneled under the scalp using a probe guide and trocar. When used with an intracranial bolt, the system measures ICP, brain tissue temperature, and $P_{bt}O_2$ saturation. It can detect early changes in ICP and $P_{bt}O_2$ so that treatment interventions can be performed before secondary brain injury occurs. Contraindications of $P_{bt}O_2$ monitoring include anticoagulation therapy, insertion site infection, and coagulopathy.

The normal value for $P_{bt}O_2$ ranges between 20 and 35 mm Hg. Decreased levels occur when there's an increased oxygen demand or a decrease in oxygen delivery. Increased levels occur when there's increased oxygen delivery or decreased oxygen demand.

Equipment

Gloves ▪ goggles ▪ face masks ▪ hair caps ▪ $P_{bt}O_2$ monitor ▪ connecting cables from the monitor to the patient ▪ $P_{bt}O_2$ probe.

Implementation

▪ Verify the doctor's order.
▪ Perform hand hygiene *to reduce the transmission of microorganisms.*[1,2,3]
▪ Confirm the patient's identity using at least two patient identifiers according to your facility's policy.[4]
▪ Ensure that the patient and his family understand the procedure. Answer any questions *to evaluate their understanding of the information provided.*
▪ Put on personal protective equipment as needed.[1,2,3]
▪ Assess the patient's neurologic status, vital signs, ICP, and $P_{bt}O_2$ every 15 minutes until the patient's condition stabilizes, then hourly or according to your facility's policy *to obtain a baseline and for ongoing assessment.*
▪ Perform an oxygen challenge test, as ordered, if the $P_{bt}O_2$ reading is unexpectedly low or if you question the probe accuracy. This can be done by placing the fraction of inspired oxygen (FIO_2) at 100% on the ventilator for 2 to 5 minutes. An accurate probe will show an increase in $P_{bt}O_2$.
▪ Obtain the patient's temperature every 1 to 2 hours and compare it to the cerebral temperature.
▪ Maintain the $P_{bt}O_2$ value between 25 and 35 mm Hg, or as ordered by the doctor.
▪ Perform a comprehensive pain assessment using techniques that are appropriate for the patient's age, condition, and ability to understand. Manage the patient's pain, as ordered.[5]
▪ Remove and discard your personal protective equipment and perform hand hygiene.[1,2,3]
▪ Document the procedure.[6]

Special considerations

▪ $P_{bt}O_2$ probes are compatible with magnetic resonance imaging machines unless they have a fiber-optic ICP device.

▪ For most patients, the goal is to have a $P_{bt}O_2$ reading of greater than 20 mm Hg.
▪ Probes may remain in place for 5 to 7 days. Check the manufacturer's guidelines and your facility's policy.

Complications

Possible complications include infection, cerebrospinal fluid leak, and bleeding.

Documentation

Document neurologic assessment findings; vital signs; ICP; temperature; teaching provided to the patient and his family and their understanding of the teaching; the patient's tolerance of the procedure; insertion site assessment; and any unexpected complications or outcomes if applicable. Record $P_{bt}O_2$ readings at least every hour or according to your facility's policy.

REFERENCES

1 The Joint Commission. (2012). Standard NPSG.07.01.01. *Comprehensive accreditation manual for hospitals: The official handbook.* Oakbrook Terrace, IL: The Joint Commission. (Level I)
2 World Health Organization. (2009). *WHO guidelines on hand hygiene in health care: First global patient safety challenge. Clean care is safer care.* Geneva, Switzerland: World Health Organization. (Level I)
3 Centers for Disease Control and Prevention. (October 2002). Guideline for hand hygiene in health-care settings. *Morbidity and Mortality Weekly Report, 51* (RR-16), 1–45. (Level I)
4 The Joint Commission. (2012). Standard NPSG.01.01.01. *Comprehensive accreditation manual for hospitals: The official handbook.* Oakbrook Terrace, IL: The Joint Commission. (Level I)
5 The Joint Commission. (2012). Standard PC.01.02.07. *Comprehensive accreditation manual for hospitals: The official handbook.* Oakbrook Terrace, IL: The Joint Commission. (Level I)
6 The Joint Commission. (2012). Standard RC.01.03.01. *Comprehensive accreditation manual for hospitals: The official handbook.* Oakbrook Terrace, IL: The Joint Commission. (Level I)

ADDITIONAL REFERENCES

Leichter, D., et al. (2005). Brain tissue oxygen practice guidelines using the LICOX® CMP monitoring system. *Journal of Neuroscience Nursing, 37*(5), 278–288.
Lynn-McHale Wiegand, D.J. (Ed.). (2011). *AACN procedure manual for critical care* (6th ed.). Philadelphia, PA: Saunders.
Siegel, J.D., et al. "2007 guideline for isolation precautions: Preventing transmission of infectious agents in healthcare settings" [Online]. Accessed June 2011 via the Web at http://www.cdc.gov/hicpac/ 2007ip/2007isolationprecautions.html

BRAIN TISSUE OXYGEN MONITORING DEVICE INSERTION, ASSISTING

Brain tissue oxygen ($P_{bt}O_2$) monitoring measures oxygen delivery to cerebral tissue. (See "Brain tissue oxygen monitoring and care," page 88.) To allow for monitoring of $P_{bt}O_2$, the doctor tunnels a $P_{bt}O_2$ probe under the patient's scalp using a probe guide and trocar. Alternatively, he may insert the probe through an intracranial bolt that he then inserts through a burr hole. When used with an intracranial bolt, the system measures $P_{bt}O_2$, brain tissue temperature, and intracranial pressure (ICP).

The doctor determines the insertion method and placement location after studying a computed tomography (CT) scan of the patient's brain and considering the patient's diagnosis. Normal values for $P_{bt}O_2$ range from 20 to 35 mm Hg. (See *Brain tissue oxygen monitoring systems.*)

Equipment

Sterile gloves, gowns, and drapes ▪ goggles, face masks, and hair caps ▪ antiseptic solution ▪ $P_{bt}O_2$ monitor ▪ connecting cables from the monitor to the patient ▪ cranial access tray ▪ $P_{bt}O_2$ probe ▪ 4″ × 4″ gauze ▪ tape ▪ sterile dry gauze ▪ intracranial bolt system ▪ central line dressing change kit ▪ sterile occlusive dressing ▪ clippers ▪ #11 scalpel blade.

Preparation of equipment

Gather the $P_{bt}O_2$ monitor and plug it into AC wall outlet. Next, attach the cables to the $P_{bt}O_2$ monitor. Some monitors and cables are color-coded.

Implementation

▪ Verify the doctor's orders.
▪ Make sure that informed consent has been obtained and is documented in the patient's medical record.[1]
▪ Conduct a preprocedure verification *to make sure that all relevant documentation, related information, and equipment are available and correctly identified to the patient's identifiers.*[2,3,4]
▪ Verify that the laboratory and imaging studies have been completed, as ordered, and that the results are in the patient's medical record. Notify the doctor of any unexpected results.
▪ Perform hand hygiene *to reduce the transmission of microorganisms.*[5,6,7]
▪ Confirm the patient's identity using at least two patient identifiers according to your facility's policy.[8]
▪ Make sure that the patient and his family understand the procedure. Answer any questions *to evaluate their understanding of the information provided.*
▪ Administer analgesia, sedation, or both as ordered before beginning the insertion procedure *to facilitate the insertion process.*
▪ Prepare the equipment, being careful not to contaminate the sterile field. Label all medications, medication containers, and other solutions on and off the sterile field while maintaining sterility of the sterile field.[9]
▪ Elevate the head of the bed to 30 to 45 degrees and place the patient's head in the neutral position. *This position helps decrease ICP by promoting jugular venous outflow, which provides for optimal insertion accessibility.*[10]
▪ Verify that the doctor has marked the insertion site with his initials or with another unambiguous mark set by your facility's policy before the procedure is performed.[2,3,4]
▪ Perform hand hygiene and assist the doctor with putting on protective eyewear, a mask, a cap, a sterile gown, and sterile gloves, as necessary. Put on the same personal protective equipment.[5,6,7]

▪ Conduct a time-out immediately before starting the procedure *to perform a final assessment that the correct patient, site, positioning, and procedure are identified and all relevant information and necessary equipment are available.*[2,3,4]
▪ Assist the doctor with site preparation, such as clipping hair and using antiseptic solution *to prepare the patient for a sterile procedure.* Use antiseptic solution according to your facility's policy. Use of chlorhexidine is disputed *because studies suggest chlorhexidine is neurotoxic.* Make sure that the antiseptic is dry before the doctor starts the incision.
▪ Assist the doctor with draping the patient's head, neck, and chest *to maintain a sterile field.*
▪ Assist the doctor with opening sterile trays, packages, probes, and other equipment *to help maintain a sterile environment and provide efficiency.*
▪ Turn on the $P_{bt}O_2$ monitor and follow the manufacturer's guidelines *to prepare the monitor.*
▪ If you are using a Licox monitor, place the smart card into the card slot located on the front of the monitor. *This monitor requires the smart card numbers to match those on the oxygen probe that the doctor will insert.*
▪ Assist the doctor with intracranial bolt insertion, which may be inserted before the $P_{bt}O_2$ probe is inserted.
▪ Assist the doctor with the oxygen and temperature probe insertions.
▪ After the doctor inserts the oxygen and temperature probes, connect them to the monitor cables.
▪ Look at the monitor for temperature and $P_{bt}O_2$ values. *Temperature values will be accurate but $P_{bt}O_2$ values may take as long as 2 hours to be accurate as brain tissue settles after the trauma of probe placement.*
▪ Depending on the beside monitor, you may be able to use a cable to capture the values from the $P_{bt}O_2$ monitor to the bedside monitor *to allow integration between monitoring systems.*
▪ Apply dry sterile gauze at the insertion site in a conical shape *to prevent an infection. A conical dressing forms a base to secure the probes to an arm board or other securing device.*
▪ Secure the $P_{bt}O_2$ monitor cables *to prevent tension at the insertion site.* Anchor cables from the patient's head and shoulder with a transparent adhesive dressing. *It's important to make sure that the entire setup is supported but allows enough slack for the patient to be turned and moved.* You may place towels or washcloths under the setup for support. Make sure that the cables aren't dragging on the ground.
▪ Discard used supplies in the appropriate containers.
▪ Remove and discard your personal protective equipment and perform hand hygiene.[5,6,7]
▪ Document the procedure.[11]

Special considerations

▪ Assess the patient's neurologic status before insertion *so that you can recognize any changes during and after insertion of the $P_{bt}O_2$ probe.*
▪ $P_{bt}O_2$ probes are compatible with magnetic resonance imaging machines unless they have a fiber-optic ICP device.

Brain tissue oxygen monitoring systems

Brain tissue oxygen ($P_{bt}O_2$) can be monitored using a tunneled system or a bolt system.

Tunneled system

With the *tunneled system,* shown at right, an oxygen catheter probe is tunneled under the scalp using a probe guide and trocar. It may be inserted during a cranial procedure at the margins of an existing bone flap or it may be inserted through a burr hole.

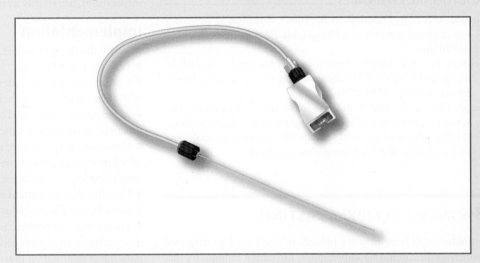

Bolt system

A *bolt system,* shown at right, is inserted through a burr hole and has the capability of monitoring $P_{bt}O_2$, brain tissue temperature, and intracranial pressure.

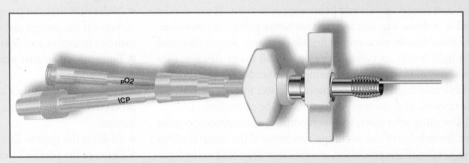

■ Probes may remain in place for 5 to 7 days. Check the manufacturer's guidelines and your facility's policy.

Complications

Possible complications include infection, cerebrospinal fluid leak, and bleeding.

Documentation

Document neurologic assessments; ICP; vital signs including temperature; teaching provided to the patient and his family and their understanding of the teaching; the patient's tolerance of the procedure; insertion site assessment; and any unexpected complications or outcomes if applicable. Record $P_{bt}O_2$ readings at least every hour.

REFERENCES

1 The Joint Commission. (2012). Standard RI.01.03.01. *Comprehensive accreditation manual for hospitals: The official handbook.* Oakbrook Terrace, IL: The Joint Commission. (Level I)

2 The Joint Commission. (2012). Standard UP.01.01.01. *Comprehensive accreditation manual for hospitals: The official handbook.* Oakbrook Terrace, IL: The Joint Commission. (Level I)

3 The Joint Commission. (2012). Standard UP.01.02.01. *Comprehensive accreditation manual for hospitals: The official handbook.* Oakbrook Terrace, IL: The Joint Commission. (Level I)

4 The Joint Commission. (2012). Standard UP.01.03.01. *Comprehensive accreditation manual for hospitals: The official handbook.* Oakbrook Terrace, IL: The Joint Commission. (Level I)

5 The Joint Commission. (2012). Standard NPSG.07.01.01. *Comprehensive accreditation manual for hospitals: The official handbook.* Oakbrook Terrace, IL: The Joint Commission. (Level I)

6 World Health Organization. (2009). *WHO guidelines on hand hygiene in health care: First global patient safety challenge. Clean care is safer care.* Geneva, Switzerland: World Health Organization. (Level I)

7 Centers for Disease Control and Prevention. (October 2002). Guideline for hand hygiene in health-care settings. *Morbidity and Mortality Weekly Report, 51* (RR-16), 1–45. (Level I)

8 The Joint Commission. (2012). Standard NPSG.01.01.01. *Comprehensive accreditation manual for hospitals: The official handbook.* Oakbrook Terrace, IL: The Joint Commission. (Level I)

9 The Joint Commission. (2012). Standard NPSG.03.04.01. *Comprehensive accreditation manual for hospitals: The official handbook.* Oakbrook Terrace, IL: The Joint Commission. (Level I)

10 Lynn-McHale Wiegand, D. J. (Ed.). (2011). *AACN procedure manual for critical care* (6th ed.). Philadelphia, PA: Saunders.

11 The Joint Commission. (2012). Standard RC.01.03.01. *Comprehensive accreditation manual for hospitals: The official handbook.* Oakbrook Terrace, IL: The Joint Commission. (Level I)

ADDITIONAL REFERENCES

Fischbach, F.T., & Dunning, M.B. (2009). *A manual of laboratory and diagnostic tests* (8th ed.). Philadelphia, PA: Lippincott Williams & Wilkins.

Leichter, D., et al. (2005). Brain tissue oxygen practice guidelines using the LICOX® CMP monitoring system. *Journal of Neuroscience Nursing, 37*(5), 278–288.

Siegel, J.D., et al. "2007 Guideline for isolation precautions: Preventing transmission of infectious agents in healthcare settings" [Online]. Accessed June 2011 via the Web at http://www.cdc.gov/hicpac/2007ip/2007isolationprecautions.html

BRONCHOSCOPY, ASSISTING

Bronchoscopy is an invasive procedure that's used to diagnose bronchogenic carcinoma, tuberculosis, interstitial pulmonary disease, and fungal or parasitic pulmonary infections. It can also be used to evaluate, manage, and treat numerous pulmonary processes. The procedure involves using a flexible fiber-optic scope connected to a light source to visualize the upper and lower airways. (See *Features of the bronchoscope.*) During the procedure, specimens can be collected from the tracheobronchial tree, foreign objects can be removed, and massive hemoptysis can be controlled.

The nurse who assists the doctor during a bronchoscopy must have knowledge of the technique, understand the complications associated with the procedure, and function according to the facility's policy. Responsibilities may include patient preparation and monitoring, handling specimens, and postprocedure care and monitoring.

Equipment

Bronchoscope ▪ suction apparatus ▪ specimen container ▪ cytology brush ▪ bite block ▪ sterile gauze sponges ▪ topical anesthetic (viscous lidocaine, 1% lidocaine, and 1% lidocaine with epinephrine) ▪ syringes (5 mL and 30 mL) ▪ pulse oximeter ▪ nebulizer equipment ▪ cardiac monitor system ▪ blood pressure monitor ▪ oxygen delivery equipment ▪ emergency equipment (code cart with cardiac medications, defibrillator, intubation equipment) ▪ personal protective equipment ▪ 150-mL bottle of normal saline solution ▪ prescribed sedative and its reversal agent (to reverse adverse effects if necessary) ▪ Optional: ventilator, capnography monitoring equipment, intubation equipment, IV insertion equipment, ventilator adapter, prescribed medications.

Preparation of equipment

Prepare intubation equipment if endotracheal intubation is necessary. Apply lidocaine to the gauze sponges for lubricating the bronchoscope. Fill five 30-mL syringes with normal saline solution, one 5-mL syringe with viscous lidocaine for local anesthesia, one 5-mL syringe with 1% lidocaine with epinephrine, and three 10-mL syringes with 1% lidocaine. Label all medications

appropriately *to prevent medication errors.*[1] Set up suction equipment and make sure it's functioning properly. Fill specimen containers with normal saline solution. Make sure other emergency equipment, such as a defibrillator and crash cart with cardiac medications, are readily available *in case complications arise.*

Implementation

- Verify the doctor's orders.
- Perform hand hygiene.[2,3,4]
- Confirm the patient's identity using at least two patient identifiers according to your facility's policy.[5]
- Make sure that informed consent has been obtained and is documented in the patient's medical record.[6]
- Conduct a preprocedure verification process *to make sure that all relevant documentation, related information, and equipment are available and correctly identified to the patient's identifiers.*[7]
- Confirm that the patient has had nothing by mouth for at least 4 hours before the procedure.
- Ensure that the patient and his family understand the procedure; answer any questions they may have *to evaluate understanding of information previously given.*
- Make sure that the patient has patent IV access. Insert an IV catheter, if the patient doesn't already have one in place. (See "IV catheter insertion and removal," page 421.)
- Ensure that a sedative was administered 30 to 45 minutes before the procedure.
- Perform hand hygiene and put on gloves and other personal protective equipment, including a mask and eye protection as needed.[2,3,4]
- Position the patient in a semi-recumbent or supine position.
- Remove the patient's dentures and eyeglasses, if applicable.
- Conduct a time-out *to ensure that the correct patient, site, positioning, and procedure are identified and that all relevant information and necessary equipment are available.*[7]
- Obtain vital signs and perform pulse oximetry *to establish a baseline for comparison.*
- Monitor the patient's respiratory status, including pulse oximetry readings, ensuring that the low saturation alarm is set at 90%.
- Connect the patient to a continuous cardiac monitor *to monitor for arrhythmias during the procedure.*
- Administer the anesthetic agent using a nebulizer or an atomizer as ordered.
- Administer oxygen therapy, as ordered, *to prevent hypoxia.*
- Administer moderate sedation, as ordered, following safe medication administration practices *to relieve the patient's anxiety and promote cooperation.* (See "Moderate sedation," page 480.)
- If the patient is intubated, insert a bite block *to prevent the patient from biting down on the endotracheal tube during the procedure.*
- Hand the bronchoscope to the doctor and turn on its light source.
- The doctor sprays a local anesthetic into the patient's mouth and throat.
- The doctor introduces the bronchoscope through the patient's mouth or nose. When the bronchoscope is just above the vocal

Features of the bronchoscope

The bronchoscope, inserted through the nostril into the bronchi, has four channels (see inset): two light channels (A), which provide a light source; one visualizing channel (B) to see through; and one open channel (C), which accommodates biopsy forceps, a cytology brush, suction apparatus, a lavage device, anesthetic, or oxygen.

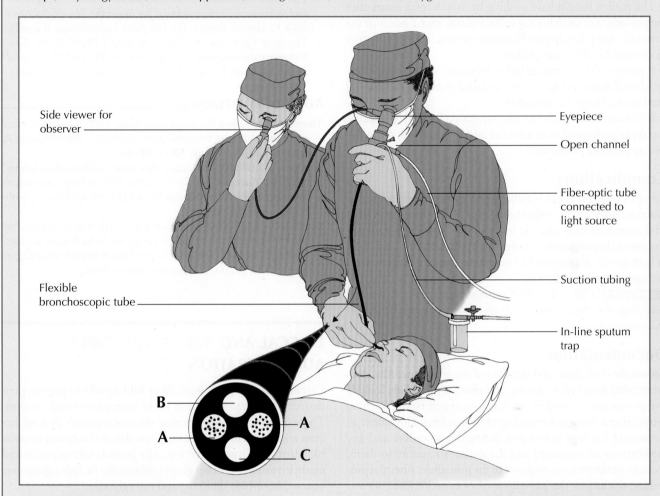

Side viewer for observer

Flexible bronchoscopic tube

B

A

C

Eyepiece

Open channel

Fiber-optic tube connected to light source

Suction tubing

In-line sputum trap

---

cords, lidocaine is flushed through the inner channel of the scope to the vocal cords *to anesthetize deeper areas.*

■ The doctor inspects the trachea and bronchi, observes the color of the mucosal lining, and notes masses or inflamed areas. The doctor may use biopsy forceps *to remove a tissue specimen from a suspect area,* a cytology brush *to obtain cells from the surface of a lesion,* or a suction apparatus *to remove foreign bodies or mucus plugs.*

■ Assist the doctor with lavage, if necessary, to remove thickened secretions.

■ Assist with specimen collection. Place the specimens in appropriate containers and then label the specimen containers in the presence of the patient *to prevent mislabeling.*

■ Assess the patient's vital signs, pulse oximetry readings, and level of consciousness during the procedure. If the patient is intubated, monitor tidal volume, peak inspiratory pressure, and inspiratory flow. Inform the doctor immediately of any abnormalities.

■ Maintain the patient's oxygen saturation (as monitored by pulse oximetry) above 90%. If needed, increase oxygen delivery according to the doctor's order.

■ Perform oral suctioning as needed *to maintain a patent airway and prevent aspiration.*

■ Make sure that the bronchoscope is properly cleaned and disinfected after the procedure according to your facility's policy.

■ Discard trash in the proper receptacles.

■ Remove personal protective equipment and perform hand hygiene.[2,3,4]

■ Document the procedure.[9]

Special considerations

■ After the procedure, if the patient is conscious, position him in semi-Fowler's position. If the patient is unconscious, position him on one side with the head of the bed slightly elevated.

■ After the procedure, encourage the patient to expectorate saliva instead of swallowing it. Notify the doctor if he develops fever, chest pain, discomfort, shortness of breath, abnormal breath sounds, or hemoptysis.

■ The doctor may order a chest X-ray after the procedure, especially after a transbronchial biopsy, to rule out a pneumothorax.

■ The patient should have nothing by mouth for 2 hours after the procedure or until his gag reflex returns; after 2 hours or the return of a gag reflex, begin offering the patient small sips of water to evaluate his ability to swallow.

■ A patient with respiratory failure who can't breathe adequately by himself may need to be intubated and placed on mechanical ventilation during the procedure.

■ If it's suspected that the patient has tuberculosis, the procedure should be performed in an airborne infection isolation room following airborne precautions.

Complications

Complications include bleeding, respiratory depression, cardiorespiratory arrest, arrhythmia, and pneumothorax. Other adverse events may include hypoxemia, hypercapnia, bronchospasm, hypotension, laryngospasm, bradycardia, epistaxis, or hemoptysis. Transbronchial biopsies are associated with hemorrhage and pneumothorax.

NURSING ALERT *The risk of complications is higher in patients with coagulopathy, refractory hypoxemia, and unstable hemodynamic status.*

Documentation

Record the date, time, and duration of the procedure. Also document vital signs before, during, and after the procedure. Include any preprocedure activities, such as patient and family teaching provided and their understanding of the teaching. Document all assessment findings before and during the procedure and any medications administered and the patient's response to them. Document the patient's response to the procedure. After the procedure, document the patient's level of consciousness, airway patency, respiratory rate and depth, pulse oximetry levels, and whether supplemental oxygen was used.

REFERENCES

1 The Joint Commission. (2012). Standard NPSG.03.04.01. *Comprehensive accreditation manual for hospitals: The official handbook.* Oakbrook Terrace, IL: The Joint Commission. (Level I)

2 The Joint Commission. (2012). Standard NPSG.07.01.01. *Comprehensive accreditation manual for hospitals: The official handbook.* Oakbrook Terrace, IL: The Joint Commission. (Level I)

3 World Health Organization. (2009). *WHO guidelines on hand hygiene in health care: First global patient safety challenge. Clean care is safer care.* Geneva, Switzerland: World Health Organization. (Level I)

4 Centers for Disease Control and Prevention. (October 2002). Guideline for hand hygiene in health-care settings. *Morbidity and Mortality Weekly Report, 51* (RR-16), 1–45. (Level I)

5 The Joint Commission. (2012). Standard NPSG.01.01.01. *Comprehensive accreditation manual for hospitals: The official handbook.* Oakbrook Terrace, IL: The Joint Commission. (Level I)

6 The Joint Commission. (2012). Standard RI.01.03.01. *Comprehensive accreditation manual for hospitals: The official handbook.* Oakbrook Terrace, IL: The Joint Commission. (Level I)

7 The Joint Commission. (2012). Standard UP.01.01.01. *Comprehensive accreditation manual for hospitals: The official handbook.* Oakbrook Terrace, IL: The Joint Commission. (Level I)

8 The Joint Commission. (2012). Standard UP.01.03.01. *Comprehensive accreditation manual for hospitals: The official handbook.* Oakbrook Terrace, IL: The Joint Commission. (Level I)

9 The Joint Commission. (2012). Standard RC.01.03.01. *Comprehensive accreditation manual for hospitals: The official handbook.* Oakbrook Terrace, IL: The Joint Commission. (Level I)

ADDITIONAL REFERENCES

American Association for Respiratory Care. (2007). AARC clinical practice guideline: Bronchoscopy assisting—2007 revision & update. *Respiratory Care, 52*(1), 74–80.

Kaufman, D. (2006). "Bronchoscopy with transbronchial biopsy" [Online]. Accessed July 2011 via the Web at http://www.medhelp.org/medical-information/show/3332/Bronchoscopy-with-transbronchial-biopsy

Siegel, J.D., et al. "2007 guideline for isolation precautions: Preventing transmission of infectious agents in healthcare settings" [Online]. Accessed June 2011 via the Web at http://www.cdc.gov/hicpac/2007ip/2007isolationprecautions.html

BUCCAL AND SUBLINGUAL DRUG ADMINISTRATION

Certain drugs are given buccally or sublingually to prevent their destruction or transformation in the stomach or small intestine. These drugs act quickly because the oral mucosa's thin epithelium and abundant vasculature allow direct absorption into the bloodstream. Drugs given buccally include nitroglycerin and methyltestosterone; drugs given sublingually include ergotamine tartrate, isosorbide dinitrate, and nitroglycerin.

Equipment

Patient's medication record and chart ■ prescribed medication ■ medication cup.

Implementation

■ Verify the order on the patient's medication record by checking it against the doctor's order on his chart.[1,2]

■ Perform hand hygiene.[3,4,5]

■ Confirm the patient's identity using at least two patient identifiers according to your facility's policy.[6]

■ If your facility uses a bar code scanning system, be sure to scan your ID badge, the patient's ID bracelet, and the medication's bar code.

■ Explain the procedure to the patient if he's never taken a drug buccally or sublingually before.

■ Check the label on the medication three times before administering it to make sure you'll be giving the prescribed medication. Verify the expiration date of all medications, especially nitroglycerin.[7]

■ For buccal administration, place the tablet in the buccal pouch, between the cheek and gum. For sublingual administration, place the tablet under the patient's tongue. (See *Placing drugs in the oral mucosa.*)

■ Instruct the patient to keep the medication in place until it dissolves completely *to ensure absorption.*

■ Caution him against chewing the tablet or touching it with his tongue *to prevent accidental swallowing.*

■ Tell him not to smoke before the drug has dissolved *because nicotine's vasoconstrictive effects slow absorption.*

■ Perform hands hygiene.[3,4,5]

■ Document the procedure.[8]

Special considerations

■ Don't give liquids to a patient who's receiving buccal medication *because some buccal tablets can take up to 1 hour to be absorbed.* Tell the patient not to rinse his mouth until the tablet has been absorbed.

■ Tell the patient with angina to wet the nitroglycerin tablet with saliva and to keep it under his tongue until it has been fully absorbed.

Complications

Some buccal medications may irritate the mucosa. Alternate sides of the mouth for repeat doses to prevent continuous irritation of the same site. Sublingual medications, such as nitroglycerin, may cause a tingling sensation under the tongue. If the patient finds this sensation bothersome, try placing the drug in the buccal pouch instead.

Documentation

Record the medication administered, dose, route, date and time, and patient's reaction, if any.

REFERENCES

1 The Joint Commission. (2012). Standard MM.06.01.01. *Comprehensive accreditation manual for hospitals: The official handbook.* Oakbrook Terrace, IL: The Joint Commission. (Level I)

2 Centers for Medicare & Medicaid Services, Department of Health and Human Services. (2006). "Conditions of Participation: Nursing Services," 42 CFR part 482.23 [Online]. Accessed November 2011 via the Web at http://cfr.vlex.com/vid/482-23-condition-participation-nursing-19811372

3 The Joint Commission. (2012). Standard NPSG.07.01.01. *Comprehensive accreditation manual for hospitals: The official handbook.* Oakbrook Terrace, IL: The Joint Commission. (Level I)

4 World Health Organization. (2009). *WHO guidelines on hand hygiene in health care: First global patient safety challenge. Clean care is safer care.* Geneva, Switzerland: World Health Organization. (Level I)

5 Centers for Disease Control and Prevention. (October 2002). Guideline for hand hygiene in health-care settings. *Morbidity and Mortality Weekly Report, 51* (RR-16), 1–45. (Level I)

6 The Joint Commission. (2012). Standard NPSG.01.01.01. *Comprehensive accreditation manual for hospitals: The official handbook.* Oakbrook Terrace, IL: The Joint Commission. (Level I)

7 Westbrook, J., et al. (2010). Association of interruptions with an increased risk and severity of medication administration errors. *Archives of Internal Medicine, 170*(8), 683–690.

Placing drugs in the oral mucosa

Buccal and sublingual administration routes allow some drugs, such as nitroglycerin and methyltestosterone, to enter the bloodstream rapidly without being degraded in the GI tract. To give a drug buccally, insert it between the patient's cheek and teeth (as shown below). Ask her to close her mouth and hold the tablet against her cheek until the tablet is absorbed.

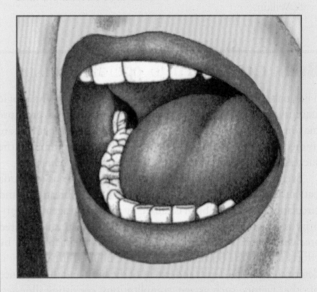

To give a drug sublingually, place it under the patient's tongue (as shown below), and ask her to leave it there until it's dissolved.

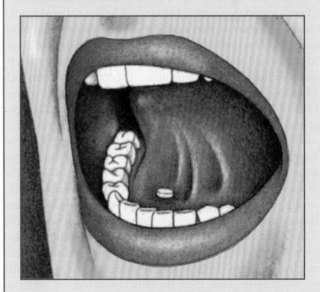

8 The Joint Commission. (2012). Standard RC.02.01.01. *Comprehensive accreditation manual for hospitals: The official handbook.* Oakbrook Terrace, IL: The Joint Commission. (Level I)

Additional references

Craven, R.F., & Hirnle, C. J. (2009). *Fundamentals of nursing: Human health and function* (6th ed.). Philadelphia, PA: Lippincott Williams & Wilkins.

Nettina, S.M. (2010). *Lippincott manual of nursing practice* (9th ed.). Philadelphia, PA: Lippincott Williams & Wilkins.

Taylor, C., et al. (2011). *Fundamentals of nursing: The art and science of nursing care* (7th ed.). Philadelphia, PA: Lippincott Williams & Wilkins.

Burn care

The goals of burn care are to maintain the patient's physiologic stability, repair skin integrity, prevent infection, and promote maximal functioning and psychosocial health. Competent care immediately after a burn occurs can dramatically improve the success of overall treatment. (See *Burn care at the scene.*)

Every burn victim should be evaluated initially as a trauma patient. Focus on maintaining the patient's airway, breathing, and circulation. When the burn is caused by a chemical agent, the priority is to remove the offending agent and irrigate the affected area with water. Next, do a head-to-toe assessment followed by efforts to stop the burn and contain the injury. Burn severity is determined by the depth and extent of the burn and the presence of other factors, such as age, complications, coexisting illnesses, and the possibility of abuse. (See *Estimating burn surfaces in adults and children* and *Evaluating burn severity,* pages 98, 99.)

To promote stability, you'll need to carefully monitor your patient's respiratory status, especially if he has suffered smoke inhalation. Be aware that a patient with burns involving more than 20% of his total body surface area usually needs fluid resuscitation, which aims to support the body's compensatory mechanisms without overwhelming them.[1] Expect to give fluids (such as lactated Ringer's solution) to keep the patient's urine output at 0.5 to 1 mL/kg/hour for children and 1 to 1.5 mL/kg/hour for adults, and expect to monitor blood pressure and heart rate.[1] You'll also need to control body temperature because skin loss interferes with temperature regulation. Use warm fluids, heat lamps, and hyperthermia blankets, as appropriate, to keep the patient's temperature above 97° F (36.1° C), if possible. Additionally, you'll frequently review laboratory values such as serum electrolyte levels to detect early changes in the patient's condition.

Infection can increase wound depth, cause rejection of skin grafts, slow healing, worsen pain, prolong hospitalization, and even lead to death. To help prevent infection, use strict sterile technique during care, dress the burn site as ordered, monitor and rotate IV lines regularly, and carefully assess the burn extent, body system functions, and the patient's emotional status.

Early positioning after a burn is extremely important to prevent contractures. Careful positioning and regular exercise for burned extremities help maintain joint function and minimize deformity. When the extremities aren't being exercised, they should be maintained in maximal extension, using splints, if necessary. Particular attention should be focused on the hands and neck because they are the most prone to rapid contracture.[2] (See *Positioning the burn patient to prevent deformity,* page 100.)

Early excision and debridement of the wound in the first 48 hours has been shown to decrease blood loss and reduce the duration of the health care facility stay; however, this procedure should be used only on wounds that are clearly full-thickness burns.

Equipment

Normal saline solution ■ sterile bowl ■ sterile scissors ■ tissue forceps ■ ordered topical medication ■ burn gauze ■ roller gauze ■ elastic netting or tape ■ fine-mesh gauze ■ elastic gauze ■ cotton-tipped applicators or sterile tongue depressor ■ ordered pain medication ■ sterile gloves ■ sterile gown ■ mask ■ surgical cap ■ heat lamps ■ impervious plastic trash bag ■ cotton bath blanket ■ 4″ × 4″ sterile gauze pad ■ Optional: moisture chambers for eyes.

A sterile field is required, and all equipment and supplies used in the dressing should be sterile.

Preparation of equipment

Warm normal saline solution by immersing unopened bottles in warm water. Gather equipment on the dressing table. Make sure the treatment area has adequate light *to allow accurate wound assessment.* Open equipment packages using sterile technique. Arrange supplies on a sterile field in order of use.

Implementation

■ Verify the doctor's orders.
■ Confirm the patient's identity using at least two patient identifiers according to your facility's policy.[3]
■ Explain the procedure to the patient and provide privacy.
■ Perform hand hygiene. Put on appropriate barrier attire, including sterile gloves.[2,4,5,6]
■ Assess the patient's pain. If ordered, administer an analgesic *to increase the patient's comfort and tolerance levels.* Oral analgesics should be given at an appropriate time before the procedure, depending on the medication's onset and peak of action. An IV analgesic may be given immediately before the procedure.[5]
■ Turn on overhead heat lamps *to keep the patient warm.* Make sure that they don't overheat the patient.
■ Pour warmed normal saline solution into the sterile bowl in the sterile field.

Removing a dressing without hydrotherapy

■ Remove old dressing layers down to the innermost layer by cutting the outer dressings with sterile blunt scissors. Lay open the dressings.
■ If the innermost layer appears dry, soak it with warm normal saline solution *to ease removal.*
■ Remove the inner dressing with sterile tissue forceps or your gloved hand.
■ Dispose of the dressings in the impervious plastic trash bag, according to your facility's policy, *because soiled dressings harbor infectious organisms.*

Burn care at the scene

By acting promptly when a burn injury occurs, you can improve a patient's chance of uncomplicated recovery. Emergency care at the scene should include steps to stop the burn from worsening; assessment of the patient's airway, breathing, and circulation (ABCs); a call for help from an emergency medical team; and emotional and physiologic support for the patient.

Stop the burning process

■ If the victim is on fire, tell him to fall to the ground and roll to put out the flames. (*If he panics and runs, air will fuel the flames, worsening the burn and increasing the risk of inhalation injury.*) Or, if you can, wrap the victim in a blanket or other large covering *to smother the flames and protect the burned area from dirt.* Keep his head outside the blanket *so that he doesn't breathe toxic fumes.* As soon as the flames are out, unwrap the patient *so that the heat can dissipate.*

■ Cool the burned area with any nonflammable liquid *to decrease pain and stop the burn from growing deeper or larger.*

■ If possible, remove any potential sources of heat, such as jewelry, belt buckles, and some types of clothing. *In addition to adding to the burning process, these items may cause constriction as edema develops.* If the patient's clothing adheres to his skin, don't try to remove it. Rather, cut around it.

■ Cover the wound with a clean, dry, sheet or other smooth, nonfuzzy material.

Assess the damage

■ Assess the patient's ABCs, and perform cardiopulmonary resuscitation, if necessary. Then check for other serious injuries, such as fractures, spinal cord injury, lacerations, blunt trauma, and head contusions.

■ Estimate the extent and depth of the burns. If flames caused the burns and the injury occurred in a closed space, assess for signs of inhalation injury: singed nasal hairs, burns on the face or mouth, soot-stained sputum, coughing or hoarseness, wheezing, or respiratory distress. Also assess for signs of carbon monoxide poisoning: dizziness, nausea, headache, and seizures.

■ Call for help as quickly as possible. Send someone to contact the emergency medical service (EMS).

■ If the patient is conscious and alert, try to get a brief medical history as soon as possible.

■ Reassure the patient that help is on the way. Provide emotional support by staying with him, answering questions, and explaining what's being done for him.

■ When help arrives, give the EMS a report on the patient's status.

■ Dispose of your gloves and perform hand hygiene. Put on new sterile gloves.[2,4,5,6]

■ Clean the wound with cotton-tipped applicators and normal saline solution, removing exudates and crusts as necessary.

■ Assess the wound condition.

■ Remove your sterile gloves and other barrier attire and discard them according to facility policy.

■ Perform hand hygiene and put on new barrier attire, including sterile gloves.[2,4,5,6]

Applying a wet dressing

■ Soak fine-mesh gauze and the elastic gauze dressing in a large sterile basin containing the ordered solution, such as silver nitrate.

■ Wring out the fine-mesh gauze until it is damp and not dripping. Apply it to the wound.

■ Wring out the elastic gauze dressing and position it to hold the fine-mesh gauze in place.

■ Roll an elastic gauze dressing over these two dressings *to keep them intact.*

■ Cover the patient with a cotton bath blanket *to prevent chills.* Change the blanket if it becomes damp. Use an overhead heat lamp, if necessary.

Applying a dry dressing with a topical medication

■ Remove the old dressing and clean the wound as described above.

■ Apply the ordered medication to the wound in thin layers (2- to 4-mm thick) with a sterile gloved hand.

■ Apply several layers of burn gauze over the wound *to contain the medication but to allow exudates to escape.*

■ Don't cover unburned areas.

■ Cover the entire dressing with roller gauze and secure it with elastic netting or tape.

Providing arm and leg care

■ Wrap burn gauze once around the arm or leg, overlapping the edges slightly, until the wound is covered. Wrap from the distal area to the proximal area *to stimulate circulation.*[2]

■ Apply a dry roller gauze dressing and secure it with elastic netting or tape.

Providing hand and foot care

■ Wrap each finger with a single layer of a 4″ × 4″ gauze pad or place gauze between the toes, as appropriate.

■ Place the patient's hand in a functional position and secure this position with a dressing.

■ Apply splints as ordered.

Estimating burn surfaces in adults and children

You need to use different formulas to compute burned body surface area (BSA) in adults and children because the proportion of BSA varies with growth.

Rule of Nines

You can quickly estimate the extent of an adult patient's burn by using the "Rule of Nines." This method quantifies BSA in percentages either in fractions of nine or in multiples of nine. To use this method, mentally assess your patient's burns by the body chart shown below. Add the corresponding percentages for each body section burned. Use the total—a rough estimate of burn extent—to calculate initial fluid replacement needs.

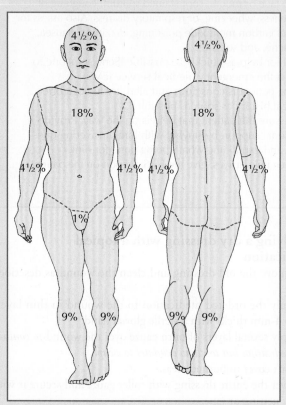

Lund and Browder chart

The Rule of Nines isn't accurate for infants and children because their body shapes differ from those of adults. An infant's head, for example, accounts for about 17% of his total BSA, compared with 7% for an adult. Instead, use the Lund and Browder chart shown here.

Percentage of burned body surface by age

	AT BIRTH	0 TO 1 YR	1 TO 4 YRS	5 TO 9 YRS	10 TO 15 YRS	ADULT
A: Half of head	9½%	8½%	6½%	5½%	4½%	3½%
B: Half of thigh	2¾%	3¼%	4%	4¼%	4½%	4¾%
C: Half of leg	2½%	2½%	2¾%	3%	3¼%	3½%

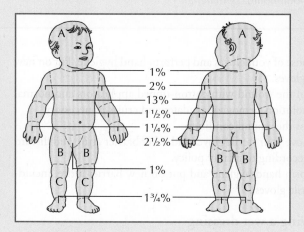

Providing arm and leg care
- Apply new sterile dressings.
- Place burn gauze on the arm or leg.
- Apply a dry roller gauze dressing and secure it.

Providing chest, abdomen, and back care
- Apply ordered medication to the wound using safe medication administration practices.
- Cover the entire burn area with sheets of burn gauze.
- Wrap the area with roller gauze or apply a specialty vest dressing.
- Secure the dressing with elastic netting or tape.
- Make sure the dressing doesn't restrict respiratory function.

Providing facial care
- If the patient has scalp burns, clip the hair around the burn, as ordered. Clip other hair until it's about 2" (5 cm) long *to prevent contamination of burned scalp areas.*
- Remove facial hair daily if it comes in contact with burned areas.
- Typically, facial burns are managed with milder topical agents (such as triple antibiotic ointment) and are left open to air. If dressings are required, make sure they don't cover the eyes, nostrils, or mouth.

Providing ear care
- Clip the hair around the affected ear.
- Place a layer of 4" × 4" gauze behind the auricle *to prevent webbing.*

Evaluating burn severity[1]

To judge a burn's severity, assess its depth and extent as well as the presence of other factors.

Superficial or epidermal (first-degree) burn

Does the burned area appear pink or red with minimal edema? Is the area sensitive to touch and temperature changes? If so, your patient most likely has a superficial or epidermal (first-degree) burn affecting only the epidermal skin layer (shown below).

Partial-thickness (second-degree) burn

Does the burned area appear pink or red, with a mottled appearance? Do red areas blanch when you touch them? Does the skin have large, thick-walled blisters with subcutaneous edema? Does touching the burn cause severe pain? Is the hair still present? If so, the person most likely has a partial-thickness (second-degree) burn (shown below), affecting the epidermal and dermal layers.

Full-thickness (third-degree) burn

Does the burned area appear red, waxy white, brown, or black? Does red skin remain red with no blanching when you touch it? Is the skin leathery with extensive subcutaneous edema? Is the skin insensitive to touch? Does the hair fall out easily? If so, your patient most likely has a full-thickness (third-degree) burn that affects all skin layers (shown below).

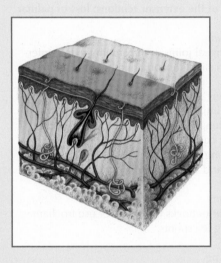 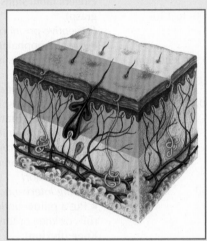 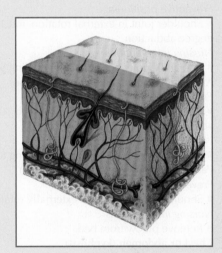

■ Apply the ordered topical medication to 4″ × 4″ gauze pads and place the pads over the burned area, or leave open to air, according to the doctor's orders. Before securing the dressing with a roller bandage, position the patient's ears normally *to avoid damaging the auricular cartilage.*

■ Assess the patient's hearing ability.

Providing eye care

■ Note that cleaning of the area should be done every 4 to 6 hours or as needed *to remove crusts and drainage.*

■ After cleaning, administer ordered eye ointments or drops using safe medication practices *to keep the eyes moist.* Use moisture chambers as needed, especially if the patient can't close his eyes completely.

■ Be sure to close the patient's eyes before applying eye pads *to prevent corneal abrasion.* Don't apply any topical ointments near the eyes without a doctor's order.

Providing nasal care

■ Check the nostrils for inhalation injury: inflamed mucosa, singed vibrissae, and soot.

■ Apply the ordered ointments using safe medication administration practices.

■ If the patient has a nasogastric tube, use tracheostomy ties to secure the tube. Be sure to check ties frequently for tightness resulting from swelling of facial tissue. Clean the area around the tube every 4 to 6 hours.[2]

Completing burn care

■ Dispose of equipment and supplies according to your facility's policy.

■ Perform hand hygiene.[4,5,6]

■ Document the procedure.[6]

Special considerations

■ *To prevent cross-contamination,* clean and dress the cleanest areas first and the dirtiest or most contaminated areas last. Make sure you remove and discard your gloves, perform hand hygiene, and put on new gloves each time you move from one area to another. *To help prevent excessive pain or cross-contamination,* you may need to perform the dressing in stages to avoid exposing all wounds at the same time.

Positioning the burn patient to prevent deformity

For each of the potential deformities listed below, you can use the corresponding positioning and interventions to help prevent the deformity.

Neck (flexion contracture of neck)
Preventive positioning
■ Extension
Nursing interventions
■ Remove pillow from bed.

Neck (extensor contracture of neck)
Preventive positioning
■ Prone with head slightly raised
Nursing interventions
■ Place pillow or rolled towel under upper chest to flex cervical spine, or apply cervical collar.

Axilla (adduction and internal rotation)
Preventive positioning
■ Shoulder joint in external rotation and 100- to 130-degree abduction
Nursing interventions
■ Use an IV pole, bedside table, or sling to suspend arm.

Axilla (adduction and external rotation)
Preventive positioning
■ Shoulder joint in forward flexion and 100- to 130-degree abduction
Nursing interventions
■ Use an IV pole, bedside table, or sling to suspend arm.

Pectoral region (shoulder protraction)
Preventive positioning
■ Shoulders abducted and externally rotated
Nursing interventions
■ Remove pillow from bed.

Chest or abdomen (kyphosis)
Preventive positioning
■ Shoulders abducted and externally rotated with hips neutral (not flexed)
Nursing interventions
■ Use no pillow under head or legs.

Lateral trunk (scoliosis)
Preventive positioning
■ Supine; affected arm abducted
Nursing interventions
■ Put pillows or blanket rolls at sides.

Elbow (flexion and pronation)
Preventive positioning
■ Arm extended and supinated
Nursing interventions
■ Use an elbow splint, arm board, or bedside table.

Wrist (flexion)
Preventive positioning
■ Splint in 15-degree extension
Nursing interventions
■ Apply a hand splint.

Wrist (extension)
Preventive positioning
■ Splint in 15-degree flexion
Nursing interventions
■ Apply a hand splint.

Fingers (adhesions of the extensor tendons; loss of palmar grasp)
Preventive positioning
■ Metacarpophalangeal joints in maximum flexion; interphalangeal joints in slight flexion; thumb in maximum abduction
Nursing interventions
■ Apply a hand splint; wrap fingers separately.

Hip (internal rotation, flexion, and adduction; possibly joint subluxation if contracture is severe)
Preventive positioning
■ Neutral rotation and abduction; maintain extension by prone position
Nursing interventions
■ Put a pillow under buttocks (if supine) or use trochanter rolls or knee or long leg splints.

Knee (flexion)
Preventive positioning
■ Extension maintained.
Nursing interventions
■ Use a knee splint with no pillows under legs.

Ankle (plantar flexion if foot muscles are weak or their tendons are divided)
Preventive positioning
■ 90-degree dorsiflexion
Nursing interventions
■ Use a footboard or ankle splint.

■ Thorough assessment and documentation of the wound's appearance are essential *to detect infection and other complications.* A purulent wound or green-gray exudate indicates infection, an overly dry wound suggests dehydration, and a wound with a swollen, red edge suggests cellulitis. Suspect a fungal infection if the wound is white and powdery. Healthy granulation tissue appears clean, pinkish, faintly shiny, and free of exudate.

■ *Blisters protect underlying tissue,* so leave them intact unless they impede joint motion, become infected, or cause patient discomfort. If ordered, they can be debrided with sterile forceps or in the shower.

■ Keep in mind that the patient with healing burns has increased nutritional needs. He'll require extra protein and carbohydrates *to accommodate an almost doubled basal metabolism.*

■ If you must manage a burn with topical medications, exposure to air, and no dressing, watch for such problems as wound adherence to bed linens, poor drainage control, and partial loss of topical medications.

Patient teaching

Begin discharge planning as soon as the patient enters the facility *to help him (and his family) make a smooth transition from facility to*

PATIENT TEACHING

Successful burn self-care after discharge

You can help the patient make a successful transition from health care facility to home by encouraging him to follow the wound care and self-care guidelines below.

To enhance healing, instruct the patient to eat well-balanced meals with adequate carbohydrates and proteins, to eat between-meal snacks, and to include at least one protein source in each meal and snack. Tell him to avoid tobacco, alcohol, and caffeine *because they constrict peripheral blood flow.*

Advise the patient to wash new skin with mild soap and water. *To prevent excessive skin dryness,* instruct him to use a lubricating lotion and to avoid lotions containing alcohol or perfume. Caution the patient to avoid bumping or scratching regenerated skin tissue.

Recommend nonrestrictive, nonabrasive clothing, which should be laundered in a mild detergent. Advise the patient

to wear protective clothing during cold weather *to prevent frostbite.*

Warn the patient not to expose new skin to strong sunlight and always to use a sunblock with a sun protection factor of 20 or higher. Also, tell him not to expose new skin to irritants, such as paint, solvent, strong detergents, and antiperspirants. Recommend cool baths or ice packs *to relieve itching.*

To minimize scar formation, the patient may need to wear a pressure garment—usually for 23 hours a day for 6 months to 1 year. Instruct him to remove it only during daily hygiene. Suspect that the garment is too tight if it causes cold, numbness, or discoloration in the fingers or toes or if its seams and zippers leave deep, red impressions for more than 10 minutes after the garment is removed.

---

home. *To encourage therapeutic compliance,* prepare him to expect scarring, teach him wound management and pain control, and urge him to follow the prescribed exercise regimen. Provide encouragement and emotional support, and urge the patient to join a burn survivor support group. Also, teach the family or caregivers how to encourage, support, and provide care for the patient. (See *Successful burn self-care after discharge.*)

Complications

Infection is the most common burn complication.

Documentation

Record the date and time of all care provided. Describe wound condition, special dressing-change techniques, topical medications administered, positioning of the burned area, and the patient's tolerance of the procedure. Record the preprocedure pain medication administered and its effectiveness. Note patient teaching provided and the patient's response to instruction.

REFERENCES

1 Pham, T.N. (2008). American Burn Association practice guidelines: Burn shock resuscitation. *Journal of Burn Care and Research, 29*(1), 257–266.
2 American Burn Association. (2009). "American Burn Association White Paper: Surgical Management of the Burn Wound and Use of Skin Substitutes" [Online]. Accessed July 2011 via the Web at http://www.ameriburn.org/WhitePaperFinal.pdf
3 The Joint Commission. (2012). Standard NPSG.01.01.01. *Comprehensive accreditation manual for hospitals: The official handbook.* Oakbrook Terrace, IL: The Joint Commission. (Level I)
4 The Joint Commission. (2012). Standard NPSG.07.01.01. *Comprehensive accreditation manual for hospitals: The official handbook.* Oakbrook Terrace, IL: The Joint Commission. (Level I)
5 World Health Organization. (2009). *WHO guidelines on hand hygiene in health care: First global patient safety challenge. Clean care is safer care.* Geneva, Switzerland: World Health Organization. (Level I)
6 Centers for Disease Control and Prevention. (October 2002). Guideline for hand hygiene in health-care settings. *Morbidity and Mortality Weekly Report, 51* (RR-16), 1–45. (Level I)
7 The Joint Commission. (2012). Standard PC.01.02.07. *Comprehensive accreditation manual for hospitals: The official handbook.* Oakbrook Terrace, IL: The Joint Commission. (Level I)
8 The Joint Commission. (2012). Standard RC.01.03.01. *Comprehensive accreditation manual for hospitals: The official handbook.* Oakbrook Terrace, IL: The Joint Commission. (Level I)

ADDITIONAL REFERENCES

Lipley, N. (2007). New guidelines for managing patients with burns. *Emergency Nurse, 14*(10), 3.
Tengvall, O.M., et al. (2006). Differences in pain patterns for infected and non-infected patients with burn injuries. *Pain Management Nursing, 7*(4), 176–182.

BURN DRESSING APPLICATION, BIOLOGICAL AND SYNTHETIC

Biological dressings provide a temporary protective covering for burn wounds and for clean granulation tissue. They also temporarily secure fresh skin grafts and protect graft donor sites. In common use are three organic materials—pigskin, cadaver skin, and amniotic membrane—and one synthetic material, Biobrane. (See *Comparing biological and synthetic dressings,* page 102.) Besides stimulating new skin growth, these dressings act like normal skin: They reduce heat loss, block infection, and minimize fluid, electrolyte, and protein losses.[1]

Comparing biological and synthetic dressings

Type	Description and uses	Nursing considerations
Cadaver (allograft)	■ Obtained at autopsy up to 24 hours after death ■ Applied in the operating room or at the bedside to debrided, untidy wounds ■ Available as fresh cryopreserved homografts in tissue banks nationwide ■ Provides protection, especially to granulation tissue after escharotomy ■ May be used in some patients as a test graft for autografting ■ Covers excised wounds immediately	■ Observe for exudate. ■ Watch for signs of rejection. ■ Keep in mind that the gauze dressing may be removed every 8 hours to observe the graft.
Pigskin (heterograft or xenograft)	■ Applied in the operating room or at the bedside ■ Comes fresh or frozen in rolls or sheets ■ Can cover and protect debrided, untidy wounds; mesh autografts; clean (eschar-free) partial-thickness burns; and exposed tendons	■ Reconstitute frozen form with normal saline solution 30 minutes before use. ■ Watch for signs of rejection. ■ Cover with gauze dressing or leave exposed to air, as ordered.
Amniotic membrane (homograft)	■ Available from the obstetric department ■ Must be sterile and come from an uncomplicated birth; serologic tests must be done ■ Bacteriostatic condition doesn't require antimicrobials ■ May be used to protect partial-thickness burns or (temporarily) granulation tissue before autografting ■ Applied by the doctor to clean wounds only	■ Change the membrane every 48 hours. ■ Cover the membrane with a gauze dressing or leave it exposed, as ordered. ■ If you apply a gauze dressing, change it every 48 hours.
Biobrane (biosynthetic membrane)	■ Comes in sterile, prepackaged sheets in various sizes and in glove form for hand burns ■ Used to cover donor graft sites, superficial partial-thickness burns, debrided wounds awaiting autograft, and meshed autografts ■ Reduces pain ■ Applied by the nurse	■ Apply taut against the skin. ■ Leave the membrane in place until the underneath tissue is healed, typically 7 to 14 days. ■ Don't use this dressing for preparing a granulation bed for subsequent autografting. ■ As the burn heals, Biobrane turns white and dry and lifts away.

Amniotic membrane or fresh cadaver skin is usually applied to the patient in the operating room, although it may be applied in a treatment room. Pigskin or Biobrane may be applied in either the operating room or a treatment room. Before applying a biological or synthetic dressing, the caregiver must clean and debride the wound. The frequency of dressing changes depends on the type of wound and the dressing's specific function.

Equipment

Ordered analgesic ■ cap ■ mask ■ two pairs of sterile gloves ■ sterile or clean gown ■ shoe covers ■ biological or synthetic dressing ■ normal saline solution ■ sterile basin ■ Xeroflo gauze ■ sterile forceps ■ sterile scissors ■ sterile hemostats ■ elastic netting.

Preparation of equipment

Place the biological dressing in the sterile basin containing sterile normal saline solution (or open the Biobrane package). Using sterile technique, open the sterile dressing packages. Arrange the equipment on the dressing cart and keep the cart readily accessible. Make sure the treatment area has adequate light *to allow accurate wound assessment and dressing placement.*

Implementation

■ Verify the doctor's order.
■ Confirm the patient's identity using at least two patient identifiers according to your facility's policy.[2]
■ If this is the patient's first treatment, explain the procedure *to allay his fears and promote cooperation.* Provide privacy.
■ Provide a warm environment.
■ Perform hand hygiene and put on a cap, a mask, a gown, shoe covers, and sterile gloves.[3,4,5,6]
■ Assess the patient's pain. If ordered, administer an analgesic *to increase the patient's comfort and tolerance levels.* Oral analgesics should be given at an appropriate time before the procedure, depending on the medication's onset and peak of action. An IV analgesic may be given immediately before the procedure.[7]

■ Assess the burn wound, noting the color, size, odor, and depth of the wound as well as the presence of drainage, bleeding, edema, and eschar. Monitor for cellulitis in the surrounding tissue.

■ Clean and debride the wound *to reduce bacteria.* (See "Sharp debridement," page 650.)

■ Remove and dispose of your gloves. Perform hand hygiene and put on a fresh pair of sterile gloves.

■ Place the dressing directly on the wound surface. Apply pigskin, dermal (shiny) side down; apply Biobrane, nylon-backed (dull) side down. Roll the dressing directly onto the skin, if applicable. Place the dressing strips so that the edges touch but don't overlap. Use sterile forceps, if necessary. Smooth the dressing. Eliminate folds and wrinkles by rolling out the dressing with the hemostat handle, the forceps handle, or your dominant hand *to cover the wound completely and ensure adherence.*

■ Use the scissors to trim the dressing around the wound *so that the dressing fits the wound without overlapping adjacent areas.*

■ Place Xeroflo gauze directly over an allograft, pigskin graft, or amniotic membrane. Place a few layers of gauze on top *to absorb exudate,* and wrap with a roller gauze dressing. Secure the dressing with tape or elastic netting. During daily dressing changes, the dressing will be removed down to the Xeroflo gauze, and the gauze will be replaced after the Xeroflo is inspected for drainage, adherence, and signs of infection.

■ Place a nonadhesive dressing (such as Exu-dry) over the Biobrane *to absorb drainage and provide stability.* Wrap the dressing with a roller gauze dressing, and secure it with tape or elastic netting. For the first 24 hours, keep the outer dressing in place and don't get it wet. After 24 hours, the dressing will be removed down to the Biobrane during daily dressing changes and you'll inspect the site for signs of infection. After the Biobrane adheres (usually in 2 to 3 days), it doesn't need to be covered with a dressing.

■ Position the patient comfortably, elevating the area if possible *to reduce edema, which may prevent the biological dressing from adhering.*

■ Assess the patient's need for additional pain medication.

■ Discard used equipment and supplies in the appropriate receptacles.

■ Remove and discard your gloves and perform hand hygiene.[3]

■ Document the procedure.[8]

Special considerations

■ Handle the biological or synthetic dressing as little as possible.

Patient teaching

Instruct the patient or caregiver to assess the site daily for signs of infection, swelling, blisters, drainage, and separation. Make sure the patient knows who to contact if these complications develop.

Complications

Infection may develop under a biological or synthetic dressing. Observe the wound carefully during dressing changes for infection signs. If wound drainage appears purulent, remove the dressing, clean the area with normal saline solution or another prescribed cleaning solution as ordered, and apply a fresh biological or synthetic dressing.

Documentation

Record the time and date of dressing changes. Note areas of application, quality of adherence, and purulent drainage or other infection signs. Also describe the patient's tolerance of the procedure.

REFERENCES

1 Demling, R.H., et al. "Use of skin substitutes" [Online]. Accessed July 2011 via the Web at http://www.burnsurgery.org/Modules/BurnWound%201/sect_VIII.htm

2 The Joint Commission. (2012). Standard NPSG.01.01.01. *Comprehensive accreditation manual for hospitals: The official handbook.* Oakbrook Terrace, IL: The Joint Commission. (Level I)

3 The Joint Commission. (2012). Standard NPSG.07.01.01. *Comprehensive accreditation manual for hospitals: The official handbook.* Oakbrook Terrace, IL: The Joint Commission. (Level I)

4 American Burn Association. (2009). "American Burn Association White Paper: Surgical Management of the Burn Wound and Use of Skin Substitutes" [Online]. Accessed July 2011 via the Web at http://www.ameriburn.org/WhitePaperFinal.pdf

5 World Health Organization. (2009). *WHO guidelines on hand hygiene in health care: First global patient safety challenge. Clean care is safer care.* Geneva, Switzerland: World Health Organization. (Level I)

6 Centers for Disease Control and Prevention. (October 2002). Guideline for hand hygiene in health-care settings. *Morbidity and Mortality Weekly Report, 51* (RR-16), 1–45. (Level I)

7 The Joint Commission. (2012). Standard PC.01.02.07. *Comprehensive accreditation manual for hospitals: The official handbook.* Oakbrook Terrace, IL: The Joint Commission. (Level I)

8 The Joint Commission. (2012). Standard RC.01.03.01. *Comprehensive accreditation manual for hospitals: The official handbook.* Oakbrook Terrace, IL: The Joint Commission. (Level I)

ADDITIONAL REFERENCES

American Burn Association. (2001). "Practice guidelines for burn care" [Online]. Accessed July 2011 via the Web at http://www.ameriburn.org/PracticeGuidelines2001.pdf

Andonovska, D., et al. (2008). The advantages of the application of amnion membrane in the treatment of burns. *Prilozi, 29*(1), 183–98.

Biobrane "Manufacturer's Instructions" [Online]. Accessed July 2011 via the Web at http://wound.smith-nephew.com/uk/node.asp?NodeId=3562

Ermolov, A.S., et al. (2008). The use of bioactive wound dressing, stimulating epithelial regeneration of IIIa-degree burn wounds. *Bulletin of Experimental Biology and Medicine, 146*(1), 153–157.

Kesting, M.R., et al. (2008). The role of allogenic amniotic membrane in burn treatment. *Journal of Burn Care and Research, 29*(6), 907–16.

Lineen, E., & Namias, N. (2008). Biologic dressing in burns. *Journal of Craniofacial Surgery, 19*(4), 923–928.

Lynn-McHale Wiegand, D.J. (Ed.). (2011). *AACN procedure manual for critical care* (6th ed.). Philadelphia, PA: Saunders.

Pham, C., et al. (2007). Bioengineered skin substitutes for the management of burns: A systematic review. *Burns, 33*(8), 946–957.

Verger, J.T., & Lebet, R.M. (Eds.). (2008). *AACN procedure manual for pediatric acute and critical care.* St. Louis, MO: Saunders.

CANES

Indicated for the patient with one-sided weakness or injury, occasional loss of balance, or increased joint pressure, a cane provides balance and support for walking and reduces fatigue and strain on weight-bearing joints. Available in various sizes, the cane should extend from the greater trochanter to the floor and have a rubber tip to prevent slipping. Canes are contraindicated for the patient with bilateral weakness; such a patient should use crutches or a walker.

Equipment

Rubber-tipped cane ■ Optional: walking belt.

Although wooden canes are available, three types of aluminum canes are used most frequently. The standard aluminum cane (used by the patient who needs only slight assistance with walking) provides the least support. The T-handle cane (used by the patient with hand weakness) has a straight-shaped handle with grips and a bent shaft. It provides greater stability than the standard cane. Three- or four-pronged (quad) canes are used by the patient with poor balance or one-sided weakness and an inability to hold onto a walker with both hands. The base of these types of canes splits into three or four short, splayed legs and provides greater stability than a standard cane but considerably less than a walker.

Preparation of equipment

Ask the patient to hold the cane on the uninvolved side 6″ (15 cm) from the base of the little toe. Adjust the aluminum cane's height by pushing in the metal button on the shaft and raising or lowering the shaft; if it's wood, the rubber tip can be removed and excess length sawed off. The handle of the cane should be level with the greater trochanter to allow approximately 30-degree flexion at the elbow. If the cane is too short, the patient will have to drop his shoulder to lean on it; if it's too long, he'll have to raise his shoulder and will have difficulty supporting his weight.

Implementation

■ Perform hand hygiene.[1,2,3]
■ Confirm the patient's identity using at least two patient identifiers according to your facility's policy.[4]
■ Tell the patient to hold the cane on the uninvolved side *to promote a reciprocal gait pattern and to distribute weight away from the involved side.*
■ Instruct the patient to hold the cane close to his body to prevent leaning and to move the cane forward 4″ to 8″ (10 to 20 cm) and simultaneously move the involved leg forward, followed by the uninvolved leg.
■ Encourage the patient to keep the stride length of each leg and the timing of each step (cadence) equal.

■ Demonstrate the technique for the patient.
■ Have the patient return the demonstration, and provide additional teaching as needed.

Negotiating stairs

■ Instruct the patient to always use a railing, if present, when going up or down stairs. Tell him to hold the cane with the other hand (as shown below). To ascend stairs, tell the patient to lead with the uninvolved leg and follow with the involved leg; to descend, tell him to lead with the involved leg and follow with the uninvolved one. Help the patient remember by telling him to use this mnemonic device: "Up with the good; down with the bad."

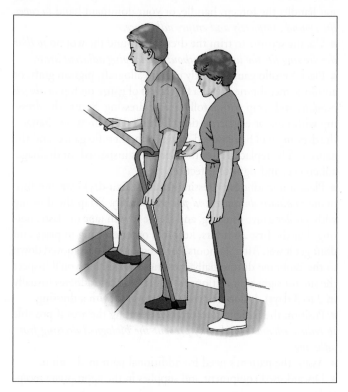

■ To negotiate stairs without a railing, tell the patient to use the walking technique to ascend and descend the stairs. Thus, to ascend stairs, tell the patient to hold the cane on the uninvolved side, step with the uninvolved leg, advance the cane, and then move the involved leg. To descend, tell him to hold the cane on the uninvolved side, lead with the cane, then advance the involved leg and then, finally, the uninvolved leg.
■ Remind the patient always to move the cane just before moving the involved leg in all stair use regardless of direction.

Using a chair

■ To teach the patient to sit down, stand by his affected side and tell him to place the backs of his legs against the edge of the chair seat. Then tell him to move the cane out from his side and to reach back with both hands to grasp the chair's armrests. Tell him to support his weight on the armrests and then lower himself onto the seat. While he's seated, he should keep the cane hooked on the armrest or the chair back.

■ To teach the patient to get up, stand by his affected side and tell him to unhook the cane from the chair and hold it in his stronger hand as he grasps the armrests. Then tell him to move his uninvolved foot slightly forward, to lean slightly forward, and to push against the armrests to raise himself upright (as shown below).

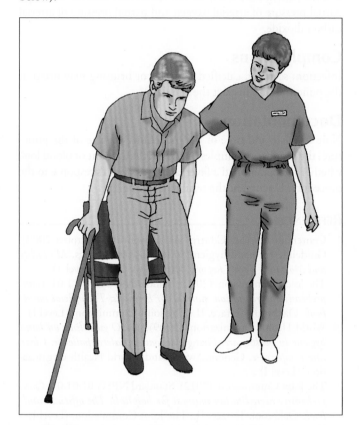

■ Instruct the patient not to lean on the cane when sitting or rising from the chair *to prevent falls.*
■ Supervise your patient each time he gets into or out of a chair until you're both certain he can do it alone.
■ Perform hand hygiene.[1,2,3]
■ Document the procedure.[5]

Special considerations

■ *To prevent falls during the learning period,* guard the patient carefully by standing behind him slightly to his stronger side and putting one foot between his feet and your other foot to the outside of the uninvolved leg. If necessary, use a walking belt.
■ Coordinate practice sessions in the physical therapy department, if necessary.

Complications

A poorly fitted cane or unclear instructions can cause the patient to lose his balance and fall.

Documentation

Record the type of cane used, the amount of guarding required, the distance walked, and the patient's understanding and tolerance of cane walking.

REFERENCES

1   The Joint Commission. (2012). Standard NPSG.07.01.01. *Comprehensive accreditation manual for hospitals: The official handbook.* Oakbrook Terrace, IL: The Joint Commission. (Level I)
2   Centers for Disease Control and Prevention. (October 2002). Guideline for hand hygiene in health-care settings. *Morbidity and Mortality Weekly Report, 51*(RR-16), 1–45. (Level 1)
3   World Health Organization. (2009). *WHO guidelines on hand hygiene in health care: First global patient safety challenge. Clean care is safer care.* Geneva, Switzerland: World Health Organization. (Level I)
4   The Joint Commission. (2012). Standard NPSG.01.01.01. *Comprehensive accreditation manual for hospitals: The official handbook.* Oakbrook Terrace, IL: The Joint Commission. (Level I)
5   The Joint Commission. (2012). Standard RC.01.03.01. *Comprehensive accreditation manual for hospitals: The official handbook.* Oakbrook Terrace, IL: The Joint Commission. (Level I)

ADDITIONAL REFERENCES

Allet, L., et al. (2009). Effect of different walking aids on walking capacity of patients with poststroke hemiparesis. *Archives of Physical Medicine and Rehabilitation, 90*(8), 1408–1413.
Craven, R.F., & Hirnle, C.J. (2009). *Fundamentals of nursing: Human health and function* (6th ed.). Philadelphia, PA: Lippincott Williams & Wilkins.
Demers, L., et al. (2008). Tracking mobility-related assistive technology in an outcomes study. *Assistive Technology, 20*(2), 73–83.

CAPILLARY BLOOD GAS SAMPLING

An alternative to arterial blood gas sampling, capillary blood gas sampling is used to help monitor a patient's respiratory status. The procedure can be performed in the presence of hypothermia and hypoperfusion (provided that hypertension isn't present) and can be easier to perform than arterial blood gas sampling in these situations. It involves a simple fingerstick and is less painful than an arterial puncture.

Capillary blood must be collected in special balanced-heparin capillary blood gas collection tubes. Transport of samples to the laboratory should occur within 30 minutes of collection; a delay may alter the results because of cellular metabolism or hemolysis.

Equipment

Sterile lancet (1.5 mm in depth) ■ antiseptic pad ■ 2″ × 2″ sterile gauze pads ■ gloves ■ preheparinized glass capillary tube ■ warming supplies (such as a chemical warmer or a warm cloth that's less than 109ϒF [42.8ϒC]) ■ sealing clay, wax sealer, or cap ■ sample collection label ■ plastic laboratory biohazard transport bag ■ Optional: ice, topical anesthetic cream.

Implementation

■ Verify the doctor's order.
■ Gather the necessary supplies, including the lancet.
■ Perform hand hygiene and put on gloves.[1,2,3]
■ Confirm the patient's identity using at least two patient identifiers according to your facility's policy.[4]

- Explain the procedure to the patient, allowing him to ask questions and express anxiety as needed *to promote better understanding of what is to be done.*
- Select the capillary puncture site. Either the earlobe or the finger is the preferred site in adults. If using a finger, select a site on the side of the finger, parallel to the side edges of the nail. Avoid the finger's tip or pad *to prevent additional discomfort.*

NURSING ALERT *Avoid using extremities with impaired circulation or localized infection.*

- Apply a topical anesthetic if indicated and time allows *to decrease discomfort.*

NURSING ALERT *Don't use lidocaine or prilocaine if the patient is receiving methemoglobin-inducing agents, such as sulfonamides and acetaminophen,* because a risk of methemoglobinemia exists.

- Apply the warming device to the puncture site for 5 to 10 minutes *to increase blood flow and reduce hemolysis and bruising.* Don't use products warmed in a microwave *because uneven heating by the microwave presents a burn risk.*
- Remove the warming device from the puncture site.
- If topical anesthetic cream was used, remove it before cleaning the puncture site.
- Clean the puncture site with an antiseptic pad and allow it to dry for 30 seconds. Then dry the site with sterile gauze.
- Place the extremity in a dependent position and grasp it firmly.
- Briskly puncture the skin with the sterile lancet and advance it at an angle so as to cut more capillary beds and generate greater blood flow. Wipe off the first drop of blood with sterile gauze *because residual alcohol or tissue fluids may contaminate the blood gas sample.*
- Continue to hold the puncture site in a dependent position while gently applying intermittent pressure to the surrounding area. *Harshly squeezing the area may produce hemolyzed samples and bruising and may contaminate the sample with tissue fluid.*
- Hold the capillary tube horizontally *to fill it by capillary action and to prevent air entrapment.*
- Fill the entire tube with blood and seal it. Label the sample in the presence of the patient *to prevent mislabeling.*[4]
- Elevate the extremity above the level of the heart and gently press dry, sterile gauze to the puncture site until the bleeding stops. Don't use bandages, *which can lead to skin maceration.*

NURSING ALERT *If the patient has a hematologic disorder or is receiving certain medications, such as warfarin, heparin, or aspirin, he may have a prolonged clotting time.*

- Discard used equipment and supplies in appropriate receptacles.[5]
- Place the sample in a laboratory biohazard transport bag and transport it to the laboratory as soon as possible.
- Place the sample on ice if analysis will be delayed longer than 10 minutes *to preserve results.*
- Evaluate the puncture site for evidence of continued bleeding.
- Keep the wound clean and dry.
- Remove and discard your gloves. Perform hand hygiene.[1,2,3]
- Document the procedure.[6]

Special considerations

- Never scoop up blood from the patient's skin *because it may be partially coagulated, which can cause hemolysis.*
- Make sure there are no air bubbles in the collected sample, *which may alter the test results.*
- If the patient has a fever, the test results may indicate false-high partial pressure of arterial oxygen and partial pressure of arterial carbon dioxide.

Complications

Infection, scarring, calcified nodules, or bruising may occur at the puncture site. Inspect the site daily.

Documentation

Note the date and time of the procedure, the site of the puncture, the number of samples obtained, the amount of blood loss, whether the patient had a fever, and the patient's response to the procedure. Document the results of testing.

REFERENCES

1 Centers for Disease Control and Prevention. (October 2002). Guideline for hand hygiene in health-care settings. *Morbidity and Mortality Weekly Report, 51*(RR-16), 1–45. (Level 1)
2 The Joint Commission. (2012). Standard NPSG.07.01.01. *Comprehensive accreditation manual for hospitals: The official handbook.* Oakbrook Terrace, IL: The Joint Commission. (Level I)
3 World Health Organization. (2009). *WHO guidelines on hand hygiene in health care: First global patient safety challenge. Clean care is safer care.* Geneva, Switzerland: World Health Organization. (Level I)
4 The Joint Commission. (2012). Standard NPSG.01.01.01. *Comprehensive accreditation manual for hospitals: The official handbook.* Oakbrook Terrace, IL: The Joint Commission. (Level I)
5 Occupational Safety and Health Administration. "Bloodborne Pathogens, Standard Number 1910.1030" [Online]. Accessed August 2011 via the Web at http://www.osha.gov/pls/oshaweb/owadisp.show_document?p_table=STANDARDS&p_id=10051 (Level I)
6 The Joint Commission. (2012). Standard RC.01.03.01. *Comprehensive accreditation manual for hospitals: The official handbook.* Oakbrook Terrace, IL: The Joint Commission. (Level I)

ADDITIONAL REFERENCES

Craven, R.F., & Hirnle, C.J. (2009). *Fundamentals of nursing: Human health and function* (6th ed.). Philadelphia, PA: Lippincott Williams & Wilkins.
Fischbach, F., & Dunning, M.B. (2009). *A manual of laboratory and diagnostic tests* (8th ed.). Philadelphia, PA: Lippincott Williams & Wilkins.

CARBON MONOXIDE OXIMETRY

Intermittent or continuous carbon monoxide oximetry can be performed noninvasively with a lightweight, portable display unit. The unit is connected to a sensor probe that's placed on the adult patient's fingertip or an infant's foot. The sensor probe collects data about the patient's carboxyhemoglobin saturation and sends that information to the oximeter, which then displays the calculated data in the form of a percentage. A carboxyhemoglobin saturation level greater than 2% for nonsmokers and greater than 9% for smokers indicates exposure to exogenous carbon monoxide.

A patient can have increased carbon monoxide levels from chronic exposure to cigarette smoke or from an acute episode, such as from exposure to a combustion heater without adequate ventilation of natural gas, fire, or vehicle exhaust. However, carbon monoxide poisoning is commonly misdiagnosed because the initial signs and symptoms—fatigue, shortness of breath, mild headache, and nausea—are similar to those of a viral-related illness. Severe symptoms include dizziness, increasingly acute headaches, weakness, drowsiness, and nausea accompanied by vomiting. Carbon monoxide poisoning can result in long-term neurologic damage, psychiatric and cardiovascular disorders, and death.

Equipment

Noninvasive pulse carbon monoxide oximeter ▪ connecting cable ▪ fingertip sensor ▪ gloves ▪ nail polish remover, if necessary ▪ flow sheet for recording data.

Preparation of equipment

Test the oximeter before attaching it to the patient *to ensure that it's in proper working order.*

Implementation

▪ Verify the doctor's order for pulse carbon monoxide oximetry, unless it is a standard of care for your facility.
▪ Review the patient's medical record for past medical history and history of present illness.
▪ Confirm the patient's identity using at least two patient identifiers according to your facility's policy.[1]
▪ Explain the procedure to the patient, encouraging him to ask questions as needed.
▪ Perform hand hygiene and put on gloves.[2,3,4]
▪ Plug the pulse carbon monoxide oximeter into an electrical source and turn on the unit.
▪ Plug the connecting cable into the oximeter unit and attach the other end to the fingertip sensor.
▪ Select a finger for the test. Although the index finger is commonly used, a smaller finger may be selected if the patient's fingers are too large for the equipment.
▪ Make sure the patient isn't wearing false fingernails or nail polish. Remove nail polish as needed.
▪ Place the sensor probe on the patient's finger so that the light beams and sensors oppose each other. If the patient has long fingernails, position the probe perpendicular to the finger, if possible, or clip the fingernail.
▪ Position the patient's hand at heart level *to eliminate venous pulsations and to promote accurate readings.*
NURSING ALERT *If you're testing a neonate or small infant, wrap the probe around the foot* so that the light beams and detec-

tors oppose each other. *For a large infant, use a probe that fits on the great toe and secure it to the foot.*
▪ Wait the time recommended by the manufacturer before obtaining the reading.
▪ During oximetry, check the patient's pulse rate and capillary refill time *to determine whether blood flow to the site is adequate.* If it isn't, loosen restraints, remove tight-fitting clothes, take off a blood pressure cuff, or check arterial and IV lines, as appropriate. If none of these interventions works, you may need to use an alternate site.
▪ Read the carbon monoxide level, displayed as a percentage.
▪ Record the measurements on the patient's flow sheet.
▪ Remove and discard your gloves. Perform hand hygiene.[2,3,4]
▪ Document the procedure.[5]

Special considerations

▪ The pulse rate on the oximeter should correspond with the patient's measured pulse. If the rates don't correspond, the saturation reading can't be considered accurate. Assess the patient, check the oximeter, and reposition the probe, if necessary.
▪ Keep the monitoring site clean and dry, and make sure that the skin doesn't become irritated from the sensor. Alternate the monitoring site daily.

Documentation

Document readings as determined by your facility's policy or by the doctor's order. Note any difficulty obtaining accurate readings. Document patient teaching provided, questions asked by the patient, and the patient's understanding.

REFERENCES

1 The Joint Commission. (2012). Standard NPSG.01.01.01. *Comprehensive accreditation manual for hospitals: The official handbook.* Oakbrook Terrace, IL: The Joint Commission. (Level I)
2 Centers for Disease Control and Prevention. (October 2002). Guideline for hand hygiene in health-care settings. *Morbidity and Mortality Weekly Report, 51*(RR-16), 1–45. (Level 1)
3 The Joint Commission. (2012). Standard NPSG.07.01.01. *Comprehensive accreditation manual for hospitals: The official handbook.* Oakbrook Terrace, IL: The Joint Commission. (Level I)
4 World Health Organization. (2009). *WHO guidelines on hand hygiene in health care: First global patient safety challenge. Clean care is safer care.* Geneva, Switzerland: World Health Organization. (Level I)
5 The Joint Commission. (2012). Standard RC.01.03.01. *Comprehensive accreditation manual for hospitals: The official handbook.* Oakbrook Terrace, IL: The Joint Commission. (Level I)

ADDITIONAL REFERENCES

Barker, S.J., & Badal, J.J. (2008). The measurement of dyshemoglobins and total hemoglobin by pulse oximetry. *Current Opinion in Anaesthesiology, 21*(6), 805–810.
Chee, K.J., et al. (2008). Finding needles in a haystack: A case series of carbon monoxide poisoning detected using new technology in the emergency department. *Clinical Toxicology, 46*(5), 461–469.

Lead selection

Your patient's clinical condition determines the leads you'll monitor. *Note:* If the monitor can detect arrhythmias, know which leads perform this function. Even if you don't continually monitor these leads, periodically check the quality of their waveforms because the arrhythmia detection algorithm will fail without adequate waveforms.

CLINICAL CONCERN	LEAD
Bundle branch block	V_1 or V_6
Ischemia based on the area of infarction or site of percutaneous coronary intervention	
Anterior	V_3, V_4
Septal	V_1, V_2
Lateral	I, aV_L, V_5, V_6
Inferior	II, III, aV_F
Right ventricle	V_{4R}
Junctional rhythm with retrograde P waves	II
Optimal view of atrial activity	I, II, or Lewis lead (positive and negative electrodes at the second and fourth intercostal spaces at the right sternal border)
Ventricular ectopy, wide complex tachycardia	V_1 (may use V_6 along with V_1)
Ventricular pacing	V_1 or II

Coulange, M., et al. (2008). Reliability of new pulse CO-oximeter in victims of carbon monoxide poisoning. *Undersea & Hyperbaric Medicine, 35*(2), 107–111.

Suner, S., et al. (2008). Non-invasive pulse CO-oximetry screening in the emergency department identifies occult carbon monoxide toxicity. *Journal of Emergency Medicine, 34*(4), 441–450.

CARDIAC MONITORING

Because it allows continuous observation of the heart's electrical activity, cardiac monitoring is used in patients with conduction disturbances or in those at risk for life-threatening arrhythmias.

Like other forms of electrocardiography, cardiac monitoring uses electrodes placed on the patient's chest to transmit electrical signals that are converted into a tracing of cardiac rhythm on an oscilloscope.

Two types of monitoring may be performed: hardwire or telemetry. With hardwire monitoring, the patient is connected to a monitor at bedside. The rhythm display appears at bedside, but it may also be transmitted to a console at a remote location. Telemetry uses a small transmitter connected to the patient to send electrical signals to another location, where they're displayed on a monitor screen. Battery powered and portable, telemetry frees the patient from cumbersome wires and cables and lets him be comfortably mobile. Telemetry is especially useful for monitoring arrhythmias that occur during sleep, rest, exercise, or stressful situations.

Regardless of the type, cardiac monitors can display the patient's heart rate and rhythm, produce a printed record of cardiac rhythm, and sound an alarm if the patient's heart rate rises above or falls below specified limits. Monitors also recognize and count abnormal heartbeats as well as changes. For example, ST-segment monitoring helps detect myocardial ischemia, electrolyte imbalance, coronary artery spasm, and hypoxic events. The ST segment represents early ventricular repolarization, and any changes in this waveform component reflect alterations in myocardial oxygenation.[1] Any monitoring lead that views an ischemic heart region will reveal ST-segment changes. The monitor's software establishes a template of the patient's normal QRST pattern from the selected leads; then the monitor displays ST-segment changes. Some monitors display such changes continuously; others, only on command. (See *Lead selection*.)

One application of bedside cardiac monitoring is a reduced-lead continuous 12-lead electrocardiogram (ECG) system (EASI system). This system uses an advanced algorithm and only five electrodes placed on the torso to derive a 12-lead ECG. The system allows all 12 leads to be simultaneously displayed and recorded. (See *Understanding the EASI system*.)

Equipment

Cardiac monitor ▪ lead wires ▪ patient cable ▪ disposable pregelled electrodes (number of electrodes varies from three to five, depending on patient's needs) ▪ washcloth, soap, and water, or alcohol pads ▪ 4″ × 4″ gauze pads ▪ gloves ▪ Optional: clippers.

For telemetry

Transmitter ▪ transmitter pouch ▪ telemetry battery pack, leads, and electrodes ▪ gloves.

Preparation of equipment

Plug the cardiac monitor into an electrical outlet and turn it on to warm up the unit while you prepare the equipment and the patient. Insert the cable into the appropriate socket in the monitor. Connect the leadwires to the cable. In some systems, the leadwires are permanently secured to the cable. Each leadwire should indicate the location for attachment to the patient: right arm (RA), left arm (LA), right leg (RL), left leg (LL), and chest (C). Leadwires may also be color-coded for placement: white (RA), black (LA), green (RL), red (LL), and brown (chest). This designation should appear on the leadwire, if it's permanently connected, or at the connection of the leadwires and cable to the patient. Then connect an electrode to each of the leadwires, carefully checking that each leadwire is in its correct outlet.

For telemetry monitoring, insert a new battery into the transmitter. Be sure to match the poles on the battery with the polar markings on the transmitter case.[2] Test the battery's charge and test the unit by pressing the button at the top of the unit; *this ensures that the battery is operational.* If the leadwires aren't permanently affixed to the telemetry unit, attach them securely. If they must be attached individually, connect each one to the correct outlet.

Implementation

- Perform hand hygiene and put on gloves.[3,4,5]
- Confirm the patient's identity using at least two patient identifiers according to your facility's policy.[6]
- Provide privacy and explain the procedure to the patient.
- Ask the patient to expose his chest.[2]
- Determine electrode positions on the patient's chest based on the system and lead you're using. (See *Positioning monitoring leads,* page 110.)
- If necessary, clip the hair in an area about 4″ (10 cm) in diameter around each electrode site *to ensure good skin contact with the electrodes.*[1,2]
- Clean the electrode area with a cleaning wipe or soap and water and dry it completely *to provide for adequate transmission of electrical impulses.*[1,2,7]
- Clean the intended sites with an alcohol pad *to remove oils from skin and improve impulse transmission.*[2]
- Gently abrade the skin at the intended sites *to remove dead skin cells and to promote better contact with living cells.*[2] (Some electrodes have a small, rough patch for abrading the skin; otherwise, use a dry washcloth or a dry gauze pad.)
- Remove the backing from the pregelled electrode. Check the gel for moistness. If the gel is dry, discard it and replace it with a fresh electrode *to ensure optimal function.*[2]
- Apply the electrode to the appropriate site by pressing one side of the electrode against the patient's skin, pulling gently, and then pressing the other side against the skin. Press your fingers in a circular motion around the electrode *to fix the gel and stabilize the electrode.* Avoid pressing directly on the gel pad *to prevent spreading of the gel and loss of adhesion and transmission.* Repeat this procedure for each electrode.

For hardwire monitoring

- When all the electrodes are in place, attach the leadwires and check for a tracing on the cardiac monitor. Assess the quality of the ECG. (See *Identifying cardiac monitor problems,* page 111.)
- To verify that each beat is being detected by the monitor, compare the digital heart rate display with your count of the patient's heart rate.
- If necessary, use the gain control to adjust the size of the rhythm tracing and the position control to adjust the waveform position on the recording paper.

Understanding the EASI system

The five-lead EASI (reduced-lead continuous 12-lead electrocardiogram [ECG]) configuration gives a three-dimensional view of the electrical activity of the heart from the frontal, horizontal, and sagittal planes to provide 12 leads of information. A mathematical calculation in the electronics of the monitoring system is applied to the information, creating a derived 12-lead ECG. Electrode placement for the EASI system is as follows:

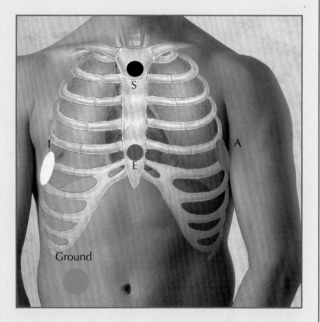

E lead	lower part of the sternum at the level of the fifth intercostal space
A lead	left midaxillary line at the level of the fifth intercostal space
S lead	upper part of the sternum
I lead	right midaxillary line at the level of the fifth intercostal space
Ground	anywhere on the torso

For telemetry monitoring

- Attach an electrode to the end of each leadwire.
- Place the transmitter in the pouch. Tie the pouch strings around the patient's neck and waist, making sure that the pouch fits snugly without causing him discomfort. If no pouch is available, place the transmitter in the patient's bathrobe pocket. Some patient gowns have a built-in pocket *to hold the transmitter and make movement easier.*

Positioning monitoring leads

The illustrations below show the electrode placement for a five-lead system and a three-lead system.

Five-lead system

With the five-lead system, the electrode positions generally remain constant. To select the leads you want to monitor, simply use the lead selection button at the central station or on the bedside monitor. If only a single lead can be monitored, the first choice is usually V_1. If dual lead monitoring is available, choose V_1 and the lead appropriate for the clinical situation.

In the five-lead system (shown at right):
- Place the right arm (RA) electrode near the right shoulder, close to the junction of the right arm and torso.
- Place the left arm (LA) electrode near the left shoulder, close to the junction of the left arm and torso.
- Place the right leg (RL) electrode below the level of the lowest rib on the right abdominal area.
- Place the left leg (LL) electrode below the level of the lowest rib on the left abdominal area.
- Place the chest (C) electrode in the fourth intercostal space to the right of the sternum for V_1 **or** in the fifth intercostal space in the left midaxillary line for V_6.[2]

Note: The chest electrode can be placed in any of the standard V_1 to V_6 locations, but V_1 and then V_6 are generally selected because of their value in arrhythmia monitoring.

Three-lead system

With the three-lead system, the electrodes may need to change position. The first choice of leads to be monitored is modified chest lead 1 (MCL_1), followed by modified chest lead 6 (MCL_6), and then lead II.

For MCL_1 or MCL_6, in the three-lead system (shown below on left):
- Place the RA electrode near the left shoulder, close to the junction of the left arm and torso.

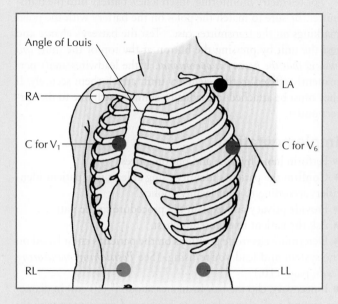

- Place the LA electrode in the fourth intercostal space to the right of the sternum.
- Place the LL electrode in the fifth intercostal space in the left midaxillary line.
- Select lead I on the monitor to obtain MCL_1 and lead II to obtain MCL_6.[2]

For lead II in the three-lead system (shown below on right):
- Place the RA electrode near the right shoulder, close to the junction of the right arm and torso.
- Place the LA electrode near the left shoulder, close to the junction of the left arm and torso.
- Place the LL electrode below the level of the lowest rib on the left abdominal area.
- Select lead II on the monitor.

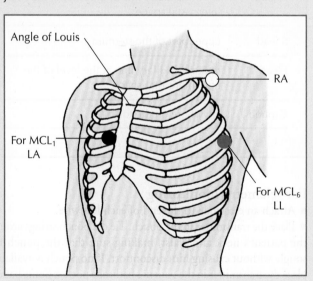

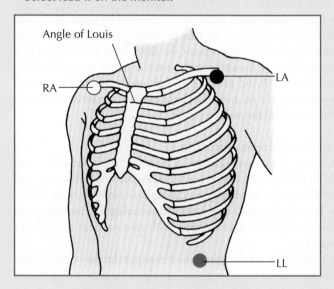

TROUBLESHOOTING

Identifying cardiac monitor problems

PROBLEM	POSSIBLE CAUSES	SOLUTIONS
False-high-rate alarm	■ Monitor interpreting large T waves as QRS complexes, which doubles the rate	■ Reposition electrodes to lead where QRS complexes are taller than T waves. Decrease gain, if necessary.
	■ Skeletal muscle activity	■ Place electrodes away from major muscle masses.
False–low-rate alarm	■ Shift in electrical axis from patient movement, making QRS complexes too small to register	■ Reapply electrodes. Set gain so height of complex is greater than 1 millivoltage.
	■ Low amplitude of QRS	■ Increase gain.
	■ Poor contact between electrode and skin	■ Reapply electrodes.
Low amplitude	■ Gain dial set too low	■ Increase gain.
	■ Poor contact between skin and electrodes; dried gel; broken or loose leadwires; poor connection between patient and monitor; malfunctioning monitor; physiologic loss of QRS amplitude	■ Check connections on all leadwires and monitoring cable. Replace electrodes as necessary.
Wandering baseline	■ Poor position or contact between electrodes and skin	■ Reposition or replace electrodes.
	■ Thoracic movement with respirations	■ Reposition electrodes.
Artifact (waveform interference)	■ Patient having seizures, chills, or anxiety	■ Notify doctor and treat patient as ordered. Keep patient warm and reassure him.
	■ Patient movement	■ Help patient relax.
	■ Electrodes applied improperly	■ Check electrodes and reapply, if necessary.
	■ Static electricity	■ Make sure cables don't have exposed connectors. Change patient's static-causing gown or pajamas.
	■ Electrical short circuit in leadwires or cable	■ Replace broken equipment. Use stress loops when applying leadwires.
	■ Interference from decreased room humidity	■ Regulate humidity to 40%.
Broken lead-wires or cable	■ Stress loops not used on leadwires	■ Replace leadwires and retape them using stress loops.
	■ Cables and leadwires cleaned with alcohol or acetone, causing brittleness	■ Clean cable and leadwires with soapy water. *Don't allow cable ends to become wet.* Replace cable as necessary.
60-cycle interference (fuzzy baseline)	■ Electrical interference from other equipment in room	■ Attach all electrical equipment to common ground. Check plugs to make sure prongs aren't loose.
	■ Patient's bed improperly grounded	■ Attach bed ground to the room's common ground.
Skin excoriation under electrode	■ Patient allergic to electrode adhesive	■ Remove electrodes and apply nonallergenic electrodes and nonallergenic tape.
	■ Electrode on skin too long	■ Remove electrode, clean site, and reapply electrode at new site.

■ Check the patient's waveform for clarity, position, and size. Adjust the gain and baseline, as needed. (If necessary, ask the patient to remain resting or sitting in his room while you locate his ECG pattern at the central station.)

Completing the procedure

■ Select the lead(s) you want to monitor based on the clinical situation. Set the upper and lower limits of the heart rate alarm, based on unit policy. Turn on the alarm. If your system has an arrhythmia and pacemaker recognition system, follow the manufacturer's directions to set individual parameters and activate the alarm.

■ To obtain a rhythm strip, press the RECORD key at the central station. Label or make sure that the strip is labeled with the patient's name, identification number, date, time, and lead(s) recorded. Also measure and record the PR interval, QRS duration, and QT interval.

■ Identify and document the rhythm. Place the rhythm strip in the appropriate location in the patient's medical record.

■ Discard the used supplies in the appropriate receptacle.

■ Remove and discard your gloves and perform hand hygiene.[3,4,5]

■ Document the procedure.[8]

Special considerations

■ Always select the best monitoring lead(s) for arrhythmia identification based on the clinical situation. Many monitors permit the monitoring of more than one lead.

■ Keep in mind that excessive alarming can cause alarm fatigue. Set alarms according to your facility's policy *to ensure a standardized approach to alarm management and to prevent unnecessary alarming, which may cause fatigue.*[9]

■ Monitor the ECG pattern continually for arrhythmias, along with the patient's response to any rhythm or heart rate change, and intervene appropriately.

■ At every shift, make sure the electrodes are properly placed *to ensure accurate interpretation of cardiac rhythm.*

■ Make sure that all electrical equipment and outlets are grounded *to avoid electric shock and interference (artifacts).* Also ensure that the patient is clean and dry *to prevent electric shock.*

■ Avoid opening the electrode packages until just before using *to prevent the gel from drying out.* Check the expiration date on the package before opening.

■ Avoid placing the electrodes on bony prominences, hairy areas, areas where defibrillator pads will be placed, or areas for chest compression.

■ Assess skin integrity, and replace and reposition the electrodes every 24 hours or as necessary.

■ If the patient is being monitored by telemetry, show him how the transmitter works. If applicable, show him the button that will produce a recording of his ECG at the central station. Teach him how to push the button whenever he has symptoms *so that the central console will print a rhythm strip.* Tell the patient to remove the transmitter if he takes a shower or bath, but stress the importance of him letting you know before he removes the unit.

Documentation

Record the date and time that monitoring begins and the monitoring lead used. Note any patient and family teaching. Document a rhythm strip at least every shift and whenever there is a change in the patient's condition (or as stated by your facility's policy). Label the strip, or make sure that the strip is labeled with the patient's name and identification number as well as the date, time, lead(s) recorded, appropriate measurements, and rhythm interpretation.

REFERENCES

1 American Heart Association. (2004). Practice standards for electrocardiographic monitoring in hospital settings. *Circulation, 110,* 2721–2746.
2 Lynn-McHale Wiegand, D. (Ed.). (2011). *AACN procedure manual for critical care* (6th ed.). Philadelphia, PA: Saunders.
3 Centers for Disease Control and Prevention. (October 2002). Guideline for hand hygiene in health-care settings. *Morbidity and Mortality Weekly Report, 51*(RR-16), 1–45. (Level I)
4 The Joint Commission. (2012). Standard NPSG.07.01.01. *Comprehensive accreditation manual for hospitals: The official handbook.* Oakbrook Terrace, IL: The Joint Commission. (Level I)
5 World Health Organization. (2009). *WHO guidelines on hand hygiene in health care: First global patient safety challenge. Clean care is safer care.* Geneva, Switzerland: World Health Organization. (Level I)
6 The Joint Commission. (2012). Standard NPSG.01.01.01. *Comprehensive accreditation manual for hospitals: The official handbook.* Oakbrook Terrace, IL: The Joint Commission. (Level I)
7 American Association of Critical-Care Nurses. (2008). "AACN Practice Alert: Dysrhythmia Monitoring" [Online]. Accessed August 2011 via the Web at http://classic.aacn.org/AACN/practiceAlert.nsf/Files/ Dysrhythmia_Monitoring_04-2008/$file/Dysrhythmia_Monitoring_04-2008.pdf (Level I)
8 The Joint Commission. (2012). Standard RC.01.03.01. *Comprehensive accreditation manual for hospitals: The official handbook.* Oakbrook Terrace, IL: The Joint Commission. (Level I)
9 Graham, K.C., & Cvach, M. (1020). Monitor alarm fatigue: Standardizing use of physiologic monitors and decreasing nuisance alarms. *American Journal of Critical Care, 19*(1), 28–34.

ADDITIONAL REFERENCES

Jevon, P. (2010). An introduction to electrocardiogram monitoring. *Nursing in Critical Care, 15*(1), 34–38.
Siegel, J.D., et al. "2007 Guideline for Isolation Precautions: Preventing Transmission of Infectious Agents in Healthcare Settings" [Online]. Accessed June 2011 via the Web at http://www.cdc.gov/hicpac/ 2007ip/2007isolationprecautions.html

CARDIAC OUTPUT MEASUREMENT

Cardiac output—the amount of blood ejected by the heart—helps evaluate cardiac function. The most widely used method of calculating this measurement is the bolus thermodilution technique. Performed at the patient's bedside, this technique evaluates the cardiac status of critically ill patients and those suspected of having cardiac disease.

Thermodilution method

This illustration shows the path of the injectant solution through the heart during thermodilution cardiac output monitoring.

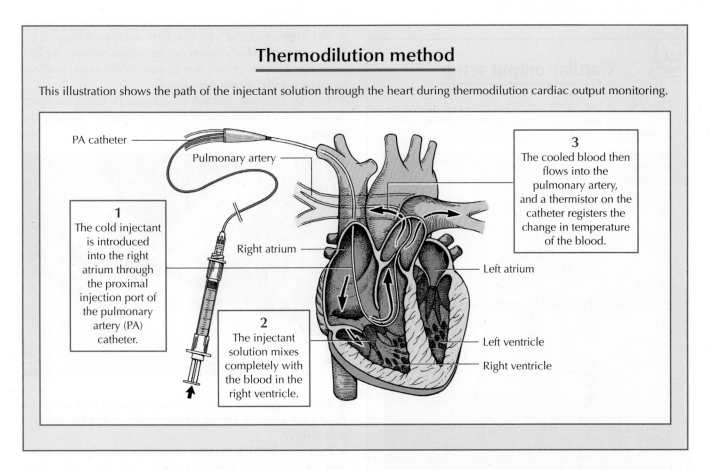

PA catheter

Pulmonary artery

1
The cold injectant is introduced into the right atrium through the proximal injection port of the pulmonary artery (PA) catheter.

2
The injectant solution mixes completely with the blood in the right ventricle.

3
The cooled blood then flows into the pulmonary artery, and a thermistor on the catheter registers the change in temperature of the blood.

Right atrium

Left atrium

Left ventricle

Right ventricle

To measure cardiac output, a quantity of solution colder than the patient's blood is injected into the right atrium through the distal port on a pulmonary artery (PA) catheter. This indicator solution mixes with the blood as it travels through the right ventricle into the pulmonary artery, and a thermistor on the catheter registers the change in temperature of the flowing blood. (See *Thermodilution method*.) A computer then plots the temperature change over time as a curve and calculates flow based on the area under the curve.

Depending on the patient's status and facility policy, iced or room-temperature injectant may be used. Although room-temperature injectant is more convenient and provides equally accurate measurements, iced injectant provides a stronger signal (because it's colder) and may be more accurate in hypothermic patients, or when smaller volumes of injectant must be used (3 to 5 mL), as in patients with volume restrictions or in children.

Equipment

Thermodilution PA catheter in position ▪ output computer and cables (or a module for the bedside cardiac monitor) ▪ closed or open injectant delivery system ▪ 10-mL syringe ▪ 500-mL bag of dextrose 5% in water or normal saline solution ▪ crushed ice and water (for iced-injectant measurement).

Some bedside cardiac monitors measure cardiac output continuously, using either an invasive or a noninvasive method. If your bedside monitor doesn't have this capability, you'll need a free-standing cardiac output computer.

Preparation of equipment

Perform hand hygiene[1,2,3] and assemble the equipment at the patient's bedside. Insert the closed injectant system tubing into the 500-mL bag of IV solution. Connect the 10-mL syringe to the system tubing, and prime the tubing with IV solution until it's free of air. Then clamp the tubing. (See *Cardiac output setup*, page 114.)

If using iced injectant, place the coiled segment into a clean container and add crushed ice and water to cover the entire coil. Let the solution cool for 15 to 20 minutes. If using room-temperature injectant, connect the primed system to the stopcock of the proximal injectant lumen of the PA catheter. Next, connect the temperature probe from the cardiac output computer to the closed injectant system's flow-through housing device. Connect the cardiac output computer cable to the thermistor connector on the PA catheter and verify the blood temperature reading. Finally, turn on the cardiac output computer and enter the correct computation constant, as provided by the catheter's manufacturer. The constant is determined by the volume and temperature of the injectant as well as the size and type of catheter. The patient's height and weight are also factored into the calculation.

Implementation

▪ Perform hand hygiene.[1,2,3]
▪ Confirm the patient's identity using at least two patient identifiers according to your facility's policy.[4]

Cardiac output setup

The photo below shows you how a cardiac output setup should look when it's put together correctly and completely.

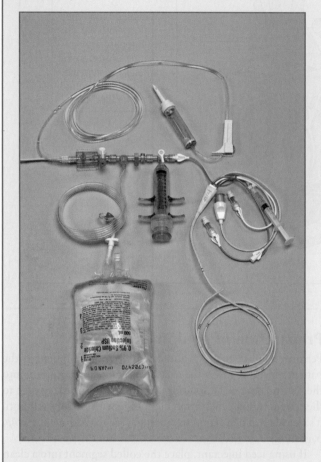

■ Explain the procedure to the patient, and tell him that it will help determine how well his heart is pumping. Reassure him that it will not cause discomfort.

■ Make sure the patient is in a comfortable, supine position with the head of the bed elevated no more than 20 degrees. If the patient's condition prevents this position, use consistent positioning *to ensure consistent cardiac output measurements.*[5] Tell him not to move during the procedure *because movement can cause an error in measurement.*

■ If the proximal line is being used for an infusion, flush the line with saline solution at an appropriate rate *to clear the line of infusing medication without bolusing the patient with medication.*

■ If using iced injectant, note the temperature of the injectant on the computer or monitoring screen; the injectant temperature should be at least 10 degree less than the patient's core temperature.[5]

■ Verify the presence of a PA waveform and observe the patient's heart rate and cardiac rhythm on the cardiac monitor; *a rapid heart rate or an arrhythmia may decrease cardiac output and lead to varying cardiac output measurements.*[5]

■ Turn the stopcock, unclamp the injectant IV tubing (as shown below), and withdraw exactly 10 mL of solution. Reclamp the tubing.[5]

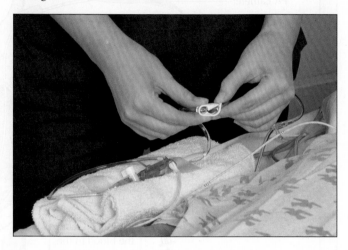

■ Turn the stopcock at the catheter injectant hub to open a fluid path between the injectant lumen of the PA catheter and syringe.

■ Press the START button on the cardiac output computer, or wait for the INJECT message to flash.

■ Observe for a steady baseline temperature before injecting the solution.

■ Inject the solution smoothly within 4 seconds at end expiration *to decrease variation in cardiac output measurements caused by the respiratory cycle* (as shown below).[5] Make sure fluid doesn't leak at the connectors.

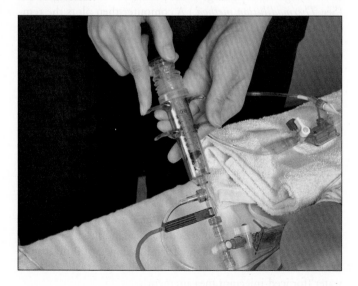

■ If available, analyze the contour of the thermodilution washout curve on a strip chart recorder for a rapid upstroke and a gradual, smooth return to baseline. (See *Analyzing thermodilution curves.*)

Analyzing thermodilution curves

The thermodilution curve provides valuable information about cardiac output, injection technique, and equipment problems. When studying the curve, keep in mind that the area under the curve is inversely proportionate to the cardiac output: The smaller the area under the curve, the higher the cardiac output; the larger the area under the curve, the lower the cardiac output.

   Besides providing a record of cardiac output, the curve may indicate problems related to technique, such as erratic or slow injectant instillations, or other problems, such as respiratory variations or electrical interference. The curves below correspond to those typically seen in clinical practice.

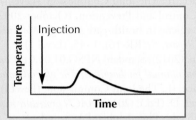

Normal thermodilution curve

With an accurate monitoring system and a patient who has adequate cardiac output, the thermodilution curve begins with a smooth, rapid upstroke and is followed by a smooth gradual downslope. The curve shown at left indicates that the injectant instillation time was within the recommended 4 seconds and that the temperature curve returned to baseline.

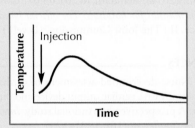

Low cardiac output curve

A thermodilution curve representing low cardiac output shows a rapid, smooth upstroke (from proper injection technique). However, because the heart is ejecting blood less efficiently from the ventricles, the injectant warms slowly and takes longer to be ejected from the ventricle. Consequently, the curve takes longer to return to baseline. This slow return produces a larger area under the curve, corresponding to low cardiac output.

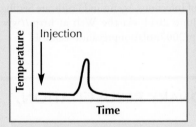

High cardiac output curve

Again, the curve has a rapid, smooth upstroke from proper injection technique. However, because the ventricles are ejecting blood too forcefully, the injectant moves through the heart quickly and the curve returns to baseline more rapidly. The smaller area under the curve suggests higher cardiac output.

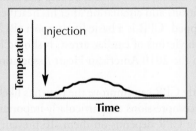

Curve reflecting poor technique

This curve results from an uneven and too-slow (taking more than 4 seconds) administration of injectant. The uneven and slower-than-normal upstroke and the larger area under the curve erroneously indicate low cardiac output. A kinked catheter, unsteady hands during the injection, or improper placement of the injectant lumen in the introducer sheath may also cause this type of curve.

■ Wait 1 minute between injections. *You'll get a better reading by allowing the temperature to return to normal.* Repeat the procedure up to three times. Compute the average of the three values within 10% of the median value, and record the patient's cardiac output.[5]

■ Return the stopcock to its original position, and make sure the injectant delivery system tubing is clamped (as shown on following page top).[5]

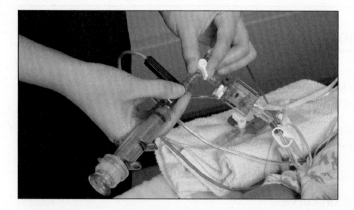

- Verify the presence of a PA waveform on the cardiac monitor.[5]
- After cardiac output measurement, make sure the clamp on the injectant bag is secured *to prevent inadvertent delivery of the injectant to the patient.*
- Perform hand hygiene.[1,2,3]
- Document the procedure.[6]

Special considerations

- Discontinue cardiac output measurements when the patient is hemodynamically stable and weaned from his vasoactive and inotropic medications, according to facility policy or doctor's order; however, you can leave the PA catheter inserted for pressure measurements.
- The normal range for cardiac output is 4 to 8 L/minute.[5] The adequacy of a patient's cardiac output is better assessed by calculating his cardiac index (CI), adjusted for his body size.
- To calculate the patient's CI, divide his cardiac output by his body surface area (BSA), a function of height and weight. For example, a cardiac output of 4 L/minute might be adequate for a 65″, 120-lb (165-cm, 54-kg) patient (normally a BSA of 1.59 and a CI of 2.5), but would be inadequate for a 74″, 230-lb (188-cm, 104-kg) patient (normally a BSA of 2.26 and a CI of 1.8). The normal CI for adults ranges from 2.5 to 4.2 L/minute/m^2; for pregnant women, 3.5 to 6.5 L/minute/m^2.

ELDER ALERT *Normal CI for elderly adults is 2 to 2.5 L/minute/m^2.*

- Monitor the patient for signs and symptoms of inadequate perfusion, including restlessness, fatigue, changes in levels of consciousness, decreased capillary refill time, diminished peripheral pulses, oliguria, and pale, cool skin.
- Add the fluid volume injected for cardiac output determinations to the patient's total intake. Injectant delivery of 30 mL/hour will contribute 720 mL to the patient's 24-hour intake.

Complications

Complications are rare from cardiac output measurement but may include bradycardia.

Documentation

Document your patient's cardiac output, CI, and other hemodynamic values and vital signs at the time of measurement. Note the patient's position during measurement and any other complications, such as bradycardia or neurologic changes. Record the date, time, and name of the doctor notified of any abnormal results, prescribed interventions, and the patient's response to those interventions. Document any patient teaching provided.

REFERENCES

1 World Health Organization. (2009). *WHO guidelines on hand hygiene in health care: First global patient safety challenge. Clean care is safer care.* Geneva, Switzerland: World Health Organization. (Level I)
2 The Joint Commission. (2012). Standard NPSG.07.01.01. *Comprehensive accreditation manual for hospitals: The official handbook.* Oakbrook Terrace, IL: The Joint Commission. (Level I)
3 Centers for Disease Control and Prevention. (October 2002). Guideline for hand hygiene in health-care settings. *Morbidity and Mortality Weekly Report, 51*(RR-16), 1–45. (Level 1)
4 The Joint Commission. (2012). Standard NPSG.01.01.01. *Comprehensive accreditation manual for hospitals: The official handbook.* Oakbrook Terrace, IL: The Joint Commission. (Level I)
5 Lynn-McHale Wiegand, D. (Ed.). (2011). *AACN procedure manual for critical care* (6th ed.). Philadelphia, PA: Saunders.
6 The Joint Commission. (2012). Standard RC.01.03.01. *Comprehensive accreditation manual for hospitals: The official handbook.* Oakbrook Terrace, IL: The Joint Commission. (Level I)

ADDITIONAL REFERENCES

Corley, A., et al. (2009). Nurse-determined assessment of cardiac output. Comparing a non-invasive cardiac output device and pulmonary artery catheter: A prospective observational study. *International Journal of Nurse Studies, 46*(10), 1291–1297.
Siegel, J.D., et al. "2007 Guideline for Isolation Precautions: Preventing Transmission of Infectious Agents in Healthcare Settings" [Online]. Accessed June 2011 via the Web at http://www.cdc.gov/hicpac/2007ip/2007isolationprecautions.html

CARDIOPULMONARY RESUSCITATION, ADULT

Cardiopulmonary resuscitation (CPR) seeks to restore and maintain the patient's respirations and circulation after his heartbeat and breathing have stopped. CPR is a basic life support (BLS) procedure performed on victims of cardiac arrest. It should be performed according to the 2010 American Heart Association (AHA) guidelines.[1]

Studies show that early CPR can improve the patient's likelihood of survival. Chest compressions are particularly important because perfusion during CPR depends on them. To prevent a delay in chest compressions, the AHA changed the sequence of CPR in the 2010 guidelines from "A-B-C" (airway, breathing, and compressions) to "C-A-B" (compressions, airway, and breathing), which gives the highest priority to chest compressions when resuscitating a patient in cardiac arrest.[1]

High-quality CPR is important not only at the onset of resuscitation but throughout the entire resuscitation process. Integrating defibrillation and other advanced cardiac life support (ACLS) measures into the resuscitation process minimizes interruptions in CPR.[1]

Equipment

Backboard or other hard surface ■ automated external defibrillator (AED) ■ gloves ■ Optional: disposable airway equipment.

Implementation

Guidelines for performing CPR vary depending on whether CPR is being performed by one or two rescuers.

One-person CPR

■ The following illustrated instructions provide a step-by-step guide for CPR as currently recommended by the AHA. (See *The AHA BLS algorithm,* page 118.)

■ As a sole rescuer, you will determine unresponsiveness, check for breathing, activate the emergency response system, check for a pulse, and begin chest compressions.[1]

■ Assess the patient to determine if he's unconscious (as shown below). Tap him on the shoulder and shout, "Are you alright?" *This helps ensure that you don't begin CPR on a conscious person.* While checking for responsiveness, check to see if the patient is apneic or only gasping. If the patient is unresponsive and apneic or only gasping, assume that he's in cardiac arrest.[1]

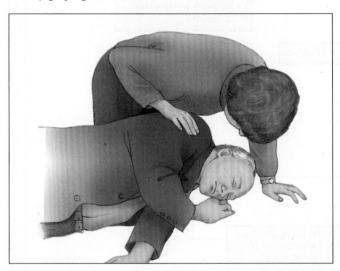

■ Immediately call out for help and have someone activate the emergency response system or call a code.[1]

■ Send someone to get the AED. If no one is available, get the AED and return to the patient.[1]

■ Put on gloves, if available, *to prevent exposure to potentially infectious blood and body fluids.*

■ Place the patient supine on a firm surface such as a backboard; if the patient is on an air-filled mattress, deflate the mattress *to maximize the effectiveness of chest compressions.* When moving him, roll his head and torso as a unit; avoid twisting or pulling his neck, shoulders, or hips (as shown in next column at top). Don't delay the initiation of CPR to place the patient on a backboard.[1]

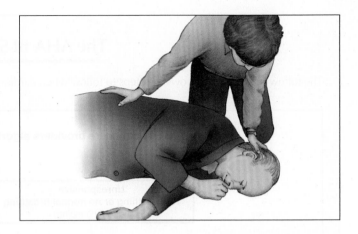

■ Kneel beside the patient's chest or stand beside his bed at his chest. Palpate the carotid artery that's closest to you. To do this, place your index and middle fingers in the groove between the trachea and the sternocleidomastoid muscle (as shown below). Palpate for no longer than 10 seconds.[1]

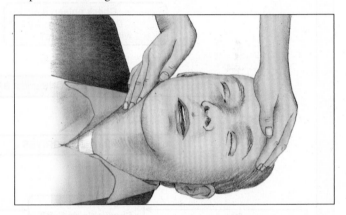

■ If you detect a strong, easily palpable pulse, don't begin chest compressions. Instead, perform rescue breathing by giving the patient 10 to 12 breaths per minute (1 breath every 5 to 6 seconds). Give each breath over 1 second; each breath should cause visible chest rise.[1]

■ If, within 10 seconds, you don't feel a pulse or you aren't sure whether you feel a pulse, start giving chest compressions. Make sure that your knees are apart *to provide a wide base of support.* Place the heel of one hand on the center of the patient's chest (over the lower half of the sternum) and the heel of the other hand on top of the first so that your hands are overlapped and parallel (as shown below).[1]

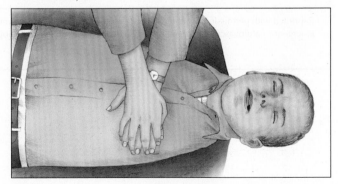

The AHA BLS algorithm[1]

The following algorithm shows the steps to follow when cardiac arrest is suspected in an adult patient.

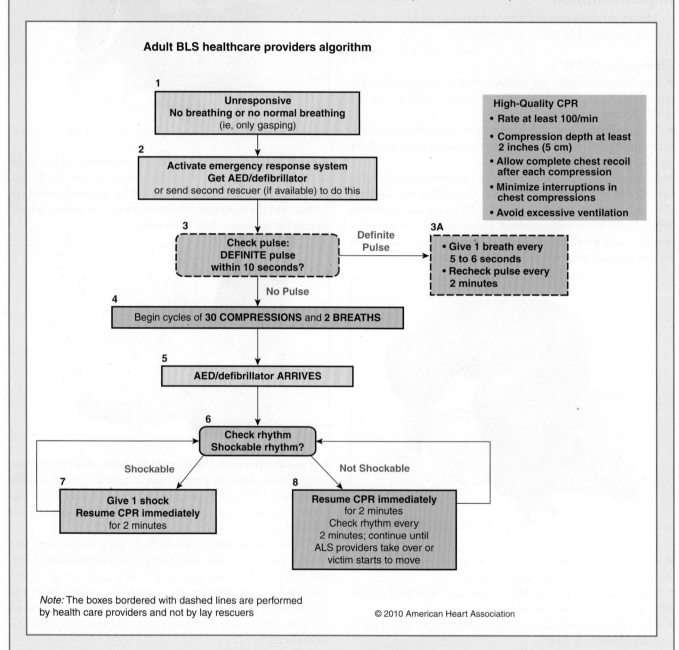

Adult BLS healthcare providers algorithm

1
Unresponsive
No breathing or no normal breathing
(ie, only gasping)

2
Activate emergency response system
Get AED/defibrillator
or send second rescuer (if available) to do this

High-Quality CPR
- Rate at least 100/min
- Compression depth at least 2 inches (5 cm)
- Allow complete chest recoil after each compression
- Minimize interruptions in chest compressions
- Avoid excessive ventilation

3
Check pulse:
DEFINITE pulse
within 10 seconds?

Definite Pulse →

3A
- Give 1 breath every 5 to 6 seconds
- Recheck pulse every 2 minutes

No Pulse

4
Begin cycles of **30 COMPRESSIONS** and **2 BREATHS**

5
AED/defibrillator ARRIVES

6
Check rhythm
Shockable rhythm?

Shockable

Not Shockable

7
Give 1 shock
Resume CPR immediately
for 2 minutes

8
Resume CPR immediately
for 2 minutes
Check rhythm every
2 minutes; continue until
ALS providers take over or
victim starts to move

Note: The boxes bordered with dashed lines are performed by health care providers and not by lay rescuers

© 2010 American Heart Association

■ With your elbows locked, arms straight, and shoulders directly over your hands (as shown below), give compressions. Using the weight of your upper body, compress the patient's chest at least 2" (5 cm), keeping chest compression and chest recoil durations equal. Allow the chest to completely recoil after each chest compression *so the heart can adequately refill with blood.*[1]

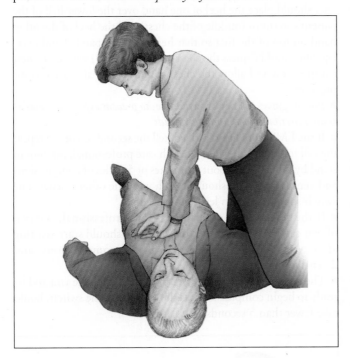

■ Give 30 compressions at a rate of at least 100 compressions per minute, pushing hard and fast. After administering 30 compressions, open the patient's airway and give 2 ventilations. If the patient doesn't appear to have a neck injury, use the head-tilt, chin-lift maneuver *to open his airway.*[1] To accomplish this, first place your hand that's closer to the patient's head on his forehead. Then apply enough pressure to tilt the patient's head back. Next, place the fingertips of your other hand under the bony part of his lower jaw near the chin; avoid placing your fingertips on the soft tissue under the patient's chin *because you may inadvertently obstruct the airway you're trying to open.* At the same time, keep his mouth partially open (as shown below).

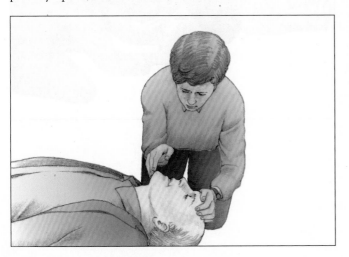

■ If you suspect a neck injury, use the jaw-thrust maneuver.[1] To perform this maneuver, kneel at the patient's head with your elbows on the ground. Rest your thumbs on his lower jaw near the corners of the mouth, pointing your thumbs toward his feet. Then place your fingertips around the lower jaw. To open the airway, lift the lower jaw with your fingertips (as shown below).

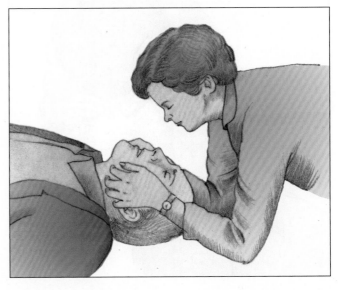

■ To begin ventilations, pinch the patient's nostrils shut with the thumb and index finger of the hand you've had on his forehead (as shown below).

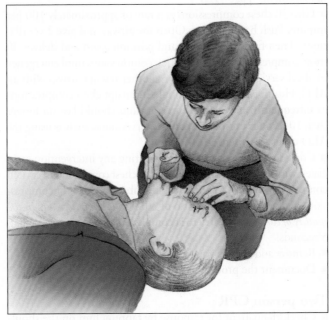

■ Take a regular breath and place your mouth over the patient's mouth, creating a tight seal (as shown below). Give 2 breaths, each over 1 second. Each ventilation should have enough volume to produce visible chest rise.[1]

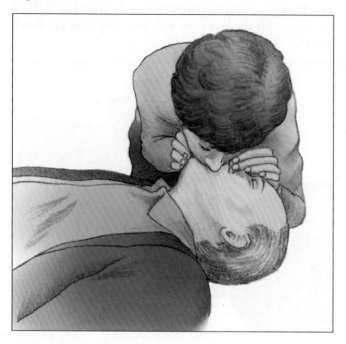

■ If the first ventilation isn't successful, reposition the patient's head and try again. If you're still unsuccessful, he may have a foreign body airway obstruction. (See "Foreign body obstruction and management," page 312.)
■ Give 30 chest compressions at a rate of approximately 100 per minute. Push hard and fast. Open the airway and give 2 ventilations. Then find the proper hand position again and deliver 30 more compressions. Continue chest compressions until emergency medical service (EMS) arrives or another rescuer arrives with an AED. Health care providers should interrupt chest compressions as infrequently as possible. Interruptions should last no longer than 10 seconds except for special interventions, such as using the AED or airway insertion.[1]
■ Consider switching compressors during any intervention associated with appropriate interruptions in chest compressions. Switch compressors every 2 minutes (or after about 5 cycles of compressions and ventilations at a ratio of 30:2) *to prevent decreases in the quality of compressions.* Try to accomplish the switch in fewer than 5 seconds.
■ Remove and discard your gloves and perform hand hygiene.[2,3,4]
■ Document the procedure.[5]

Two-person CPR
■ Check the patient for response by tapping him on the shoulder and shouting, "Are you alright?" At the same time, check to see whether the patient is apneic or only gasping.

■ In two-person rescue, if the patient is unresponsive and apneic or only gasping, one rescuer should activate EMS and get the AED, while the other rescuer checks for a pulse, taking no more than 10 seconds; if a pulse isn't present, that rescuer immediately begins chest compressions, using a compression-to-ventilation ratio of 30:2. To adequately perform chest compressions, the rescuer should place the heel of one hand over the lower half of the patient's sternum (middle of the chest) and the heel of the other hand on top of the first so that her hands are parallel and overlap. She should depress the chest at least 2″ (5 cm) with each chest compression and allow the chest to fully recoil after each compression.[1]
■ Put on gloves, if they are available, *to prevent exposure to potentially infectious blood and body fluids.*
■ If the EMS team hasn't arrived, tell the second rescuer to repeat the call for help. If he's not a health care professional, ask him to stand by. Then, after about 2 minutes or 5 cycles of compressions and ventilations, you should switch with the other rescuer. The switch should occur in less than 5 seconds.[1]
■ If the rescuer is another health care professional, the two of you can perform two-person CPR. He should start assisting after you've finished a cycle of 30 compressions and 2 ventilations.[1]
■ The second rescuer should get into place opposite you and be ready to begin compressions (as shown below); the switch should take fewer than 5 seconds.[1]

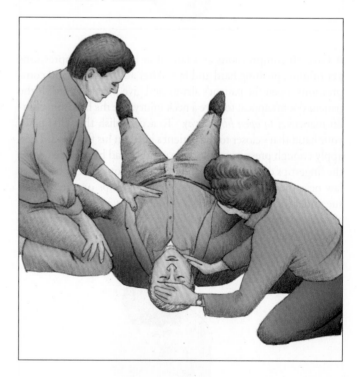

■ The second rescuer should begin delivering compressions at a rate of at least 100 per minute (as shown below). Compressions and ventilations should be administered at a ratio of 30 compressions to 2 ventilations. The compressor (at this point, the second rescuer) should count out loud so the ventilator can anticipate when to give ventilations, and compressions shouldn't be interrupted to perform ventilations. *To ensure that the ventilations are effective,* they should cause a visible chest rise and be administered over 1 second.[1]

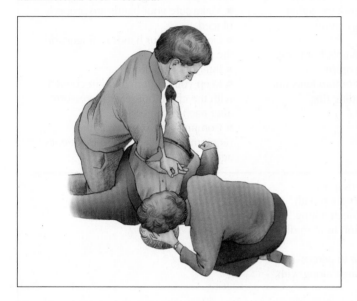

■ The compressor role should switch after 5 cycles of compressions and ventilations. The switch should occur in fewer than 5 seconds. Chest compressions shouldn't be interrupted for longer than 10 seconds unless such specific interventions as defibrillation or advanced airway placement are necessary. *Interrupting chest compressions to palpate for a pulse or to otherwise check for the return of spontaneous circulation can compromise perfusion to vital organs.*[1]
■ As shown below, both of you should continue giving CPR until an AED arrives, the ACLS providers take over, or the victim starts to move.

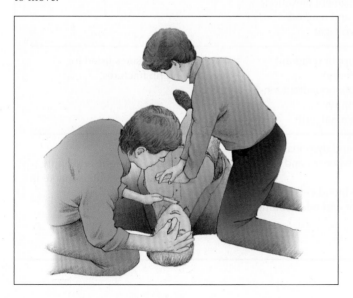

■ Remove and discard your gloves and perform hand hygiene.[2,3,4]
■ Document the procedure.[5]

Special considerations
■ Some health care professionals may hesitate to give mouth-to-mouth rescue breaths. For this reason, the AHA recommends that all health care professionals learn how to use disposable airway equipment.
■ Lay rescuers who can perform both compressions and ventilations should use the head-tilt, chin-lift maneuver to open the airway.

Complications
CPR can cause certain complications—especially if the compressor doesn't place her hands properly on the sternum. These complications include fractured ribs, a lacerated liver, and punctured lungs. Gastric distention, a common complication, results from giving too much air during ventilation. (See *Potential hazards of CPR,* page 122.)

Documentation
Whenever you perform CPR, document why you initiated it, whether the victim suffered from cardiac or respiratory arrest, when you found the victim and started CPR, and how long the victim received CPR. Note his response and any complications. Also include any interventions taken to correct complications.

If the victim also received ACLS, document which interventions were performed, who performed them, when they were performed, and what equipment was used.

REFERENCES

1 American Heart Association. (2010). 2010 American Heart Association guidelines for cardiopulmonary resuscitation and emergency cardiovascular care. *Circulation, 122*(Suppl. 3), S686–705. (Level I)
2 World Health Organization. (2009). *WHO guidelines on hand hygiene in health care: First global patient safety challenge. Clean care is safer care.* Geneva, Switzerland: World Health Organization. (Level I)
3 The Joint Commission. (2012). Standard NPSG.07.01.01. *Comprehensive accreditation manual for hospitals: The official handbook.* Oakbrook Terrace, IL: The Joint Commission. (Level I)
4 Centers for Disease Control and Prevention. (October 2002). Guideline for hand hygiene in health-care settings. *Morbidity and Mortality Weekly Report, 51*(RR-16), 1–45. (Level 1)
5 The Joint Commission. (2012). Standard RC.01.03.01. *Comprehensive accreditation manual for hospitals: The official handbook.* Oakbrook Terrace, IL: The Joint Commission. (Level I)

ADDITIONAL REFERENCES

American Association for Respiratory Care. (2004). AARC clinical practice guideline: Resuscitation and defibrillation in the health care setting—2004 revision & update. *Respiratory Care, 89*(9), 1085–1099.
Li, Y., et al. (2008). Identifying potentially shockable rhythms without interrupting cardiopulmonary resuscitation. *Critical Care Medicine, 36*(1), 198–203.

Potential hazards of CPR

Cardiopulmonary resuscitation (CPR) can cause various complications, including injury to bones and vital organs. This chart describes the causes of CPR hazards and lists preventive steps.

HAZARD	CAUSES	ASSESSMENT FINDINGS	PREVENTIVE MEASURES
Sternum and rib fractures	■ Osteoporosis ■ Malnutrition ■ Improper hand placement	■ Paradoxical chest movement ■ Chest pain or tenderness that increases with inspiration ■ Crepitus ■ Palpation of movable bony fragments over the sternum ■ On palpation, sternum feels unattached to surrounding ribs	*While performing CPR:* ■ Make sure your hands are properly placed. ■ Don't rest your hands or fingers on the patient's ribs. ■ Interlock your fingers. ■ Keep your bottom hand in contact with the chest, but release pressure after each compression. ■ Compress the sternum at the recommended depth for the patient's age.
Pneumothorax, hemothorax, or both	■ Lung puncture from fractured rib	■ Chest pain and dyspnea ■ Decreased or absent breath sounds over the affected lung ■ Tracheal deviation from midline ■ Hypotension ■ Hyperresonance to percussion over the affected area along with shoulder pain	■ Follow the measures listed for sternum and rib fractures.
Injury to the heart and great vessels (pericardial tamponade, atrial or ventricular rupture, vessel laceration, cardiac contusion, punctures of the heart chambers)	■ Improperly performed chest compressions ■ Transvenous or transthoracic pacing attempts ■ Central line placement during resuscitation ■ Intracardiac drug administration	■ Jugular vein distention ■ Muffled heart sounds ■ Pulsus paradoxus ■ Narrowed pulse pressure ■ Electrical alternans (decreased electrical amplitude of every other QRS complex) ■ Adventitious heart sounds ■ Hypotension ■ Electrocardiogram changes (arrhythmias, ST-segment elevation, T-wave inversion, and marked decrease in QRS voltage)	■ Perform chest compressions properly.
Organ laceration (primarily liver and spleen)	■ Forceful compression ■ Sharp edge of a fractured rib or xiphoid process	■ Persistent right upper quadrant tenderness (liver injury) ■ Persistent left upper quadrant tenderness (splenic injury) ■ Increasing abdominal girth	■ Follow the measures listed for sternum and rib fractures.
Aspiration of stomach contents	■ Gastric distention and an elevated diaphragm from high ventilatory pressures	■ Fever, hypoxia, and dyspnea ■ Auscultation of wheezes and crackles ■ Increased white blood cell count ■ Changes in color and odor of lung secretions	■ Intubate early. ■ Insert a nasogastric tube and apply suction, if gastric distention is marked.

Nettina, S.M. (2010). *Lippincott manual of nursing practice* (9th ed.). Philadelphia, PA: Lippincott Williams & Wilkins.

CARDIOPULMONARY RESUSCITATION, CHILD

An adult who needs cardiopulmonary resuscitation (CPR) typically suffers from a primary cardiac disorder or an arrhythmia that has stopped the heart. A child who needs CPR typically suffers from hypoxia caused by respiratory difficulty or respiratory arrest.

Most pediatric crises requiring CPR are preventable. They include motor vehicle accidents, drowning, burns, smoke inhalation, falls, poisoning, suffocation, and choking (typically from inhaling a balloon, small object, or food, such as a hot dog, rounded candy, nut, or grape).[1] Other causes of cardiopulmonary arrest in children include laryngospasm and edema from upper respiratory infections.

The goal of CPR is the return of spontaneous circulation. However, CPR techniques differ depending on whether the patient is an adult, a child, or an infant.[1]

For CPR purposes, the American Heart Association defines a patient by age. An infant is younger than age 1; a child is age 1 to puberty.[1] Survival chances improve the sooner CPR begins and the faster advanced life-support systems are implemented. However speedily you undertake CPR for a child, though, first determine whether the child's respiratory distress results from a mechanical obstruction or an infection, such as epiglottiditis or croup. These infections require immediate medical attention, not CPR. CPR is appropriate only when the child isn't breathing or is only gasping.[1]

This procedure is specific to CPR performed by health care providers.

Equipment

Backboard or other hard surface ■ automated external defibrillator (AED) ■ gloves ■ Optional: disposable child-size airway equipment.

Implementation

■ Gently tap the child and ask loudly, "Are you okay?" Call the child's name if you know it *to elicit a response.*[1] If the child is conscious but has difficulty breathing, help her into a position that best eases her breathing—if she hasn't naturally assumed this position.[1]

■ Call for help to alert others and to enlist emergency assistance. If you're alone and the child isn't breathing or is only gasping, perform CPR for 5 cycles (2 minutes) before calling for help. A single cycle for a lone rescuer is 30 chest compressions and 2 breaths.[1]

■ Put on gloves, if available, *to prevent exposure to potentially infectious blood and body fluids.*

■ Position the child in the supine position on a firm, flat surface (usually the ground).[1] The surface should provide the resistance needed for adequate chest compressions. If you must turn the

child from a prone position, support her head and neck and turn her as a unit to avoid injuring her spine (as shown below).

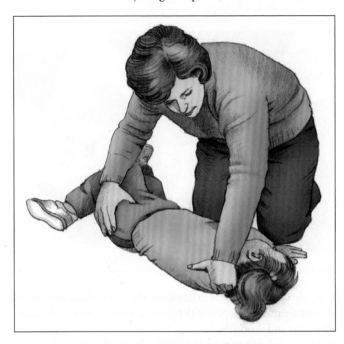

Restoring heartbeat and circulation

■ Assess circulation by palpating the carotid artery for a pulse.[1]

■ Locate the carotid artery with two or three fingers of one hand. Place your fingers in the center of the child's neck on the side closest to you, and slide your fingers into the groove formed by the trachea and the sternocleidomastoid muscles (as shown below). Palpate the artery for no more than 10 seconds to confirm the child's pulse status.[1]

■ If you feel the child's pulse, continue rescue breathing, giving 1 breath every 3 to 5 seconds (12 to 20 breaths/minute).[1]

■ If you can't feel a pulse or the pulse is less than 60 beats/minute with signs of poor perfusion, begin chest compressions.[1]

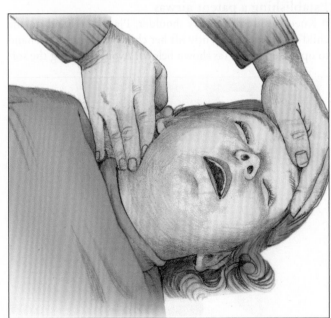

■ Kneel next to the child's chest. Place the heel of one or two hands in the center of the child's chest, directly between her nipples (as shown below).[1]

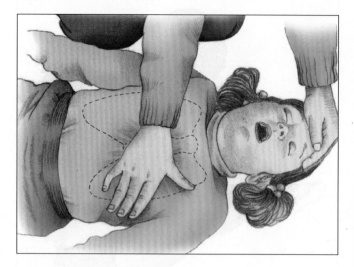

■ Apply enough pressure to compress the child's chest downward at least a third the depth of the chest. Deliver cycles of 30 compressions and 2 breaths.[1]

■ After 5 cycles (2 minutes) of CPR, call emergency medical service and get an AED, if appropriate. If you can't detect a pulse within 10 seconds, continue chest compressions and rescue breathing and use the AED after 5 cycles. Coordinate chest compressions and shock delivery to minimize the time between them. Resume CPR, beginning with chest compressions immediately after the shock is delivered.[1]

■ If you can detect a pulse, check for spontaneous respirations. If you fail to detect respirations, give 1 breath every 3 to 5 seconds (12 to 20 breaths/minute), and continue to monitor the pulse. If the child begins breathing spontaneously, keep the airway open and monitor the respirations and pulse.[1]

Establishing a patent airway

■ Kneel beside the child's shoulder. Place one hand on the child's forehead and gently lift her chin with your other hand to open her airway (as shown below). Avoid fingering the soft

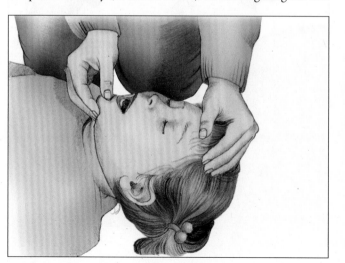

neck tissue *to avoid obstructing the airway.* Never let the child's mouth close completely.

■ If you suspect a neck injury, use the jaw-thrust maneuver to open the child's airway *to keep from moving the child's neck.*[1] To do this, kneel beside the child's head. With your elbows on the ground, rest your thumbs at the corners of the child's mouth and place two or three fingers of each hand under the lower jaw. Lift the jaw upward.

■ While maintaining an open airway, place your ear near the child's mouth and nose to evaluate her breathing status (as shown below).[1] Look for chest movement, listen for exhaled air, and feel for exhaled air on your cheek.

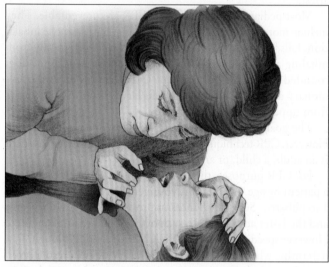

■ If the child is breathing, maintain an open airway and monitor respirations.

Restoring ventilation

■ If the child isn't breathing, maintain the open airway position and take a breath. Then pinch the child's nostrils shut and cover the child's mouth with your mouth (as shown below). Give 2 slow breaths (1 to 1½ seconds/breath) and pause between each.[1]

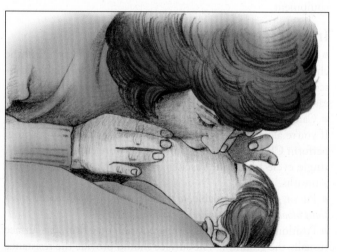

- If your first attempt at ventilation fails to restore the child's breathing, reposition the child's head to open the airway and try again.[1] If you're still unsuccessful, the airway may be obstructed by a foreign body. (See "Foreign body obstruction and management," page 312.)
- After you remove the obstruction, check for breathing and pulse. If absent, proceed with chest compressions.[1]
- Perform hand hygiene.[2,3,4]
- Document the procedure.[5]

Special considerations

- A child has a small airway that can easily be blocked by the tongue. If this occurs, simply opening the airway may eliminate the obstruction.
- When performing chest compressions, take care to ensure smooth motions. Keep your fingers off—and the heel of your hand on—the child's chest at all times. Also, time your motions so that the compression and relaxation phases are equal *to promote effective compressions.*
- If the child has breathing difficulty and a parent or guardian is present, find out whether the child recently had a fever or an upper respiratory tract infection. If so, suspect epiglottiditis. In this instance, don't attempt to manipulate the airway because laryngospasm may occur and completely obstruct the airway. Allow the child to assume a comfortable position, and monitor her breathing until additional assistance arrives.
- Persist in attempts to remove an obstruction. As hypoxia develops, the child's muscles will relax, allowing you to remove the foreign object.
- During resuscitation efforts, make sure someone communicates support and information to the parents or guardian.
- If available, use a bag-valve mask over the child's nose and mouth when performing ventilations.

Complications

CPR can cause complications if the compressor doesn't place his hands properly on the sternum. These complications include fractured ribs, a lacerated liver, and punctured lungs. Gastric distention, a common complication, results from giving too much air during ventilation.

Documentation

Document all of the events of resuscitation and the names of the individuals who were present. Record whether the child suffered cardiac or respiratory arrest. Note where the arrest occurred, the time CPR began, how long the procedure continued, and the outcome. Document any complications—for example, a fractured rib, a bruised mouth, or gastric distention—as well as nursing actions taken to correct them.

If the child received pediatric advanced life support, document which interventions were performed, who performed them, when they were performed, and what equipment was used.

References

1 American Heart Association. (2010). 2010 American Heart Association guidelines for cardiopulmonary resuscitation and emergency cardiovascular care: Pediatric basic life support. *Circulation, 122* (Suppl. 3).(Level I)
2 World Health Organization. (2009). *WHO guidelines on hand hygiene in health care: First global patient safety challenge. Clean care is safer care.* Geneva, Switzerland: World Health Organization. (Level I)
3 The Joint Commission. (2012). Standard NPSG.07.01.01. *Comprehensive accreditation manual for hospitals: The official handbook.* Oakbrook Terrace, IL: The Joint Commission. (Level I).
4 Centers for Disease Control and Prevention. (October 2002). Guideline for hand hygiene in health-care settings. *Morbidity and Mortality Weekly Report, 51*(RR-16), 1–45. (Level 1)
5 The Joint Commission. (2012). Standard RC.01.03.01. *Comprehensive accreditation manual for hospitals: The official handbook.* Oakbrook Terrace, IL: The Joint Commission. (Level I)

Cardiopulmonary resuscitation, infant

An adult who needs cardiopulmonary resuscitation (CPR) typically suffers from a primary cardiac disorder or an arrhythmia that has stopped the heart. An infant who needs CPR typically suffers from hypoxia caused by respiratory difficulty or respiratory arrest.

Most pediatric crises requiring CPR are preventable. They include motor vehicle accidents, drowning, burns, smoke inhalation, falls, poisoning, suffocation, and choking (usually from inhaling liquids).[1] Other causes of cardiopulmonary arrest in infants include laryngospasm and edema from upper respiratory infections and sudden infant death syndrome.

The goal of CPR is the return of spontaneous circulation.[1] However, CPR techniques differ depending on whether the patient is an adult, a child, or an infant.

For CPR purposes, the American Heart Association defines a patient by age. An infant is younger than age 1; a child is age 1 to puberty.[1] Survival chances improve the sooner CPR begins and the faster advanced life-support systems are implemented. No matter how speedily you undertake CPR for an infant, however, first determine whether the infant's respiratory distress results from a mechanical obstruction or an infection, such as epiglottiditis or croup. Epiglottiditis or croup requires immediate medical attention, not CPR. CPR is appropriate only when the infant isn't breathing.[1]

Equipment

Backboard or other hard surface ▪ gloves ▪ Optional: disposable infant-size airway equipment.

Implementation

- Gently tap the foot of the apparently unconscious infant and call out his name.
- Put on gloves, if available, *to prevent exposure to potentially infectious blood and body fluids.*

■ For a sudden, witnessed collapse, call for help or call emergency medical service. If you didn't witness the collapse, perform resuscitation measures for 2 minutes; then call for help.[1]
■ Place the infant supine on a hard surface.

Restoring heartbeat and circulation
■ Assess the infant's pulse by palpating the brachial artery located inside the infant's upper arm between the elbow and the shoulder (as shown below).[1] Take no more than 10 seconds to try to find a pulse. If you find a pulse and the pulse is greater than or equal to 60 beats/minute, continue rescue breathing but don't initiate chest compressions.[1]

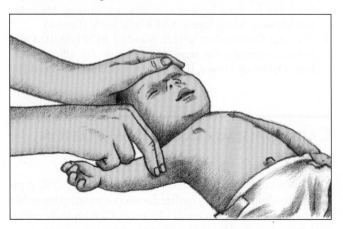

■ Begin chest compressions if you find no pulse or the pulse rate is less than 60 beats/minute with signs of poor perfusion. Place two fingers on the sternum just below the nipple line (as shown below). Use these two fingers to depress the sternum at least a third of the depth of the chest at 100 compressions per minute.[1] When performing chest compressions, take care to ensure smooth motions. Keep your fingers on the infant's chest at all times. Time your motions so that the compression and relaxation phases are equal *to promote effective compressions.*

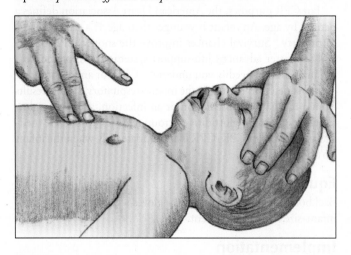

■ Supply 2 breaths after every 30 compressions if you are the lone rescuer. If two rescuers are involved, deliver 2 breaths for every 15 compressions.[1]

■ Open the airway using the head-tilt, chin-lift maneuver, unless contraindicated by trauma. Don't hyperextend the infant's neck.[1]
■ Place your ear near the infant's mouth and nose to evaluate his breathing status. Look for chest movement, listen for exhaled air, and feel for exhale air on your cheek.[1]
■ If the infant is breathing, maintain an open airway and monitor respirations.[1]

Restoring ventilation
■ If the infant isn't breathing, take a breath and tightly seal your mouth over the infant's nose and mouth (as shown below).[1]

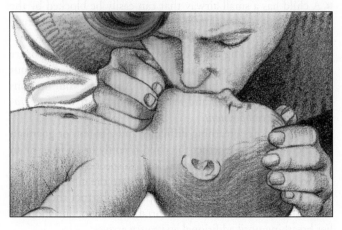

■ Deliver 2 breaths. If the infant's chest rises and falls, then the amount of air is probably adequate. If the chest doesn't rise, reposition the head, make a better seal, and try again.[1]
■ Continue rescue breathing with 1 breath every 3 to 5 seconds (12 to 20 breaths/minute) if you can detect a pulse and the pulse rate is greater than or equal to 60 beats/minute.[1]
■ Perform hand hygiene.[2,3,4]
■ Document the procedure.[5]

Special considerations
■ If two rescuers are available, the two thumb–encircling hands technique is preferred for chest compressions. Place your hands around the infant's chest with your fingers around the thorax and place your thumbs together on the lower half of the sternum.[1] Compress the sternum with your thumbs and squeeze your fingers for counterpressure.
■ An infant's tongue can easily block his small airway. If this occurs, simply opening the airway may eliminate the obstruction.
■ If the infant has breathing difficulty and a parent or guardian is present, find out whether the infant recently had a fever or an upper respiratory tract infection. If so, suspect epiglottiditis. In this instance, don't attempt to manipulate the airway because laryngospasm may occur and completely obstruct the airway. Allow the infant to assume a comfortable position, and monitor his breathing until additional assistance arrives.
■ During resuscitation efforts, make sure someone communicates support and information to the parents or guardian.
■ If available, use a bag-valve mask over the infant's nose and mouth when delivering ventilations.[1]

Elements of a nursing diagnosis

The following summary presents the key elements of a nursing diagnosis.

Human response or problem

After analyzing the patient's condition, choose a diagnostic label from a facility-sanctioned list or create a label specific to the patient. For consistency, most facilities use NANDA-I's list of nursing diagnoses. An example of a diagnostic label is *Excess fluid volume*.

Related factors

The second part of the nursing diagnosis lists factors that seem to influence the patient in a way that pertains to the diagnostic label. Connect these factors to the diagnostic label with the phrase *related to* or the abbreviation *R/T*. The previous example could read, *Excess fluid volume R/T increased sodium intake.*

Defining characteristics

To complete the nursing diagnosis, list defining characteristics, which are signs and symptoms uncovered during assessment that help define the diagnostic label. You may list them beneath the diagnosis and related factors. Or you may add them to the diagnostic statement and connect them with the phrase *as evidenced by* or the abbreviation *AEB*. The example could read, *Excess fluid volume R/T increased sodium intake AEB edema, weight gain, shortness of breath, and S₃ heart sounds.*

Complications

CPR can cause complications if the compressor doesn't place his fingers properly on the sternum. These complications include fractured ribs, a lacerated liver, and punctured lungs. Gastric distention, a common complication, results from giving too much air during ventilation.

Documentation

Document all of the events of resuscitation and the names of the individuals who were present. Record whether the infant suffered cardiac or respiratory arrest. Note where the arrest occurred, the time CPR began, how long the procedure continued, and the outcome. Document any complications—for example, a fractured rib, a bruised mouth, or gastric distention—as well as actions taken to correct them.

If the infant received pediatric advanced life support, document which interventions were performed, who performed them, when they were performed, and what equipment was used.

REFERENCES

1 American Heart Association. (2010). 2010 American Heart Association guidelines for cardiopulmonary resuscitation and emergency cardiovascular care: Pediatric basic life support. *Circulation, 122*(Suppl. 3). (Level I)
2 World Health Organization. (2009). *WHO guidelines on hand hygiene in health care: First global patient safety challenge. Clean care is safer care.* Geneva, Switzerland: World Health Organization. (Level I)
3 The Joint Commission. (2012). Standard NPSG.07.01.01. *Comprehensive accreditation manual for hospitals: The official handbook.* Oakbrook Terrace, IL: The Joint Commission. (Level I)
4 Centers for Disease Control and Prevention. (October 2002). Guideline for hand hygiene in health-care settings. *Morbidity and Mortality Weekly Report, 51*(RR-16), 1–45. (Level 1)
5 The Joint Commission. (2012). Standard RC.01.03.01. *Comprehensive accreditation manual for hospitals: The official handbook.* Oakbrook Terrace, IL: The Joint Commission. (Level I)

ADDITIONAL REFERENCES

Matshes, E.W., & Lew, E.O. (2010). Two-handed cardiopulmonary resuscitation can cause rib fractures in infants. *American Journal of Forensic and Medical Pathology, 31*(4), 3037.
Nettina, S.M. (2010). *Lippincott manual of nursing practice* (9th ed.). Philadelphia, PA: Lippincott Williams & Wilkins.
You, Y. (2009). Optimum location for chest compressions during two-rescuer infant cardiopulmonary resuscitation. *Resuscitation, 80*(12), 1378–1381.

CARE PLAN PREPARATION

A care plan directs the patient's nursing care from admission to discharge. This written action plan is based on nursing diagnoses that have been formulated after reviewing assessment findings, and it embodies the components of the nursing process: assessment, diagnosis, planning, implementation, and evaluation. (See *Elements of a nursing diagnosis.*) The care plan consists of three parts: *goals* or *expected outcomes*, which describe behaviors or results to be achieved within a specified time; appropriate *nursing actions* or *interventions* needed to achieve these goals; and *evaluations of the established goals.*

A nursing care plan should be written for each patient, preferably within 24 hours of admission. It's usually started by the patient's primary nurse or the nurse who admits the patient. If the care plan contains more than one nursing diagnosis, the nurse must assign priority to each diagnosis and implement those with the highest priority first. Nurses update and revise the plan throughout the patient's stay, and the document becomes part of the permanent patient record.

Some health care facilities use standardized care plans that can be modified to serve many patients. Others use computer programs to facilitate development of nursing care plans. Most have preprinted care plan forms that can be filled in as needed, often on the nursing Kardex.

Tips for writing an effective patient care plan

How do you write a care plan that's realistic, accurate, and helpful? Here are some guidelines.

Be systematic
Avoid setting an initial outcome that's impossible to achieve. For example, suppose the outcome for a newly admitted patient with a stroke was "Patient will ambulate without assistance." Although this outcome is certainly appropriate in the long term, several short-term outcomes, such as "Patient maintains joint range-of-motion," need to be achieved first.

Be realistic
The nursing intervention should match staff resources and capabilities. For example, "Passive range-of-motion exercises to all extremities every 2 hours" may not be reasonable given the unit's staffing pattern and care requirements. The goals you set to correct a patient's problem should reflect what is reasonably possible in your setting—for

example, "Passive range-of-motion exercises with a.m. care, p.m. care, and once at night."

Be clear
Remember, you'll use goals to evaluate the effectiveness of the care plan, so it's important to express them clearly.

Be specific
"Give plenty of fluids" doesn't indicate much; the directive is nonspecific. In contrast, an intervention that says "Encourage fluids—1,000 mL/day shift, 1,000 mL/evening shift, 500 mL/night shift" allows another nurse to carry out the intervention with some assurance of having done what you ordered.

Be brief
An intervention that says "Follow turning schedule posted at bedside" is more readable and useful than having the entire schedule written on the nursing plan.

A nursing care plan serves as a database for planning assignments, giving change-of-shift reports, conferring with the doctor or other members of the health care team, planning patient discharge, and documenting patient care. In addition, the care plan can be used as a management tool to determine staffing needs and assignments.

Equipment
Preprinted nursing care plan form ■ nursing care plan computer program if appropriate ■ patient record, including nursing assessment.

Implementation
■ Review the patient's record, especially the nursing assessment completed on admission. Obtain from the patient any additional subjective or objective information needed to complete your assessment. Review diagnostic test results, the medical plan, and other information that may affect patient care. If the patient has just been admitted, complete a nursing history and physical assessment and add it to the patient's record.
■ Based on an analysis of the data, determine which nursing diagnoses will guide your patient care.[1] Be sure to address all of the patient's significant needs when determining nursing diagnoses.
■ Work with the patient to identify individualized short-term and long-term goals (expected outcomes) for each nursing diagnosis. Short-term goals can be achieved quickly; long-term goals take more time to achieve and usually involve prevention, patient teaching, and rehabilitation. A correctly written outcome expresses the desired patient behavior, criteria for measurement, and the appropriate time and conditions under which the behavior will occur. For example, an outcome containing all these elements might read: "By Monday, using crutches, Mary Ballin will be able

to walk to the end of the hall and back." *Expected outcomes serve as the basis for evaluating the effectiveness of your nursing interventions.*
■ Select interventions that will help the patient achieve the stated outcome for each nursing diagnosis. Include specific information, such as the frequency or particular intervention technique. *Outcomes establish criteria against which you'll judge further nursing actions.* (See *Tips for writing an effective patient care plan.*)

Special considerations
■ Always fill out the nursing care plan in ink *because the document is part of the permanent medical record.* If you must revise your plan as the patient's condition changes, fill out a new care plan and add it to the medical record.
■ Sign and date the care plan whenever you make new entries *to keep the plan current and to maintain accountability for planning the patient's care.*
■ Customize a standardized care plan *to avoid "standardizing" the patient's care and to allow you to address the patient's individual concerns.*
■ Long-term goals may not be met during hospitalization, so your planning should address postdischarge and home care needs. Interventions may include coordinating home care services.
■ Some agencies use critical pathways to address standardized desired outcomes of care. Critical pathways are multidisciplinary documents that may be viewed as replacements for care plans. If nursing diagnoses are included, these agencies use only the diagnostic statements that are most frequently observed.

Documentation
Documentation of the patient's progress (or lack of it) is required by The Joint Commission and other regulatory agencies that

monitor health care quality.[1] Document all pertinent nursing diagnoses, expected outcomes, nursing interventions, and evaluations of expected outcomes. Write the care plan clearly and concisely so that other members of the health care team can understand it.

REFERENCE

1 The Joint Commission. (2012). *Standard PC.01.03.01. Comprehensive accreditation manual for hospitals: The official handbook.* Oakbrook Terrace, IL: The Joint Commission. (Level I)

ADDITIONAL REFERENCE

Carpenito-Moyet, L.J. (2008). *Nursing diagnosis: Application to clinical practice* (12th ed.). Philadelphia, PA: Lippincott Williams & Wilkins.

CAST APPLICATION

A cast is a hard mold that encases a body part, usually an extremity, to provide immobilization of bones and surrounding tissue. It can be used to treat injuries (including fractures), correct orthopedic conditions (such as deformities), or promote healing after general or plastic surgery, amputation, or nerve and vascular repair. (See *Types of cylindrical casts,* page 130.)

Casts may be constructed of cotton-polyester, plaster, fiberglass, or other synthetic materials. Typically a doctor applies a cast and a nurse prepares the patient and the equipment and assists during the procedure. With special preparation, a nurse or other practitioners may apply or change a standard cast, but an orthopedist must reduce and set the fracture.

Contraindications for casting may include the presence of skin disease, peripheral vascular disease, diabetes mellitus, open or draining wounds, extreme edema, and susceptibility to skin breakdown. These aren't strict contraindications; the doctor must weigh the potential risks and benefits for each patient.

Equipment

Tubular stockinette ▪ casting material ▪ plaster splint, if needed ▪ bucket of water ▪ sink equipped with a plaster trap ▪ linen-saver pads ▪ sheet wadding ▪ sponge or felt padding, as needed ▪ rubber gloves ▪ gloves ▪ pain medication ▪ Optional: cast stand, pillows, sterile marker.

Preparation of equipment

Gather the tubular stockinette and cast material. Tubular stockinettes range from 2″ to 12″ wide. Wear rubber gloves.

For a cotton-polyester or fiberglass cast

Gently squeeze the packaged casting material *to make sure the envelopes don't have any air leaks. Humid air penetrating the packaging can cause the casting material to fail.* To prepare the casting material, follow the manufacturer's directions for the appropriate water temperature to use. Place the equipment so that it's easily accessible during the procedure.

For a plaster cast

Gently squeeze the packaged casting material *to make sure envelopes don't have any air leaks. Humid air leaking into the envelope can cause the plaster to become stale, which could make it set too quickly, form lumps, fail to bond with lower layers, or set as a soft, friable mass.* (Baking a stale plaster roll at a medium temperature for 1 hour can make it usable.)

Follow the manufacturer's instructions for water temperature when preparing plaster. It's advisable to use water that's room temperature or slightly warmer *because it allows the cast to set in about 7 minutes without excessive exothermia.* (Cold water retards the rate at which setting occurs and may be used to facilitate molding of difficult casts. Warm water speeds the rate of cast setting and raises the temperature of the skin under the cast.) Place equipment so that it's easily accessible.

Implementation

▪ Verify the doctor's order.
▪ Make sure the doctor has obtained an informed consent and that it's documented in the medical record.[1]
▪ Gather the equipment, and check the casting packages for air leaks.
▪ Confirm the patient's identity using at least two patient identifiers according to your facility's policy.[2]
▪ Explain the procedure *to allay the patient's fears.*
▪ Perform hand hygiene and put on gloves.[3,4,5]
▪ Mark the procedure site if indicated.[6]
▪ Cover the appropriate parts of the patient's bedding with a linen-saver pad.
▪ Remove any jewelry on the limb to be casted. *Jewelry may interfere with the circulation to the limb.*
▪ Assess the condition of the skin of the affected limb, and note any areas of abnormal color, ecchymosis, open wounds, rashes, or irritation. *This will make it easier to evaluate any patient complaints after the cast is applied.*
▪ Assess the patient's baseline neurovascular status. Palpate the pulses and assess the temperature, color, capillary refill, motion, sensation, and pain in the affected and unaffected limb.
▪ Assess the patient's vital signs.
▪ Assess the patient for pain and muscle spasms and provide medication as ordered, using safe medication administration practices. Perform a follow-up pain assessment and notify the doctor if pain isn't adequately controlled.[7]
▪ If the patient has an open wound, assist the doctor with administering a local anesthetic, closing the wound, and applying dressings, as needed.
▪ Participate in a preprocedure time-out.[8]
▪ Help the doctor position the limb, as ordered. (Commonly, the limb is immobilized in the neutral position.)
▪ Support the limb in the prescribed position while the doctor applies the tubular stockinette and sheet wadding. The stockinette should extend beyond the ends of the cast to pad the edges. (If the patient has an open wound or a severe contusion, the doctor may not use the stockinette.) The limb is then wrapped in sheet wadding, beginning distally, and extra wadding is added to the proximal and distal ends of the cast

EQUIPMENT

Types of cylindrical casts

Made of cotton-polyester, fiberglass, plaster, or other synthetic material, casts may be applied almost anywhere on the body—to support a single finger or the entire body. Common casts are shown below.

Hanging arm cast

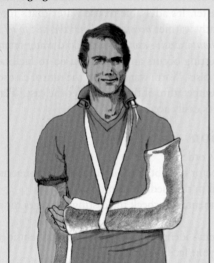

Shoulder spica

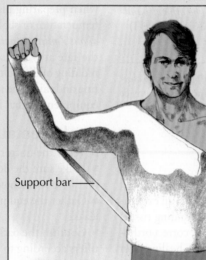

Support bar

Short arm cast

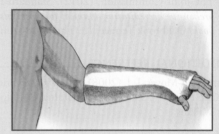

One-and-a-half hip spica

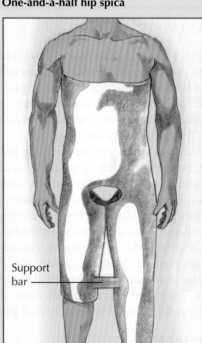

Support bar

Long leg cast

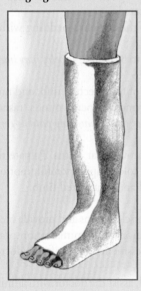

Short leg cast

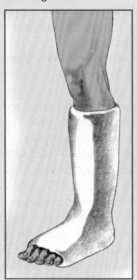

Single hip spica

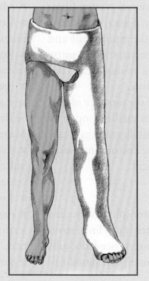

---

area as well as to any points of prominence. Smooth any wrinkles as the sheet wadding is applied.

Applying a cotton-polyester cast

■ Open the casting materials one roll at a time *because cotton and polyester casting must be applied within 3 minutes. Humidity in the air hardens the tape.*

■ Immerse the roll in cold water, and squeeze it four times *to ensure uniform saturation.*

■ Remove the material from the bucket dripping wet and hand it to the doctor.

■ Tell the patient that it will be applied immediately and will feel warm, giving off heat as it sets.

■ Prepare the necessary number of rolls in similar fashion.

Applying a fiberglass cast

■ Use a minimal amount of water to initiate the chemical reaction that causes the cast to harden. Using too much water will make the cast difficult to apply. Open one roll at a time.

■ If light-cured fiberglass material is being used, unroll the material more slowly. *This material remains soft and malleable until it's exposed to ultraviolet light, which sets it.*

Applying a plaster cast
■ Place a roll of plaster casting on its end in the bucket of water. Immerse it completely. When air bubbles stop rising from the roll, remove it, gently squeeze out the excess water, and hand it to the doctor, who will begin applying it to the extremity.
■ As the first roll is applied, prepare a second roll in the same manner. Try to stay one roll ahead during the procedure.
■ As each roll is applied, the doctor will smooth it to remove wrinkles and to spread the plaster into the cloth webbing, emptying air pockets. If plaster splints are used, they will be applied to the middle layers of the cast. Before wrapping the last roll, the ends of the tubular stockinette are pulled over the cast edges to create a padded end. *This prevents cast crumbling and reduces skin irritation.* The final roll is wrapped *to keep the ends of the stockinette in place.*

Completing the cast
■ "Petal" the edges of the cast *to reduce roughness and cushion pressure points, as needed.* (See *How to petal a cast.*)
■ Use a cast stand or your palm to support the cast in the therapeutic position until it becomes firm to touch (usually 6 to 8 minutes) *to prevent indentation in the cast.* Place the cast on a firm, smooth surface to continue drying. Place pillows under the patient's joints *to maintain flexion, if needed.*
■ Check the neurovascular status of the casted limb and compare the findings bilaterally. Palpate the patient's pulses and assess the color, temperature, capillary refill, motion, and sensation of the limbs bilaterally.
■ *To facilitate venous return and reduce edema,* elevate the limb above the level of the heart using pillows or bath blankets.
■ The doctor may order an X-ray of the limb *to ensure proper positioning.*
■ Advise the patient to maintain muscle strength by continuing any recommended exercises.
■ Remove and discard your gloves. Perform hand hygiene.[3,4,5]
■ Document the procedure.[9]

Special considerations
■ A cotton-polyester cast dries soon after application. During this drying period, the cast must be properly positioned to prevent a surface depression that could cause pressure areas or dependent edema. The patient's neurovascular status must be assessed, any drainage monitored, and the condition of the cast periodically checked.
■ After the cast dries completely, it looks shiny and no longer feels damp or soft. Nursing care consists of monitoring any drainage, preventing skin breakdown near the cast, and preventing complications resulting from immobility.
■ Patient teaching must begin immediately after the cast is applied and should continue until the patient or caregiver can effectively care for the cast.

How to petal a cast

Rough cast edges can be cushioned by petaling them with adhesive tape or moleskin. To do so, first cut several 4" × 2" (10 × 5 cm) strips. Round off one end of each strip *to keep it from curling.* Then, making sure the rounded end of the strip is on the outside of the cast, tuck the straight end just inside the cast edge.

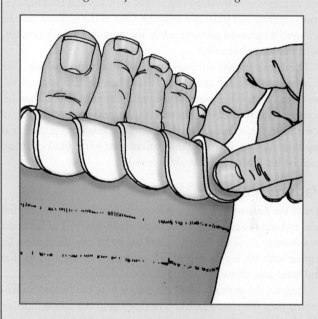

Smooth the moleskin with your finger until you're sure it's secured inside and out. Repeat the procedure, overlapping the moleskin pieces until you've gone all the way around the cast edge.

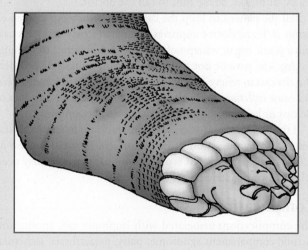

■ Never use the bed or table to support the cast as it sets *because molding can occur and cause pressure necrosis in the underlying tissue.* Also, don't use rubber- or plastic-coated pillows *because as the cast hardens, they may cause heat to be trapped under the cast.*

■ If a cast is applied after surgery or traumatic injury, remember that the most accurate way to assess for excessive bleeding is to monitor vital signs. *You can't use the amount of blood that you see on the cast as a way of telling if the patient is bleeding. A visible spot of blood on the cast can be misleading: one drop of blood can produce a circle 3" (7.6 cm) in diameter.*

■ Casts may need to be opened to assess underlying skin or pulses or to relieve pressure in a specific area. In a windowed cast, a specific area is cut out to allow inspection of the underlying skin or relieve pressure. A bivalved cast is split medially and laterally, creating anterior and posterior sections. One of the sections may be removed to prevent pressure while the remaining section maintains the immobilization.

■ The doctor usually removes the cast with a nurse assistant. (See "Cast removal.") Tell the patient that when the cast is removed, his casted limb will appear thinner with less muscle tone than his contralateral limb. His skin will also appear yellow or gray in color from the accumulated dead skin and oils from glands near the skin surface. Reassure the patient that with good care and exercise his limb will return to normal.

Patient teaching

Teach the patient to care for his cast before he goes home. Tell him to keep the casted limb elevated above the level of his heart *to minimize swelling.* Raise a casted leg by having the patient lie supine with his leg on top of pillow. Prop a casted arm so that the hand and elbow are higher than the shoulder.

Instruct the patient to call the doctor if he can't move his fingers or toes, if he has numbness or tingling in the casted limb, or if he has signs and symptoms of infection (such as fever, unusual pain, or foul odor from the cast). Advise him to maintain muscle strength by continuing any recommended exercises. If the patient has any questions about his cast care, or if the cast loosens, cracks, or breaks, advise him to call the doctor.

Tell the patient to keep the cast dry. *Moisture can weaken or destroy it.* If the doctor approves, the patient may cover his cast with a plastic bag or waterproof cast cover for showering or bathing.

Urge the patient not to insert anything (object or powder) into the cast to relieve itching. *Foreign matter can damage the skin and cause infection.* Warn the patient not to damage any area of the cast or bear weight on it unless his doctor approves.

If the patient must use crutches, instruct him to remove obstacles and throw rugs from his environment *to reduce his risk of falling.* If the patient's cast is on his dominant arm, he may need help performing activities of daily living.

Complications

The complications associated with improper cast application include compartment syndrome, palsy, paraesthesia, ischemia, ischemic myositis, pressure necrosis, deep vein thrombosis, and misalignment or nonunion of the fracture.

Documentation

Record the date and time of the cast application and the assessment of the limb both before and after the cast was applied. Note any open wounds or abnormal skin. Note the neurovascular checks before and after the cast application, and compare them to the unaffected limb. Note the location of any special devices such as felt pads or plaster splints. Note any teaching performed.

REFERENCES

1 The Joint Commission. (2012). Standard RI.01.03.01.*Comprehensive accreditation manual for hospitals: The official handbook.* Oakbrook Terrace, IL: The Joint Commission. (Level I)
2 The Joint Commission. (2012). Standard NPSG.01.01.01. *Comprehensive accreditation manual for hospitals: The official handbook.* Oakbrook Terrace, IL: The Joint Commission. (Level I)
3 World Health Organization. (2009). *WHO guidelines on hand hygiene in health care: First global patient safety challenge. Clean care is safer care.* Geneva, Switzerland: World Health Organization. (Level I)
4 The Joint Commission. (2012). Standard NPSG.07.01.01. *Comprehensive accreditation manual for hospitals: The official handbook.* Oakbrook Terrace, IL: The Joint Commission. (Level I)
5 Centers for Disease Control and Prevention. (October 2002). Guideline for hand hygiene in health-care settings. *Morbidity and Mortality Weekly Report, 51*(RR-16), 1–45. (Level 1)
6 The Joint Commission. (2012). Standard UP.01.01.01. *Comprehensive accreditation manual for hospitals: The official handbook.* Oakbrook Terrace, IL: The Joint Commission. (Level I)
7 The Joint Commission. (2012). Standard PC.01.02.07. *Comprehensive accreditation manual for hospitals: The official handbook.* Oakbrook Terrace, IL: The Joint Commission. (Level I)
8 The Joint Commission. (2012). Standard UP.01.03.01. *Comprehensive accreditation manual for hospitals: The official handbook.* Oakbrook Terrace, IL: The Joint Commission. (Level I)
9 The Joint Commission. (2012). Standard RC.01.03.01. *Comprehensive accreditation manual for hospitals: The official handbook.* Oakbrook Terrace, IL: The Joint Commission. (Level I)

ADDITIONAL REFERENCES

Boyd, A.S., et al. (2009). Splints and casts: Indications and methods. *American Family Physician, 80*(5), 491–499.
Halanski, M., & Noonan, K.J. (2008). Cast and splint immobilization: Complications. *Journal of American Academy of Orthopedic Surgeons, 16*(1), 30–40.
Nettina, S.M. (2010). *Lippincott manual of nursing practice* (9th ed.). Philadelphia, PA: Lippincott Williams & Wilkins.

CAST REMOVAL

A cast is typically removed when a fracture heals or requires further manipulation. Less common indications include cast damage, a pressure ulcer under the cast, excessive drainage or bleeding, and a constrictive cast.

Equipment

Cast spreader ■ cast saw with vacuum attachment ■ gloves ■ cast scissors ■ hearing protection for patient and staff ■ Optional: goggles, masks.

Preparation of equipment

The cast saw may be loud enough to require the use of hearing protection for the patient and staff members present during the cast removal, according to Occupational Safety and Health Administration (OSHA) standards. Follow the manufacturer's directions for use.

Implementation

- Verify the doctor's order.
- Gather the equipment.
- Confirm the patient's identity using at least two patient identifiers according to your facility's policy.[1]
- Explain the procedure to the patient. Tell him that he will feel some heat and vibration when the cast is split with the cast saw. If the patient is a child, tell him that the saw is very noisy but won't cut the skin beneath. Have the patient report any discomfort or excessive heat during the procedure. Emphasize that he must remain still during the procedure.
- Perform hand hygiene and put on gloves.[2,3,4]
- Have staff members and the patient put on hearing protective equipment and goggles or masks, if needed.
- Monitor that patient's anxiety level as the cast is removed.
- Assist the doctor, as needed, when the cast is removed. First, one side of the cast is cut and then the other (as shown below). The cast is then opened using a spreader. Cast scissors are used to cut through the cast padding.

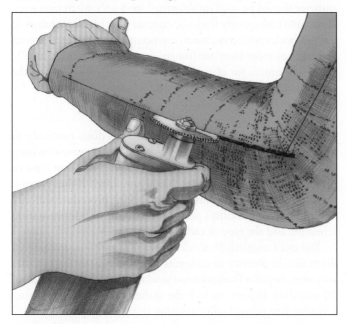

- Provide skin care to remove the accumulated dead skin.
- Remove and discard your gloves. Perform hand hygiene.[2,3,4]
- Document the procedure.[5]

Special considerations

If the cast saw doesn't have a vacuum attachment to dispose of the cast dust during removal, staff members and the patient should put on masks and eye protection during the procedure to prevent inhalation and irritation from particulate cast material.

Patient teaching

Teach the patient that when the padding is cut he will see discolored skin and signs of poor muscle tone. Instruct him in performing skin care after the cast is removed.

Complications

The doctor may accidentally injure the patient's skin with the cast saw, scissors, or spreader.

Documentation

Assess the neurovascular integrity of the limb before cast removal. Document the date and time of removal and the patient's tolerance of the procedure. Note the neurovascular assessment and condition of the patient's skin after the cast is removed. Note any complications from the procedure and nursing actions taken.

REFERENCES

1 The Joint Commission. (2012). Standard NPSG.01.01.01. *Comprehensive accreditation manual for hospitals: The official handbook.* Oakbrook Terrace, IL: The Joint Commission. (Level I)
2 World Health Organization. (2009). *WHO guidelines on hand hygiene in health care: First global patient safety challenge. Clean care is safer care.* Geneva, Switzerland: World Health Organization. (Level I)
3 The Joint Commission. (2012). Standard NPSG.07.01.01. *Comprehensive accreditation manual for hospitals: The official handbook.* Oakbrook Terrace, IL: The Joint Commission. (Level I)
4 Centers for Disease Control and Prevention. (October 2002). Guideline for hand hygiene in health-care settings. *Morbidity and Mortality Weekly Report, 51*(RR-16), 1–45. (Level 1)
5 The Joint Commission. (2012). Standard RC.01.03.01. *Comprehensive accreditation manual for hospitals: The official handbook.* Oakbrook Terrace, IL: The Joint Commission. (Level I)

ADDITIONAL REFERENCES

Nettina, S.M. (2010). *Lippincott manual of nursing practice* (9th ed.). Philadelphia, PA: Lippincott Williams & Wilkins.
Proehl, J.A. (2008). *Emergency nursing procedures* (4th ed.). Philadelphia, PA: Saunders.
Shuler, F.D., & Grisafi, F.N. (2008). Cast-saw burns: Evaluation of skin, cast, and blade temperatures generated during cast removal. *Journal of Bone and Joint Surgery, American Volume, 90*(12), 2626–2630.
Smeltzer, S.C., et al. (2010). *Brunner & Suddarth's textbook of medical-surgical nursing* (12th ed.). Philadelphia, PA: Lippincott Williams & Wilkins.

CENTRAL VENOUS ACCESS CATHETER

A central venous access catheter is a sterile catheter made of polyurethane or silicone rubber (Silastic). It may have one, two, three, or four infusion ports, which can be used for administering fluids, blood products, drugs, and total parenteral nutrition. With the addition of specialized equipment, some central venous access catheters can monitor central venous pressure, central venous oxygen saturation, arterial oxygen saturation, pulmonary artery pressure, cardiac output, and temperature.

Central venous access catheter pathways

The illustrations below show several common pathways for central venous access catheter insertion. Typically, a central venous access catheter is inserted in the subclavian vein or the internal jugular vein. The catheter typically terminates in the superior vena cava. The central venous access catheter is tunneled when long-term placement is required.

Insertion: Subclavian vein
Termination: Superior vena cava

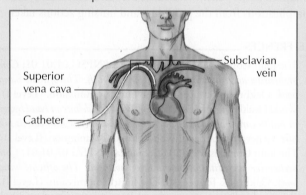

Insertion: Internal jugular vein
Termination: Superior vena cava

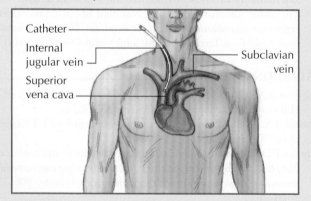

Insertion: Through a subcutaneous tunnel to the subclavian vein (a Dacron cuff helps hold catheter in place)
Termination: Superior vena cava

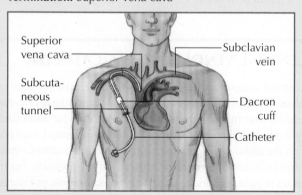

Catheters impregnated with antiseptics, such as chlorhexidine and silver sulfadiazine, and antimicrobials, such as rifampin and minocycline, are recommended for a patient whose catheter is expected to remain in place for more than 5 days.[1] Power injectable catheters are also available to enable power injection of contrast media in patients who require computed tomography and other testing.

The doctor inserts the central venous access catheter through a large vein, such as the subclavian vein or the jugular vein, and places the tip of the catheter in the superior vena cava. (See *Central venous access catheter pathways*.)

The duration of use varies depending on the type of device used. For example, standard subclavian, femoral, or internal jugular catheters are intended for short-term use (days). Other devices such as peripherally inserted central catheters (PICCs) are designed for long-term use (weeks or months). Some central venous access catheters, such as the Hickman and Broviac devices and implanted ports, can remain in place for months or years.

Central venous therapy increases the risk of complications, such as pneumothorax, sepsis, thrombus formation, and vessel and adjacent organ perforation (all life-threatening conditions).

Blood sampling

Because multiple blood samples can be drawn through a central venous access catheter without repeated venipuncture, it decreases the patient's anxiety and preserves peripheral veins. However, the catheter should be used for drawing blood only when necessary. If you don't adequately flush the catheter after blood withdrawal, a thrombotic catheter occlusion can occur. When a central venous catheter has more than one lumen, use the larger lumen, usually the distal lumen, for obtaining blood samples. Avoid using the lumen that's used for drug infusion.

Flushing

Flushing a central venous access catheter is done routinely to assess catheter patency before each infusion, to prevent mixing incompatible medications and solutions after infusion, and to prevent catheter occlusion after blood sampling.[2] If the system is for intermittent use, the flushing and locking procedure will vary according to your facility's policy, the medication administration schedule, and the type of catheter.

You must regularly flush all lumens of a multilumen catheter. To maintain patency in catheters used intermittently, facilities may use a heparin flush solution available in prefilled syringes of 10 units/mL heparin to lock the catheter. You should use preservative-free normal saline solution instead of heparin to maintain patency in two-way valved devices, such as the Groshong type, because research suggests that heparin isn't always needed to maintain patency.

The recommended frequency for flushing central venous access catheters varies. When no therapy is being infused, follow these guidelines:

■ Flush nontunneled, nonvalved catheters at least every 24 hours. Based on facility policy, you may also heparin lock the catheter with 5 mL of 10 units/mL heparin.[3]

- Flush nontunneled, valved catheters at least weekly. Based on facility policy, you may also heparin lock the catheter with 5 mL of 10 units/mL heparin.[3]
- Flush tunneled, nonvalved catheters at least one to two times per week. Based on facility policy, you may also heparin lock the catheter with 5 mL of 10 units/mL heparin.[3]
- Flush tunneled, valved catheters at least weekly. Based on facility policy, you may also heparin lock the catheter with 5 mL of 10 units/mL heparin.[3]

The flushing volume should be at least twice the internal volume of the central venous access catheter and injection cap. The size of syringe used for flushing varies according to the catheter's manufacturer instructions, although most manufacturers require a minimum of a 10-mL syringe.[2]

Dressing and injection cap changes

Despite the various designs and applications of central venous access catheters, certain aspects of dressing changes apply to all devices. Sterility and integrity of the catheter must be maintained at all times. Failure to properly maintain a central venous access catheter is associated with patient suffering, prolonged care, and increased expense. Inadequate insertion site care can lead to infection, sepsis, and death.

Most facilities have policies and procedures that address specific dressing change standards for each type of central venous access catheter. Semipermeable transparent dressings are changed at least every 7 days, and gauze dressings are changed every 2 days. Either dressing should be changed if the dressing becomes damp, loosened, or visibly soiled.[1,4,5]

Central venous access catheters used for intermittent infusions have needle-free injection caps (short luer-lock devices similar to the heparin lock adapters used for peripheral IV infusion therapy). These caps must be luer-lock types to prevent inadvertent disconnection and air embolism.[6,7] The amount of air in a cap varies, so it's important to air purge the cap before connecting it to the catheter hub.

The frequency of cap changes varies according to the manufacturer's recommendations, your facility's policy, and how often the cap is used. Change the cap if it's removed for any reason, if there's blood or debris within the cap, and before drawing a blood culture sample.[7] Change the cap with each administration set change.[1,6]

Removing a central venous access catheter

Removing a central venous access catheter is a sterile procedure that's usually performed by a doctor or nurse, either at the end of therapy or at the onset of complications.[8] (Check your facility's policy and your state's nurse practice act to determine whether removing a catheter is in your scope of practice.)

If the central venous access catheter was inserted in an emergency situation, you should remove it as soon as possible, but not longer than 48 hours after insertion.[8] Assess catheter necessity daily during multidisciplinary rounds, and remove the catheter as soon as it's no longer needed; this reduces the risk of central line–related bloodstream infection.[5,8,9,10] Consider the patient's condition and therapy, catheter position, and catheter function

when deciding whether to remove the catheter. If you suspect or confirm a central line–related bloodstream infection, base the decision to remove or salvage the catheter on blood culture results, the patient's condition, available vascular access sites, effectiveness of antimicrobial therapy, and the doctor's direction.[8]

Equipment

For insertion of a central venous access catheter

Skin preparation kit, if necessary ■ gloves ■ blanket ■ sterile gloves and gowns ■ caps ■ linen-saver pad ■ sterile towel ■ large sterile drape ■ masks ■ antiseptic solution (chlorhexidine-based is preferred, although you may use tincture of iodine, povidone iodine, or alcohol) ■ antiseptic pads (alcohol, tincture of iodine, or chlorhexidine-based) ■ preservative-free normal saline flushes in 10-mL syringes (one for each port of catheter) ■ ultrasound device with sterile probe cover ■ sterile ultrasound gel ■ IV solution with administration set as ordered or needed for monitoring equipment ■ 3-mL syringe with 25G 1" needle ■ 1% or 2% injectable lidocaine ■ suture material ■ two 14G or 16G central venous access catheters (antimicrobial impregnated, if indicated) ■ catheter securement device, sterile tape, or sterile surgical strips ■ sterile scissors ■ sterile marker ■ sterile labels ■ transparent semipermeable dressing.

The type of catheter selected depends on the type of therapy to be used. (See *Guide to central venous access catheters,* pages 136 and 137.)

Use an all-inclusive insertion kit or cart that contains all of the necessary components for maintaining sterile technique during catheter insertion to reduce the risk of catheter-related bloodstream infection.[1,5,9,10,11]

For blood sampling from a central venous access catheter

Gloves ■ protective eyewear or a face mask ■ prefilled flush syringes of normal saline solution ■ alcohol pads ■ blood collection tubes ■ label for discard blood tube or syringe ■ laboratory request forms and labels ■ laboratory biohazard transport bag ■ Optional: prefilled heparin flush syringe.

For the Vacutainer method
Vacutainer with needleless adapter needle.

For the syringe method
Appropriately sized syringes (usually 5 or 10 mL) ■ blood transfer unit.

For flushing a central venous access catheter
Prefilled 10-mL syringe with heparin or normal saline solution ■ alcohol pads.

For changing the dressing on a central venous access catheter

Gloves ■ antimicrobial skin cleaner swabs (chlorhexidine preferred) ■ sterile semipermeable transparent dressing or sterile 4" × 4" gauze pad ■ sterile drape ■ skin preparation solution (as needed to facilitate dressing adherence) ■ catheter securement device, sterile tape,

(*Text continues on page 138.*)

Guide to central venous access catheters

TYPE	DESCRIPTION	INDICATIONS	ADVANTAGES AND DISADVANTAGES	NURSING CONSIDERATIONS
Groshong catheter	■ Silicone rubber ■ About 35" (89 cm) long ■ Closed end with pressure-sensitive three-way valve ■ Dacron cuff ■ Single or double lumen ■ Tunneled	■ Long-term central venous access ■ Patient with heparin allergy	*Advantages* ■ Less thrombogenic ■ Pressure-sensitive three-way valve eliminates frequent heparin flushes ■ Dacron cuff anchors catheter and prevents bacterial migration *Disadvantages* ■ Requires surgical insertion ■ Tears and kinks easily ■ Blunt end makes it difficult to clear substances from its tip	■ Don't use a syringe smaller than 10 mL. ■ Two surgical sites require dressing after insertion. ■ Handle catheter gently. ■ Check the external portion frequently for kinks and leaks. ■ Repair kit is available. ■ Remember to flush with enough saline solution to clear the catheter, especially after drawing or administering blood. ■ Change end caps weekly.
Short-term single-lumen catheter	■ Polyurethane or silicone rubber ■ About 8" (20 cm) long ■ Lumen gauge varies ■ Percutaneously placed	■ Short-term central venous access ■ Emergency access ■ Patient who needs only one lumen	*Advantages* ■ Easily inserted at bedside ■ Easily removed ■ Stiffness aids central venous pressure monitoring *Disadvantages* ■ Limited functions	■ Assess frequently for signs of infection and clot formation.
Short-term multilumen catheter	■ Polyurethane or silicone rubber ■ Two, three, or four lumens exiting at 3/4" (2-cm) intervals ■ Lumen gauges vary ■ Percutaneously placed	■ Short-term central venous access ■ Patient with limited insertion sites who requires multiple infusions	*Advantages* ■ Same as single-lumen catheter ■ Allows infusion of multiple (even incompatible) solutions through the same catheter *Disadvantages* ■ Same as single-lumen catheter	■ Know gauge and purpose of each lumen. ■ Use the same lumen for the same task.

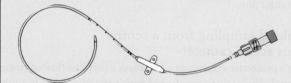

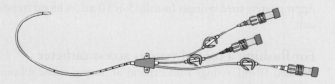

Guide to central venous access catheters *(continued)*

TYPE	DESCRIPTION	INDICATIONS	ADVANTAGES AND DISADVANTAGES	NURSING CONSIDERATIONS
Hickman catheter	■ Silicone rubber ■ About 35″ (89 cm) long ■ Open end with clamp ■ Dacron cuff 11¾″ (30 cm) from hub ■ Tunneled	■ Long-term central venous access ■ Home therapy	***Advantages*** ■ Dacron cuff prevents excess motion and migration of bacteria ■ Clamps eliminate need for Valsalva's maneuver ***Disadvantages*** ■ Requires surgical insertion ■ Open end ■ Requires doctor for removal ■ Tears and kinks easily	■ Don't use a syringe smaller than 10 mL. ■ Two surgical sites require dressing after insertion. ■ Handle catheter gently. ■ Observe frequently for kinks and tears. ■ Repair kit is available. ■ Clamp catheter with a nonserrated clamp any time it becomes disconnected or opens. ■ Flush catheter daily when not in use with 3 to 5 mL of heparin (10 units/mL) and before and after each use, using the SASH (S = Saline, A = Additive, S = Saline, H = Heparin) protocol.
Broviac catheter	■ Identical to Hickman except smaller inner lumen	■ Long-term central venous access ■ Patient with small central vessels (pediatric or geriatric)	***Advantages*** ■ Smaller lumen for better comfort ***Disadvantages*** ■ Small lumen may limit uses ■ Single lumen limits function ■ Growth in children may cause migration of catheter tip	■ Check facility policy before drawing blood or administering blood or blood products. ■ Flush catheter daily when not in use with 3 to 5 mL of heparin (10 units/mL) and before and after each use, using the SASH protocol.
Hickman/ Broviac catheter	■ Hickman and Broviac catheters combined ■ Tunneled	■ Long-term central venous access ■ Patient who needs multiple infusions	***Advantages*** ■ Double-lumen Hickman catheter allows sampling and administration of blood ■ Broviac lumen delivers IV fluids, including total parenteral nutrition ***Disadvantages*** ■ Same as Hickman catheter	■ Know the purpose and function of each lumen. ■ Label lumens to prevent confusion. ■ Flush catheter daily when not in use with 3 to 5 mL of heparin (10 units/mL) and before and after each use, using the SASH protocol.

or adhesive strips ▪ disposable surgical mask ▪ sterile gloves ▪ waterproof trash bag ▪ label ▪ Optional: chlorhexidine-impregnated sponge dressing, adhesive remover.

Commercially prepared central venous access catheter dressing change kits that include most of the equipment needed are available.

For changing an injection cap on a central venous access catheter

Gloves ▪ antiseptic pads (alcohol, tincture of iodine, chlorhexidine-based) ▪ sterile injection cap ▪ Optional: padded clamp.

For removing a central venous access catheter

Gloves ▪ sterile gloves ▪ protective eyewear ▪ mask ▪ sterile suture removal set ▪ alcohol pads ▪ sterile 2″ × 2″ gauze pads ▪ forceps ▪ tape ▪ sterile, transparent semipermeable dressing ▪ antimicrobial ointment ▪ petroleum-based ointment ▪ Optional: agar plate or specimen container, if necessary for culture.

Preparation of equipment

Gather all necessary equipment. Before insertion of a central venous access catheter, confirm catheter type and size with the doctor; usually, a 14G or 16G catheter is selected. Set up equipment for insertion, dressing change, and line removal, using strict sterile technique.[12] Check all expiration dates, and inspect packages for any tears.

Implementation

▪ For all procedures, confirm the patient's identity using at least two patient identifiers according to your facility's policy.[13]

▪ Explain the procedure to the patient and answer any questions *to decrease anxiety.*

Assisting with inserting a central venous access catheter

▪ Ensure that the patient has signed a consent form, if necessary,[14] and check his history for hypersensitivity to latex or the local anesthetic.

▪ Perform a preprocedure check and a time-out verification process with the doctor according to your facility's policy.[15,16]

▪ Place the patient in Trendelenburg's position *to dilate the veins and reduce the risk of air embolism.*

▪ Elevate the bed to a comfortable working level *to avoid back strain.*

▪ Perform hand hygiene and put on gloves.[17,18,19]

▪ For subclavian insertion, place a rolled blanket lengthwise between the shoulders *to increase venous distention.* For jugular insertion, place a rolled blanket under the opposite shoulder *to extend the neck, making anatomic landmarks more visible.* Place a linen-saver pad under the patient *to prevent soiling the bed.*

▪ Turn the patient's head away from the site *to prevent possible contamination from airborne pathogens and to make the site more accessible.* Or, if dictated by facility policy, place a mask on the patient unless doing so increases his anxiety or is contraindicated because of his respiratory status.

▪ Prepare the insertion site. Make sure the skin is free of hair *because hair can harbor microorganisms.* Clip the hair close to the skin rather than shaving *because shaving may cause skin irritation and create multiple small open wounds, increasing the risk of infection.* Clean the area with soap and water if the intended site is visibly soiled.[11]

▪ Establish a sterile field on a table, using a sterile towel or the wrapping from the instrument tray. Prepare normal saline flushes using sterile technique and drop them onto the sterile field; if using prefilled flushes, drop them onto the sterile field using sterile technique.

▪ Label all medications, medication containers, and other solutions on and off the sterile field.[20]

▪ Put on a cap, a mask, and sterile gloves and gown to comply with maximum barrier precautions.

▪ Prepare the insertion site with a chlorhexidine sponge[1,11] using a vigorous side-to-side motion for 30 seconds; allow the area to air-dry.[21]

▪ Remove and discard your gloves, perform hand hygiene,[17,18,19] and put on new sterile gloves.

▪ The doctor puts on a cap, a mask, and sterile gloves and gown. Assist with placing a large full-body sterile drape over the patient *to create a sterile field and comply with maximum barrier precautions.* Open the packaging of the 3-mL syringe and 25G needle and give it to the doctor using sterile technique.

▪ Disinfect the top of the lidocaine vial with an alcohol pad and invert it. The doctor then fills the 3-mL syringe and injects the anesthetic into the site (as shown below).

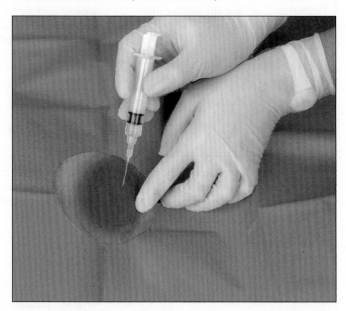

▪ Using sterile technique, give the doctor the ultrasound device with the sterile probe cover. Apply sterile ultrasound gel. The doctor locates the vessel using the device.

▪ Open the catheter package and give the catheter to the doctor using sterile technique. The doctor then inserts the catheter, flushes each port, and attaches a sterile injection cap.

■ If ordered, prepare an IV administration set for immediate attachment to the catheter hub. Ask the patient to perform Valsalva's maneuver while the doctor attaches the IV line to the catheter hub. *This maneuver increases intrathoracic pressure, reducing the possibility of an air embolus.* (See *Teaching Valsalva's maneuver.*)

■ After the doctor attaches the IV line to the catheter hub, set the flow rate at a keep-vein-open rate to maintain venous access. Trace the tubing from the patient to its point of origin to make sure that it's connected to the proper port.[22] The doctor then sutures the catheter in place.

■ Use antimicrobial solution *to remove dried blood that could harbor microorganisms.* Secure the catheter with a catheter securement device, sterile tape, or sterile surgical strips.[23] Apply a chlorhexidine-impregnated sponge dressing, if required by your facility's policy, *to reduce the risk of central line-related bloodstream infections.*[1] Apply an appropriate dressing according to your facility's policy. Expect some serosanguineous drainage during the first 24 hours.[4]

■ Label the dressing with the date, the time, and your initials (as shown below).[4]

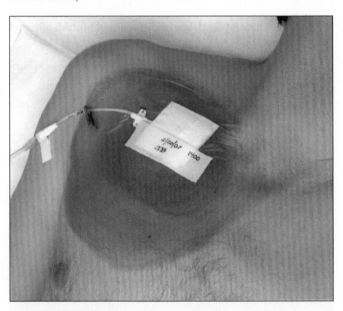

■ Remove and discard personal protective equipment and perform hand hygiene.[17,18,19]

■ Dispose of supplies in appropriate receptacles.[12,24,25]

■ Place the patient in a comfortable position and assess for signs and symptoms of complications from insertion.

■ Obtain a chest X-ray. After the X-ray confirms correct catheter placement in the superior vena cava, set the flow rate of IV fluids, as ordered, or begin medicated infusions as indicated.[11]

Blood sampling using a central venous access catheter

■ Verify the doctor's order for blood sampling.[26]

■ Place the patient in the supine position with his head slightly elevated.

Teaching Valsalva's maneuver

Increased intrathoracic pressure reduces the risk of air embolus during insertion and removal of a central venous access catheter. A simple way to achieve this pressure is to ask the patient to perform Valsalva's maneuver: forced exhalation against a closed airway. Instruct the patient to take a deep breath and hold it, and then to bear down for 10 seconds. Then tell the patient to exhale and breathe quietly.

Valsalva's maneuver raises intrathoracic pressure from its normal level of 3 to 4 mm Hg to levels of 60 mm Hg or higher. It also slows the pulse rate, decreases the return of blood to the heart, and increases venous pressure.

This maneuver is contraindicated in patients with increased intracranial pressure. It shouldn't be taught to patients who aren't alert or cooperative.

■ Label the discard blood collection tube or syringe *to prevent confusing it with the actual specimen.* If not already clearly marked, label the saline flush syringe.[20]

■ Perform hand hygiene and put on protective eyewear or a face mask (if splashing is likely) and gloves.[17,18,19]

■ Stop infusions, clamp the catheter lumen, and thoroughly disinfect the injection cap or access hub with an antiseptic pad using friction and allow it to dry.[27]

■ Attach a prefilled 10-mL normal saline solution syringe to the injection port and open the catheter clamp. Aspirate for blood return. If unable to obtain blood return, have the patient change positions, cough, move his arm above his head, or take a deep breath and hold it.

■ Instill 3 to 5 mL of saline *to check the patency of the catheter.* Reclamp the catheter and remove the syringe.[27]

■ Clean the injection cap or access hub with an alcohol pad using friction and allow it to dry.[1,6]

Vacutainer method

– Attach the needleless connector to the injection cap or access hub, release the clamp, and engage the labeled discard blood collection tube to aspirate 4 to 5 mL of blood.[21]

– Clamp the catheter and remove the labeled discard blood collection tube from the Vacutainer.

– Insert another blood collection tube, unclamp the catheter, and obtain a sample. Repeat as necessary until all blood samples are obtained.

– Clamp the catheter and remove the Vacutainer and needleless connector from the injection cap or access hub.

Syringe method
– Attach the empty discard syringe to the hub, release the clamp, and aspirate 4 to 5 mL of blood *to clear the catheter's dead space volume and remove any blood diluted by flush solution.*[21]
– Clamp the catheter, remove the discard syringe, and place it in the appropriate receptacle.
– Clean the injection cap or access hub with an alcohol pad using friction and allow it to dry.[1]
– Connect an empty syringe to the catheter, release the clamp, and withdraw the blood sample. Obtain multiple syringes of samples as necessary.
– Clamp the catheter and remove the syringe.
– Use the blood transfer unit to transfer the blood into the appropriate blood collection tube.

Completing the procedure
– Thoroughly disinfect the injection cap or access hub with an alcohol pad using friction, allow it to dry, and connect the syringe with normal saline solution.[1]
– Open the clamp and flush with solution. Close the clamp.
– If the patient doesn't have a continuous infusion prescribed, repeat the flushing procedure with a heparin flush solution according to your facility's policy.
– Change the needleless injection cap according to your facility's policy.[6,7]
– Label the samples in the presence of the patient *to prevent mislabeling.*[20]
– Place all the blood collection tubes in a laboratory biohazard transport bag and send them to the laboratory with a completed laboratory request form.[24]

Flushing a central venous access catheter
■ Perform hand hygiene and put on gloves.[17,18,19]
■ Clean the injection or access cap with an alcohol pad using friction (as shown below). Allow the cap to dry.[1]

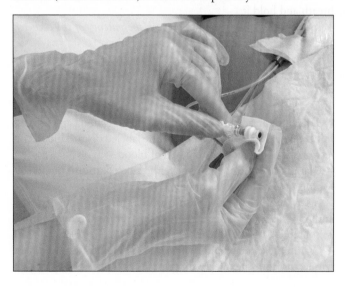

■ Attach the prefilled 10-mL flush syringe to the injection or access cap and slowly aspirate until a brisk, positive blood return is obtained *to confirm the proper function and patency of the access device* (as shown below).[2,21]

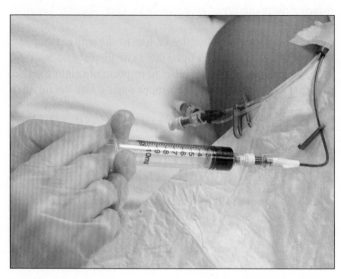

■ Inject the recommended type and amount of flush solution (as shown below).

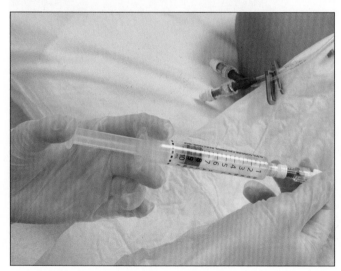

■ After flushing the catheter, follow a clamping sequence to reduce blood reflux based on the type of needleless injection cap. If using a positive-pressure needleless injection cap, clamp the catheter after syringe disconnection. For a negative-pressure needleless injection cap, maintain pressure on the syringe while clamping the catheter. For a neutral needleless injection cap, clamp the catheter before or after disconnecting the syringe.[21]

Changing the dressing on a central venous access catheter
■ Perform hand hygiene and put on gloves.[17,18,19]
■ If using a commercially prepared dressing kit, open the kit onto a sterile drape in a clean work area that's within easy reach.

■ Put on gloves and a mask if required by your facility.[4]

■ Stabilize the catheter and loosen the dressing from its outer edge toward the insertion site without putting the tension on the catheter. Adhesive remover may be used as necessary.

NURSING ALERT *If adhesive remover is needed, use one that does not contain acetone.* Acetone-based product may damage the catheter.

■ Remove the old dressing by lifting the edge of the dressing at the catheter hub and gently pulling the dressing perpendicular to the skin toward the insertion site *to prevent catheter dislodgement.* Discard it in the waterproof trash bag.

■ Remove the catheter securement device and discard it.

■ If a chlorhexidine-impregnated sponge dressing was used with the old dressing *to provide sustained antimicrobial action at the insertion site,* remove and discard it.

■ Assess the insertion site for bleeding, redness, heat, swelling, tenderness, induration, and drainage.[1,4]

■ Verify the external catheter length *to make sure that it hasn't migrated.*[4]

■ Inspect the catheter for cracks, leakage, kinking, or pinching as well as mechanical problems.

■ Remove and discard your gloves, perform hand hygiene, and put on sterile gloves.[17,18,19]

■ Clean the catheter insertion site with chlorhexidine (tincture of iodine, povidone-iodine, or alcohol may also be used, but chlorhexidine is recommended) swabs using a back-and-forth motion (as shown below).[1,4,5,9,11]

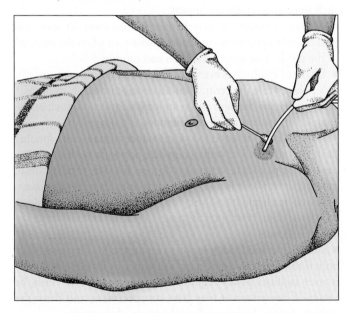

■ Allow the site to dry.[1,4,5,9] Don't blow on or fan the site.

NURSING ALERT *Don't use chlorhexidine-containing skin cleaners on patients sensitive to chlorhexidine.*

■ Apply a "window frame" of skin preparation solution around the catheter site, if needed, *to help the dressing stay in place.*

■ Secure the catheter with a catheter securement device, sterile tape, or adhesive strips.[4]

■ If applicable, place a chlorhexidine-impregnated sponge dressing at the catheter base.[1,4,5,9] *To facilitate future removal,* position the chlorhexidine-impregnated sponge dressing with the catheter resting on or near the radial slit of the dressing. The edges of the slit must touch *to maximize antimicrobial action.*

NURSING ALERT *Don't use chlorhexidine-impregnated sponge dressings on patients younger than 2 months old or on patients sensitive to chlorhexidine* because the dressing has constant contact with the skin.[1,4,5,9]

■ Secure the chlorhexidine-impregnated sponge dressing with a semipermeable transparent film dressing that has a high moisture vapor transmission rate (as shown below). There should be continuous contact between the skin and the transparent dressing or chlorhexidine-impregnated sponge dressing. Alternatively, a sterile 4″ × 4″ gauze dressing may be used in place of a semipermeable dressing.[1,4,5,9]

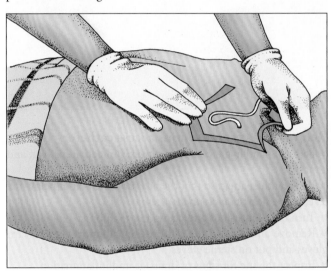

■ Label the dressing with the date, time, and your initials.[4]

Changing the injection cap on a central venous access catheter

■ Perform hand hygiene and put on gloves.[17,18,19]

■ Thoroughly disinfect the connection site with an antiseptic pad using friction and allow to dry.[1,7]

■ Air purge the injection cap *to remove the air from the cap.*

■ Close the catheter clamp or, if the catheter doesn't have a clamp, use a padded clamp to clamp the catheter to *prevent air from entering the catheter.*

■ *As an added safety measure,* instruct the patient to perform Valsalva's maneuver or exhale, if possible, while you quickly disconnect the old cap and connect the new cap using sterile technique (as shown below).

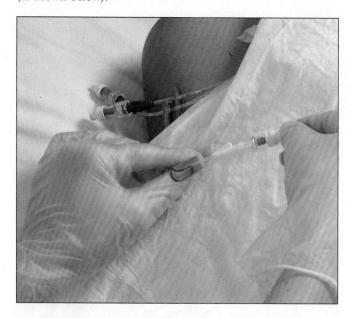

Removing a central venous access catheter
■ Perform hand hygiene. Put on gloves, protective eyewear, and a mask.[17,18,19]
■ Position the patient so that the insertion site is at or below the level of the heart *to prevent an air embolism.*[8]
■ Turn off all infusions and clamp the IV tubing.
■ Remove and discard the old dressing. Remove and discard gloves and put on sterile gloves.
■ Inspect the site for signs of drainage and inflammation.
■ Turn the patient's head to the side opposite the catheter insertion site.
■ Clip the sutures or remove the catheter securement device.
■ Have the patient perform Valsalva's maneuver or exhale as the catheter is withdrawn *to prevent an air embolism.*[21,28]
■ Using forceps, remove the catheter using gentle, even pressure.[21]
■ If you meet resistance as you remove the catheter, don't forcibly remove the catheter. Notify the doctor immediately to discuss options for successful removal.
■ Apply immediate pressure to the insertion site with a sterile gauze pad until hemostasis occurs.[21]
■ Inspect the catheter tip and measure the length of the catheter *to ensure that the catheter has been completely removed.*[8] If you suspect that the catheter hasn't been completely removed, notify the doctor immediately and monitor the patient closely for signs of distress.
■ Apply petroleum-based ointment and a sterile occlusive dressing over the insertion site *to seal the skin-to-vein tract and decrease the risk of air embolism.*[8,21]
■ Label the dressing with the date and time of the removal and your initials.
■ Change the dressing every 24 hours until healing has occurred.[21]

■ Encourage the patient to remain supine or assume a sitting position for at least 30 minutes.[21]

After the procedure
■ After all procedures, dispose of the equipment in the appropriate receptacle.[12,24,25]
■ Remove and discard any personal protective equipment and perform hand hygiene.[17,18,19]
■ Assess the patient's tolerance of the procedure.
■ Document the procedure.[29]

Special considerations
NURSING ALERT *Be alert for such signs of air embolism as sudden onset of pallor, cyanosis, dyspnea, coughing, and tachycardia, progressing to syncope and shock. If any of these signs occur, place the patient on his left side in Trendelenburg's position and notify the doctor.*[28]
■ *To prevent an air embolism,* close the catheter clamp or have the patient perform Valsalva's maneuver or exhale each time the catheter hub is open to air. (A Groshong catheter doesn't require clamping *because it has an internal valve.*) If the patient is unable to follow directions to perform Valsalva's maneuver or is on a ventilator, time opening the hub or catheter removal to coincide with end inspiration or beginning expiration.[21,28]
■ After insertion, also watch for signs and symptoms of pneumothorax, such as shortness of breath, uneven chest movement, tachycardia, and chest pain. Notify the doctor immediately if such signs and symptoms appear.
■ Change IV tubing no more frequently than every 96 hours and immediately upon suspected contamination or when the integrity of the product or system has been compromised.[1,30]
■ Change IV solutions every 24 hours or according to your facility's policy while the central venous access catheter is in place.
■ Assess the site for signs and symptoms of infection, such as discharge, inflammation, and tenderness.
■ If blood can't be aspirated or resistance is met, don't forcibly flush the catheter. The catheter tip may be poorly positioned. Ask the patient to cough, reposition him on his side, turn his head, raise his arms above his head, or put him in a sitting position.
■ Group multiple blood draws together whenever possible *to reduce the number of times the system is entered and minimize the risk of infection.*
■ Use the heparin flush solution to repeat the flushing procedure only if the patient doesn't have a continuous infusion and only if your facility's policy requires it. If using a heparin flush, be aware of any effects it may have on specimens and flush the catheter before drawing a discard sample, if necessary.
■ *Because there are different types of injection and access caps or needleless connectors,* always follow manufacturer's guidelines for flush technique and when to clamp.
■ *To prevent catheter-related blood system infections,* disinfect the injection surface with an antiseptic pad before each injection.[1]
■ Be aware of the type of solution infusing through the catheter and any effects it may have on the laboratory test results. Temporarily stop infusions if drawing blood through a multilumen

central venous catheter, or flush the line with normal saline solution before drawing a discard sample.[27]

■ Assess dressings each shift. Visually inspect or palpate the catheter-site junction through the intact dressing daily *to assess for signs of infection.*[4]

■ Application of catheter stabilization devices varies. Always follow the manufacturer's instructions.

■ When removing the catheter, if you suspect an infection, swab the catheter on a fresh agar plate or clip 1″ off the catheter tip and place it in a specimen container and send it to the laboratory for testing.

■ Monitor the patient's vital signs before and after the catheter is removed. Notify the doctor of any changes in mental status, respiratory rate, heart rate, oxygen saturation, and blood pressure.

Patient teaching

Long-term use of a central venous access catheter allows patients to receive all types of infusion therapies at home. These catheters have a much longer life *because they're less thrombogenic and less prone to infection than short-term devices.*

A candidate for home therapy must have a family member or friend who can safely and competently administer the IV fluids, a backup helper, a suitable home environment, a telephone, transportation, adequate reading skills, and the ability to prepare, handle, store, and dispose of the equipment. The care procedures used in the home are the same as those used in the facility.

The overall goal of home therapy is patient safety, so your patient teaching must begin well before discharge. After discharge, a home therapy coordinator will provide follow-up care until the patient or someone close to him can independently provide catheter care and infusion therapy. Many home therapy patients learn to care for the catheter themselves and infuse their own medications and solution.

Complications

Complications can occur at any time during infusion therapy. Traumatic complications, such as pneumothorax, typically occur on catheter insertion but may not be noticed until after the procedure is completed. Systemic complications, such as sepsis, typically occur later during infusion therapy. Other complications include phlebitis (especially in peripheral central venous therapy), thrombus formation, and air embolism. (See *Risks of central venous therapy,* pages 144 and 145.)

Occlusion of the catheter may require the placement of a new catheter. If blood can't be aspirated or resistance is met, don't forcibly flush the catheter.

Be alert for signs of air embolism, such as sudden onset of pallor, cyanosis, dyspnea, coughing, and tachycardia, progressing to syncope and shock. If any of these signs occur, place the patient on his left side in Trendelenburg's position and notify the doctor.

It's possible to accidentally dislodge or damage a catheter while performing a dressing change, which could result in catheter tip embolus, air embolus, or hemorrhage. However, the most common complication related to changing a central venous access catheter dressing is failure to maintain sterile technique during the procedure. Watch for signs of local or generalized infection.

Documentation

Record the time and date of insertion, length and location of the catheter, solution infused, doctor's name, and patient's response to the procedure. Document the time of the X-ray, its results, and your notification of the doctor.

Document the procedure performed, the date and time it was performed, and any complications that occurred.[29]

Record dressing assessment findings each shift. Document the condition of the site, dressing type, type of stabilization device used, site care given, external catheter length, and any catheter-related mechanical problems.

Record the time and date of removal and the type of antimicrobial ointment and dressing applied. Note the condition of the catheter insertion site and collection of a culture specimen. Also document the reason for discontinuation of therapy.[33]

Document patient and family teaching provided.[33]

REFERENCES

1 O'Grady, N.P., et al. (2011). "Guidelines for the Prevention of Intravascular Catheter-Related Infections" [Online]. Accessed August 2011 via the Web at http://www.cdc.gov/hicpac/pdf/guidelines/bsi-guidelines-2011.pdf

2 Standard 45. Flushing and locking: Infusion nursing standards of practice. (2011). *Journal of Infusion Nursing, 34*(1S), S59. (Level I)

3 Infusion Nurses Society. (2008). *Flushing protocols.* Boston, MA: Infusion Nurses Society.

4 Standard 46. Vascular access device site care and dressing changes. Infusion nursing standards of practice. (2011). *Journal of Infusion Nursing, 34*(1S), S63–64. (Level I)

5 Marschall, J., et al. (2008). Strategies to prevent central line-associated bloodstream infections in acute care hospitals. *Infection Control and Hospital Epidemiology, 29*(S1):S22–S30. (Level I)

6 Standard 26. Add-on devices: Infusion nursing standards of practice. (2011). *Journal of Infusion Nursing, 34*(1S), S31. (Level I)

7 Standard 27. Needleless connectors: Infusion nursing standards of practice. (2011). *Journal of Infusion Nursing, 34*(1S), S32–33. (Level I)

8 Standard 44. Vascular access device removal: Infusion nursing standards of practice. (2011). *Journal of Infusion Nursing, 34*(1S), S57–58. (Level I)

9 Association of Professionals in Infection Control and Epidemiology (APIC). (2009). "An APIC Guide 2009: Guide to the Elimination of Catheter-Related Bloodstream Infections" [Online]. Accessed August 2011 on the Web at http://www.apic.org/Content/NavigationMenu/PracticeGuidance/APICEliminationGuides/CRBSI_Elimination_Guide_logo.pdf

10 Institute for Healthcare Improvement. (2010). *5 million lives campaign getting started kit: Prevent Central line-associated bloodstream infections.* Cambridge, MA: Institute for Healthcare Improvement.

11 Standard 35. Vascular access site preparation and device placement: Infusion nursing standards of practice. (2011). *Journal of Infusion Nursing, 34*(1S), S44. (Level I)

Risks of central venous therapy

Signs and symptoms	Possible causes	Nursing interventions	Preventon
Infection			
■ Redness, warmth, tenderness, or swelling at the insertion or exit site ■ Possible exudate of purulent material ■ Local rash or pustules ■ Fever, chills, malaise ■ Leukocytosis ■ Nausea and vomiting	■ Failure to maintain sterile technique during catheter insertion or care ■ Failure to comply with dressing change protocol ■ Wet or soiled dressing remaining on the site ■ Immunosuppression ■ Irritated suture line ■ Contaminated catheter or solution ■ Frequent opening of the catheter or long-term use of a single IV access site	■ Monitor temperature frequently. ■ Monitor vital signs closely. ■ Culture the site. ■ Re-dress using sterile technique. ■ Treat systemically with antibiotics or antifungals, depending on culture results and doctor's order. ■ Catheter may be removed. ■ Collection of peripheral blood cultures is recommended.[31] ■ If cultures don't match but are positive, the catheter may be removed or the infection may be treated through the catheter. ■ Treat patients with antibiotics, as ordered. ■ If the catheter is removed, culture its tip. ■ Document interventions.[29]	■ Maintain sterile technique. Use sterile gloves, masks, and gowns when appropriate.[4] ■ Observe dressing-change protocols. ■ Change a wet or soiled dressing immediately.[30] ■ Examine the solution for cloudiness and turbidity before infusing; check the fluid container for leaks. ■ Use a 0.22-micron filter (or a 1.2-micron filter for 3-in-1 total parenteral nutrition solutions). ■ Keep the system closed as much as possible.[6]
Pneumothorax, hemothorax, chylothorax, or hydrothorax			
■ Decreased breath sounds on affected side ■ With hemothorax, decreased hemoglobin level because of blood pooling ■ Abnormal chest X-ray	■ Repeated or long-term use of the same vein ■ Preexisting cardiovascular disease ■ Lung puncture by the catheter during insertion or exchange over a guide wire ■ Large blood vessel puncture with bleeding inside or outside the lung ■ Lymph node puncture with leakage of lymph fluid ■ Infusion of solution into the chest area through an infiltrated catheter	■ Notify the doctor. ■ Remove the catheter or assist with removal. ■ Administer oxygen as ordered. ■ Set up and assist with chest tube insertion. ■ Document interventions.[29]	■ Position the patient head down with a rolled towel between his scapulae to dilate and expose the internal jugular or subclavian vein as much as possible during catheter insertion. ■ Assess for early signs of fluid infiltration (swelling in the shoulder, neck, chest, and arm). ■ Ensure that the patient is immobilized and prepared for insertion. Active patients may need to be sedated or taken to the operating room.
Air embolism			
■ Sudden onset of dyspnea ■ Breathlessness ■ Tachyarrhythmias ■ Weak pulse	■ Intake of air into the central venous system during catheter insertion or tubing changes, or inadvertent opening, cutting, or breaking of the catheter	■ Clamp, fold, or close the existing catheter or occlude the insertion site immediately.[28]	■ Purge all air from the administration sets and add-on devices before starting an infusion.

Risks of central venous therapy *(continued)*

SIGNS AND SYMPTOMS	POSSIBLE CAUSES	NURSING INTERVENTIONS	PREVENTON
AIR EMBOLISM *(continued)*			
■ Increased central venous pressure ■ Hypotension ■ Chest pain ■ Jugular vein distention ■ Wheezing ■ Altered mental status ■ Altered speech ■ Numbness ■ Paralysis ■ Loss of consciousness ■ Continued coughing		■ Place the patient in a left lateral decubitus position, if not contraindicated by other conditions.[28] ■ Administer oxygen. ■ Notify the doctor. ■ Document interventions.[29]	■ Teach the patient to perform Valsalva's maneuver during catheter insertion and tubing changes, if not contraindicated by other conditions.[28] ■ Use air-eliminating filters. ■ Use an infusion device with air detection capability. ■ Place the patient with the insertion site at or below heart level when changing administration sets or needleless connectors.[28] ■ Use luer-lock tubing and secure all connections.[6,30]
THROMBOSIS			
■ Edema at puncture site ■ Erythema ■ Ipsilateral swelling of arm, neck, and face ■ Pain along vein ■ Fever, malaise ■ Chest pain ■ Dyspnea ■ Cyanosis	■ Sluggish flow rate ■ Composition of catheter material (polyvinyl chloride catheters are more thrombogenic) ■ Hematopoietic status of patient ■ Preexisting limb edema ■ Infusion of irritating solutions	■ Notify the doctor. ■ Possibly remove the catheter. ■ Possibly infuse anticoagulant therapy, as prescribed.[32] ■ Verify thrombosis with diagnostic studies. ■ Apply warm, wet compresses locally. ■ Don't use the limb on the affected side for subsequent venipuncture. ■ Document interventions.[29]	■ Encourage early mobilization of the affected extremity.[32] ■ Maintain a steady flow rate with an infusion pump, or flush the catheter at regular intervals. ■ Use catheters made of less thrombogenic materials or catheters coated to prevent thrombosis. ■ Dilute irritating solutions. ■ Use a 0.22-micron filter for infusions.

12 Standard 18. Infection prevention: Infusion nursing standards of practice. (2011). *Journal of Infusion Nursing, 34*(1S), S25. (Level I)

13 The Joint Commission. (2012). Standard NPSG.01.01.01. *Comprehensive accreditation manual for hospitals: The official handbook.* Oakbrook Terrace, IL: The Joint Commission. (Level I)

14 The Joint Commission. (2012). Standard RI.01.03.01. *Comprehensive accreditation manual for hospitals: The official handbook.* Oakbrook Terrace, IL: The Joint Commission. (Level I)

15 The Joint Commission. (2012). Standard UP.01.01.01. *Comprehensive accreditation manual for hospitals: The official handbook.* Oakbrook Terrace, IL: The Joint Commission. (Level I)

16 The Joint Commission. (2012). Standard UP.01.03.01. *Comprehensive accreditation manual for hospitals: The official handbook.* Oakbrook Terrace, IL: The Joint Commission. (Level I)

17 The Joint Commission. (2012). Standard NPSG.07.01.01. *Comprehensive accreditation manual for hospitals: The official handbook.* Oakbrook Terrace, IL: The Joint Commission. (Level I)

18 Centers for Disease Control and Prevention. (October 2002). Guideline for hand hygiene in health-care settings. *Morbidity and Mortality Weekly Report, 51*(RR-16), 1–45. (Level 1)

19 World Health Organization. (2009). *WHO guidelines on hand hygiene in health care: First global patient safety challenge. Clean care is safer care.* Geneva, Switzerland: World Health Organization. (Level I)

20 The Joint Commission. (2012). Standard NPSG.03.04.01. *Comprehensive accreditation manual for hospitals: The official handbook.* Oakbrook Terrace, IL: The Joint Commission. (Level I)

21 Infusion Nurses Society. (2011). *Policies and procedures for infusion nursing* (4th ed.). Boston, MA: Infusion Nurses Society.

22 U.S. Food and Drug Administration. "Look. Check. Connect.: Safe Medical Device Connections Save Lives" [Online]. Accessed August 2011 via the Web at http:www.fda.gov/downloads/MedicalDevices/Safety/AlertsandNotices/UCM134873.pdf.

23 Standard 36. Vascular Access Device Stabilization: Infusion nursing standards of practice. (2011). *Journal of Infusion Nursing, 34*(1S), S46. (Level I)

24 Occupational Safety and Health Administration. "Bloodborne Pathogens, Standard Number 1910.1030" [Online]. Accessed August 2011 via the Web at http://www.osha.gov/pls/oshaweb/owadisp.show_document?p_table=STANDARDS&p_id=10051 (Level I)

25 Standard 22. Safe handling and disposal of sharps, hazardous materials, and hazardous waste: Infusion nursing standards of practice. (2011). *Journal of Infusion Nursing, 34*(1S), S286. (Level I)

26 The Joint Commission. (2012). Standard MM.04.01.01. *Comprehensive accreditation manual for hospitals: The official handbook.* Oakbrook Terrace, IL: The Joint Commission. (Level I)

27 Standard 57. Phlebotomy: Infusion nursing standards of practice. (2011). *Journal of Infusion Nursing, 34*(1S), S78–79. (Level I)

28 Standard 50. Flushing. Infusion nursing standards of practice. (2011). *Journal of Infusion Nursing, 34*(1S), S69–70. (Level I)

29 The Joint Commission. (2012). Standard RC.01.03.01. *Comprehensive accreditation manual for hospitals: The official handbook.* Oakbrook Terrace, IL: The Joint Commission. (Level I)

30 Standard 43. Administration set change: Infusion nursing standards of practice. (2011). *Journal of Infusion Nursing, 34*(1S), S55. (Level I)

31 Standard 49. Infection: Infusion nursing standards of practice. (2011). *Journal of Infusion Nursing, 34*(1S), S68. (Level I)

32 Standard 52. Catheter-associated venous thrombosis: Infusion nursing standards of practice. (2011). *Journal of Infusion Nursing, 34*(1S), S71–72. (Level I)

33 Standard 14. Catheter-associated venous thrombosis: Infusion nursing standards of practice. (2011). *Journal of Infusion Nursing, 34*(1S), S20–21. (Level I)

CENTRAL VENOUS PRESSURE MONITORING

With central venous pressure (CVP) monitoring, a catheter is inserted through a vein and advanced until its tip lies in or near the right atrium. Because no major valves lie at the junction of the vena cava and right atrium, pressure at end diastole reflects back to the catheter. When connected to a monitoring system, the catheter measures CVP—an index of right ventricular function.

CVP monitoring helps to assess cardiac function, evaluate venous return to the heart, and indirectly gauge how well the heart is pumping. The central venous (CV) catheter also provides access to a large vessel for rapid, high-volume fluid administration and allows frequent blood withdrawal for laboratory samples. CVP monitoring can be done intermittently or continuously. The catheter is inserted percutaneously or using a cutdown method. Typically, a single lumen CVP line is used for intermittent pressure readings with the use of a water manometer or a transducer and stopcock. A pulmonary artery (PA) catheter has a proximal lumen appropriate for continuous CVP monitoring.

Normal CVP ranges from 5 to 10 cm H_2O or 2 to 6 mm Hg.[1] Changes in preload status are reflected in CVP readings. Any condition that alters venous return, circulating blood volume, or cardiac performance may affect CVP. If circulating volume increases (such as with enhanced venous return to the heart from fluid overload, heart failure, and positive-pressure breathing), CVP rises. If circulating volume decreases (such as with reduced venous return from hypovolemia secondary to dehydration, interstitial fluid shift or hemorrhage, and negative pressure breathing), CVP drops.

Equipment
Leveling device ▪ IV pole ▪ IV solution ▪ gloves and other personal protective equipment, as needed.

For CVP measurement with a water manometer
Disposable CVP manometer set ▪ additional stopcock (to attach the CVP manometer to the catheter) ▪ extension tubing, if needed ▪ IV drip chamber and tubing.

For CVP measurement with a transducer
Pressure-monitoring kit with disposable pressure transducer ▪ bedside pressure module ▪ pressure bag.

Implementation
- Gather the necessary equipment.
- Perform hand hygiene and put on gloves.[2,3,4]
- Confirm the patient's identity using at least two patient identifiers according to your facility's policy.[5]
- Explain the procedure to the patient *to reduce his anxiety.*
- If one isn't already in place, assist the doctor as he inserts a CV or PA catheter. (See "Central venous access catheter," page 133.)
- With the CV catheter in place, position the patient between 0 and 45 degrees with the bed in its lowest position.[1]
- Find the right atrium by locating the fourth intercostal space at the midaxillary line. Mark the appropriate place on the patient's chest *so that all subsequent recordings will be made using the same location.* When the head of the bed is elevated, the phlebostatic axis remains constant but the midaxillary line changes. Use the same degree of elevation for all subsequent measurements.

Measuring CVP with a water manometer
- Prime the IV tubing and manometer setup. Attach the water manometer to an IV pole or place it next to the patient's chest.
- Connect the IV tubing to the CV catheter. Trace the tubing from the patient to its point of origin *to make sure that it's attached to the proper port.*
- Align the base of the manometer with the zero reference point by using a leveling device and secure the manometer in place. *Because CVP reflects right atrial pressure,* you must align the right atrium (the zero reference point) with the zero mark on the manometer. (See *Measuring CVP with a water manometer.*)

Measuring CVP with a water manometer

To ensure accurate central venous pressure (CVP) readings, make sure that the manometer base is aligned with the patient's right atrium (the zero reference point). The manometer set usually contains a leveling rod to allow you to determine this alignment quickly.

After adjusting the manometer's position, examine the three-way stopcock. By turning it to any position shown below, you can control the direction of fluid flow. Four-way stopcocks are also available.

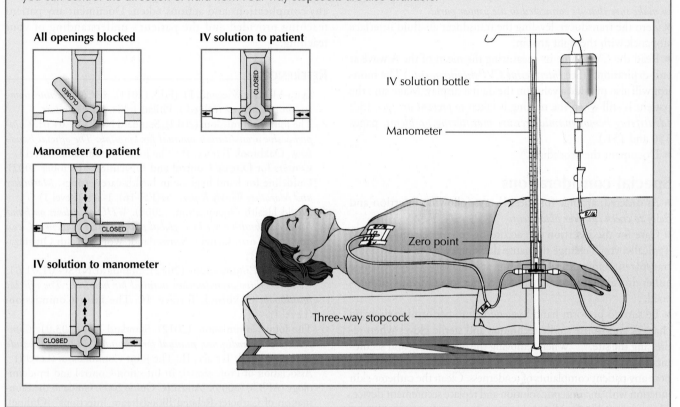

All openings blocked

IV solution to patient

Manometer to patient

IV solution to manometer

IV solution bottle

Manometer

Zero point

Three-way stopcock

■ Typically, markings on the manometer range from –2 to 38 cm H_2O. However, manufacturer's markings may differ, so be sure to read the directions before setting up the manometer and obtaining readings.

■ Turn the stopcock off to the patient and slowly fill the manometer with IV solution until the fluid level is 10 to 20 cm H_2O higher than the patient's expected CVP value. Don't overfill the tube *because fluid that spills over the top can become a source of contamination.*

Intermittent CVP readings using a water manometer

■ Turn the stopcock off to the IV solution and open to the patient. The fluid level in the manometer will drop. When the fluid level comes to rest, it will fluctuate slightly with respirations. Expect it to drop during inspiration and to rise during expiration.

■ Record CVP at the end of expiration, when intrathoracic pressure has a negligible effect and the fluctuation is at its highest point.[1] Depending on the type of water manometer used, note the value either at the bottom of the meniscus or at the midline of the small floating ball.

■ After you've obtained the CVP value, turn the stopcock to resume the IV infusion. Adjust the IV drip rate, as required.

■ Place the patient in a comfortable position.

■ Remove and discard your personal protective equipment and perform hand hygiene.[2,3,4]

■ Document the procedure.[6]

Continuous CVP readings using a water manometer

■ Make sure the stopcock is turned so that the IV solution port, CVP column port, and patient port are open. Be aware that with this stopcock position, infusion of the IV solution increases CVP. Therefore, expect higher readings than those taken with the stopcock turned off to the IV solution.

■ If the IV solution infuses at a constant rate, CVP will change as the patient's condition changes, although the initial reading will be higher. Assess the patient closely for changes.

■ Record CVP values at appropriate intervals.

■ Remove and discard your personal protective equipment and perform hand hygiene.[2,3,4]

■ Document the procedure.[6]

Measuring CVP with transducer

- Set up a pressure transducer system. (See "Transducer system setup," page 739.)
- Make sure the CV catheter or the proximal lumen of a PA catheter is attached to the system. (If the patient has a CV catheter with multiple lumens, the distal port is dedicated to continuous CVP monitoring and the other lumens used for fluid administration.) Trace the tubing from the patient to its point of origin *to make sure that it's connected to the proper port.*
- Zero the transducer, leveling the transducer air-fluid interface stopcock with the right atrium.
- Read the CVP value by measuring the mean of the A wave at end-expiration.[1] (See *Interpreting CVP measurements.*) The monitor will also provide a value on the digital display. Make sure the patient is still when the reading is taken *to prevent artifact.* (See *Identifying hemodynamic pressure-monitoring problems*, pages 150 and 151.)
- Document the procedure.[6]

Special considerations

- As ordered, arrange for chest X-rays following insertion and daily *to check catheter placement.*
- Care for the insertion site according to your facility's policy. Typically, you'll change the gauze dressing every 48 hours and a transparent semipermeable dressing at least every 7 days. Change either dressing immediately if it becomes soiled, damp, or loosened.[7,8,9]
- Be sure to perform hand hygiene before performing dressing changes and to use sterile technique and sterile gloves when re-dressing the site.[2,3,4] When removing the old dressing and securement device, observe for signs of infection, such as redness, and note any patient complaints of tenderness. Clean the catheter-skin junction with an antiseptic solution and replace securement device. Then apply a chlorhexidine-impregnated sponge dressing or a transparent semipermeable dressing.[8,9]
- After the initial CVP reading, reevaluate readings frequently *to establish a baseline for the patient.* Authorities recommend obtaining readings at 15-, 30-, and 60-minute intervals to establish a baseline. If the patient's CVP fluctuates by more than 2 cm H_2O, suspect a change in his clinical status and report this finding to the doctor.
- Change the IV solution and the IV tubing or pressure tubing every 96 hours or according to facility policy, or immediately if contamination is suspected or when integrity of the product or system has been compromised. Label the IV solution, tubing, and dressing with the date, time, and your initials.[8,10]
- Assess catheter necessity daily during multidisciplinary rounds; the catheter should be removed as soon as it's no longer needed to reduce the risk for central line–related bloodstream infections.[7,11,12]

Complications

Complications of CVP monitoring include pneumothorax (which typically occurs upon catheter insertion), sepsis, thrombus, vessel or adjacent organ puncture, and air embolism.

Documentation

Document all dressing, tubing, and solution changes, the condition of the site, and site care given. Record the patient's CVP readings, the doctor notified, prescribed interventions, and the patient's response. Document the patient's tolerance of the procedure, the date and time of catheter removal, and the type of dressing applied. Note the condition of the catheter insertion site and whether a culture specimen was collected. Note any complications and actions taken. Document any patient teaching provided and the patient's understanding of your teaching.

REFERENCES

1 Lynn-McHale Wiegand, D. (Ed.). (2011). *AACN procedure manual for critical care* (6th ed.). Philadelphia, PA: Saunders.

2 The Joint Commission. (2012). Standard NPSG.07.01.01. *Comprehensive accreditation manual for hospitals: The official handbook.* Oakbrook Terrace, IL: The Joint Commission. (Level I)

3 Centers for Disease Control and Prevention. (October 2002). Guideline for hand hygiene in health-care settings. *Morbidity and Mortality Weekly Report, 51*(RR-16), 1–45. (Level 1)

4 World Health Organization. (2009). *WHO guidelines on hand hygiene in health care: First global patient safety challenge. Clean care is safer care.* Geneva, Switzerland: World Health Organization. (Level I)

5 The Joint Commission. (2012). Standard NPSG.01.01.01. *Comprehensive accreditation manual for hospitals: The official handbook.* Oakbrook Terrace, IL: The Joint Commission. (Level I)

6 The Joint Commission. (2012). Standard RC.01.03.01. *Comprehensive accreditation manual for hospitals: The official handbook.* Oakbrook Terrace, IL: The Joint Commission. (Level I)

7 Association of Professionals in Infection Control and Epidemiology (APIC). (2009). "An APIC Guide 2009: Guide to the Elimination of Catheter-Related Bloodstream Infections" [Online]. Accessed August 2011 on the Web at http://www.apic.org/Content/NavigationMenu/PracticeGuidance/APICEliminationGuides/CRBSI_Elimination_Guide_logo.pdf

8 O'Grady, N.P., et al. (2011). "Guidelines for the Prevention of Intravascular Catheter-Related Infections" [Online]. Accessed August 2011 via the Web at http://www.cdc.gov/hicpac/pdf/guidelines/bsi-guidelines-2011.pdf

9 Standard 46. Vascular access device site care and dressing changes. Infusion nursing standards of practice. (2011). *Journal of Infusion Nursing, 34*(1S), S63–64. (Level I)

10 Standard 43. Administration set change. Infusion nursing standards of practice. (2011). *Journal of Infusion Nursing, 34*(1S), S63. (Level 1)

11 Institute for Healthcare Improvement. (2010). *5 million lives campaign getting started kit: Prevent central line-associated bloodstream infections.* Cambridge, MA: Institute for Healthcare Improvement.

12 Marschall, J. et al., (2008). Strategies to prevent central line-associated bloodstream infections in acute care hospitals. *Infection Control and Hospital Epidemiology, 29*(S1), S22–S30. (Level 1)

Interpreting CVP measurements

A pressure transducer set produces an intermittent or continuous waveform and readout that's displayed on the patient's bedside monitor, along with the patient's electrocardiogram (ECG) and other tracings. This method allows you to continually monitor for acute or gradual changes in central venous pressure (CVP).

When using a pressure transducer set, make sure the central venous (CV) catheter or the proximal lumen of a pulmonary artery catheter is attached to the system and that the patient is still when the reading is taken *to prevent artifact.*

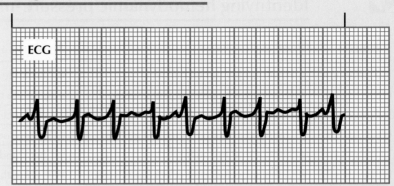

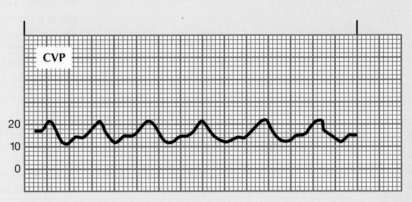

There are three waves to be aware of when interpreting a CVP waveform: the a, c, and v waves. Understanding how these waves relate to cardiac function is necessary to accurately interpret the CVP waveform.

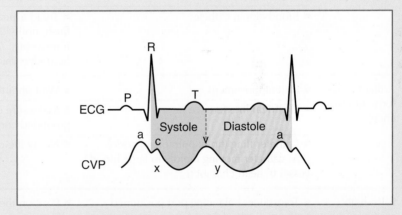

A wave (atrial contraction)

The most prominent wave is the a wave, which results from atrial contraction at end-diastole. As the right atria contracts, it forces blood into the right ventricle, causing a rise in pressure. This rise in pressure travels through the central line to the transducer and is represented by a positive inflection on the CVP waveform. When compared with the ECG waveform produced at the same time, the A wave on the CVP occurs after the P wave. To measure CVP, or right atrial pressure, measure the mean of the A wave at end-expiration.[7]

C wave (closure of the tricuspid valve)

Isovolumic right ventricular contraction, which closes the tricuspid valve and causes it to bow back toward the right atrium in early systole, produces a transient increase in atrial pressure. This increase in pressure is represented by the C wave on the waveform. The C wave, also a positive inflection on the CVP waveform, follows the onset of the QRS complex on the ECG.

V wave (ventricular contraction)

The last atrial pressure peak is the V wave, caused by a combination of atrial filling and ventricular contraction during late systole while the tricuspid valve remains closed. The V wave peaks just after the T wave on the ECG.

Identifying hemodynamic pressure-monitoring problems

PROBLEM	POSSIBLE CAUSES	NURSING INTERVENTIONS
No waveform	■ Power supply turned off	■ Check the power supply.
	■ Monitor screen pressure range set too low	■ Raise the monitor screen pressure range, if necessary.
	■ Loose connection in line	■ Rebalance and recalibrate the equipment.
	■ Transducer not connected to amplifier	■ Tighten loose connections.
	■ Stopcock off to patient	■ Check and tighten the connection.
	■ Catheter occluded or out of blood vessel	■ Position the stopcock correctly. ■ Use the fast-flush valve to flush the line, or try to aspirate blood from the catheter. If the line remains blocked, notify the doctor and prepare to replace the line.
Drifting waveforms	■ Improper warm-up	■ Allow the monitor and transducer to warm up for 10 to 15 minutes.
	■ Electrical cable kinked or compressed	■ Place the monitor's cable where it can't be stepped on or compressed.
	■ Temperature change in room air or IV flush solution	■ Routinely zero and calibrate the equipment 30 minutes after setting it up to allow IV fluid to warm to room temperature.
Line fails to flush	■ Stopcocks positioned incorrectly	■ Make sure stopcocks are positioned correctly.
	■ Inadequate pressure from pressure bag	■ Make sure the pressure bag gauge reads 300 mm Hg.
	■ Kink in pressure tubing	■ Check the pressure tubing for kinks.
	■ Blood clot in catheter	■ Try to aspirate the clot with a syringe. If the line still won't flush, notify the doctor and prepare to replace the catheter, if necessary. *Important:* Never use a syringe to flush a hemodynamic catheter.
Artifact (waveform interference)	■ Patient movement	■ Wait until the patient is quiet before taking a reading.
	■ Electrical interference	■ Make sure electrical equipment is connected and grounded correctly.
	■ Catheter fling (tip of pulmonary artery [PA] catheter moving rapidly in large blood vessel in heart chamber)	■ Notify the doctor, who may try to reposition the catheter.
False-high readings	■ Transducer balancing port positioned below patient's right atrium	■ Position the balancing port level with the patient's right atrium.
	■ Flush solution flow rate too fast	■ Check the flush solution flow rate. Maintain it at 3 to 4 mL/hour.
	■ Air in system	■ Remove air from the lines and the transducer.
	■ Catheter fling (tip of PA catheter moving rapidly in large blood vessel or heart chamber)	■ Notify the doctor, who may try to reposition the catheter.
False-low readings	■ Transducer balancing port positioned above patient's right atrium	■ Position the balancing port level with the patient's right atrium.
	■ Transducer imbalance	■ Make sure the transducer's flow system isn't kinked or occluded, and rebalance and recalibrate the equipment.
	■ Loose connection	■ Tighten loose connections.

Identifying hemodynamic pressure-monitoring problems *(continued)*

PROBLEM	POSSIBLE CAUSES	NURSING INTERVENTIONS
Damped waveform	■ Air bubbles	■ Secure all connections. ■ Remove air from the lines and the transducer. ■ Check for and replace cracked equipment.
	■ Blood clot in catheter	■ Try to aspirate the clot with a syringe. If the line still won't flush, notify the doctor and prepare to replace the catheter, if necessary. *Important:* Never use a syringe to flush a hemodynamic catheter.
	■ Blood flashback in line	■ Make sure stopcock positions are correct; tighten loose connections and replace cracked equipment; flush the line with the fast-flush valve; replace the transducer dome if blood backs up into it.
	■ Incorrect transducer position	■ Make sure the transducer is kept at the level of the right atrium at all times. Improper levels give false-high or false-low pressure readings.
	■ Arterial catheter out of blood vessel or pressed against vessel wall	■ Reposition the catheter if it's against the vessel wall. ■ Try to aspirate blood to confirm proper placement in the vessel. If you can't aspirate blood, notify the doctor and prepare to replace the line. *Note:* Bloody drainage at the insertion site may indicate catheter displacement. Notify the doctor immediately.

CEREBROSPINAL FLUID DRAINAGE MANAGEMENT

Cerebrospinal fluid (CSF) drainage aims to reduce CSF pressure to the desired level and then to maintain it at that level. Fluid can be withdrawn from the lateral ventricle (ventriculostomy) or the lumbar subarachnoid space, depending on the indication and the desired outcome, via a catheter and a closed-drainage collection system. Ventricular drainage is used to reduce increased intracranial pressure (ICP); lumbar drainage—a type of external drainage—is used to help heal the dura mater. External CSF drainage is used most commonly to manage increased ICP and facilitate spinal or cerebral dural healing after traumatic injury or surgery.

Other therapeutic uses of CSF drainage include ICP monitoring via the ventriculostomy; direct instillation of medications, contrast media, or air for diagnostic radiology; and aspiration of CSF for laboratory analysis. (See *CSF drainage,* page 152.)

This procedure focuses on ventricular drainage management.

Equipment

External drainage set (includes drainage tubing and sterile collection bag) ■ gloves ■ suture material ■ 4″ × 4″ sterile dressings ■ paper tape ■ IV pole.

Preparation of equipment

After the doctor places the catheter, connect it to the external drainage system tubing. Secure connection points with tape or a connector. Place the collection system, including drip chamber and collection bag, on an IV pole.

Implementation

■ Confirm the patient's identity using at least two patient identifiers according to your facility's policy.[1]
■ Explain the procedure to the patient and his family.
■ Perform hand hygiene and put on gloves.[2,3,4]
■ Perform a baseline neurologic assessment, including vital signs.
■ Ensure that the flow chamber of the ICP monitoring setup remains positioned as ordered. You should also correlate changes in ICP to the drainage.
■ Trace the tubing back to its point of origin *to make sure you're accessing the correct tubing.*
■ To drain CSF, as ordered, turn the main stopcock on to drainage *to allow CSF to collect in the graduated flow chamber.* Document the time and the amount of CSF obtained. Then turn the stopcock off to drainage. To drain the CSF from this chamber into the collection bag, release the clamp below the flow chamber.
■ Check the dressing frequently for drainage, *which could indicate CSF leakage.*
■ Check the tubing for patency by watching the CSF drops in the drip chamber.
■ Observe CSF for color, clarity, amount, blood, and sediment.

CSF drainage

Cerebrospinal fluid (CSF) drainage aims to control intracranial pressure (ICP) during treatment for traumatic injury or other conditions that cause a rise in ICP. A ventricular drain using a closed drainage system is detailed below.

Ventricular drain

For a ventricular drain, the doctor makes a burr hole in the patient's skull and inserts the catheter into the ventricle. The distal end of the catheter is connected to a closed drainage system.

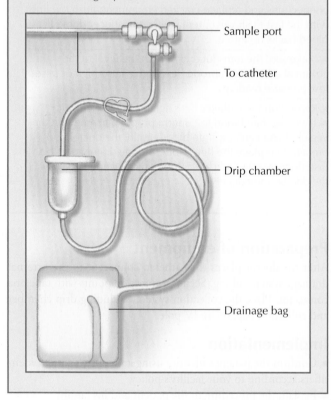

Sample port

To catheter

Drip chamber

Drainage bag

■ Change the collection bag using sterile technique when it's full or every 24 hours according to your facility's policy. Never empty the collection bag.
■ Remove and discard your gloves. Perform hand hygiene.[2,3,4]
■ Document the procedure.[5]

Special considerations

■ CSF specimens for laboratory analysis should be obtained from the collection port closest to the patient, not from the collection bag, and labeled in front of the patient.
■ Maintaining a continual hourly output of CSF is essential *to prevent overdrainage or underdrainage.* Overdrainage can occur if the drip chamber is placed too far below the catheter insertion site. Underdrainage may reflect kinked tubing, catheter displacement, or a drip chamber placed higher than the catheter insertion site.

■ Raising or lowering the head of the bed can affect the CSF flow rate. When changing the patient's position, reposition the drip chamber.
■ The patient may experience a chronic headache during continuous CSF drainage. Reassure him that this isn't unusual; administer analgesics, as appropriate.
■ Assess for signs and symptoms of hemorrhage, which may include headache.
■ Make sure ICP waveforms are monitored at all times.
■ If possible, the patient shouldn't leave his room for tests and procedures *to prevent dislodgement of catheter.* Check your facility's policy for scheduling such tests and procedures at the patient's bedside.
■ Follow strict sterile technique when connecting tubing, flushing, or taking specimens from the drainage system and during dressing changes.

Patient teaching

Teach the patient and family members about the reason for the drain. Explain to the patient that his activity level must be restricted. The patient may not sit up, stand, or walk when the drain is open and he must ask for assistance with movement. The system must be turned off when the patient is repositioned or transferred. Instruct the patient to avoid straining, coughing, and sneezing.

Complications

Signs and symptoms of excessive CSF drainage include headache, tachycardia, diaphoresis, and nausea. Acute overdrainage may result in collapsed ventricles, tonsillar herniation, and medullary compression.

NURSING ALERT *If drainage accumulates too rapidly, clamp the system, notify the doctor immediately, and perform a complete neurologic assessment.* This complication constitutes a potential neurosurgical emergency.

Cessation of drainage may indicate clot formation. If you can't quickly identify the cause of the obstruction, notify the doctor. If drainage is blocked, the patient may develop signs of increased ICP.

Infection may result from unsterile insertion technique or introduction of bacteria into the system, which may then cause meningitis. Maintain a sterile closed system and a dry, sterile dressing over the site.

Documentation

Record routine vital signs, ICP, and neurologic assessment findings at least every 4 hours or according to your facility's policy.

Document the color, clarity, and amount of CSF at least every 8 hours or according to your facility's policy. Record hourly and 24-hour CSF output, and describe the condition of the dressing.

REFERENCES

1   The Joint Commission. (2012). Standard NPSG.01.01.01. *Comprehensive accreditation manual for hospitals: The official handbook.* Oakbrook Terrace, IL: The Joint Commission. (Level I)

2 The Joint Commission. (2012). Standard NPSG.07.01.01. *Comprehensive accreditation manual for hospitals: The official handbook.* Oakbrook Terrace, IL: The Joint Commission. (Level I)

3 Centers for Disease Control and Prevention. (October 2002). Guideline for hand hygiene in health-care settings. *Morbidity and Mortality Weekly Report, 51*(RR-16), 1–45. (Level 1)

4 World Health Organization. (2009). *WHO guidelines on hand hygiene in health care: First global patient safety challenge. Clean care is safer care.* Geneva, Switzerland: World Health Organization. (Level I)

5 The Joint Commission. (2012). Standard RC.01.03.01. *Comprehensive accreditation manual for hospitals: The official handbook.* Oakbrook Terrace, IL: The Joint Commission. (Level I)

ADDITIONAL REFERENCES

Hickey, J.V. (2009). *The clinical practice of neurological and neurosurgical nursing* (6th ed.). Philadelphia, PA: Lippincott Williams & Wilkins.

Lynn-McHale Wiegand, D. (Ed.). (2011). *AACN procedure manual for critical care* (6th ed.). Philadelphia, PA: Saunders.

CERVICAL COLLAR APPLICATION

A cervical collar may be used for an acute injury (such as strained cervical muscles) or a chronic condition (such as arthritis or cervical metastasis). Or it may augment such splinting devices as a spine board to prevent potential cervical spine fracture or spinal cord damage.

Designed to hold the neck straight with the chin slightly elevated and tucked in, the collar immobilizes the cervical spine, decreases muscle spasms, and reduces pain; it also prevents further injury and promotes healing. As symptoms of an acute injury subside, the patient may gradually discontinue wearing the collar, alternating periods of wear with increasing periods of removal, until he no longer needs the collar.

Equipment

Cervical collar in the appropriate size ■ Optional: cotton (for padding). (See *Types of cervical collars.*)

Implementation

■ Verify the doctor's order.
■ Gather the equipment.
■ Confirm the patient's identity using at least two patient identifiers according to your facility's policy.[1]
■ Perform hand hygiene.[2,3,4]
■ Check the patient's neurovascular status before application.
■ Instruct the patient to position his head slowly to face directly forward.
■ With the patient upright (if possible) and facing forward, measure the height needed for the collar by measuring from the bottom of the patient's chin to the top of his sternum. Measure the circumference of the patient's neck.
■ Select the appropriate collar by applying the patient's measurements to the manufacturer's size chart.

Types of cervical collars

Cervical collars are used to support an injured or weakened cervical spine and to maintain alignment during healing.

Made of rigid plastic, the molded cervical collar holds the patient's neck firmly, keeping it straight, with the chin slightly elevated and tucked in.

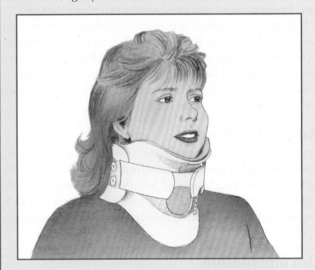

The soft cervical collar, made of spongy foam, provides gentler support and reminds the patient to avoid cervical spine motion.

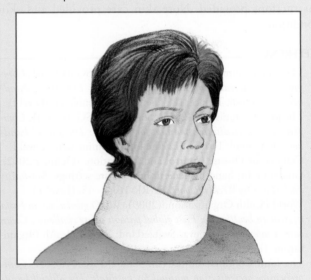

■ Place the cervical collar in front of the patient's neck *to ensure that the size is correct.*
■ Fit the collar snugly around the neck and attach the Velcro fasteners or buckles at the back of the neck.
■ Check the patient's airway and his neurovascular status *to ensure that the collar isn't too tight.*

- Perform hand hygiene.[2,3,4]
- Document the procedure.[5]

Special considerations

- Be aware that this procedure isn't adequate for acute spinal injuries.
- For a sprain or a potential cervical spine fracture, make sure the collar isn't too high in front *because this may hyperextend the neck.* In a neck sprain, such hyperextension may cause ligaments to heal in a shortened position. In a potential cervical spine fracture, hyperextension may cause serious neurologic damage.
- If the patient complains of pressure, the collar may be too tight. Remove and reapply it. If the patient complains of skin irritation or friction, the collar itself may be irritating him. Apply protective cotton padding between the irritated skin and the collar.
- Be sure to remove the collar every shift to check skin integrity and perform skin care to the neck.

Patient teaching

Teach the patient how to apply the collar and how to do a neurovascular check. Have the patient demonstrate how to apply the collar after you have instructed him. Some collars are complex and the patient (or caregiver) may need to practice if he will be responsible for application. If indicated, advise sleeping without a pillow.

Documentation

Note the type and size of the cervical collar and the time and date of application. Record the results of neurovascular checks. Document patient comfort, the collar's snugness, and all patient instructions provided. Note skin care provided and skin condition.

REFERENCES

1 The Joint Commission. (2012). Standard NPSG.01.01.01. *Comprehensive accreditation manual for hospitals: The official handbook.* Oakbrook Terrace, IL: The Joint Commission. (Level I)
2 The Joint Commission. (2012). Standard NPSG.07.01.01. *Comprehensive accreditation manual for hospitals: The official handbook.* Oakbrook Terrace, IL: The Joint Commission. (Level I)
3 Centers for Disease Control and Prevention. (October 2002). Guideline for hand hygiene in health-care settings. *Morbidity and Mortality Weekly Report, 51*(RR-16), 1–45. (Level 1)
4 World Health Organization. (2009). *WHO guidelines on hand hygiene in health care: First global patient safety challenge. Clean care is safer care.* Geneva, Switzerland: World Health Organization. (Level I)
5 The Joint Commission. (2012). Standard RC.01.03.01. *Comprehensive accreditation manual for hospitals: The official handbook.* Oakbrook Terrace, IL: The Joint Commission. (Level I)

ADDITIONAL REFERENCES

Bell, K.M., et al. (2009). Assessing range of motion to evaluate the adverse effects of ill-fitting cervical orthoses. *Spine Journal, 9*(3), 225–231.

Miller, C.P., et al. (2010). Soft and rigid collars provide similar restriction in cervical range of motion during fifteen activities of daily living. *Spine 35*(13), 1271–1278.
Proehl, J.A. (2008). *Emergency nursing procedures* (4th ed.). Philadelphia, PA: Saunders.

CHEMOTHERAPEUTIC DRUG ADMINISTRATION

Administration of chemotherapeutic drugs requires skills in addition to those used when giving other drugs.[1] For example, some drugs require specialized equipment or must be given through an unusual route. Others become unstable after a while, and still others must be protected from light. Finally, the drug dosage must be exact to avoid possibly fatal complications. For these reasons, only specially trained nurses and doctors should give chemotherapeutic drugs.

Chemotherapeutic drugs may be administered through a number of routes. Although the IV route (using peripheral or central veins) is used most commonly, these drugs may also be given orally, subcutaneously, IM, intra-arterially, into a body cavity, through a central venous catheter, through an Ommaya reservoir into the spinal canal, or through a device implanted in a vein or subcutaneously, such as through a patient-controlled analgesia device. They may also be administered into an artery, the peritoneal cavity, or the pleural space. (See *Intraperitoneal chemotherapy: An alternative approach.*)

The administration route depends on the drug's pharmacodynamics and the tumor's characteristics. For example, if a malignant tumor is confined to one area, the drug may be administered through a localized, or regional, method. Regional administration allows delivery of a high drug dose directly to the tumor. This is particularly advantageous because many solid tumors don't respond to drug levels that are safe for systemic administration.

Chemotherapy may be administered to a patient whose cancer is believed to have been eradicated through surgery or radiation therapy. This treatment, called *adjuvant chemotherapy,* helps to ensure that no undetectable metastasis exists. A patient may also receive chemotherapy before surgery or radiation therapy, called *induction chemotherapy* (or *neoadjuvant* or *synchronous chemotherapy.*) Induction chemotherapy helps improve survival rates by shrinking a tumor before surgical excision or radiation therapy.

In general, chemotherapeutic drugs prove more effective when given in higher doses, but their adverse effects often limit the dosage. An exception to this rule is methotrexate. This drug is particularly effective against rapidly growing tumors, but it's also toxic to normal tissues that are growing and dividing rapidly. However, doctors have discovered that they can give a large dose of methotrexate to destroy cancer cells and then, before the drug has had a chance to permanently damage vital organs, give a dose of folinic acid antidote. This antidote stops the effects of methotrexate, thus preserving normal tissue.

Intraperitoneal chemotherapy: An alternative approach

Intraperitoneal chemotherapy is beneficial in treating ovarian cancer that has spread within the peritoneal cavity *because much higher concentrations of the drug can be delivered directly to the peritoneal cavity when compared with the IV route of administration.*[3]

Typically, intraperitoneal chemotherapy is administered through a single-lumen implanted port that's connected to a silicone peritoneal catheter, or through a fully implanted port that's attached to a single-lumen venous silicone catheter. Peritoneal catheters designed for dialysis have been associated with an increased risk for bowel complications when used to administer chemotherapy in patients with ovarian cancer.[3]

Before administrations, the patient is typically premedicated for chemotherapy-induced nausea with an antiemetic such as ondansetron and a corticosteroid such as dexamethasone. Opioids may also be prescribed to relieve abdominal cramping. Next, the patient is positioned supine or in semi-Fowler's position with the head of the bed elevated no more than 30 degrees.[3]

The peritoneal port is accessed using a 19G or 20G 1″ to 2″ right-angled noncoring needle: patency is verified.[2,3] Chemotherapy is infused as rapidly as possible by gravitational flow;[3] an in-line fluid warmer is used to warm the solution to body temperature *to prevent abdominal cramping.* After the chemotherapy is infused, 1 L of warmed normal saline solution may be infused to help distribute the medication.

Stop the infusion if the patient becomes too uncomfortable. After the chemotherapy is infused, have the patient change position every 10 to 15 minutes for 1 to 2 hours *to help disperse the medication around the peritoneal cavity.*[2,3] Ninety percent of the administered chemotherapy drugs are absorbed within 4 hours of administration.[4]

After administering the chemotherapy drug, flush the port and catheter according to your facility's policy, remove the needle, and apply an occlusive dressing; the dressing can be safely removed after 12 hours.[3]

If the patient is pregnant, the doctor and other members of the health care team should collaborate with the patient's obstetric team before starting chemotherapy. Chemotherapy is contraindicated during the first trimester and isn't recommended after 35 weeks' gestation to avoid delivery during a period of bone marrow suppression.[2]

Equipment

Patient's medical record ■ prescribed chemotherapy drug ■ administration set ■ material safety data sheet for the prescribed chemotherapy drug ■ prescribed IV solution ■ other prescribed medications ■ syringes with luer-lock connector ■ antiseptic pads ■ infusion pump with preprogrammed dosing limits ■ low-pressure, flow-control infusion device (for vesicant administration) ■ powder-free chemotherapy gloves ■ nonlinting, nonabsorbent disposable gown ■ face shield ■ National Institute for Occupational Safety and Health (NIOSH)-approved respirator mask (if aerolization is likely) ■ chemotherapy sharps container ■ hazardous waste container approved for cytotoxic waste ■ labels ■ chemotherapy spill kit ■ extravasation equipment ■ emergency equipment ■ Optional: aluminum foil or a brown paper bag (if the drug is photosensitive), noncoring needle, IV insertion equipment.

Preparation of equipment

Make sure that a chemotherapy spill kit, extravasation equipment, and emergency equipment are readily available. Make sure that the emergency equipment is functioning properly.

Implementation

■ Verify the doctor's written order for the chemotherapy drug in the patient's medical record; verbal orders aren't permitted. Make sure the order contains the patient's complete name and a second identifier; the date; the patient's diagnosis; the patient's allergies; the regimen's name and number (if applicable), including the individual drug's generic names; treatment criteria; dosage calculation method; the patient's height and weight; and any other variables used to calculate the dosage. Also verify the route and rate of administration as well as the schedule, duration of therapy, cumulative lifetime dose (if applicable), sequence of drug administration (if applicable), and supportive care treatments that are appropriate for the regimen, such as hydration (if necessary) and premedications for hypersensitivity and nausea. Have another practitioner qualified to prepare or administer chemotherapy do the same.[2,4,5]

■ Make sure the doctor has obtained a written informed consent and that the consent form is in the patient's medical record.[2,4,6]

■ Become familiar with the information contained within the material safety data sheet specific to the drug.[7]

■ In collaboration with the patient's multidisciplinary team, review the patient's laboratory test results, specifically the complete blood count, blood urea nitrogen level, platelet count, urine creatinine level, and liver function studies.[1]

■ Check the patient's drug history for medications that might interact with chemotherapy.[8]

■ Determine whether the patient has received chemotherapy before, and note the severity of any adverse effects.

■ Check to see whether the doctor has ordered an antiemetic, fluids, a diuretic, or electrolyte supplements to be given before, during, or after chemotherapy administration. Administer them as prescribed following safe administration practices.

■ Perform hand hygiene.[9,10,11]

■ Confirm the patient's identity using at least two patient identifiers according to your facility's policy.[12]

Classifying chemotherapeutic drugs

To administer chemotherapy safely, you need to know each drug's potential for damaging tissue. In this regard, chemotherapeutic drugs are classified as vesicants, nonvesicants, or irritants.

Vesicants
- dactinomycin (Cosmegen)
- daunorubicin (Cerubidine)
- docetaxel (Taxotere)
- doxorubicin (Adriamycin)
- epirubicin (Ellence)
- idarubicin (Idamycin)
- mechlorethamine (Mustargen)
- mitomycin (Mutamycin)
- mitoxantrone (Novantrone)
- paclitaxel (Taxol)
- vinblastine (Velban)
- vincristine (Oncovin)
- vinorelbine (Navelbine)

Nonvesicants
- asparaginase (Elspar)
- cyclophosphamide (Cytoxan)
- cytarabine (Cytosar-U)
- floxuridine (FUDR)
- fluorouracil (Efudex)

Irritants
- bleomycin (Blenoxane)
- carboplatin (Paraplatin)
- carmustine (BiCNU)
- dacarbazine (DTIC-Dome)
- etoposide (VePesid)
- gemcitabine (Gemzar)
- ifosfamide (Ifex)
- irinotecan (Camptosar)
- melphalan (Alkeran)
- streptozocin (Zanosar)
- topotecan (Hycamtin)

■ Confirm that the patient received written educational material that is appropriate for his reading level and understanding and that the material includes information about his diagnosis, chemotherapy plan, possible long- and short-term adverse effects, risks associated with the regimen, reportable symptoms, monitoring, sexual relations, contraception, special precautions, and follow-up care.[2,4]

■ Assess the patient's physical condition and measure his height and weight; double-check his calculated body surface area and review his medical history.[2]

■ Recalculate the dose as ordered, using the patient's body surface area, and check your calculations against the written order.[1]

■ Make sure you understand what needs to be given and by what route, and provide the necessary teaching and support to the patient and his family.

■ Determine the best site to administer the drug. When selecting the site, consider drug compatibilities, frequency of administration, and the vesicant potential of the drug; *continuous vesicant infusions shouldn't be administered through a peripheral IV catheter because of the risk for extravasation.*[1,2] (See *Classifying chemotherapeutic drugs.*) Use a central venous access catheter or implanted access device to administer any vesicant drug infusing longer than 30 to 60 minutes.[2]

■ If a central venous access or implanted port isn't available and the drug must be given through a peripheral IV catheter, avoid using a site that's more than 24 hours old.[2] Assess the site for signs of inflammation or infiltration. If there's any doubt about the integrity of the IV site, insert a new IV catheter at another site.[2]

■ To identify an administration site, examine the patient's veins, starting with his hand and proceeding to his forearm. Veins of choice are pliable and smooth; large veins of the forearm are preferred.[2] Select the smallest gauge and shortest catheter needed to accommodate the prescribed therapy, and avoid the use of steel needles.[2,13] (See "IV catheter insertion and removal," page 421.)

■ Perform hand hygiene.[9,10,11] Put on protective equipment (two pairs of gloves, a gown, a face shield [when splashing is likely], and a respirator, if necessary). Make sure your inner glove cuff is worn under the gown cuff and the outer glove cuff extends over the gown cuff *to fully protect your skin.* Inspect your gloves *to make sure they're physically intact.*[4,7,14] Wear personal protective equipment through all stages of handling and administering the drug. Change your gloves every 30 minutes; if a drug spill occurs or your gloves become punctured or torn, remove them immediately. Wash your hands thoroughly with soap and water, and put on new gloves.

■ When you receive the drug from the pharmacy, make sure it's properly labeled with the patient's name and second identifier, full generic drug name, drug administration route, total dose to be given, total volume required to administer the dosage, date of administration, and date and time of preparation and expiration. The container should also have a label that clearly identifies the drug as hazardous.[4] If you must prepare the drug yourself, make sure to properly label it. (See "Chemotherapeutic drug preparation and handling," page 159.)

■ Establish blood return and patency, regardless of the access type *to prevent extravasation injury.*

NURSING ALERT *Never test vein patency with a chemotherapeutic drug.* If the vein isn't patent, severe tissue damage may result.

■ Avoid distractions and interruptions when preparing and administering *medication to prevent medication administration errors and protect the patient's safety.*[15]

■ Thoroughly disinfect the injection port with an antiseptic pad using friction.

■ If you're administering the drug by piggyback or short-term infusion, trace the tubing from the patient to its point of origin and attach the tubing to the appropriate injection port using a needleless, luer-lock connector. If you're administering by continuous infusion, trace the tubing from the patient to its port of origin and attach the tubing directly to the IV catheter or into a compatible maintenance IV solution, according to your facility's policy.[16] Secure all connections with luer-lock devices. If you're administering the drug by IV injection, refer to the doctor's orders and pharmacy guidelines for recommended IV injection rates, diluents, and other drug-specific details.

■ Use an electronic infusion pump for specific types of antineoplastic drugs and for all continuous infusions. When administering a vesicant, use a low-pressure, flow-control infusion device.

NURSING ALERT *Chemotherapy drugs are considered "high-alert" medications because they can cause significant patient harm when used in error. You and another practitioner who's qualified to prepare or administer chemotherapy should perform an independent double-check before chemotherapy administration.*[17]

■ Before administering the medication, have another practitioner who's qualified to prepare or administer chemotherapy perform an independent double-check according to your facility's policy *to verify the patient's identity and make sure the correct drug is prepared and in the prescribed concentrations and volume; that the drug hasn't expired; that the drug's indication corresponds with the patient's diagnosis; that the dosage calculations are correct and the dosing formula used to derive the final dose is correct; that the route of administration is safe and proper for the patient; that the drug's integrity is intact; that the infusion pump settings are correct; and that the infusion line is attached to the correct port (if applicable).* Both you and the other practitioner involved in the independent double-check should sign your names in the patient's medical record indicating that the verification took place.[1,2,4,18]

■ After comparing results of the independent double-check with the other practitioner, begin administering the drug if there are no discrepancies. If discrepancies exist, rectify them before administering the drug.[18]

■ Confirm the treatment plan, route, and symptom management plan with the patient.[4]

■ Begin administration as prescribed. Make sure that the administration tubing is clearly labeled to alert staff members that a hazardous drug is being administered through the designated line.[17]

■ During IV administration, closely monitor the patient for signs of a hypersensitivity reaction (agitation, chest tightness, shortness of breath, hypotension, rash, itching, facial edema, light-headedness, dizziness, and abdominal cramping) or extravasation (swelling, redness, stinging, burning or pain at the access site, loss of blood return from the device, and IV flow rate slowing or stoppage).[2]

■ When administering a vesicant drug by short-term infusion using a peripheral vein, stay with the patient during the infusion. Monitor the site for extravasation, and verify blood return every 5 to 10 minutes. When administering a vesicant by IV injection, verify blood return every 2 to 5 mL. When administering a vesicant through a central venous access catheter or implanted port, check for blood return periodically according to your facility's policy.[2]

■ After administration, if applicable, place a linen-saver pad underneath the connection site between the access device and administration tubing to absorb droplets that may spill. Disconnect the tubing from the access site, and then remove the IV container with the tubing attached; don't remove the spike from the IV container or reuse the tubing.[2]

■ Dispose of the IV container, tubing, and linen-saver pad in a hazardous waste receptacle. Dispose of syringes in a chemotherapy sharps container.[2,7]

■ Verify catheter patency and then flush the catheter with a compatible IV solution.[2]

Managing extravasation

Extravasation—the infiltration of a vesicant drug into the surrounding tissue—can result from a punctured vein or leakage around a venipuncture site. If vesicant drugs or fluids extravasate, blistering, peeling and sloughing of the skin, tissue necrosis, functional and sensory impairment of the affected area, disfigurement, and damage to tendons, nerves and joints may occur.[2,20]

Extravasation of vesicant drugs requires emergency treatment. Follow your facility's protocol, including the following essential steps:

■ Immediately stop administering the vesicant and other IV fluids infusing through the access device.[2,20]

■ Disconnect the IV tubing from the access device; don't remove the device or noncoring needle.[2,20]

■ Attempt to aspirate residual vesicant from the access device or noncoring needle using a small syringe (3 mL).[2,20]

■ Notify the doctor.

■ Remove the peripheral IV catheter or noncoring needle after the treatment plan has been determined.[2,20]

■ Use a standardized scale to assess and document the extent of the extravasation.

■ Estimate the amount of solution that has escaped into the tissue based on the rate of injection or infusion and the length of time since your last assessment.

■ Treat the site as prescribed; treatment may include elevating the extremity, cold or heat application, and administration of an antidote.[2,20]

■ In some cases, surgical intervention may be necessary.

■ Clean and decontaminate surfaces that might have come in contact with the drug.[2,7]

■ Remove and discard your personal protective equipment in a hazardous waste receptacle.[2,7]

■ Thoroughly wash your hands with soap and water.[2,7]

■ Document the procedure.[19]

Special considerations

■ If you suspect extravasation, stop the infusion immediately. Leave the IV catheter in place and notify the doctor. (See *Managing extravasation*.)

■ During infusion, some drugs need protection from direct sunlight *to avoid possible drug breakdown.* If this is the case, cover the container with a brown paper bag or aluminum foil.

■ Scalp veins shouldn't be used to administer vesicant drugs to a neonate or pediatric patient.[1]

■ Monitor the patient's vital signs throughout the infusion *to assess any changes during chemotherapy administration.* Assess the patient for adverse reactions to the drug.

■ Monitor the patient's cumulative chemotherapy dose *to make sure that the drug is discontinued if the maximum lifetime dose is achieved.*[1]

Complications

Common adverse effects of chemotherapy are nausea and vomiting, ranging from mild to debilitating. Another major complication, bone marrow suppression, can lead to neutropenia and thrombocytopenia. Other adverse effects include intestinal irritation, stomatitis, pulmonary fibrosis, cardiotoxicity, nephrotoxicity, neurotoxicity, hearing loss, anemia, alopecia, urticaria, radiation recall (if drugs are given with, or soon after, radiation therapy), anorexia, esophagitis, diarrhea, and constipation.

IV administration of chemotherapeutic drugs may lead to extravasation, which can cause blistering, peeling and sloughing of the skin, tissue necrosis, functional and sensory impairment of the affected area, disfigurement, and damage to tendons, nerves, and joints.

Documentation

Facilities commonly require nursing documentation on a chemotherapy flow sheet; document according to your facility's policy. Record any premedication that was administered, and note the location and description of the access site and verification of blood return. Record the drugs, dosages, route of administration, sequence of drug administration, needle type and size used, amount and type of flushing solution, and the site's condition after treatment. Document any adverse reactions, the patient's tolerance of the treatment, and patient and family teaching as well as their understanding of your teaching. Record any treatment required after chemotherapy administration.

REFERENCES

1 Standard 62. Antineoplastic therapy. Infusion nursing standards of practice. (2011). *Journal of Infusion Nursing, 34*(1S), S87–88. (Level 1)

2 Polovich, M., et al. (Eds.). (2009). *Chemotherapy and biotherapy guidelines and recommendations for practice* (3rd ed.). Pittsburgh, PA: Oncology Nursing Society.

3 Walker, J.L., & Markman, M. (2011). "Management of intraperitoneal chemotherapy for treatment of ovarian cancer" [Online]. Accessed January 2012 via the Web at http://www.uptodate.com/contents/management-of-intraperitoneal-chemotherapy-for-treatment-of-ovarian-cancer

4 Jacobson, J.O., et al. (2009). American Society of Clinical Oncology/Oncology Nursing Society chemotherapy administration safety standards. *Journal of Clinical Oncology, 27*(32), 5469–5475.

5 Centers for Medicare & Medicaid Services, Department of Health and Human Services. (2006). "Conditions of Participation: Nursing Services," 42 CFR part 482.23 [Online]. Accessed November 2011 via the Web at http://cfr.vlex.com/vid/482-23-condition-participation-nursing-19811372

6 Centers for Medicare & Medicaid Services, Department of Health and Human Services. (2006). "Conditions of Participation: Patients' Rights," 42 CFR part 482.13 [Online]. Accessed November 2011 via the Web at https://www.cms.gov/CFCsAndCoPs/downloads/finalpatientrightsrule.pdf

7 National Institute for Occupational Safety and Health. (2004). "Preventing Occupational Exposure to Antineoplastic and Other Hazardous Drugs in Health Care Settings," Publication No. 2004-165 [Online]. Accessed August 2011 via the Web at http://www.cdc.gov/ niosh/docs/2004-165#sum

8 The Joint Commission. (2012). Standard MM.06.01.01. *Comprehensive accreditation manual for hospitals: The official handbook.* Oakbrook Terrace, IL: The Joint Commission. (Level 1)

9 The Joint Commission. (2012). Standard NPSG.07.01.01. *Comprehensive accreditation manual for hospitals: The official handbook.* Oakbrook Terrace, IL: The Joint Commission. (Level 1)

10 Centers for Disease Control and Prevention. (October 2002). Guideline for hand hygiene in health-care settings. *Morbidity and Mortality Weekly Report, 51*(RR-16), 1–45. (Level 1)

11 World Health Organization. (2009). *WHO guidelines on hand hygiene in health care: First global patient safety challenge. Clean care is safer care.* Geneva, Switzerland: World Health Organization. (Level 1)

12 The Joint Commission. (2012). Standard NPSG.01.01.01. *Comprehensive accreditation manual for hospitals: The official handbook.* Oakbrook Terrace, IL: The Joint Commission. (Level 1)

13 Standard 32. Vascular access device selection. Infusion nursing standards of practice. (2011). *Journal of Infusion Nursing, 34*(1S), S37–40. (Level 1)

14 U.S. Department of Labor. Occupational Safety & Health Administration. (1999). Controlling occupational exposure to harmful drugs. In TED 1–0.15A, Section VI, Chapter 2, *OSHA Technical Manual.* Washington, DC: OSHA. Accessed August 2011 via the Web at www.osha.gov/dts/osta/otm/otm_vi/otm_vi_2.html (Level 1)

15 Westbrook, J., et al. (2010). Association of interruptions with an increased risk and severity of medication administration errors. *Archives of Internal Medicine, 170*(8), 683–690.

16 U.S. Food and Drug Administration (2009). "Look. Check. Connect.: Safe Medical Device Connections Save Lives" [Online]. Accessed August 2011 via the Web at www.fda.gov/downloads/MedicalDevices/Safety/AlertsandNotices/UCM134873.pdf

17 Institute of Safe Medication Practices. "ISMP's List of High-Alert Medications." [Online]. Accessed August 2011 via the Web at http://www.ismp.org/tools/highalertmedications.pdf

18 Institute for Safe Medication Practices. (2008). "Conducting an Independent Double-check." *ISMP Medication Safety Alert! Nurse Advise-ERR, 6*(12), 1 [Online]. Accessed July 2011 via the Web at http://www.ismp.org/newsletters/nursing/Issues/NurseAdviseERR200812.pdf

19 The Joint Commission. (2012). Standard RC.01.03.01. *Comprehensive accreditation manual for hospitals: The official handbook.* Oakbrook Terrace, IL: The Joint Commission. (Level 1)

20 Standard 48. Infiltration and extravasation. Infusion nursing standards of practice. (2011). *Journal of Infusion Nursing, 34*(1S), S66–68. (Level 1)

ADDITIONAL REFERENCES

American Society of Health System Pharmacists. (2006). "ASHP Guidelines on Handling Hazardous Drugs." *Drug Distribution and Control: Preparation and Handling Guidelines, 63*, 1172–93 [Online]. Accessed August 2011 via the Web at http://www.ashp.org/s_ashp/docs/files/BP07/Prep_Gdl_HazDrugs.pdf

Oncology Nursing Society. (2010). *Access device guidelines: Recommendations for nursing practice and education* (3rd ed.). Pittsburgh, PA: Oncology Nursing Society.

Siegel, J.D., et al. "2007 Guideline for Isolation Precautions: Preventing Transmission of Infectious Agents in Healthcare Settings" [Online]. Accessed June 2011 via the Web at http://www.cdc.gov/hicpac/2007ip/2007isolationprecautions.html

CHEMOTHERAPEUTIC DRUG PREPARATION AND HANDLING

You'll need to take extra care when preparing chemotherapeutic drugs, both for the patient's safety and for your own. Patients who receive chemotherapeutic drugs risk teratogenic, mutagenic, and carcinogenic effects, but the people who prepare and handle the drugs are at risk as well. According to the Occupational Safety and Health Administration (OSHA), no acceptable levels of exposure have been determined for these drugs. Because of this, the goal is to prevent or minimize workplace exposure.

OSHA, the National Institute for Occupational Safety and Health (NIOSH), the American Society of Health System Pharmacists, and the Oncology Nursing Society have established guidelines for handling and administering chemotherapeutic drugs. These guidelines are strongly recommended; adhering to them will help reduce the risk of contamination to both yourself and your environment.

The use of proper personal protective equipment is essential. Personal protective equipment must include chemotherapy-resistant gowns and gloves, which you should wear when handling, preparing, administering, or disposing of chemotherapeutic agents; priming administration sets; cleaning up spills; and handling excreta.[1] Gowns should be lint-free, have a full front, close in the back, and have elastic or knit cuffs. You should wear a gown once and discard of it appropriately; never hang it up after use. Also, never wear a gown for multiple patients or multiple times for the same patient. Make sure your gloves are chemotherapy-resistant. Double-gloving is recommended, and you should replace your gloves every 30 minutes or when they're visibly contaminated as well as after each individual patient contact. Wear a face mask and goggles when splashing is likely.[2] Also wear a face mask and NIOSH-approved respirator when cleaning up chemotherapy spills; surgical masks aren't effective against aerosolization of chemotherapeutic agents.

All health care workers who handle chemotherapeutic drugs must be properly educated and trained.[3] A key element of such training involves learning how to reduce exposure when handling such drugs.[4] The second requirement states that the drugs should be prepared in a class II biological safety cabinet.[4] OSHA guidelines further recommend that chemotherapeutic drugs be mixed in a properly enclosed and ventilated work area and that respiratory and skin protection be worn.[4] Smoking, drinking, applying cosmetics, and eating where these drugs are prepared, stored, or used should be strictly prohibited, and sterile technique should be used while mixing the drugs.

Gloves, gowns, syringes, or vials as well as other materials that have been used in chemotherapeutic preparation and administration present a possible source of exposure or injury to the facility's staff members, patients, and visitors. Therefore, using properly labeled, sealed, and covered containers, handled only by trained and protected personnel, should be routine practice.[4] Spills also represent a hazard, and all employees should be familiar with appropriate spill procedures for their own protection.[4]

Equipment

Prescribed drug or drugs ▪ patient's medication record and medical chart ▪ nonlint, nonabsorbent disposable gown ▪ powder-free chemotherapy gloves ▪ face shield or goggles ▪ NIOSH-approved respirator mask (if aerosolization is likely) ▪ plastic absorbent pad ▪ alcohol pads ▪ sterile gauze pads ▪ hazardous waste container ▪ IV solution ▪ compatibility reference source ▪ medication labels ▪ class II biological safety cabinet ▪ disposable towel ▪ syringes and needles of various sizes with luer-lock connectors ▪ IV tubing with luer-lock fittings ▪ infusion pump with preprogrammed dosing limits ▪ chemotherapy spill kit.

Preparation of equipment

Make sure that a chemotherapy spill kit is readily available.

Implementation

▪ Gather the appropriate equipment.
▪ Review the doctor's orders and have a second practitioner qualified to prepare or administer chemotherapy independently verify the order.[5]
▪ Make sure an informed consent form has been obtained and is in the patient's medical record.[6]
▪ Perform hand hygiene.[7,8,9] Put on protective equipment (two pairs of gloves, a gown, a face shield [when splashing is likely], and a respirator, if necessary). Make sure your inner glove cuff is worn under the gown cuff and the outer glove cuff extends over the gown cuff *to fully protect your skin.* Inspect your gloves *to make sure they're physically intact.*[1,2]
▪ Wear personal protective equipment through all stages of handling and administering the drug. Change your gloves every 30 minutes; if a drug spill occurs or your gloves become punctured or torn, remove them immediately. Wash your hands thoroughly with soap and water, and put on new gloves. Remember to perform hand hygiene before drug preparation and administration and wash thoroughly with soap and water afterward.[1,2,4,7,8,9]
▪ Maintain sterile technique when compounding these hazardous drugs.
▪ Reduce exposure when handling chemotherapy drugs *by taking care when unpacking the vials.* Wear personal protective equipment when unpacking chemotherapy vials *because vial exteriors have been found to be contaminated upon arrival from the manufacturer.*[1]
▪ Prepare the drugs in a class II biological safety cabinet.[4] Leave the hood blower on 24 hours a day, 7 days a week.[1]
▪ Before you prepare the drug (and after you finish), clean the internal surfaces of the cabinet with 70% alcohol and a disposable towel. Discard the towel in a hazardous waste container approved for cytotoxic waste.[4]
▪ Cover the work surface with a clean plastic absorbent pad *to minimize contamination by droplets or spills.* Change the pad at the end of the shift or whenever a spill occurs.[4]
▪ Consider all of the equipment used in drug preparation, as well as any unused drug, as hazardous waste.[4] Dispose of them according to your facility's policy.
▪ Always work below eye level to prevent accidental exposure to the eyes.[1]

■ Prepare the drug according to current product instructions, paying attention to compatibility, stability, and reconstitution technique. Label the prepared drug with the patient's name and second identifier, the drug's full generic name, the drug administration route, total dose to be administered, total volume required to administer the dosage, date of administration, and the date and time the drug expires.[5] Label all chemotherapeutic drugs with a hazardous drug label, such as one that states CYTOTOXIC DRUG or according to your facility's policy.[4]

■ Prime all IV bags with a compatible fluid before adding the chemotherapeutic drug.[1]

■ Wipe the exterior of the IV bag or syringe with sterile gauze before placing it in a sealed bag for transport.[1]

■ Clean and decontaminate all work surfaces that may have come in contact with the hazardous drug.[1]

■ Remove and discard your personal protective equipment before leaving the work area, and wash your hands thoroughly with soap and water.[1,7,8,9]

■ Transport syringes containing the drug in a sealed container with the luer-lock end of the syringe capped; transport IV bags and tubing in a sealed container that can contain spillage if dropped. Label the outermost container with a distinct label to alert staff members that the contents are hazardous.[1]

■ Perform hand hygiene.[7,8,9] Put on protective equipment (two pairs of gloves, a gown, a face shield [when splashing is likely], and a respirator, if necessary). Make sure your inner glove cuff is worn under the gown cuff and the outer glove cuff extends over the gown cuff *to fully protect your skin*. Inspect your gloves *to make sure they're physically intact*.[1,2]

■ Confirm the patient's identity using at least two patient identifiers according to your facility's policy.[10]

■ After administration, if applicable, place a linen-saver pad underneath the connection site between the access device and administration tubing to absorb droplets that may spill. Consider all of the equipment used in drug preparation and administration, as well as any unused drug, as hazardous waste.

■ Disconnect the tubing from the access site, and then remove the IV container with the tubing attached; don't remove the spike from the IV container or reuse the tubing. Place all chemotherapeutic waste products in a hazardous waste container.[1,4]

■ Dispose of the IV container, tubing, and the linen-saver pad in a hazardous waste receptacle. Dispose of syringes in a chemotherapy sharps container.[1,4]

■ Remove and discard your personal protective equipment in a hazardous waste receptacle.[1,4]

■ Thoroughly wash your hands with soap and water.[7,8,9]

■ Document the procedure.[11]

Special considerations

■ Take precautions to reduce your exposure to chemotherapeutic drugs. Systemic absorption can occur through ingestion of contaminated materials, contact with the skin, or inhalation. You can inhale a drug without realizing it, such as while opening a vial, clipping a needle, expelling air from a syringe, or discarding excess drug. You can also absorb a drug from handling contaminated stools or body fluids.

■ Use only syringes and IV sets that have luer-lock fittings.

■ Gloves, gowns, syringes or vials, and other materials that have been used in chemotherapeutic preparation and administration present a source of contamination to the facility's staff members, patients, visitors, and environment. Therefore, use of properly labeled, sealed, and enclosed containers for discarded equipment handled only by trained and protected personnel should be routine practice.

■ If some of the drug comes in contact with your skin, wash the involved area thoroughly with soap (not a germicidal agent) and water. If eye contact occurs, flood the eye with water or saline solution for at least 15 minutes while holding the eyelid open. Obtain a medical evaluation as soon as possible after accidental exposure.[1]

■ If a spill occurs, use a chemotherapeutic spill kit to clean the area. Wear all personal protective equipment (double gloves and a gown), including a respirator mask, goggles, and booties. Post a sign to warn others. Follow you facility's procedure for hazardous spills. Report and document the spill according to your facility's policy.[1]

■ Don't place any food or drinks in the same refrigerator as chemotherapeutic drugs. For accidental ingestion, don't induce vomiting unless indicated by the material safety data sheet. Seek emergency treatment.[1]

■ Become familiar with drug excretion patterns, and use chemotherapeutic-resistant personal protective equipment (double gloves, a gown, and a face shield) when handling a chemotherapy patient's body fluids and excreta for the first 48 hours after the patient has received chemotherapy.[1]

■ Provide male patients with a urinal with a tight-fitting lid. Wear disposable latex surgical gloves when handling body fluids. Before flushing the toilet, place a waterproof pad over the toilet bowl *to avoid splashing*. Wear chemotherapy-resistant gloves and a gown when handling linens soiled with body fluids. Place soiled linens in isolation linen bags designated for separate laundering.

■ Women who are pregnant, trying to conceive, or breast-feeding should exercise caution when handling chemotherapeutic drugs.[1,3,4]

Patient teaching

When teaching your patient about handling chemotherapeutic drugs, discuss appropriate safety measures. If the patient will be receiving chemotherapy at home, teach him how to dispose of contaminated equipment. Tell the patient and his family to wear gloves whenever handling chemotherapy equipment or contaminated linens or gowns and pajamas. Instruct them to place soiled linens in a separate washable pillowcase and to launder the pillowcase twice, with the soiled linens inside, separately from other linens.

When providing home care, empty waste products into the toilet close to the water *to minimize splashing*. Close the lid and flush two or three times.

All materials used for treatment should be placed in a leak-proof container and taken to a designated disposal area. The patient or his family should make arrangements with either a health care facility or a private company for pickup and proper disposal of contaminated waste.

Complications

Chemotherapeutic drugs may be mutagenic. Chronic exposure to chemotherapeutic drugs may damage the liver or chromosomes. Direct exposure to these drugs may burn and damage the skin.

Documentation

Document each incident of exposure according to your facility's policy.

REFERENCES

1 Polovich, M., et al. (Eds.). (2009). *Chemotherapy and biotherapy guidelines and recommendations for practice* (3rd ed.). Pittsburgh, PA: Oncology Nursing Society.

2 National Institute for Occupational Safety and Health. (2004). "Preventing Occupational Exposure to Antineoplastic and Other Hazardous Drugs in Health Care Settings," Publication No. 2004-165 [Online]. Accessed August 2011 via the Web at http://www.cdc.gov/ niosh/docs/2004-165#sum

3 Standard 62. Antineoplastic therapy. Infusion nursing standards of practice. (2011). *Journal of Infusion Nursing, 34*(1S), S87–88. (Level 1)

4 U.S. Department of Labor. Occupational Safety & Health Administration. (1999). "Controlling Occupational Exposure to Harmful Drugs." In TED 1–0.15A, Section VI, Chapter 2. OSHA Technical Manual. Washington, D.C.: OSHA. Accessed August 2011 via the Web at www.osha.gov/dts/osta/otm_vi/otm_vi_2.html (Level 1)

5 Jacobson, J.O., et al. (2009). American Society of Clinical Oncology/Oncology Nursing Society chemotherapy administration safety standards, *Journal of Clinical Oncology, 27*(32), 5469–75.

6 The Joint Commission. (2012). Standard RI.01.03.01. *Comprehensive accreditation manual for hospitals: The official handbook.* Oakbrook Terrace, IL: The Joint Commission. (Level 1)

7 World Health Organization. (2009). *WHO guidelines on hand hygiene in health care: First global patient safety challenge. Clean care is safer care.* Geneva, Switzerland: World Health Organization. (Level 1)

8 Centers for Disease Control and Prevention. (October 2002). Guideline for hand hygiene in health-care settings. *Morbidity and Mortality Weekly Report, 51*(RR-16), 1–45. (Level 1)

9 The Joint Commission. (2012). Standard NPSG.07.01.01. *Comprehensive accreditation manual for hospitals: The official handbook.* Oakbrook Terrace, IL: The Joint Commission. (Level 1)

10 The Joint Commission. (2012). Standard NPSG.01.01.01. *Comprehensive accreditation manual for hospitals: The official handbook.* Oakbrook Terrace, IL: The Joint Commission. (Level 1)

11 The Joint Commission. (2012). Standard RC.01.03.01. *Comprehensive accreditation manual for hospitals: The official handbook.* Oakbrook Terrace, IL: The Joint Commission. (Level 1)

ADDITIONAL REFERENCES

American Society of Health System Pharmacists. (2006). "ASHP Guidelines on Handling Hazardous Drugs." *Drug Distribution and Control: Preparation and Handling Guidelines, 63,* 1172–1193 [Online]. Accessed August 2011 via the Web at http://www.ashp.org/s_ashp/ docs/files/BP07/Prep_Gdl_HazDrugs.pdf

Siegel, J.D., et al. "2007 Guideline for Isolation Precautions: Preventing Transmission of Infectious Agents in Healthcare Settings" [Online]. Accessed June 2011 via the Web at http://www.cdc.gov/ hicpac/ 2007ip/2007isolationprecautions.html

CHEST PHYSIOTHERAPY

Chest physiotherapy (PT) includes postural drainage, chest percussion and vibration, and coughing and deep-breathing exercises. Together, these techniques mobilize secretions, help to reexpand lung tissue, and promote efficient use of respiratory muscles. Of critical importance to the bedridden patient, chest PT helps prevent or treat atelectasis and may also help prevent pneumonia—two respiratory complications that can seriously impede recovery.

Postural drainage performed in conjunction with percussion and vibration encourages peripheral pulmonary secretions to empty by gravity into the major bronchi or trachea and is accomplished by sequential repositioning of the patient. Usually, secretions drain best with the patient positioned so that the bronchi are perpendicular to the floor. Lower and middle lobe bronchi usually empty best with the patient in the head-down position; upper lobe bronchi, in the head-up position. (See *Positioning patients for postural drainage*, pages 162 and 163.)

Percussing the chest with cupped hands mechanically dislodges thick, tenacious secretions from the bronchial walls. Vibration can be used with percussion to enhance secretion mobility or as an alternative to it in a patient who is frail, in pain, or recovering from thoracic surgery or trauma.

Candidates for chest PT include patients who produce large amounts of sputum, such as those with bronchiectasis and cystic fibrosis.[1,2] The procedure hasn't proved effective in treating patients with status asthmaticus, lobar pneumonia, or acute exacerbations of chronic bronchitis when the patient has scant secretions and is being mechanically ventilated. Chest PT has little value for treating patients with stable, chronic bronchitis.

Contraindications may include active pulmonary bleeding with hemoptysis and the immediate posthemorrhage stage, fractured ribs or an unstable chest wall, lung contusions, pulmonary tuberculosis, untreated pneumothorax, acute asthma or bronchospasm, lung abscess or tumor, bony metastasis, head injury, and recent myocardial infarction.[1]

Equipment

Stethoscope ■ pillows or folded towels for positioning ■ tilt or postural drainage table (if available) or adjustable hospital bed ■ gloves ■ emesis basin ■ facial tissues ■ suction equipment ■ equipment for oral care ■ trash bag ■ Optional: sterile specimen container, mechanical ventilator, supplemental oxygen.

Preparation of equipment

Gather the equipment at the patient's bedside. Set up suction equipment and test its function.

Positioning patients for postural drainage

The following illustrations show the various postural drainage positions and the areas of the lungs affected by each.

Lower lobes: Posterior basal segments
Elevate the foot of the bed 30 degrees. Have the patient lie prone with his head lowered. Position pillows under his chest and abdomen. Percuss his lower ribs on both sides of his spine.

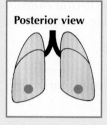

Posterior view

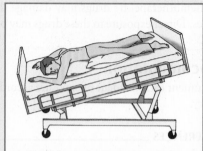

Lower lobes: Lateral basal segments
Elevate the foot of the bed 30 degrees. Instruct the patient to lie on his abdomen with his head lowered and his upper leg flexed over a pillow for support. Then have him rotate a quarter turn upward. Percuss his lower ribs on the uppermost portion of his lateral chest wall.

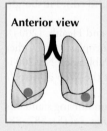

Anterior view

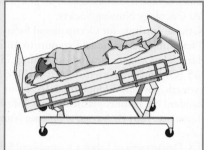

Lower lobes: Anterior basal segments
Elevate the foot of the bed 30 degrees. Instruct the patient to lie on his side with his head lowered. Then place pillows as shown. Percuss with a slightly cupped hand over his lower ribs just beneath the axilla. If an acutely ill patient has trouble breathing in this position, adjust the bed to an angle he can tolerate. Then begin percussion.

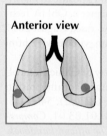

Anterior view

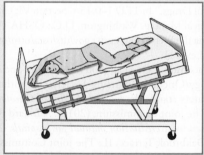

Lower lobes: Superior segments
With the bed flat, have the patient lie on his abdomen. Place two pillows under his hips. Percuss on both sides of his spine at the lower tip of his scapulae.

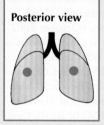

Posterior view

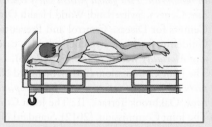

Right middle lobe: Medial and lateral segments
Elevate the foot of the bed 15 degrees. Have the patient lie on his left side with his head down and his knees flexed. Then have him rotate a quarter turn backward. Place a pillow beneath him. Percuss with your hand moderately cupped under the right nipple. For a woman, cup your hand so that its heel is under the armpit and your fingers extend forward beneath the breast.

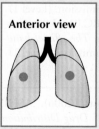

Anterior view

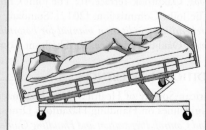

Positioning patients for postural drainage (continued)

Left upper lobe: Superior and inferior segments, lingular portion

Elevate the foot of the bed 15 degrees. Have the patient lie on his right side with his head down and knees flexed. Then have him rotate a quarter turn backward. Place a pillow behind him, from shoulders to hips. Percuss with your hand moderately cupped over his left nipple. For a woman, cup your hand so that its heel is beneath the armpit and your fingers extend forward beneath the breast.

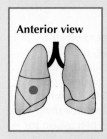

Anterior view

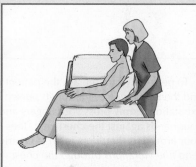

Upper lobes: Anterior segments

Make sure the bed is flat. Have the patient lie on his back with a pillow folded under his knees. Then have him rotate slightly away from the side being drained. Percuss between his clavicle and nipple.

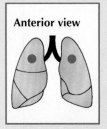

Anterior view

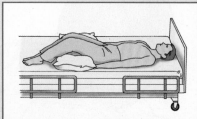

Upper lobes: Apical segments

Keep the bed flat. Have the patient lean back at a 30-degree angle against you and a pillow. Percuss with a cupped hand between his clavicles and the top of each scapula.

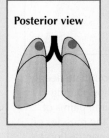

Posterior view

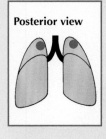

Upper lobes: Posterior segments

Keep the bed flat. Have the patient lean over a pillow at a 30-degree angle. Percuss and clap his upper back on each side.

Posterior view

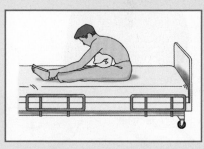

Implementation

■ Confirm the patient's identity using at least two patient identifiers according to your facility's policy.[3]
■ Verify the doctor's order.
■ Explain the procedure to the patient.
■ Provide privacy.
■ Perform hand hygiene, put on gloves, and follow standard precautions.[4,5,6]
■ Auscultate the patient's lungs *to determine baseline respiratory status*.[1]
■ Position the patient as ordered. In generalized disease, drainage usually begins with the lower lobes, continues with the middle lobes, and ends with the upper lobes. In localized disease, drainage begins with the affected lobes and then proceeds to the other lobes *to avoid spreading the disease to uninvolved areas*.
■ Instruct the patient to remain in each position for 3 to 15 minutes. During this time, perform percussion and vibration as ordered. (See *Performing percussion and vibration*, page 164.)
■ After postural drainage, percussion, or vibration, instruct the patient to cough *to remove loosened secretions*. First, tell him to inhale deeply through his nose and then exhale in three short huffs. Then have him inhale deeply again and cough through a slightly open mouth. Three consecutive coughs are highly effective.

Performing percussion and vibration

To perform percussion, instruct the patient to breathe slowly and deeply, using the diaphragm, *to promote relaxation*. Hold your hands in a cupped shape, with fingers flexed and thumbs pressed tightly against your index fingers. Percuss each segment for 1 to 2 minutes by alternating your hands against the patient in a rhythmic manner. Listen for a hollow sound on percussion *to verify correct performance of the technique*.

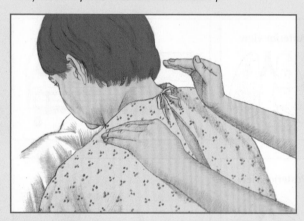

To perform vibration, ask the patient to inhale deeply and then exhale slowly through pursed lips. During exhalation, firmly press your fingers and the palms of your hands against the chest wall. Tense the muscles of your arms and shoulders in an isometric contraction *to send fine vibrations through the chest wall*. Vibrate during five exhalations over each chest segment.

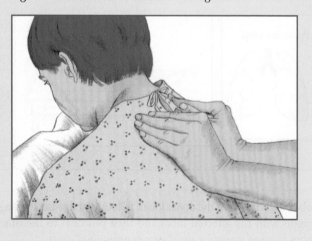

An effective cough sounds deep, low, and hollow; an ineffective one, high-pitched.

■ Have the patient perform coughing exercises for about 1 minute and then rest for 2 minutes. Gradually progress to a 10-minute exercise period four times daily. Try to schedule the last session just before bedtime *to help maximize the patient's oxygenation while he's sleeping*.

■ If the patient's cough is ineffective, suction the patient.
■ Monitor the patient's response to the treatment.[1] Be alert for significant color changes, particularly if the patient becomes dusky, which may indicate poor oxygenation.
■ Dispose of secretions appropriately.
■ Provide oral hygiene *because secretions may have a foul taste or a stale odor.*
■ Auscultate the patient's lungs *to evaluate the effectiveness of therapy.*[1]
■ Remove and discard gloves. Perform hand hygiene.[4,5,6]
■ Document the procedure.[7]

Special considerations

■ *For optimal effectiveness and safety,* modify chest PT according to the patient's condition. For example, initiate or increase the flow of supplemental oxygen, if indicated. If the patient tires quickly during therapy, shorten the sessions *because fatigue leads to shallow respirations and increased hypoxia.*
■ Maintain adequate hydration in the patient receiving chest PT *to prevent mucus dehydration and promote easier mobilization of secretions.* Avoid performing postural drainage immediately before or within 1½ hours after meals *to avoid nausea, vomiting, and aspiration of food or vomitus.*
■ *Because chest percussion can induce bronchospasm,* any adjunct treatment (for example, intermittent positive-pressure breathing or aerosol or nebulizer therapy) should precede chest PT.
■ Refrain from percussing over the spine, liver, kidneys, or spleen *to avoid injury to the spine or internal organs.* Also avoid performing percussion on bare skin or the female patient's breasts. Percuss over soft clothing (but not over buttons, snaps, or zippers), or place a thin towel over the chest wall. Remember to remove jewelry that might scratch or bruise the patient.
■ Teach coughing and deep-breathing exercises preoperatively *so that the patient can practice them when he's pain-free and better able to concentrate.*
■ Postoperatively, splint the patient's incision using your hands or, if possible, teach the patient to splint it himself *to minimize pain during coughing.*

Complications

During postural drainage in head-down positions, pressure on the diaphragm by abdominal contents can impair respiratory excursion and lead to hypoxia or orthostatic hypotension. The head-down position also may lead to increased intracranial pressure, which precludes the use of chest PT in a patient with acute neurologic impairment. Vigorous percussion or vibration can cause rib fracture, especially in a patient with osteoporosis. In an emphysematous patient with blebs, coughing could lead to pneumothorax.

Documentation

Record the date and time of chest PT. Note the positions used for secretion drainage and the length of time each was maintained. Note which chest segments were percussed or vibrated. Record the color, amount, odor, and viscosity of any secretions produced and the presence of any blood. Record any complications and nursing actions taken. Document the patient's tolerance of treatment.

REFERENCES

1 American Association for Respiratory Care. (1991). AARC clinical practice guideline: Postural drainage therapy. *Respiratory Care, 36*(12), 1418–1426. (Level I)

2 McCool, F.D., et al. (2006). Nonpharmacologic airway clearance therapies: ACCP evidence-based clinical practice guidelines. *Chest, 129*(1 Suppl.), 250S–259S.

3 The Joint Commission. (2012). Standard NPSG.01.01.01. *Comprehensive accreditation manual for hospitals: The official handbook.* Oakbrook Terrace, IL: The Joint Commission. (Level I)

4 The Joint Commission. (2012). Standard NPSG.07.01.01. *Comprehensive accreditation manual for hospitals: The official handbook.* Oakbrook Terrace, IL: The Joint Commission. (Level I)

5 Centers for Disease Control and Prevention. (October 2002). Guideline for hand hygiene in health-care settings. *Morbidity and Mortality Weekly Report, 51*(RR-16), 1–45. (Level 1)

6 World Health Organization. (2009). *WHO guidelines on hand hygiene in health care: First global patient safety challenge. Clean care is safer care.* Geneva, Switzerland: World Health Organization. (Level 1)

7 The Joint Commission. (2012). Standard RC.01.03.01. *Comprehensive accreditation manual for hospitals: The official handbook.* Oakbrook Terrace, IL: The Joint Commission. (Level I)

ADDITIONAL REFERENCES

Freynet, A., & Falcoz, P.E. (2008). Does non-invasive ventilation associated with chest physiotherapy improve outcome after lung resection? *Interactive Cardiovascular and Thoracic Surgery, 7*(6), 1152–1154.

Nettina, S.M. (2010). *Lippincott manual of nursing practice* (9th ed.). Philadelphia, PA: Lippincott Williams & Wilkins.

Ries, A.L. (2008). Pulmonary rehabilitation: Summary of an evidence-based guideline. *Respiratory Care, 53*(9), 1203–1207.

Taylor, C., et al. (2011). *Fundamentals of nursing: The art and science of nursing care* (7th ed.). Philadelphia, PA: Lippincott Williams & Wilkins.

Yang, M., et al. (2010). Chest physiotherapy for pneumonia in adults. *Cochrane Database of Systematic Reviews, 2*, CD006338.

CHEST TUBE DRAINAGE SYSTEM MONITORING AND CARE

Maintaining and troubleshooting a patient's chest tube keeps the chest tube functioning properly and prevents infection. As part of this process, the nurse is responsible for making respiratory and thoracic assessments, obtaining vital signs that reflect effectiveness of therapy or impending complications, and knowing the appropriate interventions to perform in response to changes in the patient's therapy.

Equipment

Sterile gloves ■ personal protective equipment (gown, gloves, goggles, face shield) ■ single-use, disposable, sterile chest tube drainage collection unit ■ sterile water ■ suction source ■ suction connec-

tion tubing ■ two sterile 4″ × 4″ drain dressings ■ sterile 4″ × 4″ or 2″ × 2″ gauze pads ■ 3″ to 4″ (7.5 to 10 cm) sturdy elastic tape ■ 1″ adhesive tape for connections ■ two rubber-tipped clamps for each chest tube inserted ■ Optional: sterile petroleum gauze, sterile nonadherent gauze, sterile transparent dressing.

Implementation

■ Review the doctor's orders regarding chest tube care.

■ Confirm the patient's identity using at least two patient identifiers according to your facility's policy.[1]

■ Explain the procedure to the patient.

■ Perform hand hygiene before providing patient care.[2,3,4]

■ Maintain sterile technique whenever you make changes in the system or alter any of the connections *to avoid introducing pathogens into the pleural space.*[5]

For all drainage systems

■ Repeatedly note the character, consistency, and amount of drainage in the drainage collection chamber.

■ Mark the drainage level by writing the time and date at the drainage level on the drainage collection chamber every shift (or more often if there's a large amount of drainage).

■ Observe the integrity of the drainage tubing and chest tube every 2 to 4 hours as well as with a change in the patient's condition *to ensure that the system is intact, with no air leaks, and to help prevent kinks or clots from forming.*[6]

■ Periodically check that the air vent in the system is working properly (if applicable). *Occlusion of the air vent results in a buildup of pressure in the system that could cause the patient to develop a tension pneumothorax.*

■ Coil the system's tubing and secure it to the edge of the bed. Be sure the tubing remains at the level of the patient. Avoid creating dependent loops, kinks, or pressure on the tubing. Avoid lifting the drainage system above the patient's chest *because fluid may flow back into the pleural space.*[5]

■ Keep two rubber-tipped clamps at the bedside *to clamp the chest tube if the commercially prepared system cracks or to help locate an air leak in the system.*

NURSING ALERT *Never clamp the tube to get the patient out of bed or during transportation of the patient.* Whenever the chest tube is clamped, air or fluid can't escape from the pleural space, which puts the patient at risk for a tension pneumothorax.

■ Encourage the patient to cough frequently and breathe deeply *to help drain the pleural space and expand the lungs.*[5]

■ Instruct the patient to sit upright for optimal lung expansion and to splint the insertion site while coughing *to minimize pain.*

■ Check the rate and quality of the patient's respirations and auscultate his lungs periodically *to assess air exchange in the affected lung.*[5] Diminished or absent breath sounds may indicate that the lung hasn't reexpanded.

■ Tell the patient to report any breathing difficulty immediately. Notify the doctor immediately if the patient develops cyanosis, decreased oxygen saturation, rapid or shallow breathing, subcutaneous emphysema, chest pain, or excessive bleeding.

■ When clots are visible, after carefully assessing the patient, you may be able to milk the tubing, depending on your facility's policy. Gently milk the tubing in the direction of the drainage chamber as needed.[5]

■ Check the chest tube dressing at least every shift. Palpate the area surrounding the dressing for crepitus or subcutaneous emphysema, *which indicates that air is leaking into the subcutaneous tissue surrounding the insertion site.* Change the dressing when soiled or according to the doctor's order or your facility's policy.[5]

■ Encourage active or passive range-of-motion (ROM) exercises for the patient's arm or the affected side if he has been splinting the arm. Usually, the thoracotomy patient will splint his arm *to decrease his discomfort.*[5]

■ Assess the patient for pain and administer ordered pain medication, using safe medication administration practices, as needed for comfort and *to help with deep breathing, coughing, and ROM exercises.*[6]

■ Remind the ambulatory patient to keep the drainage system below chest level and to be careful not to disconnect the tubing, *which would disrupt the water seal.*

■ Troubleshoot the system as needed when problems arise. (See *Troubleshooting chest tubes.*) *Early and prompt attention to system difficulties will minimize the patient's complications.*

■ Document the procedure.[7]

Additional steps for a water-seal–wet suction system

■ Check the water-seal level every shift and maintain the proper level *to ensure that the system is being used properly and to maintain the patient's safety.*

■ Check for fluctuations in the water-seal chamber as the patient breathes. Normal fluctuations of 2″ to 4″ (about 5 to 10 cm) reflect pressure changes in the pleural space during respiration. To check for fluctuation when a suction system is being used, momentarily disconnect the suction system so the air vent is opened, and observe for fluctuation.

■ Check for intermittent bubbling in the water-seal chamber. *This bubbling occurs normally when the system is removing air from the pleural cavity.* If bubbling isn't readily apparent during quiet breathing, have the patient take a deep breath or cough. *Absence of bubbling indicates that the pleural space has sealed.*[5]

■ Check the water level in the suction-control chamber. Detach the chamber or bottle from the suction source; when bubbling ceases, observe the water level. If necessary, add sterile water to bring the level to the 20-cm line or to the ordered level.

■ Check for gentle bubbling in the suction-control chamber, *which indicates that the proper suction level has been reached. Vigorous bubbling in this chamber increases the rate of water evaporation.*

Additional steps for a water-seal–dry suction system

■ Check the water-seal level every shift and maintain the proper level *to ensure that the system is being used properly and to maintain the patient's safety.*

■ Check for fluctuation in the water-seal chamber as the patient breathes. Normal fluctuations of 2″ to 4″ (about 5 to 10 cm) reflect pressure changes in the pleural space during respiration. To check for fluctuation when a suction system is being used, momentarily disconnect the suction system so the air vent is opened, and observe for fluctuation.

■ Check for intermittent bubbling in the water-seal chamber. *This bubbling occurs normally when the system is removing air from the pleural cavity.* If bubbling isn't readily apparent during quiet breathing, have the patient take a deep breath or cough. *Absence of bubbling indicates that the pleural space has sealed.*

■ Check that the rotary dry suction control dial is turned to the ordered suction mark, usually −20 cm suction, and verify that the appropriate indicator is present, indicating the desired amount of suction is applied. In some models, an orange float appears in an indicator window. Other models indicate that the correct amount of suction is being delivered when the bellows reach the calibrated triangular mark in the suction monitor bellows window. Always refer to the manufacturer's instructions.

Additional steps for a dry seal–dry suction system

■ Check the air leak monitor for right-to-left bubbling and fluctuation every shift (or more often as symptoms warrant). *Fluctuation of water in the air-leak chamber is a normal reflection of pressure changes in the pleural cavity during respirations. Bubbling indicates that air is leaving the system and is normal for the patient with a pneumothorax, but it could indicate an air leak.*

■ Check that the rotary dry suction control dial is turned to the ordered suction mark, usually −20 cm suction, and verify that the appropriate indicator is present, indicating the desired amount of suction is applied. In some models, an orange float appears in an indicator window. Other models indicate that the correct amount of suction is being delivered when the bellows reach the calibrated triangular mark in the suction monitor bellows window. Always refer to the manufacturer's instructions.

Changing the dressings

■ Change the dressings around the chest tube according to the doctor's orders, if permitted by facility policy.

■ Perform hand hygiene and put on nonsterile gloves.[2,3,4]

■ Confirm the patient's identity using at least two patient identifiers according to facility policy.[1]

■ Explain the procedure to the patient.

■ Remove the dressings around the chest tube insertion site and dispose of them in the appropriate receptacle.[8] Examine the site for signs of infection or subcutaneous emphysema.

■ Remove your gloves and perform hand hygiene.[2,3,4]

■ Open the packages containing the petroleum gauze, 4″ × 4″ drain dressings, and gauze pads.

■ Put on sterile gloves.

■ Place the petroleum gauze and two 4″ × 4″ drain dressings around the insertion site, one from the top and the other from the bottom, *to seal the insertion site from any air entry or escape.*[5]

■ Place several 4″ × 4″ gauze pads on top of the drain dressings.[5]

TROUBLESHOOTING

Troubleshooting chest tubes

Use this table to determine possible causes of and interventions for common chest tube problems.

PROBLEM	POSSIBLE CAUSES	INTERVENTION
Water level in the water-seal chamber not rising and falling with breathing	Clot in chest tubing or patient's chest	Gently pinch the tubing around the clot and gingerly milk fluid to move it into the collection chamber; repeat as needed. Unless absolutely necessary, don't strip the tubing *because doing so creates high negative pressure and can damage lung tissue.*
	Dependent loop or kink in patient's tube with fluid occlusion	Straighten the catheter and tubing along its length to its connection with the collection device.
	Dislodgment of catheter from patient	If tube accidentally pulls out, immediately cover the site with gauze pads and tape them in place. Stay with the patient, and monitor his vital signs every 10 minutes. Observe him for signs and symptoms of tension pneumothorax (hypotension, distended jugular veins, absent or decreased breath sounds, tracheal shift, hypoxemia, weak and rapid pulse, dyspnea, tachypnea, diaphoresis, and chest pain). Notify the doctor immediately. If another staff member is present, have that person gather the equipment needed to reinsert the tube.
	Disconnection of patient's tube from chest tube connector	Keep rubber-tipped clamps at the bedside. If the drainage system cracks or a tube disconnects, clamp the chest tube momentarily as close to the insertion site as possible. Alternately, you can clamp the chest tube with a gauze-wrapped Kelly clamp to prevent puncturing or tearing the tube. *Because no air or liquid can escape from the pleural space while the tube is clamped,* observe the patient closely for signs and symptoms of tension pneumothorax while the clamp is in place. As an alternative to clamping the tube, you can submerge the distal end of the tube in a container of normal saline solution to create a temporary water seal while you replace the drainage system. Notify the doctor immediately.
	Patient's tube clamp closed	Clamp only when indicated; otherwise, leave tube open.
	Chest drain not positioned sufficiently below patient's chest	Lower chest tube to allow for gravity drainage.
	In-line connectors not properly secured, allowing for an air leak	Ensure that in-line connectors are properly secured and sealed at all times; check for loose connections periodically.
Constant bubbling in the water-seal chamber	Air leak	To determine the source of an air leak (patient or catheter connection), momentarily clamp the chest tube close to the chest drain and observe the water seal. If the bubbling stops, the air leak may be from the catheter connections or the patient's chest. Check the catheter connections and patient's dressing for a partially withdrawn catheter. If catheter is dislodged, follow the procedure for a dislodged catheter, described above. Bubbling that continues after temporarily clamping the patient's tube indicates a system leak requiring system replacement.

(continued)

TROUBLESHOOTING

Troubleshooting chest tubes *(continued)*

PROBLEM	POSSIBLE CAUSES	INTERVENTION
Overfilled water-seal level (water above 2-cm limit line) or over-filled suction-control chamber	Too much water in the chamber	Press and hold the negative-pressure relief valve at the top of the chest drainage system to vent excess negative pressure in the water-seal chamber. Release the valve when the level of the water returns to the 2-cm mark. To remove water from the suction-control chamber, insert a syringe and withdraw excess water.
Not enough water in the water-seal or suction-control chamber	Evaporation, underfilling, or spillage	Add more water to the suction-control chamber by temporarily turning off the suction source, removing the rubber stopper, and adding water to the desired level. More water may be added to the water-seal chamber with a syringe by quickly and temporarily clamping the patient's tube and injecting water to the desired level.
Suction-control chamber isn't bubbling or is bubbling too vigorously	Possible disconnection of suction source or too much suction-source pressure in the system	Ensure that the suction tubing is connected and the suction source is turned on. A constant, gentle bubbling is normal. Vigorous bubbling causes quicker evaporation. Adjust the suction-control source for gentle bubbling.
Chest drainage system accidentally knocked over	Human error	Set the system upright and check the fluid levels in the water-seal and suction-control chambers for proper volumes. Adjust accordingly. Most units have a baffle system that prevents fluids from mixing between chambers, allowing for proper function after setting upright again.
Patient being transported or leaving the unit	As the situation indicates	Don't clamp the catheter tubing; disconnect the suction tubing from the suction source. The system continues to collect fluid (by gravity) or air (by water seal).
Specimen collection required	Doctor's orders for laboratory analysis	Remove fluid with needle and syringe from the self-sealing portion of the drainage tubing after following facility policy for cleaning the tubing fluid collection site.

■ Tape the dressings, covering them completely, forming an occlusive dressing.
■ Mark the dressing with the date, time, and your initials.
■ Remove your gloves and perform hand hygiene.[2,3,4]
■ Document the procedure.[7]

Replacing the chest tube drainage system collection device
■ Replace the chest tube drainage system collection device as ordered or as needed. Notify the doctor if the device must be changed because of a leak.
■ Gather the necessary supplies.
■ Perform hand hygiene.[2,3,4]
■ Confirm the patient's identity using at least two patient identifiers according to facility policy.[1]
■ Explain the procedure to the patient.
■ Open a new single-use sterile chest drainage unit.

■ If using a chest drainage system that has a water seal, use sterile water to fill the water-seal chamber to the specified level according to the manufacturer's instructions.
■ If using a dry-seal chest drainage system, use sterile water to fill the air leak monitor to the specified level according to the manufacturer's instructions.
■ If using a wet-suction chest drainage system, fill the suction-control chamber with sterile water to 20 cm of water or as ordered by the doctor. *The addition of suction (usually 20 cm of water) increases the negative intrapleural pressure and helps overcome air leakage by improving the rate of airflow out of the patient and improving fluid removal.* If using a dry-suction chest drainage system, turn the rotary dry suction control dial to the ordered suction mark, usually –20 cm.
■ Maintain a sterile patient connection tube, with cap in place *to allow for later connection of a chest tube catheter to the chest tube drainage system collection device after the existing device is removed.*

■ Place the chest tube drainage system collection device at the bedside in the upright position, at least 1′ (30 cm) below the patient's chest. Avoid accidentally knocking over the device by hanging it on the bed frame with the hangers provided or by securing the base of the device to the floor with tape. Ensure that the device is ready when the existing device is removed.

■ If suction is being used, turn off the suction to the current drainage system.

■ Undo the tape on the connections from the existing chest tube drainage system to the chest tube catheter *to allow access to the chest tube catheter for drainage device replacement.*

■ Cross-clamp the chest tube catheter with two padded clamps (so as not to rip or tear the catheter) about 1½″ to 2½″ (4 to 6.5 cm) from the insertion site *to minimize dead space and stop air from entering or exiting catheter.*

■ Put on sterile gloves and appropriate personal protective equipment.

■ Instruct the patient to exhale and hold his breath *to allow for maximum positive pressure in the pleural space.*

■ Using sterile technique, disconnect the old drainage system and connect the new one.

■ Remove the clamp or clamps and instruct the patient to breathe normally *to allow fluid and air removal to begin again.*

■ Secure the chest tube and drainage tube so that there's no tension pulling on the insertion site *to help prevent accidental tube dislodgment.*

■ Securely tape the junction of the chest tube and the drainage tube *to prevent their separation.*

■ Dispose of equipment and waste in the appropriate receptacle.[8]

■ Remove your gloves and perform hand hygiene.[2,3,4]

■ Ensure that all clamps are open and that the drainage tubing has a straight flow to the chest tube drainage collection device and has no dependent loops or kinks.

■ Ensure that the chest tube drainage system is correctly connected to the patient's chest tube; then, if appropriate, connect the suction tubing to the drainage system and the suction regulator.

■ If using a wet-suction chest drainage system, adjust the suction until gentle bubbling appears in the suction-control chamber. If using a dry-suction chest drainage system, adjust the suction regulator and verify that the appropriate indicator is present, indicating that the desired amount of suction is applied. Verify suction operation according to the manufacturer's instructions.

■ Check the status of the drainage tubing.

■ Reassess the patient after the procedure. Obtain vital signs and assess skin color, perfusion, level of consciousness, oxygen requirements, hemodynamic stability, comfort and pain levels, and respiratory rate, pattern, and effort *to identify the patient's response to and tolerance of the procedure.*

■ Document the procedure.[7]

Special considerations

■ Instruct staff members and visitors to avoid touching the equipment *to prevent complications from separated connections.*

■ If excessive continuous bubbling is present in the water-seal chamber—especially if suction is being used—rule out a leak in the drainage system.[9] Try to locate the leak by clamping the tube momentarily at various points along its length. Begin clamping at the tube's proximal end and work down toward the drainage system, paying special attention to the seal around the connections. If any connection is loose, push it back together and tape it securely. The bubbling will stop when a clamp is placed between the air leak and the water seal. If you clamp along the tube's entire length and the bubbling doesn't stop, the drainage unit may be cracked and need replacement.

NURSING ALERT *Never leave the tubes clamped for more than 1 minute to prevent a tension pneumothorax from forming, which may occur when clamping stops air and fluid from escaping.*

■ If the system cracks, clamp the chest tube momentarily with the two rubber-tipped clamps at the bedside (placed there at the time of tube insertion). Place the clamps close to each other near the insertion site; they should face in opposite directions to provide a more complete seal. Observe the patient for altered respirations while the tube is clamped. Then replace the damaged equipment. (Prepare the new unit before clamping the tube.) For the patient on a ventilator with positive end-expiratory pressure (PEEP), continuous bubbling typically occurs because PEEP maintains positive pressure in the alveoli; thus, air will continually flow through the lungs. However, lack of continuous bubbling for patients on PEEP isn't abnormal.

NURSING ALERT *Don't routinely strip a chest drain (occluding the chest tube with one hand while quickly squeezing and moving the other hand down the tube to move fluid down the tube into the drainage chamber) because intraluminal pressures can rise dangerously high, which may convert a simple pneumothorax to life-threatening pneumothorax and cause tissue trauma and unnecessary discomfort.* Only in special circumstances, such as hemorrhaging, should the chest tube be stripped to maintain patency.

■ Remember that routine clamping of the chest tube isn't recommended *because of the risk of tension pneumothorax.*

■ During patient transport, keep the chest tube drainage system below chest level. Don't clamp the chest tube during transport.

■ Don't tip the chest tube drainage system.

■ If you hear air leaking from the site, tape the dressing on only two or three sides *to allow air to escape and to prevent a tension pneumothorax.* Closely monitor the patient and prepare for insertion of a new chest tube.

If the chest tube comes out accidentally, immediately cover the site with gauze pads, and tape three of the pads' sides *to allow air to escape.* Stay with the patient, and monitor his vital signs every 10 minutes. Tension pneumothorax may result from excessive accumulation of air, drainage, or both and eventually may exert pressure on the heart and aorta, causing a fall in cardiac output. Observe the patient for signs and symptoms of tension pneumothorax, including hypotension, distended jugular veins, absent or decreased breath sounds, tracheal shift, hypoxemia, weak and rapid pulse, dyspnea, tachypnea, diaphoresis, and chest pain. If possible, have another staff member notify the doctor and gather equipment needed to reinsert the tube.

Complications

Tension pneumothorax may result from excessive accumulation of air, drainage, or both in the chest cavity and eventually may exert pressure on the heart and aorta, causing a precipitous fall in cardiac output.

Documentation

Routine care

Record the date and time thoracic drainage began, type of system used, amount of suction applied to the pleural cavity, presence or absence of bubbling or fluctuation in the water-seal or air-leak monitor chamber (if applicable), initial amount and type of drainage, and the patient's respiratory status.

At the end of each shift, record the frequency of system inspection; amount, color, and consistency of drainage; presence or absence of bubbling or fluctuation in the water-seal or air-leak monitor chamber (if applicable); the patient's respiratory status; condition of the chest dressings; pain medication, if given; any complications and nursing actions taken; and any patient teaching provided.

Dressing change

Record the date, time, and reasons for changing the dressings. Document your assessment findings before and after the procedure and the patient's response to the procedure. Record the condition of the insertion site, the patient's respiratory status, and vital signs as well as any teaching provided.

Drainage system collection device change

Record the date, time, and reasons for changing the chest tube drainage system. Document your assessment findings before and after the procedure and the patient's response to the procedure. Note the type of drainage system used, the amount of suction applied to the pleural cavity (if applicable), the presence or absence of bubbling or fluctuation in the water-seal or air-leak monitor chamber (if applicable), the patient's respiratory status, and the amount, color, and consistency of drainage. Record the patient's respiratory status, vital signs, amount of drainage and its color and consistency, and any teaching provided.

REFERENCES

1 The Joint Commission. (2012). Standard NPSG.01.01.01. *Comprehensive accreditation manual for hospitals: The official handbook.* Oakbrook Terrace, IL: The Joint Commission. (Level I)

2 The Joint Commission. (2012). Standard NPSG.07.01.01. *Comprehensive accreditation manual for hospitals: The official handbook.* Oakbrook Terrace, IL: The Joint Commission. (Level I)

3 Centers for Disease Control and Prevention. (October 2002). Guideline for hand hygiene in health-care settings. *Morbidity and Mortality Weekly Report, 51*(RR-16), 1–45. (Level 1)

4 World Health Organization. (2009). *WHO guidelines on hand hygiene in health care: First global patient safety challenge. Clean care is safer care.* Geneva, Switzerland: World Health Organization. (Level 1)

5 Lynn-McHale Wiegand, D. (Ed.). (2011). *AACN procedure manual for critical care* (6th ed.). Philadelphia, PA: Saunders.

6 The Joint Commission. (2012). Standard PC.01.02.07. *Comprehensive accreditation manual for hospitals: The official handbook.* Oakbrook Terrace, IL: The Joint Commission. (Level I)

7 The Joint Commission. (2012). Standard RC.01.03.01. *Comprehensive accreditation manual for hospitals: The official handbook.* Oakbrook Terrace, IL: The Joint Commission. (Level I)

8 Occupational Safety and Health Administration. "Bloodborne Pathogens, Standard Number 1910.1030" [Online]. Accessed August 2011 via the Web at http://www.osha.gov/pls/oshaweb/owadisp. show_document?p_table=STANDARDS&p_id=10051 (Level I)

ADDITIONAL REFERENCE

Nettina, S.M. (2010). *Lippincott manual of nursing practice* (9th ed.). Philadelphia, PA: Lippincott Williams & Wilkins.

CHEST TUBE DRAINAGE SYSTEM SETUP

Chest tube drainage uses gravity and, possibly, suction to restore negative pressure and remove material that collects in the pleural cavity. The disposable drainage system combines drainage collection, a wet or dry seal, and suction control. The seal in the drainage system allows air and fluid to escape from the pleural cavity but doesn't allow air to reenter. Patient safety features on the device include a pressure relief valve and an air-leak indicator. There are three types of chest tube drainage systems: a water-seal–wet suction system, a water-seal–dry suction system, and a dry seal–dry suction system.

Chest tube drainage may be ordered to remove accumulated air, fluids (blood, pus, chyle, and serous fluids), or solids (blood clots) from the pleural cavity; to restore negative pressure in the pleural cavity; or to reexpand a partially or totally collapsed lung.

Equipment

Single-use, disposable, sterile chest drainage collection unit (water-seal–wet suction system, water-seal–dry suction system, or dry seal–dry suction system) ■ sterile water ■ gloves ■ suction source ■ wall-mounted or portable suction-control device ■ suction connection tubing ■ chest tube clamp (one per chest tube placed).

Implementation

■ Check the doctor's order to determine the type of drainage system to be used and other procedural details.

■ Gather the necessary supplies.

■ Confirm the patient's identity using at least two patient identifiers according to your facility's policy.[1]

■ Explain the procedure to the patient.

■ Perform hand hygiene and put on gloves *to reduce the transmission of microorganisms.*[2,3,4]

■ Maintain sterile technique throughout the procedure and whenever you make changes in the system or alter the connections *to avoid introducing pathogens into the pleural space.*

■ Open the single-use sterile chest drainage unit. Use the floor stand to set the unit on the floor or use the hangers to hang it level on the bed.

Water-seal–wet suction system

■ Use sterile water to fill the water-seal chamber to the specified level according to the manufacturer's instructions. The water-seal chamber acts as a one-way valve to allow air to pass out of the lung, down through a narrow channel, and bubble out through the bottom of the water seal.

■ Fill the suction-control chamber with sterile water or normal saline solution to the prescribed level (usually –10 to –20 cm of water).

■ Connect the patient's chest tube to the chest tube drainage system.

■ Connect the suction tubing to the drainage system and the suction regulator (as shown below). Adjust the suction until gentle bubbling appears in the suction-control chamber. *The addition of suction increases the negative intrapleural pressure and helps overcome air leakage by improving the rate of airflow out of the patient and improving fluid removal.*

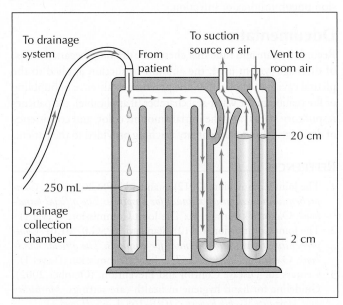

Water-seal–dry suction system

■ Use sterile water to fill the water-seal chamber to the specified level according to the manufacturer's instructions. The water-seal chamber acts as a one-way valve to allow air to pass out of the lung, down through a narrow channel, and bubble out through the bottom of the water seal.

■ If suction is ordered, turn the rotary dry suction control dial to the ordered suction mark, usually –20 cm.

■ Connect the patient's chest tube to the chest tube drainage system.

■ Connect the suction tubing to the drainage system and adjust the suction regulator. Verify suction operation according to the manufacturer's instructions. An indicator appears when the desired negative pressure is achieved. In some models, an orange float appears in an indicator window. Other models indicate that the correct amount of suction is being delivered when the bellows reach the calibrated triangular mark in the suction monitor bellows window (as shown below). *The addition of suction increases the negative intrapleural pressure and helps overcome air leakage by improving the rate of airflow out of the patient and improving fluid removal.*

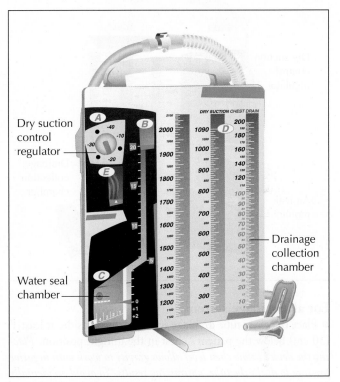

Dry seal–dry suction system

■ Use sterile water to fill the air leak monitor to the specified level according to the manufacturer's instructions.

■ If suction is ordered, turn the rotary dry suction control dial to the ordered suction mark, usually –20 cm.

■ Connect the patient's chest tube to the chest tube drainage system.

■ Connect the suction tubing to the drainage system and adjust the suction regulator. Verify suction operation according to the manufacturer's instructions. An indicator appears when the desired negative pressure is achieved. In some models, an orange float appears in an indicator window. Other models indicate that the correct amount of suction is being delivered when the bellows reach the calibrated triangular mark in the suction monitor bellows window (as shown below). *The addition of suction increases the negative intrapleural pressure and helps overcome air leakage by improving the rate of airflow out of the patient and improving fluid removal.*

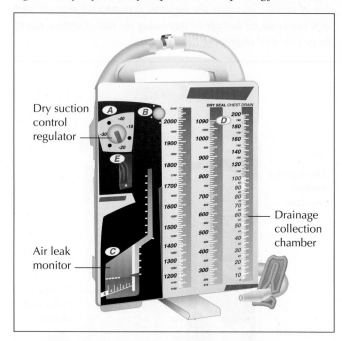

For all drainage systems
■ Place the chest tube drainage system at the bedside, at least 1' (30 cm) below the patient's chest in the upright position. *Placing the device below chest level allows gravity to work with negative pressure to drain the tube, optimizing results. To avoid accidentally knocking over the device,* hang it on the bed frame with the hangers provided or by securing the base of the collection device to the floor with tape.
■ Remove and discard your gloves. Perform hand hygiene.[2,3,4]
■ Document the procedure.[5]

Special considerations
■ Don't overfill the water-seal chamber. *A fluid level greater than 2 cm makes breathing more difficult.* If you accidentally overfill the chamber, aspirate the excess water with a needle and syringe. Many models have a grommet to access the water-seal chamber.
■ Some systems have a stopcock that can be gradually closed *to limit the suction flow into the drainage* system.
■ Don't block the pressure relief valve, typically located on the top of the unit, at any time.
■ Instruct staff members and visitors to avoid touching the equipment *to prevent complications from separated connections.*
■ If excessive continuous bubbling is present in the water-seal chamber, especially if suction is being used, rule out a leak in the

drainage system. Try to locate the leak by cross-clamping the tube momentarily at various points along its length. (The bubbling will stop when a clamp is placed between the air leak and the water seal.) Begin clamping at the tube's proximal end and work down toward the drainage system, paying special attention to the seal around the connections. If a connection is loose, push it back together and tape it securely. If you clamp along the tube's entire length and the bubbling doesn't stop, the drainage system may be cracked and need replacement.
■ If the chest tube comes out accidentally, immediately cover the site with gauze pads, and tape three of the pads' sides *to allow air to escape.* Stay with the patient, and monitor his vital signs every 10 minutes. Tension pneumothorax may result from excessive accumulation of air, drainage, or both and eventually may exert pressure on the heart and aorta, causing a fall in cardiac output. Observe the patient for signs and symptoms of tension pneumothorax, including hypotension, distended jugular veins, absent or decreased breath sounds, tracheal shift, hypoxemia, weak and rapid pulse, dyspnea, tachypnea, diaphoresis, and chest pain. If possible, have another staff member notify the doctor and gather equipment needed to reinsert the tube.

Complications
Incorrect setup of a chest tube drainage system may result in tension pneumothorax or infection.

Documentation
Record the date and time that chest tube drainage began, the type of drainage system used, the amount of suction applied to the pleural cavity (if applicable), the presence or absence of bubbling or fluctuation in the water-seal chamber (if applicable), the patient's respiratory status, and the initial amount, color, and consistency of drainage. Also document any teaching provided to the patient.

REFERENCES

1 The Joint Commission. (2012). Standard NPSG.01.01.01. *Comprehensive accreditation manual for hospitals: The official handbook.* Oakbrook Terrace, IL: The Joint Commission. (Level 1)
2 The Joint Commission. (2012). Standard NPSG.07.01.01. *Comprehensive accreditation manual for hospitals: The official handbook.* Oakbrook Terrace, IL: The Joint Commission. (Level 1)
3 Centers for Disease Control and Prevention. (October 2002). Guideline for hand hygiene in health-care settings. *Morbidity and Mortality Weekly Report, 51*(RR-16), 1–45. (Level 1)
4 World Health Organization. (2009). *WHO guidelines on hand hygiene in health care: First global patient safety challenge. Clean care is safer care.* Geneva, Switzerland: World Health Organization. (Level 1)
5 The Joint Commission. (2012). Standard RC.01.03.01. *Comprehensive accreditation manual for hospitals: The official handbook.* Oakbrook Terrace, IL: The Joint Commission. (Level 1)

ADDITIONAL REFERENCES

Lynn-McHale Wiegand, D. (Ed.). (2011). *AACN procedure manual for critical care* (6th ed.). Philadelphia, PA: Saunders.
Nettina, S.M. (2010). *Lippincott manual of nursing practice* (9th ed.). Philadelphia, PA: Lippincott Williams & Wilkins.

CHEST TUBE INSERTION

The pleural space normally contains a thin layer of lubricating fluid that allows the visceral and parietal pleura to move without friction during respiration. An excess of fluid (hemothorax or pleural effusion), air (pneumothorax), or both in this space alters intrapleural pressure and causes partial or complete lung collapse.

Chest tube insertion allows drainage of air or fluid from the pleural space. Usually performed by a doctor with a nurse assisting, this procedure requires sterile technique. The insertion site varies, depending on the patient's condition. For pneumothorax, the second to third intercostal space is the usual site because air rises to the top of the intrapleural space. For hemothorax or pleural effusion, the fourth to sixth intercostal spaces are common sites because fluid settles to the lower levels of the intrapleural space. For removal of air and fluid, a chest tube is inserted into a high and a low site.

After insertion, one or more chest tubes are connected to a thoracic drainage system that removes air, fluid, or both from the pleural space and prevents backflow into that space, thus promoting lung reexpansion. (See "Chest tube drainage system monitoring and care," page 165.)

Equipment

Lidocaine local anesthetic (0.5% or 1%) ■ sterile gowns, gloves, and masks ■ eye goggles or face mask with eye shield ■ alcohol wipes ■ rolled towels or a blanket ■ sterile drapes ■ chlorhexidine-based antiseptic swabs ■ sterile syringes (assortment of sizes: 3 mL, 5 mL, and TB) ■ 22G and 25G needles ■ sterile chest tube tray, which includes hemostats, forceps, trocar, scalpel, Kelly clamps, scissors, skin expanders, and sponges ■ sterile chest tube catheter (#16 to #20 French catheter for air or serous fluid; #28 to #40 French catheter for blood, pus, or thick fluid) ■ suture material (usually 2-0 to 3-0 silk with cutting needle) ■ sterile petrolatum gauze ■ two sterile 4″ × 4″ drain dressings (gauze pads with slits) ■ sterile 4″ × 4″ or 2″ × 2″ gauze pads ■ 3″ to 4″ (7.6 to 10 cm) sturdy elastic tape ■ 1″ (2.5 cm) adhesive tape for connections ■ two rubber-tipped clamps for each chest tube inserted ■ sterile chest tube drainage system with tubing and connector ■ sterile marker ■ sterile labels ■ Optional: sterile nonadherent gauze and transparent dressing, sterile water, Y connector (for more than one chest tube).

Prepackaged sterile chest tube trays are commercially available and contain most of the equipment listed.

Preparation of equipment

Check the expiration date on the sterile packages, and inspect for tears. Then gather all equipment in the patient's room. Set up the drainage system according to the manufacturer's instructions and your facility's policy. (See "Chest tube drainage system setup," page 170.) Place the system next to the patient's bed below chest level *to facilitate drainage.* Label all medications, medication containers, and other solutions on and off the sterile field.[1]

Implementation

■ Verify the doctor's order for chest tube insertion and the number and sizes of chest tubes needed.

■ Perform hand hygiene.[2,3,4]
■ Gather the necessary supplies.
■ Conduct a preprocedure verification process *to make sure that all relevant documentation, related information, and equipment are available and correctly identified to the patient's identifiers.*[5]
■ Confirm the patient's identity using at least two patient identifiers according to your facility's policy.[6]
■ Explain the procedure to the patient and provide privacy.
■ Make sure the patient has a signed informed consent form in his chart, unless the procedure is being performed in an emergency.[7]
■ Verify that the doctor has marked the insertion site with his initials or with another unambiguous mark set by your facility's policy before the procedure is performed.[6]
■ Assess the patient for signs and symptoms of respiratory distress, including tachypnea, decreased or absent breath sounds, dyspnea, cyanosis, asymmetrical chest expansion, anxiety, restlessness, shortness of breath, tachycardia, hypotension, arrhythmias, and sudden sharp chest pain.
■ Review the patient's chart for abnormal chest X-ray or blood gas results.
■ Assess the patient for a history of previous chronic lung disease, spontaneous pneumothorax, and pulmonary disease or procedures that may have included the need for chest tube placement.
■ Obtain the patient's baseline data, including vital signs, skin color, perfusion, level of consciousness, oxygen requirements, hemodynamic stability, and respiratory rate, pattern, and effort *to help identify and document acute changes that may occur during and after the procedure.*
■ Participate in a time-out immediately before starting the procedure *to perform a final assessment that the correct patient, site, positioning, and procedure are identified and that, as applicable, all relevant information and necessary equipment are available during and after the procedure.*[8]
■ Administer sedation and pain medication as ordered. The doctor may request sedation (benzodiazepines) and opioid analgesia *to reduce pain and to help the patient remain calm.*
■ Position the patient for chest tube insertion. (Typically, the doctor places the chest tube in the midaxillary to anterior axillary line.) It's easiest to lay the patient supine, using rolled towels or a blanket to slightly rotate the upper body in a side-lying position, with the arm of the affected side raised above the head.
■ Perform hand hygiene and put on sterile gloves and attire, including eyewear, *to maintain standard precautions for a sterile surgical procedure.*[2,3,4]
■ Ask the patient to take a deep breath just before tube insertion, if the patient can cooperate. *A deep breath displaces the diaphragm downward, minimizing the risk for injury.*
■ Assist the doctor as needed with the procedure while continually assessing the patient for vital sign changes. (See *Inserting the chest tube,* page 175.)
■ Remove and discard your gloves and perform hand hygiene.[2,3,4]
■ Open the packages containing the petroleum gauze, 4″ × 4″ drain dressings, and gauze pads.
■ Put on new sterile gloves.[2,3,4]

■ Place two 4″ × 4″ drain dressings around the insertion site, one from the top and the other from the bottom, to seal the insertion site from any air entry or escape (as shown below).

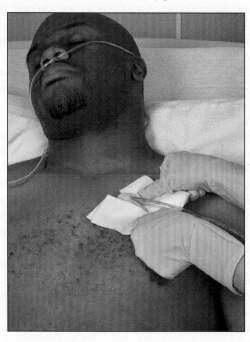

■ Place several 4″ × 4″ sterile gauze pads on top of the drain dressings.
■ Tape the dressings, covering them completely to form an occlusive dressing.
■ Place the date and time on the dressing.
■ Secure the chest tube and drainage tube so that there's no tension pulling on the insertion site *to help prevent accidental tube dislodgment.*
■ Securely tape the junction of the chest tube and the drainage tube (as shown below) *to prevent their separation.*

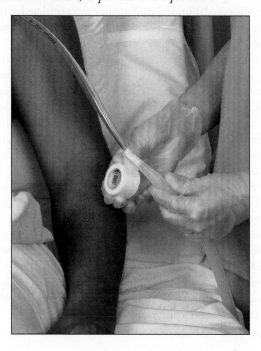

■ Dispose of equipment and waste in the appropriate biohazard receptacles.[9]
■ Remove and discard your gloves, take off other protective attire, and perform hand hygiene.[2,3,4]
■ Ensure that all clamps are open and that the drainage tubing has a straight flow to the chest tube drainage collection device and has no dependent loops or kinks.
■ Ensure that the chest tube drainage system is correctly connected to the patient's chest tube; then, if ordered, connect the suction tubing to the drainage system and the suction regulator.
■ Adjust the suction until gentle bubbling appears in the suction-control chamber of a wet-suction system or that the appropriate indicator appears when the desired negative pressure is achieved in a dry-suction system.
■ Check the status of the drainage tubing.
■ Reassess the patient after the procedure. Obtain vital signs and assess skin color, perfusion, level of consciousness, oxygen requirements, hemodynamic stability, comfort level, pain level, and respiratory rate, pattern, and effort *to identify the patient's tolerance of the procedure and response to chest tube placement.*
■ Arrange for a portable chest X-ray, as ordered, to check tube position, air or fluid evacuation, and lung reexpansion.
■ Obtain the patient's vital signs every 15 minutes for 1 hour, then every 2 hours as his condition indicates. Auscultate his lungs at least every 4 hours *to assess air exchange in the affected lung. Diminished or absent breath sounds indicate that the lung hasn't reexpanded.*
■ Record the type, color, and amount of drainage in the drainage collection chamber.
■ Mark the drainage level on the disposable chest drainage collection device every 2 to 4 hours or as needed.
■ Perform hand hygiene.[2,3,4]
■ Document the procedure.[10]

Special considerations

NURSING ALERT *Don't routinely strip a chest drain (occluding the chest tube with one hand while quickly squeezing and moving the other hand down the tube to move fluid down the tube into the drainage chamber)* because intraluminal pressures can rise dangerously high, which may convert a simple pneumothorax to life-threatening pneumothorax and cause tissue trauma and unnecessary discomfort. *Only in special circumstances, such as hemorrhaging, should the chest tube be stripped to maintain patency.*[11]

NURSING ALERT *Drain large effusions slowly.* Rapid removal during the first 30 minutes after chest tube insertion may cause post-thoracentesis pulmonary edema.

■ Routine clamping of the chest tube isn't recommended *because of the risk of tension pneumothorax.*
■ During patient transport, keep the chest tube drainage system below chest level. Don't clamp the chest tube during transport.
■ Don't tip the chest tube drainage system.
■ If you hear air leaking from the site, tape the dressing on only two or three sides *to allow air to escape and to prevent a tension*

pneumothorax. Closely monitor the patient and prepare for insertion of a new chest tube.

Documentation

Record the date and time of chest tube insertion, who inserted the tube, the insertion site, the size of the chest tube used, medications given, chest tube drainage system used, presence of drainage and bubbling, associated complications and nursing actions taken, and patient teaching provided. Record your assessment findings before and after the procedure and the patient's response to the procedure. Record the patient's respiratory status, vital signs, amount of drainage and its color and consistency, and any teaching provided to the family every 2 to 4 hours.

REFERENCES

1 The Joint Commission. (2012). Standard NPSG.03.04.01. *Comprehensive accreditation manual for hospitals: The official handbook.* Oakbrook Terrace, IL: The Joint Commission. (Level I)
2 The Joint Commission. (2012). Standard NPSG.07.01.01. *Comprehensive accreditation manual for hospitals: The official handbook.* Oakbrook Terrace, IL: The Joint Commission. (Level I)
3 Centers for Disease Control and Prevention. (October 2002). Guideline for hand hygiene in health-care settings. *Morbidity and Mortality Weekly Report, 51*(RR-16), 1–45. (Level 1)
4 World Health Organization. (2009). *WHO guidelines on hand hygiene in health care: First global patient safety challenge. Clean care is safer care.* Geneva, Switzerland: World Health Organization. (Level I)
5 The Joint Commission. (2012). Standard UP.01.01.01. *Comprehensive accreditation manual for hospitals: The official handbook.* Oakbrook Terrace, IL: The Joint Commission. (Level I)
6 The Joint Commission. (2012). Standard NPSG.01.01.01. *Comprehensive accreditation manual for hospitals: The official handbook.* Oakbrook Terrace, IL: The Joint Commission. (Level I)
7 The Joint Commission. (2012). Standard RI.01.03.01. *Comprehensive accreditation manual for hospitals: The official handbook.* Oakbrook Terrace, IL: The Joint Commission. (Level I)
8 The Joint Commission. (2012). Standard UP.01.03.01. *Comprehensive accreditation manual for hospitals: The official handbook.* Oakbrook Terrace, IL: The Joint Commission. (Level I)
9 Occupational Safety and Health Administration. "Bloodborne Pathogens, Standard Number 1910.1030" [Online]. Accessed August 2011 via the Web at http://www.osha.gov/pls/oshaweb/owadisp.show_document?p_table=STANDARDS&p_id=10051
10 The Joint Commission. (2012). Standard RC.01.03.01. *Comprehensive accreditation manual for hospitals: The official handbook.* Oakbrook Terrace, IL: The Joint Commission. (Level I)
11 Haim, M. (2007). To strip or not to strip? Physiological effects of chest tube manipulation. *American Journal of Critical Care, 16*(6), 609–612.

ADDITIONAL REFERENCES

Lynn-McHale Wiegand, D. (Ed.). (2011). *AACN procedure manual for critical care* (6th ed.). Philadelphia, PA: Saunders.
Nettina, S.M. (2010). *Lippincott manual of nursing practice* (9th ed.). Philadelphia, PA: Lippincott Williams & Wilkins.

Inserting the chest tube

Chest tube insertion involves these steps:
■ The doctor puts on a cap, a mask, eye protection, a sterile gown, and sterile gloves and prepares a sterile field using sterile drapes.
■ The doctor completes sterile preparation of the patient, using sterile towels and a chlorhexidine-based antiseptic swab to clean the insertion site.
■ The nurse wipes the rubber stopper of the lidocaine vial with an alcohol pad. Then she inverts the bottle and holds it for the doctor to withdraw the anesthetic.
■ The doctor injects a local anesthetic at the site to reduce the pain of the procedure and waits for the anesthetic to take effect.
■ The doctor makes a skin incision about 1″ (2.5 cm) long and then inserts a hemostat through the opening to enter the pleural space. Typically, when the pleural space is entered, there will be a return of pleural contents, confirming penetration.
■ The hemostat is spread open slightly to enlarge the opening enough to accommodate the chest tube.
■ Using his finger, the doctor creates a track for the chest tube. He then clamps the chest tube with the hemostat and inserts them through the incision, guiding the hemostat and tube along his inserted finger.
■ The doctor removes the hemostat and immediately connects the chest tube to the drainage system.
■ The nurse assists the doctor in attaching the disposable sterile chest tube drainage system to the chest tube, using a Y connector if more than one chest tube is placed.
■ The doctor sutures the chest tube securely into place and wraps sterile petrolatum gauze around the chest tube where it enters the chest.

CHEST TUBE REMOVAL, ASSISTING

The pleural space normally contains a thin layer of lubricating fluid that allows the visceral and parietal pleura to move without friction during respiration. An excess of fluid, air, or both in this space alters intrapleural pressure and causes partial or complete lung collapse. A chest tube allows drainage of the air or fluid from the pleural space and enables lung reexpansion and the restoration of negative pressure to the pleural space.[1]

After the patient's lung has reexpanded and any drainage has been controlled, the doctor may order a chest tube to be clamped or have suction discontinued, with the tube left to water-seal drainage for several hours before removal to assess the patient's tolerance. This waiting period allows time to observe the patient for signs and symptoms of respiratory distress, an indication that air or fluid remains trapped in the pleural space. The doctor may also order a chest X-ray before removal.

A chest tube is usually removed within 7 days of insertion to prevent infection along the tube tract.[1] Chest tube removal is the responsibility of the doctor, nurse practitioner, advance practice nurse, or physician's assistant, according to scope of practice.

Equipment

Gloves ▪ sterile gloves ▪ chest tube clamp ▪ topical analgesic cream ▪ personal protective equipment ▪ suture removal kit ▪ sterile forceps ▪ linen-saver pad ▪ sterile petroleum gauze ▪ 4″ × 4″ sterile gauze dressing ▪ tape.

Implementation

▪ Verify the doctor's order for chest tube removal.
▪ Gather the appropriate equipment.
▪ Confirm the patient's identity using at least two patient identifiers according to your facility's policy.[2]
▪ Explain the procedure to the patient *to ensure his cooperation and decrease anxiety.*
▪ Perform hand hygiene.[3,4,5]
▪ Premedicate the patient, as ordered, *to reduce the patient's discomfort.*
▪ Obtain vital signs and perform a respiratory assessment.
▪ As ordered, apply topical analgesic cream to the chest tube wound site.
▪ Place the patient in semi-Fowler's position or on his unaffected side.
▪ Place a linen-saver pad under the affected side *to protect the linen from drainage and to provide a place to put the chest tube after removal.*
▪ Put on gloves and appropriate personal protective equipment.[3,4,5]
▪ Prepare a sterile airtight dressing with petroleum gauze and 4″ × 4″ sterile gauze dressings *so that the doctor can cover the insertion site with it immediately after quickly and smoothly removing the tube.*
▪ If instructed by the doctor, remove the existing chest tube dressings and discard them appropriately.[6] Be careful not to dislodge the chest tube prematurely.
▪ Trace the chest tube from the point of origin to the patient *to make sure that you're removing the proper tube.*[7] Clamp the chest tube catheter (if not already done) *to minimize dead space and stop air from entering or exiting catheter.*
▪ Assist the doctor as necessary. The doctor will instruct the patient to perform Valsalva's maneuver by exhaling and bearing down *to increase intrathoracic pressure and prevent air from entering the pleural space* as he removes the chest tube and covers the insertion site with the airtight dressing.
▪ Help secure the dressing with tape. Make it as airtight as possible *to seal the insertion site from air entry.*
▪ Instruct the patient to breathe normally.
▪ Mark the dressing with the date, time, and your initials.
▪ Dispose of equipment and waste in an appropriate receptacle.[6]
▪ Remove and discard your gloves and other personal protective equipment, and perform hand hygiene.[3,4,5]
▪ Closely monitor the patient after the procedure *to determine the patient's response to and tolerance of the procedure.*

▪ Obtain vital signs, including respiratory rate, pattern, and effort. Monitor the patient's color, perfusion, level of consciousness, oxygen requirements, and hemodynamic stability. Assess the patient carefully for signs and symptoms of pneumothorax, subcutaneous emphysema, or infection.
▪ Obtain a chest X-ray, as ordered.

NURSING ALERT *Notify the doctor immediately if the patient develops acute respiratory distress* because a new chest tube may be indicated.

▪ Position the patient for comfort and raise the bed's side rails.
▪ Encourage coughing and deep breathing. (See *Instructions for coughing and deep breathing.*)
▪ Assess the chest tube site and dressing for drainage and re-dress as ordered or according to your facility's policy.
▪ Document the procedure.[8]

Special considerations

▪ The doctor may elect to physiologically simulate tube removal by placing the tube to water seal (removing suction) before removing the tube *to evaluate the patient's tolerance.*

Complications

Complications of chest tube removal can include infection at the site, tension pneumothorax, and redevelopment of the pneumothorax, hemothorax, or chylothorax that was present before tube placement.

Documentation

Record the date and time of chest tube removal, your preparation procedures, the patient's vital signs and respiratory status, medications given and their effectiveness, and the patient's tolerance of the procedure. Document the condition of the insertion site, complications and nursing actions taken, and any teaching provided.

REFERENCES

1 Lynn-McHale Wiegand, D. (Ed.). (2011). *AACN procedure manual for critical* care (6th ed.). Philadelphia, PA: Saunders.
2 The Joint Commission. (2012). Standard NPSG.01.01.01. *Comprehensive accreditation manual for hospitals: The official handbook.* Oakbrook Terrace, IL: The Joint Commission. (Level I)
3 The Joint Commission. (2012). Standard NPSG.07.01.01. *Comprehensive accreditation manual for hospitals: The official handbook.* Oakbrook Terrace, IL: The Joint Commission. (Level I)
4 Centers for Disease Control and Prevention. (October 2002). Guideline for hand hygiene in health-care settings. *Morbidity and Mortality Weekly Report, 51*(RR-16), 1–45. (Level 1)
5 World Health Organization. (2009). *WHO guidelines on hand hygiene in health care: First global patient safety challenge. Clean care is safer care.* Geneva, Switzerland: World Health Organization. (Level I)
6 Occupational Safety and Health Administration. "Bloodborne Pathogens, Standard Number 1910.1030" [Online]. Accessed August 2011 via the Web at http://www.osha.gov/pls/oshaweb/owadisp.show_document?p_table=STANDARDS&p_id=10051 (Level I)

Instructions for coughing and deep breathing

Coughing or "huffing" helps break up secretions in the lungs so that the mucus can be suctioned out or expectorated. Deep-breathing exercises help to expand the lungs and force better distribution of the air into all areas. The patient may initially need to lie down to do these exercises, but eventually they're done while sitting upright, then while walking.

Coughing

Have the patient sit upright and drink a glass of water. For a controlled cough, the patient purses his lips and takes a deep breath. He should hold the breath for several seconds and then make two brief, gentle coughs. For huffing, the patient purses his lips and takes a deep breath. After holding the breath for several seconds, the patient exhales, using his stomach muscles to push out the air. The vocal chords remain open so that the cough has almost a whispery sound. Coughing and huffing are repeated several times per day as needed.

Deep-breathing exercises

The patient starts by taking a deep breath through the nose, and then purses his lips as if to whistle. He then exhales the air slowly through pursed lips. The exhalation should take twice as long as the inhalation. For example, the patient may start by inhaling for 2 seconds and then exhaling for 4 seconds. After taking several deep breaths, he should breathe at a normal rhythm and then begin another cycle of deep breathing.

Usually, coughing and deep-breathing exercises are performed together. To do this, first tell the patient to breathe in deeply through his nose and then exhale in three short huffs. Then have him inhale deeply again and cough through a slightly open mouth. Three consecutive coughs are highly effective. An effective cough sounds deep, low, and hollow; an ineffective cough is high-pitched. If possible, have the patient perform this exercise for about 1 minute and then rest for 2 minutes.

7 U.S. Food and Drug Administration. (2009). "Look. Check. Connect. Safe Medical Device Connections Save Lives" [Online]. Accessed August 2011 via the Web at http://www.fda.gov/downloads/MedicalDevices/Safety/AlertsandNotices/UCM134873.pdf
8 The Joint Commission. (2012). Standard RC.01.03.01. *Comprehensive accreditation manual for hospitals: The official handbook.* Oakbrook Terrace, IL: The Joint Commission. (Level I)

ADDITIONAL REFERENCES

Hunter, J. (2008). Chest drain removal. *Nursing Standard, 22*(45), 35–38.
Nettina, S.M. (2010). *Lippincott manual of nursing practice* (9th ed.). Philadelphia, PA: Lippincott Williams & Wilkins.

CLAVICLE STRAP APPLICATION

Also called a *figure-eight strap,* a clavicle strap reduces and immobilizes fractures of the clavicle. It does this by elevating, extending, and supporting the shoulders in position for healing, known as the *position of attention.* A commercially available figure-eight strap or a 4″ elastic bandage may serve as a clavicle strap. (See *Types of clavicle straps,* page 178.) This strap is contraindicated for an uncooperative patient.

Equipment

Powder or cornstarch ▪ figure-eight clavicle strap or 4″ elastic bandage ▪ safety pins, if necessary ▪ tape ▪ cotton batting or padding ▪ marking pen ▪ analgesics, as ordered ▪ Optional: scissors.

Implementation

▪ Verify the doctor's order.
▪ Gather the equipment.
▪ Confirm the patient's identity using at least two patient identifiers according to your facility's policy.[1]
▪ Explain the procedure to the patient and provide privacy.
▪ Perform hand hygiene.[2,3,4]
▪ Help the patient take off his shirt or cut off the shirt if movement is too painful.
▪ Assess arm neurovascular integrity by palpating skin temperature; noting the color and temperature of the hand and fingers; palpating the radial, ulnar, and brachial pulses bilaterally; and then comparing the affected with the unaffected side. Ask the patient about any numbness or tingling distal to the injury, and assess his motor function.
▪ Determine the patient's degree of comfort and administer analgesics as ordered, using safe medication administration practices. Perform a follow-up pain assessment and notify the doctor if pain isn't adequately controlled.[5]
▪ Demonstrate how to assume the position of attention. Instruct the patient to sit upright and assume this position gradually *to minimize pain.*
▪ Gently apply powder or cornstarch, as appropriate, to the axillae and shoulder area *to reduce friction from the clavicle strap.* You can use cornstarch if the patient is allergic to powder.

Applying a commercially made figure-eight strap

▪ Place the apex of the triangle between the scapulae and drape the straps over the shoulders. Bring the strap with the Velcro or

EQUIPMENT

Types of clavicle straps

Clavicle straps provide support to the shoulder to help heal a fractured clavicle. These straps are available ready-made. They can also be made from a bandage.

Commercially made clavicle straps have a short back panel and long straps that extend around the patient's shoulders and axillae. They have Velcro pads or buckles on the ends for easy fastening.

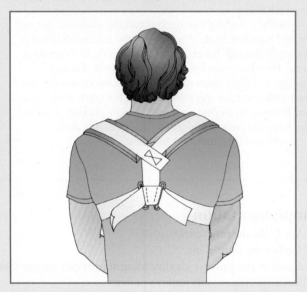

When making a clavicle strap with a wide elastic bandage, start in the middle of the patient's back. After wrapping the bandage around the shoulders, fasten the ends with safety pins.

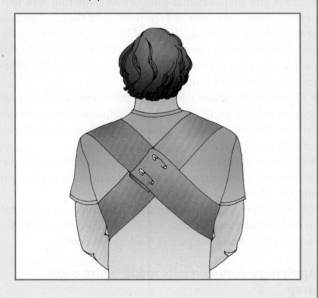

buckle end under one axilla and through the loop; then pull the other strap under the other axilla and through the loop.

■ Gently adjust the straps so they support the shoulders in the position of attention.

■ Bring the straps back under the axillae toward the anterior chest, making sure they maintain the position of attention.

Applying a 4″ elastic bandage strap

■ Roll both ends of the elastic bandage toward the middle, leaving between 12″ to 18″ (30.5 to 45.7 cm) unrolled.

■ Place the unrolled portion diagonally across the patient's back, from right shoulder to left axilla.

■ Bring the lower end of the bandage under the left axilla and back over the left shoulder; loop the upper end over the right shoulder and under the axilla.

■ Pull the two ends together at the center of the back *so the bandage supports the position of attention.*

Completing a commercially made figure-eight strap or an elastic bandage application

■ Secure the ends using safety pins, Velcro pads, or a buckle, depending on the equipment. Make sure a buckle or any sharp edges face away from the skin. Tape the secured ends to the underlying strap or bandage.

■ Place cotton batting or padding under the straps, as well as under the buckle or pins, *to prevent skin irritation.*

■ Use a pen to mark the strap at the site of the loop of the figure-eight strap, or the site where the elastic bandage crosses on the patient's back. *If the strap loosens, this mark helps you tighten it to the original position.*

■ Assess neurovascular integrity, *which may be impaired by a strap that's too tight.* If neurovascular integrity is compromised when the strap is correctly applied, notify the doctor. *He may want to change the treatment.*

■ Perform hand hygiene.[2,3,4]

■ Document the procedure.[6]

Special considerations

■ If possible, perform the procedure with the patient standing. However, this may not be feasible, because the pain from the fracture can cause syncope. If the patient can't stand, have him sit upright.

■ An adult with a clavicle strap made from an elastic bandage may require a triangular sling *to help support the weight of the arm, enhance immobilization, and reduce pain. Inadequate immobilization can cause improper healing.*

■ For a hospitalized patient, monitor the position of the strap by checking the pen markings every shift. Also assess neurovascular integrity. Teach the outpatient how to assess his own neurovascular integrity and to recognize symptoms he should report promptly to the doctor.

■ Clavicle straps are typically worn for 4 to 8 weeks.

Patient teaching

Instruct the patient not to remove the clavicle strap until his doctor orders him to do so. Explain that, with help, he can maintain proper hygiene by lifting segments of the strap to remove the cotton and by washing and powdering the skin daily. Explain that fresh cotton should be applied after cleaning.

Documentation

In the appropriate section of the emergency department sheet or in your notes, record the date and time of strap application, type of clavicle strap, use of powder and padding, bilateral neurovascular integrity before and after the procedure, analgesia administered, and instructions given to the patient.

REFERENCES

1 The Joint Commission. (2012). Standard NPSG.01.01.01. *Comprehensive accreditation manual for hospitals: The official handbook.* Oakbrook Terrace, IL: The Joint Commission. (Level I)
2 The Joint Commission. (2012). Standard NPSG.07.01.01. *Comprehensive accreditation manual for hospitals: The official handbook.* Oakbrook Terrace, IL: The Joint Commission. (Level I)
3 Centers for Disease Control and Prevention. (October 2002). Guideline for hand hygiene in health-care settings. *Morbidity and Mortality Weekly Report, 51*(RR-16), 1–45. (Level 1)
4 World Health Organization. (2009). *WHO guidelines on hand hygiene in health care: First global patient safety challenge. Clean care is safer care.* Geneva, Switzerland: World Health Organization. (Level I)
5 The Joint Commission. (2012). Standard PC.01.02.07. *Comprehensive accreditation manual for hospitals: The official handbook.* Oakbrook Terrace, IL: The Joint Commission. (Level I)
6 The Joint Commission. (2012). Standard RC.01.03.01. *Comprehensive accreditation manual for hospitals: The official handbook.* Oakbrook Terrace, IL: The Joint Commission. (Level I)

ADDITIONAL REFERENCE

Wheeless, C.R. III, et al. (Eds.). (2010). "Wheeless' Textbook of Orthopaedics" [Online]. Accessed November 2011 via the Web at http://www.wheelessonline.com

CLOSED-WOUND DRAIN MANAGEMENT

Typically inserted during surgery in anticipation of postoperative drainage, a closed-wound drain promotes healing and prevents swelling by suctioning the exudate that accumulates at the wound site. By removing this fluid, the closed-wound drain helps reduce the risk of infection and skin breakdown as well as the number of dressing changes. The drain is usually emptied every shift and as needed. Jackson-Pratt and Hemovac closed drainage systems are used most commonly. (See *Types of closed drainage systems.*)

A closed-wound drain consists of perforated tubing connected to a portable vacuum unit. The distal end of the tubing lies within the wound and usually leaves the body from a site other than the primary suture line to preserve the integrity of the surgical wound. The tubing exit site is treated as an additional surgical wound; the drain is usually sutured to the skin.

If the wound produces heavy drainage, the closed-wound drain may be left in place for longer than 1 week. Drainage must be

Types of closed drainage systems

There are two common types of closed drainage systems. The Jackson-Pratt drain collects exudate in a bulblike device that's typically used with breast and abdominal surgery.

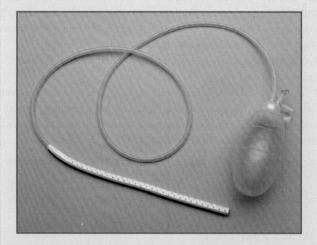

The Hemovac drain is used when blood drainage is expected after surgery, such as in abdominal and orthopedic surgeries.

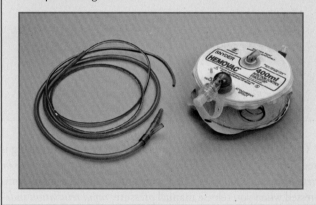

emptied and measured frequently to maintain maximum suction and prevent strain on the suture line.

Equipment

Graduated cylinder ▪ alcohol pads ▪ gloves and other personal protective equipment as needed ▪ sterile gauze pads ▪ antiseptic cleaning agent or antimicrobial swabs ▪ sterile laboratory container, if needed ▪ Optional: label.

Implementation

▪ Verify the doctor's order.
▪ Confirm the patient's identity using at least two patient identifiers according to your facility's policy.[1]

- Explain the procedure to the patient and provide privacy.
- Perform hand hygiene and put on gloves and other personal protective equipment.[2,3,4]
- Assess the patient's condition.
- Unclip the vacuum unit from the patient's bed or gown.
- Using sterile technique, release the vacuum by removing the spout plug on the collection chamber. The container expands completely as it draws in air.
- Empty the unit's contents into a graduated cylinder, and note the amount and appearance of the drainage. If diagnostic tests will be performed on the fluid specimen, pour the drainage directly into a sterile laboratory container, note the amount and appearance, label the specimen and send it to the laboratory.
- Maintaining sterile technique, use an alcohol pad to clean the unit's spout and plug.
- *To reestablish the vacuum that creates the drain's suction power,* fully compress the vacuum unit. With one hand holding the compressed unit *to maintain the vacuum,* replace the spout plug with your other hand (as shown below).

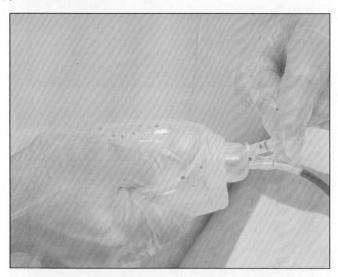

- Check the patency of the equipment. Make sure the tubing is free of twists, kinks, and leaks *because the drainage system must be airtight to work properly.* The vacuum unit should remain compressed when you release manual pressure; *rapid reinflation indicates an air leak.* If this occurs, recompress the unit and make sure the spout plug is secure.
- Secure the vacuum unit to the patient's gown. Fasten it below wound level *to promote drainage.* Don't apply tension on drainage tubing when fastening the unit *to prevent possible dislodgment.*
- Observe the sutures that secure the drain to the patient's skin; look for signs of pulling or tearing and for swelling or infection of surrounding skin. Gently clean the sutures with sterile gauze pads soaked in an antiseptic cleaning agent or with an antimicrobial swab.
- Properly dispose of drainage and solutions, and clean or dispose of soiled equipment and supplies.[5]
- Remove and discard your gloves and perform hand hygiene.[2,3,4]
- Document the procedure.[6]

Special considerations

- Empty the drain and measure its contents once during each shift if drainage has accumulated, more often if drainage is excessive. *Removing excess drainage maintains maximum suction and avoids straining the drain's suture line.*
- Empty the drain and measure its contents before the patient ambulates *to prevent the weight of drainage from pulling on the drain as the patient ambulates.*
- If the patient has more than one closed drain, number the drains *so you can record drainage from each site.*
- **NURSING ALERT** *Be careful not to mistake chest tubes for closed-wound drains because the vacuum of a chest tube should never be released.*

Complications

Occlusion of the tubing by fibrin, clots, or other particles can reduce or obstruct drainage. Infection may develop at the tubing exit site.

Documentation

Record the date and time you empty the drain, appearance of the drain site and presence of swelling or signs of infection, equipment malfunction and consequent nursing action, and the patient's tolerance of the treatment. On the intake and output sheet, record drainage color, consistency, type, and amount. If the patient has more than one closed-wound drain, number the drains and record the information above separately for each drainage site.

REFERENCES

1 The Joint Commission. (2012). Standard NPSG.01.01.01. *Comprehensive accreditation manual for hospitals: The official handbook.* Oakbrook Terrace, IL: The Joint Commission. (Level I)
2 The Joint Commission. (2012). Standard NPSG.07.01.01. *Comprehensive accreditation manual for hospitals: The official handbook.* Oakbrook Terrace, IL: The Joint Commission. (Level I)
3 Centers for Disease Control and Prevention. (October 2002). Guideline for hand hygiene in health-care settings. *Morbidity and Mortality Weekly Report, 51*(RR-16), 1–45. (Level 1)
4 World Health Organization. (2009). *WHO guidelines on hand hygiene in health care: First global patient safety challenge. Clean care is safer care.* Geneva, Switzerland: World Health Organization. (Level I)
5 Occupational Safety and Health Administration. "Bloodborne Pathogens, Standard Number 1910.1030" [Online]. Accessed August 2011 via the Web at http://www.osha.gov/pls/oshaweb/owadisp.show_document?p_table=STANDARDS&p_id=10051 (Level I)
6 The Joint Commission. (2012). Standard RC.01.03.01. *Comprehensive accreditation manual for hospitals: The official handbook.* Oakbrook Terrace, IL: The Joint Commission. (Level I)

ADDITIONAL REFERENCE

Nettina, S.M. (2010). *Lippincott manual of nursing practice* (9th ed.). Philadelphia, PA: Lippincott Williams & Wilkins.

CODE MANAGEMENT

The goals of any code are to restore the patient's spontaneous heartbeat and respirations and also to prevent hypoxic damage to the brain and other vital organs. Fulfilling these goals requires a team approach. Ideally, the team should consist of health care workers trained in advanced cardiac life support (ACLS), although health care workers trained in basic life support (BLS) may also be a part of the team. Sponsored by the American Heart Association (AHA), the ACLS course incorporates BLS skills with advanced resuscitation techniques. BLS and ACLS should be performed according to the 2010 AHA guidelines.

In most health care facilities, ACLS-trained nurses provide the first resuscitative efforts to cardiac arrest patients, often administering cardiopulmonary resuscitation (CPR) and performing defibrillation before the doctor's arrival. Ventricular fibrillation commonly precedes sudden cardiac arrest; initial resuscitative efforts should focus on early CPR, rapid recognition of arrhythmias and, when indicated, defibrillation. If monitoring equipment isn't available, you should simply perform BLS measures. Of course, the scope of your responsibilities in any situation depends on your facility's policies and procedures and your state's nurse practice act.

A code may be called for patients with absent pulse, apnea or inadequate breathing, ventricular fibrillation, ventricular tachycardia, and asystole. Family members may be present during a code if your facility's policy supports it. The Emergency Nurses Association supports the option of family presence during invasive procedures and CPR in its 2005 position statement.[1]

According to the 2010 AHA guidelines for CPR and emergency cardiovascular care, ACLS interventions build on the foundation of basic life support, which includes immediate recognition and activation of the emergency response system, early high-quality CPR, and rapid defibrillation to increase the patient's chance for survival. The recommended priority of the 2010 AHA guidelines is performing high-quality CPR chest compressions of adequate rate and depth that allow complete chest recoil after each compression, with minimal interruptions and avoiding excessive ventilation.

To prevent a delay in chest compressions, the AHA changed the sequence of CPR in the 2010 guidelines from "A-B-C" (airway, breathing, and compressions) to "C-A-B" (compressions, airway, and breathing), which gives the highest priority to chest compressions when resuscitating a patient in cardiac arrest. In addition to high-quality CPR, the only rhythm-specific therapy known to increase survival is defibrillation. As such, defibrillation remains of primary importance in the CPR cycle when a rhythm check reveals ventricular fibrillation or ventricular tachycardia. Establishing vascular access, administering medications, and inserting an advanced airway are important, but they shouldn't cause significant interruptions in CPR or delay defibrillation.[2]

Equipment

Oral, nasal, and endotracheal (ET) airways ▪ one-way valve masks ▪ oxygen source ▪ oxygen flowmeter ▪ intubation supplies ▪ handheld resuscitation bag ▪ suction supplies ▪ end-tidal carbon dioxide detector ▪ nasogastric (NG) tube ▪ goggles, masks, gloves, other personal protective equipment as indicated by the patient's condition ▪ cardiac arrest board ▪ peripheral IV supplies ▪ central IV supplies ▪ IV administration sets (including macrodrip and microdrip) ▪ IV fluids (normal saline and lactated Ringer's solutions) ▪ electrocardiogram (ECG) monitor and leads ▪ automated external defibrillator (AED), if available ▪ cardioverter-defibrillator (monophasic or biphasic) ▪ defibrillator pads ▪ cardiac drugs, including adenosine, amiodarone, atropine, calcium chloride, dobutamine, dopamine, epinephrine, isoproterenol, lidocaine, procainamide, sodium bicarbonate, and vasopressin ▪ tape ▪ marker ▪ Optional: transcutaneous pacemaker, percutaneous transvenous pacer, cricothyrotomy kit, and waveform capnography.

Preparation of equipment

Because effective emergency care depends on reliable and accessible equipment, the equipment, as well as the personnel, must be ready for a code at any time. You also should be familiar with the cardiac drugs you may have to administer. (See *Common emergency cardiac drugs*, pages 182 and 183.)

Always be aware of your patient's code status as defined by the doctor's orders, the patient's advance directives, and family wishes. If the doctor has ordered a "no code," make sure the doctor has written and signed the order. If possible, have the patient or a responsible family member cosign the order.

For some patients, you may need to consider whether the family wishes to be present during a code. If they do want to be present, see if another nurse, social worker, or clergy member can remain with them.

Implementation

▪ Perform hand hygiene and put on gloves (if possible).[3,4,5]
▪ If you're the first to arrive at the scene of a code, tap the patient on the shoulder and shout, "Are you all right?" If the patient is unresponsive, check to see if the patient is apneic or only gasping.[2]
▪ If the patient is unresponsive and apneic or only gasping, assume the patient is in cardiac arrest and immediately activate the emergency response system.[2]
▪ Take no longer than 10 seconds to check for a pulse; if you don't feel a pulse within that time (or are unsure of a pulse), begin chest compressions. Depress the adult sternum at least 2″ (5 cm), allowing the chest to completely recoil after each compression. Perform compressions at a rate of at least 100 compressions per minute.[2] After 30 compressions, provide 2 ventilations.
▪ When a second person arrives with the emergency equipment, have that person apply the AED. In many facilities, the AED is a function of the defibrillator. Follow the directions provided by the AED. Then have the second person assist with placing the cardiac arrest board under the patient and with providing CPR.
▪ The second person should get into position on the other side of the patient and begin chest compressions at a rate of at least 100 compressions per minute. You provide ventilations after every 30 compressions. After 5 cycles of compressions and ventilations,

(*Text continues on page 184.*)

Common emergency cardiac drugs

You may be called on to administer several cardiac drugs during a code. This chart lists the most common emergency cardiac drugs, along with their actions, indications, and dosages.

DRUG	ACTIONS	INDICATIONS	TYPICAL ADULT DOSAGE
adenosine (Adenocard)	■ Slows conduction through atrioventricular (AV) node; may interrupt reentry through AV node ■ Shortens duration of atrial action potential during supraventricular tachycardia	■ Stable narrow complex regular tachycardia ■ Unstable narrow complex regular tachycardia ■ Stable regular monomorphic wide complex tachycardia	■ 6 mg IV push over 1 to 3 seconds initially; may be increased to 12 mg if conversion hasn't occurred within 2 minutes; may repeat 12 mg in 1 to 2 minutes if needed. Reduce initial dose to 3 mg when administered through a central venous catheter, in patients receiving dipyridamole or carbamazepine, and in heart transplant recipients. Each dose should be followed by a 20-mL saline flush.[2] ■ *Caution:* Slower-than-recommended administration decreases the drug's effectiveness. ■ Avoid use in patients with asthma.[2]
amiodarone	■ Thought to prolong refractory period and action potential duration	■ Cardiac arrest caused by persistent ventricular tachycardia (VT) or ventricular fibrillation (VF) ■ Stable irregular narrow complex tachycardia (atrial fibrillation) ■ Stable regular narrow complex tachycardia	■ For narrow complex tachycardia, 150 mg over 10 minutes, followed by 1 mg/minute infusion for 6 hours, then 0.5 mg/minute.[2] ■ For cardiac arrest, 300 mg IV push or intraosseously (I.O.); repeat 150 mg IV push in 3 to 5 minutes. Dilute in 20 to 30 mL of dextrose 5% in water (D_5W). Maximum dose: 2.2 g IV/24 hour.[2]
atropine	■ Accelerates AV conduction and heart rate by blocking the vagal nerve	■ Symptomatic bradycardia	■ 0.5 mg IV push repeated every 3 to 5 minutes until the heart rate reaches 60 beats/minute; can give up to 3 mg total.[2]
diltiazem	■ Slows AV node conduction and increases AV node refractoriness	■ Stable narrow complex tachycardia ■ Atrial fibrillation or atrial flutter with rapid ventricular response	■ Initially, 15 to 20 mg IV over 2 minutes, followed by 20 to 25 mg IV in 15 minutes, if needed. Maintenance: 5 to 15 mg/hour titrated to ventricular response.[2]
dobutamine	■ Increases myocardial contractility without raising oxygen demand	■ Heart failure ■ Cardiogenic shock after cardiac arrest	■ 5 to 10 mcg/kg/minute by continuous IV infusion. Titrate as needed to optimize blood pressure, cardiac output, and systemic perfusion.[2]
dopamine	■ Produces inotropic effect, increasing cardiac output, blood pressure, and renal perfusion	■ Symptomatic bradycardia associated with hypotension (except when caused by hypovolemia)	■ Continuous IV infusion at 2 to 20 mcg/kg/minute. *Note:* Always dilute and give IV drip, never IV push. Titrate to patient response. ■ *Caution:* Don't administer in the same IV line with alkaline solutions.[2]

Common emergency cardiac drugs *(continued)*

DRUG	ACTIONS	INDICATIONS	TYPICAL ADULT DOSAGE
epinephrine (Adrenalin)	■ Increases heart rate, peripheral resistance, and blood flow to heart (enhancing myocardial and cerebral oxygenation) ■ Strengthens myocardial contractility ■ Increases coronary perfusion pressure during cardiopulmonary resuscitation	■ VF ■ Pulseless VT ■ Pulseless electrical activity ■ Asystole ■ Severe hypotension (secondary agent) ■ Symptomatic bradycardia	■ 10 mL of 1:10,000 solution (1 mg) IV push or I.O. initially; may be repeated every 3 to 5 minutes, as needed. After each dose, flush 20 mL of IV fluid if administered peripherally.[2] ■ 2 to 2½ times the IV dose given endotracheally if no IV line is available.[2] (*Note:* 1:1,000 solution contains 1 mg/mL, so it must be diluted in 9 mL of normal saline solution to provide 1 mg/10 mL.)[2] ■ For hypotension, 1 mg/500 mL of D_5W by continuous infusion; titrate to desired effect (2 to 10 mcg/minute).[2] ■ *Caution:* Don't administer in the same IV line with alkaline solutions.
isoproterenol (Isuprel)	■ Enhances automaticity and accelerates conduction ■ Increases heart rate and cardiac contractility, but exacerbates ischemia and arrhythmias in patients with ischemic heart disease	■ Symptomatic bradycardia unresponsive to atropine (while awaiting pacemaker insertion) ■ Torsades de pointes (polymorphic VT) when accompanied by bradycardia ■ Brugada syndrome	■ Continuous IV infusion at 2 to 10 mcg/minute titrated according to heart rate and rhythm response.[2] Monitor heart rate and blood pressure carefully. Doses that increase heart rate to greater than 130 beats/minute may induce ventricular arrhythmias. ■ *Caution:* Avoid use in patients with torsades de pointes associated with familial long QT syndrome.[2]
lidocaine (Xylocaine)	■ Depresses automaticity and conduction of ectopic impulses in ventricles, especially in ischemic tissue ■ Raises fibrillation threshold, especially in an ischemic heart	■ Cardiac arrest from VF or VT when amiodarone isn't available	■ 1 to 1.5 mg/kg IV push or I.O. initially; may be followed by a 0.5 to 0.75 mg/kg bolus dose every 5 to 10 minutes, up to a total of 3 mg/kg.[2] ■ Maintenance: Continuous IV infusion of 2 g/500 mL of D_5W (at 1 to 4 mg/minute) to prevent recurrence of lethal arrhythmias.[1]
magnesium sulfate	■ Mechanism of action is unclear but may help in cardiac arrest associated with refractory VT or VF	■ Cardiac arrest associated with torsades de pointes ■ Torsades de pointes associated with a long QT interval	■ For cardiac arrest associated with torsades de pointes, 1 to 2 g IV in 10 mL of D_5W.[2] ■ For torsades de pointes without cardiac arrest, 1 to 2 g in 50 to 100 mL of D_5W over 15 minutes.[2]
procainamide	■ Depresses automaticity and conduction ■ Prolongs refraction in atria and ventricles	■ Premature ventricular contractions (PVCs) ■ Stable monomorphic VT ■ Supraventricular arrhythmias	■ 20 to 50 mg/minute IV infusion up to a total of 17 mg/kg, followed by a maintenance dose of 1 to 4 mg/minute by IV infusion. Administration is limited by the need for slow infusion.
vasopressin	■ Causes peripheral vasoconstriction	■ Cardiac arrest	■ 40 units IV or I.O. as a single dose, one time only; may replace first or second dose of epinephrine.[2]
verapamil (Isoptin)	■ Slows conduction through AV node ■ Causes vasodilation ■ Produces negative inotropic effect on heart, depressing myocardial contractility	■ Paroxysmal supraventricular tachycardia with narrow QRS complex and rate control in atrial fibrillation	■ 2.5 to 5 mg IV push over 2 minutes initially (over 3 minutes in older adults). Repeat dose of 5 to 10 mg every 15 to 30 minutes, if needed. Total dose: 20 mg. Monitor electrocardiogram and blood pressure.[2] ■ *Caution:* Don't use drug to treat preexcited atrial fibrillation or flutter.[2]

switch roles. The switch should take fewer than 5 seconds *because interruptions in chest compressions can compromise vital organ perfusion.* The compressor should be relieved every 2 minutes *to prevent rescuer fatigue that could lead to inadequate compression rates or depth.*[2]

■ Ask the nurse assigned to the patient to relate the patient's medical history and describe the events leading to cardiac arrest.

■ A third person, either a nurse certified in BLS or a respiratory therapist, will then attach the handheld resuscitation bag to the oxygen source.

■ Ideally, a fourth person will be available to open the patient's airway and seal the mask to the patient's face. After the mask is in place, the other person will squeeze the resuscitation bag to deliver 2 ventilations (each over 1 second) during a brief pause after 30 compressions. Both people will watch for the chest to rise. If a fourth person isn't available, the other person will open the patient's airway, seal the mask to the patient's face using one hand and then, with the other hand, squeeze the resuscitation bag to deliver 2 ventilations during a brief pause after 30 compressions.[2]

■ When the ACLS-trained nurse arrives, she'll expose the patient's chest and apply defibrillator pads if not already in place. The patient's cardiac rhythm will appear on the defibrillator monitor. If the patient is in ventricular fibrillation, ACLS protocol calls for defibrillation as soon as possible with 360 joules (monophasic energy) or 120 to 200 joules (biphasic energy) according to the manufacturer's recommendations. Be sure to continue CPR while the defibrillator is charging. Then resume CPR immediately after the shock is delivered. Perform a rhythm check after five cycles of CPR; if a rhythm is detected, perform a pulse check. The ACLS-trained nurse will act as code leader until the doctor arrives.[2]

■ After five cycles of CPR, check the patient's rhythm and, if necessary, administer another shock at the same or higher rate if using a biphasic defibrillator or at the same rate if using a monophasic defibrillator. Be sure to continue CPR while the defibrillator is charging. After another five cycles of CPR, check the patient's rhythm and give another shock at the same rate.

■ As CPR and defibrillation continue, you or an ACLS-trained nurse will then start two peripheral IV lines with large-bore IV catheters.[2] Avoid interrupting chest compressions for IV insertion. Be sure to use only a large vein, such as the antecubital vein, *to allow for rapid fluid administration and to prevent drug extravasation.*

■ As soon as the IV catheter is in place, begin an infusion of normal saline solution or lactated Ringer's solution *to help prevent circulatory collapse.*

■ Another team member will set up portable or wall suction equipment and suction the patient's oral secretions, as necessary, *to maintain an open airway.*

■ The ACLS-trained nurse will then prepare and administer emergency cardiac drugs, as needed. (See *AHA algorithm.*) Keep in mind that drugs administered through a central venous access catheter reach the myocardium more quickly than those administered through a peripheral line. Drugs administered should be followed by a 20-mL bolus of IV fluid *to facilitate the flow of the drug to central circulation.*[2]

■ The AHA algorithm shows the timing of both drug and shock administration. Drug doses should be given immediately after a rhythm check.[2]

■ If IV or intraosseous access can't be established, you may administer medications such as epinephrine, lidocaine, and vasopressin through an ET tube during cardiac arrest. To do so, dilute the drugs in 5 to 10 mL of normal saline solution or sterile water and then instill them into the patient's ET tube. *Studies have shown that dilution with sterile water, instead of normal saline solution, may improve absorption of epinephrine and lidocaine.* Afterward, ventilate the patient manually *to improve absorption by distributing the drug throughout the bronchial tree.*[2]

■ The ACLS-trained nurse will also prepare for, and assist with, ET intubation or other advanced airway placement. Compression interruption should be minimized during advanced airway placement.[2]

■ Suction the patient as needed. After the patient has been intubated, the health care provider should use a clinical assessment and a confirmation device such as an end-tidal carbon dioxide detector, continuous quantitative waveform capnography, or an esophageal detector. However, continuous quantitative waveform capnography is recommended[2] to confirm ET tube placement. Assessment includes visualization of chest expansion, auscultation for equal breath sounds, and auscultation for absent breath sounds over the epigastrium. When the tube is correctly positioned, tape it securely. *To serve as a reference,* mark the point on the tube that is level with the patient's lips. Document the tube location on the code record.[2]

■ Meanwhile, another member of the code team should keep a written record of the events. Other duties of the recorder include prompting participants about when to perform certain activities (such as when to check a pulse or take vital signs), overseeing the effectiveness of CPR, and keeping track of the time between therapies. Each team member should know what the other participant's role is *to prevent duplicating effort.* Finally, someone from the team should make sure that the primary nurse's other patients are reassigned to another nurse and that any family members present are cared for appropriately.

■ When the code is finished, remove and discard your gloves and perform hand hygiene.[3,4,5]

■ Document the procedure.[6]

Special considerations

■ If the family is at the facility during the code, have someone, ideally a clergy member or social worker, remain with them. Keep the family informed of the patient's status.

■ If the family isn't at the facility, contact them as soon as possible. Encourage them not to drive to the facility, but offer to call someone who can give them a ride.

■ When the patient's condition has stabilized, assess his level of consciousness, breath sounds, heart sounds, peripheral perfusion, bowel sounds, and urine output. Take his vital signs every 15 minutes, and monitor his cardiac rhythm continuously.[2]

■ Make sure the patient receives an adequate supply of oxygen, whether through a mask or a ventilator.[2]

AHA algorithm[2]

This American Heart Association (AHA) algorithm shows the guidelines for treating an adult in cardiac arrest.

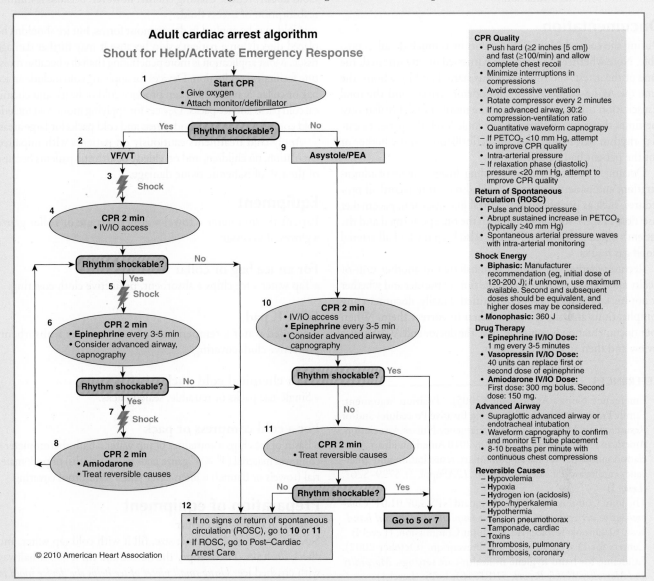

Adult cardiac arrest algorithm

Shout for Help/Activate Emergency Response

1
Start CPR
• Give oxygen
• Attach monitor/defibrillator

Rhythm shockable? — Yes / No

2 **VF/VT**

3 **Shock**

4 **CPR 2 min**
• IV/IO access

Rhythm shockable? — No / Yes

5 **Shock**

6 **CPR 2 min**
• **Epinephrine** every 3-5 min
• Consider advanced airway, capnography

Rhythm shockable? — No / Yes

7 **Shock**

8 **CPR 2 min**
• **Amiodarone**
• Treat reversible causes

9 **Asystole/PEA**

10 **CPR 2 min**
• IV/IO access
• **Epinephrine** every 3-5 min
• Consider advanced airway, capnography

Rhythm shockable? — Yes / No

11 **CPR 2 min**
• Treat reversible causes

Rhythm shockable? — No / Yes

Go to 5 or 7

12
• If no signs of return of spontaneous circulation (ROSC), go to **10** or **11**
• If ROSC, go to Post–Cardiac Arrest Care

© 2010 American Heart Association

CPR Quality
• Push hard (≥2 inches [5 cm]) and fast (≥100/min) and allow complete chest recoil
• Minimize interrruptions in compressions
• Avoid excessive ventilation
• Rotate compressor every 2 minutes
• If no advanced airway, 30:2 compression-ventilation ratio
• Quantitative waveform capnograpy
– If PETCO$_2$ <10 mm Hg, attempt to improve CPR quality
• Intra-arterial pressure
– If relaxation phase (diastolic) pressure <20 mm Hg, attempt to improve CPR quality

Return of Spontaneous Circulation (ROSC)
• Pulse and blood pressure
• Abrupt sustained increase in PETCO$_2$ (typically ≥40 mm Hg)
• Spontaneous arterial pressure waves with intra-arterial monitoring

Shock Energy
• **Biphasic:** Manufacturer recommendation (eg, initial dose of 120-200 J); if unknown, use maximum available. Second and subsequent doses should be equivalent, and higher doses may be considered.
• **Monophasic:** 360 J

Drug Therapy
• **Epinephrine IV/IO Dose:** 1 mg every 3-5 minutes
• **Vasopressin IV/IO Dose:** 40 units can replace first or second dose of epinephrine
• **Amiodarone IV/IO Dose:** First dose: 300 mg bolus. Second dose: 150 mg.

Advanced Airway
• Supraglottic advanced airway or endotracheal intubation
• Waveform capnography to confirm and monitor ET tube placement
• 8-10 breaths per minute with continuous chest compressions

Reversible Causes
– **H**ypovolemia
– **H**ypoxia
– **H**ydrogen ion (acidosis)
– **H**ypo-/hyperkalemia
– **H**ypothermia
– **T**ension pneumothorax
– **T**amponade, cardiac
– **T**oxins
– **T**hrombosis, pulmonary
– **T**hrombosis, coronary

■ Assist with transfer to the intensive care unit (if not there already). Check the infusion rates of all IV fluids, and use infusion pumps (preferably smart pumps with dose-range alerts) to deliver vasoactive drugs. *To evaluate the effectiveness of fluid therapy,* insert an indwelling catheter if the patient doesn't already have one. Also insert an NG tube *to relieve or prevent gastric distention.*

■ If appropriate, reassure the patient and explain what is happening. Allow the patient's family to visit as soon as possible. If the patient expires, notify the family and allow them to see the patient as soon as possible.

■ *To make sure your code team performs optimally,* schedule a time to review the code.

Complications

Even when performed correctly, CPR can cause fractured ribs, liver laceration, lung puncture, and gastric distention. Defibrillation can cause burns to the skin, and emergency intubation can result in esophageal or tracheal laceration, subcutaneous emphysema, or accidental right mainstem bronchus intubation. (Decreased or absent breath sounds on the left side of the chest and normal breath sounds on the right may signal accidental right mainstem bronchus intubation.)

Documentation

During the code, document the events in as much detail as possible. Note whether the arrest was witnessed or unwitnessed, the time of the arrest, the time CPR was started and by whom, the time the ACLS-trained nurse and doctor arrived, and the total resuscitation time. Also document the number of defibrillations, the times they were performed, the joule level, the patient's cardiac rhythm before and after the defibrillation, and whether or not the patient had a pulse.

Document all drug therapy, including dosages, routes of administration, and patient response. You'll also want to record all procedures, such as peripheral and central line insertion, pacemaker insertion, and ET tube insertion with the time performed and the patient's tolerance of the procedure. Also keep track of all arterial blood gas results.

Record whether the patient is transferred to another unit or facility along with his condition at the time of transfer and whether or not his family was present or notified. Finally, document any complications and the measures taken to correct them. When your documentation is complete, have the doctor and ACLS nurse review and then sign the document.

REFERENCES

1 Emergency Nurses Association. (2005). "Position Statement: Family Presence at the Bedside during Invasive Procedures and/or Resuscitation." Des Plaines, IL: Emergency Nurses Association.
2 American Heart Association. (2010). 2010 American Heart Association guidelines for cardiopulmonary resuscitation and emergency cardiovascular care. *Circulation, 122*(Suppl. 3), S729–S767. (Level I)
3 The Joint Commission. (2012). Standard NPSG.07.01.01. *Comprehensive accreditation manual for hospitals: The official handbook.* Oakbrook Terrace, IL: The Joint Commission. (Level I)
4 Centers for Disease Control and Prevention. (October 2002). Guideline for hand hygiene in health-care settings. *Morbidity and Mortality Weekly Report, 51*(RR-16), 1–45. (Level 1)
5 World Health Organization. (2009). *WHO guidelines on hand hygiene in health care: First global patient safety challenge. Clean care is safer care.* Geneva, Switzerland: World Health Organization. (Level I)
6 The Joint Commission. (2012). Standard RC.01.03.01. *Comprehensive accreditation manual for hospitals: The official handbook.* Oakbrook Terrace, IL: The Joint Commission. (Level I)

COLD APPLICATION

The application of cold constricts blood vessels; inhibits local circulation, suppuration, and tissue metabolism; relieves vascular congestion; slows bacterial activity in infections; reduces body temperature; and may act as a temporary anesthetic during brief, painful procedures. (See *Reducing pain with ice massage.*) Because treatment with cold also relieves inflammation, reduces edema, and slows bleeding, it may provide effective initial treatment after eye injuries, strains, sprains, bruises, muscle spasms, and burns. Cold doesn't reduce existing edema, however, because it inhibits reabsorption of excess fluid.

Cold may be applied in dry or moist forms, but ice shouldn't be placed directly on a patient's skin because it may further damage tissue. Moist application is more penetrating than dry because moisture facilitates conduction. Devices for applying cold include an ice bag or collar, K pad (which can produce cold or heat), and chemical cold packs and ice packs. Devices for applying moist cold include cold compresses for small body areas and cold packs for large areas.

Apply cold treatments cautiously on patients with impaired circulation, on children, and on elderly or arthritic patients because of the risk of ischemic tissue damage.

Equipment

Patient thermometer ▪ towel ▪ adhesive tape or roller gauze ▪ gloves, if necessary.

For an ice bag or collar

▪ Tap water ▪ ice chips ▪ absorbent, protective cloth covering.

For a K pad

▪ distilled water ▪ temperature-adjustment key ▪ absorbent, protective cloth covering.

For a chemical cold pack

▪ Single-use packs or reusable, sealed packs.

For a cold compress or pack

▪ Basin of ice chips ▪ container of tap water ▪ bath thermometer ▪ compress material (4″ × 4″ gauze pads or washcloths) or pack material (towels or flannel) ▪ linen-saver pad ▪ waterproof covering.

Preparation of equipment
For an ice bag or collar

Select a device of the correct size, fill it with cold tap water, and check for leaks. Then empty the device and fill it about halfway with crushed ice. *Using small pieces of ice helps the device mold to the patient's body.* Squeeze the device *to expel air that might reduce conduction.* Fasten the cap and wipe any moisture from the outside of the device. Wrap the bag or collar in a cloth covering, and secure the cover with tape or roller gauze. *The protective cover prevents tissue trauma and absorbs condensation.*

For a K pad

Check the cord for damage. Then fill the control unit two-thirds full with distilled water or to the level recommended by the manufacturer. Don't use tap water *because it leaves mineral deposits in the unit.* Check for leaks, and then tilt the unit several times *to clear the pad's tubing of air.* Tighten the cap. After ensuring that the hoses between the control unit and pad are free of tangles, place the unit on the bedside table, slightly above the patient *so gravity can assist water flow.* If the central supply department hasn't preset the temperature, use the temperature-adjustment key to adjust the control unit to the lowest temperature. Cover the pad with an absorbent, protective cloth and secure the cover with tape or roller gauze. Plug in the unit and turn it on. Allow the pad to cool for 2 minutes before placing it on the patient.

For a chemical cold pack
Select a pack of the appropriate size, and follow the manufacturer's directions (strike, squeeze, or knead) *to activate the cold-producing chemicals.* Make certain that the container hasn't been broken during activation. Remove a reusable pack from the freezer. Wrap the pack in a cloth cover, and secure the cover with tape or roller gauze.

For a cold compress or pack
Cool a container of tap water by placing it in a basin of ice or by adding ice to the water. Using a bath thermometer for guidance, adjust the water temperature to 59ϒF (15ϒC) or as ordered. Immerse the compress material or pack material in the water.

Implementation
- Verify the doctor's order.
- Gather the equipment.
- Confirm the patient's identity using at least two patient identifiers according to your facility's policy.[1]
- Explain the procedure to the patient, provide privacy, and make sure the room is warm and free from drafts.
- Perform hand hygiene and put on gloves, if appropriate.[2,3,4]
- Record the patient's temperature, pulse, and respirations *to serve as a baseline.*
- Expose only the treatment site *to avoid chilling the patient.*

Applying an ice bag or collar, a K pad, or a chemical cold pack
- Place the covered cold device on the treatment site and begin timing the application.
- Observe the site frequently for signs of tissue intolerance, such as blanching, mottling, cyanosis, maceration, or blisters. Also, be alert for shivering and complaints of burning or numbness. If these signs or symptoms develop, discontinue treatment and notify the doctor.
- Refill or replace the cold device as necessary *to maintain the correct temperature.* Change the protective cover if it becomes wet.
- Remove the device after the prescribed treatment period (usually 30 minutes).

Applying a cold compress or pack
- Place a linen-saver pad under the site.
- Remove the compress or pack from the water, and wring it out *to prevent dripping.* Apply it to the treatment site and begin timing the application.
- Cover the compress or pack with a waterproof covering *to provide insulation and to keep the surrounding area dry.* Secure the covering with tape or roller gauze *to prevent it from slipping.*
- Check the application site frequently for signs of tissue intolerance, and note any complaints of burning or numbness. If these issues develop, discontinue treatment and notify the doctor.

Reducing pain with ice massage

Normally, ice shouldn't be applied directly to a patient's skin *because it risks damaging the skin surface and underlying tissues.* However, when carefully performed, this technique—called ice massage—may help patients tolerate brief, painful procedures such as bone marrow aspiration, catheterization, chest tube removal, injection into joints, lumbar puncture, and suture removal.

Prepare for ice massage by gathering the ice, a porous covering to hold it in (if desired), and a cloth for wiping water from the patient as the ice melts. Water may be frozen in a paper cup ahead of time. The paper is removed from half the cup, exposing the ice to be used for the procedure.

Just before the procedure begins, rub the ice over the appropriate area *to numb it.* Assess the site frequently; stop rubbing immediately if you detect signs of tissue intolerance.

As the procedure begins, rub the ice over a point near but not at the site. *This action distracts the patient from the procedure itself and gives him another stimulus on which to concentrate.* If the procedure lasts longer than 10 minutes or if you think tissue damage may occur, move the ice to a different site and continue massage.

If you know in advance that the procedure probably will last longer than 10 minutes, massage the site intermittently—2 minutes of massage alternating with a rest period until the skin regains its normal color. Alternatively, you can divide the area into several sites and apply ice to each one for several minutes at a time.

- Change the compress or pack as needed *to maintain the correct temperature.* Remove it after the prescribed treatment period (usually 20 minutes).

Concluding all cold applications
- Remove the cold device, dry the patient's skin if needed, and re-dress the treatment site according to the doctor's orders. Then position the patient comfortably and take his temperature, pulse, and respirations *for comparison with baseline.*
- Dispose of liquids and soiled materials properly. If treatment will be repeated, clean and store the equipment in the patient's room, out of his reach; otherwise, return it to storage.
- Document the procedure.[5]

Special considerations
- Apply cold immediately after an injury *to minimize edema.* (See *Using cold for a muscle sprain,* page 188.) Although colder temperatures can be tolerated for a longer time when the treatment site is small, don't continue any application for longer than 1 hour *to avoid reflex vasodilation.* The application of temperatures below 59ϒF (15ϒC) also causes local reflex vasodilation.
- Use sterile technique when applying cold to an open wound or to a lesion that may open during treatment. Also, maintain

Using cold for a muscle sprain

Cold can help relieve pain and reduce edema during the first 24 to 72 hours after a sprain occurs. Tell the patient to apply cold to the area four times daily for 20 to 30 minutes each time.

For each application, instruct the patient to obtain enough crushed ice to cover the painful area, place it in a plastic bag, and place the bag inside a pillowcase or large piece of cloth, as shown at right.

For later applications, the patient may want to fill a paper cup with water, stand a tongue blade in the cup, and place it in the freezer. After the water freezes, he can peel the paper off the ice and hold it with the protruding handle. If he chooses this method, tell him to first cover the area with a cloth. *Applying ice directly to the skin can cause frostbite or cold shock.*

Instruct the patient to rub the ice over the painful area for the specified treatment time. Warn him that although ice eases pain in a joint that has begun to stiffen, he shouldn't let the analgesic effect encourage overuse of the joint.

After 24 to 72 hours, when heat and swelling have subsided or when cold no longer helps, the patient should switch to heat application.

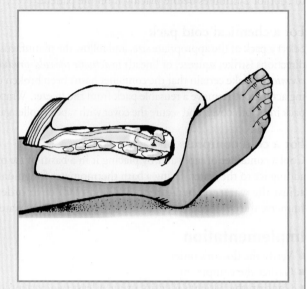

sterile technique during eye treatment, with separate sterile equipment for each eye *to prevent cross-contamination.*

■ Avoid securing cooling devices with pins *because an accidental puncture could allow extremely cold fluids to leak out and burn the patient's skin.*

■ If the patient is unconscious, anesthetized, neurologically impaired, irrational, or otherwise insensitive to cold, stay with him throughout the treatment and check the application site frequently for complications.

■ Warn the patient against placing ice directly on his skin *because the extreme cold can cause burns.*

Complications

Hemoconcentration may cause thrombi. Intense cold may cause pain, burning, or numbness.

Documentation

Record the time, date, and duration of cold application; type of device used (ice bag or collar, K pad, chemical cold pack, or cold compress or pack); site of application; temperature or temperature setting; patient's temperature, pulse, and respirations before and after application; skin appearance before, during, and after application; signs of complications; and the patient's tolerance of treatment.

REFERENCES

1 The Joint Commission. (2012). Standard NPSG.01.01.01. *Comprehensive accreditation manual for hospitals: The official handbook.* Oakbrook Terrace, IL: The Joint Commission. (Level I)

2 The Joint Commission. (2012). Standard NPSG.07.01.01. *Comprehensive accreditation manual for hospitals: The official handbook.* Oakbrook Terrace, IL: The Joint Commission. (Level I)

3 Centers for Disease Control and Prevention. (October 2002). Guideline for hand hygiene in health-care settings. *Morbidity and Mortality Weekly Report, 51*(RR-16), 1–45. (Level 1)

4 World Health Organization. (2009). *WHO guidelines on hand hygiene in health care: First global patient safety challenge. Clean care is safer care.* Geneva, Switzerland: World Health Organization. (Level I)

5 The Joint Commission. (2012). Standard RC.01.03.01. *Comprehensive accreditation manual for hospitals: The official handbook.* Oakbrook Terrace, IL: The Joint Commission. (Level I)

ADDITIONAL REFERENCES

Craven, R.F., & Hirnle, C.J. (2009). *Fundamentals of nursing: Human health and function* (6th ed.). Philadelphia, PA: Lippincott Williams & Wilkins.

Nettina, S.M. (2010). *Lippincott manual of nursing practice* (9th ed.). Philadelphia, PA: Lippincott Williams & Wilkins.

Taylor, C., et al. (2011). *Fundamentals of nursing: The art and science of nursing care* (7th ed.). Philadelphia, PA: Lippincott Williams & Wilkins.

COLOSTOMY AND ILEOSTOMY CARE

A patient with an ascending, transverse, or descending colostomy or an ileostomy must wear an external pouch to collect emerging fecal matter, which may be watery, pasty, or formed, depending on location of the stoma. Besides collecting waste matter, the pouch helps to control odor and protect the stoma and peristomal skin. Most disposable pouching systems can be used for

3 to 7 days; however, single-use, closed-end pouches should be changed more frequently.

All pouching systems need to be changed immediately if a leak develops, and every pouch needs emptying when it's one-third to one-half full. The patient with an ileostomy may need to empty his pouch four or five times daily.

The best time to change the pouching system is when the bowel is least active, usually in the morning before breakfast. After a few months, most patients can predict the best changing time.

The selection of a pouching system should take into consideration which system provides the best adhesive seal and skin protection for the individual patient. The type of pouch selected also depends on the stoma's location and structure, availability of supplies, wear time, consistency of effluent, personal preference, and finances.

Equipment

For appliance care
Pouching system ▪ scissors ▪ stoma measuring guide ▪ stoma paste or moldable barrier ring (if drainage is watery to pasty or if stoma secretes excess mucus) ▪ plastic bag ▪ water ▪ washcloth and towel ▪ closure clamp, if needed ▪ water or pouch cleaning solution ▪ gloves ▪ Optional: paper tape, clippers, liquid skin sealant, pouch deodorant.

Pouching systems may be drainable or closed-ended, disposable or reusable, adhesive-backed, and one-piece or two-piece. (See *Comparing ostomy pouching systems,* page 190.)

For pouch emptying
Bedpan, toilet, or measuring device ▪ gloves ▪ tissue ▪ Optional: pouch deodorant.

Implementation
▪ Gather the appropriate equipment.
▪ Confirm the patient's identity using at least two patient identifiers according to your facility's policy.[1]
▪ Perform hand hygiene and put on gloves.[2,3,4]
▪ Explain the procedure to the patient and answer any questions *to decrease anxiety and ensure cooperation.* As you perform each step, explain what you are doing and why *because the patient will eventually perform the procedure himself.*
▪ Provide privacy and emotional support.

Fitting the skin barrier and pouch
▪ For a pouch with an attached skin barrier, measure the stoma with the measuring guide. Select the opening size that matches the stoma.
▪ For an adhesive-backed pouch with a separate skin barrier, measure the stoma with the measuring guide and select the opening that matches the stoma. Trace the selected size opening onto the paper back of the skin barrier's adhesive side. Cut out the opening. (If the pouch has precut openings, which can be handy for a round stoma, select an opening that's ⅛″ larger than the stoma. If the pouch comes without an opening, cut the hole ⅛″ wider than the measured tracing.) The cut-to-fit system works best for an irregularly shaped stoma. (See *Applying a skin barrier and pouch,* page 191.)

Applying or changing the pouch
▪ Empty, remove, and discard the old pouch, if applicable (as shown below).

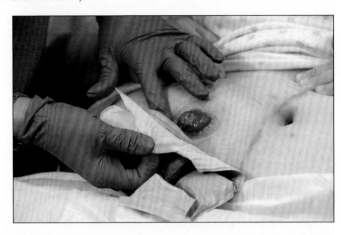

▪ Wipe the stoma and peristomal skin gently with a soft cloth or gauze (as shown below).

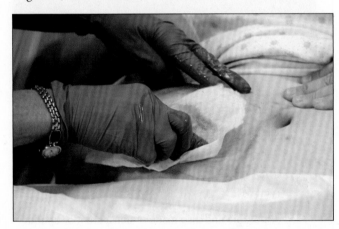

▪ Carefully wash with water and dry the peristomal skin by patting gently. Allow the skin to dry thoroughly. Inspect the peristomal skin and stoma (as shown below). If necessary, clip surrounding hair (in a direction away from the stoma) *to promote a better seal and avoid skin irritation from hair pulling against the adhesive.*

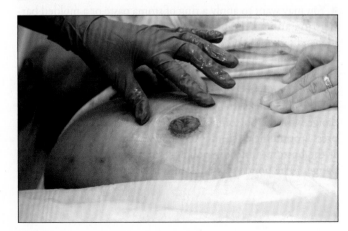

Comparing ostomy pouching systems

Manufactured in many shapes and sizes, ostomy pouches are fashioned for comfort, safety, and easy application. For example, a disposable closed-end pouch may meet the needs of a patient who irrigates his ostomy, who wants added security, or who wants to discard the pouch after each bowel movement. Another patient may prefer a reusable, drainable pouch. Some commonly available pouches are described below.

Disposable pouches

The patient who must empty his pouch often (because of diarrhea or a new colostomy or ileostomy) may prefer a one-piece, drainable, disposable pouch with a closure clamp attached to a skin barrier (as shown below). These transparent or opaque, odor-proof plastic pouches come with attached adhesive backing. Some pouches have microporous adhesive or belt tabs. The bottom opening allows for easy draining. This pouch may be used permanently or temporarily, until stoma size stabilizes.

A two-piece, drainable, disposable pouch with separate skin barrier (as shown below) permits more frequent pouch changes. Also made of transparent or opaque odor-proof plastic, this style comes with belt tabs and usually snaps to the skin barrier with a flange mechanism. Newer, two-piece pouches have an adhesive coupling. The pouch sticks to the wafer, allowing greater flexibility and comfort.

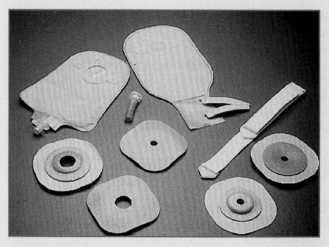

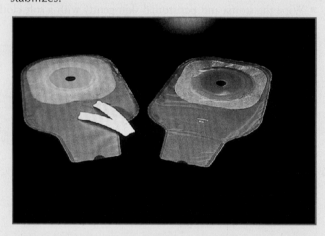

Also disposable and also made of transparent or opaque odor-proof plastic, a one-piece, disposable, closed-end pouch may come with a filter. A patient with a regular bowel elimination pattern may choose this style for additional security and confidence.

Reusable pouches

Typically manufactured from sturdy, opaque, hypoallergenic plastic, the reusable pouch comes with a separate custom-made faceplate and O-ring. The device has a 1- to 3-month life span, depending on how frequently the patient empties the pouch. Reusable equipment may benefit a patient who needs a firm faceplate or who wishes to minimize cost.

■ You may want to apply a ring of stoma paste or a molded barrier ring around the opening on the back of the skin barrier (depending on the product) *to provide extra skin protection.*

■ If applying a separate skin barrier, peel off the paper backing of the prepared skin barrier, center the barrier over the stoma, and press gently *to ensure adhesion.*

■ For a pouching system with flanges, align the lip of the pouch flange with the bottom edge of the skin barrier flange. Gently press around the circumference of the pouch flange, beginning at the bottom, until the pouch securely adheres to the barrier flange. (The pouch will click into its secured position.) Hold-

ing the barrier against the skin, gently pull on the pouch *to confirm the seal between flanges.*

■ Encourage the patient to stay quietly in position for about 5 minutes *to improve adherence. The patient's body warmth helps to improve adherence and soften a rigid skin barrier.*

■ Leave a bit of air in the pouch *to allow drainage to fall to the bottom.*

■ Apply the closure clamp, if necessary.

■ If desired, apply paper tape in a picture-frame fashion to the pouch edges *for additional security.*

Applying a skin barrier and pouch

Fitting a skin barrier and ostomy pouch properly can be done in a few steps. Shown below is a two-piece pouching system with flanges.

1. Measure the stoma using a measuring guide.

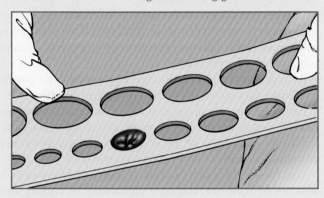

2. Trace the appropriate circle carefully on the back of the skin barrier.

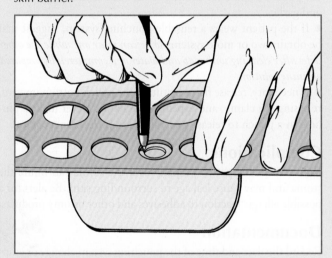

3. Cut the circular opening in the skin barrier. Smooth any rough edges with your finger.

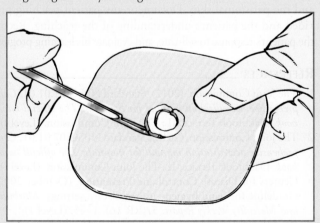

4. Remove the backing from the skin barrier and apply barrier paste or moldable barrier ring, as needed, along the edge of the circular opening.

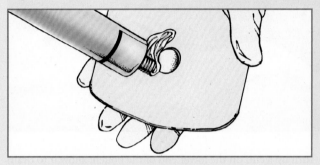

5. Center the skin barrier over the stoma, adhesive side down, and gently press it to the skin. When using a two-piece system, gently press the pouch opening onto the ring until it snaps into place.

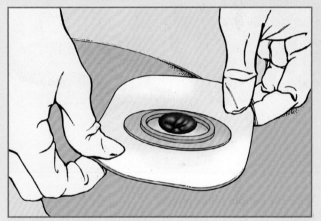

6. Close the bottom of the pouch by folding the end upward and using the clip that comes with the product or close the integrated closure system.

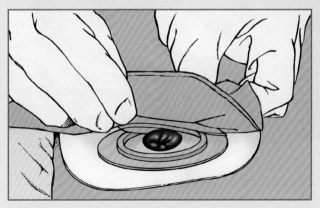

Emptying the pouch

■ Tilt the bottom of the pouch upward and remove the closure clamp or undo the integrated closure system (as shown below).

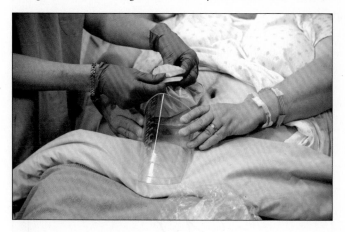

■ Turn up a cuff on the lower end of the pouch; allow it to drain into the toilet, bedpan, or measuring device (as shown below).

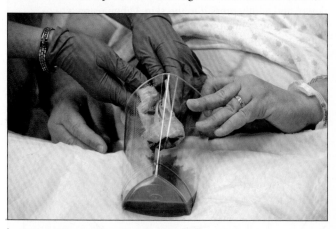

■ Wipe the bottom of the pouch.
■ Reapply the closure clamp or secure the integrated closure system (as shown below).

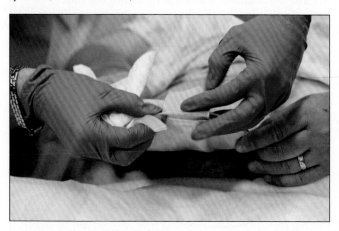

■ Discard the fecal material and clean the bedpan or measuring container appropriately.

Completing the procedure

■ Remove and discard your gloves and perform hand hygiene.[2,3,4]
■ Document the procedure.[6]

Special considerations

■ Avoid cutting the opening too big. *A large opening may expose the skin to fecal matter and moisture.*
■ Between 6 and 8 weeks after surgery, the stoma will shrink to its permanent size. At that point, pattern-making preparations will be unnecessary unless the patient gains weight, has additional surgery, or injures the stoma.
■ After performing and explaining the procedure to the patient, encourage the patient's increasing involvement in self-care.
■ Remove the pouching system if the patient reports burning or itching beneath it or purulent drainage around the stoma. Notify the doctor or therapist of any skin irritation, breakdown, rash, or unusual appearance of the stoma or peristomal area.
■ Use commercial pouch deodorants, if desired. However, most pouches are odor-free, and odor should only be evident when you empty the pouch or if it leaks. Before discharge, suggest that the patient avoid odor-causing foods such as fish, eggs, onions, and garlic.
■ If the patient wears a reusable pouching system, suggest that he obtain two or more systems *so he can wear one while the other dries after cleaning with soap and water or a commercially prepared cleaning solution.*
■ If necessary, release flatus by tilting the pouch bottom upward, releasing the clamp, and expelling the flatus. Never make a pinhole in a pouch to release gas. *This destroys the odor-proof seal.*

Complications

Failure to fit the pouch properly over the stoma can injure the stoma and may cause leakage to surrounding skin. Be alert for a possible allergic reaction to adhesives and other ostomy products.

Documentation

Record the date and time of the pouching system change or emptying; note the character of drainage, including color, amount, type, and consistency. Also describe the appearance of the stoma and the peristomal skin. Document any patient teaching provided and the patient's understanding of the teaching. Record the patient's response to self-care, and evaluate his learning progress.

REFERENCES

1 The Joint Commission. (2012). Standard NPSG.01.01.01. *Comprehensive accreditation manual for hospitals: The official handbook.* Oakbrook Terrace, IL: The Joint Commission. (Level I)
2 The Joint Commission. (2012). Standard NPSG.07.01.01. *Comprehensive accreditation manual for hospitals: The official handbook.* Oakbrook Terrace, IL: The Joint Commission. (Level I)
3 Centers for Disease Control and Prevention. (October 2002). Guideline for hand hygiene in health-care settings. *Morbidity and Mortality Weekly Report, 51*(RR-16), 1–45. (Level 1)
4 World Health Organization. (2009). *WHO guidelines on hand hygiene in health care: First global patient safety challenge. Clean care is safer care.* Geneva, Switzerland: World Health Organization. (Level I)

5 Occupational Safety and Health Administration. "Bloodborne Pathogens, Standard Number 1910.1030" [Online]. Accessed August 2011 via the Web at http://www.osha.gov/pls/oshaweb/owadisp.show_document?p_table=STANDARDS&p_id=10051

6 The Joint Commission. (2012). Standard RC.01.03.01. *Comprehensive accreditation manual for hospitals: The official handbook.* Oakbrook Terrace, IL: The Joint Commission. (Level I)

ADDITIONAL REFERENCES

Black, P. (2009). Choosing the correct stoma appliance. *British Journal of Nursing, 18*(4), S10, S12–S14.

Burch, J. (2009). An update on stoma appliance flanges and baseplates. *British Journal of Community Nursing, 14*(8), 338, 340–342.

Hocevar, B., & Gray, M. (2008). Intestinal diversion (colostomy or ileostomy) in patients with severe bowel dysfunction following spinal cord injury. *Journal of Wound, Ostomy, and Continence Nursing, 35*(2), 159–166.

Nettina, S.M. (2010). *Lippincott manual of nursing practice* (9th ed.). Philadelphia, PA: Lippincott Williams & Wilkins.

Pittman, J., et al. (2008). Demographic and clinical factors related to ostomy complication and quality of life in veterans with an ostomy. *Journal of Wound, Ostomy, and Continence Nursing, 35*(5), 493–503.

Taylor, C., et al. (2011). *Fundamentals of nursing: The art and science of nursing care* (7th ed.). Philadelphia, PA: Lippincott Williams & Wilkins.

COLOSTOMY IRRIGATION

Irrigation of a colostomy can serve two purposes: It allows a patient with a descending or sigmoid colostomy to regulate bowel function, and it cleans the large bowel before and after tests, surgery, or other procedures.

Colostomy irrigation may begin as soon as bowel function resumes after surgery. However, most clinicians recommend waiting until bowel movements are more predictable. Initially, the nurse or the patient irrigates the colostomy at the same time every day, recording the amount of output and any spillage between irrigations. Between 4 and 6 weeks may pass before colostomy irrigation establishes a predictable elimination pattern.

Colostomy irrigation is contraindicated in patients with bowel disease, irritable bowel syndrome, or severe heart or kidney disease.

Equipment

Colostomy irrigation set (contains an irrigation drain or sleeve, an ostomy belt [if needed] to secure the drain or sleeve, water-soluble lubricant, drainage pouch clamp, and irrigation bag with clamp, tubing, and cone tip) ▪ 1,000-mL (1 quart) of tap water irrigant warmed to about 105°F (40.6°C) ▪ IV pole or wall hook ▪ washcloth and towel ▪ water ▪ ostomy pouching system ▪ linen-saver pad ▪ gloves ▪ Optional: bedpan or chair, clip, small dressing or bandage, stoma cap.

Preparation of equipment

Set up the irrigation bag, tubing, and cone tip. If irrigation will take place with the patient in bed, place the bedpan beside the bed and elevate the head of the bed between 45 and 90 degrees, if allowed. If irrigation will take place in the bathroom, have the patient sit on the toilet or on a chair facing the toilet, whichever he finds more comfortable.

Fill the irrigation bag with warmed tap water. Hang the bag on the IV pole or wall hook. The bottom of the bag should be at the patient's shoulder level *to prevent the fluid from entering the bowel too quickly.* Most irrigation sets also have a clamp that regulates the flow rate.

Prime the tubing with irrigant *to prevent air from entering the colon and possibly causing cramps and gas pains.*

Implementation

▪ Verify the doctor's order.
▪ Confirm the patient's identity using at least two patient identifiers according to your facility's policy.[1]
▪ Explain every step of the procedure to the patient *because he'll eventually be irrigating the colostomy himself.*
▪ Provide privacy.
▪ Perform hand hygiene and put on gloves.[2,3,4]
▪ If the patient is in bed, place a linen-saver pad under him *to protect the sheets.*
▪ Remove the ostomy pouch if the patient uses one.
▪ Place the irrigation sleeve over the stoma. If the sleeve doesn't have an adhesive backing, secure the sleeve with an ostomy belt. If the patient has a two-piece pouching system with flanges, snap off the pouch and save it. Snap on the irrigation sleeve.
▪ Place the open-ended bottom of the irrigation sleeve in the bedpan or toilet *to promote drainage by gravity.*
▪ Lubricate your gloved small finger with water-soluble lubricant and insert the finger into the stoma. If you're teaching the patient, have him do this step *to determine the bowel angle at which to insert the cone safely.* Expect the stoma to tighten when the finger enters the bowel and then to relax in a few seconds.
▪ Lubricate the cone with water-soluble lubricant *to prevent it from irritating the mucosa.*
▪ Insert the cone into the top opening of the irrigation sleeve and then into the stoma. Angle the cone to match the bowel angle. Insert it gently but snugly; never force it in place.
▪ Unclamp the irrigation tubing and allow the water to flow slowly. If you don't have a clamp to control the irrigant's flow rate, pinch the tubing *to control the flow.* The water should enter the colon over 5 to 10 minutes.
▪ If the patient reports cramping, slow or stop the flow, keep the cone in place, and have the patient take a few deep breaths until the cramping stops. Cramping during irrigation may result from a bowel that's ready to empty, water that's too cold, a rapid flow rate, or air in the tubing.
▪ Have the patient remain stationary for 15 or 20 minutes *so that the initial effluent can drain.*
▪ If the patient is ambulatory, he can stay in the bathroom until all effluent empties, or he can clamp the bottom of the drainage sleeve with a clip and return to bed. Explain that *ambulation and activity stimulate elimination.* Suggest that the nonambulatory patient lean forward or massage his abdomen *to stimulate elimination.*

- Wait about 45 minutes for the bowel to finish eliminating the irrigant and effluent. Then remove the irrigation sleeve.
- Using a washcloth and water, gently clean the area around the stoma. Rinse and dry the area thoroughly with a clean towel.
- Inspect the skin and stoma for changes in appearance. Usually dark pink to red, stoma color may change with the patient's status. Notify the doctor of marked stoma color changes *because a pale hue may result from anemia, and substantial darkening suggests a change in blood flow to the stoma.*
- Apply a clean pouch. If the patient has a regular bowel elimination pattern, he may prefer a small dressing, bandage, or commercial stoma cap.
- Discard a disposable irrigation sleeve. Rinse a reusable irrigation sleeve and hang it to dry along with the irrigation bag, tubing, and cone.
- Remove and dispose of gloves and perform hand hygiene.[2,3,4]
- Document the procedure.[5]

Special considerations

- Irrigating a colostomy to establish a regular bowel elimination pattern doesn't work for all patients. If the bowel continues to move between irrigations, try decreasing the volume of irrigant. *Increasing the irrigant won't help because it serves only to stimulate peristalsis.* Keep a record of results. Also consider irrigating every other day.
- Irrigation may help to regulate bowel function in patients with a descending or sigmoid colostomy *because this is the bowel's stool storage area.* However, a patient with an ascending or transverse colostomy won't benefit from irrigation. Also, a patient with descending or sigmoid colostomy who's missing part of the ascending or transverse colon may not be able to irrigate successfully *because his ostomy may function like an ascending or transverse colostomy.*
- If diarrhea develops, discontinue irrigations until stools form again. Keep in mind that irrigation alone won't achieve regularity for the patient. He must also observe a complementary diet and exercise regimen.
- If the patient has a strictured stoma that prohibits cone insertion, remove the cone from the irrigation tubing and replace it with a soft silicone catheter. Angle the catheter gently 2″ to 4″ (5 to 10 cm) into the bowel to instill the irrigant. Don't force the catheter into the stoma, and don't insert it further than the recommended length *because you may perforate the bowel.*

Complications

Bowel perforation may result if a catheter is incorrectly inserted into the stoma. Fluid and electrolyte imbalances may result from using too much irrigant.

Documentation

Record the date and time of irrigation and the type and amount of irrigant. Note the stoma's color and the character of drainage, including the color, consistency, and amount. Record any patient teaching. Describe teaching content and the patient's response to self-care instruction. Evaluate the patient's learning progress.

REFERENCES

1 The Joint Commission. (2012). Standard NPSG.01.01.01. *Comprehensive accreditation manual for hospitals: The official handbook.* Oakbrook Terrace, IL: The Joint Commission. (Level I)
2 The Joint Commission. (2012). Standard NPSG.07.01.01. *Comprehensive accreditation manual for hospitals: The official handbook.* Oakbrook Terrace, IL: The Joint Commission. (Level I)
3 Centers for Disease Control and Prevention. (October 2002). Guideline for hand hygiene in health-care settings. *Morbidity and Mortality Weekly Report, 51*(RR-16), 1–45. (Level 1)
4 World Health Organization. (2009). *WHO guidelines on hand hygiene in health care: First global patient safety challenge. Clean care is safer care.* Geneva, Switzerland: World Health Organization. (Level I)
5 The Joint Commission. (2012). Standard RC.01.03.01. *Comprehensive accreditation manual for hospitals: The official handbook.* Oakbrook Terrace, IL: The Joint Commission. (Level I)

ADDITIONAL REFERENCES

Craven, R.F., & Hirnle, C.J. (2009). *Fundamentals of nursing: Human health and function* (6th ed.). Philadelphia, PA: Lippincott Williams & Wilkins.
Nettina, S.M. (2010). *Lippincott manual of nursing practice* (9th ed.). Philadelphia, PA: Lippincott Williams & Wilkins.
Salvadalena, G. (2008). Incidence of complications of the stoma and peristomal skin among individuals with colostomy, ileostomy, and urostomy: A systematic review. *Journal of Wound, Ostomy, and Continence Nursing, 35*(6), 596–607.
Taylor, C., et al. (2011). *Fundamentals of nursing: The art and science of nursing care* (7th ed.). Philadelphia, PA: Lippincott Williams & Wilkins.
Varma, S. (2009). Issues in irrigation for people with a permanent colostomy: A review. *British Journal of Nursing, 18*(4), S15–S18.

CONTACT LENS CARE

Illness or emergency treatment may require that you insert or remove and store a patient's contact lenses. Proper handling and lens care techniques help prevent eye injury and infection as well as lens loss or damage. Appropriate lens-handling techniques depend in large part on what type of lenses the patient wears.

All contact lenses float on the corneal tear layer. Soft lenses have diameters typically exceeding the diameter of the cornea; rigid lenses have diameters that are typically smaller than the cornea. Because they're larger and more pliable, soft lenses tend to mold themselves more closely to the eye for a more stable fit than rigid lenses.

Modes of lens wear vary widely. Although most patients remove and clean their lenses daily, some wear lenses overnight or for several days (sometimes up to a month) without removing them for cleaning. Still other patients wear disposable lenses, which means that they replace old lenses with new ones at regular intervals (a few days to a few months), possibly without removing them for cleaning between replacements.

Keep in mind that handling contact lenses improperly can provide a direct source of contamination or injury to the eye.

Equipment

Patient's own equipment for contact lens care, if available ■ towel ■ lens storage case or two small medicine cups ■ adhesive tape ■ gloves ■ sterile normal saline solution or soaking solution ■ flashlight, if needed.

Preparation of equipment

If a commercial lens storage case isn't available, place enough sterile normal saline solution into two small medicine cups to submerge a lens in each one. *To avoid confusing the left and right lenses,* which may have different prescriptions, mark one cup "L" and the other cup "R" and place the corresponding lens in each cup.

Implementation

■ Confirm the patient's identity using at least two patient identifiers according to your facility's policy.[1]
■ Tell the patient what you're about to do, perform hand hygiene, and put on gloves *to help prevent ocular infection.*[2,3,4]
■ Place a towel on the patient's chest.

Inserting soft lenses

■ *To see if the lens is inside out,* bend it between your thumb and index finger or fill it with saline or soaking solution. If the lens tends to roll inward or the edge points slightly inward, it's oriented correctly. If the edge points outward or the lens tends to collapse over your fingertip, it's probably inside out and should be reversed.
■ Wet the lens with fresh normal saline solution and rub it gently between your thumb and index finger, or place it on your palm and rub it with your opposite index finger. Rinse well.
■ Place the lens, convex side down, on the tip of the index finger of your dominant hand.
■ Instruct the patient to gaze upward slightly.
■ Separate the eyelids with your other thumb and index finger, and place the lens on the sclera, just below the cornea. Then, slide the lens gently upward with your finger until it centers on the cornea.
■ Using the same procedure, insert the opposite lens.

Inserting rigid lenses

■ Wet one lens with solution and gently rub it between your thumb and index finger, or place it on your palm and rub it with your opposite index finger. Rinse well with the solution, leaving a small amount in the lens.
■ Place the lens, convex side down, on the tip of the index finger of your dominant hand.
■ Instruct the patient to gaze upward slightly.
■ Separate the eyelids with your other thumb and index finger, and place the lens directly and gently on the cornea. You need not press it to the eye; the tear film will attract it naturally at the first touch. Using the same procedure, insert the opposite lens.

Removing soft lenses

■ Place the patient in the supine position.
■ Tell the patient what you're about to do.

■ Using your nondominant hand, raise the patient's upper eyelid and hold it against the orbital rim (as shown below).

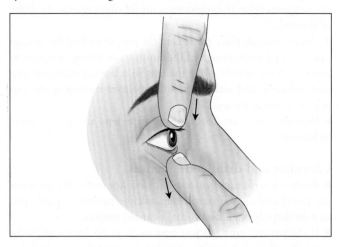

■ Lightly place the forefinger of your other hand on the lens and move it down onto the sclera below the cornea.
■ Pinch the lens between your forefinger and thumb; it should pop off (as shown below).

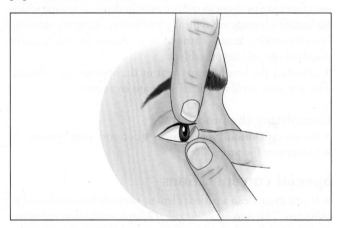

■ Place the lens in the proper well of the storage case with enough of the appropriate storage solution to cover it. Alternatively, place the lens in a labeled medicine cup with solution, and secure adhesive tape over the top of the cup *to prevent loss of the lens.*
■ Remove and care for the other lens using the same technique.

Removing rigid lenses

■ Before removing a lens, position the patient supine *to prevent the lens from popping out onto the floor, risking loss or damage.*
■ Tell the patient what you're about to do.
■ Place one thumb against the patient's upper eyelid and the other thumb against the lower eyelid.
■ Move the eyelids toward each other while gently pressing inward against the eye to trap the lens edge and break the suction. Extract the lens from the patient's eyelashes.
■ Depending on the lens type and thickness, it may pop out when the suction breaks. You may want to try to break the suction with one hand while cupping the other hand below the patient's eye to catch the lens as it falls.

■ Sometimes the lens will pop out on its own if you ask the patient to blink after stretching the corner of the eyelids toward the temporal bone, thus tightening the lid edges against the globe of the eye.

■ After removal, place the lens in the proper well of the storage case (L or R) with enough of the appropriate storage solution to cover it. Alternatively, place the lens in a labeled medicine cup with solution, and secure adhesive tape over the top of the cup *to prevent loss of the lens.*

■ Remove and care for the opposite lens using the same technique.

Cleaning and disinfecting lenses

■ *Because lens-cleaning steps vary with lens type and with each manufacturer's and doctor's instructions,* ask the patient to guide you step-by-step through his normal cleaning routine.

■ If the patient can't tell you how to clean his lenses properly, remember that all lens types require two steps: cleaning and disinfection.

■ Clean the lens by rubbing it with a surfactant solution designed to remove most surface deposits. For most patients, especially those who wear soft lenses, the cleaning step may also include use of an enzyme agent to remove protein deposits against which surfactant cleaners are typically ineffective. Enzyme cleaning involves soaking lenses overnight in a solution in which you've dissolved special enzyme tablets.

■ Disinfect the lens by using heat or the appropriate solution. *This step aims to rid the lens of infectious organisms.*

Completing the procedure

■ Remove and discard your gloves and perform hand hygiene.[2,3,4]

■ Document the procedure.[5]

Special considerations

■ If you must clean a patient's lenses, use only his own brand of solutions. *This minimizes the risk of allergic reactions to substances included in other solution brands.* Never touch the nozzle of a solution bottle to the lens, to your fingers, or to anything else *to avoid contaminating the solution in the bottle.*

■ If the patient's eyes appear dry or you have trouble moving the lens on the eye, instill several drops of sterile normal saline solution and wait a few minutes before trying again to remove the lens *to prevent corneal damage.* If you still can't remove the lens easily, notify the doctor. Avoid instilling eye medication while the patient is wearing lenses. *The lenses could trap the medication, possibly causing eye irritation or lens damage.*

■ Don't allow soft lenses, which are 40% to 60% water, to dry out. If they do, soak them in sterile normal saline solution and they may return to their natural shape.

■ If an unconscious patient is admitted to the emergency department, check for contact lenses by opening each eyelid and searching with a small flashlight. If you detect lenses, remove them immediately *because tears can't circulate freely beneath the lenses with eyelids closed, possibly leading to corneal oxygen depletion or infection.*

■ If a patient can't provide adequate care for his lenses during hospitalization, encourage him to send them home with a family member. If you aren't sure how to care for the lenses in the interim, store them in sterile normal saline solution until the family member can take them home.

Patient teaching

Advise contact lens wearers to carry appropriate identification *to speed lens removal and ensure proper care in an emergency.*

Documentation

Record eye condition before and after removal of lenses; the time of lens insertion, removal, and cleaning; the location of stored lenses; and, if applicable, the removal of lenses from the facility by a family member.

REFERENCES

1 The Joint Commission. (2012). Standard NPSG.01.01.01. *Comprehensive accreditation manual for hospitals: The official handbook.* Oakbrook Terrace, IL: The Joint Commission. (Level I)

2 The Joint Commission. (2012). Standard NPSG.07.01.01. *Comprehensive accreditation manual for hospitals: The official handbook.* Oakbrook Terrace, IL: The Joint Commission. (Level I)

3 Centers for Disease Control and Prevention. (October 2002). Guideline for hand hygiene in health-care settings. *Morbidity and Mortality Weekly Report, 51*(RR-16), 1–45. (Level 1)

4 World Health Organization. (2009). *WHO guidelines on hand hygiene in health care: First global patient safety challenge. Clean care is safer care.* Geneva, Switzerland: World Health Organization. (Level I)

5 The Joint Commission. (2012). Standard RC.01.03.01. *Comprehensive accreditation manual for hospitals: The official handbook.* Oakbrook Terrace, IL: The Joint Commission. (Level I)

ADDITIONAL REFERENCE

Craven, R.F., & Hirnle, C.J. (2009). *Fundamentals of nursing: Human health and function* (6th ed.). Philadelphia, PA: Lippincott Williams & Wilkins.

CONTACT PRECAUTIONS

Contact precautions are used to prevent the spread of microorganisms that are spread by direct or indirect contact with the patient or the patient's environment. (See *Conditions requiring contact precautions.*) Effective contact precautions require a single room, if possible, and the use of gloves and gowns by anyone having contact with the patient, the patient's support equipment, or items that have come in contact with the patient or the patient's environment.[1] Proper hand hygiene and handling and disposal of articles that have come in contact with the patient and his environment are essential.

Equipment

Gloves ■ gowns ■ isolation sign ■ plastic bags ■ any additional supplies needed for patient care, such as a thermometer, stethoscope, blood pressure cuff, and clean dressings.

(*Text continues on page 201.*)

Conditions requiring contact precautions[1]

The Centers for Disease Control and Prevention recommends contact precautions for patients who are infected or colonized (positive for the microorganism without clinical signs or symptoms of infection) with epidemiologically important organisms that can be transmitted by direct or indirect contact.

CONDITION	PRECAUTIONARY PERIOD	SPECIAL CONSIDERATIONS (IF APPLICABLE)
Abscess, major draining	■ Duration of illness or until drainage stops or can be contained by a dressing	■ Droplet precautions should be added for the first 24 hours of appropriate antibiotic therapy if invasive group A streptococcal disease is suspected.
Acute viral (acute hemorrhagic) conjunctivitis	■ Duration of illness	
Adenovirus gastroenteritis in a diapered or incontinent patient	■ Duration of illness or a duration that's appropriate to control a facility outbreak	
Adenovirus pneumonia	■ Duration of illness	■ Droplet precautions should also be instituted. ■ Precautions should be extended in immunocompromised patients because viral shedding is prolonged.
Avian influenza	■ For 14 days after onset of signs and symptoms or until an alternate diagnosis is confirmed	■ Airborne precautions should also be implemented. ■ Eye protection should be worn by individuals within 3″ (1 m) of the patient.
Bronchiolitis	■ Duration of illness	
Burkholderia cepacia pneumonia in a patient with cystic fibrosis	■ Unknown	■ Contact precautions should also be instituted for patients with cystic fibrosis whose respiratory tracts are colonized with bacteria. ■ Exposure to other patients with cystic fibrosis should be avoided.
Campylobacter species gastroenteritis in a diapered or incontinent patient	■ Duration of illness or a duration that's appropriate to control a facility outbreak	
Cholera gastroenteritis in a diapered or incontinent patient	■ Duration of illness or a duration that's appropriate to control a facility outbreak	
Clostridium difficile gastroenteritis	■ Duration of illness	■ Discontinue antibiotic use, if appropriate. *Antibiotics change the normal intestinal flora, making it more susceptible to* C. difficile. ■ Environmental cleaning and disinfection should be done consistently; a hypochlorite solution may be required if transmission continues. ■ Hand washing with soap and water is preferred because alcohol-based hand rubs aren't effective against *C. difficile* spores.

(continued)

Conditions requiring contact precautions (continued)

CONDITION	PRECAUTIONARY PERIOD	SPECIAL CONSIDERATIONS (IF APPLICABLE)
Cryptosporidium species gastroenteritis in a diapered or incontinent patient	■ Duration of illness or a duration that's appropriate to control a facility outbreak	
Diphtheria, cutaneous	■ Until two cultures (obtained 24 hours apart) are negative	
Escherichia coli gastroenteritis (0157:H7 and other Shiga toxin–producing strains, other species) in a diapered or incontinent patient	■ Duration of illness or a duration that's appropriate to control a facility outbreak	
Enteroviral infection in a diapered or incontinent patient	■ Duration of illness	
Giardia lamblia gastroenteritis in a diapered or incontinent patient	■ Duration of illness or a duration that's appropriate to control a facility outbreak	
Hepatitis type A	■ Duration of hospitalization in infants and children younger than age 3 years ■ For 2 weeks after the onset of signs and symptoms in children ages 3 to 14 years ■ For 1 week after the onset of signs and symptoms in children older than age 14 years	
Hepatitis type E in a diapered or incontinent patient	■ Duration of illness	
Herpes simplex, neonatal	■ Until lesions are dry and crusted ■ For asymptomatic, exposed neonates, until cultures obtained at 24 and 36 hours of age are negative; incubation required for 48 hours	
Herpes zoster, disseminated disease or localized disease in an immunocompromised patient	■ Duration of illness or until disseminated disease is ruled out in the immunocompromised patient	■ Airborne precautions should also be implemented. ■ Susceptible health care workers shouldn't enter the room if immune staff members are available.
Human metapneumovirus	■ Duration of illness	
Impetigo	■ For 24 hours after initiation of effective therapy	
Monkeypox	■ Until lesions are crusted	■ Airborne precautions should also be implemented until monkeypox is confirmed and smallpox is ruled out.

Conditions requiring contact precautions *(continued)*

CONDITION	PRECAUTIONARY PERIOD	SPECIAL CONSIDERATIONS (IF APPLICABLE)
Multidrug-resistant organism (MDRO) infection or colonization (such as with methicillin-resistant *Staphylococcus aureus,* vancomycin-resistant enterococcus, vancomycin intermediate-resistant *S. aureus,* vancomycin-resistant *S. aureus,* extended beta-lactamase producers, and resistant *Streptococcus pneumoniae*)	■ Duration specified by your facility's infection control program, which is based on local, state, regional, and national recommendations	■ Following standard precautions only may be permitted in some areas. ■ For guidance concerning new or emerging MDROs, consult your state or local health department.
Mycobacterium tuberculosis, draining extrapulmonary lesion	■ Until patient improves clinically and drainage has stopped or until three consecutive drainage cultures test negative	■ Airborne precautions should also be implemented. ■ Active pulmonary tuberculosis should be ruled out.
Norovirus gastroenteritis in a diapered or incontinent patient	■ Duration of illness or a duration that's appropriate to control a facility outbreak	■ Those who clean areas that are heavily contaminated with feces or vomitus should wear a mask. ■ Environmental cleaning and disinfection should be done consistently, with special attention given to restrooms; a hypochlorite solution may be required if transmission continues.
Parainfluenza virus infection in an infant or young child	■ Duration of illness	■ Viral shedding may be prolonged in immunocompromised patients. ■ Antigen testing to determine when contact precautions can be discontinued may be unreliable.
Pediculosis (head lice infestation)	■ For 4 hours after the initiation of effective therapy	
Poliomyelitis	■ Duration of illness	
Pressure ulcer; major, draining	■ Duration of illness ■ Until drainage stops or wound drainage can be contained	
Respiratory syncytial virus infection in an infant, young child, or immunocompromised adult	■ Duration of illness	■ Viral shedding may be prolonged in immunocompromised patients. ■ Antigen testing to determine when contact precautions can be discontinued may be unreliable.
Ritter's disease (staphylococcal scaled skin syndrome)	■ Duration of illness	■ Health care workers may be a source of nursery or neonatal intensive care unit outbreaks.
Rotavirus gastroenteritis	■ Duration of illness	■ Environmental cleaning and disinfection should be done consistently. ■ Soiled diapers should be changed and disposed of frequently. ■ Viral shedding may be prolonged in children and the elderly.

(continued)

Conditions requiring contact precautions *(continued)*

CONDITION	PRECAUTIONARY PERIOD	SPECIAL CONSIDERATIONS (IF APPLICABLE)
Rubella, congenital syndrome	■ Until the child is 1 year old or until nasopharyngeal and urine cultures are repeatedly negative after age 3 months	
Salmonella species gastroenteritis, diapered or incontinent patient	■ Duration of illness or a duration that's appropriate to control a facility outbreak	
Scabies	■ For 24 hours following initiation of effective therapy	
Severe acute respiratory syndrome	■ Duration of illness plus 10 days after fever resolves (provided respiratory signs and symptoms have improved or resolved)	■ Airborne precautions should also be implemented.
Shigella species gastroenteritis in a diapered or incontinent patient	■ Duration of illness or a duration that's appropriate to control a facility outbreak	
Staphylococcus aureus enterocolitis in a diapered or incontinent child	■ Duration of illness	
Staphylococcus aureus–infected draining major skin wound or burn	■ Duration of illness	
Streptococcus group A–infected draining major skin wound or burn	■ For 24 hours following initiation of effective therapy	■ Droplet precautions should also be initiated.
Vaccinia, eczema; fetal, generalized, or progressive	■ Until lesions are dry and crusted and scabs are separated	
Vaccinia blepharitis or conjunctivitis with copious drainage	■ Until drainage ceases	
Vibrio parahaemolyticus gastroenteritis in a diapered or incontinent patient	■ Duration of illness or a duration that's appropriate to control a facility outbreak	
Yersinia enterocolitica gastroenteritis in a diapered or incontinent patient	■ Duration of illness or a duration that's appropriate to control a facility outbreak	
Zoster (chickenpox, disseminated zoster, or localized zoster in an immunodeficient patient)	■ Until all lesions are crusted; requires airborne precautions	

Preparation of equipment

Place contact precaution supplies outside the patient's room in a wall- or door-mounted cabinet, a cart, or an anteroom.

Implementation

- Perform hand hygiene and put on a gown and gloves before entering the patient's room. Instruct any visitors to do the same according to your facility's policy.[2,3,4]
- Confirm the patient's identity using at least two patient identifiers according to your facility's policy.[5]
- Situate the patient in a single room with private toilet facilities and an anteroom, if possible. If necessary, two patients with the same infection may share a room; however, consult with your facility's infection preventionist before placing two patients together.[1]
- Explain isolation procedures to the patient and his family *to ease patient anxiety and promote cooperation.*
- Place a contact precautions sign on the door according to your facility's policy *to notify anyone entering the room of the situation.*
- Always change gloves after contact with a contaminated body site or contact with body fluids, excretions, mucous membranes, nonintact skin, and wound dressings. Perform hand hygiene after removing used gloves and before putting on new gloves.[2,3,4]
- Handle all items that have come in contact with the patient as you would for a patient on standard precautions.[1]
- Limit the patient's movement from the room. If the patient must be moved, cover any infected areas with clean dressings.[1] Notify the receiving department or area of the patient's isolation precautions *so that the precautions will be maintained and the patient can be returned to the room promptly.*
- Remove and discard your gown and gloves before leaving the room.[1]
- Perform hand hygiene after leaving the patient's room.[2,3,4]
- Document initiating contact precautions.[6]

Special considerations

- Clean and disinfect equipment that must be used for different patients in between each patient use according to your facility's policy *to prevent cross-contamination.* Clean and disinfect the patient's room when he has been discharged.[1]
- Try to dedicate certain reusable equipment (thermometer, stethoscope, blood pressure cuff) for the patient in contact precautions *to reduce the risk of transmitting infection to other patients.*[1]
- Hand washing with soap and water is required for *Clostridium difficile* enteric infection *because alcohol-based hand rubs don't have sporicidal activity.* Alcohol-based hand rubs are also less effective with noroviruses.[1]

Patient teaching

Teach the patient and his family about the importance of hand hygiene in preventing the spread of infection and about other measures to prevent the spread of multidrug-resistant organisms.

Complications

Social isolation is a complication of contact precautions. Ineffective contact precautions may result in the spread of an organism.

Documentation

Record the need for contact precautions on the nursing care plan and as otherwise indicated by your facility. Document initiation and maintenance of the precautions, the patient's tolerance of the procedure, and any patient or family teaching provided and their understanding of your teaching. Also document the date contact precautions were discontinued.

REFERENCES

1 Siegel, J.D., et al. "2007 Guideline for Isolation Precautions: Preventing Transmission of Infectious Agents in Healthcare Settings" [Online]. Accessed June 2011 via the Web at http://www.cdc.gov/hicpac/2007ip/2007isolationprecautions.html (Level I)
2 The Joint Commission. (2012). Standard NPSG.07.01.01. *Comprehensive accreditation manual for hospitals: The official handbook.* Oakbrook Terrace, IL: The Joint Commission. (Level I)
3 Centers for Disease Control and Prevention. (October 2002). Guideline for hand hygiene in health-care settings. *Morbidity and Mortality Weekly Report, 51*(RR-16), 1–45. (Level 1)
4 World Health Organization. (2009). *WHO guidelines on hand hygiene in health care: First global patient safety challenge. Clean care is safer care.* Geneva, Switzerland: World Health Organization. (Level I)
5 The Joint Commission. (2012). Standard NPSG.01.01.01. *Comprehensive accreditation manual for hospitals: The official handbook.* Oakbrook Terrace, IL: The Joint Commission. (Level I)
6 The Joint Commission. (2012). Standard RC.01.03.01. *Comprehensive accreditation manual for hospitals: The official handbook.* Oakbrook Terrace, IL: The Joint Commission. (Level I)

ADDITIONAL REFERENCES

Craven, R.F., & Hirnle, C.J. (2009). *Fundamentals of nursing: Human health and function* (6th ed.). Philadelphia, PA: Lippincott Williams & Wilkins.
The Joint Commission. (2012). Standard IC.02.01.01. *Comprehensive accreditation manual for hospitals: The official handbook.* Oakbrook Terrace, IL: The Joint Commission.

CONTINENT ILEOSTOMY CARE

An alternative to conventional ileostomy, a continent, or pouch, ileostomy (also called a *Koch ileostomy* or an *ileal pouch*) features an internal reservoir fashioned from the terminal ileum. This procedure may be used for a patient who requires proctocolectomy for chronic ulcerative colitis or multiple polyposis. Other patients may have a traditional ileostomy converted to a continent ileostomy. This procedure is contraindicated in Crohn's disease or gross obesity. Patients who need emergency surgery and those who can't care for the pouch are also unlikely to have this procedure.

The length of preoperative hospitalization varies with the patient's condition. Nursing responsibilities include providing bowel preparation, antibiotic therapy, and emotional support. After surgery, nursing responsibilities include ensuring patency of the drainage catheter, assessing GI function, caring for the stoma and peristomal skin, managing pain resulting from surgery, and, if necessary, perineal skin care.

Understanding pouch construction

Depending on the patient and related factors during intestinal surgery, the doctor may construct a pouch to collect fecal matter internally. To make such a pouch, the doctor loops about 12″ (30.5 cm) of ileum and sutures the inner sides together.

He opens the loop with a U-shaped cut and seams the inside to create a smooth lining. Then he fashions a nipple or valve between what is becoming the pouch and what will be the stoma. He folds the open ileum over, sews the pouch closed, and fixes the pouch to the abdominal wall.

Because the pouch holds fecal matter in reserve, the patient benefits from not having to change and empty ostomy equipment. Instead, he empties and irrigates the pouch as needed by inserting a catheter though the stoma and into the pouch.

Initially after surgery, the nurse performs this procedure until the patient can do it himself.

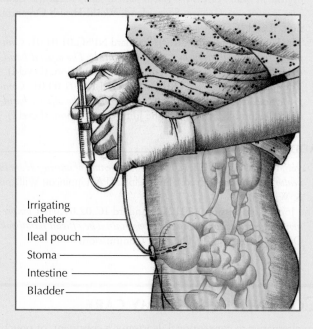

Irrigating catheter

Ileal pouch

Stoma

Intestine

Bladder

Patient teaching on pouch intubation and drainage usually begins soon after surgery. Continuous drainage is maintained for about 2 to 6 weeks to allow the suture lines to heal. During this period, a drainage catheter is attached to low intermittent suction. After the suture line heals, the patient learns how to drain the pouch himself.

Equipment

Leg drainage bag ▪ bedside drainage bag ▪ normal saline solution ▪ 50-mL catheter-tip syringe ▪ continent ileostomy catheter ▪ 20-mL syringe with adapter ▪ 4″ × 4″ × 1″ foam dressing and Montgomery straps ▪ precut drain dressing ▪ gloves ▪ water-soluble lubricant ▪ graduated container ▪ skin sealant ▪ Optional: commercial catheter securement device, gown.

Implementation

Preoperative care
▪ Confirm the patient's identity using at least two patient identifiers according to your facility's policy.[1]
▪ Perform hand hygiene.[2,3,4]
▪ Reinforce and, if necessary, supplement the doctor's explanation of a continent ileostomy and its implications for the patient. (See *Understanding pouch construction.*)
▪ Assess patient and family attitudes related to the operation and to the forthcoming changes in the patient's body image.
▪ Provide encouragement and support. Answer all questions as completely as possible.

Postoperative care
▪ Perform hand hygiene and put on gloves.[2,3,4]
▪ Confirm the patient's identity using at least two patient identifiers according to your facility's policy.[1]
▪ Attach the drainage catheter emerging from the ileostomy to continuous gravity drainage. (Attach a leg drainage bag to the patient's thigh during ambulation.)
▪ Irrigate the catheter with 30 mL of normal saline solution, as ordered and needed, *to prevent catheter obstruction and allow fluid return by gravity.* During the early postoperative period, keep the pouch empty; drainage will be serosanguineous.
▪ Monitor fluid intake and output.
▪ Check the catheter frequently once the patient begins eating solid food *to ensure that neither mucus nor undigested food particles block it.*
▪ If the patient complains of abdominal cramps, distention, and nausea—signs and symptoms of bowel obstruction—the catheter may be clogged. Gently irrigate with 20 to 30 mL of water or normal saline solution until the catheter drains freely. Then move the catheter slightly or rotate it gently *to help clear the obstruction.* Finally, try milking the catheter. If these measures fail, notify the doctor.
▪ Check the stoma frequently for color, edema, and bleeding. Normally pink to red, a stoma that turns dark red or blue-red may have a compromised blood supply.
▪ Provide stoma and peristomal skin care.
▪ Remove the dressing, gently clean the peristomal area with water, and pat dry. Use a skin sealant around the stoma *to prevent skin irritation.*
▪ Remove and discard gloves. Perform hand hygiene and put on new gloves.[2,3,4]
▪ Apply a new stoma dressing. One technique is to slip a precut drain dressing around the catheter to cover the stoma. Cut a hole slightly larger than the lumen of the catheter in the center of a 4″ × 4″ × 1″ piece of foam.
▪ Disconnect the catheter from the drainage bag and insert the distal end of the catheter through the hole in the foam. Slide the foam pad onto the dressing.
▪ Secure the foam in place with Montgomery straps. Secure the catheter by wrapping the strap ties around it or by using a commercial catheter securement device. Then reconnect the catheter to the drainage bag. (The drainage catheter will be removed by the surgeon when he determines that the suture line has healed.)
▪ Assess the peristomal skin for irritation from moisture.

- Remove and discard gloves. Perform hand hygiene.[2,3,4]
- Document the procedure.[5]

Draining the pouch
- Confirm the patient's identity using at least two patient identifiers according to your facility's policy.[1]
- Provide privacy and explain the procedure to the patient.
- Perform hand hygiene and put on gloves.[2,3,4]
- Have the patient with a pouch conversion sit on the toilet *to help him feel more at ease during the procedure.*
- Remove the stoma dressing.
- Encourage the patient to relax his abdominal muscles *to allow the catheter to slide easily into the pouch.*
- Lubricate the drainage catheter tip with the water-soluble lubricant and insert it in the stoma. Gently push the catheter downward. (The direction of insertion may vary depending on the patient.)
- When the catheter reaches the nipple valve of the internal pouch or reservoir (after about 2″ or 2½″ [5 or 6.5 cm]), you'll feel resistance. Instruct the patient to take a deep breath as you exert gentle pressure on the catheter to insert it through the valve. If this fails, have the patient lie supine and rest for a few minutes. Then, with the patient still supine, try to insert the catheter again.
- Gently advance the catheter to the suture marking made by the surgeon.
- Let the pouch drain completely. This usually takes 5 to 10 minutes. With thick drainage or a clogged catheter, the process may take 30 minutes.
- If the tube clogs, irrigate with 30 mL of water or normal saline using the 50-mL catheter-tip syringe. Also, rotate and milk the tube. If these steps fail, remove, rinse, and reinsert the catheter.
- Remove the catheter after completing drainage.
- Rinse the catheter thoroughly with warm water.
- Clean the peristomal area and apply a fresh stoma dressing.
- Remove and discard your gloves. Perform hand hygiene.[2,3,4]
- Document the procedure.[5]

Special considerations
- Never aspirate fluid from the catheter *because the resulting negative pressure may damage inflamed tissue.*
- The first few times you intubate the pouch, the patient may be tense, making insertion difficult. Encourage relaxation. *To shorten drainage time,* have the patient cough, press gently on his abdomen over the pouch, or suddenly tighten his abdominal muscles and then relax them.
- Keep an accurate record of intake and output *to ensure fluid and electrolyte balance.* The average daily output should be 1,000 mL. Report inadequate or excessive output (more than 1,400 mL daily).
- *To reduce discomfort from gas pains,* encourage ambulation. Also recommend that the patient avoid swallowing air *to minimize gas pains* by chewing food well, limiting conversation while eating, and not drinking from a straw.

Patient teaching
Make sure the patient can properly intubate and drain the pouch himself. Provide the patient with the appropriate equipment. If the postoperative drainage catheter is still in place, teach the patient how to care for it properly. Make sure the patient has a pouch-draining schedule, and give him appropriate pamphlets or video instructions on pouch care. Make sure he feels comfortable calling the doctor, nurse, or other appropriate caregivers to ask questions or discuss problems. Tell the patient where to obtain supplies. Refer the patient to a local ostomy group. Provide dietary counseling.

Complications
Common postoperative complications include obstruction, fistula, pouch perforation, nipple valve dysfunction, abscesses, diarrhea, skin irritation, stenosis of the stoma, and bacterial overgrowth in the pouch.

Documentation
Record the date, time, and all aspects of preoperative and postoperative care. Include the condition of the stoma and peristomal skin, diet, medications, intubations, patient teaching, and discharge planning. Document the patient's tolerance and understanding of all procedures and teaching.

REFERENCES
1 The Joint Commission. (2012). Standard NPSG.01.01.01. *Comprehensive accreditation manual for hospitals: The official handbook.* Oakbrook Terrace, IL: The Joint Commission. (Level I)
2 The Joint Commission. (2012). Standard NPSG.07.01.01. *Comprehensive accreditation manual for hospitals: The official handbook.* Oakbrook Terrace, IL: The Joint Commission. (Level I)
3 Centers for Disease Control and Prevention. (October 2002). Guideline for hand hygiene in health-care settings. *Morbidity and Mortality Weekly Report, 51*(RR-16), 1–45. (Level 1)
4 World Health Organization. (2009). *WHO guidelines on hand hygiene in health care: First global patient safety challenge. Clean care is safer care.* Geneva, Switzerland: World Health Organization. (Level I)
5 The Joint Commission. (2012). Standard RC.01.03.01. *Comprehensive accreditation manual for hospitals: The official handbook.* Oakbrook Terrace, IL: The Joint Commission. (Level I)

ADDITIONAL REFERENCES
Craven, R.F., & Hirnle, C.J. (2009). *Fundamentals of nursing: Human health and function* (6th ed.). Philadelphia, PA: Lippincott Williams & Wilkins.
Deitz, D., & Gates, J. (2010). Basic ostomy management, part 1. *Nursing, 40*(2), 61–62.
Nettina, S.M. (2010). *Lippincott manual of nursing practice* (9th ed.). Philadelphia, PA: Lippincott Williams & Wilkins.
Rathnayake, M.M., et al. (2008). Complications of loop ileostomy and ileostomy closure and their implications for extended enterostomal therapy: A prospective clinical study. *International Journal of Nursing Studies, 45*(8), 1118–1121.
Taylor, C., et al. (2011). *Fundamentals of nursing: The art and science of nursing care* (7th ed.). Philadelphia, PA: Lippincott Williams & Wilkins.

How peritoneal dialysis works

Peritoneal dialysis works through a combination of diffusion and osmosis.

Diffusion

In diffusion, particles move through a semipermeable membrane from an area of high-solute concentration to an area of low-solute concentration.

In peritoneal dialysis, the water-based dialysate being infused contains glucose, sodium chloride, calcium, magnesium, acetate or lactate, and no waste products. Therefore, the waste products and excess electrolytes in the blood cross through the semipermeable peritoneal membrane into the dialysate. Removing the waste-filled dialysate and replacing it with fresh solution keeps the waste concentration low and encourages further diffusion.

Osmosis

In osmosis, fluids move through a semipermeable membrane from an area of low-solute concentration to an area of high-solute concentration. In peritoneal dialysis, dextrose is added to the dialysate to give it a higher solute concentration than the blood, creating a high osmotic gradient. Water migrates from the blood through the membrane at the beginning
of each infusion, when the osmotic gradient is highest.

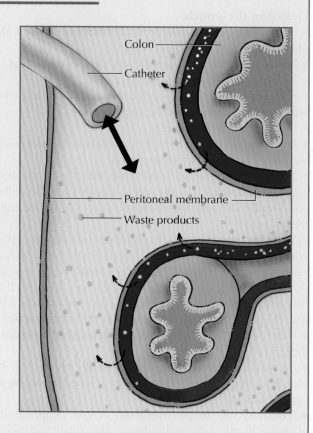

Colon
Catheter
Peritoneal membrane
Waste products

CONTINUOUS AMBULATORY PERITONEAL DIALYSIS

Continuous ambulatory peritoneal dialysis (CAPD) requires insertion of a permanent peritoneal catheter (such as a Tenckhoff catheter) to circulate dialysate in the peritoneal cavity constantly. Inserted under local anesthetic, the catheter is sutured in place and its distal portion is tunneled subcutaneously to the skin surface. There it serves as a port for the dialysate, which flows in and out of the peritoneal cavity by gravity. (See *How peritoneal dialysis works*.)

CAPD is used most commonly for patients with end-stage renal disease who are looking for an alternative to renal replacement therapy. It can also be used in patients with vascular access issues, chronic heart failure, and ischemic heart disease. This procedure can be a welcome alternative to hemodialysis because it gives the patient more independence and requires less travel for treatments. CAPD also provides more stable fluid and electrolyte levels than conventional hemodialysis.

Patients or family members can usually learn to perform CAPD after appropriate training. And because the patient can resume normal daily activities between solution changes, CAPD helps promote independence and a return to a near-normal lifestyle. It also costs less than hemodialysis.

Conditions that may prohibit CAPD include recent abdominal surgery, abdominal adhesions, an infected abdominal wall, diaphragmatic tears, ileus, and respiratory insufficiency.

Equipment
To infuse dialysate

Prescribed amount of dialysate (usually in 2-L bags) ▪ heating pad or commercial warmer ▪ three face masks ▪ 42″ (106.7 cm) connective tubing with drain clamp ▪ six to eight packages of sterile 4″ × 4″ gauze pads ▪ medication, if ordered ▪ antiseptic pads ▪ hypoallergenic tape ▪ plastic snap-top container ▪ antiseptic solution ▪ sterile basin ▪ container of alcohol ▪ gloves ▪ sterile gloves ▪ belt or fabric pouch ▪ two sterile, waterproof paper drapes (one fenestrated) ▪ Optional: syringes, labeled specimen container.

To discontinue dialysis temporarily

Three sterile, waterproof paper barriers (two fenestrated) ▪ 4″ × 4″ gauze pads (for cleaning and dressing the catheter) ▪ two face masks ▪ sterile basin ▪ hypoallergenic tape ▪ antiseptic solution ▪ gloves ▪ sterile gloves ▪ sterile rubber catheter cap.

All equipment for infusing the dialysate and discontinuing the procedure must be sterile. Commercially prepared sterile CAPD kits are available.

Preparation of equipment

Check the concentration of the dialysate against the doctor's order. Also check the expiration date and appearance of the solution—it should be clear, not cloudy. Warm the solution to body temperature with a heating pad set on low or a commercial warmer. Don't warm the solution in a microwave oven *because the temperature is unpredictable.*

To minimize the risk of contaminating the bag's port, leave the dialysate container's wrapper in place during warming. This also keeps the bag dry, which makes examining it for leakage easier after you remove the wrapper.

Perform hand hygiene[1,2,3] and put on a surgical mask and follow standard precautions. Remove the dialysate container from the warming setup, and remove its protective wrapper. Squeeze the bag firmly *to check for leaks.*

If ordered, use a syringe to add any prescribed medication to the dialysate, using sterile technique *to avoid contamination.* (The ideal approach is to add medication under a laminar flow hood.) Disinfect multiple-dose vials in a 5-minute antiseptic soak. Insert the connective tubing into the dialysate container. Open the drain clamp to prime the tube. Then close the clamp.

Place an antiseptic pad on the dialysate container's port. Cover the port with a dry gauze pad, and secure the pad with tape. Remove and discard the surgical mask. Tear the tape so it will be ready to secure the new dressing. Commercial devices with antiseptic pads are available for covering the dialysate container and tubing connection.

Implementation

- Verify the doctor's order and that an informed consent was signed.[4]
- Confirm the patient's identity using at least two patient identifiers according to your facility's policy.[5]
- Explain the procedure to the patient and answer any questions.
- Weigh the patient *to establish a baseline level.* Weigh him at the same time every day *to help monitor fluid balance.*

Infusing dialysate

- Gather all equipment at the patient's bedside. Prepare the sterile field by placing a waterproof, sterile paper drape on a dry surface near the patient. Take care to maintain the drape's sterility.
- Perform hand hygiene and put on sterile gloves.[1,2,3]
- Fill the snap-top container with antiseptic solution, label it,[6] and place it on the sterile field. Place the basin on the sterile field. Then place four pairs of sterile gauze pads in the sterile basin and saturate them with the antiseptic solution. Drop the remaining gauze pads on the sterile field. Loosen the cap on the alcohol container and place it next to the sterile field.
- Remove your gloves and perform hand hygiene.[1,2,3]
- Put on gloves and a surgical mask and provide one for the patient.
- Carefully remove the dressing covering the peritoneal catheter and discard it.[7] Be careful not to touch the catheter or skin. Check skin integrity at the catheter site, and look for signs of infection, such as purulent drainage, redness, or edema. If drainage is present, obtain a swab specimen, put it in a labeled specimen container, and notify the doctor.

- Palpate the insertion site and subcutaneous tunnel route for tenderness or pain. If these symptoms occur, notify the doctor.
NURSING ALERT *If the patient has drainage, tenderness, or pain, don't proceed with the infusion without specific orders.*
- Remove and discard gloves. Perform hand hygiene.[1,2,3] Put on sterile gloves.
- Wrap one gauze pad saturated with antiseptic solution around the distal end of the catheter and leave it in place for 5 minutes.
- Clean the catheter and insertion site with the rest of the gauze pads, moving in concentric circles away from the insertion site. Use straight strokes to clean the catheter, beginning at the insertion site and moving outward. Use a clean area of the pad for each stroke. Loosen the catheter cap one notch and clean the exposed area. Place each used pad at the base of the catheter *to help support it.* After using the third pair of pads, place the fenestrated paper drape around the base of the catheter. Continue cleaning the catheter for another minute with one of the remaining pads soaked with antiseptic.
- Remove the antiseptic pad on the catheter cap, remove the cap, and use the remaining antiseptic pad to clean the end of the catheter hub.
- Attach the connective tubing from the dialysate container to the catheter. Be sure to secure the luer-lock connector tightly.
- Open the drain clamp on the dialysate container *to allow solution to enter the peritoneal cavity by gravity* over a period of 5 to 10 minutes. Leave a small amount of fluid in the bag *to make folding it easier.* Close the drain clamp.
- Fold the bag and secure it with a belt, or tuck it in the patient's clothing or a small fabric pouch.
- After the prescribed dwell time (usually 4 to 6 hours), unfold the bag, open the clamp, and allow peritoneal fluid to drain back into the bag by gravity.
- When drainage is complete, attach a new bag of dialysate and repeat the infusion.

Discontinuing dialysis temporarily

- Perform hand hygiene, put on gloves and a surgical mask, and provide one for the patient.[1,2,3]
- Explain the procedure to the patient and answer any questions.
- Remove and discard the dressing over the peritoneal catheter.
- Remove and discard gloves. Perform hand hygiene.[1,2,3]
- Put on sterile gloves. Set up a sterile field next to the patient by covering a clean, dry surface with a waterproof drape. Be sure to maintain the drape's sterility. Place all equipment on the sterile field, and place the 4" × 4" gauze pads in the basin. Saturate them with the antiseptic solution. Open the 4" × 4" gauze pads to be used as the dressing, and drop them onto the sterile field. Tear pieces of tape as needed.
- Tape the dialysate tubing to the side rail of the bed *to keep the catheter and tubing off the patient's abdomen.*
- Remove and discard gloves. Perform hand hygiene.[1,2,3] Put on another pair of sterile gloves.
- Place one of the fenestrated drapes around the base of the catheter.

Three major steps of continuous ambulatory peritoneal dialysis

A bag of dialysate is attached to the tube entering the patient's abdominal area so the fluid flows into the peritoneal cavity.

While the dialysate remains in the peritoneal cavity, the patient can roll up the bag, place it under his shirt, and go about his normal activities. Or, the patient may cap off the catheter using sterile technique so only a small amount of tubing is taped to the body. After the dwell time, a new bag is applied.

Unrolling the bag and suspending it below the pelvis allows the dialysate to drain from the peritoneal cavity back into the bag.

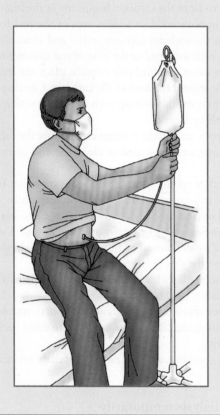

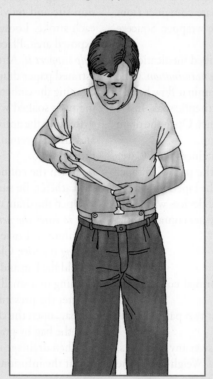

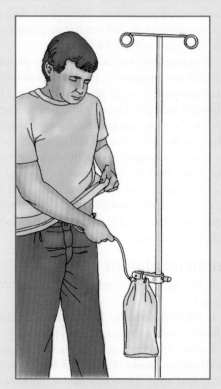

■ Use a pair of antiseptic pads to clean about 6″ (15 cm) of the dialysis tubing. Clean for 1 minute, moving in one direction only, away from the catheter. Then clean the catheter, moving from the insertion site to the junction of the catheter and dialysis tubing. Place used pads at the base of the catheter *to prop it up.* Use two more pairs of pads to clean the junction for a total of 3 minutes.

■ Place the second fenestrated paper drape over the first at the base of the catheter.

■ With another pair of antiseptic pads, clean the junction of the catheter and 6″ of the dialysate tubing for another minute.

■ Disconnect the dialysate tubing from the catheter. Pick up the catheter cap and fasten it to the catheter, making sure it fits securely over both notches of the hard plastic catheter tip.

■ Clean the insertion site and a 2″ (5 cm) radius around it with antiseptic pads, working from the insertion site outward. Let the skin air-dry before applying the dressing.

Completing the procedure
■ Remove gloves and discard used supplies appropriately. Perform hand hygiene.[1,2,3]
■ Document the procedure.[8]

Special considerations
■ If inflow and outflow are slow or absent, check the tubing for kinks. You can also try raising the solution or repositioning the patient *to increase the inflow rate.* Repositioning the patient or applying manual pressure to the lateral aspects of the patient's abdomen may also help increase drainage.

Patient teaching
Teach the patient and family how to use sterile technique throughout the procedure, especially for cleaning and dressing changes, *to prevent complications such as peritonitis.* (See *Three major steps of continuous ambulatory peritoneal dialysis.*)

Inform the patient about the advantages of an automated continuous cycle system for home use. (See *Continuous-cycle peritoneal dialysis.*) Teach them the signs and symptoms of peritonitis—cloudy fluid, fever, abdominal pain, and tenderness—and stress the importance of notifying the doctor immediately if such signs or symptoms arise. Also tell them to call the doctor if redness and drainage occur; these are also signs of infection.

Instruct the patient to record his weight and blood pressure daily and to check regularly for swelling of the extremities. Teach him to keep an accurate record of intake and output.

Complications

Peritonitis is the most frequent complication of CAPD. Although treatable, it can permanently scar the peritoneal membrane, decreasing its permeability and reducing the efficiency of dialysis. Untreated peritonitis can cause septicemia and death.

Excessive fluid loss may result from a concentrated (4.25%) dialysate solution, improper or inaccurate monitoring of inflow and outflow, or inadequate oral fluid intake. Excessive fluid retention may result from improper or inaccurate monitoring of inflow and outflow as well as from excessive salt or oral fluid intake.

Documentation

Record the type and amount of fluid instilled and returned for each exchange, the time and duration of the exchange, and any medications added to the dialysate. Note the color and clarity of the returned exchange fluid, and check it for mucus, pus, and blood. Also note any discrepancy in the balance of fluid intake and output, as well as any signs of fluid imbalance, such as weight changes, decreased breath sounds, increased dyspnea, peripheral edema, ascites, and changes in skin turgor. Record the patient's weight, blood pressure, and pulse rate after his last fluid exchange for the day.

REFERENCES

1 The Joint Commission. (2012). Standard NPSG.07.01.01. *Comprehensive accreditation manual for hospitals: The official handbook.* Oakbrook Terrace, IL: The Joint Commission. (Level I)
2 Centers for Disease Control and Prevention. (October 2002). Guideline for hand hygiene in health-care settings. *Morbidity and Mortality Weekly Report, 51*(RR-16), 1–45. (Level 1)
3 World Health Organization. (2009). *WHO guidelines on hand hygiene in health care: First global patient safety challenge. Clean care is safer care.* Geneva, Switzerland: World Health Organization. (Level I)
4 The Joint Commission. (2012). Standard RI.01.03.01. *Comprehensive accreditation manual for hospitals: The official handbook.* Oakbrook Terrace, IL: The Joint Commission. (Level I)
5 The Joint Commission. (2012). Standard NPSG.01.01.01. *Comprehensive accreditation manual for hospitals: The official handbook.* Oakbrook Terrace, IL: The Joint Commission. (Level I)
6 The Joint Commission. (2012). Standard NPSG.03.04.01. *Comprehensive accreditation manual for hospitals: The official handbook.* Oakbrook Terrace, IL: The Joint Commission. (Level I)
7 Occupational Safety and Health Administration. "Bloodborne Pathogens, Standard Number 1910.1030" [Online]. Accessed August 2011 via the Web at http://www.osha.gov/pls/oshaweb/owadisp.show_document?p_table=STANDARDS&p_id=10051

Continuous-cycle peritoneal dialysis

Continuous ambulatory peritoneal dialysis is easier for the patient who uses an automated continuous-cycle system. When set up, the system runs the dialysis treatment automatically until all the dialysate is infused. The system remains closed throughout the treatment, which cuts the risk of contamination. Continuous-cycle peritoneal dialysis (CCPD) can be performed while the patient is awake or asleep. The system's alarms warn about general system, dialysate, and patient problems.

The cycler can be set to an intermittent or continuous dialysate schedule at home or in a health care facility. The patient typically initiates CCPD at bedtime and undergoes three to seven exchanges depending on individual prescriptions. Upon awakening, the patient infuses the prescribed dialysis volume, disconnects himself from the unit, and carries the dialysate in his peritoneal cavity during the day.

The continuous cycler follows the same aseptic care and maintenance procedures as the manual method.

8 The Joint Commission. (2012). Standard RC.01.03.01. *Comprehensive accreditation manual for hospitals: The official handbook.* Oakbrook Terrace, IL: The Joint Commission. (Level I)

ADDITIONAL REFERENCES

Mehrotra, R. (2009). Long-term outcomes in automated peritoneal dialysis: Similar or better than in continuous ambulatory peritoneal dialysis? *Peritoneal Dialysis International, 29*(Suppl. 2), S111–S114.
National Kidney Foundation/KDOQI. (2006). "Clinical Practice Guidelines for Peritoneal Dialysis Adequacy, Update 2006" [Online]. Accessed August 2010 via the Web at http://www.kidney.org/professionals/KDOQI/guideline_upHD_PD_VA/index.htm
Nettina, S.M. (2010). *Lippincott manual of nursing practice* (9th ed.). Philadelphia, PA: Lippincott Williams & Wilkins.

CONTINUOUS BLADDER IRRIGATION

Continuous bladder irrigation can help prevent urinary tract obstruction by flushing out small blood clots that form after prostate or bladder surgery. It may also be used to treat an irritated, inflamed, or infected bladder lining.

This procedure requires placement of a three-way bladder catheter. One lumen controls balloon inflation, one allows irrigant inflow, and one allows irrigant outflow. The continuous flow of irrigating solution through the bladder creates a mild tamponade that may help prevent venous hemorrhage. (See *Setup for continuous bladder irrigation.*) Although the catheter is inserted

Setup for continuous bladder irrigation

With continuous bladder irrigation, a three-way catheter allows irrigating solution to flow into the bladder through one lumen and flow out through another, as shown in the inset. The third lumen is used to inflate the balloon that holds the catheter in place.

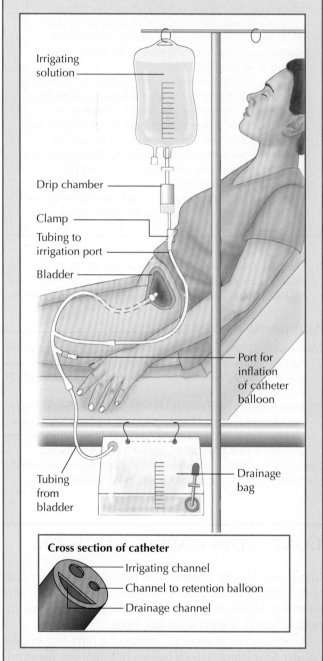

Irrigating solution

Drip chamber

Clamp

Tubing to irrigation port

Bladder

Port for inflation of catheter balloon

Tubing from bladder

Drainage bag

Cross section of catheter

Irrigating channel

Channel to retention balloon

Drainage channel

in the operating room during prostate or bladder surgery, it may also be inserted at bedside.

Unless specified otherwise, the patient should remain on bed rest throughout continuous bladder irrigation.

Equipment

Sterile irrigating solution (usually normal saline solution) ▪ sterile tubing for use with bladder irrigation system ▪ drainage bag and tubing ▪ gloves ▪ antiseptic pad ▪ IV pole.

Normal saline solution is usually prescribed for bladder irrigation after prostate or bladder surgery. Large volumes of irrigating solution are usually required during the first 24 to 48 hours after surgery. If medication solution is ordered, it's usually prepared by a pharmacist before use.

Preparation of equipment

Check the solution bag for leakage. If the solution contains an antibiotic, check the patient's chart *to make sure he isn't allergic to the drug.* Make sure that the irrigating solution is at room temperature *to prevent bladder spasm.*

Implementation

▪ Verify the doctor's order.
▪ Confirm the patient's identity using at least two patient identifiers according to your facility's policy.[1]
▪ Assemble all equipment at the patient's bedside.
▪ Provide privacy, explain the procedure, and answer any questions.
▪ Perform hand hygiene and put on gloves.[2,3,4]
▪ Insert the spike of the tubing into the container of irrigating solution.
▪ Squeeze the drip chamber on the spike of the tubing.
▪ Open the flow clamp and flush the tubing *to remove air, which could cause bladder distention.* Then close the clamp.
▪ Hang the bag of irrigating solution on the IV pole.
▪ Clean the opening to the inflow lumen of the catheter with the antiseptic pad.
▪ Insert the distal end of the tubing securely into the inflow lumen of the catheter.
▪ Make sure the catheter's outflow lumen is securely attached to the drainage bag tubing.
▪ Open the flow clamp under the container of irrigating solution, and set the drip rate as ordered.
▪ Remove and discard gloves. Perform hand hygiene.[2,3,4]
▪ Monitor urine output at least hourly for the first 4 hours. Check for bladder distention or abdominal pain.
▪ Check the inflow and outflow lines periodically for kinks *to make sure the solution is running freely.* If the solution flows rapidly, check the lines frequently.
▪ Document the procedure.[5]

Special considerations

▪ *To prevent air from entering the system,* don't allow the primary container to empty completely before replacing it.

- Empty the drainage bag about every 4 hours, or as often as needed. Use sterile technique *to avoid the risk of contamination.*
- Measure the outflow volume accurately. It should equal or, allowing for urine production, slightly exceed inflow volume. If inflow volume exceeds outflow volume postoperatively, suspect bladder rupture at the suture lines or renal damage, and notify the doctor immediately.
- Assess outflow for changes in appearance and for blood clots, especially if irrigation is being performed postoperatively to control bleeding. If drainage is bright red, irrigating solution should usually be infused rapidly with the clamp wide open until drainage clears. Notify the doctor immediately if you suspect hemorrhage. If drainage is clear, the solution is usually given at a rate of 40 to 60 drops/minute. The doctor typically specifies the rate for antibiotic solutions.
- Monitor vital signs at least every 4 hours during irrigation; increase the frequency if the patient becomes unstable.
- Encourage oral fluid intake of 2 to 3 L/day unless contraindicated by another medical condition.

Complications

Interruptions in a continuous irrigation system can predispose the patient to infection. Obstruction in the catheter's outflow lumen can cause bladder distention or spasm.

Documentation

Each time you finish a container of solution, record the date, time, and amount of fluid given on the intake and output record. Also record the time and amount of fluid each time you empty the drainage bag. Note the appearance of the drainage and any complaints the patient has. Note the patient's tolerance of the procedure.

REFERENCES

1   The Joint Commission. (2012). Standard NPSG.01.01.01. *Comprehensive accreditation manual for hospitals: The official handbook.* Oakbrook Terrace, IL: The Joint Commission. (Level I)
2   The Joint Commission. (2012). Standard NPSG.07.01.01. *Comprehensive accreditation manual for hospitals: The official handbook.* Oakbrook Terrace, IL: The Joint Commission. (Level I)
3   Centers for Disease Control and Prevention. (October 2002). Guideline for hand hygiene in health-care settings. *Morbidity and Mortality Weekly Report, 51*(RR-16), 1–45. (Level 1)
4   World Health Organization. (2009). *WHO guidelines on hand hygiene in health care: First global patient safety challenge. Clean care is safer care.* Geneva, Switzerland: World Health Organization. (Level I)
5   The Joint Commission. (2012). Standard RC.01.03.01. *Comprehensive accreditation manual for hospitals: The official handbook.* Oakbrook Terrace, IL: The Joint Commission. (Level I)

ADDITIONAL REFERENCES

Gould, C.V., et al. (2009). "Guideline for Prevention of Catheter-associated Urinary Tract Infections, 2009" [Online]. Accessed November 2011 via the Web at http://www.cdc.gov/hicpac/cauti/001_cauti.html

Smeltzer, S.C., et al. (2010). *Brunner & Suddarth's textbook of medical-surgical nursing* (12th ed.). Philadelphia, PA: Lippincott Williams & Wilkins.

CONTINUOUS PASSIVE MOTION DEVICE USE

A continuous passive motion (CPM) device is frequently used after joint surgery—particularly after total knee arthroplasty. The device increases range of motion in the joint as the flexion and extension settings are adjusted during therapy. The device also minimizes the negative effects of immobility because it increases passive range of movement of the limb. The CPM device also stimulates healing within the articular cartilage and reduces adhesions and swelling. The doctor determines the amount of flexion and extension of the joint and the cycle rate (the number of revolutions per minute) as well as the length of time it's to be used.

Although the CPM device is usually used on the knee, it may be appropriate for other joints as well.

Equipment

CPM device ▪ single-patient-use soft-goods kit ▪ tape measure ▪ goniometer ▪ gloves, if indicated ▪ pain medication.

Preparation of equipment

Apply the soft-goods padding to the CPM device. Turn the unit on at the main power switch and set the controls to the level prescribed by the doctor *to ensure that the unit is functioning.*

Implementation

- Verify the doctor's order for the CPM settings, frequency, and duration.[1]
- Gather the appropriate equipment.
- Confirm the patient's identity using at least two patient identifiers according to your facility's policy.[1]
- Explain the procedure to the patient and answer any questions *to reduce anxiety and encourage compliance.*
- Assess the patient's pain level and administer a prescribed analgesic, if needed, following safe medication administration practices.[2] Allow time for the full effect of the analgesic to occur before starting the machine. Perform a follow-up pain assessment and notify the doctor if pain isn't adequately controlled.[3]
- Perform hand hygiene and put on gloves, if indicated, *to prevent possible contact with blood or body fluids.*[4,5,6]
- Provide privacy. Place the bed at a comfortable working height.
- Determine the distance between the gluteal crease and the popliteal space using the measuring tape.
- Measure the length of the lower leg from the knee to ¼" (0.6 cm) beyond the bottom of the foot.
- Adjust the thigh length and foot plate position on the CPM machine based on your measurements.
- Position the patient in the middle of the bed.

■ Support the affected extremity, elevating it to allow placement of the padded CPM device on the bed. Gently lower the leg onto the device (as shown below).

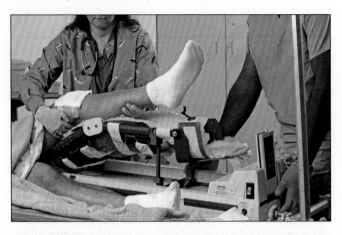

■ Make sure the knee is resting at the hinged joint of the CPM machine and that the leg is slightly abducted.
■ Adjust the footplate to maintain a neutral position for the patient's foot (as shown below). Assess the patient's position to make sure the leg isn't internally or externally rotated *to prevent injury*.

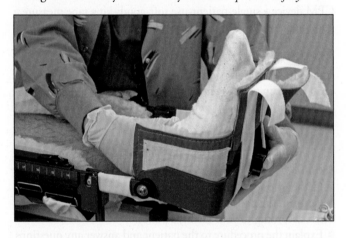

■ Secure the restraining straps under the CPM device and around the leg *to hold the leg in position*. Check that two fingers fit between the strap and the leg (as shown below) *to prevent injury from excessive pressure from the strap*.

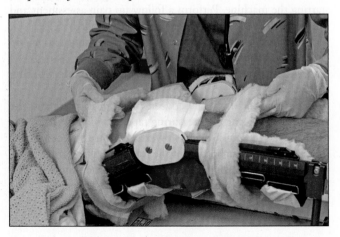

■ Teach the patient how to use the STOP/GO button.
■ Set the device to ON and start the therapy by pressing the GO button. Monitor the patient and the device through the first few cycles. Verify the angle of flexion when the device reaches its greatest height by measuring with a goniometer (as shown below) *to ensure the device is set to the prescribed parameters*.

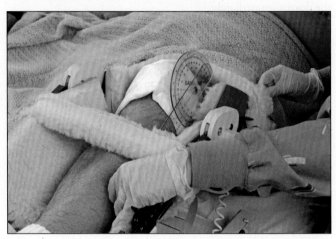

■ Return the bed to the lowest position *for patient safety*. Make sure the call bell and other necessary items are within easy reach.
■ Check the patient's level of comfort frequently and perform skin and neurovascular assessments at least every 8 hours or according to facility policy.
■ Remove and discard your gloves and perform hand hygiene.[4,5,6]
■ Document the procedure.[7]

Special considerations

■ The use of the CPM device is in addition to physical therapy during the rehabilitation process.
■ Encourage the patient to use the CPM device, as prescribed, *to promote healing and function of the joint*.

Patient teaching

Instruct the patient how to use the device and patient controls. Make the patient aware of setting changes and the goals of CPM therapy. Teach him signs and symptoms of neurovascular impairment to report, such as numbness or tingling, sudden pain, or coolness of the affected limb.

Documentation

Record settings and the patient's tolerance of the CPM device. Note skin and incision condition and your neurovascular assessment. Document your pain assessment, nursing actions taken, and outcomes. Also record any patient teaching provided and the patient's response to the teaching.

REFERENCES

1. The Joint Commission. (2012). Standard NPSG.01.01.01. *Comprehensive accreditation manual for hospitals: The official handbook.* Oakbrook Terrace, IL: The Joint Commission. (Level I)

2 The Joint Commission. (2012). Standard MM.06.01.01. *Comprehensive accreditation manual for hospitals: The official handbook.* Oakbrook Terrace, IL: The Joint Commission. (Level I)

3 The Joint Commission. (2012). Standard PC.01.02.01. *Comprehensive accreditation manual for hospitals: The official handbook.* Oakbrook Terrace, IL: The Joint Commission. (Level I)

4 The Joint Commission. (2012). Standard NPSG.07.01.01. *Comprehensive accreditation manual for hospitals: The official handbook.* Oakbrook Terrace, IL: The Joint Commission. (Level I)

5 Centers for Disease Control and Prevention. (October 2002). Guideline for hand hygiene in health-care settings. *Morbidity and Mortality Weekly Report, 51*(RR-16), 1–45. (Level 1)

6 World Health Organization. (2009). *WHO guidelines on hand hygiene in health care: First global patient safety challenge. Clean care is safer care.* Geneva, Switzerland: World Health Organization. (Level I)

7 The Joint Commission. (2012). Standard RC.01.03.01. *Comprehensive accreditation manual for hospitals: The official handbook.* Oakbrook Terrace, IL: The Joint Commission. (Level I)

Additional references

Bruun-Olsen, V., et al. (2009). Continuous passive motion as an adjunct to active exercises in early rehabilitation following total knee arthroplasty: A randomized controlled trial. *Disability and Rehabilitation, 31*(4), 277–283.

Harvey, L.A., et al. (2010). Continuous passive motion following total knee arthroplasty in people with arthritis. *Cochrane Database of Systematic Reviews, 3*:CD004260.

Taylor, C., et al. (2011). *Fundamentals of nursing: The art and science of nursing care* (7th ed.). Philadelphia, PA: Lippincott Williams & Wilkins.

Continuous positive airway pressure use

Continuous positive airway pressure (CPAP) provides constant low-flow pressure into the airways to help hold the airway open, mobilize secretions, treat atelectasis and, generally, ease the work of breathing. CPAP is also used to treat chronic obstructive sleep apnea because it prevents the palate and tongue from collapsing and obstructing the airway.[1]

Nonintubated patients receive CPAP through a high-flow generating system, which may eliminate the need for intubation. Many patients are started on CPAP in the health care facility and then continue therapy at home. Intubated patients may receive CPAP through a ventilator setting. Although CPAP has traditionally been administered through a face mask, other, more comfortable methods include the face pillow and nasal mask.

Because of the increase in thoracic pressure, CPAP is contraindicated in patients with increased intracranial pressure, hemodynamic instability, or recent facial, oral, or skull trauma.[1]

Equipment

Nasal mask, nasal pillows, or face mask (properly sized) ■ permanent marker ■ CPAP machine ■ oxygen source ■ oxygen delivery tubing ■ washcloth ■ water ■ personal protective equipment ■ Optional: oxygen source, pulse oximeter.

Preparation of equipment

Set up the CPAP machine according to manufacturer's instructions. Position the CPAP machine so that the tubing easily reaches the patient and plug in the machine. Don't plug the CPAP machine into an outlet with another plug in it, and don't use an extension cord to reach the outlet. Connect the CPAP machine to the oxygen source; then connect the oxygen delivery tubing to the air outlet valve on the CPAP unit, if ordered. Check the nasal mask, nasal pillow, or face mask to make sure the cushion isn't hard or broken. If it is, replace it.

Implementation

■ Verify the doctor's order.

■ Confirm the patient's identity using at least two patient identifiers according to your facility's policy.[2]

■ Explain the procedure to the patient and answer any questions *to decrease anxiety and increase compliance.*

■ Perform hand hygiene and use personal protective equipment, as appropriate, *to prevent bacterial contamination.*[3,4,5]

■ Wash the patient's face with a washcloth and water *to remove facial oils and help achieve a better fit.*

Applying a nasal mask

■ Place the nasal mask so that the longer straps are located at the top of the mask (as shown below).

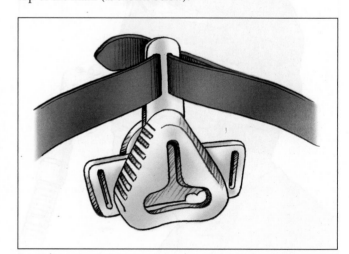

■ Make sure that the Velcro is facing away from you, and thread the four tabs through the slots on the sides and top of the mask (as shown below).

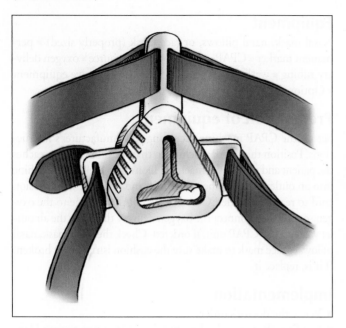

■ Pull the straps through the slots and fasten them using the Velcro.
■ Place the mask over the patient's nose and position the headgear over the patient's head.
■ Gradually tighten all the straps on the mask until a seal is obtained. The mask doesn't have to be very tight to fit correctly—it just has to have a seal (as shown below).

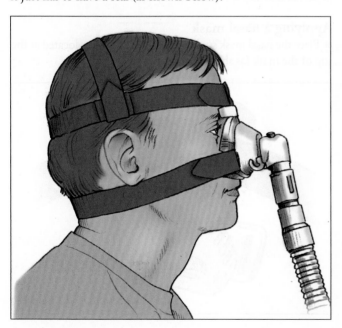

■ Use the permanent marker to mark the straps with the final position *to eliminate having to fit the mask each time the patient wears it.*

Applying a nasal pillow
■ Insert the nasal pillows into the shell making sure they fit correctly and that there's no air leaking around them (as shown below).

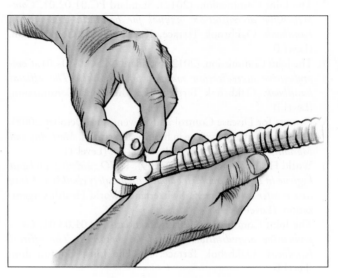

■ Place the headgear around the patient's head and use the Velcro straps to achieve the proper fit. After the straps are in the correct place, remove the headgear without undoing the straps.
■ Attach the nasal pillow to the headgear by wrapping the Velcro around the tubing, leaving room for rotation (as shown below).

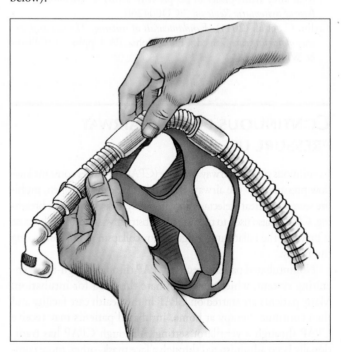

- Place the completely assembled headgear back on the patient and position the nasal pillows comfortably.
- Attach the shell strap across the shell and adjust the tension of the strap until there's a seal in both nostrils (as shown below).

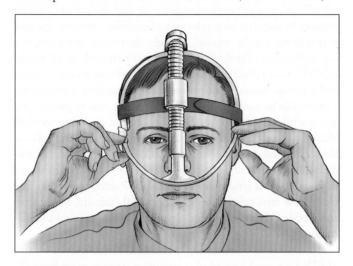

- Be careful not to block the exhalation port on the backside of the shell.

Applying a face mask
- Hold the mask against the patient's face and position the headgear over his head.
- Using the Velcro straps, adjust the straps (as with the nasal mask) until there are no leaks present (as shown below).

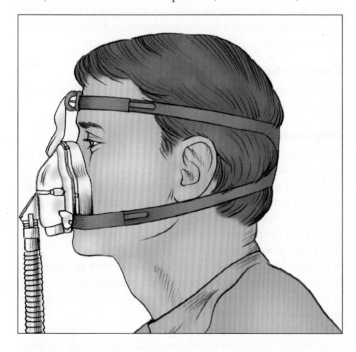

- Connect the flexible tubing to the mask.

Administering CPAP
- After the administration device is correctly fitted on the patient, turn on the pressure generator.

- Turn on the CPAP unit before turning on the oxygen flow to the ordered level.
- If ordered, monitor the patient's pulse oximetry during the treatment.
- When the treatment is over—in the morning or upon discontinuation of the order—turn off the pressure generator and remove the headgear and appliance from the patient.
- Clean the equipment according to facility policy and store it properly.
- Remove and discard personal protective equipment. Perform hand hygiene.[3,4,5]
- Document the procedure.[6]

Special considerations
- If the mask isn't properly fitted, the patient may complain of dry or sore eyes. If this is the case, remove the mask and headgear and readjust them to minimize leaks.
- The patient may need to use a humidifier with the CPAP unit if he complains of a runny nose or dryness or burning in his nose and throat. Discuss this option with the doctor and obtain an order for humidification.
- Always make sure there's air coming out of the unit when the power is turned on.
- *Because CPAP via a mask can cause nausea and vomiting, it shouldn't be used in a patient who's unresponsive or at risk for aspiration.*
- Remove the mask and perform oral care every 2 to 4 hours and as needed *to prevent drying and thickening of oral secretions.*
- Remove the mask and perform skin care at least every shift and as needed *to prevent or identify skin breakdown caused by the pressure of the mask.*

Patient teaching
Teach the patient how to use the machine at home, including fitting the mask and taking care of the equipment. Make sure the patient has the name and phone number of the company that will be supplying the machine for home use. Also provide a contact number for him to ask questions.

Complications
Most complications, such as dry eyes, runny or dry nose, or burning in the throat or nose, result from ill-fitting masks. Some patients may be allergic to the mask or develop skin irritation from the contact of the mask to their face. If this complication happens, apply a barrier between the mask and the skin.

CPAP can also cause decreased cardiac output as the result of increased intrathoracic pressure. Other complications include nosebleeds, abdominal bloating, headaches, and nightmares.

Documentation
Document CPAP settings, the length of time the patient was on CPAP, how the patient tolerated CPAP, and if there were any complications. Also record any patient teaching provided.

REFERENCES

1 American Association for Respiratory Care. (1993). AARC clinical practice guideline: Use of positive airway pressure adjuncts to bronchial hygiene therapy. *Respiratory Care, 28*(5), 516–521. (Level I)

2 The Joint Commission. (2012). Standard NPSG.01.01.01. *Comprehensive accreditation manual for hospitals: The official handbook*. Oakbrook Terrace, IL: The Joint Commission. (Level I)

3 The Joint Commission. (2012). Standard NPSG.07.01.01. *Comprehensive accreditation manual for hospitals: The official handbook*. Oakbrook Terrace, IL: The Joint Commission. (Level I)

4 Centers for Disease Control and Prevention. (October 2002). Guideline for hand hygiene in health-care settings. *Morbidity and Mortality Weekly Report, 51*(RR-16), 1–45. (Level 1)

5 World Health Organization. (2009). *WHO guidelines on hand hygiene in health care: First global patient safety challenge. Clean care is safer care.* Geneva, Switzerland: World Health Organization. (Level I)

6 The Joint Commission. (2012). Standard RC.01.03.01. *Comprehensive accreditation manual for hospitals: The official handbook*. Oakbrook Terrace, IL: The Joint Commission. (Level I)

ADDITIONAL REFERENCES

Abe, H., et al. (2010). Efficacy of continuous positive airway pressure on arrhythmias in obstructive sleep apnea patients. *Heart Vessels, 25*(1), 63–69.

Broström, A., et al. (2010). Putative facilitators and barriers for adherence to CPAP treatment in patients with obstructive sleep apnea syndrome: A qualitative content analysis. *Sleep Medicine, 11*(2), 126–130.

Dernaika, T.A., et al. (2009). Effects of nocturnal continuous positive airway pressure therapy in patients with resistant hypertension and obstructive sleep apnea. *Journal of Clinical Sleep Medicine, 5*(2), 103–107.

Gilman, M.P. (2008). Continuous positive airway pressure increases heart rate variability in heart failure patients with obstructive sleep apnea. *Clinical Science (London, England), 114*(3), 243–249.

Johnson, C.B., et al. (2008). Acute and chronic effects of continuous positive airway pressure therapy on left ventricular systolic and diastolic function in patients with obstructive sleep apnea and congestive heart failure. *Canadian Journal of Cardiology, 24*(9), 697–704.

Nettina, S.M. (2010). *Lippincott manual of nursing practice* (9th ed.). Philadelphia, PA: Lippincott Williams & Wilkins.

Ruttanaumpawan, P., et al. (2008). Sustained effect of continuous positive airway pressure on baroreflex sensitivity in congestive heart failure patients with obstructive sleep apnea. *Journal of Hypertension, 26*(6), 1163–1168.

CONTINUOUS RENAL REPLACEMENT THERAPY

Continuous renal replacement therapy (CRRT) is an extracorporeal purification therapy used to treat patients who suffer from acute renal failure. Unlike the more traditional hemodialysis, CRRT is administered around the clock, providing patients with continuous therapy and sparing them the destabilizing hemodynamic and electrolytic changes characteristic of traditional hemodialysis. For patients who can't tolerate traditional hemodialysis—such as those who have hypotension—CRRT is often the only choice for treatment.

The techniques used vary in complexity. Slow continuous ultrafiltration uses arteriovenous access and the patient's blood pressure to circulate blood through a hemofilter. Because the goal of this therapy is the removal of fluids, the patient doesn't receive any replacement fluids. Continuous venovenous hemofiltration (CVVH) uses a double-lumen catheter to provide access to a vein, and a pump moves blood through the hemofilter. Continuous venovenous hemodialysis (CVVH-D) uses a vein to provide the access while a pump moves dialysate solution concurrently with blood flow; this process continuously removes fluid and solutes. Slow extended daily dialysis (SLEDD) is a modification of traditional intermittent hemodialysis. SLEDD is usually performed in 6- to 12-hour treatment sessions, 5 to 7 days each week. The blood flow rates range from 100 to 250 mL/minute, resulting in an extended dialysis time and decreased solute rate and ultrafiltration.

For treatment of critically ill patients, CVVH, CVVH-D, and SLEDD are used instead of continuous arteriovenous hemofiltration (CAVH). CVVH, in particular, has several advantages over CAVH: It doesn't require arterial access, it can be performed in patients with low mean arterial pressures, and it has better solute clearance than CAVH.

Equipment

CRRT equipment ▪ heparin flush solution ▪ occlusive dressings for catheter insertion sites ▪ gloves ▪ sterile gloves ▪ mask and gown, as needed ▪ antiseptic solution ▪ sterile gauze pads ▪ hypoallergenic adhesive tape ▪ filtration replacement fluid, as ordered ▪ infusion pump.

Preparation of equipment

Prime the hemofilter and tubing according to the manufacturer's instructions.

Implementation

▪ Verify the doctor's order and verify that informed consent has been obtained.[1]

▪ Gather and assemble the equipment at the patient's bedside according to the manufacturer's recommendations and your facility's policy. (See *Setup for CVVH*.)

▪ Confirm the patient's identity using at least two patient identifiers according to your facility's policy.[2]

▪ Perform hand hygiene, put on gloves and other personal protective equipment, and follow standard precautions.[3,4,5]

▪ Explain the procedure to the patient and family and answer any questions *to decrease anxiety*.

▪ If necessary, assist with inserting the catheters, using strict sterile technique. Common catheter insertion sites include the internal jugular, subclavian, and femoral veins. The internal jugular vein is the preferred site; the subclavian site is associated with an increased risk of stenosis and the femoral site is associated with an increased risk of infection.[6] (In some cases, an arteriovenous fistula or double-lumen catheter may be used.)

EQUIPMENT

Setup for CVVH

Continuous renal replacement therapy is typically performed using continuous venous hemofiltration (CVVH). For this technique, the doctor inserts a special double-lumen catheter into a large vein—commonly the internal jugular, subclavian, or femoral vein. Because the catheter is in a vein, an external pump is used to move blood through the system. The patient's venous blood moves through the "arterial" lumen to the pump, which then pushes the blood through the catheter to the hemofilter. Here, water and toxic solutes (ultrafiltrate) are removed from the patient's blood and drain into a collection device. Blood cells aren't removed because they are too large to pass through the filter. As the blood exits the hemofilter, it's then pumped through the "venous" lumen back to the patient.

Several components of the pump provide safety mechanisms. Pressure monitors on the pump maintain the flow of blood through the circuit at a constant rate. An air detector traps air bubbles before the blood returns to the patient. A venous trap collects any blood clots that may be in the blood. A blood-leak detector signals when blood is found in the dialysate. A venous clamp operates if air is detected in the circuit or if there is any disconnection in the blood line.

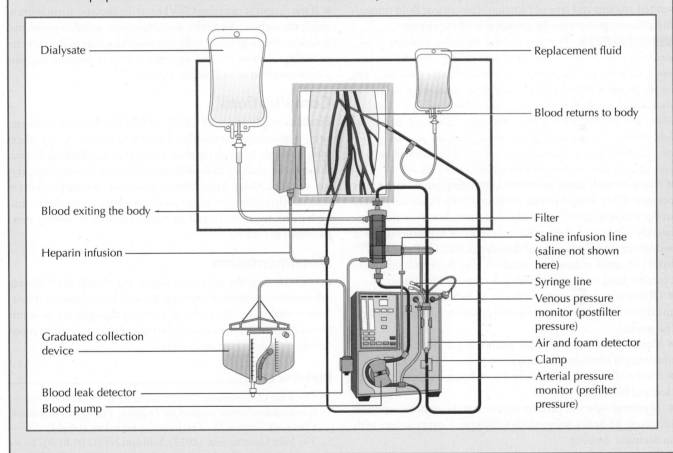

- If ordered, flush both catheter lumens with the heparin flush solution *to prevent clotting*.
- Apply an occlusive dressing to the insertion site, and mark the dressing with the date and time. Secure the tubing and connections with tape *to prevent accidental dislodgment*.
- Weigh the patient, take baseline vital signs, and make sure all necessary laboratory studies have been done (usually, electrolyte levels, coagulation factors, complete blood count, blood urea nitrogen, and creatinine studies). Monitor the patient's condition and vital signs frequently, according to the patient's condition.

- Remove and discard your gloves, and perform hand hygiene.[3,4,5]
- Put on sterile gloves and a mask.
- Prepare the connection sites by cleaning them with gauze pads soaked in antiseptic solution; then connect them to the exit port of each catheter.
- Using sterile technique, connect the arterial and venous lines to the hemofilter.
- Turn on the hemofilter and monitor the blood-flow rate through the circuit. The flow rate is typically between 150 and 300 mL/ minute.

- Inspect the ultrafiltrate during the procedure. It should remain clear yellow, with no gross blood. *Pink-tinged or bloody ultrafiltrate may signal a membrane leak in the hemofilter, which permits bacterial contamination and possible exsanguination.* Notify the doctor, and discontinue the procedure immediately.
- If femoral access is used, assess all pulses—dorsalis pedis, posterior tibial, popliteal, and femoral—in the affected leg every hour for the first 4 hours, then every 2 hours afterward. Also, assess the affected leg for signs of obstructed blood flow, such as pain, coolness, pallor, weak pulse, and paraesthesia. Check the groin area on the affected side for signs of hematoma or pseudoaneurysm. Ask the patient whether he has pain at the insertion site. Check for significant limb edema.
- Calculate the amount of filtration replacement fluid every hour, as ordered, or according to your facility's policy. Infuse the prescribed amount and type of filtration replacement fluid through the infusion pump into the arterial side of the circuit.

NURSING ALERT *The targeted net fluid loss amount is prescribed by the doctor. To calculate the amount of filtration replacement fluid to administer, determine the patient's total fluid loss in the previous hour. Add the total fluid amount in the collection device in the past hour plus any other fluid losses (such as blood loss, emesis, or nasogastric drainage). From the total fluid loss, subtract the patient's fluid intake from the past hour plus the net fluid loss prescribed by the doctor. This calculation will give you the filtration replacement fluid to be infused.*

- Assess hemodynamic parameters, including pulmonary artery pressure (PAP), central venous pressure (CVP), pulmonary artery wedge pressure (PAWP), and blood pressure, hourly or more frequently if indicated. Be alert for indications of hypovolemia (such as dropping blood pressure and decreases in PAP, CVP, and PAWP) from too-rapid removal of ultrafiltrate or hypervolemia form excessive fluid replacement with a decrease in ultrafiltrate.
- Obtain serum electrolyte levels every 4 to 6 hours or as ordered; anticipate adjustments in replacement fluid or dialysate based on the results.
- Maintain continuous cardiac monitoring *to detect arrhythmias indicative of electrolyte imbalances.*
- Inspect the site dressing every 4 to 8 hours for signs of infection and bleeding.
- *To prevent infection,* perform skin care at the catheter insertion sites every 48 hours, using sterile technique. Cover the sites with an occlusive dressing.
- Remove and discard personal protective equipment. Perform hand hygiene.[3,4,5]
- Document the procedure.[7]

Special considerations

- *Because blood flows through an extracorporeal circuit during CVVH,* the blood in the hemofilter may need to be anticoagulated. To do this, infuse heparin in low doses (usually starting at 500 units/hour) into an infusion port on the arterial side of the setup. Measure thrombin clotting time or the activated clotting time (ACT). *Doing so ensures that the circuit, not the patient, is anticoagulated.* A normal ACT is 100 seconds; during CRRT, keep it between 100 and 300 seconds, depending on the patient's clotting times.

If the ACT is too high or too low, the doctor will adjust the heparin dose accordingly.
- Another way to prevent clotting in the hemofilter is to infuse medications or blood through another venous access rather than the venous line, if possible.
- A third way to help prevent clots in the hemofilter, and also to prevent kinks in the catheter, is to make sure the patient doesn't bend the affected leg more than 30 degrees at the hip.
- If the ultrafiltrate flow rate decreases, raise the bed *to increase the distance between the collection device and the hemofilter.* Lower the bed *to decrease the flow rate.*

NURSING ALERT *Clamping the ultrafiltrate line is contraindicated with some types of hemofilters* because pressure may build up in the filter, clotting it and collapsing the blood compartment.
- If the patient is receiving CVVH and the pressure alarm sounds, check the catheter for kinks, disconnections, or other problems. A sudden rise in pressure indicates some blockage in the catheter or tubing. A dramatic and significant drop in pressure suggests a disconnection or opening of a port.

Complications

Possible complications of CRRT include bleeding from catheter sites, hemorrhage, hemofilter occlusion, infection, hypothermia, unstable hemodynamics, vascular access limb ischemia, thrombosis, dialysis disequilibrium (decreased neurologic status, seizure activity, hypertensory nausea or vomiting), dialyzer reaction (hypotension, anaphylaxis, pruritus, angioedema, and back pain), hypoxemia, and air embolism. (See *Preventing complications of CRRT.*)

Documentation

Record the time the treatment began and ended; fluid balance information; neurologic, respiratory, and hemodynamic assessments; vital signs; the times of dressing changes; medications given; the patient's tolerance of the procedure; any complications noted; and nursing actions taken.

REFERENCES

1 The Joint Commission. (2012). Standard RI.01.03.01. *Comprehensive accreditation manual for hospitals: The official handbook.* Oakbrook Terrace, IL: The Joint Commission. (Level I)
2 The Joint Commission. (2012). Standard NPSG.01.01.01. *Comprehensive accreditation manual for hospitals: The official handbook.* Oakbrook Terrace, IL: The Joint Commission. (Level I)
3 The Joint Commission. (2012). Standard NPSG.07.01.01. *Comprehensive accreditation manual for hospitals: The official handbook.* Oakbrook Terrace, IL: The Joint Commission. (Level I)
4 Centers for Disease Control and Prevention. (October 2002). Guideline for hand hygiene in health-care settings. *Morbidity and Mortality Weekly Report, 51*(RR-16), 1–45. (Level 1)
5 World Health Organization. (2009). *WHO guidelines on hand hygiene in health care: First global patient safety challenge. Clean care is safer care.* Geneva, Switzerland: World Health Organization. (Level I)
6 Lynn-McHale Wiegand, D. (Ed.). (2011). *AACN procedure manual for critical care* (6th ed.). Philadelphia, PA: Saunders.

7 The Joint Commission. (2012). Standard RC.01.03.01. *Comprehensive accreditation manual for hospitals: The official handbook.* Oakbrook Terrace, IL: The Joint Commission. (Level I)

ADDITIONAL REFERENCES

Baldwin, I., & Fealy, N. (2009). Clinical nursing for the application of continuous renal replacement therapy in the intensive care unit. *Seminars in Dialysis, 22*(2), 189–193.

Ghahramani, N., et al. (2008). A systematic review of continuous renal replacement therapy and intermittent haemodialysis in management of patients with acute renal failure. *Nephrology (Carlton), 13*(7), 570–578.

Hussain, S., et al. (2009). Outcome among patients with acute renal failure needing continuous renal replacement therapy: A single center study. *Hemodialysis International, 13*(2), 205–214.

Rauf, A.A., et al. (2008). Intermittent hemodialysis versus continuous renal replacement therapy for acute renal failure in the intensive care unit: An observational outcomes analysis. *Journal of Intensive Care Medicine, 23*(3), 195–203.

Susla, G.M. (2009). The impact of continuous renal replacement therapy on drug therapy. *Clinical Pharmacology and Therapeutics, 86*(5), 562–565.

CREDE'S MANEUVER

When lower motor neuron damage impairs the voiding reflex, the bladder may become flaccid or areflexic. Because the bladder fails to contract properly, urine collects inside it, causing distention. Crede's maneuver—application of manual pressure over the lower abdomen—promotes complete emptying of the bladder. After appropriate instruction, the patient can perform the maneuver himself, unless he can't reach his lower abdomen or lacks sufficient strength and dexterity. Even when performed properly, however, Crede's maneuver isn't always successful and doesn't always eliminate the need for catheterization.

Crede's maneuver can't be used after abdominal surgery if the incision isn't completely healed. When using Crede's maneuver, close monitoring of urine output is necessary to help detect possible infection from accumulation of residual urine.

Equipment

Gloves ■ bedpan, urinal, or bedside commode.

Implementation

■ Verify the doctor's order, if needed.
■ Perform hand hygiene and put on gloves, if appropriate.[1,2,3]
■ Confirm the patient's identity using at least two patient identifiers according to your facility's policy.[4]
■ Explain the procedure to the patient and answer any questions *to decrease anxiety.*
■ Place the patient in Fowler's position and position the bedpan or urinal, or if the patient's condition permits, assist into the bathroom or onto the bedside commode. A male patient may benefit from standing, if possible.
■ Place your hands flat on the patient's abdomen just below the umbilicus. Ask the female patient to bend forward from the hips.

Preventing complications of CRRT

The measures listed below help avoid complications of continuous renal replacement therapy (CRRT).

Hypotension
■ Monitor blood pressure.
■ Temporarily decrease the blood pump's speed for transient hypotension.
■ Increase the vasopressor support.

Hypothermia
■ Use an inline fluid warmer placed on the blood return line to the patient or an external warming blanket.

Fluid and electrolyte imbalances
■ Monitor the patient's fluid levels every 4 to 6 hours.
■ Monitor the patient's sodium, lactate, potassium, and calcium levels and replace as necessary.

Acid-base imbalances
■ Monitor the patient's bicarbonate and arterial blood gas levels.

Air embolism
■ Observe for air in the system.
■ Use luer-lock devices on catheter openings.

Hemorrhage
■ Check all connections and keep the dialysis lines visible.

Infection
■ Perform sterile dressing changes.

Then firmly stroke downward toward the bladder about six times *to stimulate the voiding reflex.*
■ Place one hand on top of the other above the pubic arch. Press firmly inward and downward *to compress the bladder and expel residual urine.* (See *Crede's maneuver,* page 218.)
■ Remove and discard your gloves and perform hand hygiene.[1,2,3]
■ Document the procedure.[5]

Special considerations

■ Some facilities require a doctor's order for performance of Crede's maneuver. This procedure should not be performed on patients with normal bladder tone or bladder spasms.
■ An ultrasound bladder scanner, if available, may be used to document urine volume before and after the procedure.
■ After the patient has learned the procedure and can use it successfully, measuring the expelled urine may not be necessary. The patient may then use the maneuver to void directly into the toilet.

Patient teaching

Explain to the patient that Crede's maneuver is a simple exercise that can be done at home. Tell the patient that he can start a

Crede's maneuver

To perform this maneuver, place one hand on top of the other above the pubic arch and press firmly inward and downward to compress the bladder.

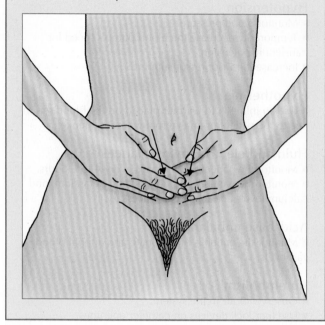

stream of urine from his bladder by performing this easy-to-do maneuver. Tell the male patient to void directly into the toilet from a standing position if possible. The female patient should sit on the toilet as she normally would.

Show the female patient how to lean forward, bending at the hips, *to increase pressure on the bladder.*

Have the patient place one hand on top of the other in a return demonstration. *Explain that the stroking movement compresses the bladder and expels urine.*

Documentation

Record the date and time of the procedure, the amount and characteristics of urine expelled, and the patient's tolerance of the procedure. Document any patient teaching provided and the patient's understanding of the teaching.

REFERENCES

1 The Joint Commission. (2012). Standard NPSG.07.01.01. *Comprehensive accreditation manual for hospitals: The official handbook.* Oakbrook Terrace, IL: The Joint Commission. (Level I)
2 Centers for Disease Control and Prevention. (October 2002). Guideline for hand hygiene in health-care settings. *Morbidity and Mortality Weekly Report, 51*(RR-16), 1–45. (Level 1)
3 World Health Organization. (2009). *WHO guidelines on hand hygiene in health care: First global patient safety challenge. Clean care is safer care.* Geneva, Switzerland: World Health Organization. (Level I)
4 The Joint Commission. (2012). Standard NPSG.01.01.01. *Comprehensive accreditation manual for hospitals: The official handbook.* Oakbrook Terrace, IL: The Joint Commission. (Level I)
5 The Joint Commission. (2012). Standard RC.01.03.01. *Comprehensive accreditation manual for hospitals: The official handbook.* Oakbrook Terrace, IL: The Joint Commission. (Level I)

ADDITIONAL REFERENCE

National Diabetes Information Clearinghouse (NDIC). (2009). "Diabetic Neuropathies: The Nerve Damage of Diabetes" [Online]. Accessed August 2011 via the Web at http://diabetes.niddk.nih.gov/dm/pubs/neuropathies

CRICOTHYROTOMY, ASSISTING

When endotracheal intubation or a tracheotomy can't be performed quickly to establish an airway, an emergency cricothyrotomy may be necessary. Performed rarely, this procedure involves puncturing the trachea through the cricothyroid membrane.

Usually, your role will be to assist a doctor with this procedure, but if you have received special training, you may have to perform the procedure in an emergency. Ideally, cricothyrotomy is performed using sterile technique but, in an emergency, this may not be possible.

Equipment

Have one person stay with the patient while another collects the necessary equipment.

For scalpel or needle cricothyrotomy

Sterile gloves ■ goggles ■ antiseptic cleaning solution ■ sterile 4" × 4" gauze pads ■ sterile drapes or towels ■ dilator ■ tape ■ oxygen source.

For scalpel cricothyrotomy

Scalpel ■ #6 or smaller tracheostomy tube (if available) ■ handheld resuscitation bag or T tube and wide-bore oxygen tubing.

For needle cricothyrotomy

14G (or larger) through-the-needle or over-the-needle catheter ■ 10-mL syringe ■ tape ■ IV extension tubing ■ hand-operated release valve or pressure-regulating adjustment valve.

Implementation

■ Confirm the patient's identity using at least two patient identifiers according to your facility's policy.[1]
■ Perform hand hygiene and put on sterile gloves and personal protective equipment.[2,3,4]
■ Place the patient in the supine position.
■ Hyperextend the patient's neck *to expose the area of the incision site.*
■ The doctor cleans the patient's neck with a gauze pad soaked in antiseptic cleaning solution. *To reduce the risk of contamination, he should use a circular motion, working outward from the incision site.*

- Assist with draping the patient's neck with sterile towels.
- The doctor locates the precise insertion site by sliding his thumb and fingers down to the thyroid gland. He'll know he's located its outer borders when the space between his fingers and thumb widens.
- The doctor assesses for hematomas, which may displace the trachea to the unaffected side.
- The doctor then moves his fingers across the center of the gland, over the anterior edge of the cricoid ring (as shown below).

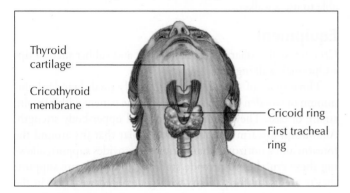

Using a scalpel
- Hand the doctor a scalpel so he can make a horizontal incision, less than ½″ (1.3 cm) long, in the cricothyroid membrane just above the cricoid ring.
- The doctor inserts a dilator *to prevent tissue from closing around the incision*. If a dilator isn't available, he inserts the handle of the scalpel and rotates it 90 degrees (as shown below).

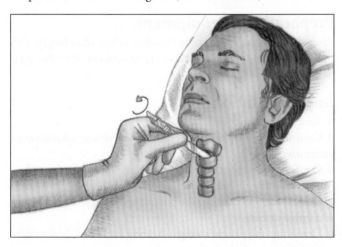

- If a small tracheostomy tube (#6 or smaller) is available, the doctor inserts it into the opening and secures it *to help maintain a patent airway*. If a tracheostomy tube isn't available, he may tape the dilator or scalpel handle in place until a tracheostomy tube is available.
- If the patient can breathe spontaneously, attach a humidified oxygen source to the tracheostomy tube with a T tube; if he can't, attach a handheld resuscitation bag. You'll need to inflate the cuff of the tracheostomy tube with a syringe *to provide positive-pressure ventilation*.

Using a needle
- Attach a 10-mL syringe to a 14G (or larger) through-the-needle or over-the-needle catheter. Hand the catheter to the doctor, who inserts the catheter into the cricothyroid membrane just above the cricoid ring.
- The doctor directs the catheter downward at a 45-degree angle (as shown below) to the trachea *to avoid damaging the vocal cords*. He maintains negative pressure by pulling back the syringe plunger as he advances the catheter. He'll know the catheter has entered the trachea when air enters the syringe.

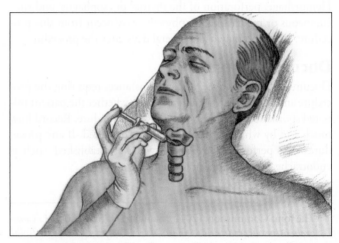

- When the catheter reaches the trachea, the doctor advances it and removes the needle and syringe.
- Tape the catheter in place.
- Attach the catheter hub to one end of the IV extension tubing. At the other end, attach a hand-operated release valve or a pressure-regulating adjustment valve. Connect the entire assembly to an oxygen source.
- Press the release valve to introduce oxygen into the trachea and inflate the lungs. When you can see that they're inflated, release the valve to allow passive exhalation. Adjust the pressure-regulating valve to the minimum pressure needed for adequate lung inflation.

Completing the procedure
- Auscultate bilaterally for breath sounds, and take the patient's vital signs.
- Check the patient's end-tidal carbon dioxide level.
- Check for bleeding at the insertion site, subcutaneous emphysema or inadequate ventilation, and tracheal or vocal cord damage.
- Remove and discard your gloves and perform hand hygiene.[2,3,4]
- Anticipate a chest X-ray to evaluate tube placement.
- Document the procedure.[5]

Special considerations
PEDIATRIC ALERT *Scalpel cricothyrotomy isn't recommended for children younger than age 12 because it could damage the cricoid cartilage—the only circumferential support to the upper trachea.*

■ Whenever possible, use an ultrasound machine *to visualize the patient's anatomy* before starting the procedure.

■ If your facility indicates that cricothyrotomy falls within universal protocol guidelines and time allows, follow the necessary steps, including conducting a time-out immediately before starting the procedure, *to ensure that the correct patient, site, positioning, and procedure are identified and that (as applicable) all relevant information and necessary equipment are available.*[6,7]

Complications

Hemorrhage, perforation of the thyroid or esophagus, and subcutaneous or mediastinal emphysema may occur from this procedure. Infection may occur several days after the procedure.

Documentation

Document the date, time, and circumstances requiring the procedure and the patient's vital signs. Note whether the patient initiated spontaneous respirations after the procedure. Record how much and by what method oxygen was delivered. If any procedures were performed after the airway was established, such as endotracheal intubation, note them.

REFERENCES

1 The Joint Commission. (2012). Standard NPSG.01.01.01. *Comprehensive accreditation manual for hospitals: The official handbook.* Oakbrook Terrace, IL: The Joint Commission. (Level I)

2 The Joint Commission. (2012). Standard NPSG.07.01.01. *Comprehensive accreditation manual for hospitals: The official handbook.* Oakbrook Terrace, IL: The Joint Commission. (Level I)

3 Centers for Disease Control and Prevention. (October 2002). Guideline for hand hygiene in health-care settings. *Morbidity and Mortality Weekly Report, 51*(RR-16), 1–45. (Level 1)

4 World Health Organization. (2009). *WHO guidelines on hand hygiene in health care: First global patient safety challenge. Clean care is safer care.* Geneva, Switzerland: World Health Organization. (Level I)

5 The Joint Commission. (2012). Standard RC.01.03.01. *Comprehensive accreditation manual for hospitals: The official handbook.* Oakbrook Terrace, IL: The Joint Commission. (Level I)

6 The Joint Commission. (2012). Standard UP.01.01.01. *Comprehensive accreditation manual for hospitals: The official handbook.* Oakbrook Terrace, IL: The Joint Commission. (Level I)

7 The Joint Commission. (2012). Standard UP.01.03.01. *Comprehensive accreditation manual for hospitals: The official handbook.* Oakbrook Terrace, IL: The Joint Commission. (Level I)

ADDITIONAL REFERENCES

Lynn-McHale Wiegand, D. (Ed.). (2011). *AACN procedure manual for critical care* (6th ed.). Philadelphia, PA: Saunders.

Mace, S.E., & Khan, N. (2008). Needle cricothyrotomy. *Emergency Medical Clinics of North America, 26*(4), 1085–1101.

Vissers, R.J., & Bair, A.E. (2008). Surgical airway techniques. In R.M. Walls & M.F. Murphy (Eds.), *Manual of emergency airway management* (3rd ed.). Philadelphia, PA: Lippincott Williams & Wilkins.

CRUTCH USE

Crutches remove weight from one or both legs, enabling the patient to support himself with his hands and arms. Typically prescribed for the patient with lower-extremity injury or weakness or one who has had a surgical procedure on the lower limbs, crutches require balance, stamina, and upper-body strength for successful use. Crutch selection and walking gait depend on the patient's condition. The patient who can't use crutches may be able to use a walker.

Equipment

Crutches with axillary pads, handgrips, and rubber suction tips
■ Optional: walking belt.

Three types of crutches are commonly used. Standard aluminum or wooden crutches are used by the patient with a sprain, strain, or cast. They require stamina and upper-body strength. Aluminum forearm crutches have a collar that fits around the forearm and a horizontal handgrip that provides support, allowing these crutches to provide stability and moderate support; they're are useful for patients with generalized weakness in the lower extremities, such as those with paraplegia or cerebral palsy. The patient using forearm crutches generally uses the swing-through gait.

Platform crutches are used by a patient who has an upper-extremity deficit that prevents weight bearing through the wrist, such as in those with arthritis or an upper-extremity fracture. These crutches provide padded surfaces for the upper extremities.

Preparation of equipment

After choosing the appropriate crutches, adjust their height with the patient standing or, if necessary, recumbent. (See *Fitting a patient for a crutch.*)

Implementation

■ Verify the doctor's order.

■ Consult with the physical therapist *to coordinate rehabilitation orders and teaching.*

■ Confirm the patient's identity using at least two patient identifiers according to your facility's policy.[1]

■ Explain the procedure to the patient and answer any questions *to decrease anxiety.*

■ Determine the patient's weight-bearing status *to help determine which gait to teach the patient.*

■ Describe the gait you will teach and the reason for your choice.

■ Perform hand hygiene.[2,3,4]

■ Place a walking belt around the patient's waist, if necessary, *to help prevent falls.* Tell the patient to position the crutches and to shift his weight from side to side.

■ Place the patient in front of a full-length mirror *to facilitate learning and coordination.*

■ Teach the four-point gait to the patient who can bear weight on both legs. Although this is the safest gait *because three points are always in contact with the floor,* it requires greater coordination than others *because of its constant shifting of weight.* Use this

Fitting a patient for a crutch

Axilla crutch

1. To measure for an axilla crutch, position the crutch so that it extends from a point 4″ to 6″ (10 to 15 cm) to the side and 4″ to 6″ in front of the patient's feet to 1″ to 1½″ (2.5 to 4 cm) below the axillae (about the width of two fingers).

2. Adjust the handgrips so that the patient's elbows are flexed at a 30-degree angle and the wrists are at a 15-degree angle when he's standing with the crutches in the resting position. The handgrips should be even with the top of the hip line. Check that the vinyl padding on the arm cuffs, the rubber handgrips, and the rubber tips at the end of the crutches are securely placed.

Forearm crutch

To fit a forearm crutch, have the patient flex his elbow so the crease in his wrist is at his hip. Measure his forearm from 3″ (7.5 cm) below the elbow to his wrist (A). Then measure the distance between his wrist and the floor (B). Then add the two distances (A & B) to establish the correct height (C).

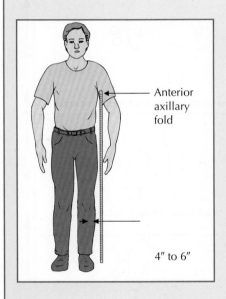

Anterior axillary fold

4″ to 6″

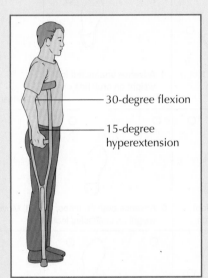

30-degree flexion

15-degree hyperextension

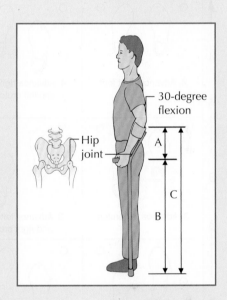

30-degree flexion

Hip joint

A

C

B

sequence: right crutch, left foot, left crutch, right foot. Suggest counting *to help develop rhythm,* and make sure each short step is of equal length. If the patient gains proficiency at this gait, teach him the faster two-point gait. (See *Crutch gaits,* page 222.)

■ Teach the three-point gait to the patient who can bear only partial or no weight on one leg. Instruct him to advance both crutches 6″ to 8″ (15 to 20 cm) along with the involved leg. Then tell him to bring the uninvolved leg forward and to bear the bulk of his weight on the crutches but some of it on the involved leg, if possible. Stress the importance of taking steps of equal length and duration with no pauses.

■ Teach the two-point gait to the patient with weak legs but good coordination and arm strength. This is the most natural crutch-walking gait *because it mimics walking,* with alternating swings of the arms and legs. Instruct the patient to advance the right crutch and left foot simultaneously, followed by the left crutch and right foot.

■ Teach the swing-to or swing-through gaits—the fastest ones—to the patient with complete paralysis of the hips and legs. Instruct the patient to advance both crutches simultaneously and to swing the legs parallel to (swing-to) or beyond the crutches (swing-through).

■ Teach the patient to sit down in a chair by supporting himself with the crutches in one hand and lowering himself with the other.

■ Teach the patient to get up from a chair by holding both crutches in one hand, with the tips resting firmly on the floor. Instruct him to push up from the chair with his free hand, supporting himself with the crutches.

■ Teach the patient to ascend stairs using the three-point gait, leading with the good leg and following with both crutches and the involved leg. Teach him to descend stairs by leading with the crutches and the involved leg and following with the good leg.

■ Observe the patient as he provides return demonstrations of using the appropriate gait, using a chair, and negotiating stairs.

■ Perform hand hygiene.[2,3,4]

■ Document the procedure.[5]

Crutch gaits

This is a guide for using the four-point, three-point, and two-point swing-to or swing-through gaits. Start at the bottom and move upward. *Note:* Shaded areas indicate weight bearing.

FOUR-POINT GAIT	TWO-POINT GAIT	THREE-POINT GAIT	THREE-POINT-PLUS-ONE GAIT
• Partial weight bearing both feet • Maximal support provided • Requires constant shift of weight	• Partial weight bearing both feet • Provides less support • Faster than a four-point gait	• Non-weight bearing on one foot • Requires good balance • Requires arm strength • Faster gait • Non-weight bearing foot moves with crutches • Can use this gait with a walker	• Partial weight bearing on one foot and full weight bearing on the second • Crutches and affected leg move together • Requires good balance • Faster than three-point gait • Dashed line indicates partial weight bearing
4. Advance right foot	4. Advance right foot and left crutch	4. Advance unaffected foot, weight on crutches only.	4. Advance unaffected leg beyond crutches again
3. Advance left crutch	3. Advance left foot and right crutch	3. Advance both crutches, weight on unaffected foot.	3. Move crutches and affected leg forward
2. Advance left foot	2. Advance right foot and left crutch	2. Advance unaffected foot, weight on crutches only.	2. Move unaffected leg forward beyond crutches
1. Advance right crutch	1. Advance left foot and right crutch	1. Advance both crutches, weight on unaffected foot.	1. Full weight on crutches and partial weight on affected leg; move crutches and affected leg forward
Beginning stance	Beginning stance	Beginning stance	Beginning stance

Special considerations

■ If possible, consult physical therapy to teach two techniques—one fast and one slow—*so the patient can alternate between them to prevent excessive muscle fatigue and can adjust more easily to various walking conditions.*

Complications

When used with chronic conditions, the swing-to and swing-through gaits can lead to atrophy of the hips and legs if appropriate therapeutic exercises aren't performed routinely. Instruct the patient to avoid habitually leaning on his crutches *because prolonged pressure on the axillae can damage the brachial nerves, causing brachial nerve palsy.*

Patient teaching

Instruct the patient not to move too fast or swing his leg too far forward *because this could cause a loss of balance.*

Tell the patient to check the wing nuts or locking mechanisms daily *to make sure they're tightened securely.*

Advise the patient to remove rugs and clutter from the floor *to decrease the risk of falls.*

Tell the patient to wear a tennis shoe or other flat rubber-soled shoe on the unaffected foot *to avoid slipping.*

Documentation

Record the type of gait the patient used, the amount of assistance required, the distance walked, and the patient's tolerance of the crutches and gait.

REFERENCES

1 The Joint Commission. (2012). Standard NPSG.01.01.01. *Comprehensive accreditation manual for hospitals: The official handbook.* Oakbrook Terrace, IL: The Joint Commission. (Level I)
2 The Joint Commission. (2012). Standard NPSG.07.01.01. *Comprehensive accreditation manual for hospitals: The official handbook.* Oakbrook Terrace, IL: The Joint Commission. (Level I)
3 Centers for Disease Control and Prevention. (October 2002). Guideline for hand hygiene in health-care settings. *Morbidity and Mortality Weekly Report, 51*(RR-16), 1–45. (Level 1)
4 World Health Organization. (2009). *WHO guidelines on hand hygiene in health care: First global patient safety challenge. Clean care is safer care.* Geneva, Switzerland: World Health Organization. (Level I)
5 The Joint Commission. (2012). Standard RC.01.03.01. *Comprehensive accreditation manual for hospitals: The official handbook.* Oakbrook Terrace, IL: The Joint Commission. (Level I)

ADDITIONAL REFERENCES

Craven, R.F., & Hirnle, C.J. (2009). *Fundamentals of nursing: Human health and function* (6th ed.). Philadelphia, PA: Lippincott Williams & Wilkins.
Salminen, A.L., et al. (2009). Mobility devices to promote activity and participation: A systematic review. *Journal of Rehabilitation Medicine, 41*(9), 697–706.

DEFIBRILLATION

The standard treatment for ventricular fibrillation, defibrillation involves using external pads or paddles to direct an electrical current through the patient's heart. The current causes the myocardium to depolarize; this, in turn, encourages the sinoatrial node to resume control of the heart's electrical activity. This current can be delivered by a monophasic or biphasic defibrillator.

Defibrillators with monophasic waveforms deliver current in one direction (as shown below). Few monophasic defibrillators are being manufactured, but some are still in use. For monophasic defibrillation to be effective, a high amount of electrical current is required.

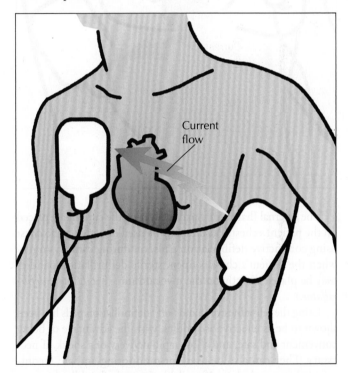

Current flow

With biphasic defibrillation, the electrical current discharged from the pads or paddles travels in a positive direction for a specified duration and then reverses and flows in a negative direction for the remaining time of the electrical discharge (as shown on next page). It delivers two currents of electricity and lowers the defibrillation threshold of the heart muscle, making it possible to successfully defibrillate ventricular fibrillation with smaller amounts of energy. The biphasic defibrillator can adjust for differences in impedance or the resistance of the current through the chest. This helps reduce the number of shocks needed to terminate ventricular fibrillation. Biphasic technology uses lower energy levels and fewer shocks, thus reducing the damage to the myocardial muscle. Biphasic defibrillators, when used at the clinically appropriate energy level, may be used for defibrillation and, when placed in the synchronized mode, may be used for synchronized cardioversion.

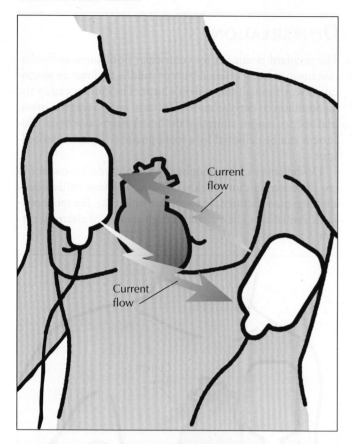

Current flow

Current flow

The external (hands-off) pads delivering the current are placed on the patient's chest. Paddles may be used directly on the chest using conductive defibrillation pads, or, during cardiac surgery when the patient's chest is open, sterile defibrillation paddles may be placed directly on the myocardium. (See *Using a defibrillator.*)

Using the self-adhesive (hands-off) defibrillation pads has been shown to be as effective as paddles, with the advantage of being convenient and safe, and allow rapid delivery of a shock, if necessary. They can also be used for monitoring and are recommended for routine use, if available, instead of paddles.[1]

Patients with a history of ventricular fibrillation may be candidates for an implantable cardioverter-defibrillator (ICD), a sophisticated device that automatically discharges an electrical current when it senses a ventricular tachyarrhythmia. (See *Understanding the ICD,* page 226.)

Equipment

Gloves ▪ defibrillator with electrocardiogram (ECG) monitor and recorder ▪ self-adhesive defibrillation pads and connector cable or defibrillation paddles with conductive gel, or prepackaged gelled conductive pads ▪ bag-mask device with mask and oxygen delivery equipment ▪ emergency suction and intubation equipment ▪ blood pressure monitoring equipment ▪ pulse oximeter ▪ IV infusion pumps.

Preparation of equipment

Connect the defibrillation pads or paddles to the defibrillator and check that the defibrillator battery is adequately charged or the defibrillator electrical cord is plugged into the wall. Ensure that resuscitation equipment and medications are immediately available.

Implementation

▪ Perform hand hygiene.[4,5,6]
▪ Confirm the patient's identity using at least two patient identifiers, according to your facility's policy.[7]
▪ If time allows, make sure the patient and family understand the procedure.
▪ Put on gloves and follow standard precautions throughout the procedure.[8]
▪ Assess the patient to determine that he's unresponsive and not breathing (or only gasping).[3]
▪ If the patient is unresponsive and not breathing, call for help and then take up to 10 seconds to attempt to feel for a pulse (carotid or femoral). If you're alone and don't feel a pulse or you're unsure whether you feel a pulse, begin chest compressions. After 30 compressions, open the patient's airway using a head tilt–chin lift and give two breaths. If there is evidence of trauma that suggests spinal injury, use a jaw thrust without head tilt to open the airway. Continue cardiopulmonary resuscitation (CPR) until the defibrillator and emergency equipment arrive.[3]

NURSING ALERT *Remove any transdermal medication patches from the chest (and back if using anteroposterior placement) and wipe the area clean, if possible,* because the medication may interfere with the conduction of the current or produce a chest burn.[3]

Defibrillation using self-adhesive defibrillation pads

NURSING ALERT *If the patient is wet, dry the chest quickly before attempting to apply self-adhesive defibrillation pads* to prevent inappropriate conduction of electrical current.[3]

NURSING ALERT *Remove metallic objects that the patient may be wearing* because they are excellent conductors of electrical current and could cause a burn.[3]

▪ Expose the patient's chest and apply the self-adhesive defibrillation pads.
▪ For anterolateral placement, position one pad to the right of the upper sternum, just below the right clavicle, and the other over the fifth or sixth intercostal space at the left anterior axillary line (as shown on next page top).

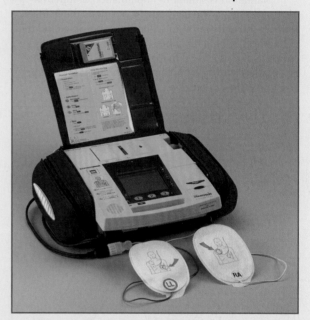

■ For anteroposterior placement, position the anterior pad directly over the heart at the precordium, to the left of the lower sternal border (as shown below, top illustration). Place the posterior pad under the patient's body beneath the heart and immediately below the scapula but not on the vertebral column (as shown below, bottom illustration).

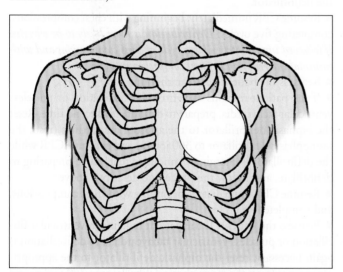

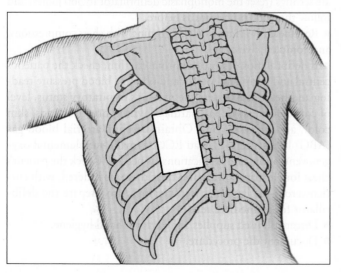

Using a defibrillator

Because ventricular fibrillation leads to death if not corrected, the success of defibrillation depends on early recognition and quick treatment of this arrhythmia.[2] In addition to treating ventricular fibrillation, defibrillation may also be used to treat ventricular tachycardia that doesn't produce a pulse.[3] To help treat your patient as quickly as possible, you should familiarize yourself with the defibrillator available at your facility. Use the defibrillators below as a guide to help familiarize yourself with the parts of a defibrillator.

Defibrillator with self-adhesive defibrillation pads

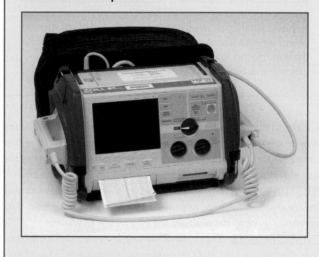

Defibrillator with paddles

Understanding the ICD

The implantable cardioverter-defibrillator (ICD) has a programmable pulse generator and lead system that monitors the heart's activity, detects ventricular brad-yarrhythmias and tachyarrhythmias, and responds to each with different interventions. These interventions include antitachycardia pacing, cardioversion, defibril-lation, and bradycardia pacing. Some ICDs can be pro-grammed to pace both the atrium and ventricle or both ventricles (known as *cardiac resynchronization therapy*). Some models can also detect and correct atrial arrhythmias.

Implantation is similar to implantation of a perma-nent pacemaker. The cardiologist positions the lead or leads in the endocardium of the right ventricle (and the right atrium if both chambers require pacing) and then connects the other end to the generator (about the size of a wallet), which is implanted in the right or left upper chest near the collarbone.

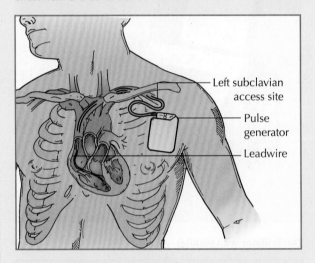

Left subclavian access site

Pulse generator

Leadwire

New, smaller devices can be installed through the blood vessels. These newer devices can also store infor-mation related to the arrhythmic event and perform electrophysiology testing.

■ Make sure you position the pads correctly. *Defibrillation occurs when an electrical current passes through the cardiac muscle to restore a single source of impulse production. Appropriate positioning of the pads maximizes the flow of electrical current through the heart.*[1]
NURSING ALERT *Always keep the self-adhesive defibrillation pads in a sealed package* to prevent them from drying out. *The expiration date of the pads should be checked routinely.*
NURSING ALERT *Don't place the self-adhesive defibrillation pads directly over an ICD or implanted pacemaker.* This place-ment may damage the device. Position the pad at least 1″ (2.5 cm) from the implanted device.[1]
■ Turn on the defibrillator and, if performing external defibril-lation using a biphasic defibrillator, use clinically appropriate

energy levels (usually 120 to 200 joules) following the manufac-turer's recommended dose.[3] Few monophasic defibrillators are manufactured. If using a monophasic defibrillator, set the energy level for 360 joules for an adult patient.
■ Connect the monitoring leads of the defibrillator to the patient *to assess his cardiac rhythm.*
■ Turn on the ECG recorder *to provide a visual recording of the patient's ECG as well as his response to interventions.*[1]
■ Charge the device by pressing the appropriate button on the defibrillator. Continue compressions while the defibrillator is charging.
■ Reassess the patient's cardiac rhythm.
■ Turn off or remove the oxygen source during actual defibrilla-tion *to decrease the chance of combustion caused by arcing of the electrical current in the presence of oxygen.*[1]
■ If the patient remains in ventricular fibrillation or pulseless ventricular tachycardia, instruct all personnel to stand clear of the patient and the bed. Visually verify that all personnel are clear of the patient and the bed before discharging the electrical cur-rent. *Electrical current can be conducted from the patient to any-one in contact with the patient.*[1]
■ Discharge the current by pressing the appropriate button on the defibrillator.
■ Resume CPR immediately, beginning with chest compressions, completing five cycles. *Defibrillation is more likely to be effective if followed immediately with a cycle of chest compressions and with minimal interruption in chest compressions.*[3]
■ Reassess the patient's cardiac rhythm.
■ If the patient remains in ventricular fibrillation or pulseless ventricular tachycardia, prepare to defibrillate a second time. Reset the biphasic defibrillator to the appropriate settings (reset the monophasic defibrillator to 360 joules) and continue CPR while the defibrillator is charging. Announce that you're preparing to defibrillate, and follow the procedure described above.[3]
■ Resume CPR immediately, beginning with chest compressions, and complete five cycles.[3]
■ Reassess the patient. If the patient remains in ventricular fib-rillation or pulseless ventricular tachycardia and defibrillation is again necessary, reset the biphasic defibrillator to the appropri-ate settings (reset the monophasic defibrillator to 360 joules) and follow the same procedure as before.
■ Resume CPR immediately, beginning with chest compressions, and complete five cycles.[3]
■ If defibrillation restores a normal rhythm, check the patient's central and peripheral pulses and obtain a blood pressure read-ing and heart rate. Assess the patient's respiratory status, level of consciousness (LOC), cardiac rhythm, breath sounds, skin color, and urine output. Obtain baseline arterial blood gas (ABG) levels and a 12-lead ECG. Provide supplemental oxy-gen, ventilation, and medications, as needed. Check the patient's chest for electrical burns and treat them, as ordered, with cor-ticosteroid- or lanolin-based creams. Also prepare the defib-rillator for immediate reuse.
■ Discard all used supplies and perform hand hygiene.[4,5,6]
■ Document the procedure.[9]

Defibrillation using defibrillator paddles

NURSING ALERT *If the patient is wet, dry the chest quickly before attempting to defibrillate* to prevent inappropriate conduction of electrical current.

■ If the defibrillator can monitor the patient's rhythm using the paddles, turn on the defibrillator, expose the patient's chest, and apply the gelled conductive pads on the patient's chest. For anterolateral placement, position one gelled conductive pad to the right of the upper sternum, just below the right clavicle, and the other over the fifth or sixth intercostal space at the left anterior axillary line. For anteroposterior placement, position the anterior gelled conductive pad directly over the heart at the precordium to the left of the lower sternal border. Place the posterior gelled conductive pad under the patient's body beneath the heart and immediately below the scapula but not on the vertebral column. *Defibrillation occurs when an electrical current passes through the cardiac muscle to restore a single source of impulse production. Appropriate positioning of the pads maximizes the flow of electrical current through the heart.*[1]

■ Press the paddles firmly against the patient's chest on top of the gelled conductive pads, using 25 lb/in^2 (11 kg) of pressure to quickly view the cardiac rhythm (as shown below).[10]

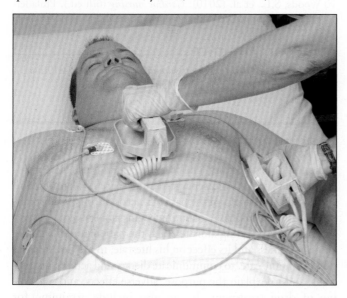

NURSING ALERT *Avoid placing the paddles directly over an ICD or implanted pacemaker.* This placement may damage the device.[3]

■ Connect the monitoring leads of the defibrillator to the patient, and assess his cardiac rhythm.

■ Turn on the ECG recorder to provide a visual recording of the patient's ECG as well as his response to interventions.

■ Charge the paddles by pressing the charge buttons, located either on the defibrillator or on the paddles themselves or by using the appropriate button on the machine.

■ Reassess the patient's cardiac rhythm.

■ Turn off or remove the oxygen source during actual defibrillation. *This decreases the chance of combustion caused by arcing of the electrical current in the presence of oxygen.*[3]

■ If the patient remains in ventricular fibrillation or pulseless ventricular tachycardia, instruct all personnel to stand clear of the patient and the bed. Visually verify all personnel are clear of the patient and the bed before discharging the current. *Electrical current can be conducted from the patient to anyone in contact with the patient.*[3]

■ Discharge the current by pressing both paddle charge buttons simultaneously, maintaining 25 lb/in^2 (11 kg) of pressure on both paddles.[9] *Using this pressure decreases transthoracic resistance.* Hold until the defibrillator delivers the electrical current.[1]

■ Resume CPR immediately, beginning with chest compressions, giving five cycles. *Defibrillation is more likely to be effective if followed immediately with a cycle of chest compressions and with minimal interruption in chest compressions.*[3]

■ Reassess the patient's cardiac rhythm.

■ If the patient remains in ventricular fibrillation or pulseless ventricular tachycardia, prepare to defibrillate a second time. Reset the biphasic defibrillator to the appropriate settings (reset the monophasic defibrillator to 360 joules) and continue CPR while the defibrillator is charging. Announce that you're preparing to defibrillate, and follow the procedure described above.[3]

■ Resume CPR immediately, starting with chest compressions, and complete five cycles.[3]

■ Reassess the patient. If the patient remains in ventricular fibrillation or pulseless ventricular tachycardia and defibrillation is again necessary, reset the biphasic defibrillator to the appropriate settings (reset the monophasic defibrillator to 360 joules). Then follow the same procedure as before.

■ Resume CPR immediately, starting with chest compressions, and give five cycles.[3]

■ If defibrillation restores a normal rhythm, check the patient's central and peripheral pulses and obtain a blood pressure reading and heart rate. Assess the patient's respiratory status, LOC, cardiac rhythm, breath sounds, skin color, and urine output. Obtain baseline ABG levels and a 12-lead ECG. Provide supplemental oxygen, ventilation, and medications, as needed. Check the patient's chest for electrical burns and treat them, as ordered, with corticosteroid- or lanolin-based creams. Also prepare the defibrillator for immediate reuse.

■ Discard all used supplies appropriately and perform hand hygiene.[4,5,6]

■ Provide support and information to the patient's family, as appropriate. After the procedure, if possible, inform the patient about what happened.

■ Document the procedure.[9]

Special considerations

■ Additional defibrillation should be done 30 seconds to 1 minute after administering medications.

■ Defibrillators vary from one manufacturer to the next, so familiarize yourself with your facility's equipment. Defibrillator operation should be checked according to your facility's policy (usually once per shift).

■ If gelled conductive pads aren't available, defibrillator paddles require that a conductive gel be placed on the paddles before use. Place the gel on one paddle, and rub the two paddles together to spread the gel evenly between them. Ensure that the surface of the paddle is completely covered.

■ Defibrillation can be affected by several factors, including paddle size and placement, condition of the patient's myocardium, duration of the arrhythmia, chest resistance, and the number of countershocks.[2]

■ Avoid placing the defibrillator pad or paddle over a female patient's breast. Instead, place the apex of the pad or paddle at the fifth to sixth intercostal space, with the middle of the pad or paddle at the midaxillary line.

■ If the patient has a hairy chest, remove the hair from necessary locations for pad or paddle placement. If using self-adhesive defibrillation pads, you can remove the hair by placing the pads on the chest in the proper location and then removing them quickly. Use a second set of pads for defibrillation.

Complications

Defibrillation can cause accidental electrical shock to those providing care. Using dry self-adhesive defibrillation pads or applying an insufficient amount of conductive medium can lead to skin burns.

Documentation

Document the procedure, including the patient's ECG rhythm both before and after defibrillation; the number of times defibrillation was performed; the energy used with each attempt; whether a pulse returned; the dosage, route, and time of drug administration; whether CPR was performed; how the airway was maintained; and the patient's outcome. Document any patient or family teaching.

References

1 Lynn-McHale Wiegand, D. (Ed.). (2011). *AACN procedure manual for critical care* (6th ed.). Philadelphia, PA: Saunders.

2 Chan, P. S., et al. (2008). Delayed time to defibrillation after in-hospital cardiac arrest. *NEJM, 358*(1), 9–17. (Level VI)

3 American Heart Association. (2010). 2010 American Heart Association guidelines for cardiopulmonary resuscitation and emergency cardiovascular care. *Circulation, 122* (Suppl. 3), S685–S719. (Level I)

4 The Joint Commission. (2012). Standard NPSG.07.01.01. *Comprehensive accreditation manual for hospitals: The official handbook.* Oakbrook Terrace, IL: The Joint Commission.. (Level I)

5 World Health Organization. (2009). *WHO guidelines on hand hygiene in health care: First global patient safety challenge. Clean care is safer care.* Geneva, Switzerland: World Health Organization. (Level I)

6 Centers for Disease Control and Prevention. (October 2002). Guideline for hand hygiene in health-care settings. *Morbidity and Mortality Weekly Report, 51*(RR-16), 1–45. (Level 1)

7 The Joint Commission. (2012). Standard NPSG.01.01.01. *Comprehensive accreditation manual for hospitals: The official handbook.* Oakbrook Terrace, IL: The Joint Commission. (Level I)

8 Siegel, J.D., et al. "2007 Guideline for Isolation Precautions: Preventing Transmission of Infectious Agents in Healthcare Settings" [Online]. Accessed August 2011 via the Web at http://www.cdc.gov/hicpac/2007ip/2007isolationprecautions.html

9 The Joint Commission. (2012). Standard RC.01.03.01. *Comprehensive accreditation manual for hospitals: The official handbook.* Oakbrook Terrace, IL: The Joint Commission. (Level I)

10 Woods, S.L., et al. (2010). *Cardiac nursing* (6th ed.). Philadelphia, PA: Lippincott Williams & Wilkins.

Additional reference

Nettina, S.M. (2010). *Lippincott manual of nursing practice* (9th ed.). Philadelphia, PA: Lippincott Williams & Wilkins.

Discharge

Although discharge from a health care facility is usually considered routine, effective discharge requires careful planning and continuing assessment of the patient's needs during his hospitalization. Ideally, discharge planning begins at admission.[1,2]

Discharge planning aims to teach the patient and his family about his illness and its effect on his lifestyle, to provide instructions for home care, to communicate dietary and activity instructions, and to explain the purpose, adverse effects, and scheduling of drug treatment. It can also include arranging for transportation; follow-up care; coordination of outpatient or home health care services, if necessary; and information about support services, if appropriate.

Equipment

Wheelchair, unless the patient leaves by ambulance ■ patient's chart ■ patient instruction sheet and medication list ■ discharge summary sheet ■ plastic bag or patient's suitcase for personal belongings.

Implementation

■ Verify a written discharge order from the doctor, along with medication reconciliation information. If the patient discharges himself against medical advice, obtain the appropriate form. (See *Dealing with a discharge against medical advice.*)[3]

- Perform hand hygiene.[4,5,6]
- Confirm the patient's identity using at least two patient identifiers according to your facility's policy.[7]
- Inform the patient's family of the time and date of discharge as soon as it's known. If the patient's family can't arrange transportation, notify the social services department. (Always confirm arranged transportation on the day of discharge.)[1,2]
- If the patient requires home medical care, confirm arrangements with the appropriate facility department or community agency.
- Review the patient's discharge care plan, initiated on admission and modified during his hospitalization, with the patient and his family.[2] (See *Discharge teaching goals.*) List prescribed drugs on the patient instruction sheet along with the dosage, prescribed time schedule, and adverse reactions that he should report to the doctor.[8] Ensure that the drug schedule is consistent with the patient's lifestyle *to prevent improper administration and to promote patient compliance.* Remind the patient to discard old medication lists when he returns home.
- Review procedures the patient or family will perform at home. If necessary, demonstrate these procedures, provide written instructions, and check performance with a return demonstration.
- List dietary and activity instructions on the patient instruction sheet, if applicable, and review the reasons for them. If the doctor orders bed rest, make sure the patient's family can provide daily care and will obtain necessary equipment.
- Check with the doctor about the patient's follow-up office appointment; if the doctor hasn't yet done so, inform the patient of the date, time, and location. If scheduling is your responsibility, make an appointment with the doctor, outpatient clinic, physical therapy, X-ray department, or other health services, as needed. If the patient can't arrange transportation to these appointments, notify the social services department *to help the patient comply with the treatment plan.*[1]
- Have the patient or family member sign the discharge instructions to verify receipt of written discharge instructions.
- Retrieve the patient's valuables from the facility's safe and review each item with him. Then obtain the patient's signature *to verify receipt of his valuables.*
- Obtain from the pharmacy any drugs the patient brought with him. Return these to the patient if drug therapy is unchanged. If giving a new prescription, provide an explanation of the dosage, schedule, and adverse effects.
- If the patient is being discharged to another facility, such as an assisted living or long-term care facility, or if the patient will be followed up at home by a home care agency, make sure that a complete list of his medications is communicated to the next provider *to comply with Joint Commission standards.*[8]
- If appropriate, perform hand hygiene and take and record the patient's vital signs on the discharge summary form. Notify the doctor if any signs are abnormal, such as an elevated temperature. *If necessary, the doctor may alter the patient's discharge plan.*
- Help the patient get dressed if necessary.

PATIENT TEACHING

Discharge teaching goals

Your discharge teaching should aim to ensure that the patient:
- understands his illness
- complies with his drug therapy
- follows his diet
- manages his activity level
- understands his treatments
- recognizes his need for rest
- knows about possible complications
- knows when to seek follow-up care.

Remember that your discharge teaching must include the patient's family or other caregivers *to ensure that the patient receives proper home care.*

- Collect the patient's personal belongings from his room, compare them with the admission inventory of belongings, and help place them in his suitcase or a plastic bag.
- After checking the room for misplaced belongings, help the patient into the wheelchair, and escort him to the exit; if the patient is leaving by ambulance, help him onto the stretcher.
- After the patient has left the area, strip the bed linens and notify the housekeeping staff that the room is ready for cleaning. Be sure to identify to housekeeping if the room was an isolation room that requires terminal cleaning.
- Perform hand hygiene.[4,5,6]
- Document the procedure.[9]

Special considerations

- Whenever possible, involve the patient's family in discharge planning *so they can better understand and perform patient care procedures.*
- If patient or his family seeks discharge against medical advice, take the appropriate steps. (See *Dealing with a discharge against medical advice.*)
- Before the patient is discharged, perform a physical assessment. If you detect abnormal signs or the patient develops new symptoms, notify the doctor and delay discharge until he has seen the patient.

Documentation

Although your facility's policy determines the extent and form of discharge documentation, you'll usually record the time and date of discharge and family members or caregivers present for teaching. You'll also include details of instructions given to the patient, including medications, activity, diet, treatments and the use of medical equipment, signs and symptoms to report to the doctor, and the date, time, and location of follow-up appointments. Place the signed copy of the discharge instructions given to the patient in the medical record.

REFERENCES

1 The Joint Commission. (2012). Standard PC.04.01.03. *Comprehensive accreditation manual for hospitals: The official handbook.* Oakbrook Terrace, IL: The Joint Commission. (Level I)

2 The Joint Commission. (2012). Standard PC.04.01.05. *Comprehensive accreditation manual for hospitals: The official handbook.* Oakbrook Terrace, IL: The Joint Commission. (Level I)

3 The Joint Commission. (2012). Standard MM.04.01.01. *Comprehensive accreditation manual for hospitals: The official handbook.* Oakbrook Terrace, IL: The Joint Commission. (Level I)

4 The Joint Commission. (2012). Standard NPSG.07.01.01. *Comprehensive accreditation manual for hospitals: The official handbook.* Oakbrook Terrace, IL: The Joint Commission. (Level I)

5 Centers for Disease Control and Prevention. (October 2002). Guideline for hand hygiene in health-care settings. *Morbidity and Mortality Weekly Report, 51*(RR-16), 1–45. (Level 1)

6 World Health Organization. (2009). *WHO guidelines on hand hygiene in health care: First global patient safety challenge. Clean care is safer care.* Geneva, Switzerland: World Health Organization. (Level I)

7 The Joint Commission. (2012). Standard NPSG.01.01.01. *Comprehensive accreditation manual for hospitals: The official handbook.* Oakbrook Terrace, IL: The Joint Commission. (Level I)

8 The Joint Commission. (2012). Standard PC.04.02.01. *Comprehensive accreditation manual for hospitals: The official handbook.* Oakbrook Terrace, IL: The Joint Commission. (Level I)

9 The Joint Commission. (2012). Standard RC.01.03.01. *Comprehensive accreditation manual for hospitals: The official handbook.* Oakbrook Terrace, IL: The Joint Commission. (Level I)

DOCUMENTATION

Documentation is the process of preparing a complete record of a patient's care and is a vital tool for communication among health care team members. Accurate, detailed charting shows the extent and quality of the care that nurses provide, the outcomes of that care, and treatment and education that the patient still needs. Thorough, accurate documentation decreases the potential for miscommunication and errors.

Documentation is a valuable method for demonstrating that the nurse has applied nursing knowledge, skills, and judgment according to professional nursing standards. In a court of law, the patient's health record serves as the legal record of the care provided to that patient. Accrediting agencies and risk managers use the medical record to evaluate the quality of care a patient receives. Insurance companies use documentation systems to verify the care received. Nursing documentation in the medical record may also be used for research and education as well as for quality improvement programs.

Equipment

Medical record (electronic or written) ■ pen with black or blue ink, if using a written medical record.

Preparation of equipment

There are various systems used for documentation. Because each documentation system follows specific policies and procedures for charting, you should familiarize yourself with the requirements of each system. (See *Comparing charting systems.*)

Implementation

■ Write legibly *because illegible entries can result in misinterpretation of information and possible patient harm.*

■ Use ink *because the medical record is a permanent document and ink can't be erased.*

■ Sign all entries using your first and last name and title *to clearly identify who wrote the entry.*

■ When signing your initials on a form, use your full signature in the appropriate place on the form *to identify yourself as the care provider.*

■ Ensure that each sheet of the medical record contains the patient's identifying information *to avoid documenting on the wrong patient or mistaking the patient for another.*

■ Use correct spelling and grammar in your entries *because misspelled words and poor grammar look unprofessional and can lead to errors.*

■ If you make an error, draw a single line through the mistake and make a notation, such as "documentation error," and initial it along with the date and time according to facility policy. Then, record the correct entry. Don't use correction fluid, erasures, or entries between lines.

■ Don't leave blank lines within and between entries. Draw a line through the blank line *to ensure that no further entries may be made.*

■ Document in chronological order using the correct time and date. Avoid block documentation, *which is vague, implies inattention to the patient, and makes it hard to determine when specific events occurred.*[1]

■ Document time according to your facility policy using 24-hour military time or including a.m. or p.m.

■ Document information as soon as possible *to ensure the accuracy of the information and to reflect ongoing care. Delayed documentation increases the potential for omissions, error, and inaccuracy due to memory lapse.*[2]

■ Describe observations and behavior of the patient rather than "label" the patient. Don't offer opinions or use subjective statements or judgments.

■ Use only approved abbreviations.[3] (See *Abbreviations to avoid,* page 232.)

Special considerations

■ If your facility uses computerized documentation, most computer systems record the date and time that entries are made, so you should specifically state in the body of your note the time that events occurred and the action taken.

■ Maintain the confidentiality of the medical record at all times. Keep the medical record closed when not in use and store it in a secure place. If documenting on a computer, be sure that no one else can read the screen, and log off when you are finished documenting or if you need to leave the area. Never share your password with anyone else.

■ At times, you may need to add a late entry, such as an event that you forgot to document earlier or when the medical

Comparing charting systems

SYSTEM	USEFUL SETTINGS	PARTS OF RECORD	ASSESSMENT	CARE PLAN	OUTCOMES AND EVALUATIONS	PROGRESS NOTES FORMAT
Narrative	■ Acute care ■ Long-term care ■ Home care ■ Ambulatory care	■ Progress notes ■ Flow sheets to supplement care plan	■ Initial: history and admission form ■ Ongoing: progress notes	■ Care plan	■ Progress notes ■ Discharge summaries	■ Narration at time of entry
Problem-oriented medical record (POMR)	■ Acute care ■ Long-term care ■ Home care ■ Rehabilitation ■ Mental health facilities	■ Database ■ Care plan ■ Problem list ■ Progress notes ■ Discharge summary	■ Initial: database and care plan ■ Ongoing: progress notes	■ Database ■ Nursing care plan based on problem list	■ Progress notes (section E of SOAPIE and SOAPIER)	■ SOAP, SOAPIE, SOAPIER
Problem-intervention-evaluation (PIE)	■ Acute care	■ Assessment flow sheets ■ Progress notes ■ Problem list	■ Initial: assessment form ■ Ongoing: assessment form every shift	■ None; included in progress notes (section P)	■ Progress notes (section E of PIE)	■ Problem ■ Intervention ■ Evaluation
FOCUS	■ Acute care ■ Long-term care	■ Progress notes ■ Flow sheets ■ Checklists	■ Initial: patient history and admission assessment ■ Ongoing: assessment form	■ Nursing care plan based on problems or nursing diagnoses	■ Progress notes	■ Data ■ Action ■ Response
Charting by exception (CBE)	■ Acute care ■ Long-term care	■ Care plan ■ Flow sheets, including patient-teaching records and patient-discharge notes ■ Graphic record ■ Progress notes	■ Initial: database assessment sheet ■ Ongoing: nursing and medical order flow sheets	■ Nursing care plan based on nursing diagnoses	■ Progress notes (section E of CBE)	■ SOAPIE or SOAPIER
Flow sheet, assessment, concise, timely (FACT)	■ Acute care ■ Long-term care	■ Assessment sheet ■ Flow sheets ■ Progress notes	■ Initial: baseline assessment ■ Ongoing: flow sheets and progress notes	■ Nursing care plan based on nursing diagnoses	■ Flow sheets	■ Data ■ Action ■ Response
Core (with DAE)	■ Acute care ■ Long-term care	■ Kardex ■ Flow sheets ■ Progress notes	■ Initial: baseline assessment ■ Ongoing: progress notes	■ Care plan	■ Progress notes (section E of DAE)	■ Data ■ Action ■ Evaluation
Computerized	■ Acute care ■ Long-term care ■ Home care ■ Ambulatory care	■ Progress notes ■ Flow sheets ■ Nursing care plan ■ Database ■ Teaching plan	■ Initial: baseline assessment ■ Ongoing: progress notes	■ Database ■ Care plan	■ Outcome-based care plan	■ Evaluative statements ■ Expected outcomes ■ Learning outcomes

Abbreviations to avoid

To reduce the risk of medical errors, The Joint Commission has created a "Do Not Use" list of abbreviations.[3] The list applies to all orders and medication-related documentation that's handwritten, part of free-text computer entry, or on preprinted forms.

ABBREVIATION	POTENTIAL PROBLEM	PREFERRED TERM
U (for "unit")	Mistaken as zero, four, or cc.	Write "unit."
IU (for "international unit")	Mistaken as IV (intravenous) or 10 (ten).	Write "international unit."
Q.D., Q.O.D, QD, QOD, q.d., q.o.d., qd, qod (Latin abbreviations for "once daily" and "every other day")	Mistaken for each other. The period after the "Q" can be mistaken for an "I" and the "O" can be mistaken for "I."	Write "daily" and "every other day."
Trailing zero (X.0 mg) (Note: Prohibited only for medication-related notations); lack of leading zero (.X mg)	Decimal point is missed.	Never write a zero by itself after a decimal point (X mg), and always use a zero before a decimal point (0.X mg).
MS MSO4 MgSO4	Confused for one another. Can mean "morphine sulfate" or "magnesium sulfate."	Write "morphine sulfate" or "magnesium sulfate."

© The Joint Commission. Reprinted with permission.

record wasn't available. Late entries, however, can look suspicious. Add the entry on the next available line and label it as a "late entry" to show it's out of sequence. Then record the date and time of the entry as well as the date and time when the entry should have been made. Follow facility policy for documenting late entries.

■ When documentation continues from one page to the next, sign the bottom of the first page. At the top of the next page, write the date, time, and "continued from previous page."

■ If information listed on a form doesn't apply to your patient, write N/A (not applicable) rather than leaving the space blank. *This notation shows that you read the question and that it doesn't apply instead of you forgetting to write down the information. It also prevents someone else from adding the information later.*

■ If your facility uses computerized records, know that most software programs establish an electronic signature based on your personal user password.

REFERENCES

1 The Joint Commission. (2012). Standard RC.01.01.01. *Comprehensive accreditation manual for hospitals: The official handbook.* Oakbrook Terrace, IL: The Joint Commission. (Level I)

2 The Joint Commission. (2012). Standard RC.01.03.01. *Comprehensive accreditation manual for hospitals: The official handbook.* Oakbrook Terrace, IL: The Joint Commission. (Level I)

3 The Joint Commission. "Official 'Do Not Use' List and 'Additional Abbreviations, Acronyms, and Symbols'" [Online]. Accessed August 2011 via the Web at www.jointcommission.org/assets/1/18/Official_Do%20Not%20Use_List_%206_10.pdf

ADDITIONAL REFERENCE

Westra, B.L., et al. (2008). Nursing standards to support the electronic health record. *Nursing Outlook, 56*(5), 258–266.

DOPPLER USE

More sensitive than palpation for determining pulse rate, the Doppler ultrasound blood flow detector is especially useful when a pulse is faint or weak. Unlike palpation, which detects arterial wall expansion and retraction, this instrument detects the motion of red blood cells (RBCs).

Equipment

Doppler ultrasound blood flow detector ■ coupling or transmission gel ■ soft cloth ■ antiseptic solution or soapy water.

Implementation

■ Verify the doctor's order.

■ Confirm the patient's identity using at least two patient identifiers.[1]

■ Explain the procedure to the patient and answer any questions *to decrease anxiety.*

■ Perform hand hygiene.[2,3,4]

■ Apply a small amount of coupling gel or transmission gel (not water-soluble lubricant) to the ultrasound probe.

■ Position the probe on the skin directly over the selected artery.

■ Turn the instrument on and, moving counterclockwise, set the volume control to the lowest setting. If your model doesn't have a speaker, plug in the earphones and slowly raise the volume.
■ Tilt the probe 45 degrees from the artery *to obtain the best signals with either device.* Be sure to put gel between the skin and the probe.
■ Slowly move the probe in a circular motion *to locate the center of the artery and the Doppler signal—a hissing noise at the heartbeat.* Avoid moving the probe rapidly *because it distorts the signal.*
■ Count the signals for 60 seconds *to determine the pulse rate.*
■ After you've located and measured the pulse rate, clean the probe with a soft cloth soaked in antiseptic solution or soapy water. Don't immerse the probe or bump it against a hard surface.
■ Perform hand hygiene.[2,3,4]
■ Document the procedure.[5]

Documentation

Record the location and quality of the pulse as well as the pulse rate and time of measurement.

REFERENCES

1 The Joint Commission. (2012). Standard NPSG.01.01.01. *Comprehensive accreditation manual for hospitals: The official handbook.* Oakbrook Terrace, IL: The Joint Commission. (Level I)
2 The Joint Commission. (2012). Standard NPSG.07.01.01. *Comprehensive accreditation manual for hospitals: The official handbook.* Oakbrook Terrace, IL: The Joint Commission. (Level I)
3 Centers for Disease Control and Prevention. (October 2002). Guideline for hand hygiene in health-care settings. *Morbidity and Mortality Weekly Report, 51*(RR-16), 1–45. (Level 1)
4 World Health Organization. (2009). *WHO guidelines on hand hygiene in health care: First global patient safety challenge. Clean care is safer care.* Geneva, Switzerland: World Health Organization. (Level I)
5 The Joint Commission. (2012). Standard RC.01.03.01. *Comprehensive accreditation manual for hospitals: The official handbook.* Oakbrook Terrace, IL: The Joint Commission. (Level I)

ADDITIONAL REFERENCE

Rutala, W.A., et al. (2008). "Guideline for Disinfection and Sterilization in Healthcare Facilities, 2008" [Online]. Accessed September 2011 via the Web at http://www.cdc.gov/hicpac/pdf/guidelines/Disinfection_Nov_2008.pdf

DROPLET PRECAUTIONS

Droplet precautions prevent infectious pathogens from traveling from the respiratory tract of an infectious person to the mucous membranes of a susceptible host.[1] These pathogens, which are carried by respiratory droplets, spread when an infected individual coughs, sneezes, or talks or during procedures such as suctioning or endotracheal intubation. (See *Conditions requiring droplet precautions*, page 234.)

Ideally, a patient requiring droplet precautions should be placed in a single-patient room.[1] People having direct contact with the patient and those who will be within 3' (0.9 m) of him should wear a surgical mask covering the nose and mouth. When exposure to a highly virulent pathogen is likely, it may be prudent to wear a mask when within 6' to 10' (2 to 3 m) of the patient or upon entering the patient's room.[1]

As a general precaution, instruct anyone who enters your health care facility with signs of a respiratory infection (such as cough, congestion, rhinorrhea, or increased respiratory secretions) to cover his mouth and nose with a tissue when coughing and have him dispose of soiled tissues promptly. Have him wear a surgical mask, if tolerated, and instruct him to perform hand hygiene after contact with respiratory secretions. If possible, separate him by at least 3' from other people in common waiting areas to prevent the spread of infection.[1] These actions can help prevent the spread of infectious pathogens until appropriate isolation precautions are established.

Equipment

Mask ■ plastic bags ■ tissues ■ droplet precautions sign ■ hospital-grade disinfectant ■ Optional: gowns, gloves.

Preparation of equipment

Keep all droplet precaution supplies outside the patient's room in a cart or anteroom.

Implementation

■ Verify the patient's condition requiring droplet precautions. Put a droplet precautions sign on the door, according to your facility's policy, *to notify anyone entering the room of the situation.*
■ Perform hand hygiene.[2,3,4]
■ Just before entering the patient's room, put on a mask and secure the ties or elastic band at the middle of the back of your head and neck. Fit the flexible metal nose strip to your nose bridge so it fits firmly but comfortably. Make sure the mask fits snugly to your face and below your chin.[1]
■ Put on gloves and a gown if necessary, according to standard precautions.[1]
■ Confirm the patient's identity using at least two patient identifiers according to your facility's policy.[5]
■ Situate the patient in a single room with private toilet facilities and an anteroom if possible. If necessary, at least two patients with the same infection may share a room if approved by your facility's infection preventionist.[1]
■ Explain isolation procedures to the patient and his family *to ease patient anxiety and promote cooperation.*
■ If the patient is wearing a mask during transport to the room, remove his mask.
■ Instruct the patient to cover his nose and mouth with a facial tissue while coughing or sneezing, dispose of the tissue immediately, and then perform hand hygiene *to prevent the spread of infectious droplets.*[1,2,3,4]
■ Tape a plastic bag to the patient's bedside *so the patient can dispose of facial tissues correctly.*
■ When finished providing patient care, remove your gloves and gown (if worn) in the anteroom or at the patient's doorway just before leaving the room, if an anteroom isn't available.[1]

Conditions requiring droplet precautions[1]

Because these conditions may be transmitted by respiratory droplets from infectious patients, they require droplet precautions.

PEDIATRIC ALERT *When handling infants or young children who require droplet precautions, you may also need to institute contact precautions and wear gloves and a gown to prevent soiling of clothing from nasal and oral secretions.*

CONDITION	PRECAUTIONARY PERIOD	SPECIAL CONSIDERATIONS (AS APPLICABLE)
Adenovirus infection in infants and young children	■ Duration of illness	■ Institute contact precautions in addition to droplet precautions. ■ Prolonged viral shedding occurs in immunocompromised patients.
Diphtheria (pharyngeal)	■ Until off antibiotics and two cultures taken at least 24 hours apart are negative	
Haemophilus influenzae type b disease, including epiglottitis, meningitis, pneumonia, and sepsis	■ Until 24 hours after initiation of effective therapy	
Influenza (seasonal)	■ For 5 days after onset of symptoms ■ For the duration of illness in immunocompromised patients	■ Viral shedding is prolonged in immunocompromised patients.
Mumps	■ For 9 days after onset of swelling	■ Susceptible health care workers shouldn't provide care if immune caregivers are available.
Mycoplasma pneumoniae infection	■ Duration of illness	
Neisseria meningitidis disease, including meningitis, pneumonia, and sepsis	■ Until 24 hours after initiation of effective therapy	■ Household contacts should receive postexposure prophylactic antibiotic therapy. ■ Health care workers exposed to respiratory secretions should receive postexposure prophylactic antibiotic therapy. ■ Postexposure vaccine may be given to control outbreaks.
Parvovirus B19	■ When chronic disease occurs in an immunocompromised patient: duration of hospitalization ■ In patients with transient aplastic crisis or red-cell crisis: 7 days	■ Duration of precautions for immunosuppressed patients with persistently positive polymerase chain reaction is unknown, but transmission has occurred.
Pertussis (whooping cough)	■ Until 5 days after initiation of effective therapy	■ Household contacts should receive postexposure prophylaxis. ■ Health care workers with prolonged exposure to respiratory secretions should receive postexposure prophylaxis.
Pneumonic plague	■ Until 48 hours after initiation of effective therapy	■ Exposed health care workers should receive postexposure prophylactic antibiotics.
Rhinovirus	■ Duration of illness	■ Also institute contact precautions if contact with copious moist secretions is likely.

Conditions requiring droplet precautions *(continued)*

CONDITION	PRECAUTIONARY PERIOD	SPECIAL CONSIDERATIONS (AS APPLICABLE)
Rubella (German measles)	■ Until 7 days after onset of rash	■ Susceptible health care workers shouldn't enter the room if immune caregivers are available. ■ Administer vaccine to nonpregnant susceptible individuals within 3 days of exposure. ■ Place exposed susceptible patients on droplet precautions.
Severe acute respiratory distress syndrome	■ Duration of illness plus 10 days after resolution of fever	■ Airborne precautions are preferred. ■ Institute contact precautions in addition to airborne or droplet precautions. ■ Wear eye protection. ■ Vigilant environmental disinfection is required.
Streptococcal group A disease, including pharyngitis (in infants and young children), pneumonia, serious invasive wounds, and scarlet fever (in infants and young children)	■ Until 24 hours after initiation of effective therapy	■ Also institute contact precautions if skin lesions are present.
Viral hemorrhagic infection (Ebola, Lassa, Marburg, and Crimean-Congo hemorrhagic fever viruses)	■ Duration of illness	■ Also institute contact precautions. ■ Wear eye protection. ■ Handle wastes appropriately. ■ Use an N-95 (or higher) respirator mask when performing aerosol-generating procedures. ■ Make sure public health officials are notified, according to your facility's policy, if Ebola is suspected.

After leaving the patient's room
■ Perform hand hygiene.[2,3,4]
■ Untie the strings or remove the elastic bands and dispose of the mask, handling it by the strings or elastic bands only *because the front of the mask is considered contaminated*, and then perform hand hygiene again.[1,2,3,4]
■ Clean and disinfect equipment that isn't dedicated for single-patient use with a hospital-grade disinfectant after use *to prevent the spread of infection to other patients.*[6]
■ Perform hand hygiene.[2,3,4]
■ Document the procedure.[7]

Special considerations
■ Make sure all visitors wear masks when in close proximity to the patient (within 3′ [0.9 m]) and, if necessary, gowns and gloves.[1]
■ If the patient must leave the room for essential procedures, place a surgical mask over his nose and mouth and instruct the patient to use respiratory hygiene and proper cough etiquette.[1] It isn't necessary for health care workers to wear masks when transporting a patient on droplet precautions *because the patient is wearing a mask.*[1] Notify the receiving department or area of the patient's isolation precautions *so that the precautions will be maintained and the patient can be returned to the room promptly.*
■ *Because pathogens in respiratory droplets don't remain infectious over long distances (they generally drop to the ground within 3′),* special air handling and ventilation systems and an airborne infection isolation room with negative airflow aren't necessary.

Complications
Social isolation is a complication of droplet precautions.

Documentation
Record the need for droplet precautions on the nursing care plan and as otherwise indicated by your facility. Document initiation and maintenance of the precautions, the patient's compliance with droplet precautions, any patient or family teaching performed, and their understanding of the teaching. Also document the date and time droplet precautions were discontinued.

REFERENCES

1 Siegel, J.D., et al. "2007 Guideline for Isolation Precautions: Preventing Transmission of Infectious Agents in Healthcare Settings" [Online]. Accessed June 2011 via the Web at http://www.cdc.gov/hicpac/2007ip/2007isolationprecautions.html (Level I)

2 The Joint Commission. (2012). Standard NPSG.07.01.01. *Comprehensive accreditation manual for hospitals: The official handbook.* Oakbrook Terrace, IL: The Joint Commission. (Level I)

3 Centers for Disease Control and Prevention. (October 2002). Guideline for hand hygiene in health-care settings. *Morbidity and Mortality Weekly Report, 51*(RR-16), 1–45. (Level 1)

4 World Health Organization. (2009). *WHO guidelines on hand hygiene in health care: First global patient safety challenge. Clean care is safer care.* Geneva, Switzerland: World Health Organization. (Level I)

5 The Joint Commission. (2012). Standard NPSG.01.01.01. *Comprehensive accreditation manual for hospitals: The official handbook.* Oakbrook Terrace, IL: The Joint Commission. (Level I)

6 Rutala, W. A., et al. (2008). "Guideline for Disinfection and Sterilization in Healthcare Facilities, 2008" [Online]. Accessed September 2011 via the Web at http://www.cdc.gov/hicpac/pdf/guidelines/Disinfection_Nov_2008.pdf (Level I)

7 The Joint Commission. (2012). Standard RC.01.03.01. *Comprehensive accreditation manual for hospitals: The official handbook.* Oakbrook Terrace, IL: The Joint Commission. (Level I)

ADDITIONAL REFERENCES

Craven, R.F., & Hirnle, C.J. (2009). *Fundamentals of nursing: Human health and function* (6th ed.). Philadelphia, PA: Lippincott Williams & Wilkins.

The Joint Commission. (2012). Standard IC.02.01.01. *Comprehensive accreditation manual for hospitals: The official handbook.* Oakbrook Terrace, IL: The Joint Commission.

DRUG AND ALCOHOL SPECIMEN COLLECTION

Specimen collection for drug and alcohol testing is performed to identify a patient's drug or alcohol use. It's performed for several reasons, including obtaining evidence for a possible criminal charge (for instance, after an accident), helping to determine a cause of death, and screening for employment suitability or adherence to an ongoing drug addiction rehabilitation program. It's also used to establish a differential diagnosis for a patient who's experiencing an altered mental state or has such signs and symptoms as slurred speech, dizziness, confusion, blurred vision, anxiety, hallucinations, memory impairment, lack of muscle coordination, or hyperthermia. The collection method and source of the specimens vary, based on the reason for testing. Because of the variability in local and state laws, nurses must strictly follow all facility guidelines, policies, and procedures.

Drug testing that's performed to determine employment suitability and rehabilitation program adherence usually involves a urine sample collected under highly controlled conditions. Although collection requirements may vary slightly, depending on the employer and type of employment or rehabilitation program, most include a designated collection site, security for the collection site, use of authorized personnel, privacy during collection, integrity and identity of the specimen, and chain-of-custody documentation. Some rehabilitation programs and employment circumstances may require the specimen collection to be observed. Testing is usually limited to five drug types: marijuana, cocaine, opiates, amphetamines, and phencyclidine. In the case of employment screening, if the results of the initial test are positive, a confirmatory test is performed using gas chromatography–mass spectrometry.

Depending on the reason for collection and your state laws, you should ensure that informed consent has been obtained from the patient or a family member before obtaining the sample. Consent may not be required if it's an emergency, if results will be used only for a differential diagnosis in an acute crisis, or if the patient is not in a condition to grant permission. In a criminal case, a law enforcement officer can't order blood to be drawn and doesn't have the legal right to grant permission if the patient refuses consent.

Blood samples, when needed, are collected in 10-mL gray-top blood collection tubes that contain a preservative (100 mg of sodium fluoride) *to help prevent deterioration of the specimen,* including changes in alcohol concentration and the breakdown of cocaine, and an anticoagulant (20 mg of potassium oxalate) *to prevent the sample from clotting.* The integrity and identity of the specimen must be maintained and, if indicated, chain-of-custody documentation preserved.

In general, prescription and over-the-counter drugs can be detected in blood in 4 to 24 hours and in urine for 2 to 4 days. Detection times for alcohol and other drugs vary. (See *Drug detection times.*)

This procedure focuses on drug and alcohol specimen collection for medicolegal reasons. When specimens are collected for a patient who's experiencing an altered mental state or other signs and symptoms, be sure to use the appropriate collection tubes. (See "Venipuncture," page 781.)

Equipment

Gloves ■ Optional: Shipping containers (if samples are to be sent to an outside laboratory), sphygmomanometer, stethoscope, thermometer, pulse oximeter.

Urine sample

Urine collection cup with temperature measurement device attached in sealed covering ■ 90-mL plastic, screw-top specimen container in sealed covering ■ adhesive label ■ plastic sealable pouch ■ absorbent material ■ chain-of-custody labels ■ chain-of-custody form with multiple copies ■ bluing agent for toilet water.

Blood sample

Two 10-mL gray-top Vacutainer blood tubes containing sodium fluoride and potassium oxalate with adhesive labels ■ venipuncture supplies ■ nonalcohol swab (povidone-iodine) ■ 2″ × 2″ sterile gauze pads ■ evidence seals ■ padded transport box ■ biohazard laboratory transport bag ■ chain-of-custody labels ■ chain-of-custody form with multiple copies ■ evidence tape.

Note: Prepackaged blood and urine collection kits for such specimens are commercially available and contain everything necessary to collect and preserve the chain of custody for the specimens.

Drug detection times

DRUG	BLOOD	URINE
Ethanol	3 to 12 hours	3 to 12 hours
Amphetamines	1 to 3 days	1 to 5 or more days
Marijuana	Infrequent user: 1 to 4 hours Frequent user: 3 to 6 hours	Not found in urine
Marijuana metabolite	Infrequent user: Typically, 2 to 3 days (sometimes longer) Frequent user: 2 or more weeks	Infrequent user: 2 weeks Frequent user: 3 to 6 weeks
Cocaine	5 to 6 hours (will break down in unrefrigerated blood)	12 hours
Cocaine metabolite	Varies	2 to 4 days
Opiates	1 to 4 hours	3 to 4 days
Phencyclidine	1 to 3 days	Typically, 3 to 7 days (sometimes longer)

Implementation

■ Verify the doctor's order for drug and alcohol specimen collection, if appropriate.
■ If required, verify that informed consent has been obtained and is included in the patient's medical record.[1]
■ Perform hand hygiene.[2,3,4]
■ Gather the necessary supplies.
■ Confirm the patient's identity using at least two patient identifiers according to your facility's policy.[5]
■ Explain the appropriate procedure to the patient, allowing him to ask questions as needed.
■ Assess the patient's level of consciousness and behavior.
■ If applicable, obtain the patient's vital signs, including heart rate, respiratory rate, blood pressure, temperature, and pulse oximetry.

Urine sample collection

■ Prepare the collection site by turning off the water supply or securing water sources.
■ Add bluing agent to the toilet and water tank to prevent undetected specimen dilution by the donor.
■ Remove the waste container, soap dispenser, and any unnecessary items from the bathroom.
■ Perform hand hygiene and put on gloves.[2,3,4]
■ Instruct the patient to remove any unnecessary outer clothing, such as a coat, hat, or extra shirt.
■ Instruct the patient to empty his pockets into a lockable cabinet or box, and have him turn his pockets inside out to ensure that they're emptied and that he doesn't have anything that could be used to adulterate the specimen.

■ Have the patient wash and dry his hands.
■ Provide the patient with the sealed collection kit or container, and have him unwrap or break the seal on the kit or collection container.
■ Have the patient enter the bathroom and instruct him to provide a urine specimen of at least 30-mL into the collection cup, to not flush the toilet, to not wash his hands until told to do so after delivering the specimen to you and watching the specimen being sealed with the labels, and to immediately leave the bathroom with the specimen and hand it to you when he's finished urinating.
■ Check the specimen's temperature by reading the temperature strip and note it on the chain-of-custody form.
■ Check the specimen volume to ensure that the specimen contains the required amount of urine.
■ Open the sealed screw-top specimen container and transfer the urine into the container.
■ Label the specimen container in the presence of the patient *to prevent mislabeling* with the patient's name and identification number and the date and time.[5]
■ Complete the required information on the chain-of-custody seal, initial the seal, have the patient initial the seal, and place it over the top of the specimen container.
■ Turn the water on and allow the patient to wash his hands.
■ Complete the chain-of-custody form and have the patient sign the form.
■ Give the patient a copy of the chain-of-custody form.
■ Place the specimen, absorbent material, and completed chain-of-custody form in the shipping bag.
■ Seal the bag in the presence of the patient.

■ Remove and discard your gloves and perform hand hygiene.[2,3,4]
■ Place the specimen in a secure refrigerator if it won't be immediately transported to the laboratory.
■ Make sure the person who removes the specimen for transport signs the chain-of-custody form. Retain a copy and place it in the patient's medical record.
■ Document the procedure.[6]

Blood sample collection

■ If applicable, ensure that the collection is observed by a law enforcement officer, according to facility policy and state law.
■ Perform hand hygiene and put on gloves.[2,3,4]
■ Choose a venipuncture site. The most common sites are the veins in the antecubital space of the arms; however, if the patient has scarring in this area from self-injected drugs, you may need to find an alternate venipuncture site.
■ Clean the skin at the venipuncture site with a nonalcohol swab such as povidone-iodine. If a nonalcohol antiseptic isn't available, use a gauze pad with a solution of soap and water, making sure that the soap doesn't contain any alcohol.
■ Use proper venipuncture technique to collect the blood sample. (See "Venipuncture," page 781.)
■ Fill the collection tubes completely *to minimize the air space above the specimen, which can change the testing results.*
■ Slowly invert the tubes completely at least five times *to ensure proper mixing of the additives.* Don't shake them vigorously.
■ Label the specimen tubes in the presence of the patient *to prevent mislabeling*[6] with the patient's name and identification number and the date and time. Obtain the officer's initials on the tubes, if applicable.
■ Complete the required information on the evidence seals, initial the seals, and have the patient initial the seals.
■ Place a completed evidence seal across the top of each tube.
■ Complete the chain-of-custody labels and form, and have the patient sign the form.
■ Place the tubes into a padded transport box and then into a biohazard laboratory transport bag.
■ Seal the bag with the chain-of-custody and evidence labels.
■ Remove and discard your gloves and perform hand hygiene.[2,3,4]
■ Attach the chain-of-custody form.
■ Document the procedure.[6]

NURSING ALERT *Complete all of the above steps in full view of the patient and, if applicable, the appropriate law enforcement officer.*

■ Place the specimen in a secure refrigerator if it won't be immediately transported to the laboratory.
■ Make sure the person who removes the specimen for transport signs the chain-of-custody form. Retain a copy and place it in the patient's medical record.

Special considerations

■ If the specimen is being collected for a law enforcement agency, make sure that an officer has notified the patient of his rights and explained the procedure before you obtain the sample.
■ If the patient is a minor, permission must be obtained from the parent or legal guardian, unless superseded by state laws.

■ Temperature strips attached to urine collection containers allow temperature certification between 90° and 100° F (32.2° and 37.8° C), which are acceptable under most standards. However, some testing standards require that the urine's temperature be taken with a digital thermometer and be between 96° and 99° F (35.6° and 37.2° C).
■ If the specimen volume is inadequate, discard any specimen collected and the specimen collection container used for that attempt, have the patient sit in a waiting area where you can continuously observe him, and provide the patient with up to 40 ounces of water to drink (which should be evenly spread out over a 3-hour period or until he can provide an adequate specimen). Instruct the patient to tell you when he feels he can provide the specimen. If, after 3 hours, the patient can't provide a specimen, the collection should be terminated and you should notify the person who requested the test.

Complications

If specimen collection is performed with no subsequent medical follow-up, serious medical conditions may be overlooked, causing the patient to experience adverse effects. Mishandling of the specimen or improper documentation of the chain of custody may lead to the evidence being inaccurate or inadmissible in court.

Documentation

Record the date and time, the test being performed, the reason for the test, and the type of specimen that was obtained. Note whether a law enforcement officer was present for the specimen collection, including the agency he represented and his badge number. Document that the chain of custody was preserved.[6]

REFERENCES

1 The Joint Commission. (2012). Standard RI.01.03.01. *Comprehensive accreditation manual for hospitals: The official handbook.* Oakbrook Terrace, IL: The Joint Commission. (Level I)
2 The Joint Commission. (2012). Standard NPSG.07.01.01. *Comprehensive accreditation manual for hospitals: The official handbook.* Oakbrook Terrace, IL: The Joint Commission. (Level I)
3 Centers for Disease Control and Prevention. (October 2002). Guideline for hand hygiene in health-care settings. *Morbidity and Mortality Weekly Report, 51*(RR-16), 1–45. (Level 1)
4 World Health Organization. (2009). *WHO guidelines on hand hygiene in health care: First global patient safety challenge. Clean care is safer care.* Geneva, Switzerland: World Health Organization. (Level I)
5 The Joint Commission. (2012). Standard NPSG.01.01.01. *Comprehensive accreditation manual for hospitals: The official handbook.* Oakbrook Terrace, IL: The Joint Commission. (Level I)
6 The Joint Commission. (2012). Standard RC.01.03.01. *Comprehensive accreditation manual for hospitals: The official handbook.* Oakbrook Terrace, IL: The Joint Commission. (Level I)

ADDITIONAL REFERENCES

Moeller, K.E., et al. (2008). Urine drug screening: Practical guide for clinicians. *Mayo Clinic Proceedings, 83*(1), 66–76.

Five stages of dying

According to Elisabeth Kübler-Ross, author of *On Death and Dying*, the dying patient may progress through five psychological stages in preparation for death. Although each patient experiences these stages differently, and not necessarily in this order, understanding them will help you meet your patient's needs.

Denial

When the patient first learns of his terminal illness, he may refuse to accept the diagnosis. He may experience physical symptoms similar to a stress reaction—shock, fainting, pallor, sweating, tachycardia, nausea, and GI disorders. During this stage, be honest with the patient but not blunt or callous. Maintain communication with him so he can discuss his feelings when he accepts the reality of death. Don't force the patient to confront this reality.

Anger

Once the patient stops denying his impending death, he may show deep resentment toward those who will live on after he dies—to you, to the facility staff, and to his own family. Although you may instinctively draw back from the patient or even resent this behavior, remember that he is dying and has a right to be angry. After you accept his anger, you can help him find different ways to express it and can help his family to understand it.

Bargaining

Although the patient acknowledges his impending death, he may attempt to bargain for more time with God or fate. He will probably strike this bargain secretly. If he does confide in you, don't urge him to keep his promises.

Depression

In this stage, the patient may first experience regrets about his past and then grieve about his current condition. He may withdraw from his friends, his family, the doctor, and you. He may suffer from anorexia, increased fatigue, or self-neglect. You may find him sitting alone, in tears. Accept the patient's sorrow, and if he talks to you, listen. Provide comfort by touch, as appropriate. Resist the temptation to make optimistic remarks or cheerful small talk.

Acceptance

The patient who reaches this last stage accepts the inevitability and imminence of his death. The patient may simply desire the quiet company of a family member or friend. If, for some reason, a family member or friend can't be present, stay with the patient to satisfy his final need. Remember, however, that many patients die before reaching this stage.

National Institutes of Health; National Institute on Drug Abuse. "Drugs of Abuse Information" [Online]. Accessed December 2011 via the Web at http://www.drugabuse.gov/drugpages.html

Yelland, L.N., et al. (2008). Inter- and intra-subject variability in ethanol pharmacokinetic parameters: Effects of testing interval and dose. *Forensic Science International, 175*(1), 65–72.

DYING PATIENT CARE

A patient needs intensive physical support and emotional comfort as he approaches death. Signs and symptoms of impending death include reduced respiratory rate and depth, decreased or absent blood pressure, weak or erratic pulse rate, lowered skin temperature (although occasional spikes in core temperature may occur), decreased level of consciousness (LOC), diminished sensorium and neuromuscular control, diaphoresis, pallor, cyanosis, and mottling. Emotional support for the dying patient and his family most often means reassurance and your physical presence to help ease fear and loneliness. More intense emotional support is important at much earlier stages, especially for patients with long-term progressive illnesses, who can work through the stages of dying. (See *Five stages of dying*.)

The patient may have made clear his wishes about extraordinary means of supporting life and may have signed a living will. This document, legally binding in most states, declares the patient's desire for a death unimpeded by such artificial support as defibrillators, respirators, and life-sustaining drugs. If the patient has signed such a document, you must respect his wishes and communicate the doctor's "no code" order to all staff members.

Equipment

Clean bed linens ▪ gowns ▪ gloves ▪ water-filled basin ▪ soap ▪ washcloth ▪ towels ▪ lotion ▪ linen-saver pads ▪ petroleum jelly ▪ sponge-tipped swab ▪ suction equipment, as necessary ▪ Optional: indwelling urinary catheter.

Implementation

▪ Gather equipment at the patient's bedside, as needed.
▪ Confirm the patient's identity using at least two patient identifiers according to your facility's policy.[1]

Meeting physical needs

▪ Perform hand hygiene and put on gloves. Put on new gloves and perform hand hygiene whenever moving from a contaminated to a clean area during patient care.[2,3,4]
▪ Observe for pallor, diaphoresis, and decreased LOC. Take vital signs as warranted, based on the patient's requested resuscitation status.

Understanding organ and tissue donation

A federal regulation was enacted in 1998 and revised in 2004 that requires facilities to report individuals whose death is imminent or have died in the health care facility to a regional organ procurement organization in a timely manner.[6] This regulation was enacted so that no potential donor is missed. The regulation ensures that the family of every potential donor will understand the option to donate. According to the American Medical Association, about 25 kinds of organs and tissues are transplanted. Although donor organ requirements vary, the typical donor must be between ages of newborn and 60 years and free from transmissible disease. Tissue donations are less restrictive, and some tissue banks will accept skin from donors up to age 75.

Collection of most organs, such as the heart, liver, kidney, or pancreas, requires that the patient be pronounced brain dead and kept physically alive until the organs are harvested. Tissue, such as eyes, skin, bone, and heart valves, may be taken after death. Contact your regional organ procurement organization for specific organ donation criteria or to identify a potential donor. If you don't know the regional organ procurement organization in your area, call the United Network for Organ Sharing at 804-782-4800.

■ Reposition the patient in bed at least every 2 hours *because sensation, reflexes, and mobility diminish first in the legs and gradually in the arms.* Make sure the bedsheets cover him loosely *to reduce discomfort caused by pressure on arms and legs.*

■ When the patient's vision and hearing start to fail, turn his head toward the light and speak to him from near the head of the bed. *Because hearing may be acute despite loss of consciousness,* avoid whispering or speaking inappropriately about the patient in his presence.

■ Change the bed linens and the patient's gown as needed. Provide skin care during gown changes, and adjust the room temperature for patient comfort, if necessary.

■ Observe for incontinence or anuria, *the result of diminished neuromuscular control or decreased renal function.* If necessary, obtain an order to catheterize the patient, or place linen-saver pads beneath the patient's buttocks. Provide perineal care with soap, a washcloth, and towels *to prevent irritation.*

■ Suction the patient's mouth and upper airway *to remove secretions.* Elevate the head of the bed *to decrease respiratory resistance.* As the patient's condition deteriorates, he may breathe mostly through his mouth.

■ Lubricate the patient's lips and mouth with petroleum jelly and a sponge-tipped swab *to counteract dryness.* Offer fluids, as appropriate, *because the patient may have a decreased gag reflex and may aspirate oral fluids.*

■ Provide eye care to the comatose patient *to prevent corneal ulceration. Such ulceration can cause blindness and prevent the use of*

these tissues for transplantation after the patient dies (if the patient or family has consented to cornea donation).

■ Administer pain medication as ordered following safe medication administration practices. Keep in mind that, as circulation diminishes, medications given IM will be poorly absorbed. Medications should be given IV, if possible, *for optimum results and comfort.*

Meeting emotional needs

■ Fully explain all care and treatments to the patient even if he's unconscious *because he may still be able to hear.* Answer any questions as honestly as possible.

■ Allow the patient to express his feelings, which may range from anger, to fear, to loneliness. Provide time for the patient to verbalize.

■ Notify family members, if they're absent, when the patient wishes to see them. Let the patient and family members discuss death at their own pace.

■ Offer to contact a member of the clergy or social services department, if appropriate.

■ Perform hand hygiene.[2,3,4]

■ Document your actions.[5]

Special considerations

■ If the patient has signed a living will, the doctor will write a "no code" order on his progress notes and order sheets. Know your state's policy regarding living wills. If it's legal, transfer the "no code" order to the patient's chart or Kardex and, at the end of your shift, inform incoming staff members of this order.

■ If family members remain with the patient, explain the patient's needs, treatments, and care plan to them. If appropriate, offer to teach them specific skills so they can take part in caring for the patient. Emphasize that their efforts are important and effective. As the patient's death approaches, provide emotional support. Educate the family about signs and symptoms of impending death.

■ Obtain a palliative care or hospice care consultation, if requested.

■ If permitted by your local organ and tissue donor network and if appropriate, respectfully approach the patient's family to inquire if they have considered organ and tissue donation. Check the patient's records *to determine whether he completed an organ donor card.* (See *Understanding organ and tissue donation.*)

Documentation

Record changes in the patient's vital signs, intake and output, and LOC. Note the times of cardiac arrest and the end of respiration, and notify the doctor when these occur. Document interactions with the patient and family members. Document notification of the local organ and tissue donor network.

References

1 The Joint Commission. (2012). Standard NPSG.01.01.01. *Comprehensive accreditation manual for hospitals: The official handbook.* Oakbrook Terrace, IL: The Joint Commission. (Level I)

2 The Joint Commission. (2012). Standard NPSG.07.01.01. *Comprehensive accreditation manual for hospitals: The official handbook.* Oakbrook Terrace, IL: The Joint Commission. (Level I)

3 Centers for Disease Control and Prevention. (October 2002). Guideline for hand hygiene in health-care settings. *Morbidity and Mortality Weekly Report, 51*(RR-16), 1–45. (Level 1)

4 World Health Organization. (2009). *WHO guidelines on hand hygiene in health care: First global patient safety challenge. Clean care is safer care.* Geneva, Switzerland: World Health Organization. (Level I)

5 The Joint Commission. (2012). Standard RC.01.03.01. *Comprehensive accreditation manual for hospitals: The official handbook.* Oakbrook Terrace, IL: The Joint Commission. (Level I)

6 Centers for Medicare & Medicaid Services, Department of Health and Human Services. (2010). "Conditions for Participation: Organ, Tissue, and Eye Procurement," 42 CFR part 482.45 [Online]. Accessed December 2011 via the Web at http://cfr.vlex.com/vid/482-condition-participation-organ-eye-19811462

ADDITIONAL REFERENCES

Craven, R.F., & Hirnle, C.J. (2009). *Fundamentals of nursing: Human health and function* (6th ed.). Philadelphia, PA: Lippincott Williams & Wilkins.

Taylor, C., et al. (2011). *Fundamentals of nursing: The art and science of nursing care* (7th ed.). Philadelphia, PA: Lippincott Williams & Wilkins.

Truog, R.D., et al. (2008). Recommendations for end-of-life care in the intensive care unit: A consensus statement by the American College of Critical Care Medicine. *Critical Care Medicine, 36*(3), 953–963.

EARDROP INSTILLATION

Eardrops may be instilled to treat infection and inflammation, soften cerumen for later removal, produce local anesthesia, or facilitate removal of an insect trapped in the ear by immobilizing and smothering it.

Instillation of eardrops is usually contraindicated if the patient has a perforated eardrum, but it may be permitted with certain medications and adherence to sterile technique. Other conditions may also prohibit instillation of certain medications into the ear. For instance, instillation of drops containing hydrocortisone is contraindicated if the patient has herpes, another viral infection, or a fungal infection.

Equipment

Prescribed eardrops ■ patient's medication record and chart ■ light source ■ facial tissue or cotton-tipped applicator ■ gloves ■ Optional: cotton ball, bowl of warm water.

Implementation

■ Verify the doctor's order.[1]
■ Avoid distractions and interruptions when preparing and administering the medication *to prevent medication errors.*[2]
■ Compare the medication label to the order and verify that the medication is correct. Confirm in which ear you must administer the medication.[2]
■ Check the expiration date on the medication, and don't give if the medication is expired.[2]
■ Check the patient's medical record for an allergy or other contraindication to the prescribed medication. If an allergy or other contraindication exists, notify the doctor and hold the medication.
■ Perform hand hygiene and put on gloves.[3,4,5]
■ Confirm the patient's identity using at least two patient identifiers according to your facility's policy.[6]
■ Provide privacy if possible. Explain the procedure to the patient.
■ Have the patient lie on the side opposite the affected ear.
■ Straighten the patient's ear canal. For an adult, pull the auricle of the ear up and back. (See *Positioning the patient for eardrop instillation,* page 242.)
■ Using a light source, examine the ear canal for drainage. If you find any, clean the canal with the tissue or cotton-tipped applicator *because drainage can reduce the medication's effectiveness.*
■ *To avoid damaging the ear canal with the dropper,* gently support the hand holding the dropper against the patient's head. Straighten the patient's ear canal once again and instill the ordered number of drops. *To avoid patient discomfort,* aim the dropper so that the drops fall against the sides of the ear canal, not on the eardrum. Hold the ear canal in position until you see the medication disappear down the canal. Then release the ear.
■ Massage the tragus (fleshy part in front of the ear canal) with your finger.
■ Instruct the patient to remain on his side for 5 to 10 minutes *to allow the medication to run down into the ear canal.*
■ If ordered, tuck a cotton ball loosely into the opening of the ear canal *to prevent the medication from leaking out.* Be careful not to insert it too deeply into the canal *because this would prevent drainage of secretions and increase pressure on the eardrum.*
■ Clean and dry the outer ear.
■ If ordered, repeat the procedure in the other ear after 5 to 10 minutes.
■ Assist the patient into a comfortable position.
■ Remove and discard your gloves and perform hand hygiene.[3,4,5]
■ Document the procedure.[7]

Special considerations

■ Don't administer cold otic medication *because cold medication may cause discomfort, vomiting, and vertigo.* Allow the medication to reach room temperature before administration. Warm the solution by gently rotating the bottle in your hands.
■ *Because some conditions make the normally tender ear canal even more sensitive,* be especially gentle when performing this procedure.
■ Never insert a cotton-tipped applicator into the ear canal past the point where you can see the tip *to prevent injury to the eardrum.*

Positioning the patient for eardrop instillation

Before instilling eardrops, have the patient lie on his side. Then straighten the patient's ear canal to help the medication reach the eardrum. For an adult, gently pull the auricle *up and back;* for an infant or young child, gently pull *down and back* (as shown here).

Adult

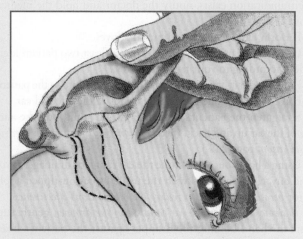

Child

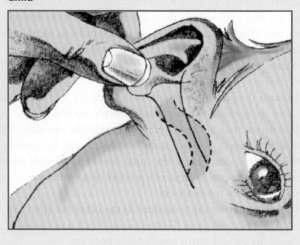

After instilling eardrops to soften cerumen, irrigate the ear as ordered *to facilitate removal of cerumen.*

■ If the patient develops vertigo, keep the side rails of his bed up and assist him during the procedure, as necessary. Also, move slowly and unhurriedly *to avoid exacerbating his vertigo.*

Patient teaching

Teach the patient to instill the eardrops correctly so that he can continue treatment at home, if necessary. Review the procedure and let the patient try it himself while you observe.

Documentation

Record the medication, ear treated, and date, time, and number of eardrops instilled. Also note any signs or symptoms that arise during the procedure, such as drainage, redness, vertigo, nausea, and pain. Document any patient teaching and the patient's understanding of that teaching.

REFERENCES

1 The Joint Commission. (2012). Standard MM.04.01.01. *Comprehensive accreditation manual for hospitals: The official handbook.* Oakbrook Terrace, IL: The Joint Commission. (Level I)

2 The Joint Commission. (2012). Standard MM.06.01.01. *Comprehensive accreditation manual for hospitals: The official handbook.* Oakbrook Terrace, IL: The Joint Commission. (Level I)

3 The Joint Commission. (2012). Standard NPSG.07.01.01. *Comprehensive accreditation manual for hospitals: The official handbook.* Oakbrook Terrace, IL: The Joint Commission. (Level I)

4 Centers for Disease Control and Prevention. (October 2002). Guideline for hand hygiene in health-care settings. *Morbidity and Mortality Weekly Report, 51*(RR-16), 1–45. (Level I)

5 World Health Organization. (2009). *WHO guidelines on hand hygiene in health care: First global patient safety challenge. Clean care is safer care.* Geneva, Switzerland: World Health Organization. (Level I)

6 The Joint Commission. (2012). Standard NPSG.01.01.01. *Comprehensive accreditation manual for hospitals: The official handbook.* Oakbrook Terrace, IL: The Joint Commission. (Level I)

7 The Joint Commission. (2012). Standard RC.01.03.01. *Comprehensive accreditation manual for hospitals: The official handbook.* Oakbrook Terrace, IL: The Joint Commission. (Level I)

ADDITIONAL REFERENCE

Taylor, C., et al. (2011). *Fundamentals of nursing: The art and science of nursing care* (7th ed.). Philadelphia, PA: Lippincott Williams & Wilkins.

EAR IRRIGATION

Irrigating the ear involves washing the external auditory canal with a stream of solution to clean the canal of discharges, soften and remove impacted cerumen, or dislodge a foreign body. Sometimes, irrigation aims to relieve localized inflammation and discomfort. The procedure must be performed carefully so that it doesn't cause discomfort or vertigo, or increase the risk of otitis externa. Because irrigation may contaminate the middle ear if the tympanic membrane is ruptured, an otoscopic examination always precedes ear irrigation.

NURSING ALERT *This procedure is contraindicated when a vegetable (such as a pea) obstructs the auditory canal* because this type of foreign body attracts and absorbs moisture. In contact with an irrigant or other solution, the foreign body swells, causing intense pain and complicating removal of the object by irrigation. *Ear irrigation is also contraindicated if the patient has a cold, a fever, an ear infection, or an injured or ruptured tympanic membrane. The presence of a battery (or a battery part) in the ear contraindicates* irrigation because battery acid could leak, and irrigation would spread caustic material throughout the canal.

Equipment

Ear irrigation syringe (rubber bulb) ▪ otoscope with aural speculum ▪ prescribed irrigant ▪ large basin ▪ emesis basin ▪ gloves ▪ linen-saver pad and bath towel ▪ cotton balls or cotton-tipped applicators ▪ 4″ × 4″ gauze pad ▪ Optional: adjustable light (such as a gooseneck lamp).

Preparation of equipment

Select the appropriate syringe, and obtain the prescribed irrigant. Put the container of irrigant into the large basin filled with hot water *to warm the solution to body temperature: 98.6° F (37° C)*. Avoid extreme temperature changes *because they can affect inner ear fluids, causing nausea and dizziness.*

Test the temperature of the solution by sprinkling a few drops on your inner wrist. Inspect equipment for breaks or cracks.

Implementation

▪ Verify the doctor's order.
▪ Perform hand hygiene and put on gloves.[1,2,3]
▪ Confirm the patient's identity using at least two patient identifiers according to your facility's policy.[4]
▪ Provide privacy and explain the procedure to the patient. Answer all questions *to decrease anxiety and improve cooperation.*
▪ If you haven't already done so, inspect the auditory canal that will be irrigated with an otoscope.
▪ Help the patient to a sitting position and tilt his head slightly forward and toward the affected side *to prevent the solution from running down his neck.* If he can't sit, have him lie on his back and tilt his head slightly forward and toward the affected ear.
▪ Make sure that you have adequate lighting.
▪ If the patient is sitting, place the linen-saver pad (covered with the bath towel) on his shoulder and upper arm, under the affected ear. If he's lying down, cover his pillow and the area under the affected ear.
▪ Have the patient hold the emesis basin close to his head under the affected ear (as shown below).

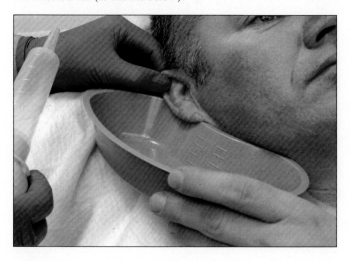

▪ Clean the auricle and the meatus of the auditory canal with a cotton-tipped applicator moistened with normal saline or the prescribed irrigating solution *to avoid getting foreign matter into the ear canal.*
▪ Draw the irrigant into the syringe and expel any air.
▪ Straighten the auditory canal; then insert the syringe tip and start the flow. (See *How to irrigate the ear canal,* page 244.)
▪ Observe the patient for signs of pain or dizziness during irrigation. If he reports either, stop the procedure, recheck the temperature of the irrigant, inspect the patient's ear with the otoscope, and resume irrigation, as indicated.
▪ Remove the syringe when it's empty and inspect the return flow for cloudiness, cerumen, blood, or foreign matter. Then, refill the syringe, and continue the irrigation until the return flow is clear. Never use more than 500 mL of irrigant during this procedure.
▪ Remove the syringe, and inspect the ear canal for cleanliness with the otoscope.
▪ Dry the patient's auricle and neck.
▪ Remove the bath towel and linen-saver pad. Help the seated patient lie on his affected side with the 4″ × 4″ gauze pad under his ear *to promote drainage of residual debris and solution.*
▪ Remove and discard your gloves and perform hand hygiene.[1,2,3]
▪ Document the procedure.[5]

Special considerations

▪ Avoid dropping or squirting irrigant on the tympanic membrane, *which may startle the patient and cause discomfort.*
▪ If the doctor directs you to place a cotton pledget in the ear canal *to retain some of the solution,* pack the cotton loosely. Instruct the patient not to remove it.
▪ If irrigation doesn't dislodge impacted cerumen, the doctor may order you to instill several drops of glycerin, carbamide peroxide (Debrox), or a similar preparation two to three times daily for 2 to 3 days, and then to irrigate the ear again.

Complications

Possible complications include pain, vertigo, nausea, otitis externa, and otitis media (if the patient has a perforated or ruptured tympanic membrane). *Forceful instillation of irrigant can rupture the tympanic membrane.*

Documentation

Record the date and time of irrigation. Note which ear you irrigated. Also note the volume and the solution used, the appearance of the canal before and after irrigation, the appearance of the return flow, the patient's tolerance of the procedure, and any comments he made about his condition, especially related to his hearing acuity.

REFERENCES

1   The Joint Commission. (2012). Standard NPSG.07.01.01. *Comprehensive accreditation manual for hospitals: The official handbook.* Oakbrook Terrace, IL: The Joint Commission. (Level I)

How to irrigate the ear canal

Follow these guidelines for irrigating the ear canal.
■ Gently pull the auricle up and back *to straighten the ear canal.*
■ Have the patient hold an emesis basin beneath the ear *to catch returning irrigant.* Position the tip of the irrigating syringe at the meatus of the auditory canal. Don't block the meatus *because you'll impede backflow and raise pressure in the canal.*

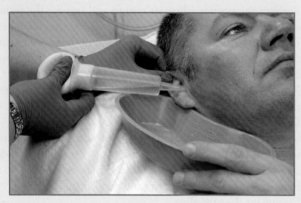

■ Tilt the patient's head toward the opposite ear, and point the syringe tip upward and toward the posterior ear canal. *This angle prevents damage to the tympanic membrane and guards against pushing debris farther into the canal.*

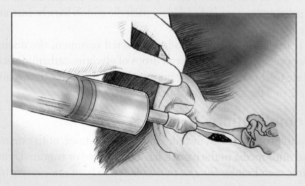

■ Direct a steady stream of irrigant against the upper wall of the ear canal.
■ Inspect return fluid for cloudiness, cerumen, blood, or foreign matter.

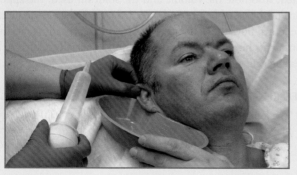

2 Centers for Disease Control and Prevention. (October 2002). Guideline for hand hygiene in health-care settings. *Morbidity and Mortality Weekly Report, 51*(RR-16), 1–45. (Level I)
3 World Health Organization. (2009). *WHO guidelines on hand hygiene in health care: First global patient safety challenge. Clean care is safer care.* Geneva, Switzerland: World Health Organization. (Level I)
4 The Joint Commission. (2012). Standard NPSG.01.01.01. *Comprehensive accreditation manual for hospitals: The official handbook.* Oakbrook Terrace, IL: The Joint Commission. (Level I)
5 The Joint Commission. (2012). Standard RC.01.03.01. *Comprehensive accreditation manual for hospitals: The official handbook.* Oakbrook Terrace, IL: The Joint Commission. (Level I)

ADDITIONAL REFERENCES

Kraszewski, S. (2008). Safe and effective ear irrigation. *Nursing Standard, 22*(43), 45–48.
Nettina, S.M. (2010). *Lippincott manual of nursing practice* (9th ed.). Philadelphia, PA: Lippincott Williams & Wilkins.
Roland, P.S., et al. (2008). Clinical practice guideline: Cerumen impaction. *Otolaryngology: Head Neck Surgery, 139*(3 Suppl. 2) S1–S21.
Taylor, C., et al. (2011). *Fundamentals of nursing: The art and science of nursing care* (7th ed.). Philadelphia, PA: Lippincott Williams & Wilkins.

ELASTIC BANDAGE APPLICATION

Elastic bandages exert gentle, even pressure on a body part. By supporting blood vessels, these rolled bandages promote venous return and prevent pooling of blood in the legs. They're typically used in place of antiembolism stockings to prevent thrombophlebitis and pulmonary embolism in postoperative or bedridden patients who can't stimulate venous return by muscle activity.

Elastic bandages also minimize joint swelling after trauma to the musculoskeletal system. Used with a splint, they immobilize a fracture during healing. They can provide hemostatic pressure and anchor dressings over a fresh wound or after surgical procedures such as vein stripping.

Equipment

Elastic bandage of appropriate width ■ tape, pins, or self-closures ■ gauze pads or absorbent cotton ■ Optional: gloves.

Bandages usually come in 2″ to 6″ (5- to 15-cm) widths and 4′ and 6′ (1.2- and 1.8-m) lengths. The 3″ (7.6-cm) width is adaptable to most applications. An elastic bandage with self-closures is also available.

Preparation of equipment

Select a bandage that wraps the affected body part completely but isn't excessively long. Generally, use a narrower bandage for wrapping the foot, lower leg, hand, or arm and a wider bandage for the thigh or trunk. The bandage should be clean and rolled before application.

Implementation

- Verify the doctor's order.
- Perform hand hygiene and put on gloves, if indicated.[1,2,3]
- Confirm the patient's identity using at least two patient identifiers according to your facility's policy.[4]
- Examine the area to be wrapped for lesions or skin breakdown. If these conditions are present, consult the doctor before applying the elastic bandage.
- Explain the procedure to the patient, provide privacy, and answer any questions *to decrease anxiety and increase cooperation.*
- Position the patient with the body part to be bandaged in normal functioning position *to promote circulation and prevent deformity and discomfort.*
- Avoid applying a bandage to a dependent extremity. If you're wrapping an extremity, elevate it for 15 to 30 minutes before application *to facilitate venous return.*
- Apply the bandage so that two skin surfaces don't remain in contact when wrapped. Place gauze pads or absorbent cotton as needed between skin surfaces, such as between toes and fingers and under breasts and arms, *to prevent skin irritation.*
- Hold the bandage with the roll facing upward in one hand and the free end of the bandage in the other hand. Hold the bandage roll close to the part being bandaged *to ensure even tension and pressure.*
- Unroll the bandage as you wrap the body part in a spiral or spiral-reverse method. Never unroll the entire bandage before wrapping *because this could produce uneven pressure, which interferes with blood circulation and cell nourishment.*
- Overlap each layer of bandage by one-half to two-thirds the width of the strip. (See *Bandaging techniques,* page 246.)
- Begin wrapping an extremity at the most distal part and work proximally *to promote venous return.* Wrap firmly but not too tightly. As you wrap, ask the patient to tell you if the bandage feels comfortable. If he complains of tingling, itching, numbness, or pain, loosen the bandage.
- When wrapping an extremity, anchor the bandage initially by circling the body part twice. *To prevent the bandage from slipping out of place on the foot,* wrap it in a figure eight around the foot, the ankle, and then the foot again before continuing. The same technique works on any joint, such as the knee, wrist, or elbow. Include the heel when wrapping the foot, but never wrap the toes (or fingers) unless absolutely necessary *because the distal extremities are used to detect impaired circulation.*
- When you're finished wrapping, secure the end of the bandage with tape, pins, or self-closures. Be careful not to scratch or pinch the patient. Avoid using metal clips *because they typically come loose when the patient moves and can get lost in the bed linens and injure the patient.*
- Check distal circulation after the bandage is in place *because the elastic may tighten as you wrap.*
- Elevate a wrapped extremity for 15 to 30 minutes *to facilitate venous return.*
- Check distal circulation once or twice every 8 hours *because an elastic bandage that's too tight may result in neurovascular damage.* Lift the distal end of the bandage and assess the skin underneath for color, temperature, and integrity.
- Remove the bandage every 8 hours or whenever it's loose and wrinkled. Roll it up as you unwrap *to ready it for reuse.* Observe the area and provide skin care before rewrapping the bandage.
- Change the bandage at least once daily. Bathe the skin, dry it thoroughly, and observe for irritation and breakdown before applying a fresh bandage.
- Remove and discard gloves and perform hand hygiene.[1,2,3]
- Document the procedure.[5]

Special considerations

- Don't leave gaps in bandage layers or exposed skin surfaces *because doing so may result in uneven pressure on the body part.*
- Observe the patient for an allergic reaction *because some patients can't tolerate the sizing in a new bandage.* Laundering the bandage reduces this risk.
- Launder the bandage daily or whenever it becomes limp; *laundering restores its elasticity.* Always keep two bandages handy *so one can be applied while the other bandage is being laundered.*
- When using an elastic bandage after a surgical procedure on an extremity (such as vein stripping) or with a splint to immobilize a fracture, remove it only as ordered rather than every 8 hours.

Patient teaching

If the patient will be using an elastic bandage at home, teach him or a family member how to apply it correctly and how to assess for restricted circulation. Tell him to keep two bandages available *so he'll have one while the other is being laundered.*

If the patient or a family member must apply the elastic bandage at home, demonstrate the procedure and observe a return demonstration before the patient's discharge. Make sure the patient has the information needed to obtain additional supplies.

Complications

Arterial obstruction—characterized by a decreased or absent distal pulse, blanching or bluish discoloration of the skin, dusky nail beds, numbness and tingling or pain and cramping, and cold skin—can result from elastic bandage application. Edema can occur from obstruction of venous return. Less serious complications include allergic reaction and skin irritation.

Documentation

Record the date and time of bandage application and removal, application site, bandage size, skin condition before application, skin care provided after removal, any complications, the patient's tolerance of the treatment, any patient teaching, and the patient's understanding of the teaching.

REFERENCES

1   The Joint Commission. (2012). Standard NPSG.07.01.01. *Comprehensive accreditation manual for hospitals: The official handbook.* Oakbrook Terrace, IL: The Joint Commission. (Level I)
2   Centers for Disease Control and Prevention. (October 2002). Guideline for hand hygiene in health-care settings. *Morbidity and Mortality Weekly Report, 51*(RR-16), 1–45. (Level I)

Bandaging techniques

Circular

Each turn encircles the previous one, covering it completely. Use this technique to anchor a bandage.

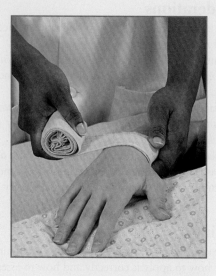

Spiral

Each turn partially overlaps the previous one. Use this technique to wrap a long, straight body part or one of increasing circumference.

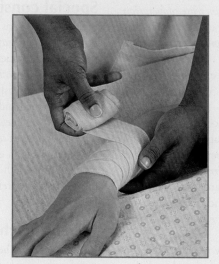

Spiral-reverse

Anchor the bandage and then reverse direction halfway through each spiral turn. Use this technique to accommodate the increasing circumference of a body part.

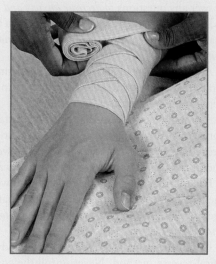

Figure eight

Anchor below the joint, and then use alternating ascending and descending turns to form a figure eight. Use this technique around joints.

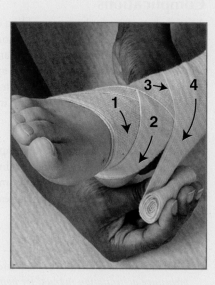

Recurrent

This technique includes a combination of recurrent and circular turns. Hold the bandage as you make each recurrent turn and then use the circular turns as a final anchor. Use this technique for a stump, a hand, or the scalp.

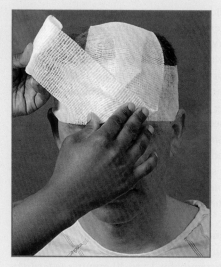

Methods of electrical bone growth stimulation

Electrical bone growth stimulation may be invasive or noninvasive.

Invasive system

An invasive system involves placing a spiral cathode inside the bone at the fracture site. A wire leads from the cathode to a battery-powered generator, also implanted in local tissues. The patient's body completes the circuit.

Noninvasive system

A noninvasive system may include a cufflike transducer or fitted ring that wraps around the patient's limb at the level of the injury. Electrical current penetrates the limb.

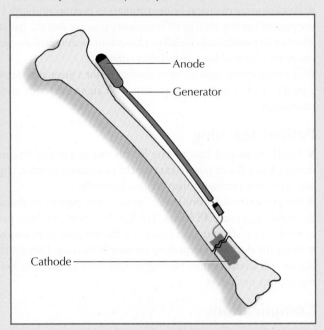

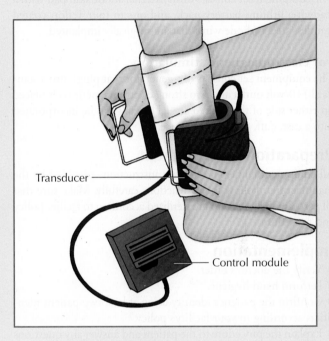

---

3 World Health Organization. (2009). *WHO guidelines on hand hygiene in health care: First global patient safety challenge. Clean care is safer care.* Geneva, Switzerland: World Health Organization. (Level I)

4 The Joint Commission. (2012). Standard NPSG.01.01.01. *Comprehensive accreditation manual for hospitals: The official handbook.* Oakbrook Terrace, IL: The Joint Commission. (Level I)

5 The Joint Commission. (2012). Standard RC.01.03.01. *Comprehensive accreditation manual for hospitals: The official handbook.* Oakbrook Terrace, IL: The Joint Commission. (Level I)

ADDITIONAL REFERENCES

Craven, R.F., & Hirnle, C.J. (2009). *Fundamentals of nursing: Human health and function* (6th ed.). Philadelphia, PA: Lippincott Williams & Wilkins.

Mosti, G., et al. (2008). Influence of different materials in multi-component bandages on pressure and stiffness of the final bandage. *Dermatologic Surgery, 34*(5), 631–639.

Partsch, H., et al. (2008). Classification of compression bandages: Practical aspects. *Dermatologic Surgery, 34*(5), 600–609.

Taylor, C., et al. (2011). *Fundamentals of nursing: The art and science of nursing care* (7th ed.). Philadelphia, PA: Lippincott Williams & Wilkins.

ELECTRICAL BONE GROWTH STIMULATION

By imitating the body's natural electrical forces, this procedure initiates or accelerates the healing process in a fractured bone that fails to heal. About 1 in 20 fractures may fail to heal properly, possibly as a result of infection, insufficient reduction or fixation, pseudarthrosis, or severe tissue trauma around the fracture. Electrical bone growth stimulation is also used to help bones grow together after such procedures as spinal fusion.

Three basic electrical bone stimulation techniques are available: fully implantable direct current stimulation; semi-invasive percutaneous stimulation; and noninvasive electromagnetic coil stimulation. (See *Methods of electrical bone growth stimulation.*) The choice of technique depends on the fracture type and location, the doctor's preference, and the patient's ability and willingness to comply. The invasive device requires little or no patient involvement. With the other two methods, however, the patient must manage his own treatment schedule and maintain the equipment. Treatment time averages 3 to 6 months.

Equipment
Clippers.

For direct current stimulation
The equipment set consists of a small generator and leadwires that connect to a titanium cathode wire that's surgically implanted into the nonunited bone site.

For percutaneous stimulation
The equipment set consists of an external anode skin pad with a leadwire, lithium battery pack, and one to four Teflon-coated stainless steel cathode wires that are surgically implanted.

For electromagnetic stimulation
The equipment set consists of a generator that plugs into a standard 110-volt outlet and two strong electromagnetic coils placed on either side of the injured area. The coils can be incorporated into a cast, cuff, or orthotic device.

Preparation of equipment
All equipment comes in sets with instructions provided by the manufacturer. Follow the instructions carefully. Make sure that all parts are included and are sterilized according to facility policy and procedure.

Implementation
- Verify the doctor's order.
- Perform hand hygiene.[1,2,3]
- Confirm the patient's identity using at least two patient identifiers according to your facility's policy.[4]
- Explain the procedure to the patient and answer any questions to decrease anxiety.
- Tell the patient whether he'll have an anesthetic and, if possible, which kind.

Direct current stimulation
- Implantation is performed with the patient under general anesthesia. Afterward, the doctor may apply a cast or external fixator to immobilize the limb. The patient is usually hospitalized for 2 to 3 days after implantation. Weight bearing may be ordered as tolerated.
- After the bone fragments join, the generator and leadwire can be removed under local anesthesia. The titanium cathode remains implanted.

Percutaneous stimulation
- Remove excessive body hair from the injured site using clippers. Apply the anode pad. Avoid stressing or pulling on the anode wire.

Electromagnetic stimulation
- Demonstrate to the patient where to place the coils, and tell him to apply them for 3 to 10 hours each day, as ordered by his doctor. Urge the patient not to interrupt the treatments for more than 10 minutes at a time. Many patients find it most convenient to perform the procedure at night.

Completing the procedure
- Perform hand hygiene.[1,2,3]
- Document the procedure.[5]

Special considerations
- A patient being treated with direct current electrical bone stimulation shouldn't undergo electrocauterization, diathermy, or magnetic resonance imaging (MRI). *Electrocautery may "short" the system; diathermy may potentiate the electrical current, possibly causing tissue damage; and MRI will interfere with or stop the current.*
- Percutaneous electrical bone stimulation is contraindicated if the patient has any kind of inflammatory process. Ask the patient whether he's sensitive to nickel or chromium *because both are present in the electrical bone stimulation system.*
- Electromagnetic coils are contraindicated for a pregnant patient, a patient with a tumor, or a patient with an arm fracture and a pacemaker.

Patient teaching
- Teach the patient how to care for his cast or external fixation device. Also tell him how to care for the electrical generator. Urge him to follow treatment instructions faithfully.
- For percutaneous stimulation, instruct the patient to change the anode pad every 48 hours. Tell him to report any local pain to his doctor and not to bear weight for the duration of treatment.
- Relay the doctor's instructions for weight bearing. Usually, the doctor will advise against bearing weight until evidence of healing appears on X-rays.

Complications
Complications associated with any surgical procedure, including increased risk of infection, may occur with direct current electrical bone stimulation equipment. Local irritation or skin ulceration may occur around cathode pin sites with percutaneous devices. No complications are associated with use of electromagnetic coils.

Documentation
Record the type of electrical bone stimulation equipment provided, including date, time, and location, as appropriate. Note the patient's skin condition and tolerance of the procedure. Also record teaching provided to the patient and family members, as well as their ability to understand and act on those instructions.

REFERENCES
1 The Joint Commission. (2012). Standard NPSG.07.01.01. *Comprehensive accreditation manual for hospitals: The official handbook.* Oakbrook Terrace, IL: The Joint Commission. (Level I)
2 Centers for Disease Control and Prevention. (October 2002). Guideline for hand hygiene in health-care settings. *Morbidity and Mortality Weekly Report, 51*(RR-16), 1–45. (Level I)
3 World Health Organization. (2009). *WHO guidelines on hand hygiene in health care: First global patient safety challenge. Clean care is safer care.* Geneva, Switzerland: World Health Organization. (Level I)
4 The Joint Commission. (2012). Standard NPSG.01.01.01. *Comprehensive accreditation manual for hospitals: The official handbook.* Oakbrook Terrace, IL: The Joint Commission. (Level I)

Reviewing ECG waveforms and components

An electrocardiogram (ECG) waveform has three basic components: the P wave, QRS complex, and T wave. These elements can be further divided into the PR interval, J point, ST segment, U wave, and QT interval.

P wave and PR interval

The P wave represents atrial depolarization. The PR interval represents the time it takes an impulse to travel from the atria through the AV nodes and bundle of His. The PR interval measures from the beginning of the P wave to the beginning of the QRS complex.

QRS complex

The QRS complex represents ventricular depolarization (the time it takes for the impulse to travel through the bundle branches to the Purkinje fibers). The Q wave appears as the first negative deflection in the QRS complex; the R wave, as the first positive deflection. The S wave appears as the second negative deflection or the first negative deflection after the R wave.

J point and ST segment

Marking the end of the QRS complex, the J point also indicates the beginning of the ST segment. The ST segment represents part of ventricular repolarization.

T wave and U wave

Usually following the same deflection pattern as the P wave, the T wave represents ventricular repolarization. The U wave follows the T wave, but isn't always seen.

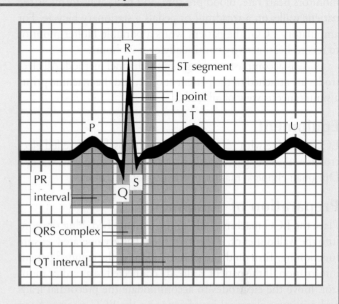

QT interval

The QT interval represents ventricular depolarization and repolarization. It extends from the beginning of the QRS complex to the end of the T wave.

---

5 The Joint Commission. (2012). Standard RC.01.03.01. *Comprehensive accreditation manual for hospitals: The official handbook.* Oakbrook Terrace, IL: The Joint Commission. (Level I)

ADDITIONAL REFERENCES

Goldstein, C., et al. (2010). Electrical stimulation for fracture healing: Current evidence. *Journal of Orthopedic Trauma, 24* (Suppl. 1), S62–S65.

Haddad, J.B., et al. (2007). The biologic effects and the therapeutic mechanism of action of electric and electromagnetic field stimulation on bone and cartilage: New findings and a review of earlier work. *Journal of Alternative and Complementary Medicine, 13*(5), 485–490.

Ramanujam, C.L., et al. (2009). Bone growth stimulation for foot and ankle nonunions. *Clinics in Podiatric Medicine and Surgery, 26*(4), 607–618.

ELECTROCARDIOGRAM, 12-LEAD

One of the most valuable and frequently used diagnostic tools, an electrocardiogram (ECG) can display the heart's electrical activity as waveforms. Impulses moving through the heart's conduction system create electrical currents that can be monitored on the body's surface. Electrodes attached to the skin can detect these electrical currents and transmit them to an instrument that produces a record (the ECG) of cardiac activity.

An ECG can be used to identify myocardial ischemia and infarction, rhythm and conduction disturbances, chamber enlargement, electrolyte imbalances, and drug toxicity.[1,2] The standard 12-lead ECG uses a series of electrodes placed on the extremities and the chest wall to assess the heart from 12 different views (leads). The 12 leads consist of 3 standard bipolar limb leads (designated I, II, III), 3 unipolar augmented leads (aV$_R$, aV$_L$, aV$_F$), and 6 unipolar precordial leads (V$_1$ to V$_6$). The limb leads and augmented leads show the heart from the frontal plane. The precordial leads show the heart from the horizontal plane.

The ECG device measures and averages the differences between the electrical potential of the electrode sites for each lead and graphs them over time. This creates the standard ECG complex, made up of *P-QRS-T.* The P wave represents atrial depolarization; the QRS complex, ventricular depolarization; and the T wave, ventricular repolarization. (See *Reviewing ECG waveforms and components.*)

Variations of the standard ECG include exercise ECG (stress ECG) and ambulatory ECG (Holter monitoring). Exercise ECG monitors heart rate, blood pressure, and ECG waveforms as the patient walks on a treadmill or pedals a stationary bicycle. For ambulatory ECG, the patient wears a portable Holter monitor to record heart activity continually over 24 hours.

ECG is accomplished using a multichannel method. All electrodes are attached to the patient at once, and the machine prints a simultaneous view of all leads.

Equipment

ECG machine with recording paper ■ disposable pregelled electrodes ■ 4″ × 4″ gauze pads or washcloth ■ soap and water ■ Optional: clippers, marking pen, alcohol pad, gloves.

Preparation of equipment

Place the ECG machine close to the patient's bed. Plug the cord into the wall outlet or, if the machine is battery operated, ensure functioning. Turn on the machine, and input the required patient information. If the patient is already connected to a cardiac monitor, move the electrodes to accommodate the precordial leads and minimize electrical interference on the ECG tracing. Keep the patient away from electrical fixtures and power cords.

Implementation

■ Verify the doctor's order.
■ Perform hand hygiene and follow standard precautions.[3,4,5]
■ Confirm the patient's identity using at least two patient identifiers according to your facility's policy.[6]
■ Explain the procedure to the patient and answer any questions *to decrease anxiety and increase cooperation.* Tell the patient that the test records the heart's electrical activity and that it may be repeated at certain intervals. Emphasize that no electrical current will enter his body. Also, tell him that the test typically takes just a few minutes.
■ Position the patient so that he's lying supine in the center of the bed with his arms at his sides.[1,2] Raise the head of the bed *to promote comfort.* Expose his arms and legs, and cover him appropriately. His arms and legs should be relaxed *to minimize muscle trembling, which can cause electrical interference.*[2]
■ If the patient is shivering or trembling, place his hands under his buttocks *to prevent muscle tension.* Make sure his feet aren't touching the bed board.
■ Place the limb lead electrodes on flat, fleshy areas. Avoid muscular and bony areas. If the patient has an amputated limb, choose a site on the stump.
■ Clip excessive hair. Clean the skin with soap and water, drying it thoroughly *to enhance electrode contact.* Then clean oils from the skin with an alcohol pad and allow the skin to dry.[7]
■ Apply electrodes to the patient's wrists and to the medial aspects of his ankles. Apply the electrode directly to the prepared site, as recommended by the manufacturer's instructions. Position electrodes on the legs with the lead connection pointing superiorly *to guarantee the best connection to the leadwire.*
■ Expose the patient's chest. Put an electrode at each electrode position. Place the chest electrodes below the breast tissue. For a

large-breasted woman, you may need to displace the breast tissue laterally. (See *Positioning chest electrodes.*)
■ Connect the leadwires to the electrodes.
■ You'll see that the tip of each leadwire is lettered and color-coded for easy identification. The white (RA) leadwire goes to the right arm; the green (RL) leadwire, to the right leg; the red (LL) leadwire, to the left leg; the black (LA) leadwire, to the left arm; and the brown (V_1 to V_6) leadwires, to the chest electrodes.
■ Check to see that the paper speed selector is set to the standard 25 mm/second and that the machine is set to full voltage. The machine will record a normal standardization mark—a square that's the height of 2 large squares or 10 small squares on the recording paper.
■ If any part of the waveform height extends beyond the paper when you record the ECG, adjust the normal standardization to half-standardization. Note this adjustment on the ECG strip *because this will need to be considered in interpreting the results.*[2]

Ask the patient to relax and breathe normally. Tell him to lie still and not to talk when you record his ECG. Begin the recording by pressing the AUTO or START button (as shown below).

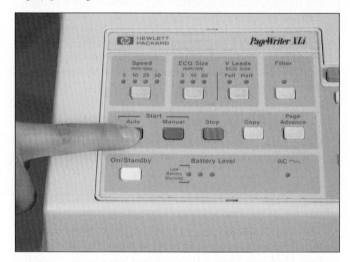

■ Observe the tracing quality. The machine will record all 12 leads automatically, recording 3 consecutive leads simultaneously. Some machines have a display screen so you can preview waveforms before the machine records them on paper.
■ Remove the electrodes when the machine finishes recording the 12-lead ECG. Then clean the patient's skin. After disconnecting the leadwires from the electrodes, dispose of the electrodes, as indicated.
■ Perform hand hygiene.[3,4,5]
■ Document the procedure.[8]

Special considerations

■ Small areas of hair on the patient's chest or extremities may be clipped, but this usually isn't necessary.
■ If the patient's skin is exceptionally oily or diaphoretic, rub the electrode site with an alcohol pad before applying the electrode *to help reduce interference in the tracing.* During the procedure, ask

the patient to breathe normally. If his respirations distort the recording, ask him to hold his breath briefly *to reduce baseline wander in the tracing.*

■ If the patient has a pacemaker, you can perform an ECG with or without a magnet, according to the doctor's orders. Be sure to note the presence of a pacemaker and the use of the magnet on the strip.

Documentation

Document in your notes the test's date and time and significant responses by the patient. Verify the date, time, patient's name, and assigned identification number on the ECG itself. Note any appropriate clinical information on the ECG.

REFERENCES

1 Kligfield, P., et al. (2007). Recommendations for the standardization and interpretation of the electrocardiogram: Part I: The electrocardiogram and its technology. A scientific statement from the American Heart Association Electrocardiography and Arrhythmias Committee, Council on Clinical Cardiology; the American College of Cardiology Foundation; and the Heart Rhythm Society. *Circulation, 115*(10), 1306–1324.

2 American College of Cardiology and American Heart Association. (2001). ACC/AHA clinical competence statement on electrocardiography and ambulatory electrocardiography. *Circulation, 104*, 3169–3178. (Level I)

3 The Joint Commission. (2012). Standard NPSG.07.01.01. *Comprehensive accreditation manual for hospitals: The official handbook.* Oakbrook Terrace, IL: The Joint Commission. (Level I)

4 Centers for Disease Control and Prevention. (October 2002). Guideline for hand hygiene in health-care settings. *Morbidity and Mortality Weekly Report, 51*(RR-16), 1–45. (Level I)

5 World Health Organization. (2009). *WHO guidelines on hand hygiene in health care: First global patient safety challenge. Clean care is safer care.* Geneva, Switzerland: World Health Organization. (Level I)

6 The Joint Commission. (2012). Standard NPSG.01.01.01. *Comprehensive accreditation manual for hospitals: The official handbook.* Oakbrook Terrace, IL: The Joint Commission. (Level I)

7 Lynn-McHale Wiegand, D. (Ed.). (2011). *AACN procedure manual for critical care* (6th ed.). Philadelphia, PA: Saunders.

8 The Joint Commission. (2012). Standard RC.01.03.01. *Comprehensive accreditation manual for hospitals: The official handbook.* Oakbrook Terrace, IL: The Joint Commission. (Level I)

ADDITIONAL REFERENCES

American Heart Association. (2010). 2010 American Heart Association guidelines for cardiopulmonary resuscitation and emergency cardiovascular care. *Circulation, 122*(Suppl. 3), S640–S656.

Nettina, S.M. (2010). *Lippincott manual of nursing practice* (9th ed.). Philadelphia, PA: Lippincott Williams & Wilkins.

Positioning chest electrodes

To ensure accurate test results, position chest electrodes as follows:

V_1: Fourth intercostal space at right border of sternum
V_2: Fourth intercostal space at left border of sternum
V_3: Halfway between V_2 and V_4
V_4: Fifth intercostal space at midclavicular line
V_5: Fifth intercostal space at anterior axillary line (halfway between V_4 and V_6)
V_6: Fifth intercostal space at midaxillary line, level with V_4

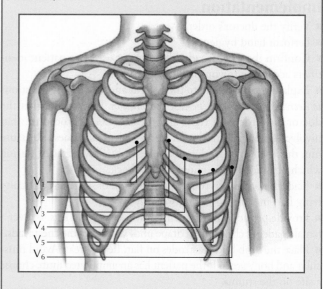

ELECTROCARDIOGRAM, RIGHT CHEST LEAD

Unlike a standard 12-lead electrocardiogram (ECG), used primarily to evaluate left ventricular function, a right chest lead ECG reflects right ventricular function and provides clues to damage or dysfunction in this chamber. You might need to perform a right chest lead ECG for a patient with an inferior wall myocardial infarction (MI) and suspected right ventricular involvement. Between 25% and 50% of patients with this type of MI have right ventricular involvement.

Early identification of a right ventricular MI is essential because its treatment differs from treatment for other MIs. For instance, in left ventricular MI, treatment involves administering IV fluids judiciously to prevent heart failure. Conversely, in right ventricular MI, treatment typically requires administration of IV fluids to maintain adequate filling pressures on the right side of the heart. This helps the right ventricle eject an adequate volume of blood at an adequate pressure.

Equipment

Multichannel ECG machine with recording paper ■ disposable pregelled electrodes ■ dry washcloth or 4″ × 4″ gauze pads ■ Optional: clippers, moist cloth, soap, alcohol pad, marking pen.

Preparation of equipment

Place the ECG machine close to the patient's bed. Plug the cord into the wall outlet or, if the machine is battery operated, ensure functioning. Turn on the machine, and input the required patient information. Keep the patient away from electrical fixtures and power cords.

Implementation

■ Verify the doctor's order.
■ Perform hand hygiene.[1,2,3]
■ Confirm the patient's identity using at least two patient identifiers according to your facility's policy.[4]
■ Explain the procedure to the patient and answer any questions *to decrease anxiety and increase cooperation.* Inform him that the doctor has ordered a right chest lead ECG, a procedure that involves placing electrodes on his arms, legs, and chest. Reassure him that the test is painless and takes only a few minutes, during which he'll need to lie quietly on his back.
■ Place the patient in the supine position or, if he has difficulty lying flat, in semi-Fowler's position.
■ Provide privacy and expose his arms, chest, and legs. (Cover a female patient's chest with a drape until you apply the chest leads.)
■ Place the limb lead electrodes on flat, fleshy areas. Avoid muscular and bony areas. If the patient has an amputated limb, choose a site on the stump.
■ Prepare the application sites by washing them with soap and water and drying them thoroughly *to enhance limb lead electrode contact,* If the patient is diaphoretic or if the skin is oily or has lotion on it, you may use an alcohol pad. Clip excessive hair.[5]
■ Rub the electrode sites briskly with a dry washcloth or gauze pad.[5]
■ Apply electrodes to the patient's arms and legs, distal to the shoulders and hips.[6] Position them in approximately the same location on each limb. Apply the electrode directly to the prepared site, as recommended by the manufacturer's instructions. Position electrodes on the legs with the lead connection pointing superiorly *to guarantee the best connection to the leadwire.*
■ Connect the leadwires to the electrodes. The leadwires are color-coded and lettered. Place the white or right arm (RA) wire on the right arm; the black or left arm (LA) wire on the left arm; the green or right leg (RL) wire on the right leg; and the red or left leg (LL) wire on the left leg.

■ Examine the patient's chest *to locate the correct sites for chest lead placement* (as shown below). Place the electrodes under the breast tissue on a woman. Prepare the electrode application sites as done for the limb leads.

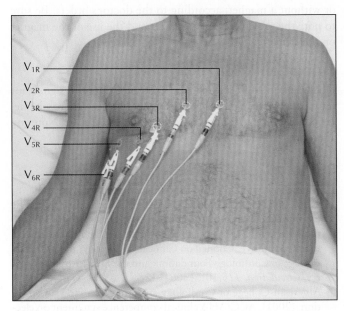

■ Feel between the patient's ribs (the intercostal spaces) using your fingertips. Start at the second intercostal space on the left (the notch felt at the top of the sternum, where the manubrium joins the body of the sternum). Count down two spaces to the fourth intercostal space at the left sternal border. Then apply an electrode to the site and attach lead wire V_{1R} to that electrode.
■ Move your fingers across the sternum to the fourth intercostal space at the right sternal border. Apply an electrode to that site and attach lead V_{2R}.
■ Move your finger down to the fifth intercostal space and over to the midclavicular line. Place an electrode here and attach lead V_{4R}. Apply an electrode midway on this line from V_{2R} and attach lead V_{3R}.
■ Move your finger horizontally from V_{4R} to the right midaxillary line. Apply an electrode to this site and attach lead V_{6R}.
■ Move your fingers along the same horizontal line to the midpoint between V_{4R} and V_{6R}. This is the right anterior midaxillary line. Apply an electrode to this site and attach lead V_{5R}.
■ Turn on the ECG machine. Ask the patient to breathe normally but not to talk during the recording *so that muscle movement won't distort the tracing.*
■ Make sure that the paper speed is set at 25 mm/second and the amplitude at 1 mV/10 mm.[6]
■ Press the AUTO or START key. The ECG machine will record all 12 leads automatically. Check your facility's policy for the number of readings to obtain. (Some facilities require at least two ECGs so that one copy can be sent out for interpretation while the other remains at the bedside.)
■ Observe the tracing quality. If any part of the waveform height extends beyond the paper when you record the ECG, adjust the

normal standardization to half-standardization. Note this adjustment on the ECG strip *because this will need to be considered in interpreting the results.*[6]

- Turn off the machine when you're finished recording the ECG. Make sure that the ECG is clearly labeled with the patient's name, identification number, date, and time. Also label the tracing as "RIGHT CHEST ECG" to distinguish it from a standard 12-lead ECG. Make sure that the tracings are correctly labeled: V_{1R} through V_{6R}.
- If you think you may need more than one right chest lead ECG, use a marking pen to mark the electrode sites on the patient's skin. *This permits accurate comparisons for future tracings.*
- Remove and discard the electrodes.
- Perform hand hygiene.[1,2,3]
- Document the procedure.[7]

Special considerations

- For best results, place the electrodes symmetrically on the limbs. If the patient's wrist or ankle is covered by a dressing or if the patient is an amputee, choose an area that's available on both sides.

Documentation

Document the procedure in the nurse's notes, and document the patient's tolerance to the procedure. Place a copy of the tracing on the patient's chart. Verify the date, time, patient's name, and assigned identification number on the ECG itself.

REFERENCES

1 The Joint Commission. (2012). Standard NPSG.07.01.01. *Comprehensive accreditation manual for hospitals: The official handbook.* Oakbrook Terrace, IL: The Joint Commission. (Level I)
2 Centers for Disease Control and Prevention. (October 2002). Guideline for hand hygiene in health-care settings. *Morbidity and Mortality Weekly Report, 51*(RR-16), 1–45. (Level I)
3 World Health Organization. (2009). *WHO guidelines on hand hygiene in health care: First global patient safety challenge. Clean care is safer care.* Geneva, Switzerland: World Health Organization. (Level I)
4 The Joint Commission. (2012). Standard NPSG.01.01.01. *Comprehensive accreditation manual for hospitals: The official handbook.* Oakbrook Terrace, IL: The Joint Commission. (Level I)
5 Kligfield, P., et al. (2007). Recommendations for the standardization and interpretation of the electrocardiogram: Part I: The electrocardiogram and its technology. A scientific statement from the American Heart Association Electrocardiography and Arrhythmias Committee, Council on Clinical Cardiology; the American College of Cardiology Foundation; and the Heart Rhythm Society. *Circulation, 115*(10), 1306–1324.
6 American College of Cardiology and American Heart Association. (2001). ACC/AHA clinical competence statement on electrocardiography and ambulatory electrocardiography. *Circulation, 104*, 3169–3178. (Level I)
7 The Joint Commission. (2012). Standard RC.01.03.01. *Comprehensive accreditation manual for hospitals: The official handbook.* Oakbrook Terrace, IL: The Joint Commission. (Level I)

ADDITIONAL REFERENCES

Lynn-McHale Wiegand, D. (Ed.). (2011). *AACN procedure manual for critical care* (6th ed.). Philadelphia, PA: Saunders.
Nettina, S.M. (2010). *Lippincott manual of nursing practice* (9th ed.). Philadelphia, PA: Lippincott Williams & Wilkins.

ELECTROCARDIOGRAM, POSTERIOR CHEST LEAD

Because of the location of the heart's posterior surface, changes associated with myocardial damage may not be apparent on a standard 12-lead electrocardiogram (ECG). To help identify posterior involvement, some practitioners recommend using posterior chest leads in addition to the limb leads of the 12-lead ECG. Despite lung and muscle barriers, posterior leads may provide clues to posterior wall infarction so that appropriate treatment can begin.

Equipment

Multichannel ECG machine with recording paper ▪ disposable pregelled electrodes ▪ dry washcloth or 4″ × 4″ gauze pads ▪ Optional: clippers, moist cloth, soap, alcohol pad, marking pen.

Preparation of equipment

Place the ECG machine close to the patient's bed. Plug the cord into the wall outlet or, if the machine is battery operated, ensure functioning. Turn on the machine, and input the required patient information. Keep the patient away from electrical fixtures and power cords.

Implementation

- Verify the doctor's order.
- Perform hand hygiene.[1,2,3]
- Confirm the patient's identity using at least two patient identifiers according to your facility's policy.[4]
- Provide privacy and explain the procedure to the patient. Answer all questions *to decrease anxiety and increase cooperation.* Tell him that the test records the heart's electrical activity and that it may be repeated at certain intervals. Emphasize that no electrical current will enter his body. Also, tell him that the test typically takes about 5 minutes.
- Position the patient supine in the center of the bed with his arms at his sides. You may raise the head of the bed *to promote comfort.* Expose the patient's arms and legs, and cover him appropriately. His arms and legs should be relaxed *to minimize muscle trembling, which can cause electrical interference.*
- Place the limb lead electrodes on flat, fleshy areas. Avoid muscular and bony areas. If the patient has an amputated limb, choose a site on the stump.
- Prepare the application sites by washing them with soap and water and drying them thoroughly *to enhance limb lead electrode contact.* If the patient is diaphoretic or if the skin is oily or has lotion on it, you may use an alcohol pad. Clip excessive hair.[5]

Placing electrodes for posterior ECG

To ensure an accurate electrocardiogram (ECG) reading, make sure that the posterior leads V_7, V_8, and V_9 are placed at the same level horizontally as the V_6 lead at the fifth intercostal space. Place lead V_7 at the posterior axillary line, lead V_9 at the paraspinal line, and lead V_8 halfway between leads V_7 and V_9.

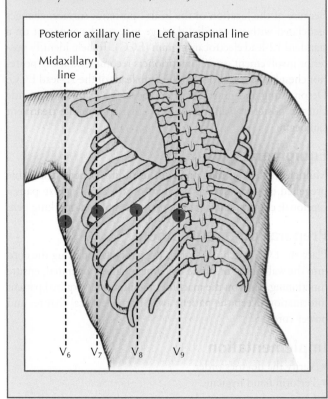

Posterior axillary line   Left paraspinal line

Midaxillary line

V_6 V_7 V_8 V_9

■ Rub the electrode sites briskly with a dry washcloth or gauze pad.[5]

■ Apply electrodes to the patient's arms and legs, distal to the shoulders and hips.[7] Position them in approximately the same location on each limb. Apply the electrode directly to the prepared site, as recommended by the manufacturer's instructions. Position electrodes on the legs with the lead connection pointing superiorly *to guarantee the best connection to the leadwire.*

■ Help the patient turn onto his right side and expose the left side of his back.

■ Prepare the posterior electrode application sites as described for the limb leads.

■ Attach an electrode to the V_7 position on the left posterior axillary line, fifth intercostal space, at the same level as V_6. Then attach the V_4 leadwire to the V_7 electrode.

■ Attach an electrode to the patient's back at the V_9 position, just left of his spinal column at the left paraspinal line, at the same level as V_6 and V_7. Then, attach the V_6 leadwire to the V_9 electrode.

■ Attach an electrode to the patient's back at the V_8 position, halfway between leads V_7 and V_9, at the same level as V_6 and V_7, and attach the V_5 leadwire to this electrode. (See *Placing electrodes for posterior ECG.*)

■ Turn on the machine and make sure that the paper speed is set for 25 mm/second. If necessary, standardize the machine. Press AUTO or START.

■ Observe the tracing quality. If any part of the waveform height extends beyond the paper when you record the ECG, adjust the normal standardization to half-standardization. Note this adjustment on the ECG strip *because this adjustment will need to be considered in interpreting the results.*[6]

■ When using a multichannel ECG machine, the unattached leads will print out as straight lines. Relabel the leads labeled V_4, V_5, and V_6 to leads V_7, V_8, and V_9, respectively.

■ Turn off the machine when the ECG is complete.

■ Label the tracing with the patient's name and the date and time. Note whether the tracing is a right or left posterior chest lead ECG. Make sure the leads are correctly labeled V_7 through V_9.

■ Remove and discard the electrodes. Then clean the patient's skin with a gauze pad or a moist cloth. If you think you may need more than one posterior lead ECG, use a marking pen to mark the electrode sites on the patient's skin *to permit accurate comparison for future tracings.*

■ Place the ECG in the patient's chart for the doctor to interpret.

■ Perform hand hygiene.[1,2,3]

■ Document the procedure.[7]

Documentation

Document in your notes the test's date and time and significant responses by the patient. Verify the date, time, patient's name, and assigned identification number on the ECG itself. Note any appropriate clinical information on the ECG.

REFERENCES

1 The Joint Commission. (2012). Standard NPSG.07.01.01. *Comprehensive accreditation manual for hospitals: The official handbook.* Oakbrook Terrace, IL: The Joint Commission. (Level I)

2 Centers for Disease Control and Prevention. (October 2002). Guideline for hand hygiene in health-care settings. *Morbidity and Mortality Weekly Report, 51*(RR-16), 1–45. (Level I)

3 World Health Organization. (2009). *WHO guidelines on hand hygiene in health care: First global patient safety challenge. Clean care is safer care.* Geneva, Switzerland: World Health Organization. (Level I)

4 The Joint Commission. (2012). Standard NPSG.01.01.01. *Comprehensive accreditation manual for hospitals: The official handbook.* Oakbrook Terrace, IL: The Joint Commission. (Level I)

5 American College of Cardiology and American Heart Association. (2001). ACC/AHA clinical competence statement on electrocardiography and ambulatory electrocardiography. *Circulation, 104,* 3169–3178. (Level I)

6 Kligfield, P., et al. (2007). Recommendations for the standardization and interpretation of the electrocardiogram: Part I: The electrocardiogram and its technology. A scientific statement from the American Heart Association Electrocardiography and Arrhythmias Committee, Council on Clinical Cardiology; the American College of Cardiology Foundation; and the Heart Rhythm Society. *Circulation, 115*(10), 1306–1324.

7 The Joint Commission. (2012). Standard RC.01.03.01. *Comprehensive accreditation manual for hospitals: The official handbook.* Oakbrook Terrace, IL: The Joint Commission. (Level I)

ADDITIONAL REFERENCES

Aqel, R.A., et al. (2009). Usefulness of three posterior chest leads for the detection of posterior wall acute myocardial infarction. *American Journal of Cardiology. 103*(2), 159–164.

Lettina, S.M. (2010). *Lippincott manual of nursing practice* (9th ed.). Philadelphia, PA: Lippincott Williams & Wilkins.

Lynn-McHale Wiegand, D. (Ed.). (2011). *AACN procedure manual for critical care* (6th ed.). Philadelphia, PA: Saunders.

ELECTROCARDIOGRAM, SIGNAL-AVERAGED

Signal-averaged electrocardiography (ECG) helps to identify patients at risk for sustained ventricular tachycardia. Because this cardiac arrhythmia can be a precursor of sudden death after a myocardial infarction (MI), the results of signal-averaged ECG can allow appropriate preventive measures.[1]

Using a computer-based ECG, signal averaging detects low-amplitude signals or late electrical potentials, which reflect slow conduction or disorganized ventricular activity through abnormal or infarcted regions of the ventricles. The signal-averaged ECG is developed by recording the noise-free surface ECG in three specialized leads for several hundred beats. (See *Placing electrodes for signal-averaged ECG.*) Signal averaging enhances signals that would otherwise be missed because of increased amplitude and sensitivity to ventricular activity. For instance, on the standard 12-lead ECG, "noise" created by muscle tissue, electronic artifacts, and electrodes masks late potentials, which have a low amplitude. This procedure identifies the risk for sustained ventricular tachycardia in patients with malignant ventricular tachycardia, a history of MI, unexplained syncope, nonischemic congestive cardiomyopathy, or nonsustained ventricular tachycardia.

Equipment

Signal-averaged ECG machine ▪ signal-averaged computer ▪ record of patient's surface ECG for 200 to 300 QRS complexes ▪ three bipolar electrodes or leads ▪ Optional: moist cloth, soap, clippers, gloves.

Implementation

▪ Verify the doctor's order.
▪ Perform hand hygiene and put on gloves, if necessary.[2,3,4]

Placing electrodes for signal-averaged ECG

To prepare your patient for a signal-averaged electrocardiogram (ECG), place the electrodes in the X, Y, and Z orthogonal positions, as shown here. These positions bisect one another to provide a three-dimensional, composite view of ventricular activation.

Anterior chest

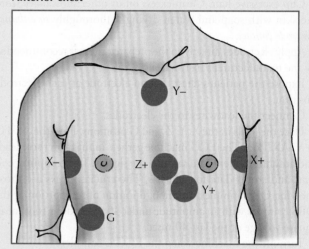

Posterior chest

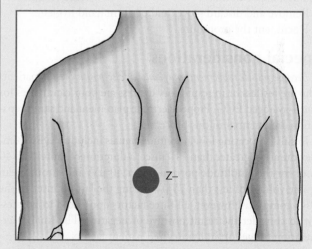

KEY

X+	Fourth intercostal space, midaxillary line, left side
X−	Fourth intercostal space, midaxillary line, right side
Y+	Standard V_3 position (or proximal left leg)
Y−	Superior aspect of manubrium
Z+	Standard V_2 position
Z−	V_2 position, posterior
G	Ground; eighth rib on right side

- Confirm the patient's identity using at least two patient identifiers according to your facility's policy.[5]
- Explain the procedure and answer any questions *to decrease anxiety and increase cooperation.* Inform the patient that this procedure will take 10 to 30 minutes and will help the doctor determine his risk for a certain type of arrhythmia. If appropriate, mention that it may be done along with other tests, such as echocardiography, Holter monitoring, or stress testing.
- Place the patient in the supine position, and tell him to lie as still as possible. Tell him he should not speak and should breathe normally during the procedure.
- Clip excessive hair. Clean excess oil or other substances from the skin with soap and water, drying it thoroughly *to enhance electrode contact.*[6]
- Apply electrodes directly to the prepared sites, as recommended by the manufacturer's instructions.
- Expose the patient's chest. Put an electrode at each electrode position.
- Connect the leadwires to the electrodes.
- Place the leads in the X, Y, Z, and G positions. Press the AUTO or START key. The ECG machine gathers input from these leads and amplifies, filters, and samples the signals. The computer collects and stores data for analysis. The crucial values are those showing QRS complex duration, duration of the portion of the QRS complex with an amplitude under 40 μV, and the root mean square voltage of the last 40 msec.
- Turn off the machine when the ECG is complete.
- Remove the electrodes and clean the patient's skin with a gauze pad or a moist cloth.
- Remove and discard gloves and perform hand hygiene.[2,3,4]
- Document the procedure.[7]

Special considerations

- *Because muscle movements may cause a false-positive result,* patients who are restless or in respiratory distress are poor candidates for signal-averaged ECG. Proper electrode placement and skin preparation are essential to this procedure.
- Results indicating low-amplitude signals include a QRS complex duration greater than 110 msec; a duration of more than 40 msec for the amplitude portion under 40 μV; and a root mean square voltage of less than 25 μV during the last 40 msec of the QRS complex. However, all three factors don't need to be present to consider the result positive or negative. The final interpretation hinges on individualized patient factors.
- Results of signal-averaged ECG help the doctor determine whether the patient is a candidate for invasive procedures, such as electrophysiologic testing or angiography.
- Keep in mind that the significance of signal-averaged ECG results in patients with bundle-branch heart block is unknown *because myocardial activation doesn't follow the usual sequence in these patients.*

Documentation

Document the time of the procedure, why the procedure was done, and how the patient tolerated it.

REFERENCES

1 American College of Cardiology and American Heart Association. (2001). ACC/AHA clinical competence statement on electrocardiography and ambulatory electrocardiography. *Circulation, 104,* 3169–3178.
2 The Joint Commission. (2012). Standard NPSG.07.01.01. *Comprehensive accreditation manual for hospitals: The official handbook.* Oakbrook Terrace, IL: The Joint Commission. (Level I)
3 Centers for Disease Control and Prevention. (October 2002). Guideline for hand hygiene in health-care settings. *Morbidity and Mortality Weekly Report, 51*(RR-16), 1–45. (Level I)
4 World Health Organization. (2009). *WHO guidelines on hand hygiene in health care: First global patient safety challenge. Clean care is safer care.* Geneva, Switzerland: World Health Organization. (Level I)
5 The Joint Commission. (2012). Standard NPSG.01.01.01. *Comprehensive accreditation manual for hospitals: The official handbook.* Oakbrook Terrace, IL: The Joint Commission. (Level I)
6 Kligfield, P., et al. (2007). Recommendations for the standardization and interpretation of the electrocardiogram: Part I: The electrocardiogram and its technology. A scientific statement from the American Heart Association Electrocardiography and Arrhythmias Committee, Council on Clinical Cardiology; the American College of Cardiology Foundation; and the Heart Rhythm Society. *Circulation, 115*(10), 1306–1324.
7 The Joint Commission. (2012). Standard RC.01.03.01. *Comprehensive accreditation manual for hospitals: The official handbook.* Oakbrook Terrace, IL: The Joint Commission. (Level I)

ADDITIONAL REFERENCES

Andrikopoulos, G.K., et al. (2009). Correlation of mechanical dyssynchrony with QRS duration measured by signal-averaged electrocardiography. *Annals of Noninvasive Electrocardiography, 14*(3), 234–241.
Huang, Z., et al. (2009). Role of signal-averaged electrocardiograms in arrhythmic risk stratification of patients with Brugada syndrome: A prospective study. *Heart Rhythm, 6*(8), 1156–1162.
Marcus, F.I., et al. (2007). Evaluation of the normal values for signal-averaged electrocardiogram. *Journal of Cardiovascular Electrophysiology, 18*(2), 231–233.
Nettina, S.M. (2010). *Lippincott manual of nursing practice* (9th ed.). Philadelphia, PA: Lippincott Williams & Wilkins.
Schueller, P.O., et al. (2007). Signal-averaged P-wave ECG as a marker of atrial electrical instability in patients with right ventricular dysfunction. *Journal of Physiology and Pharmacology, 58*(Suppl. 5, Pt. 2), 627–632.

ENDOSCOPIC THERAPY, ASSISTING

Endoscopic therapy allows visualization of the upper GI tract to help diagnose, control, or prevent bleeding and evacuate blood and clots. During this procedure, the doctor advances a fiberoptic endoscope through the patient's esophagus and into the stomach and duodenum to help look for a bleeding site. After locating the bleeding site, he may inject a sclerosing agent through an injector needle, which is inserted through a port in the endoscope. The doctor injects the sclerosing agent into the bleeding vessel or tissue surrounding the vessel; he may also apply a band to stop bleeding.

Equipment

Topical anesthetic ▪ oral airway ▪ water-soluble lubricant ▪ oxygen administration equipment ▪ suction apparatus ▪ sterile normal saline solution or sterile water for irrigation ▪ endoscope (rigid or flexible) ▪ endoscopic injector needle (23G to 26G, 2- to 5-mm needle) ▪ three 10-mL syringes filled with prescribed sclerosing agent ▪ tonsil-tip suction device ▪ gloves, gowns, masks, and goggles or face shields ▪ two 30- to 60-mL syringes ▪ cardiac monitor ▪ pulse oximeter ▪ automatic blood pressure cuff ▪ prescribed IV fluid ▪ emergency equipment (cardiac medications, intubation equipment, defibrillator) ▪ Optional: esophageal bands, specimen containers, laboratory biohazard transport bag, laboratory request form.

Preparation of equipment

Set up the suction apparatus and make sure it's functioning properly.[1] Prepare and label sedatives for administration, as ordered. Gather the emergency equipment and make sure it's functioning properly.

Implementation

▪ Verify the doctor's orders.
▪ Confirm that written informed consent was obtained and that the consent is in the patient's medical record.[2]
▪ Conduct a preprocedure verification *to make sure that all relevant documentation, related information, and equipment are available and correctly identified to the patient's identifiers.*[3]
▪ Review baseline coagulation studies *because abnormal results increase the potential for bleeding.*[1]
▪ Review baseline hematocrit and hemoglobin levels.[1]
▪ Perform hand hygiene and put on gloves and other personal protective equipment, as appropriate.[4,5,6]
▪ Confirm the patient's identity using at least two patient identifiers according to your facility's policy.[7]
▪ Make sure that the patient and his family understand the procedure. Answer any questions *to evaluate their understanding of the information provided.*
▪ Make sure that the patient has had nothing by mouth for at least 4 hours before the procedure or according to your facility's policy.[1]
▪ Remove the patient's dentures, if appropriate.
▪ Verify that the patient has an adequate-sized, patent IV catheter (an 18G catheter is preferred) *to administer sedation and any emergency medications or IV fluid, if necessary.* If an adequate catheter isn't in place, insert one. (See "IV catheter insertion and removal," page 421.) Begin an IV infusion, as prescribed.
▪ Provide goggles or a waterproof covering for the patient's eyes *to protect him against accidental exposure to blood or sclerosing agents.*[8]
▪ Attach the patient to the cardiac monitor, pulse oximeter, and automatic blood pressure cuff *for continuous monitoring during the procedure.*

Double-checking high-alert medications[10]

When administering high-alert medications such as moderate sedation agents, another nurse must perform an independent double-check of your preparation of the drug *to ensure safe administration.* The second nurse must:
▪ verify the patient's identity[7]
▪ make sure that the correct medication is being given and in the prescribed concentration[12]
▪ make sure that the medication's indication corresponds with the patient's diagnosis
▪ verify that the dosage calculations are correct and the dosing formula used to derive the final dose is correct[11]
▪ verify that the route of administration is safe and appropriate for the patient[11]
▪ ensure that pump settings are correct and that the infusion line is attached to the correct port, if appropriate.

▪ Obtain baseline vital signs and pulse oximetry and assess the patient's neurologic, cardiac, and respiratory status.
▪ Determine the patient's sedation score based on vital signs, level of consciousness (LOC), and respiratory status using a scoring system according to your facility's policy.
▪ Position the patient in a left lateral position. *This position is the position of choice to prevent aspiration and allows predictable views of the stomach as the scope is advanced. This position also allows secretions to collect in the dependent areas of the mouth for easy suctioning.*[1]
▪ Administer analgesia, sedation, or both as ordered, following safe medication administration practices, before endoscope insertion *to facilitate the insertion process.*
NURSING ALERT *Moderate sedation agents are considered high-alert medications* because they can cause significant patient harm when used in error. *Another nurse must double-check certain preparation steps to ensure safe medication administration.*[9] (See Double-checking high-alert medications.)
▪ Conduct a time-out immediately before starting the procedure *to perform a final assessment that the correct patient, site, positioning, and procedure are identified and, as applicable, all relevant information and necessary equipment are available.*[12]
▪ Monitor the patient's heart rhythm, vital signs, oxygen saturation, neurologic status, and sedation score every 5 minutes during the procedure. *A vagal response, causing a drop in heart rate, may occur during insertion and advancement of the probe; secretions may obstruct the patient's airway causing a decrease in oxygen saturation levels; and sedation may cause hypotension, respiratory depression, and decreased LOC.*
▪ Assist the doctor as necessary during the procedure.[13] The doctor will anesthetize the posterior pharynx with a topical anesthetic agent. He'll insert an oral airway *to prevent the patient from biting down on the endoscope.*[1]

■ The doctor will lubricate the distal end of the endoscope with a water-soluble lubricant *to facilitate passage of the endoscope.*[1] Instruct the patient to swallow while the endoscope is being advanced *to help facilitate endoscope passage into the esophagus.*[1]

■ Suction the oropharynx, as needed, using a tonsil-tip suction catheter *to prevent aspiration of secretions.*[1]

■ Prepare the equipment for thermal or laser coagulation therapy, as needed, *which will be used to control bleeding.*

■ Assist with irrigation using sterile normal saline solution or sterile water through the endoscope *to improve visualization.*[1]

■ If the site requires sclerosing, assist with the sclerosing needle and inject sclerosant, as requested.[1]

■ Provide the doctor with endoscopic bands as requested if endoscopic variceal ligation (the treatment of choice for controlling variceal hemorrhage) is necessary.

■ If the doctor obtains a specimen for testing, place it in the proper specimen container, label the container in the presence of the patient *to prevent mislabeling,* and place the container in a laboratory transport bag.[14] Send specimens to the laboratory in the laboratory biohazard transport bag along with a completed laboratory request form.

■ The doctor will then carefully remove the endoscope.

■ Insert a nasogastric tube, if ordered, *to assess for recurrent bleeding.*[1] (See "Nasogastric tube insertion and removal," page 498.)

■ Position the patient in the left lateral position until his gag, swallow, and cough reflexes return. After these reflexes return, reposition the patient *to promote comfort.*

■ Remove and discard your personal protective equipment and place it in the appropriate receptacle.

■ Perform hand hygiene.[4,5,6]

■ Monitor the patient's heart rhythm, vital signs, pulse oximetry, neurologic status, and sedation score every 15 minutes until the patient's condition returns to baseline for at least 30 minutes, or according to your facility's policy.[1]

■ Send the endoscope for cleaning and disinfecting according to your facility's policy.[15]

■ Perform hand hygiene.[4,5,6]

■ Document the procedure.[16]

Special considerations

■ Endoscope insertion and advancement may stimulate a vagal response in the patient, causing bradycardia. Close monitoring of the patient is necessary.[1]

■ Keep in mind that sedatives and topical anesthetics interfere with the patient's gag reflex, placing the patient at risk for aspiration.[1]

Complications

Complications include respiratory depression, hypotension, bradycardia, anaphylactic reaction to sclerosing agent and premedications, aspiration, bleeding, temporary dysphagia, esophageal perforation, and decreased LOC.

Documentation

Record the patient's vital signs, pulse oximetry, and other assessment findings during and after the procedure. Document the date and time of the procedure, sclerosing agents administered (if applicable), and the patient's tolerance of the procedure. If any unexpected complications occurred, document the necessary interventions and the patient's response to such interventions. Also document any patient and family teaching.

REFERENCES

1 Lynn-McHale Wiegand, D. (Ed.). (2011). *AACN procedure manual for critical care* (6th ed.). Philadelphia, PA: Saunders.

2 The Joint Commission. (2012). Standard RI.01.03.01. *Comprehensive accreditation manual for hospitals: The official handbook.* Oakbrook Terrace, IL: The Joint Commission. (Level I)

3 The Joint Commission. (2012). Standard UP.01.01.01. *Comprehensive accreditation manual for hospitals: The official handbook.* Oakbrook Terrace, IL: The Joint Commission. (Level I)

4 The Joint Commission. (2012). Standard NPSG.07.01.01. *Comprehensive accreditation manual for hospitals: The official handbook.* Oakbrook Terrace, IL: The Joint Commission. (Level I)

5 Centers for Disease Control and Prevention. (October 2002). Guideline for hand hygiene in health-care settings. *Morbidity and Mortality Weekly Report, 51*(RR-16), 1–45. (Level I)

6 World Health Organization. (2009). *WHO guidelines on hand hygiene in health care: First global patient safety challenge. Clean care is safer care.* Geneva, Switzerland: World Health Organization. (Level I)

7 The Joint Commission. (2012). Standard NPSG.01.01.01. *Comprehensive accreditation manual for hospitals: The official handbook.* Oakbrook Terrace, IL: The Joint Commission. (Level I)

8 Siegel, J.D., et al. "2007 Guideline for Isolation Precautions: Preventing Transmission of Infectious Agents in Healthcare Settings" [Online]. Accessed September 2011 via the Web at http://www.cdc.gov/hicpac/2007ip/2007isolationprecautions.html

9 Institute of Safe Medication Practices. "ISMP's List of High-Alert Medications" [Online]. Accessed August 2011 via the Web at http://www.ismp.org/tools/highalertmedications.pdf

10 Institute for Safe Medication Practices. (2008). "Conducting an Independent Double-check." *ISMP Medication Safety Alert! Nurse Advise-ERR, 6*(12), 1 [Online]. Accessed July 2011 via the Web at http://www.ismp.org/newsletters/nursing/Issues/NurseAdviseERR200812.pdf

11 The Joint Commission. (2012). Standard MM.06.01.01. *Comprehensive accreditation manual for hospitals: The official handbook.* Oakbrook Terrace, IL: The Joint Commission. (Level I)

12 The Joint Commission. (2012). Standard UP.01.03.01. *Comprehensive accreditation manual for hospitals: The official handbook.* Oakbrook Terrace, IL: The Joint Commission. (Level I)

13 Society of Gastroenterological Nurses and Associates, Inc. (2009). "Position Statement: Manipulation of Endoscopes during Endoscopic Procedures" [Online]. Accessed September 2011 via the Web at http://www.sgna.org/Portals/0/Education/Position%20Statements/ManipulationofEndoscopesPositionStatements.pdf

14 The Joint Commission. (2012). Standard NPSG.03.04.01. *Comprehensive accreditation manual for hospitals: The official handbook.* Oakbrook Terrace, IL: The Joint Commission. (Level I)

15 Rutala, W.A., et al. (2008). "Guideline for Disinfection and Sterilization in Healthcare Facilities, 2008" [Online]. Accessed September 2011 via the Web at http://www.cdc.gov/ncidod/dhqp/pdf/guidelines/Disinfection_Nov_2008.pdf (Level I)

16 The Joint Commission. (2012). Standard RC.01.03.01. *Comprehensive accreditation manual for hospitals: The official handbook.* Oakbrook Terrace, IL: The Joint Commission. (Level I)

ENDOTRACHEAL DRUG ADMINISTRATION

When an IV line isn't readily available, drugs can be administered into the respiratory system through an endotracheal (ET) tube. This route allows uninterrupted resuscitation efforts and avoids such complications as coronary artery laceration, cardiac tamponade, and pneumothorax, which can occur when emergency drugs are administered intracardially.

However, a drug given endotracheally typically produces lower blood levels of the drug than the same dose of the drug given IV. According to the 2010 American Heart Association guidelines for cardiopulmonary resuscitation (CPR) and emergency cardiovascular care, studies show that these lower blood levels may actually be detrimental to the patient. For example, epinephrine administered endotracheally may produce transient beta-adrenergic effects, causing vasodilation and subsequent hypotension and reducing the patient's chances of survival. Because of this, the IV or intraosseous (I.O.) routes are preferred because they provide more predictable drug delivery and pharmacologic effect, even though some resuscitation drugs can be administered endotracheally.[1]

When IV or I.O. access can't be established, epinephrine, vasopressin, and lidocaine may be administered endotracheally during cardiac arrest. Typically, the dose given by the ET route is 2 to 2½ times the recommended IV dose. The drug should be diluted in 5 to 10 mL of sterile water or normal saline solution and then injected directly into the ET tube. Better absorption may occur when epinephrine and lidocaine are diluted in sterile water instead of normal saline solution.[1]

Drugs given endotracheally are usually administered in an emergency situation by a doctor, an emergency medical technician, or a critical care nurse. Although guidelines may vary with state, county, or city regulations, the basic administration method is the same. The drugs may be given using either the syringe method or the adapter method. Usually used for bronchoscopy suctioning, the swivel adapter can be placed on the end of the tube and, while ventilation continues through a bag-valve device, the drug can be delivered through the closed stopcock. (See *Administering drugs endotracheally.*)

Equipment

ET tube or swivel adapter ■ gloves ■ end-tidal carbon dioxide (CO_2) detector, esophageal detection device, or continuous waveform capnography device ■ handheld resuscitation bag ■ prescribed drug ■ syringe or adapter ■ sterile water or normal saline solution ■ personal protective equipment as needed.

Preparation of equipment

Verify the order on the patient's medication administration record by checking it against the doctor's order.[2,3] Perform hand hygiene.[4,5,6] Check ET tube placement by using an end-tidal CO_2

Administering drugs endotracheally

In an emergency, some drugs can be given through an endotracheal (ET) tube if IV access isn't available. They may be given using the syringe method or the adapter method. Before injecting any drug, check for proper placement of the ET tube using an end-tidal carbon dioxide detector, an esophageal detection device, or continuous waveform capnography. Make sure the patient is in a supine position with the head level with or slightly higher than the body.

Syringe method
Remove the needle before injecting medication into the ET tube. Insert the tip of the syringe into the ET tube, and inject the drug deep into the tube (as shown).

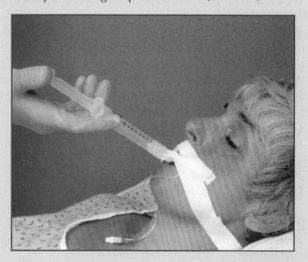

Adapter method
An adapter device for ET drug administration provides a more closed system of drug delivery than the syringe method. A special adapter placed on the end of the ET tube (as shown) allows drug delivery through the closed stopcock.

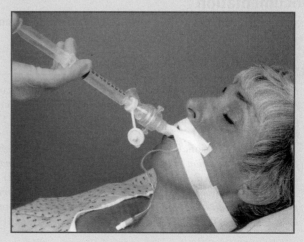

detector, esophageal detection device, or waveform capnography device.

Calculate the drug dose. Keep in mind that adult advanced cardiac life support guidelines recommend that drugs be administered at 2 to 2½ times the recommended IV dose.[1,7] Next, draw the drug up into a syringe. Dilute it in 5 to 10 mL of sterile water or normal saline solution.[1] *Dilution increases drug volume and contact with lung tissue.*

Implementation

- Verify the doctor's order.[2]
- Confirm the patient's identity using at least two patient identifiers according to your facility's policy.[8]
- Put on gloves and any other personal protective equipment needed, according to the clinical situation.[4,5,6,9]
- Move the patient into the supine position, and make sure his head is level with or slightly higher than his trunk.
- If CPR is in progress, interrupt chest compressions briefly to administer the medication.[1]
- Remove the needle from the syringe and insert the tip of the syringe into the ET tube or swivel adapter. Inject the drug deep into the tube.
- After injecting the drug, reattach the resuscitation bag and ventilate the patient briskly. *This propels the drug into the lungs, oxygenates the patient, and clears the tube.*
- Discard the syringe in an appropriate sharps container.
- Remove and discard your gloves and other personal protective equipment.
- Perform hand hygiene.[4,5,6]
- Document the procedure.[10]

Special considerations

- Keep in mind that during cardiac arrest, drug administration should only briefly interrupt chest compressions.[1]

Complications

Potential complications of drugs administered endotracheally generally result from the prescribed drug, not the administration route.

Documentation

Record the date and time of drug administration, the drug administered, and the patient's response.

REFERENCES

1 American Heart Association. (2010). 2010 American Heart Association guidelines for cardiopulmonary resuscitation and emergency cardiovascular care. *Circulation, 122*(Suppl. 3), S729–S767. (Level I)
2 The Joint Commission. (2012). Standard MM.04.01.01. *Comprehensive accreditation manual for hospitals: The official handbook.* Oakbrook Terrace, IL: The Joint Commission. (Level I)
3 The Joint Commission. (2012). Standard MM.06.01.01. *Comprehensive accreditation manual for hospitals: The official handbook.* Oakbrook Terrace, IL: The Joint Commission. (Level I)
4 The Joint Commission. (2012). Standard NPSG.07.01.01. *Comprehensive accreditation manual for hospitals: The official handbook.* Oakbrook Terrace, IL: The Joint Commission. (Level I)
5 Centers for Disease Control and Prevention. (October 2002). Guideline for hand hygiene in health-care settings. *Morbidity and Mortality Weekly Report, 51*(RR-16), 1–45. (Level I)
6 World Health Organization. (2009). *WHO guidelines on hand hygiene in health care: First global patient safety challenge. Clean care is safer care.* Geneva, Switzerland: World Health Organization. (Level I)
7 American Association for Respiratory Care. (2004). AARC clinical practice guideline: Resuscitation and defibrillation in the health care setting—2004 revision & update. *Respiratory Care, 89*(9), 1085–1099. (Level I)
8 The Joint Commission. (2012). Standard NPSG.01.01.01. *Comprehensive accreditation manual for hospitals: The official handbook.* Oakbrook Terrace, IL: The Joint Commission. (Level I)
9 Siegel, J. D., et al. (2007). "2007 Guideline for Isolation Precautions: Preventing Transmission of Infectious Agents in Healthcare Settings" [Online]. Accessed September 2011 via the Web at http://www.cdc.gov/hicpac/2007ip/2007isolationprecautions.html
10 The Joint Commission. (2012). Standard RC.01.03.01. *Comprehensive accreditation manual for hospitals: The official handbook.* Oakbrook Terrace, IL: The Joint Commission. (Level I)

ADDITIONAL REFERENCES

Nettina, S.M. (2010). *Lippincott manual of nursing practice* (9th ed.). Philadelphia, PA: Lippincott Williams & Wilkins.
Taylor, C., et al. (2011). *Fundamentals of nursing: The art and science of nursing care* (7th ed.). Philadelphia, PA: Lippincott Williams & Wilkins.

ENDOTRACHEAL INTUBATION

Endotracheal (ET) intubation involves the oral or nasal insertion of a flexible tube through the larynx into the trachea for the purposes of controlling the airway and mechanically ventilating the patient. Performed by a doctor, anesthetist, respiratory therapist, or nurse educated in the procedure, ET intubation typically occurs in emergencies, such as cardiopulmonary arrest or in diseases such as epiglottitis. However, intubation may also occur under more controlled circumstances, such as just before surgery or in patients who can't clear their secretions effectively. In these situations, ET intubation requires patient teaching and preparation.

Advantages of the procedure include establishing and maintaining a patent airway, protecting against aspiration by sealing off the trachea from the digestive tract, permitting removal of tracheobronchial secretions in patients who can't cough effectively, and providing a route for mechanical ventilation. Disadvantages include bypassing normal respiratory defenses against infection, reducing cough effectiveness, and preventing verbal communication.

The two routes for ET intubation are the oral or nasotracheal routes. Oral ET intubation allows direct visualization of the vocal cords, which the ET tube must pass through to be in correct position. It's preferred over nasotracheal intubation because nasotracheal intubation increases the risk for sinusitis, which may increase the risk of ventilator-associated pneumonia.[1] Nasotracheal intubation is more comfortable than oral intubation, but it's also more difficult to perform because the vocal cords—which the ET tube needs to pass through to be in correct position—can't be directly visualized. Because ET the tube passes blindly through the nasal cavity, the procedure causes greater tissue trauma, increases the risk of infection by nasal bacteria introduced into the trachea, and risks pressure necrosis of the nasal mucosa. However, exact tube placement is easier, and the risk of dislodgment is lower. The cuff on the ET tube maintains a closed system that permits positive-pressure ventilation and protects the airway from aspiration of secretions and gastric contents.

Nasotracheal intubation is contraindicated in patients with facial fractures or suspected basilar skull fractures and after cranial surgery, such as transsphenoidal hypophysectomy.[2]

Equipment

Two ET tubes (one spare) in appropriate size (normal female size is 7 to 8 mm; normal male size is 8 to 9 mm) ▪ 10-mL syringe ▪ stethoscope ▪ sedative ▪ paralytic agent ▪ local anesthetic spray ▪ overbed or other table ▪ water-soluble lubricant ▪ adhesive or other strong tape or commercial tube holder ▪ skin preparation product ▪ sterile gloves ▪ gloves ▪ goggles and other personal protective equipment ▪ suction equipment ▪ handheld resuscitation bag with sterile swivel adapter ▪ humidified oxygen source ▪ carbon dioxide detector or waveform capnography ▪ oral care equipment.

For direct visualization intubation

Lighted laryngoscope with a handle and blades of various sizes, both curved and straight ▪ oral airway or bite block ▪ Optional: prepackaged intubation tray, stylet.

For blind nasotracheal intubation

Mucosal vasoconstricting agent.

Preparation of equipment

Gather the individual supplies or use a prepackaged intubation tray, which will contain most of the necessary supplies. Select an ET tube of the appropriate size.

Perform hand hygiene and put on sterile gloves.[3,4,5] Using sterile technique, open the package containing the ET tube and, if desired, open the other supplies on an overbed table. Then, *to ease insertion,* you may lubricate the first 1″ (2.5 cm) of the distal end of the ET tube with the water-soluble lubricant, using sterile technique. Do this by squeezing the lubricant directly on the tube. Use only water-soluble lubricant *because it can be absorbed by mucous membranes.*

Next, attach the syringe to the port on the tube's exterior pilot cuff. Slowly inflate the cuff, observing for uniform inflation. Then use the syringe to deflate the cuff.

A stylet may be used *to stiffen the tube.* The entire stylet may be lubricated. Insert the stylet into the tube so that its distal tip lies about ½″ (1.3 cm) inside the distal end of the tube. Make sure the stylet doesn't protrude from the tube *to avoid vocal cord trauma.* Prepare the humidified oxygen source and the suction equipment for immediate use. If the patient is in bed, remove the headboard *to provide easier access.*

Before direct visualization intubation, check the light in the laryngoscope by snapping the appropriate-sized blade into place; if the bulb doesn't light, replace the batteries or the laryngoscope (whichever will be quicker). Remove and discard your gloves and perform hand hygiene.[3,4,5]

Implementation

NURSING ALERT *Intubation performed during cardiac arrest shouldn't delay initial cardiopulmonary resuscitation (CPR) and defibrillation for ventricular fibrillation.*[6]

▪ Verify the doctor's order, if appropriate.

▪ Confirm the patient's identity using at least two patient identifiers, if possible, according to your facility's policy.[7]

▪ Assess the patient's immediate history to see whether he has a suspected spinal cord injury or underwent cranial surgery *to make sure the proper intubation method is chosen.*[2]

▪ Determine when the patient last had something to eat. *Using a handheld resuscitation bag may further increase abdominal distention and increase the risk of aspiration.*[2]

▪ Assess the patient's level of consciousness, level of anxiety, and respiratory status *to determine whether the patient needs sedation, a paralytic agent, or both.*[2]

▪ Assess the patient's oral cavity for dentures or any loose teeth; remove them if possible *because they might obstruct the airway.*[2]

▪ Explain the procedure to the patient or his family, if able, *to allay the patient's and family's anxiety.*

▪ Perform hand hygiene and put on gloves and other personal protective equipment.[3,4,5]

▪ If the patient doesn't already have an IV catheter established, insert one *to administer sedation or other emergency medications if needed.*[2] (See "IV catheter insertion and removal," page 421.)

▪ Administer the sedative, as ordered, *to decrease respiratory secretions, induce amnesia or analgesia, and help calm and relax the conscious patient.*

▪ Administer the paralytic agent, as ordered, *to stop muscle movement and ease insertion of the ET tube.*

▪ Hyperventilate the patient with 100% oxygen using a handheld resuscitation bag for at least 3 to 5 minutes; continue until the tube is inserted *to prevent hypoxia.*[2]

For direct visualization intubation

▪ Place the patient supine in the sniffing position so that the mouth, pharynx, and trachea are extended. If cervical spine injury is suspected, have an assistant maintain the patient's head in a neutral position with the spine immobilized.[2]

▪ A local anesthetic (such as lidocaine) may be sprayed deep into the posterior pharynx *to diminish the gag reflex and reduce patient discomfort.*

▪ If necessary, suction the patient's pharynx just before tube insertion *to improve visualization of the patient's pharynx and vocal cords and to prevent aspiration of secretions.*

- Be prepared to time each intubation attempt, limiting attempts to less than 20 seconds *to prevent hypoxia.* Hyperventilate the patient between attempts, if necessary.
- Stand at the head of the patient's bed. Using your right hand, hold the patient's mouth open by crossing your index finger over your thumb and placing your thumb on the patient's upper teeth and your index finger on the lower teeth. *This technique provides greater leverage.*
- Grasp the laryngoscope handle in your left hand, and gently slide the blade into the right side of the patient's mouth. Center the blade, and push the patient's tongue to the left. Hold the patient's lower lip away from the teeth *to prevent the lip from being traumatized.*
- Advance the blade *to expose the epiglottis.* When using a straight blade, insert the tip under the epiglottis; when using a curved blade, insert the tip between the base of the tongue and the epiglottis.
- Lift the laryngoscope handle upward and away from your body at a 45-degree angle *to reveal the vocal cords.* Avoid pivoting the laryngoscope against the patient's teeth *to avoid damaging them.*
- If desired, have an assistant apply pressure to the cricoid ring *to occlude the esophagus and minimize gastric regurgitation,* although this procedure is no longer recommended by the American Heart Association for patients in cardiac arrest.
- Insert the ET tube into the right side of the patient's mouth.
- Guide the tube into the vertical openings of the larynx between the vocal cords, being careful not to mistake the horizontal opening of the esophagus for the larynx. If the vocal cords are closed because of a spasm, wait a few seconds for them to relax; then gently guide the tube past them *to avoid traumatic injury.*
- Advance the tube until the cuff disappears beyond the vocal cords. Avoid advancing the tube farther *to avoid occluding a major bronchus and precipitating lung collapse.*
- Holding the ET tube in place, quickly remove the stylet, if present.
- Remove the laryngoscope. Insert an oral airway or a bite block, if necessary, *to prevent the patient from obstructing airflow or puncturing the tube with the teeth.*

For blind nasotracheal intubation

- Place the patient with his head and neck in a neutral position.
- Spray a local anesthetic and a mucosal vasoconstrictor into the nasal passages *to anesthetize the nasal turbinates and reduce the chance of bleeding.*
- Pass the ET tube along the floor of the nasal cavity. If necessary, use gentle force to pass the tube through the nasopharynx and into the pharynx.
- Listen and feel for air movement through the tube as it's advanced *to ensure that the tube is properly placed in the airway.*
- Slip the tube between the vocal cords when the patient inhales *because the vocal cords separate on inhalation.*
- When the tube is past the vocal cords, the breath sounds should become louder. If, at any time during tube advancement, breath sounds disappear, withdraw the tube until they can be heard.

After intubation

- Inflate the tube's cuff with 5 to 10 mL of air until you feel resistance. When the patient is mechanically ventilated, you'll use the minimal-leak technique or the minimal–occlusive volume technique *to establish correct inflation of the cuff.* (See "Tracheal cuff pressure measurement," page 708.)
- Confirm ET tube placement using physical and nonphysical examination techniques, as recommended by the 2010 American Heart Association guidelines for CPR and emergency care. Physical examination techniques include auscultating for bilateral breath sounds, observing for bilateral chest expansion, and listening over the epigastrium (where breath sounds shouldn't be heard). The preferred nonphysical examination technique to confirm and monitor placement is continuous quantitative waveform capnography.[6]

NURSING ALERT *If ET tube insertion is occurring during resuscitation, avoid interrupting chest compressions when confirming tube placement. Be prepared to time each intubation attempt, limiting attempts to less than 15 to 20 seconds to prevent hypoxia. Hyperventilate the patient between attempts, if necessary.*[6]

- Stomach distention, belching, or a gurgling sound indicates esophageal intubation. If these signs occur, immediately deflate the cuff and remove the tube. After reoxygenating the patient to prevent hypoxia, repeat insertion using a sterile tube *to prevent contamination of the trachea.*
- Auscultate bilaterally *to exclude the possibility of endobronchial intubation.* If you fail to hear breath sounds on both sides of the chest, you may have inserted the tube into one of the mainstem bronchi (usually the right one because of its wider angle at the bifurcation); such insertion occludes the other bronchus and lung and results in atelectasis on the obstructed side. Or the tube may be resting on the carina, resulting in dry secretions that obstruct both bronchi. (The patient's coughing and fighting the ventilator will alert you to the problem.) To correct these situations, deflate the cuff, withdraw the tube 1 to 2 cm, auscultate for bilateral breath sounds, and reinflate the cuff.
- When you've confirmed correct tube placement, administer oxygen or initiate mechanical ventilation and suction, if indicated. During CPR, deliver ventilations using a handheld resuscitation bag at a rate of one breath every 6 to 8 seconds.[6]
- Measure the distance from the edge of the lip or nose to the end of the tube and document the distance on the flow sheet or emergency sheet. If the tube has measurement markings on it, record the measurement where the tube exits at the lips or nose. *By periodically monitoring this mark, you can detect tube displacement.*[6]
- *To secure the tube,* apply skin preparation product to each cheek and let it dry. Tape the tube firmly with adhesive or other strong tape or use a commercial tube holder. (See *Methods to secure an ET tube.*)
- Make sure a chest X-ray is taken *to verify tube position.*[6]
- Place a swivel adapter between the tube and the humidified oxygen source *to allow for intermittent suctioning and to reduce tube tension.*
- Elevate the patient's head 30 to 45 degrees *to reduce the risk of ventilator-associated pneumonia.*[1,8]

Methods to secure an ET tube

An endotracheal (ET) tube should be secured with a tracheal tube holder for either the adult or infant patient, as recommended by The American Heart Association and American Pediatric Association. Alternatively, the tube may be taped in place *to prevent dislodgment.*

To secure the tube, use one of the following methods.

Method 1

An ET tube holder, available in hard plastic or of softer materials, is a convenient way to secure an ET tube in place. The tube holder is available in adult and pediatric sizes, and some models come with bite blocks attached. The strap is placed around the patient's neck and secured around the tube with Velcro fasteners. *Because each model is different,* check with the manufacturer's guidelines for correct placement and care.

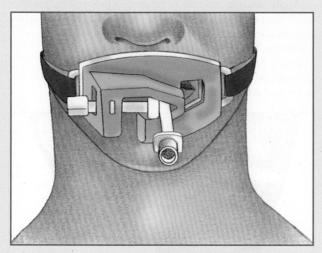

Method 2

Cut two 2″ (5-cm) strips and two 15″ (38-cm) strips of 1″ cloth adhesive tape. Then cut a 13″ (33-cm) slit in one end of each 15″ strip (as shown below). (Some facilities require the tape to encircle the patient's head; check your facility's policy and procedure manual.)

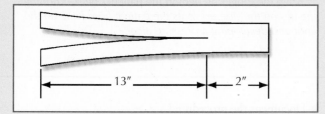

Apply compound benzoin tincture or other skin preparation product to the patient's cheeks. Place the 2″ strips on his cheeks, creating a new surface on which to anchor the tape securing the tube. *When frequent retaping is necessary, this step helps preserve the patient's skin integrity.* If the patient's skin is excoriated or at risk, you can use a transparent semipermeable dressing to protect the skin.

Apply the benzoin tincture or other skin preparation product to the part of the tube where you'll be applying the tape. On the side of the mouth where the tube will be anchored, place the unslit end of the long tape on top of the tape on the patient's cheek.

Wrap the top half of the tape around the tube twice, pulling the tape tightly around the tube. Then, directing the tape over the patient's upper lip, place the end of the tape on his other cheek. Cut off any excess tape. Use the lower half of the tape to secure an oral airway, if necessary (as shown below).

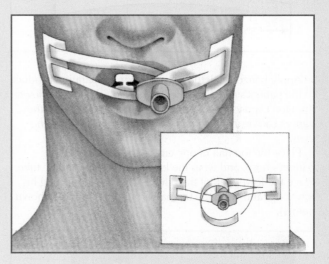

Alternatively, twist the lower half of the tape around the tube twice, and attach it to the original cheek. *Taping in opposite directions places equal traction on the tube.*

If you've taped in an oral airway or are concerned about the tube's stability, apply the other 15″ strip of tape in the same manner, starting on the other side of the patient's face (as shown below). If the tape around the tube is too bulky, use only the upper part of the tape and cut off the lower part. If the patient has copious oral secretions, seal the tape by cutting a 1″ piece of paper tape, coating it with benzoin tincture, and placing the paper tape over the adhesive tape.

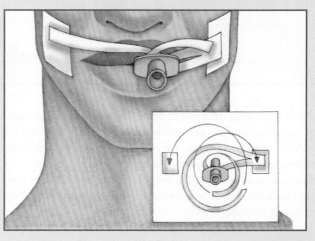

(continued)

Methods to secure an ET tube *(continued)*

Method 3

Cut one piece of 1″ cloth adhesive tape long enough to wrap around the patient's head and overlap in front. Then cut an 8″ (20-cm) piece of tape and center it on the longer piece, sticky sides together. Next, cut a 5″ (12.7-cm) slit in each end of the longer tape (as shown below).

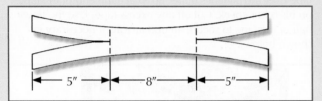

Apply benzoin tincture or other skin preparation product to the patient's cheeks, under his nose, and under his lower lip. Don't spray benzoin directly on his face *because the vapors can be irritating if inhaled and can also harm the eyes.*

Place the top half of one end of the tape under the patient's nose, and wrap the lower half around the ET tube. Place the lower half of the other end of the tape along his lower lip, and wrap the top half around the tube (as shown below).

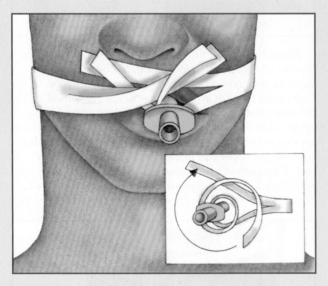

Method 4

Cut a tracheostomy tie in two pieces, one a few inches longer than the other, and cut two 6″ (15-cm) pieces of 1″ cloth adhesive tape. Then cut a 2″ slit in one end of both pieces of tape. Fold back the other end of the tape ½″ (1.3 cm) so that the sticky sides are together, and cut a small hole in it (as shown below).

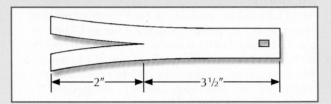

Apply benzoin tincture or other skin preparation product to the part of the ET tube that will be taped. Wrap the split ends of each piece of tape around the tube, one piece on each side. Overlap the tape to secure it.

Apply the free ends of the tape to both sides of the patient's face. Then insert tracheostomy ties through the holes in the tape and knot the ties (as shown below).

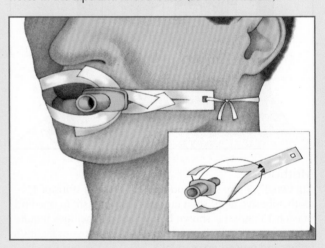

Bring the longer tie behind the patient's neck. *Knotting the ties on the side prevents the patient from lying on the knot and developing a pressure ulcer.*

■ Provide frequent nasal and oral care (use a chlorhexidine-based oral care solution daily, as prescribed), and reposition an oral ET tube daily *to prevent formation of pressure ulcers and to avoid excessive pressure on the sides of the mouth.*

■ Suction secretions through the ET tube as the patient's condition indicates *to clear secretions and to prevent mucus plugs from obstructing the tube.*

■ Remove and discard your gloves, remove other personal protective equipment, and perform hand hygiene.[3,4,5]

■ Document the procedure.[9]

Special considerations

■ Orotracheal intubation is preferred in emergencies *because insertion is easier and faster than it is with nasotracheal intubation.* However, maintaining exact tube placement is more difficult, and the tube must be well secured *to avoid kinking and to prevent bronchial obstruction or accidental extubation.*

Retrograde intubation: An alternative form of airway maintenance

When a patient's airway can't be secured using conventional oral or nasal intubation, retrograde intubation should be considered. In this technique, a wire is inserted through the trachea and out the mouth and is then used to guide the insertion of an endotracheal (ET) tube (as shown). Only doctors, nurses, and paramedics who've been specially trained may perform retrograde intubation.

The procedure has numerous advantages: It requires little or no head movement, it's less invasive than cricothyrotomy or tracheotomy and doesn't leave a permanent scar, and it doesn't require direct visualization of the vocal cords.

Retrograde intubation is contraindicated in patients with complete airway obstruction, thyroid tumor, enlarged thyroid gland that overlies the cricothyroid ligament, or coagulopathy as well as in those whose mouths can't open wide enough to allow the guide wire to be retrieved. Possible complications include minor bleeding and hematoma formation at the puncture site, subcutaneous emphysema, hoarseness, and bleeding into the trachea.

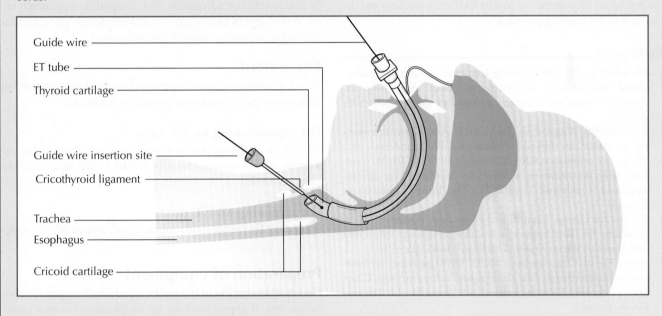

Guide wire
ET tube
Thyroid cartilage
Guide wire insertion site
Cricothyroid ligament
Trachea
Esophagus
Cricoid cartilage

■ Although low-pressure cuffs have significantly reduced the incidence of tracheal erosion and necrosis caused by cuff pressure on the tracheal wall, overinflation of a low-pressure cuff can negate the benefit. Use the minimal-leak technique to avoid these complications. Inflating the cuff a bit more to make a complete seal with the least amount of air is the next most desirable method.

■ Always record the volume of air needed to inflate the cuff. A gradual increase in this volume indicates tracheal dilatation or erosion. A sudden increase in volume indicates rupture of the cuff and requires immediate reintubation if the patient is being ventilated or if he requires continuous cuff inflation to maintain a high concentration of delivered oxygen. When the cuff has been inflated, measure its pressure at least every 8 hours to avoid overinflation. Normal cuff pressure is about 18 mm Hg.

■ If the patient requires mechanical ventilation, using a multidisciplinary approach, interrupt the patient's sedation daily and assess the patient's readiness to wean. *Doing so reduces the amount of time the patient spends on a ventilator and reduces the risk of ventilator-associated pneumonia.*[1,8]

■ If the patient requires mechanical ventilation, make sure he receives deep venous thrombosis prophylaxis (unless contraindicated), as prescribed, as well as peptic ulcer disease prophylaxis. *When combined with head-of-bed elevation, oral care, daily sedation interruption, and assessment of the readiness to wean, these measures reduce the incidence of ventilator-associated pneumonia.*[1,8]

■ When ET intubation isn't possible, consider the alternative of retrograde intubation. (See *Retrograde intubation: An alternative form of airway maintenance.*)

Patient teaching

Teach the patient and his family about home measures to prevent ventilator-associated pneumonia, including performing hand hygiene regularly and keeping the head of bed elevated 30 to 45 degrees.

Complications

ET intubation can result in apnea caused by reflex breath-holding or interruption of oxygen delivery; bronchospasm; aspiration of blood, secretions, or gastric contents; tooth damage or loss; and injury to the lips, mouth, pharynx, or vocal cords. It can also result in laryngeal edema and erosion and in tracheal stenosis, erosion, and necrosis. The patient is at risk for ventilator-associated pneumonia. Nasotracheal intubation can result in nasal bleeding, laceration, sinusitis, and otitis media.

Documentation

Record the date and time of the procedure; its indication and success or failure; tube type and size; cuff size and location in centimeters at the lip or nose, amount of inflation, and inflation technique; administration of medication; initiation of supplemental oxygen or ventilation therapy; results of physical and nonphysical examination techniques used to confirm tube placement; complications and nursing actions taken; and the patient's tolerance of the procedure. Document any patient and family teaching and the response to the teaching provided.

REFERENCES

1 Marschall, J. et al. (2008). Strategies to prevent central line-associated bloodstream infections in acute care hospitals. *Infection Control and Hospital Epidemiology, 29*(S1), S22–S30. (Level I)

2 Lynn-McHale Wiegand, D. (Ed.). (2011). *AACN procedure manual for critical care* (6th ed.). Philadelphia, PA: Saunders.

3 The Joint Commission. (2012). Standard NPSG.07.01.01. *Comprehensive accreditation manual for hospitals: The official handbook.* Oakbrook Terrace, IL: The Joint Commission. (Level I)

4 Centers for Disease Control and Prevention. (October 2002). Guideline for hand hygiene in health-care settings. *Morbidity and Mortality Weekly Report, 51*(RR-16), 1–45. (Level I)

5 World Health Organization. (2009). *WHO guidelines on hand hygiene in health care: First global patient safety challenge. Clean care is safer care.* Geneva, Switzerland: World Health Organization. (Level I)

6 American Heart Association. (2010). 2010 American Heart Association guidelines for cardiopulmonary resuscitation and emergency cardiovascular care. *Circulation, 122*(Suppl. 3), S729–S767. (Level I)

7 The Joint Commission. (2012). Standard NPSG.01.01.01. *Comprehensive accreditation manual for hospitals: The official handbook.* Oakbrook Terrace, IL: The Joint Commission. (Level I)

8 Institute for Healthcare Improvement. (2010). *5 million lives campaign getting started kit: Prevent ventilator-associated pneumonia how-to guide.* Cambridge, MA: Institute for Healthcare Improvement. (Level I)

9 The Joint Commission. (2012). Standard RC.01.03.01. *Comprehensive accreditation manual for hospitals: The official handbook.* Oakbrook Terrace, IL: The Joint Commission. (Level I)

ADDITIONAL REFERENCES

American Association of Critical-Care Nurses. (2008). "AACN Practice Alert: Ventilator Associated Pneumonia" [Online]. Accessed August 2011 via the Web at http://classic.aacn.org/AACN/practiceAlert.nsf/ Files/VAP/$file/Ventilator%20Associated%20Pneumonia%2011-2007.pdf

Nettina, S.M. (2010). *Lippincott manual of nursing practice* (9th ed.). Philadelphia, PA: Lippincott Williams & Wilkins.

ENDOTRACHEAL TUBE CARE

The intubated patient requires meticulous care to ensure airway patency and prevent complications. Care includes repositioning the endotracheal (ET) tube daily to prevent skin and mucosal injury and repositioning the ET tube if it becomes partially dislodged or a chest X-ray shows improper placement.

After a patient has been successfully weaned from mechanical ventilation, the ET tube is usually removed. The patient should be able to ventilate adequately, with acceptable oxygenation levels, and be able to clear secretions independently. The condition that led to intubation should also be resolved.

Equipment

10-mL syringe ■ suction equipment ■ handheld resuscitation bag with mask ■ gloves ■ personal protective equipment.

For repositioning an ET tube

Washcloth ■ skin preparation ■ stethoscope ■ adhesive or hypoallergenic tape or commercial tube holder ■ sedative or 2% lidocaine, as needed.

For removing an ET tube

Equipment for reintubation ■ supplemental oxygen delivery equipment.

Preparation of equipment

Gather all equipment at the patient's bedside. Set up the suction equipment. If appropriate, set up supplemental oxygen equipment. Have a handheld resuscitation bag with a mask available.

Implementation

■ Explain the procedure to the patient and provide privacy.
■ Perform hand hygiene and put on gloves and personal protective equipment.[1,2,3]
■ Confirm the patient's identity using at least two patient identifiers according to your facility's policy.[4]

For repositioning an ET tube

■ Obtain assistance from a respiratory therapist or another nurse *to prevent accidental extubation during the procedure if the patient coughs.*
■ Suction the patient's trachea through the ET tube *to remove any secretions, which can cause the patient to cough during the procedure. Coughing increases the risk of trauma and tube dislodgment.* Then suction the patient's pharynx *to remove any secretions that may have accumulated above the tube cuff, which helps to prevent aspiration of secretions during cuff deflation.*[5,6]

■ *To prevent traumatic manipulation of the tube,* instruct the assisting nurse to hold the tube as you carefully untape it or unfasten the commercial tube holder (as shown below). When freeing the tube, locate a landmark, such as a number on the tube, or measure the distance from the patient's mouth to the top of the tube *so that you have a reference point when moving the tube.*[5]

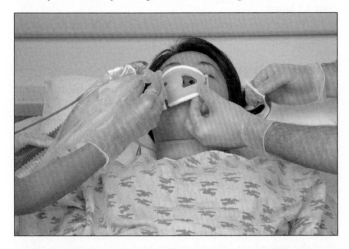

■ Next, deflate the cuff by attaching a 10-mL syringe to the pilot balloon port and aspirating air until you meet resistance and the pilot balloon deflates. Deflate the cuff before moving the tube (as shown below) *because the cuff forms a seal within the trachea and movement of an inflated cuff can damage the tracheal wall and vocal cords.*

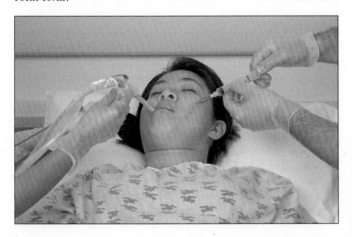

■ Reposition the tube, as necessary, noting new landmarks or measuring the length. Then immediately reinflate the cuff. To do this, instruct the patient to inhale (if appropriate), and slowly inflate the cuff using a 10-mL syringe attached to the pilot balloon port. As you do this, use your stethoscope to auscultate the patient's neck *to determine the presence of an air leak.* When air leakage ceases, stop cuff inflation and, while still auscultating the patient's neck, aspirate a small amount of air until you detect a slight leak (as shown at top of next column). *This maneuver creates a minimal air leak, which indicates that the cuff is inflated at the lowest pressure possible to create an adequate seal.* If the patient is being mechanically ventilated, aspirate to create a minimal air leak during the inspiratory phase of respiration *because the positive*

pressure of the ventilator during inspiration will create a larger leak around the cuff.[5] Note the number of cubic centimeters of air required to achieve a minimal air leak.

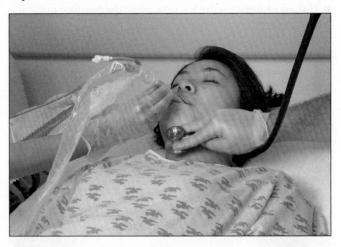

■ Measure cuff pressure, and compare the reading with previous pressure readings *to prevent overinflation.*
■ Wash around the patient's mouth with the wash cloth *to remove any crusting and provide comfort.* Assess the skin and mouth for any breakdown.
■ Apply skin preparation and tape to secure the tube in place, or attach a commercial tube holder.
■ Obtain a chest X-ray for tube position verification, if appropriate.

For removing an ET tube
■ Verify the doctor's order.
■ Obtain assistance from a respiratory therapist or another nurse *to prevent traumatic manipulation of the tube when it's untaped or unfastened.*
■ Position the patient in semi-Fowler's position (as shown below).

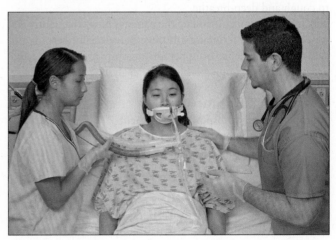

■ Suction the ET tube and the patient's oropharynx *to remove any accumulated secretions and to help prevent aspiration of secretions when the cuff is deflated.*[5,6]

■ Using a handheld resuscitation bag or the mechanical ventilator, give the patient several deep breaths through the ET tube *to hyperinflate the lungs and increase oxygen reserve.*[5,6]

■ Untape or unfasten the ET tube while the assisting nurse stabilizes the tube.

■ Attach a 10-mL syringe to the pilot balloon port, and aspirate air until you meet resistance and the pilot balloon deflates. If you fail to detect an air leak around the deflated cuff, notify the doctor immediately and don't proceed with extubation. *Absence of an air leak may indicate marked tracheal edema, which can result in total airway obstruction if the ET tube is removed.*[5]

■ Instruct the patient to take a deep breath. At the peak of inspiration remove the ET tube, following the natural curve of the patient's mouth (as shown below).

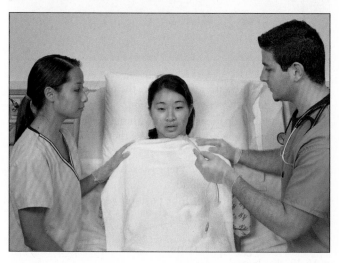

■ Give the patient supplemental humidified oxygen *to promote oxygenation and help decrease airway irritation, patient discomfort, and laryngeal edema.*

■ Suction the oropharynx, if needed, and encourage the patient to cough and deep-breathe.

■ After extubation, auscultate the patient's lungs frequently and watch for signs of respiratory distress. Be especially alert for stridor or other evidence of upper airway obstruction. If ordered, draw an arterial sample for blood gas analysis.[5]

Completing the procedure

■ Properly clean or dispose of equipment.

■ Remove and dispose of personal protective equipment and perform hand hygiene.[1,2,3]

■ Document the procedure.[7]

Special considerations

■ When repositioning an ET tube, be especially careful in patients with highly sensitive airways. Sedation or direct instillation of 2% lidocaine *to numb the airway* may be indicated in such patients. *Because lidocaine is absorbed systemically,* you must have a doctor's order to use it.

■ If you inadvertently cut the pilot balloon on the cuff, immediately call the person responsible for intubation in your facility, who will remove the damaged ET tube and replace it with one that's

intact. Don't remove the tube *because a tube with an air leak is better than no airway.*

■ Measure cuff pressure at least every 8 hours *to avoid overinflation.*[6] (See "Tracheal cuff pressure measurement," page 708.)

■ After extubation of a patient who has been intubated for an extended time, keep reintubation supplies readily available for at least 12 hours.

■ Never extubate a patient unless someone skilled at intubation is readily available.

Complications

Traumatic injury to the larynx or trachea may result from tube manipulation, accidental extubation, or tube slippage into the right bronchus. Ventilatory failure and airway obstruction, from laryngospasm or marked tracheal edema, are the gravest possible complications of extubation.

Documentation

After tube repositioning, record the date and time of the procedure, reason for repositioning (such as malpositioning shown by chest X-ray), new tube position, total amount of air in the cuff after the procedure, complications and nursing actions taken, and the patient's tolerance of the procedure.

After extubation, record the date and time of extubation, presence or absence of stridor or other signs of upper airway edema, type of supplemental oxygen administered, complications and required subsequent therapy, and the patient's tolerance of the procedure.

REFERENCES

1 The Joint Commission. (2012). Standard NPSG.07.01.01. *Comprehensive accreditation manual for hospitals: The official handbook.* Oakbrook Terrace, IL: The Joint Commission. (Level I)

2 Centers for Disease Control and Prevention. (October 2002). Guideline for hand hygiene in health-care settings. *Morbidity and Mortality Weekly Report, 51*(RR-16), 1–45. (Level I)

3 World Health Organization. (2009). *WHO guidelines on hand hygiene in health care: First global patient safety challenge. Clean care is safer care.* Geneva, Switzerland: World Health Organization. (Level I)

4 The Joint Commission. (2012). Standard NPSG.01.01.01. *Comprehensive accreditation manual for hospitals: The official handbook.* Oakbrook Terrace, IL: The Joint Commission. (Level I)

5 American Association for Respiratory Care. (2007). AARC clinical practice guideline: Removal of the endotracheal tube—2007 revision and update. *Respiratory Care, 52*(1), 81–93. (Level I)

6 American Association of Critical-Care Nurses. (2008). "AACN Practice Alert: Ventilator Associated Pneumonia" [Online]. Accessed August 2011 via the Web at http://classic.aacn.org/ AACN/practiceAlert.nsf/Files/VAP/$file/Ventilator%20Associated%20Pneumonia%2011-2007.pdf (Level I)

7 The Joint Commission. (2012). Standard RC.01.03.01. *Comprehensive accreditation manual for hospitals: The official handbook.* Oakbrook Terrace, IL: The Joint Commission. (Level I)

ADDITIONAL REFERENCES

Lynn-McHale Wiegand, D. (Ed.). (2011). *AACN procedure manual for critical care* (6th ed.). Philadelphia, PA: Saunders.

Nettina, S.M. (2010). *Lippincott manual of nursing practice* (9th ed.). Philadelphia, PA: Lippincott Williams & Wilkins.

END-TIDAL CARBON DIOXIDE MONITORING

End-tidal carbon dioxide ($ETCO_2$) determines the carbon dioxide (CO_2) concentration in exhaled gas to provide information about a patient's pulmonary, cardiac, and metabolic status. Such information aids patient management and helps prevent clinical compromise.

In $ETCO_2$ monitoring, a photodetector measures the amount of infrared light absorbed by airway gas during inspiration and expiration. (Light absorption increases along with the CO_2 concentration.) A monitor converts these data to a CO_2 value and a corresponding waveform, or capnogram, if capnography is used. (See *How $ETCO_2$ monitoring works*.) The sensor is positioned at one of two sites in the monitoring setup. With a mainstream monitor, it's positioned directly at the patient's airway with an airway adapter, between the endotracheal (ET) tube and the breathing circuit tubing. With a sidestream monitor, the airway adapter is positioned at the airway (regardless of whether or not the patient is intubated) to allow aspiration of gas from the patient's airway back to the sensor, which lies either within or close to the monitor.

Some CO_2 detection devices provide semiquantitative indications of CO_2 concentrations, supplying an approximate range rather than a specific value for $ETCO_2$. Other devices simply indicate whether CO_2 is present during exhalation. (See *Analyzing CO_2 levels*, page 270.)

The 2010 American Heart Association guidelines for cardiopulmonary resuscitation and emergency cardiovascular care recommend $ETCO_2$ monitoring in combination with clinical assessment to confirm initial ET tube placement in the patient in cardiac arrest when continuous quantitative waveform capnography isn't available.[1]

$ETCO_2$ monitoring has become standard during anesthesia administration, such as in patients who are undergoing moderate sedation. It may also be used in those receiving epidural or patient-controlled analgesia for pain control. The $ETCO_2$ measurements can alert the nurse to hypoventilation from oversedation.[2]

When $ETCO_2$ is detected during cardiac arrest, it's a good indicator that the ET tube is properly placed in the trachea. However, such conditions as pulmonary embolus, pulmonary edema, status asthmaticus, or gastric content contamination of the $ETCO_2$ detector may produce false results. Therefore, if CO_2 isn't detected, a second method should be used to confirm ET tube placement, such as direct visualization or use of an esophageal detector device.[1]

Equipment

Gloves ▪ mainstream or sidestream CO_2 monitor ▪ CO_2 sensor ▪ airway adapter, as recommended by the manufacturer (a neona-

How $ETCO_2$ monitoring works

The optical portion of an end-tidal carbon dioxide ($ETCO_2$) monitor contains an infrared light source, a sample chamber, a special carbon dioxide (CO_2) filter, and a photodetector. The infrared light passes through the sample chamber and is absorbed in varying amounts, depending on the amount of CO_2 the patient has just exhaled. The photodetector measures CO_2 content and relays this information to the microprocessor in the monitor, which displays the CO_2 value and waveform.

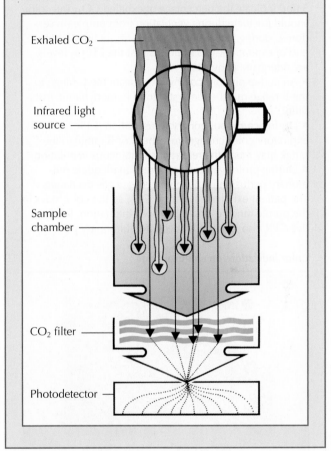

Exhaled CO_2

Infrared light source

Sample chamber

CO_2 filter

Photodetector

tal adapter may have a much smaller dead space, making it appropriate for a smaller patient) ▪ $ETCO_2$ sensor.

Preparation of equipment

If the monitor you're using isn't self-calibrating, calibrate it as the manufacturer directs. If you're using a sidestream CO_2 monitor, be sure to replace the water trap between patients, if directed. *The trap allows humidity from exhaled gases to be condensed into an attached container.* Newer sidestream models don't require water traps.

Implementation

▪ Verify the doctor's order, if appropriate.

EQUIPMENT

Analyzing CO₂ levels

Depending on which end-tidal carbon dioxide (ETCO₂) detector you use, the meaning of color changes within the detector dome may differ from the analysis for the Easy Cap detector described below.

■ The rim of the Easy Cap is divided into four segments (clockwise from the top): CHECK, A, B, and C. The CHECK segment is solid purple, signifying the absence of carbon dioxide (CO₂).

■ The numbers in the other sections range from 0.03 to 5 and indicate the percentage of exhaled CO₂. The color should fluctuate during ventilation from purple (in section A) during inspiration to yellow (in section C) at the end of expiration. This indicates that the ETCO₂ levels are adequate: above 2%.

■ An end-expiratory color change from the C range to the B range may be the first sign of hemodynamic instability.

■ During cardiopulmonary resuscitation (CPR), an end-expiratory color change from the A or B range to the C range may mean the return of spontaneous ventilation.

■ During prolonged cardiac arrest, inadequate pulmonary perfusion leads to inadequate gas exchange. The patient exhales little or no CO₂, so the color stays in the purple range even with proper intubation. Ineffective CPR also leads to inadequate pulmonary perfusion.

Color indications on end-expiration

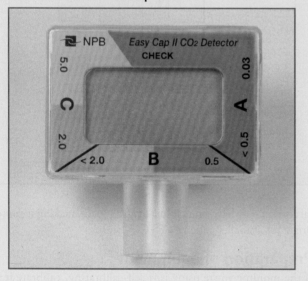

■ Confirm the patient's identity using at least two patient identifiers according to your facility's policy.[3]

■ If the patient requires ET intubation, an ETCO₂ detector or monitor is usually applied immediately after the tube is inserted. If he doesn't require intubation or is already intubated and alert, explain the purpose and expected duration of monitoring. Tell the patient that the monitor will painlessly measure the amount of

CO₂ he exhales and track his CO₂ concentration to make sure his breathing is effective.

■ Perform hand hygiene and put on gloves *to prevent cross-contamination.*[4,5,6]

■ After turning on the monitor and calibrating it (if necessary), position the airway adapter and sensor as the manufacturer directs. For an intubated patient, position the adapter directly on the ET tube. For a nonintubated patient, place the adapter at or near the patient's airway.

■ Turn on all alarms and adjust alarm settings as appropriate for your patient. Make sure the alarm volume is loud enough to hear.

■ Remove and discard your gloves and perform hand hygiene.[4,5,6]

■ Document the procedure.[7]

Special considerations

■ Make sure the adapter is changed with every breathing circuit and ET tube change.

■ Place the adapter on the ET tube *to avoid contaminating exhaled gases with fresh gas flow from the ventilator.* If you're using a heat and moisture exchanger, you may be able to position the airway adapter between the exchanger and breathing circuit.

■ If your patient's ETCO₂ values differ from his partial pressure of arterial carbon dioxide, assess him for factors that can influence ETCO₂—especially when the differential between arterial and ETCO₂ values (the arterial absolute difference of carbon dioxide [a-ADCO₂]) is above normal.

■ The a-ADCO₂ value, if correctly interpreted, provides useful information about your patient's status. For example, an increased a-ADCO₂ may mean that your patient has worsening dead space, especially if his tidal volume remains constant.

■ Remember that ETCO₂ monitoring doesn't replace arterial blood gas (ABG) measurements *because it doesn't assess oxygenation or blood pH.* Supplementing ETCO₂ monitoring with pulse oximetry may provide more complete information.

■ If the CO₂ waveform is available, assess it for height, frequency, rhythm, baseline, and shape *to help evaluate gas exchange.* Make sure you know how to recognize a normal waveform and can identify any abnormal waveforms in the patient's medical record. (See *CO₂ waveform.*)

■ In a nonintubated patient, use ETCO₂ values to establish trends. Be aware that in such a patient, exhaled gas is more likely to mix with ambient air, and exhaled CO₂ may be diluted by fresh gas flow from the nasal cannula.

■ ETCO₂ monitoring commonly is discontinued when the patient has been weaned effectively from mechanical ventilation or when he's no longer at risk for respiratory compromise. Carefully assess your patient's tolerance for weaning. After extubation, continuous ETCO₂ monitoring may detect the need for reintubation.

■ Disposable ETCO₂ detectors are available. When using a disposable ETCO₂ detector, always check its color under fluorescent or natural light *because the dome looks pink under incandescent light.* (See *Using a disposable ETCO₂ detector: Some do's and don'ts,* page 272.)

Complications

Inaccurate measurements, such as from poor sampling technique, calibration drift, contamination of optics with moisture or

CO$_2$ waveform

The carbon dioxide (CO$_2$) waveform, or capnogram, produced in end-tidal carbon dioxide (ETCO$_2$) monitoring reflects the course of CO$_2$ elimination during exhalation. A normal capnogram (shown below) consists of several segments, which reflect the various stages of exhalation and inhalation.

Normally, any gas eliminated from the airway during early exhalation is dead-space gas, which hasn't undergone exchange at the alveolocapillary membrane. Measurements taken during this period contain no CO$_2$.

As exhalation continues, CO$_2$ concentration rises sharply and rapidly. The sensor now detects gas that has undergone exchange, producing measurable quantities of CO$_2$.

The final stages of alveolar emptying occur during late exhalation. During the alveolar plateau phase, CO$_2$ concentration rises more gradually because alveolar emptying is more constant.

The point at which the ETCO$_2$ value is derived is the end of exhalation, when CO$_2$ concentration peaks. Unless an alveolar plateau is present, this value doesn't accurately estimate alveolar CO$_2$. During inhalation, the CO$_2$ concentration declines sharply to zero.

Continuous waveform capnography, combined with clinical assessment, is the most reliable method for confirming and monitoring correct ET tube placement. Continuous quantitative waveform capnography can help monitor the quality of cardiopulmonary resuscitation in an intubated patient and help detect fatigue in the person performing chest compressions.[1]

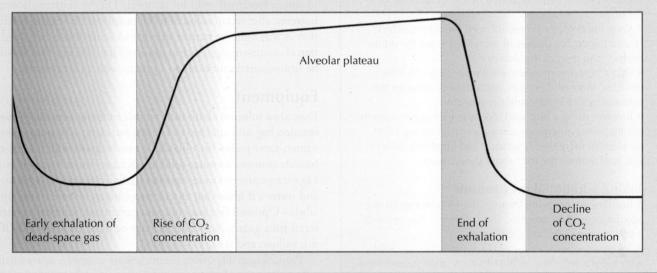

Alveolar plateau

Early exhalation of dead-space gas

Rise of CO$_2$ concentration

End of exhalation

Decline of CO$_2$ concentration

---

secretions, or equipment malfunction, can lead to misdiagnosis and improper treatment.

The effects of manual resuscitation or ingestion of alcohol or carbonated beverages can alter the detector's findings. Color changes detected after fewer than six ventilations can be misleading.[1]

Documentation

Document the initial ETCO$_2$ value and all ventilator settings. Describe the waveform if one appears on the monitor. If the monitor has a printer, you may want to print out a sample waveform and include it in the patient's medical record.

Document ETCO$_2$ values at least as often as vital signs, whenever significant changes in waveform or patient status occur, and before and after weaning, respiratory procedures, and other interventions. Periodically obtain samples for ABG analysis as the patient's condition dictates, and document the corresponding ETCO$_2$ values.

REFERENCES

1 American Heart Association. (2010). 2010 American Heart Association guidelines for cardiopulmonary resuscitation and emergency cardiovascular care. *Circulation, 122*(Suppl. 3), S729–S767. (Level I)

2 Deitch, K., et al. (2010). Does end tidal CO2 monitoring during emergency department procedural sedation and analgesia with propofol decrease the incidence of hypoxic events? A randomized, controlled trial. *Annals of Emergency Medicine, 55*(3), 258–264. (Level II)

3 The Joint Commission. (2012). Standard NPSG.01.01.01. *Comprehensive accreditation manual for hospitals: The official handbook.* Oakbrook Terrace, IL: The Joint Commission. (Level I)

4 The Joint Commission. (2012). Standard NPSG.07.01.01. *Comprehensive accreditation manual for hospitals: The official handbook.* Oakbrook Terrace, IL: The Joint Commission. (Level I)

5 Centers for Disease Control and Prevention. (October 2002). Guideline for hand hygiene in health-care settings. *Morbidity and Mortality Weekly Report, 51*(RR-16), 1–45. (Level I)

Using a disposable ETCO$_2$ detector: Some do's and don'ts

When using a disposable end-tidal carbon dioxide (ETCO$_2$) detector, check the instructions and ensure ideal working conditions for the device. Here are some additional guidelines.

Avoiding high humidity, moisture, and heat

▪ Watch for changes indicating that the ETCO$_2$ detector's life span is decreasing—for example, sluggish color changes from breath to breath. A detector may be used for about 2 hours. However, using it with a ventilator that delivers high-humidity ventilation may shorten its usefulness to no more than 15 minutes.

▪ Don't use the detector with a heated humidifier or a nebulizer.

▪ Keep the detector protected from secretions, which render the device useless. If secretions enter the dome, remove and discard the detector.

▪ Use a heat and moisture exchanger to protect the detector. In some detectors, this filter fits between the endotracheal (ET) tube and the detector.

▪ If you're using a heat and moisture exchanger, remember that it may increase your patient's breathing effort. Be alert for increased resistance and breathing difficulties, and remove the exchanger if necessary.

Taking additional precautions

▪ Instilling epinephrine through the ET tube can damage the detector's indicator (the color may stay yellow). If this happens, discard the device.

▪ Take care when using an ETCO$_2$ detector in a child who weighs less than 30 lb (14 kg). A small patient who rebreathes air from the dead air space (about 38 mL) will inhale too much of his own carbon dioxide.

▪ Frequently spot-check the ETCO$_2$ detector you're using for effectiveness. If you must transport the patient to another area for testing or treatment, use another method to verify the tube's placement.

▪ Never reuse a disposable ETCO$_2$ detector. It's intended for one-time, one-patient use only.

6 World Health Organization. (2009). *WHO guidelines on hand hygiene in health care: First global patient safety challenge. Clean care is safer care.* Geneva, Switzerland: World Health Organization. (Level I)

7 The Joint Commission. (2012). Standard RC.01.03.01. *Comprehensive accreditation manual for hospitals: The official handbook.* Oakbrook Terrace, IL: The Joint Commission. (Level I)

ADDITIONAL REFERENCES

Lynn-McHale Wiegand, D. (Ed.). (2011). *AACN procedure manual for critical care* (6th ed.). Philadelphia, PA: Saunders.

Nagler, J., & Krauss, B. (2008). Capnography: A valuable tool for airway management. *Emergency Medical Clinics of North America, 26*(4), 881–897.

ENEMA ADMINISTRATION

Enema administration involves instilling a solution into the rectum and colon. In a retention enema, the patient holds the solution within the rectum or colon for 30 minutes to 1 hour. With a cleansing enema, the patient expels the solution almost completely within 15 minutes. Both types of enema stimulate peristalsis by mechanically distending the colon and stimulating rectal wall nerves.

Enemas are used to clean the lower bowel in preparation for diagnostic or surgical procedures; to relieve distention and promote expulsion of flatus; to lubricate the rectum and colon; and to soften hardened stool for removal. They're contraindicated, however, after recent colon or rectal surgery or myocardial infarction as well as in the patient who has an acute abdominal condition of unknown origin such as suspected appendicitis. They should be administered cautiously to a patient with an arrhythmia.

Equipment

Prescribed solution ▪ bath (utility) thermometer ▪ enema administration bag with attached rectal tube and clamp ▪ IV pole ▪ gloves ▪ linen-saver pads ▪ bath blanket ▪ two bedpans with covers, or bedside commode ▪ water-soluble lubricant ▪ toilet tissue ▪ plastic bag for equipment ▪ water ▪ gown ▪ stethoscope ▪ washcloth ▪ soap and water ▪ if observing enteric precautions: plastic trash bags, labels ▪ Optional (for patients who can't retain solution): plastic rectal tube guard, indwelling urinary or rectal catheter with 30-mL balloon and syringe.

Prepackaged disposable enema sets are available, as are small-volume enema solutions in both irrigating and retention types and in pediatric sizes.

Preparation of equipment

Prepare the prescribed type and amount of solution, as indicated. (See *Commonly used enema solutions.*) Standard irrigating enema volume is 750 to 1,000 mL for an adult.

PEDIATRIC ALERT *Standard irrigating enema volumes for pediatric patients are 500 to 750 mL for a school-age child; 250 to 500 mL for a toddler or preschooler; and 250 mL or less for an infant.*

Because some ingredients may be mucosal irritants, make sure the proportions are correct and the agents are thoroughly mixed *to avoid localized irritation.* Warm the solution *to reduce patient discomfort.* Administer an adult's enema at 105° to 110° F (41° to 43° C). Check the temperature with a bath thermometer.

PEDIATRIC ALERT *Administer a child's enema at 100° F (38° C) to avoid burning rectal tissues.*

Clamp the tubing and fill the solution bag with the prescribed solution. Unclamp the tubing, flush the solution through the tubing, and then reclamp it. *Flushing detects leaks and removes air, which could cause discomfort if introduced into the colon.*

Commonly used enema solutions

SOLUTION	AMOUNT	ACTION	TIME TO TAKE EFFECT	ADVERSE EFFECTS
Tap water (hypotonic)	500 to 1,000 mL	■ Distends intestine ■ Increases peristalsis ■ Softens stool	15 min	Fluid and electrolyte imbalance, water intoxication
Normal saline solution (isotonic)	500 to 1,000 mL	■ Distends intestine ■ Increases peristalsis ■ Softens stool	15 min	Fluid and electrolyte imbalance, sodium retention
Soap	500 to 1,000 mL (concentrate at 3 to 5 mL/ 1,000 mL of tap water)	■ Distends intestine ■ Irritates intestinal mucosa ■ Softens stool	10 to 15 min	Rectal mucosa irritation or damage
Hypertonic solution	70 to 130 mL	■ Distends intestine ■ Irritates intestinal mucosa	5 to 10 min	Sodium retention
Oil (mineral, olive, or cottonseed oil)	150 to 200 mL	■ Lubricates stool and intestinal mucosa	30 min	Rectal mucosa irritation

Hang the solution container on the IV pole and take all supplies to the patient's room. If you're using an indwelling urinary or rectal catheter, fill the syringe with 30 mL of water.

Implementation

■ Verify the doctor's order.
■ Confirm the patient's identity using at least two patient identifiers according to your facility's policy.[1]
■ Perform hand hygiene and put on gloves.[2,3,4]
■ Assess the patient, paying special attention to his abdomen. Auscultate for bowel sounds; a cleansing enema will increase peristalsis.
■ Provide privacy and explain the procedure. If you're administering an enema to a child, familiarize him with the equipment and allow a parent, another relative, or guardian to remain with him during the procedure *to provide reassurance.*
■ Ask the patient if he's had previous difficulty retaining an enema *to determine whether you need to use a rectal tube guard or a catheter.*
■ Assist the patient as necessary in putting on a hospital gown. *The gown makes enema administration easier, and the patient worries less about soiling it.*
■ Assist the patient into the left-lateral Sims' position. *This position will facilitate the solution's flow by gravity into the descending colon.* If contraindicated or if the patient reports discomfort, reposition him on his back or right side.
■ Place linen-saver pads under the patient's buttocks *to prevent soiling the linens.* Replace the top bed linens with a bath blanket *to provide privacy and warmth.*
■ Have a bedpan or commode nearby for the patient to use. If the patient may use the bathroom, make sure it will be available

when the patient needs it. Have toilet tissue within the patient's reach.
■ Lubricate the distal tip of the rectal tube with water-soluble lubricant *to facilitate rectal insertion and reduce irritation.*
■ Separate the patient's buttocks and touch the anal sphincter with the rectal tube *to stimulate contraction.* Then, as the sphincter relaxes, tell the patient to breathe deeply through the mouth as you gently advance the tube.
■ Advance the tube 2″ to 4″ (5 to 10 cm), aiming it toward the umbilicus. Avoid forcing the tube *to prevent rectal wall trauma.* If it doesn't advance easily, allow a little solution to flow in *to relax the inner sphincter enough to allow passage* (as shown below).

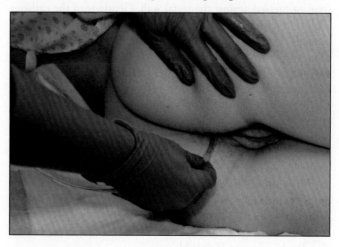

PEDIATRIC ALERT *For a child, insert the tube only 2″ to 3″ (5 to 7.5 cm); for an infant, insert it only 1″ to 1¹/₂″ (2.5 to 3.5 cm).*

■ If the patient feels pain or the tube meets continued resistance, notify the doctor. *These issues may signal an unknown stricture or abscess.* If the patient has poor sphincter control, use a plastic rectal tube guard.

■ If you're using an indwelling urinary or rectal catheter (as permitted by your facility's policy), insert the lubricated catheter as you would a rectal tube. Then gently inflate the catheter's balloon with 20 to 30 mL of water. Gently pull the catheter back against the patient's internal anal sphincter *to seal off the rectum.* If leakage still occurs with the balloon in place, add more water to the balloon in small amounts. When using either catheter, avoid inflating the balloon above 45 mL *because overinflation can compromise blood flow to the rectal tissues and cause possible necrosis from pressure on the rectal mucosa.*

■ If you're using a rectal tube, hold it in place throughout the procedure *because bowel contractions and the pressure of the tube against the anal sphincter can promote tube displacement.*

■ Hold the solution container slightly above bed level and release the tubing clamp. Then raise the container gradually to start the flow, usually at a rate of 75 to 100 mL/minute for an irrigating enema, but at the slowest possible rate for a retention enema *to avoid stimulating peristalsis and to promote retention.* Adjust the flow rate of an irrigating enema by raising or lowering the solution container according to the patient's retention ability and comfort. However, don't raise it higher than 18″ (46 cm) for an adult, 12″ (31 cm) for a child, and 8″ (20 cm) for an infant *because excessive pressure can force colon bacteria into the small intestine or rupture the colon.*

■ Assess the patient's tolerance frequently during instillation. If he complains of discomfort, cramps, or the need to defecate, stop the flow by pinching or clamping the tubing. Then hold the patient's buttocks together. Instruct him to gently massage his abdomen and breathe slowly and deeply through his mouth *to help relax abdominal muscles and promote retention.* Resume administration at a slower flow rate after a few minutes when discomfort passes, but interrupt the flow any time the patient feels uncomfortable.

■ If the flow slows or stops, the catheter tip may be clogged with feces or pressed against the rectal wall. Gently turn the catheter slightly *to free it without stimulating defecation.* If the catheter tip remains clogged, withdraw the catheter, flush it with solution, and reinsert it.

■ After administering most of the prescribed amount of solution, clamp the tubing. Stop the flow before the container empties completely *to avoid introducing air into the bowel.*

■ For a flush enema, stop the flow by lowering the solution container below bed level and allowing gravity to siphon the enema from the colon. Continue to raise and lower the container until gas bubbles cease or the patient feels more comfortable and abdominal distention subsides. Don't allow the solution container to empty completely before lowering it *because this may introduce air into the bowel.*

■ For a cleansing enema, instruct the patient to retain the solution for 15 minutes, if possible.

■ For a retention enema, instruct the patient not to defecate for the prescribed time or as follows: 30 minutes or longer for oil retention, and 15 to 30 minutes for an anthelmintic or emollient enema. If you're using an indwelling catheter, leave the catheter in place *to promote retention.*

■ If the patient is apprehensive, position him on the bedpan and allow him to hold toilet tissue or a rolled washcloth against his anus. Place the call signal within his reach. If he'll be using the bathroom or the commode, instruct him to call for help before attempting to get out of bed *because the procedure may make the patient, particularly an elderly patient, feel weak or faint.* Also instruct him to call you if he feels weak at any time.

■ When the solution has remained in the colon for the recommended time or for as long as the patient can tolerate it, assist the patient onto a bedpan or to the commode or bathroom, as required.

■ If an indwelling catheter is in place, deflate the balloon and remove the catheter, if applicable.

■ Provide privacy while the patient expels the solution. Instruct the patient not to flush the toilet.

■ While the patient uses the bathroom, remove and discard any soiled linen and linen-saver pads.

■ Assist the patient with cleaning, if necessary, and help him to bed. Make sure he feels clean and comfortable and can easily reach the call signal. Place a clean linen-saver pad under him *to absorb rectal drainage,* and tell him that he may need to expel additional stool or flatus later. Encourage him to rest *because the procedure may be tiring.*

■ Cover the bedpan or commode and take it to the utility room for observation, or observe the contents of the toilet, as applicable. Carefully note fecal color, consistency, amount (minimal, moderate, or generous), and foreign matter, such as blood, rectal tissue, worms, pus, mucus, or other unusual matter.

■ Send specimens to the laboratory, if ordered.

■ Rinse the bedpan or commode with cold water, and then wash it in hot, soapy water. Return it to the patient's bedside.

■ Properly dispose of the enema equipment. If additional enemas are scheduled, store clean, reusable equipment in a closed plastic bag in the patient's bathroom.

■ Discard your gloves and perform hand hygiene.[2,3,4]

■ Ventilate the room or use an air freshener, if necessary.

■ Document the procedure.[5]

Special considerations

■ *Because patients with salt-retention disorders, such as heart failure, may absorb sodium from the saline enema solution,* administer the solution to such patients cautiously and monitor electrolyte status.

■ Schedule a retention enema before meals *because a full stomach may stimulate peristalsis and make retention difficult.* Follow an oil-retention enema with a soap-and-water enema 1 hour later *to help expel the softened feces completely.*

■ Administer less solution when giving a hypertonic enema *because osmotic pull moves fluid into the colon from body tissues, increasing the volume of colon contents.* Alternative means of instilling the solution include using a bulb syringe or a funnel with the rectal tube.

■ For the patient who can't tolerate a flat position (for example, a patient with shortness of breath), administer the enema with the head of the bed in the lowest position he can safely and comfortably maintain. For a bedridden patient who needs to expel the enema into a bedpan, raise the head of the bed to approximate a sitting or squatting position. Don't give an enema to a patient who's in a sitting position, unless absolutely necessary, *because the solution won't flow high enough into the colon and will only distend the rectum and trigger rapid expulsion.*

■ If the patient has hemorrhoids, instruct him to bear down gently during tube insertion. *This action causes the anus to open and facilitates insertion.*

■ If the patient fails to expel the solution within 1 hour because of diminished neuromuscular response, you may need to remove the enema solution. First, review your facility's policy *because you may need a doctor's order.* Inform the doctor when a patient can't expel an enema spontaneously because of possible bowel perforation or electrolyte imbalance. To siphon the enema solution from the patient's rectum, assist him to a side-lying position on the bed. Place a bedpan on a bedside chair so it rests below mattress level. Disconnect the tubing from the solution container, place the distal end in the bedpan, and reinsert the rectal end into the patient's anus. If gravity fails to drain the solution into the bedpan, instill 30 to 50 mL of warm water through the tube (105° F [41° C] for an adult patient; 100° F [38° C] for a child or infant). Then quickly direct the distal end of the tube into the bedpan. In both cases, measure the return *to make sure all of the solution has drained.*

■ For patients with fluid and electrolyte disturbances, measure the amount of expelled solution *to assess for retention of enema fluid.*

■ Double-bag all enema equipment and label it as isolation equipment if the patient is on enteric precautions.

■ If the doctor orders enemas until returns are clear, give no more than three *to avoid excessive irritation of the rectal mucosa.* Notify the doctor if the returned fluid isn't clear after three administrations.

■ To administer a commercially prepared, small-volume enema, first remove the cap from the rectal tube. Insert the rectal tube into the rectum and squeeze the bottle *to deposit the contents in the rectum.* Remove the rectal tube, replace the used enema unit in its original container, and discard.

Patient teaching

If the patient will have to repeat the enema at home, describe the procedure to the patient and his family. Emphasize that administering an enema to a person in a sitting position or on the toilet could injure the rectal wall. Tell the patient how to prepare and care for the equipment. Discuss relaxation techniques, and review measures for preventing constipation, including regular exercise, dietary modifications, and adequate fluid intake.

Complications

Enemas may produce dizziness or faintness, excessive irritation of the colonic mucosa resulting from repeated administration or from sensitivity to the enema ingredients, hyponatremia or hypokalemia from repeated administration of hypotonic solutions,

and cardiac arrhythmias resulting from vasovagal reflex stimulation after insertion of the rectal catheter. Colonic water absorption may result from prolonged retention of hypotonic solutions, which may, in turn, cause hypervolemia or water intoxication.

Documentation

Record the date and time of enema administration; special equipment used; type and amount of solution; retention time; approximate amount returned; color, consistency, and amount of the return; abnormalities within the return; any complications that occurred; and the patient's tolerance of the treatment. Document any patient teaching.

REFERENCES

1 The Joint Commission. (2012). Standard NPSG.01.01.01. *Comprehensive accreditation manual for hospitals: The official handbook.* Oakbrook Terrace, IL: The Joint Commission. (Level I)
2 The Joint Commission. (2012). Standard NPSG.07.01.01. *Comprehensive accreditation manual for hospitals: The official handbook.* Oakbrook Terrace, IL: The Joint Commission. (Level I)
3 Centers for Disease Control and Prevention. (October 2002). Guideline for hand hygiene in health-care settings. *Morbidity and Mortality Weekly Report, 51*(RR-16), 1–45. (Level I)
4 World Health Organization. (2009). *WHO guidelines on hand hygiene in health care: First global patient safety challenge. Clean care is safer care.* Geneva, Switzerland: World Health Organization. (Level I)
5 The Joint Commission. (2012). Standard RC.01.03.01. *Comprehensive accreditation manual for hospitals: The official handbook.* Oakbrook Terrace, IL: The Joint Commission. (Level I)

ADDITIONAL REFERENCES

Kyle G. (2007). Bowel care part 4. Administering an enema. *Nursing Times, 103*(45), 26–27.
Nettina, S.M. (2010). *Lippincott manual of nursing practice* (9th ed.). Philadelphia, PA: Lippincott Williams & Wilkins.

EPICARDIAL PACING AND CARE

Epicardial pacing wires are commonly positioned on the epicardial (outer) surface of the heart after cardiac surgery to diagnose and treat arrhythmias, which may be caused by electrolyte imbalances, inflammation, injury, edema, and hypothermia. Depending on the needs of the patient, the surgeon usually places positive and negative electrodes on both the right atrium and the right ventricle. These electrodes are loosely sutured to the epicardial surface and brought out through the chest wall through small incisions.

In the event that pacing is required, epicardial pacing wires are connected to the pulse generator of a temporary pacemaker. When the patient becomes hemodynamically stable, the wires can be removed. Complications following epicardial pacing wire removal occur more frequently in patients with a history of heart failure and repeat heart surgery. Historically, only doctors or

Sensitivity and stimulation threshold testing[10]

Sensitivity and stimulation threshold testing help determine the appropriate pacemaker rate and the amount of electrical current needed to initiate depolarization of the myocardium. Testing should occur on both chambers, as appropriate. Sensitivity threshold testing isn't necessary if the patient has no intrinsic rhythm. In some facilities, critical care nurses are permitted to perform sensitivity and stimulation threshold testing; in other facilities, the doctor must perform the testing. Follow your facility's policy regarding who can perform testing as well as the frequency of testing. Commonly, testing occurs at least every 24 hours to make sure that the pacemaker is functioning properly and that it isn't delivering high levels of energy to the myocardium.

Performing sensitivity threshold testing

- Slowly turn the sensitivity dial counterclockwise to a higher setting until the sensing indicator light stops flashing; the light will stop flashing when the device no longer senses the patient's intrinsic rhythm.
- Gradually turn the sensitivity dial clockwise to a lower setting until the sensing light begins flashing with each complex and the pacing light stops flashing; this setting is the sensing threshold.
- Set the sensitivity dial to the setting that's half the value of the sensing threshold.

Performing stimulation threshold testing

- Set the pacing rate about 10 beats/minute above the patient's intrinsic rate.
- Beginning at 20 milliamperes, slowly decrease the output until capture is lost.
- Gradually increase the milliamperes until you see a 1:1 capture and the pacing light flashes; this is the stimulation threshold.
- Set the milliamperes at least two times higher than the stimulation threshold.

physician assistants were allowed to remove epicardial pacing wires; however, specially trained critical care nurses can now safely remove them.

Equipment
For insertion
Pacemaker generator with new battery ▪ extra batteries ▪ connecting cable ▪ atrial epicardial wires ▪ ventricular epicardial wires ▪ sterile rubber finger cot, glove, or plastic cap ▪ sterile dressing materials (if the wires won't be connected to a pulse generator) ▪ antiseptic solution such as a chlorhexidine-based solution ▪ gloves ▪ tape ▪ electrocardiogram (ECG) monitoring equipment. (See "Cardiac monitoring," page 108.)

For removal
Gloves ▪ gown ▪ goggles or a face shield with a mask ▪ sterile gauze pads ▪ antiseptic solution such as a chlorhexidine-based solution ▪ tape ▪ suture removal kit ▪ cardiac monitor ▪ emergency cart, including temporary transcutaneous or transvenous pacing equipment and IV catheter.

Preparation of equipment
For insertion
Insert a new battery into the pulse generator and make sure it's functioning properly.

For removal
Check that the emergency cart with temporary transcutaneous or transvenous pacing equipment is readily available.

Implementation
For insertion and care
- Confirm that a written informed consent has been obtained and that the consent is in the patient's medical record.[1,2,3]
- Perform hand hygiene.[4,5,6]
- Confirm the patient's identity using at least two patient identifiers according to your facility's policy. [7]
- Perform a preprocedure verification *to make sure that all relevant documentation, related information, and equipment is available and correctly identified to the patient's identifiers.*[8]
- The surgical team will conduct a time-out immediately before starting the procedure *to perform a final assessment that the correct patient, site, positioning, and procedure are identified and all relevant information and necessary equipment are available.*[9]
- The doctor will hook epicardial wires into the epicardium just before the end of surgery. Depending on the patient's condition, the doctor may insert atrial wires, ventricular wires, or both.
- Perform hand hygiene and put on gloves.[4,5,6]
- After insertion, attach the patient to the bedside cardiac monitor *to monitor the patient's heart rhythm and evaluate pacemaker function.*
- If indicated, attach the connecting cable to the pulse generator by connecting the positive pole on the cable to the positive pole on the pulse generator and the negative pole on the cable to the negative pole on the pulse generator.[10]
- Expose the epicardial pacing wires and identify the atrial and ventricular wires if both are present. Epicardial wires that exit the chest to the right of the sternum originate in the atrium; wires that exit to the left of the sternum originate in the ventricle.[10]
- Using the connecting cable, connect the epicardial wires to the pulse generator. Connect the positive electrode to the positive terminal on the pulse generator through the connecting cable; connect the negative electrode to the negative terminal.[10]
- Set the pacing mode, rate, and energy level (output or milliamperes) according to the doctor's order, or as determined by sensitivity (how sensitive the pacemaker is to intrinsic cardiac depolarization) and stimulation threshold testing (the minimum amount of voltage necessary to capture the heart consistently).[10] (See *Sensitivity and stimulation threshold testing.*)

■ After adjustment of pacemaker settings, place the protective plastic cover over the pacemaker controls or lock the controls.

■ Apply a sterile occlusive dressing over the insertion site and label it with the date, the time, and your initials *to prevent infection at the insertion site.*

■ Secure the pulse generator *to prevent it from falling or becoming inadvertently detached.*

■ Insulate exposed wires using a plastic cap, glove, or finger cot.[10]

■ Assess the patient's vital signs, skin color, level of consciousness, and peripheral pulses *to determine the effectiveness of the paced rhythm.* Perform a 12-lead ECG to serve as a baseline, and then perform additional ECGs daily or with clinical changes. Also, if possible, obtain a rhythm strip before, during, and after pacemaker placement; after any adjustment in pacemaker settings; and whenever the patient receives treatment because of a pacemaker complication.

■ Assess the patient for pain using techniques appropriate for the patient's age, condition, and ability to understand. Respond to the patient's pain appropriately.[11]

For removal

■ Verify the order in the patient's medical record for epicardial wire removal.

■ Check laboratory data for coagulation and electrolyte results to make sure they're within normal limits *to reduce the risk of bleeding and cardiac arrhythmias.* Notify the doctor of abnormal values.

■ Check the medication record to ensure that the patient isn't receiving anticoagulants *to reduce the risk of hemorrhage following the procedure.*[12]

■ Administer an analgesic, following safe medication administration practices, 20 to 30 minutes before the procedure *to promote patient comfort.*

■ Bring the equipment to the patient's bedside.

■ Perform hand hygiene.[4,5,6]

■ Confirm the patient's identity using two patient identifiers according to your facility's policy.[7]

■ Explain the procedure to the patient *to reduce anxiety and enhance cooperation* and tell him that he may feel a slightly painful pulling sensation.

■ Obtain vital signs and an ECG rhythm strip, and assess the patient's cardiovascular status *to ensure the patient is stable before removing pacing wires and to provide a baseline for comparison.*

■ Confirm that the patient has patent IV access *in case emergency fluids or medications are required.* Insert an IV catheter if patent access isn't available. (See "IV catheter insertion and removal," page 421.)

■ Perform hand hygiene and put on goggles, a mask, gloves, and a gown.[4,5,6,13]

■ Place the patient in the supine position *so that the wires are readily accessible and the patient is properly positioned if emergency measures become necessary.*

■ Using sterile technique, open the suture removal kit and gauze packages and place them within reach.

■ Carefully remove and discard the dressing covering the exit site.

■ Remove and discard your gloves, perform hand hygiene, and put on a new pair of gloves.[4,5,6]

■ Clean the exit sites with antiseptic solution.[10]

■ Cut the sutures at the appropriate place and remove them. (See "Suture removal," page 688.)

■ Grasp a wire and slowly and gently pull to uncoil it from the epicardium. If you feel resistance, stop and notify the doctor.

■ While pulling each wire, observe the cardiac monitor for arrhythmias.

■ Inspect the pacing wire for a small piece of tissue at the tip, which indicates that you've removed the entire wire intact.

■ Observe the site, noting drainage, redness, or skin breakdown. If you note bleeding at the exit site, apply pressure.

■ Place sterile gauze pads over the exit sites and secure them with tape.

■ Dispose of soiled supplies in the appropriate receptacles.

■ Monitor vital signs and cardiac rhythm, and assess for signs of cardiac tamponade according to your facility's policies (usually every 15 minutes for the first hour, every 30 minutes for the next 2 hours, and then hourly for the following 2 hours) *to assess hemodynamic stability.*

■ Assess the patient for pain and respond appropriately.

Completing the procedure

■ Discard your gloves and perform hand hygiene.[4,5,6]

■ Document the procedure.[14]

Special considerations

■ Take care to prevent microshock, including warning the patient not to use any electrical equipment that isn't grounded, such as telephones, electric shavers, televisions, and lamps.

■ If the patient needs emergency defibrillation, make sure the pacemaker can withstand the procedure. If you're unsure, disconnect the pulse generator *to avoid damage.*

■ Continuously monitor the ECG reading, noting capture, sensing, rate, intrinsic beats, and competition of paced and intrinsic rhythms. If the pacemaker is sensing correctly, the sense indicator on the pulse generator should flash with each beat. (See *Handling pacemaker malfunction,* pages 278 and 279.)

■ Clean the insertion site with an antiseptic solution, and change the dressing according to your facility's policy and label it with the date, time, and your initials. Inspect the site for signs of infection.

■ Assess and document sensitivity and stimulation thresholds (commonly every 24 hours) according to your facility's policy *to make sure the pacemaker is functioning properly.*[10]

■ Monitor the pulse generator's battery light indicator and change the battery when necessary; battery life varies according to the pacing energy needed.

■ If the pulse generator is no longer needed, disconnect it from the pacing wires and insulate the wires using a plastic cap, glove, or finger cot *to prevent microshocks.*

■ Remove pacing wires at least 24 hours before discharge so the patient can be monitored for complications.

TROUBLESHOOTING

Handling pacemaker malfunction

Occasionally, a temporary pacemaker may fail to function appropriately. When this occurs, you need to take immediate action to correct the problem. Follow these steps when your patient's pacemaker fails to pace, capture, or sense intrinsic beats.

Failure to pace

This problem happens when the pacemaker either doesn't fire or fires too often. The pulse generator may not be working properly, or it may not be conducting the impulse to the patient.

Nursing interventions
■ If the pacing or sensing indicator flashes, check the patient, all connections, and the battery. Check the position of the pacing electrode in the patient by X-ray if ordered.
■ If the pulse generator is turned on but the indicators still aren't flashing, change the battery. If that doesn't help, use a different pulse generator.
■ Position the patient on his left side.
■ Check the settings if the pacemaker is firing too rapidly. If they're correct, or if altering them (according to your facility's policy or the doctor's order) doesn't help, change the pulse generator.

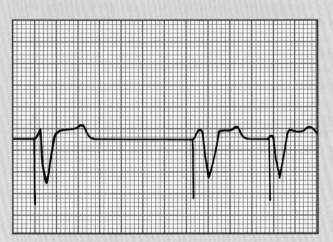

Failure to capture

Here, the pacemaker spikes but the heart isn't responding. This malfunction may be caused by changes in the pacing threshold from ischemia, swelling at the insertion site, an electrolyte imbalance (high or low potassium or magnesium levels), acidosis, an adverse reaction to a medication, a perforated ventricle, fibrosis, or the electrode position.

Nursing interventions
■ If the patient's condition has changed, notify the doctor and ask him for new settings.
■ If pacemaker settings are altered by the patient or others, return them to their correct positions. Then make sure that the face of the pacemaker is covered with a plastic shield. Also, tell the patient or others not to touch the dials.
■ If the heart isn't responding, try any or all of these suggestions: Carefully check all connections; increase the milliamperes slowly (according to your facility's policy or the doctor's order); turn the patient on his left side, then on his right (if turning him to the left didn't help); reverse the

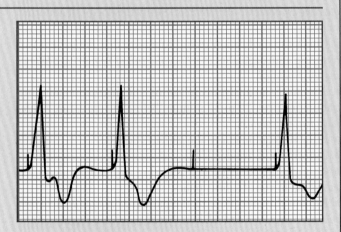

cable in the pulse generator so the positive electrode wire is in the negative terminal and the negative electrode wire is in the positive terminal; or schedule an anteroposterior or lateral chest X-ray to determine the electrode position.

■ *Because pacing wires provide a direct electrical route to the heart, you should wear gloves when handling the wires to prevent microshocks.*[10]

Complications

Complications associated with pacemaker therapy include microshock, equipment failure, and competitive or fatal arrhythmias. Epicardial pacemakers carry a risk of infection, cardiac arrest, and diaphragmatic stimulation.

After removal, monitor for signs and symptoms of life-threatening cardiac tamponade, such as Beck's triad (hypotension, muffled heart tones, and jugular vein distention), tachycardia, decreased peripheral pulses, and dyspnea. Cardiac tamponade may not be immediately evident if the bleeding is slow; therefore, you may need to monitor the patient closely for up to 2 hours. Other complications include infection, hemorrhage, hematoma, arrhythmias, hemodynamic instability, myocardial ischemia, and graft site trauma.

TROUBLESHOOTING

Handling pacemaker malfunction *(continued)*

Failure to sense intrinsic beats

This problem could cause ventricular tachycardia or ventricular fibrillation if the pacemaker fires on the vulnerable T wave. Possible causes include the pacemaker sensing an external stimulus as a QRS complex, which could lead to asystole, or the pacemaker not being sensitive enough, which means it could fire anywhere within the cardiac cycle.

Nursing interventions

■ If the pacing is undersensing, increase the sensitivity by turning down the millivoltage, usually to 2 to 5 mV. If it's oversensing, decrease the sensitivity by turning up the millivoltage to 5 mV or greater.

■ If the pacemaker isn't functioning correctly, change the battery or the pulse generator.

■ Remove items in the room causing electromechanical interference (razors, radios, cautery devices). Check the ground wires on the bed and other equipment for obvious damage. Unplug each piece and see if the interference stops. When you locate the cause, notify the staff engineer and ask him to check it.

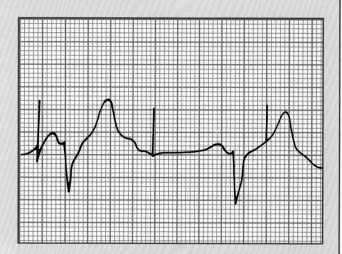

■ If the pacemaker is still firing on the T wave and all else has failed, turn off the pacemaker. Make sure that atropine is available in case the patient's heart rate drops. Be prepared to call a code and start cardiopulmonary resuscitation, if necessary.

Documentation

Record the reason for pacing, the time it started, the locations of the electrodes, and the pacemaker settings. Note the patient's response to the procedure, along with any complications and interventions taken. If possible, obtain rhythm strips before, during, and after pacemaker placement and whenever pacemaker settings are changed or when the patient receives treatment for a complication caused by the pacemaker. As you monitor the patient, record his response to temporary pacing and note any changes in his condition.

Record the date, time, and name of the person removing the wires. If an analgesic was administered, record the name, dose, route, and time it was given and the patient's rating of his pain level (on a 0 to 10 scale).

Describe the condition of the insertion sites, the ease with which you removed the wires, and whether you noted tissue at the end of the wires. Include vital signs, ECG strip, and patient assessment before, during, and after the procedure. Record how you dressed the site. Note the patient's tolerance of the procedure.

If any adverse effects occurred, note the time, name of the doctor notified, orders given, nursing interventions, and patient's response. Document frequent assessments on a frequent vital sign assessment sheet, according to your facility's policy. Include patient and family teaching provided.

REFERENCES

1 The Joint Commission. (2012). Standard RI.01.03.01. *Comprehensive accreditation manual for hospitals: The official handbook.* Oakbrook Terrace, IL: The Joint Commission. (Level I)

2 Centers for Medicare and Medicaid Services, Department of Health and Human Services. (2006). "Conditions of Participation: Patients' Rights," 42 CFR part 482.13 [Online]. Accessed January 2012 via the Web at https://www.cms.gov/CFCsAndCoPs/downloads/finalpatientrightsrule.pdf

3 Centers for Medicare and Medicaid Services, Department of Health and Human Services. (2006). "Conditions of Participation: Surgical Services," 42 CFR part 482.51 [Online]. Accessed January 2012 via the Web at http://cfr.vlex.com/vid/482-51-condition-participation-surgical-19811471

4 The Joint Commission. (2012). Standard NPSG.07.01.01. *Comprehensive accreditation manual for hospitals: The official handbook.* Oakbrook Terrace, IL: The Joint Commission. (Level I)

5 World Health Organization. (2009). *WHO guidelines on hand hygiene in health care: First global patient safety challenge. Clean care is safer care.* Geneva, Switzerland: World Health Organization. (Level I)

6 Centers for Disease Control and Prevention. (October 2002). Guideline for hand hygiene in health-care settings. *Morbidity and Mortality Weekly Report, 51*(RR-16), 1–45. (Level I)

7 The Joint Commission. (2012). Standard NPSG.01.01.01. *Comprehensive accreditation manual for hospitals: The official handbook.* Oakbrook Terrace, IL: The Joint Commission. (Level I)

8 The Joint Commission. (2012). Standard UP.01.01.01. *Comprehensive accreditation manual for hospitals: The official handbook.* Oakbrook Terrace, IL: The Joint Commission. (Level I)

Understanding intrathecal injections

An intrathecal injection allows the doctor or specially trained nurse to inject medication into the subarachnoid space of the spinal canal. Certain drugs, such as anti-infectives or antineoplastics used to treat meningeal leukemia, are administered by this route because they can't readily penetrate the blood-brain barrier through the bloodstream. Intrathecal injection may also be used to deliver anesthetics such as lidocaine hydrochloride, to achieve regional anesthesia (as in spinal anesthesia), or to administer pain-management medications such as preservative-free morphine.

An invasive procedure performed under sterile conditions by a doctor or specially trained nurse with nursing assistance, intrathecal injection requires the patient's informed consent. The injection site is usually between the third and fourth (or fourth and fifth) lumbar vertebrae, well below the spinal cord, to avoid the risk of paralysis. Aspiration of spinal fluid for laboratory analysis may precede intrathecal injection.

Contraindications to this procedure include inflammation or infection at the puncture site, septicemia, and spinal deformities (especially when considered as an anesthesia route).

9 The Joint Commission. (2012). Standard UP.01.03.01. *Comprehensive accreditation manual for hospitals: The official handbook.* Oakbrook Terrace, IL: The Joint Commission. (Level I)
10 Lynn-McHale Wiegand, D. (Ed.). (2011). *AACN procedure manual for critical care* (6th ed.). Philadelphia, PA: Saunders.
11 The Joint Commission. (2012). Standard PC.01.02.07. *Comprehensive accreditation manual for hospitals: The official handbook.* Oakbrook Terrace, IL: The Joint Commission. (Level I)
12 The Joint Commission. (2012). Standard MM.06.01.01. *Comprehensive accreditation manual for hospitals: The official handbook.* Oakbrook Terrace, IL: The Joint Commission. (Level I)
13 Siegel, J. D., et al. "2007 Guideline for Isolation Precautions: Preventing Transmission of Infectious Agents in Healthcare Settings" [Online]. Accessed September 2011 via the Web at http://www.cdc.gov/hicpac/2007ip/2007isolationprecautions.html
14 The Joint Commission. (2012). Standard RC.01.03.01. *Comprehensive accreditation manual for hospitals: The official handbook.* Oakbrook Terrace, IL: The Joint Commission. (Level I)

ADDITIONAL REFERENCES

American Heart Association. (2010). 2010 American Heart Association guidelines for cardiopulmonary resuscitation and emergency cardiovascular care. *Circulation, 122*(Suppl. 3), S685–S719. (Level I)
Reade, M.C. (2007) Temporary epicardial pacing after cardiac surgery: A practical review. Part 1: General considerations in the management of epicardial pacing. *Anaesthesia, 62*(3), 264–271.
Woods, S., et al. (2010). *Cardiac nursing* (6th ed.). Philadelphia, PA: Lippincott Williams & Wilkins.

EPIDURAL ANALGESIC ADMINISTRATION

When administering an epidural analgesic, the doctor or specially trained nurse injects or infuses medication into the epidural space, which lies just outside the subarachnoid space where cerebrospinal fluid (CSF) flows. The drug diffuses slowly into the subarachnoid space of the spinal canal and then into the CSF, which carries it directly into the spinal area, bypassing the blood-brain barrier. In some cases, medication is injected directly into the subarachnoid space. (See *Understanding intrathecal injections.*)

Epidural analgesia helps manage acute or chronic pain, including moderate to severe postoperative pain. It's especially useful in patients with cancer or degenerative joint disease. This procedure works well because opioid receptors are located along the entire spinal cord. Opioid drugs act directly on the receptors of the dorsal horn to produce localized analgesia without motor blockage. Opioids, such as preservative-free morphine, fentanyl, and hydromorphone, are administered as a bolus dose or by continuous infusion, either alone or in combination with a local anesthetic. Infusion through an epidural catheter is preferred because it allows a smaller drug dosage to be given continuously. The epidural catheter, inserted into the epidural space, eliminates the risks of multiple IM injections, minimizes adverse cerebral and systemic effects, and eliminates the analgesic peaks and valleys that usually occur with intermittent IM injections. (See *Placement of an epidural catheter.*)[1]

Typically, epidural catheter insertion is performed by an anesthesiologist using sterile technique. Once the catheter has been inserted, the nurse is responsible for monitoring the infusion and assessing the patient.[1]

Epidural analgesia is contraindicated in patients who have local or systemic infection, neurologic disease, coagulopathy, spinal arthritis or deformity, hypotension, marked hypertension, or an allergy to the prescribed drug as well as in those who are undergoing anticoagulant therapy.

Equipment

Volume infusion device and epidural infusion tubing (depending on your facility's policy) ■ patient's medication record and prescribed epidural solutions (preservative-free) ■ sterile transparent semipermeable dressing ■ sterile tape measure ■ epidural tray ■ label ■ labels for epidural infusion line ■ silk tape ■ sterile gloves ■ gloves ■ mask ■ Optional: monitoring equipment for blood pressure and pulse, apnea monitor, pulse oximeter, chlorhexidine-impregnated sponge dressing.

Have on hand the following drugs and equipment for emergency use: 0.4 mg of IV naloxone, 50 mg of IV ephedrine, oxygen, an intubation set, and a handheld resuscitation bag.

Preparation of equipment

Prepare the infusion device according to the manufacturer's instructions and your facility's policy. Obtain an epidural tray. Make sure the pharmacy has been notified ahead of time about the medication order *because epidural solutions require special preparation.* Avoid distractions and interruptions when preparing and administering medication.[2] Check the medication concentration and infusion rate against the doctor's order.[3] Inspect the medication for particulates, discoloration, or other loss of integrity. Verify that the medication hasn't expired and that no contraindications to the medication exist. Discuss any unresolved issues with the doctor.[3]

Implementation

■ Verify the doctor's order.[4]
■ Perform hand hygiene.[5,6,7]
■ Confirm the patient's identity using at least two patient identifiers according to your facility's policy.[8]
■ Perform a comprehensive pain assessment using techniques that are appropriate for the patient's age, condition, and ability to understand.[9]
■ Explain the procedure and its possible complications to the patient. Tell him that he'll feel some pain as the catheter is inserted. Answer any questions he has.
■ Verify that a consent form has been properly signed and that the form is in the patient's medical record.[10]
■ Put on gloves and a mask.[11]
■ Position the patient on his side in the knee-chest position, or have him sit on the edge of the bed and lean over a bedside table while the catheter is being inserted.
■ After the catheter is in place, prime the infusion device, confirm the appropriate medication and infusion rate, and then adjust the device for the correct rate.
■ If your facility uses a bar code scanning system, scan your identification badge, the patient's identification band, and the medication's bar code according to your facility's policy.

NURSING ALERT *Epidural medications are considered high-alert medications* because they can cause significant patient harm when used in error.[12] *Before beginning an epidural infusion, have another nurse perform an independent double-check according to your facility's policy* to verify the patient's identity and make sure that the correct medication is hanging in the prescribed concentration, the medication's indication corresponds with the patient's diagnosis, the dosage calculations are correct and the dosing formula used to derive the final dose is correct, the route of administration is safe and proper for the patient, the pump settings are correct, and the infusion line is attached to the correct port.[13]

■ After the anesthesiologist aspirates the device to make sure cerebrospinal fluid or blood isn't present, help him connect the infusion tubing to the epidural catheter. Trace the tubing from the patient to its point of origin *to make sure it's connected to the proper port.*[14] Then connect the tubing to the infusion pump.
■ Bridge-tape all connection sites, and apply an EPIDURAL INFUSION label to the catheter, infusion tubing, and infusion pump *to prevent accidental infusion of other drugs.* Compare the results of the independent double-check with the other nurse. If there are no discrepancies, move forward with medication administration. If discrepancies exist, rectify them before administering the medication.[13] Then start the infusion.
■ Remove and discard your gloves, perform hand hygiene, and put on sterile gloves.[5,6,7,15]

Placement of an epidural catheter

An epidural catheter is implanted beneath the patient's skin and inserted near the spinal cord at the first lumbar (L1) interspace.

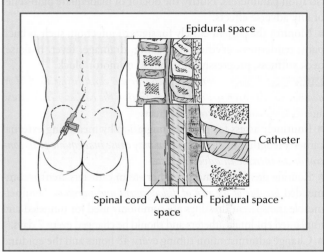

Epidural space

Catheter

Spinal cord   Arachnoid   Epidural space
space

■ Measure the external catheter length with a tape measure *to serve as a baseline for comparison to assess for catheter migration.*[15]
■ Clean the insertion site with povidone-iodine solution, and then allow it to dry completely.[15]
■ Place a chlorhexidine-impregnated sponge dressing around the insertion site according to your facility's policy *to reduce the risk for central nervous system infection.*
■ Secure the catheter to the skin with sterile tape, as needed. Place a transparent semipermeable dressing over the chlorhexidine-impregnated sponge dressing, if used; center the transparent dressing over the catheter insertion site.[15]
■ Label the dressing with the date, the time, and your initials.[15]
■ Discard all used supplies in the appropriate receptacle.
■ Remove and discard your mask and gloves.
■ Perform hand hygiene.[5,6,7]
■ Tell the patient to report any pain immediately. Instruct him to use a pain scale from 0 to 10, with 0 denoting no pain and 10 denoting the worst pain imaginable. A response of 3 or less typically indicates tolerable pain. If the patient reports a higher pain score, the infusion rate may need to be increased. If the patient is unable to use a numerical pain scale, use an assessment tool that's appropriate for the patient.[9] Call the doctor or change the rate within prescribed limits.
■ If ordered, place the patient on a pulse oximeter or cardiac monitor for the first 24 hours after beginning the infusion.[16]
■ Perform hand hygiene.[5,6,7]
■ Document the procedure.[17]

Special considerations

■ Assess the patient's vital signs, oxygen saturation level, sedation level (if an opioid is being administered), and pain status hourly for the first 24 hours, and then every 4 hours thereafter. Also assess for such adverse effects as pruritus, nausea, urinary retention, orthostatic hypotension, or motor block; catheter and administration set disconnections; and dressing intactness. Check the infusion pump for history of analgesic use and correct administration parameters. Notify the doctor of inadequate pain relief or any adverse effects.[16]

■ Monitor the patient closely for signs of infection, such as back pain, tenderness, erythema, swelling, drainage, fever, malaise, neck stiffness, progressive numbness, or motor block.[16]

NURSING ALERT *Don't use preparations containing alcohol or acetone for site preparation or disinfecting the catheter hub; these agents may cause neurotoxic effects.*[16]

■ Routinely assess for catheter migration by measuring external catheter length; *catheter migration may cause inadequate pain control or an increase in adverse effects.*

■ Routine dressing changes on short-term catheters aren't recommended *because of the risk of dislodgement and infection.* Semipermeable transparent dressings are commonly used for tunneled and implanted epidural catheters and should be changed every 7 days.[16]

■ Change administration tubing every 48 hours and the epidural solution every 24 hours, or as specified by your facility's policy.

■ A change in sedation level (the patient becoming somnolent) is an early indicator of the respiratory depressant effects of the opioid. Respiratory depression usually occurs during the first 24 hours and is treated with IV naloxone. Nausea, vomiting, and pruritus may be treated with low-dose IV naloxone.

■ If sensorimotor loss occurs (numbness and leg weakness), large motor nerve fibers have been affected and dosage may need to be decreased. Notify the doctor *because he may need to titrate the dosage in order to identify the dose that provides adequate pain control without causing excessive numbness and weakness.*

■ Keep in mind that drugs given epidurally diffuse slowly and may cause adverse effects, including excessive sedation, up to 12 hours after epidural infusion has been discontinued.

■ The patient should always have a peripheral IV catheter (either continuous infusion or saline lock) open *to allow immediate administration of emergency drugs.*

■ Postdural puncture headache may result from accidental puncture of the dura during an attempted epidural insertion. The anesthesiologist will stop the procedure and may attempt the epidural again at a different lumbar interspace. If CSF leaks into the dura mater at the initial puncture site, the patient usually experiences a headache. This postanalgesia headache worsens with postural changes, such as standing or sitting. The headache can be treated with a "blood patch," in which the patient's own blood (about 10 mL) is withdrawn from a peripheral vein and then injected into the epidural space. When the epidural needle is withdrawn, the patient is instructed to sit up. Because the blood clots seal off the leaking area, the blood patch should relieve the patient's headache immediately. The patient need not restrict his activity after this procedure.

■ Typically, the anesthesiologist orders analgesics and removes the catheter. However, your facility's policy may allow a specially trained nurse to remove the catheter.[16] If you feel resistance when removing the catheter, stop and call the doctor for further orders. Be sure to save the catheter. *The doctor will want to examine the catheter tip to rule out any damage during removal.*

Patient teaching

Home use of epidural analgesia is possible only if the patient or a family member is willing and able to learn the care needed. The patient also must be willing and able to abstain from alcohol and illegal drugs *because these substances potentiate opioid action.*

Complications

Potential complications of epidural analgesic administration include adverse reactions from opioids or local anesthetics as well as catheter-related problems, such as infection, epidural hematoma, and catheter migration. Infection is treated with antibiotics. Insertion site hematomas should be observed and any increase in size reported to the doctor.

Catheter migration occurs when the epidural catheter migrates out of the epidural space toward the skin. If migration occurs, the patient will have decreased pain relief and leaking at the catheter site. Notify the doctor because the infusion needs to be stopped and the catheter removed. Contact the doctor for further pain management orders. The catheter can also migrate through the dura into the subarachnoid space. If the epidural dose is too high for the smaller subarachnoid space, the dose may eventually be toxic in high concentrations (the patient may show signs of increasing somnolence and eventually a decrease in respirations). Assess the patient and notify the doctor immediately. The infusion needs to be stopped and the catheter removed; the patient may need to be treated with IV naloxone and oxygen therapy.

Documentation

Document the infusion device type, gauge, external catheter length, specific site preparation, infection prevention and safety precautions taken, drug dose, and rate of infusion. Record the patient's response to treatment, catheter patency, condition of the dressing and insertion site, vital signs, and assessment results. Also document the labeling of the epidural catheter, changing of the infusion bags, and the patient's response.

References

1 American Society of Pain Management Nurses. (2007). "Registered Nurse Management and Monitoring of Analgesia by Catheter Techniques: A Position Statement" [Online]. Accessed September 2011 via the Web at www.aspmn.org/Organization/documents/RegisteredNurseManagementandMonitoringofAnalgesiaByCatheterTechniquesPMNversion.pdf (Level I)

2 Westbrook, J., et al. (2010). Association of interruptions with an increased risk and severity of medication administration errors. *Archives of Internal Medicine, 170*(8), 683–690.

3 The Joint Commission. (2012). Standard MM.06.01.01. *Comprehensive accreditation manual for hospitals: The official handbook.* Oakbrook Terrace, IL: The Joint Commission. (Level I)

4 The Joint Commission. (2012). Standard MM.04.01.01. *Comprehensive accreditation manual for hospitals: The official handbook.* Oakbrook Terrace, IL: The Joint Commission. (Level I)

5 The Joint Commission. (2012). Standard NPSG.07.01.01. *Comprehensive accreditation manual for hospitals: The official handbook.* Oakbrook Terrace, IL: The Joint Commission. (Level I)

6 World Health Organization. (2009). *WHO guidelines on hand hygiene in health care: First global patient safety challenge. Clean care is safer care.* Geneva, Switzerland: World Health Organization. (Level I)

7 Centers for Disease Control and Prevention. (October 2002). Guideline for hand hygiene in health-care settings. *Morbidity and Mortality Weekly Report, 51*(RR-16), 1–45. (Level I)

8 The Joint Commission. (2012). Standard NPSG.01.01.01. *Comprehensive accreditation manual for hospitals: The official handbook.* Oakbrook Terrace, IL: The Joint Commission. (Level I)

9 The Joint Commission. (2012). Standard PC.01.02.07. *Comprehensive accreditation manual for hospitals: The official handbook.* Oakbrook Terrace, IL: The Joint Commission. (Level I)

10 The Joint Commission. (2012). Standard RI.01.03.01. *Comprehensive accreditation manual for hospitals: The official handbook.* Oakbrook Terrace, IL: The Joint Commission. (Level I)

11 Siegel, J.D., et al. "2007 Guideline for Isolation Precautions: Preventing Transmission of Infectious Agents in Healthcare Settings" [Online]. Accessed September 2011 via the Web at http://www.cdc.gov/hicpac/2007ip/2007isolationprecautions.html

12 Institute for Safe Medication Practices. "ISMP's List of High-Alert Medications" [Online]. Accessed September 2011 via the Web at http://www.ismp.org/tools/highalertmedications.pdf.

13 Institute for Safe Medication Practices. (2008). "Conducting an Independent Double-check." *ISMP Medication Safety Alert! Nurse Advise-ERR, 6*(12), 1 [Online]. Accessed September 2011 via the Web at http://www.ismp.org/newsletters/nursing/Issues/NurseAdviseERR200812.pdf

14 U.S. Food and Drug Administration. "Look. Check. Connect.: Safe Medical Device Connections Save Lives" [Online]. Accessed August 2011 via the Web at http:www.fda.gov/downloads/MedicalDevices/Safety/AlertsandNotices/UCM134873.pdf

15 Infusion Nurses Society. (2011). *Policies and procedures for infusion nursing* (4th ed.). Boston, MA: Infusion Nurses Society.

16 Standard 58. Intraspinal access devices. Infusion nursing standards of practice . (2011). *Journal of Infusion Nursing, 34*(1S), S81–82. (Level I)

17 The Joint Commission. (2012). Standard RC.01.03.01. *Comprehensive accreditation manual for hospitals: The official handbook.* Oakbrook Terrace, IL: The Joint Commission. (Level I)

ADDITIONAL REFERENCES

Förster, J.G., et al. (2009). An evaluation of the epidural catheter position by epidural nerve stimulation in conjunction with continuous epidural analgesia in adult surgical patients. *Anesthesia and Analgesia, 108*(1), 351–358.

Konigsrainer, I., et al. (2009). Audit of motor weakness and premature catheter dislodgement after epidural analgesia in major abdominal surgery. *Anaesthesia, 64*(1), 27–31.

Pöpping, D.M. (2008). Protective effects of epidural analgesia on pulmonary complications after abdominal and thoracic surgery: A meta-analysis. *Archives of Surgery, 143*(10), 990–999; discussion 1000.

ESOPHAGEAL TUBE CARE

Used to control hemorrhage from esophageal or gastric varices, an esophageal tube is inserted nasally or orally and advanced into the esophagus or stomach. (See *Types of esophageal tubes*, page 284.)

Although the doctor inserts an esophageal tube, the nurse cares for the patient during and after intubation. Typically, the patient with an esophageal tube is in the intensive care unit for close observation and constant care. Sedatives may be contraindicated, especially for a patient with portal systemic encephalopathy.

A patient who has an esophageal tube in place to control variceal bleeding (typically from portal hypertension) must be observed closely for possible esophageal rupture because varices weaken the esophagus. Possible traumatic injury from intubation or esophageal balloon inflation also increases the chance of rupture. If a rupture occurs, emergency surgery is typically performed, although the operation has a low success rate.

Equipment

Manometer ▪ two 2-liter bottles of normal saline solution ▪ irrigation set ▪ water-soluble lubricant ▪ several cotton-tipped applicators ▪ oral care equipment (see "Oral care," page 524) ▪ nasopharyngeal suction apparatus ▪ several #12 French suction catheters ▪ intake-and- output record sheets ▪ gloves ▪ goggles ▪ traction weights, football helmet, or tape ▪ scissors ▪ Optional: sedatives.

Implementation

▪ Verify the doctor's order.
▪ Confirm the patient's identity using at least two patient identifiers according to your facility's policy.[1]
▪ Provide privacy and explain the care that you'll give *to ease the patient's anxiety.*
▪ Perform hand hygiene and put on gloves and goggles.[2,3,4]
▪ Monitor the patient's vital signs every 5 minutes to 1 hour, as ordered. *A change in vital signs may signal complications or recurrent bleeding.*
▪ If the patient has a Sengstaken-Blakemore or Minnesota tube, check the pressure gauge on the manometer every hour. Maintain esophageal balloon pressures at 25 to 45 mm Hg.[5]
▪ Reduce esophageal balloon pressure by 5 mm Hg every 3 hours, as ordered, until pressure is 25 mm Hg and the patient shows no signs of bleeding.[5]
▪ Assist the doctor with completely deflating the esophageal balloon for 30 minutes every 8 hours, as ordered, *to prevent esophageal necrosis.*[5]
▪ Maintain drainage and suction on gastric and esophageal aspiration ports, as ordered. *Fluid accumulating in the stomach may cause the patient to regurgitate the tube, and fluid accumulating in the esophagus may lead to vomiting and aspiration.*
▪ Trace the tube from the patient to the point of origin. Then irrigate the gastric aspiration port, as ordered, using the irrigation set and normal saline solution. *Frequent irrigation keeps the tube from clogging. Obstruction in the tube can lead to regurgitation of the tube and vomiting.*

EQUIPMENT

Types of esophageal tubes

When working with a patient who has an esophageal tube, remember the advantages of the most common types.

Sengstaken-Blakemore tube

A Sengstaken-Blakemore tube is a triple-lumen, double-balloon tube that has a gastric aspiration port, which allows you to obtain drainage from below the gastric balloon and also to instill medication.

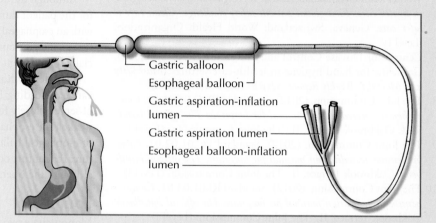

Gastric balloon
Esophageal balloon
Gastric aspiration-inflation lumen
Gastric aspiration lumen
Esophageal balloon-inflation lumen

Linton tube

A Linton tube is a triple-lumen, single-balloon tube that has a port for gastric aspiration and one for esophageal aspiration, too. Additionally, the Linton tube reduces the risk of esophageal necrosis because it doesn't have an esophageal balloon.

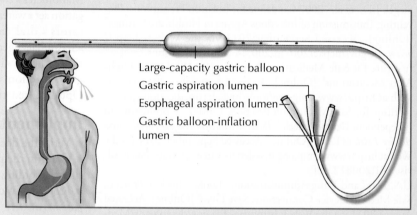

Large-capacity gastric balloon
Gastric aspiration lumen
Esophageal aspiration lumen
Gastric balloon-inflation lumen

Minnesota esophagogastric tamponade tube

A Minnesota esophagogastric tamponade tube is an esophageal tube that has four lumens and two balloons. The device provides pressure-monitoring ports for both balloons without the need for Y connectors. One port is used for gastric suction, the other for esophageal suction.

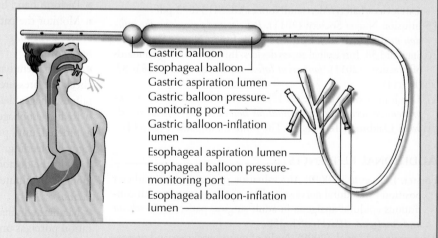

Gastric balloon
Esophageal balloon
Gastric aspiration lumen
Gastric balloon pressure-monitoring port
Gastric balloon-inflation lumen
Esophageal aspiration lumen
Esophageal balloon pressure-monitoring port
Esophageal balloon-inflation lumen

■ *To prevent pressure ulcers,* clean the patient's nostrils, and apply water-soluble lubricant frequently. Use warm water *to loosen crusted nasal secretions* before applying the lubricant with cotton-tipped applicators.

■ Provide oral care often *to rid the patient's mouth of foul-tasting matter and to prevent hospital-associated pneumonia.*

■ Use #12 French catheters to provide gentle oral suctioning, if necessary, *to help remove secretions.*

■ Offer emotional support. Keep the patient as quiet as possible, and administer sedatives, if ordered.

■ Make sure the tube is secured. A football helmet, gentle traction using a 1-lb weight, or tape may be used. If a weight is used, make sure that the weight hangs from the foot of the bed at all times. Never rest it on the bed. Instruct housekeepers and other coworkers not to move the weight *because reduced traction may change the position of the tube*. If using tape, tape the tube to the patient's face, *which provides traction*.

■ Keep the patient on complete bed rest *because exertion, such as coughing or straining, increases intra-abdominal pressure, which may trigger further bleeding*.

■ Observe the patient carefully for esophageal rupture, indicated by signs and symptoms of shock, increased respiratory difficulties, and increased bleeding.

■ Keep the head of the patient's bed elevated 30 to 45 degrees *to minimize aspiration and to prevent ventilator-associated pneumonia if the patient is intubated*.[5]

■ Monitor intake and output, as ordered.

■ Remove and discard your gloves and goggles. Perform hand hygiene.[2,3,4]

■ Document the procedure.[6]

Special considerations

■ Keep scissors at the bedside *so you can cut the tube quickly to deflate the balloons if asphyxia develops*. When performing this emergency intervention, hold the tube firmly close to the nostril before cutting.

■ If using traction, be sure to release the tension before deflating any balloons. If a weight is being used, remove the weight. If a football helmet or tape supplies traction, untape the esophageal tube from the face guard or face before deflating the balloons. *Deflating the balloon under tension triggers a rapid release of the entire tube from the nose, which may injure mucous membranes, initiate recurrent bleeding, and obstruct the airway.*

■ If the doctor orders an X-ray study to check the tube's position or to view the chest, lift the patient in the direction of the pulley, and then place the X-ray film behind his back. Never roll him from side to side *because pressure exerted on the tube in this way may shift the tube's position*. Lift the patient in a similar manner to make the bed or to assist him with the bedpan.

Complications

Esophageal rupture, the most life-threatening complication associated with esophageal balloon tamponade, can occur at any time, but it's most likely to occur during intubation or inflation of the esophageal balloon. Asphyxia may result if the balloon moves up the esophagus and blocks the airway. Aspiration of pooled esophageal secretions may also complicate this procedure.

Documentation

Read the manometer hourly, and record the esophageal pressures. Note when the balloons are deflated and by whom. Document vital signs, the condition of the patient's nostrils, routine care provided, and any drugs administered. Also note the color, consistency, and amount of gastric returns. Record any signs and symptoms of complications and the nursing actions taken. Document gastric port irrigations. Maintain accurate intake and output records.

References

1 The Joint Commission. (2012). Standard NPSG.01.01.01. *Comprehensive accreditation manual for hospitals: The official handbook*. Oakbrook Terrace, IL: The Joint Commission. (Level I)

2 The Joint Commission. (2012). Standard NPSG.07.01.01. *Comprehensive accreditation manual for hospitals: The official handbook*. Oakbrook Terrace, IL: The Joint Commission. (Level I)

3 World Health Organization. (2009). *WHO guidelines on hand hygiene in health care: First global patient safety challenge. Clean care is safer care*. Geneva, Switzerland: World Health Organization. (Level I)

4 Centers for Disease Control and Prevention. (October 2002). Guideline for hand hygiene in health-care settings. *Morbidity and Mortality Weekly Report, 51*(RR-16), 1–45. (Level I)

5 Lynn-McHale Wiegand, D. (Ed.). (2011). *AACN procedure manual for critical care* (6th ed.). Philadelphia, PA: Saunders.

6 The Joint Commission. (2012). Standard RC.01.03.01. *Comprehensive accreditation manual for hospitals: The official handbook*. Oakbrook Terrace, IL: The Joint Commission. (Level I)

ESOPHAGEAL TUBE INSERTION AND REMOVAL

Used to control hemorrhage from esophageal or gastric varices, an esophageal tube is inserted nasally or orally and advanced into the esophagus and stomach. Ordinarily, a doctor inserts and removes the tube. However, in an emergency situation, a nurse may remove it.

Once the tube is in place, a gastric balloon secured at the end of the tube can be inflated and drawn tightly against the cardia of the stomach. The inflated balloon secures the tube and exerts pressure on the cardia. The pressure, in turn, controls the bleeding varices.

Most tubes also contain an esophageal balloon to control esophageal bleeding. The esophageal balloon should be used to control bleeding for no longer than 36 hours; the gastric balloon, for no longer than 72 hours. Pressure necrosis may develop and cause further hemorrhage or perforation.

Other procedures to control bleeding include irrigation with tepid or iced saline solution, drug therapy with a vasopressor, variceal banding, and transjugular intrahepatic portosystemic shunts. Used with the esophageal tube, these procedures provide effective, temporary control of acute variceal hemorrhage.

Equipment
For insertion

Esophageal tube ■ nasogastric (NG) tube (if using a Sengstaken-Blakemore tube) ■ two suction sources ■ irrigation set ■ 2 L of normal saline solution ■ two 60-mL syringes ■ water-soluble lubricant ■ ½″ or 1″ adhesive tape ■ stethoscope ■ foam nose guard ■ four rubber-shod clamps (two clamps and two plastic plugs for a Minnesota tube) ■ traction equipment (football helmet or a basic frame with traction rope, pulleys, and a 1-lb [0.5-kg] weight) ■ manometer ■ Y-connector tube (for Sengstaken-Blakemore or Linton tube) ■ basin of water ■ cup of water with straw ■ scissors

■ gloves ■ gown ■ waterproof marking pen ■ goggles ■ sphygmomanometer ■ anesthetic spray.

For removal
60-mL syringe ■ gloves ■ gown ■ goggles ■ sphygmomanometer.

Preparation of equipment
For insertion
Keep the football helmet at the bedside or attach traction equipment to the bed *so that either is readily available after tube insertion.* Place the suction machines nearby and plug them in. Open the irrigation set and fill the container with normal saline solution. Place all equipment within reach.

Test the balloons on the esophageal tube for air leaks by inflating them and submerging them in the basin of water. If no bubbles appear in the water, the balloons are intact. Remove them from the water and deflate them. Clamp the tube lumens so that the balloons stay deflated during insertion.

To prepare the Minnesota tube, connect the manometer to the gastric pressure monitoring port. Note the pressure when the balloon fills with 100, 200, 300, 400, and 500 mL of air.

Check the aspiration lumens for patency, and make sure they're labeled according to their purpose. If they aren't identified, label them carefully with the waterproof marking pen.

Implementation
■ Verify the doctor's order.
■ Confirm the patient's identity using at least two patient identifiers according to your facility's policy.[1]
■ Explain the procedure and its purpose to the patient, and provide privacy. Answer all questions to decrease anxiety and increase cooperation.
■ Perform hand hygiene, and put on gloves, gown, and goggles *to protect yourself from splashing blood.*[2,3,4]
■ Assist the patient into semi-Fowler's position, and turn him slightly toward his left side. *This position promotes stomach emptying and helps prevent aspiration.*

For insertion
■ Explain that the doctor will inspect the patient's nostrils *for patency.*
■ *To determine the length of tubing needed,* hold the balloon at the patient's xiphoid process and then extend the tube to the patient's ear and forward to his nose. Using a waterproof pen, mark this point on the tubing.
■ Inform the patient that the doctor will spray his throat (posterior pharynx) and nostril with an anesthetic *to minimize discomfort and gagging during intubation.*
■ After lubricating the tip of the tube with water-soluble lubricant *to reduce friction and facilitate insertion,* the doctor will pass the tube through the more patent nostril. As he does this, he'll direct the patient to tilt his chin toward his chest and to swallow when he senses the tip of the tube in the back of his throat. *Swallowing helps to advance the tube into the esophagus and prevents intubation of the trachea.* (If the doctor introduces the tube orally,

he'll direct the patient to swallow immediately.) As the patient swallows, the doctor quickly advances the tube at least ½″(1.3 cm) beyond the previously marked point on the tube.
■ *To confirm tube placement,* the doctor will aspirate stomach contents through the gastric port. After partially inflating the gastric balloon with 50 to 100 mL of air, he'll order an X-ray of the abdomen *to confirm correct placement of the balloon.* Before fully inflating the balloon, he'll use the 60-mL syringe to irrigate the stomach with normal saline solution and empty the stomach as completely as possible. *This irrigation helps the patient avoid regurgitating gastric contents when the balloon inflates.*
■ After confirming tube placement, the doctor will fully inflate the gastric balloon (250 to 500 mL of air for a Sengstaken-Blakemore tube; 700 to 800 mL of air for a Linton tube) and clamp the tube. If he's using a Minnesota tube, he'll connect the pressure-monitoring port for the gastric balloon lumen to the manometer and then inflate the balloon in 100-mL increments until it fills with up to 500 mL of air. As he introduces the air, he'll monitor the intragastric balloon pressure *to make sure the balloon stays inflated.* Then he'll clamp the ports. For the Sengstaken-Blakemore or Minnesota tube, the doctor will gently pull on the tube until he feels resistance, *which indicates that the gastric balloon is inflated and exerting pressure on the cardia of the stomach.* When he senses that the balloon is engaged, he'll place the foam nose guard around the area where the tube emerges from the nostril.
■ Be ready to tape the nose guard in place around the tube *to help minimize pressure on the nostril from the traction and decrease the risk of necrosis.*
■ With the nose guard secured, apply traction to the tube using the method preferred by your facility's policy. Use a traction rope and a 1-lb weight, or pull the tube gently and tape it tightly to the face guard of a football helmet. (See *Securing an esophageal tube with a football helmet.*) Alternatively, some facilities tape the tube to the side of the patient's face as a method of providing traction, *which helps eliminate any issues that may occur with weights or a helmet.*
■ Lavage the stomach through the gastric aspiration lumen with normal saline solution (iced or tepid) until the return fluid is clear. *The vasoconstriction from the lavage stops the hemorrhage; the lavage empties the stomach. Any blood detected later in the gastric aspirate indicates that bleeding remains uncontrolled.*
■ Attach one of the suction sources to the gastric aspiration lumen *to empty the stomach, help prevent nausea and possible vomiting, and allow continuous observation of the gastric contents for blood.*
■ If the doctor inserted a Sengstaken-Blakemore or a Minnesota tube, he'll inflate the esophageal balloon as he inflates the gastric balloon *to compress the esophageal varices and control bleeding.*
■ With a Sengstaken-Blakemore tube, the Y-connector tube is attached to the esophageal lumen. Then a sphygmomanometer inflation bulb is attached to one end of the Y-connector and the manometer to the other end. The esophageal balloon is inflated until the pressure gauge ranges from 30 to 40 mm Hg and the tube is clamped.
■ With a Minnesota tube, the manometer is attached directly to the esophageal pressure-monitoring outlet. Then, using the

60-mL syringe and pushing the air slowly into the esophageal balloon port, the balloon is inflated until the pressure gauge ranges from 35 to 45 mm Hg.

■ Set up esophageal suction *to prevent accumulation of secretions that may cause vomiting and pulmonary aspiration.* This is important because swallowed secretions can't pass into the stomach if the patient has an inflated esophageal balloon in place. If the patient has a Linton or a Minnesota tube, attach the suction source to the esophageal aspiration port. If the patient has a Sengstaken-Blakemore tube, advance an NG tube through the other nostril into the esophagus to the point where the esophageal balloon begins, and attach the suction source, as ordered.

■ Assess the patient for signs of airway obstruction.

For removal

■ The doctor will deflate the esophageal balloon by aspirating the air with a syringe. (He may order the esophageal balloon to be deflated at 5-mm Hg increments every 30 minutes for several hours.) Then, if bleeding doesn't recur, he'll remove the traction from the gastric tube and deflate the gastric balloon (also by aspiration). The gastric balloon is always deflated just before removing the tube *to prevent the balloon from riding up into the esophagus or pharynx and obstructing the airway or, possibly, causing asphyxia or rupture.*

■ After disconnecting all suction tubes, the doctor will gently remove the esophageal tube. If he feels resistance, he'll aspirate the balloons again. (To remove a Minnesota tube, he'll grasp it near the patient's nostril and cut across all four lumens approximately 3″ [7.5 cm] below that point *to ensure deflation of all balloons.*)

■ Discard equipment in the appropriate receptacles.

■ After the tube has been removed, assist the patient with oral care.

Completing the procedure

■ Remove and discard your gloves and protective equipment. Perform hand hygiene.[2,3,4]

■ Document the procedure.[5]

Special considerations

■ If the patient appears cyanotic or if other signs of airway obstruction develop during tube placement, remove the tube immediately *because it may have entered the trachea instead of the esophagus.*

■ Many doctors will intubate a patient before inserting an esophageal tube *to help eliminate the possibility of aspiration pneumonia during tube insertion and while the tube is in place.*

■ After intubation, keep scissors at the bedside. If respiratory distress occurs, cut across all lumens while holding the tube at the nares, and remove the tube quickly.

■ Unless contraindicated, the patient can sip water through a straw during intubation *to facilitate tube advancement.*

■ Keep in mind that the intraesophageal balloon pressure varies with respirations and esophageal contractions. Baseline pressure is the important pressure to use when monitoring for complications.

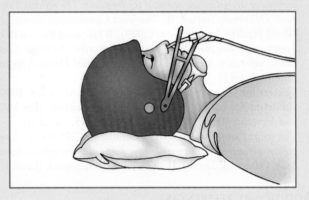

Securing an esophageal tube with a football helmet

An esophageal tube can be secured using traction or by taping the tube either to the patient's face or to the face guard of a football helmet *to reduce the risk of the gastric balloon's slipping down or away from the cardia of the stomach.* To secure the tube to a football helmet, tape the tube to the face guard, as shown, and fasten the chin strap.

To remove the tube quickly, unfasten the chin strap and pull the helmet slightly forward. Cut the tape and the gastric balloon and esophageal balloon lumens. Be sure to hold onto the tube near the patient's nostril.

■ The balloon on the Linton tube should stay inflated no longer than 24 hours *because necrosis of the cardia may result.* Usually, the doctor removes the tube only after a trial period (lasting at least 12 hours) with the esophageal balloon deflated or with the gastric balloon tension released from the cardia *to check for rebleeding.* In some facilities, the doctor may deflate the esophageal balloon for 5 to 10 minutes every hour *to temporarily relieve pressure on the esophageal mucosa.*

Complications

Erosion and perforation of the esophagus and gastric mucosa may result from the tension placed on these areas by the balloons during traction. Esophageal rupture may result if the gastric balloon accidentally inflates in the esophagus. Acute airway occlusion may result if the balloon dislodges and moves upward into the trachea. Other erosions, nasal tissue necrosis, and aspiration of oral secretions may complicate the patient's condition.

Documentation

Record the date and time of insertion and removal, the type of tube used, and the name of the doctor who performed the procedure. Also document the intraesophageal balloon pressure (for the Sengstaken-Blakemore and Minnesota tubes), intragastric balloon pressure (for the Minnesota tube), or amount of air injected (for the Sengstaken-Blakemore and Linton tubes). Record the amount of fluid used for gastric irrigation and the color, consistency, and amount of gastric returns, both before and after lavage.

Record the date and time of removal and the name of the doctor who performed the procedure.

REFERENCES

1 The Joint Commission. (2012). Standard NPSG.01.01.01. *Comprehensive accreditation manual for hospitals: The official handbook.* Oakbrook Terrace, IL: The Joint Commission. (Level I)
2 The Joint Commission. (2012). Standard NPSG.07.01.01. *Comprehensive accreditation manual for hospitals: The official handbook.* Oakbrook Terrace, IL: The Joint Commission. (Level I)
3 World Health Organization. (2009). *WHO guidelines on hand hygiene in health care: First global patient safety challenge. Clean care is safer care.* Geneva, Switzerland: World Health Organization. (Level I)
4 Centers for Disease Control and Prevention. (October 2002). Guideline for hand hygiene in health-care settings. *Morbidity and Mortality Weekly Report, 51*(RR-16), 1–45. (Level I)
5 The Joint Commission. (2012). Standard RC.01.03.01. *Comprehensive accreditation manual for hospitals: The official handbook.* Oakbrook Terrace, IL: The Joint Commission. (Level I)

ADDITIONAL REFERENCES

Collyer, T.C., et al. (2008). Acute upper airway obstruction due to displacement of a Sengstaken-Blakemore tube. *European Journal of Anesthesiology, 25*(4), 341–342.
Lynn-McHale Wiegand, D. (Ed.). (2011). *AACN procedure manual for critical care* (6th ed.). Philadelphia, PA: Saunders.
Nettina, S.M. (2010). *Lippincott manual of nursing practice* (9th ed.). Philadelphia, PA: Lippincott Williams & Wilkins.

EXTERNAL FIXATION MANAGEMENT

With external fixation, a doctor inserts metal pins and wires through skin and muscle layers into the broken bones and affixes them to an adjustable external frame that maintains their proper alignment during healing. (See *Types of external fixation devices.*) This procedure is used most commonly to treat open, unstable fractures with extensive soft-tissue damage, comminuted closed fractures, and septic, nonunion fractures and to facilitate surgical immobilization of a joint. Specialized types of external fixators may be used to lengthen leg bones or immobilize the cervical spine.

An advantage of external fixation over other immobilization techniques is that it stabilizes the fracture while allowing full visualization and access to open wounds. It also facilitates early ambulation, which reduces the risk of complications from immobilization.

The Ilizarov fixator is a special type of external fixation device. This device is a combination of rings and tensioned transosseous wires used primarily in limb lengthening, bone transport, and limb salvage. Highly complex, it provides gradual distraction that results in good-quality bone formation with a minimum of complications.

Equipment

Sterile gloves ■ sterile cotton-tipped applicators ■ prescribed antiseptic cleaning solution ■ ice bag ■ sterile gauze pads ■ pain medication.

Equipment varies with the type of fixator and the type and location of the fracture. Typically, sets of pins, stabilizing rods, and clips are available from manufacturers. Don't reuse pins.

Preparation of equipment

Make sure that the external fixation set includes all the equipment it's supposed to include and that the equipment has been sterilized according to your facility's procedure.

Implementation

■ Verify the doctor's order.
■ Confirm that a written informed consent is obtained and that the consent is in the patient's medical record.[1]
■ Confirm the patient's identity using at least two patient identifiers according to your facility's policy.[2]
■ Explain the procedure to the patient and answer all questions *to reduce his anxiety.* Emphasize that he'll feel little pain after the fixation device is in place. Assure him that his feelings of anxiety are normal and that he'll be able to adjust to the apparatus.
■ Tell the patient that he'll be able to move about with the apparatus in place, which may help him resume normal activities more quickly.
■ Perform hand hygiene.[3,4,5]
■ Assess the patient for pain and provide medication, as ordered, using safe medication administration practices. Perform a follow-up pain assessment and notify the doctor if pain isn't adequately controlled.[6]
■ After the fixation device is in place, perform neurovascular checks every 2 to 4 hours for 24 hours, then every 4 to 8 hours, according to your facility policy, *to assess for possible neurologic damage.* Assess color, warmth, motion, sensation, digital movement, edema, capillary refill, and pulses of the affected extremity. Compare with the unaffected side.
■ Apply an ice bag to the surgical site, as ordered, *to reduce swelling, relieve pain, and lessen bleeding.*
■ Assess the patient's pain and administer pain medication, as ordered, 30 minutes to 1 hour before exercising or mobilizing the affected extremity *to promote comfort.*
■ Monitor the patient for pain not relieved by analgesics and for burning, tingling, or numbness, *which may indicate nerve damage or circulatory impairment.*
■ Elevate the affected extremity, if appropriate, *to minimize edema.*
■ Perform pin site care, as ordered, *to prevent infection.*
■ Perform hand hygiene and put on sterile gloves.[3,4,5]
■ Using sterile technique, clean the pin site with a sterile cotton-tipped applicator dipped in the prescribed antiseptic solution (chlorhexidine-based solution may be the most effective solution).

EQUIPMENT

Types of external fixation devices

The doctor's selection of an external fixation device depends on the severity of the patient's fracture and on the type of bone alignment needed. Here are some examples of external fixation devices.

Universal day frame
This device is used to manage tibial fractures. The frame allows the doctor to readjust the position of bony fragments by angulation and rotation. The compression-distraction device allows compression and distraction of bony fragments.

Portsmouth external fixation bar
This device is used to manage complicated tibial fractures. The locking nut adjustment on the mobile carriage only allows bone compression, so the doctor must accurately reduce bony fragments before applying the device.

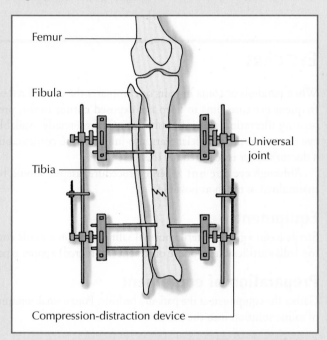

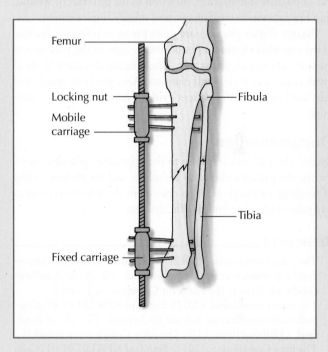

■ If ordered, apply a loose sterile dressing.

■ Remove and discard your gloves and perform hand hygiene.[3,4,5]

■ Perform pin site care, daily or weekly, after the first 48 to 72 hours, depending on the amount of drainage.

■ Check for redness, tenting of the skin, prolonged or purulent drainage from the pin site, swelling, elevated body or pin site temperature, and any bowing or bending of pins, which may stress the skin.

■ Document the procedure.[7]

Special considerations
■ The National Association of Orthopaedic Nurses recommends using chlorhexidine 2-mg/mL solution for pin site care.

■ Because external fixation is commonly used in adolescents, pay special attention to their psychosocial needs. Assess for depression, social issues, body image concerns, and sleep deprivation. Design a care plan with the patient and family to address these issues.

■ If the patient smokes, encourage him to stop smoking and provide smoking-cessation materials *because smoking delays bone healing.*

For the patient with an Ilizarov fixator
■ When the device has been placed and preliminary calluses have begun to form at the insertion sites (in 5 to 7 days), gentle distraction is initiated by turning the appropriate screws one-quarter turn (1 mm) every 4 to 6 hours, as ordered.

■ Nonsteroidal anti-inflammatory drugs are usually contraindicated *because they may decrease the necessary inflammation caused by the distraction, resulting in delayed bone formation.*

Patient teaching
■ Teach the patient with an Ilizarov fixator that he must be consistent in turning the screws every 4 to 6 hours around the clock. Make sure he understands that he must be strongly committed to compliance with the protocol for the procedure to be successful. *Because the treatment period may be prolonged (4 to 10 months),*

discuss with the patient and family members the psychological effects of long-term care.

■ Before discharge, teach the patient and family members how to provide pin site care. This is a sterile procedure in the hospital, but the patient can use clean technique at home. Provide him with written instructions and have him demonstrate the procedure before leaving the hospital. Teach him to recognize signs of pin site infection. Tell him to keep the affected limb elevated when sitting or lying down.

Complications

Complications of external fixation include loosening of pins and loss of fracture stabilization, infection of the pin tract or wound, skin breakdown, nerve damage, and muscle impingement.

Ilizarov fixator pin sites are more prone to infection because of the extended treatment period and because of the pins' movement to accomplish distraction. The pins are also more likely to break because of their small diameter. Also, the large number of pins used increases the patient's risk of neurovascular compromise.

Documentation

Record the patient's response to the apparatus, pin site assessments, the patient's ability to ambulate, and his understanding of teaching instructions. Also document the administration of any pain medication and its effectiveness.

REFERENCES

1 The Joint Commission. (2012). Standard RI.01.03.01. *Comprehensive accreditation manual for hospitals: The official handbook.* Oakbrook Terrace, IL: The Joint Commission. (Level I)
2 The Joint Commission. (2012). Standard NPSG.01.01.01. *Comprehensive accreditation manual for hospitals: The official handbook.* Oakbrook Terrace, IL: The Joint Commission. (Level I)
3 The Joint Commission. (2012). Standard NPSG.07.01.01. *Comprehensive accreditation manual for hospitals: The official handbook.* Oakbrook Terrace, IL: The Joint Commission. (Level I)
4 World Health Organization. (2009). *WHO guidelines on hand hygiene in health care: First global patient safety challenge. Clean care is safer care.* Geneva, Switzerland: World Health Organization. (Level I)
5 Centers for Disease Control and Prevention. (October 2002). Guideline for hand hygiene in health-care settings. *Morbidity and Mortality Weekly Report, 51*(RR-16), 1–45. (Level I)
6 The Joint Commission. (2012). Standard PC.01.02.07. *Comprehensive accreditation manual for hospitals: The official handbook.* Oakbrook Terrace, IL: The Joint Commission. (Level I)
7 The Joint Commission. (2012). Standard RC.01.03.01. *Comprehensive accreditation manual for hospitals: The official handbook.* Oakbrook Terrace, IL: The Joint Commission. (Level I)

ADDITIONAL REFERENCES

Bibbo, C., & Brueggeman, J. (2010). Prevention and management of complications arising from external fixation pin sites. *Journal of Foot and Ankle Surgery, 49*(1), 87–92.

Lee, D.K., et al. (2010). The Ilizarov method of external fixation: Current intraoperative concepts. *AORN, 91*(3), 326–337; quiz 338–340.
Lethaby, A., et al. (2008). Pin site care for preventing infections associated with external bone fixators and pins. *Cochrane Database of Systematic Reviews,* (4):CD004551.
MedLine Plus. (2009). "External Fixation Device" [Online]. Accessed September 2011 via the Web at http://www.nlm.nih.gov/medlineplus/ency/imagepages/18021.htm
Solomon, L.B., et al. (2009). The subcristal pelvic external fixator: Technique, results, and rationale. *Journal of Orthopedic Trauma, 23*(5), 365–369.
Spiegelberg, B., et al. (2010). Ilizarov principles of deformity correction. *Annals of the Royal College of Surgery, 92*(2), 101–105.

EYE CARE

When paralysis or coma impairs or eliminates the corneal reflex, frequent eye care aims to keep the exposed cornea moist, preventing ulceration and inflammation. Commercially available eye ointments and artificial tears also lubricate the corneas, but a doctor's order is required for their use.

Although eye care isn't a sterile procedure, asepsis should be maintained as much as possible.

Equipment

Sterile basin ■ gloves ■ sterile normal saline solution ■ sterile cotton balls ■ artificial tears or eye ointment (if ordered) ■ paper tape.

Preparation of equipment

Gather the equipment at the patient's bedside. Pour a small amount of saline solution into the basin.

Implementation

■ Perform hand hygiene and put on gloves.[1,2,3]
■ Confirm the patient's identity using at least two patient identifiers according to your facility's policy.[4]
■ Tell the patient what you're about to do, even if he is comatose or appears unresponsive.
■ *To remove secretions or crusts adhering to the eyelids and eyelashes,* first soak a cotton ball in sterile normal saline solution. Then gently wipe the patient's eye with the moistened cotton ball, working from the inner canthus to the outer canthus *to prevent debris and fluid from entering the nasolacrimal duct.*
■ *To prevent cross-contamination,* use a fresh cotton ball for each wipe until the eye is clean. *To prevent irritation,* avoid using soap for cleaning the eyes. Repeat the procedure for the other eye.
■ After cleaning the eyes, instill artificial tears or apply eye ointment, as ordered, following safe medication administration practices, *to keep them moist.*
■ Close the patient's eyelids. Use paper tape to close the eyes, as needed.
■ Dispose of the supplies, remove your gloves, and perform hand hygiene.[1,2,3]
■ Document the procedure.[5]

Documentation

Record the time and type of eye care in your notes. If applicable, chart administration of eyedrops or ointment in the patient's medication record. Document unusual crusting or excessive or colored drainage.

REFERENCES

1 The Joint Commission. (2012). Standard NPSG.07.01.01. *Comprehensive accreditation manual for hospitals: The official handbook.* Oakbrook Terrace, IL: The Joint Commission. (Level I)
2 World Health Organization. (2009). *WHO guidelines on hand hygiene in health care: First global patient safety challenge. Clean care is safer care.* Geneva, Switzerland: World Health Organization. (Level I)
3 Centers for Disease Control and Prevention. (October 2002). Guideline for hand hygiene in health-care settings. *Morbidity and Mortality Weekly Report, 51*(RR-16), 1–45. (Level I)
4 The Joint Commission. (2012). Standard NPSG.01.01.01. *Comprehensive accreditation manual for hospitals: The official handbook.* Oakbrook Terrace, IL: The Joint Commission. (Level I)
5 The Joint Commission. (2012). Standard RC.01.03.01. *Comprehensive accreditation manual for hospitals: The official handbook.* Oakbrook Terrace, IL: The Joint Commission. (Level I)

ADDITIONAL REFERENCES

Craven, R.F., & Hirnle, C.J. (2009). *Fundamentals of nursing: Human health and function* (6th ed.). Philadelphia, PA: Lippincott Williams & Wilkins.
Marshall, A.P., et al. (2008). Eyecare in the critically ill: Clinical practice guideline. *Australian Critical Care, 21*(2), 97–109.
Taylor, C., et al. (2011). *Fundamentals of nursing: The art and science of nursing care* (7th ed.). Philadelphia, PA: Lippincott Williams & Wilkins.

EYE COMPRESS APPLICATION

Whether applied warm or cold, eye compresses are soothing and therapeutic. Because heat increases circulation which enhances absorption and decreases inflammation, warm compresses may relieve discomfort and promote drainage of superficial infections.

Typically, a cold compress should be applied for 20-minute periods, four to six times per day. Ocular infection requires the use of sterile technique.

Equipment

Gloves ■ prescribed solution, usually sterile water or normal saline solution ■ sterile basin ■ sterile 4″ × 4″ gauze pads ■ towel ■ Optional: ophthalmic ointment, eye patch.

Additional equipment for a cold compress

Small plastic bag (such as a sandwich bag) or latex-free glove ■ ice chips ■ ½″ hypoallergenic tape.

Preparation of equipment

Gather appropriate equipment and label all medications, medication containers, and other solutions.[1]

For a warm compress

Place a capped bottle of sterile water or normal saline solution in a basin of hot water or under a stream of hot tap water. Allow the solution to become warm (no higher than 120° F [49° C]). Pour the warm water or saline solution into a sterile basin, filling the basin about halfway. Place some sterile gauze pads in the basin.

For a cold compress

Place ice chips in a plastic bag (or a glove, if necessary) to make an ice pack. Keep the ice pack small *to avoid excessive pressure on the eye.* Remove excess air from the bag or glove, and seal or knot the open end. Cut a piece of hypoallergenic tape *to secure the ice pack.* Place all equipment on the bedside stand near the patient.

Implementation

■ Check the doctor's order for solution, frequency, and duration of treatment.[2]
■ Confirm the patient's identity using at least two patient identifiers according to your facility's policy.[3]
■ Explain the procedure to the patient, make him comfortable, and provide privacy. Answer all questions *to decrease anxiety and increase cooperation.*
■ Perform hand hygiene.[4,5,6]
■ If the patient has an eye patch, put on gloves and remove and discard the eye patch. Then remove the gloves and perform hand hygiene.[4,5,6]
■ Help the patient into a supine position. Support his head with a pillow, and turn his head slightly to the unaffected side. *This position will help hold the compress in place.*
■ Drape a towel around the patient's shoulders *to catch any spills.*
■ Perform hand hygiene and put on gloves.[4,5,6]

For a warm compress

■ Take two 4″ × 4″ gauze pads from the basin of warm solution. Squeeze out the excess solution.
■ Instruct the patient to close his eyes. Gently apply the pads, one on top of the other, to the affected eye. (If the patient complains that the compress feels too hot, remove it immediately.)
■ Change the compress every few minutes, as necessary, for the prescribed length of time. After removing each compress, check the patient's skin for signs that the compress solution is too hot.

For a cold compress

■ Moisten the center of one of the sterile 4″ × 4″ gauze pads with the sterile water, normal saline solution, or ophthalmic irrigating solution *to help conduct the cold from the ice pack.* Keep the edges dry *so that they can absorb excess moisture.*
■ Tell the patient to close his eyes; then place the moist gauze pad over the affected eye.
■ Place the ice pack on top of the gauze pad, and tape it in place. If the patient complains of pain, remove the ice pack. *Some patients may have an adverse reaction to cold.*
■ Remove your gloves and perform hand hygiene.[4,5,6]
■ After 15 to 20 minutes, or as ordered, perform hand hygiene and put on gloves.[4,5,6]
■ Remove the tape, ice pack, and gauze pad and discard them.

For all compresses

■ Use the remaining sterile 4″ × 4″ gauze pads to clean and dry the patient's face.
■ If ordered, apply ophthalmic ointment or an eye patch. (See "Eye medication administration," page 295.)
■ Discard used supplies in appropriate receptacle.
■ Remove and discard your gloves and perform hand hygiene.[4,5,6]
■ Document the procedure.[7]

Special considerations

■ When applying warm compresses, change the compress as frequently as necessary *to maintain a constant* temperature, usually every 5 to 10 minutes.
■ Don't use a microwave to warm the solution *because of the risk of overheating the solution and causing a burn.*
■ If ordered to apply moist, cold compresses directly to the patient's eyelid, fill a basin with ice and water and soak the 4″ × 4″ gauze pads in it. Place a compress directly on the lid; change compresses every 2 to 3 minutes.
■ Cold compresses are contraindicated in treating eye inflammation, such as keratitis and iritis, *because the capillary constriction inhibits delivery of nutrients to the cornea.*

Patient teaching

When teaching a patient to apply compresses at home, explain that he can substitute a clean basin and washcloth for the sterile equipment. If both eyes are infected, emphasize the importance of using separate equipment for each eye. Inform the patient that this approach will keep him from passing infection back and forth between the eyes. Direct him to wash his hands thoroughly before and after treating each eye. Teach the patient how to instill eyedrops or ophthalmic ointment correctly and without contaminating the medication container. Direct him to wash his hands thoroughly before and after treating each eye.

Documentation

Record the time and duration of the procedure. Describe the eye's appearance before and after treatment, any drainage, and the patient's comfort level. Note any ointments or dressings applied to the eye. Record the patient's tolerance of the procedure. Document any patient teaching provided and the patient's understanding of the teaching.

REFERENCES

1 The Joint Commission. (2012). Standard NPSG.03.04.01. *Comprehensive accreditation manual for hospitals: The official handbook.* Oakbrook Terrace, IL: The Joint Commission. (Level I)
2 The Joint Commission. (2012). Standard MM.04.01.01. *Comprehensive accreditation manual for hospitals: The official handbook.* Oakbrook Terrace, IL: The Joint Commission. (Level I)
3 The Joint Commission. (2012). Standard NPSG.01.01.01. *Comprehensive accreditation manual for hospitals: The official handbook.* Oakbrook Terrace, IL: The Joint Commission. (Level I)
4 The Joint Commission. (2012). Standard NPSG.07.01.01. *Comprehensive accreditation manual for hospitals: The official handbook.* Oakbrook Terrace, IL: The Joint Commission. (Level I)
5 World Health Organization. (2009). *WHO guidelines on hand hygiene in health care: First global patient safety challenge. Clean care is safer care.* Geneva, Switzerland: World Health Organization. (Level I)
6 Centers for Disease Control and Prevention. (October 2002). Guideline for hand hygiene in health-care settings. *Morbidity and Mortality Weekly Report, 51*(RR-16), 1–45. (Level I)
7 The Joint Commission. (2012). Standard RC.01.03.01. *Comprehensive accreditation manual for hospitals: The official handbook.* Oakbrook Terrace, IL: The Joint Commission. (Level I)

ADDITIONAL REFERENCE

Smeltzer, S.C., et al. (2010). *Brunner & Suddarth's textbook of medical surgical-nursing* (12th ed.). Philadelphia, PA: Lippincott Williams & Wilkins.

EYE IRRIGATION

Used mainly to flush secretions, chemicals, and foreign bodies from the eye, eye irrigation also provides a way to administer medications for corneal and conjunctival disorders. In an emergency, tap water may serve as an irrigant.

The amount of solution needed to irrigate an eye depends on the contaminant. Secretions require a moderate volume; major chemical burns require a copious amount. Usually, an IV bottle or bag of normal saline solution (with IV tubing attached) supplies enough solution for continuous irrigation of a chemical burn. (See *Three devices for eye irrigation.*)

Equipment

Gloves ■ goggles ■ towels ■ eyelid retractor ■ sterile gauze pads ■ 60-mL sterile syringe ■ sterile basin ■ emesis basin ■ Optional: proparacaine hydrochloride topical anesthetic.

For moderate-volume irrigation
Prescribed sterile ophthalmic irrigant.

For copious irrigation
One or more 1,000-mL bottles or bags of normal saline solution ■ standard IV infusion set without needle ■ IV pole.

Commercially prepared bottles of sterile ophthalmic irrigant are available. All solutions should be at body temperature: 98.6° F (37° C).

Preparation of equipment

Read the label on the sterile ophthalmic irrigant. Double-check its sterility, strength, and expiration date.

For moderate-volume irrigation
Pour the sterile irrigant into the sterile basin. Fill the syringe with 30 to 60 mL of irrigant. If you're using a commercially prepared bottle of sterile irrigant, remove the cap from the irrigant container and place the container within easy reach. (Be sure to keep the tip of the container sterile.)

Three devices for eye irrigation

Depending on the type and extent of injury, the patient's eye may need to be irrigated using different devices.

Squeeze bottle

For moderate-volume irrigation—to remove eye secretions, for example—apply sterile ophthalmic irrigant to the eye directly from the squeeze bottle container. Direct the stream at the inner canthus, and position the patient so the stream washes across the cornea and exits at the outer canthus.

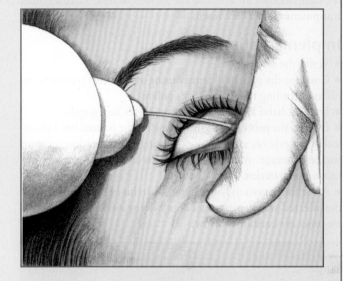

IV tube

For copious irrigation—to treat chemical burns, for example—set up an IV bag and tubing without a needle. Use the procedure described for moderate irrigation to flush the eye for at least 15 minutes. Alkali burns may require irrigation for several hours.

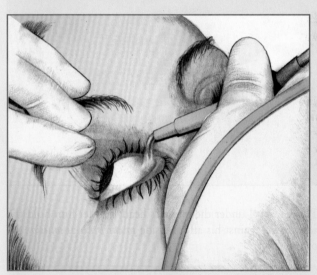

Morgan lens

Connected to irrigation tubing, a Morgan lens permits continuous lavage and also delivers medication to the eye. Use an adapter to connect the lens to the IV tubing and the solution container. Begin the irrigation at the prescribed flow rate. To insert the device, ask the patient to look down as you insert the lens under the upper eyelid. Then have him look up as you retract and release the lower eyelid over the lens.

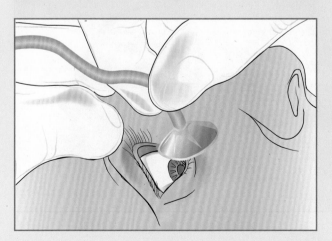

For copious irrigation

Use aseptic technique to set up the IV tubing and the bag or bottle of normal saline solution. Hang the container on an IV pole, fill the IV tubing with the solution, and adjust the drip regulator valve *to ensure an adequate but not forceful flow.* Place all other equipment within easy reach.

Implementation

- Verify the doctor's order.[1]
- Confirm the patient's identity using at least two patient identifiers according to your facility's policy.[2]
- Perform hand hygiene and put on gloves and goggles.[3,4,5]
- Explain the procedure to the patient. If the patient has a chemical burn, ease his anxiety by explaining that irrigation prevents further damage. Answer all questions *to decrease anxiety and increase cooperation.*
- Assist the patient in lying supine. Turn his head slightly toward the affected side *to prevent solution flowing over his nose and into the other eye* (as shown below).

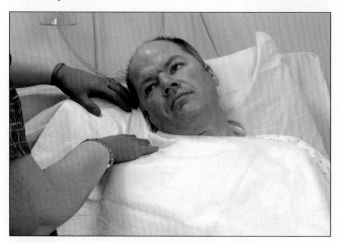

- Place a towel under the patient's head, and let him hold the emesis basin against his affected side *to catch excess solution* (as shown below).

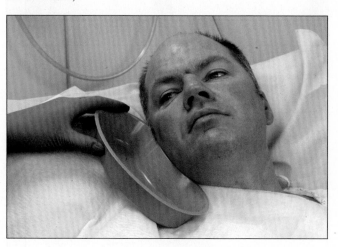

- Using the thumb and index finger of your nondominant hand, separate the patient's eyelids (as shown below).

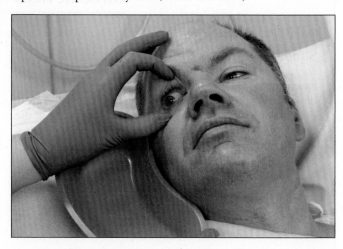

- If ordered, instill ophthalmic anesthetic eyedrops *as a comfort measure.* Use them only once *because repeated use retards healing.*
- *To irrigate the conjunctival cul-de-sac,* continue holding the eyelids apart with your thumb and index finger.
- *To irrigate the upper eyelid (the superior fornix)* use an eyelid retractor. Steady the hand holding the retractor by resting it on the patient's forehead. *The retractor prevents the eyelid from closing involuntarily when solution touches the cornea and conjunctiva.*

Moderate irrigation

- Holding the syringe or sterile ophthalmic irrigant about 1″ (2.5 cm) from the eye, direct a constant, gentle stream at the inner canthus *so that the solution flows across the cornea to the outer canthus* (as shown below).

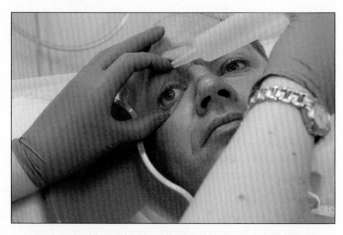

- Evert the lower eyelid and then the upper eyelid *to inspect for retained foreign particles.*
- Remove any foreign particles by gently touching the conjunctiva with a wet, sterile gauze pad. Don't touch the cornea.
- Resume irrigating the eye until it's clean of all visible foreign particles.

Copious irrigation

- Hold the control valve on the IV tubing about 1″ (2.5 cm) above the eye, and direct a constant, gentle stream of normal saline solution at the inner canthus *so that the solution flows across the cornea to the outer canthus.*
- Ask the patient to rotate his eye periodically while you continue the irrigation. *This action may dislodge foreign particles.*
- Evert the lower eyelid and then the upper eyelid *to inspect for retained foreign particles.* (This inspection is especially important when the patient has caustic lime in his eye.)

Aftercare

- After eye irrigation, gently dry the eyelids with a sterile gauze pad, wiping from the inner to the outer canthus. Use a new sterile gauze pad for each wipe. *This reduces the patient's need to rub his eye.*
- Remove and discard your gloves and goggles.
- Perform hand hygiene *to avoid burning from residual chemical contaminants.*[3,4,5]
- Document the procedure.[6]

Special considerations

- Arrange for follow-up care, when necessary.
- When irrigating both eyes, have the patient tilt his head toward the side being irrigated *to avoid cross-contamination.*
- For chemical burns, irrigate each eye for at least 15 minutes with normal saline solution *to dilute and wash the harsh chemical.* (After irrigating any chemical, note the time, date, and chemical for your own reference *in case you develop contact dermatitis.*)
- If an ophthalmic anesthetic agent was used, instruct the patient to avoid touching his eye. *Touching the eye before the anesthetic has worn off may damage the cornea or conjunctiva.*
- Studies have shown that the most comfortable method of irrigation for patients is the use of the Morgan lens in combination with a lidocaine-saline solution.[7]

Documentation

Note the duration of irrigation, the type and amount of solution, and characteristics of the drainage. Record your assessment of the patient's eye before and after irrigation. Also note his response to the procedure.

REFERENCES

1 The Joint Commission. (2012). Standard MM.04.01.01. *Comprehensive accreditation manual for hospitals: The official handbook.* Oakbrook Terrace, IL: The Joint Commission. (Level I)
2 The Joint Commission. (2012). Standard NPSG.01.01.01. *Comprehensive accreditation manual for hospitals: The official handbook.* Oakbrook Terrace, IL: The Joint Commission. (Level I)
3 The Joint Commission. (2012). Standard NPSG.07.01.01. *Comprehensive accreditation manual for hospitals: The official handbook.* Oakbrook Terrace, IL: The Joint Commission. (Level I)
4 World Health Organization. (2009). *WHO guidelines on hand hygiene in health care: First global patient safety challenge. Clean care is safer care.* Geneva, Switzerland: World Health Organization. (Level I)
5 Centers for Disease Control and Prevention. (October 2002). Guideline for hand hygiene in health-care settings. *Morbidity and Mortality Weekly Report, 51*(RR-16), 1–45. (Level I)
6 The Joint Commission. (2012). Standard RC.01.03.01. *Comprehensive accreditation manual for hospitals: The official handbook.* Oakbrook Terrace, IL: The Joint Commission. (Level I)
7 O'Malley, G.F., et al. (2008). Eye irrigation is more comfortable with a lidocaine-containing irrigation solution compared with normal saline. *Journal of Trauma, 64*(5), 1360–1362.

ADDITIONAL REFERENCES

Khodabukus, R., & Tallouzi, M. (2009). Chemical eye injuries. 1: Presentation, clinical features, treatment and prognosis. *Nursing Times, 105*(22), 28–29.
Nettina, S.M. (2010). *Lippincott manual of nursing practice* (9th ed.). Philadelphia, PA: Lippincott Williams & Wilkins.
Rodrigues, Z. (2009). Irrigation of the eye after alkaline and acidic burns. *Emergency Nurse, 17*(8), 26–29.
Taylor, C., et al. (2011). *Fundamentals of nursing: The art and science of nursing care* (7th ed.). Philadelphia, PA: Lippincott Williams & Wilkins.

EYE MEDICATION ADMINISTRATION

During an eye examination, eyedrops can be used to anesthetize the eye, dilate the pupil to facilitate examination, and stain the cornea to identify corneal abrasions, scars, and other anomalies. Eye medications can also be used to lubricate the eye, treat certain eye conditions (such as glaucoma and infections), protect the vision of neonates, and lubricate the eye socket for insertion of a prosthetic eye.

Understanding the ocular effects of medications is important because certain drugs may cause eye disorders or have serious ocular effects. For example, anticholinergics, which are commonly used during eye examinations, can precipitate acute glaucoma in patients with a predisposition to the disorder.

Equipment

Prescribed eye medication ∎ patient's medication record and chart ∎ gloves ∎ warm water or normal saline solution ∎ sterile gauze pads ∎ facial tissues ∎ Optional: ocular dressing.

Preparation of equipment

Make sure the medication is labeled for ophthalmic use.[1] Then check the expiration date. Remember to date the container the first time you use the medication.[2] Follow your facility's policy or manufacturer's recommendations on when to discard an opened eye medication.

If the tip of an eye ointment tube has crusted, turn the tip on a sterile gauze pad *to remove the crust.*

Implementation

- Verify the order on the patient's medication record by checking it against the doctor's order as written in the medical record.[1]
- Perform hand hygiene and put on gloves.[3,4,5]

Instilling eyedrops

To instill eyedrops, pull the lower lid down to expose the conjunctival sac. Have the patient look up and away, and then squeeze the prescribed number of drops into the sac. Release the patient's eyelid, and have him blink to distribute the medication.

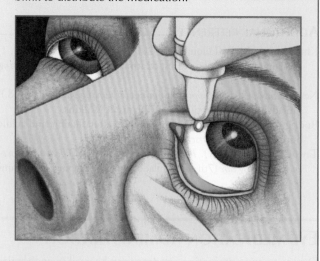

■ Compare the medication label to the doctor's order to verify the correct medication, indication, dose, route, and time of administration.[1]
■ Confirm the patient's identity using at least two patient identifiers according to your facility's policy.[6]
■ Check the patient's medical record for an allergy or other contraindication to the prescribed medication. If an allergy or other contraindication is present, don't administer the medication; notify the doctor.[1]
■ Visually inspect the medication for discoloration or any other loss of integrity. Don't give the medication if its integrity is compromised.[1]
■ If the patient is receiving the medication for the first time, inform the patient or his family about possible significant adverse reactions or other concerns related to administering the medication.
NURSING ALERT *Confirm which eye is being treated because different medications or doses may be ordered for each eye.*
■ If your facility uses a bar code scanning system, be sure to scan your ID badge, the patient's ID bracelet, and the medication's bar code.
■ Explain the procedure to the patient and provide privacy. Answer all questions *to decrease anxiety and increase cooperation.*
■ If the patient is wearing an eye dressing, remove it by gently pulling it down and away from his forehead. Take care not to contaminate your hands.
■ Remove any discharge by cleaning around the eye with sterile gauze pads moistened with warm water or normal saline solution. With the patient's eye closed, clean from the inner to the outer canthus, using a fresh sterile gauze pad for each stroke.

■ *To remove crusted secretions around the eye,* moisten a gauze pad with warm water or normal saline solution. Ask the patient to close the eye, and then place the gauze pad over it for 1 or 2 minutes. Remove the pad, and then reapply moist sterile gauze pads, as necessary, until the secretions are soft enough to be removed without traumatizing the mucosa.
■ Remove and discard gloves. Perform hand hygiene and put on gloves.[3,4,5]
■ Have the patient sit or lie in the supine position. Instruct him to tilt his head back and toward the side of the affected eye *so that excess medication can flow away from the tear duct, minimizing systemic absorption through the nasal mucosa.*

For eyedrop administration
■ Remove the dropper cap from the medication container, if necessary, and draw the medication into it. Be careful to avoid contaminating the dropper tip or bottle top.
■ Before instilling the eyedrops, instruct the patient to look up and away. *This position moves the cornea away from the lower lid and minimizes the risk of touching the cornea with the dropper if the patient blinks.*
■ You can steady the hand holding the dropper by resting it against the patient's forehead. Then, with your other hand, gently pull down the lower lid of the affected eye and instill the drops in the conjunctival sac. Try to avoid placing the drops directly on the eyeball *to prevent the patient from experiencing discomfort.* (See *Instilling eyedrops.*) If you're instilling more than one medication, you should wait 5 or more minutes between instillations.

For eye ointment
■ Squeeze a small ribbon of medication on the edge of the conjunctival sac from the inner to the outer canthus. Cut off the ribbon by turning the tube. You can steady the hand holding the medication tube by bracing it against the patient's forehead or cheek. If you're applying more than one ribbon of medication, wait 10 minutes before applying the second medication.

For all eye medication
■ After instilling the medication, instruct the patient to close his eyes gently, without squeezing the lids shut. Tell the patient to blink.
■ Use a clean tissue to remove any excess solution or ointment leaking from the eye. Remember to use a fresh tissue for each eye *to prevent cross-contamination.*
■ Apply a new eye dressing, if necessary.
■ Return the medication to the storage area. Make sure you store it according to the label's instructions.
■ Remove and discard gloves. Perform hand hygiene.[3,4,5]
■ Document the procedure.[7]

Special considerations
■ When administering an eye medication that may be absorbed systemically (such as atropine), gently press your thumb on the inner canthus for 1 to 2 minutes after instilling drops while the patient closes his eyes. *Doing so helps prevent medication from flowing into the tear duct.*

■ *To maintain the drug container's sterility,* never touch the tip of the bottle or dropper to the patient's eyeball, lids, or lashes. Discard any solution remaining in the dropper before returning the dropper to the bottle. If the dropper or bottle tip has become contaminated, discard it and obtain another sterile dropper. *To prevent cross-contamination,* never use a container of eye medication for more than one patient.

■ If an ointment and drops have been ordered, the drops should be instilled first.

Complications

Instillation of some eye medications may cause transient burning, itching, and redness. Rarely, systemic effects may occur.

Patient teaching

Teach the patient to instill eye medications *so that he can continue treatment at home, if necessary.* Review the procedure and ask for a return demonstration.

Documentation

Record the medication instilled or applied, eye or eyes treated, and date, time, and dose. Note any adverse effects and the patient's response. Document any patient teaching.

REFERENCES

1 The Joint Commission. (2012). Standard MM.06.01.01. *Comprehensive accreditation manual for hospitals: The official handbook.* Oakbrook Terrace, IL: The Joint Commission. (Level I)
2 The Joint Commission. (2012). Standard MM.04.01.01. *Comprehensive accreditation manual for hospitals: The official handbook.* Oakbrook Terrace, IL: The Joint Commission. (Level I)
3 The Joint Commission. (2012). Standard NPSG.07.01.01. *Comprehensive accreditation manual for hospitals: The official handbook.* Oakbrook Terrace, IL: The Joint Commission. (Level I)
4 World Health Organization. (2009). *WHO guidelines on hand hygiene in health care: First global patient safety challenge. Clean care is safer care.* Geneva, Switzerland: World Health Organization. (Level I)
5 Centers for Disease Control and Prevention. (October 2002). Guideline for hand hygiene in health-care settings. *Morbidity and Mortality Weekly Report, 51*(RR-16), 1–45. (Level I)
6 The Joint Commission. (2012). Standard NPSG.01.01.01. *Comprehensive accreditation manual for hospitals: The official handbook.* Oakbrook Terrace, IL: The Joint Commission. (Level I)
7 The Joint Commission. (2012). Standard RC.01.03.01. *Comprehensive accreditation manual for hospitals: The official handbook.* Oakbrook Terrace, IL: The Joint Commission. (Level I)

ADDITIONAL REFERENCES

Nettina, S.M. (2010). *Lippincott manual of nursing practice* (9th ed.). Philadelphia, PA: Lippincott Williams & Wilkins.
Taylor, C., et al. (2011). *Fundamentals of nursing: The art and science of nursing care* (7th ed.). Philadelphia, PA: Lippincott Williams & Wilkins.

FALL PREVENTION AND MANAGEMENT

Falls are a major cause of injury and death among elderly people. In fact, the older the person, the more likely he is to die of a fall or its complications. In people age 75 or older, falls account for three times as many accidental deaths as motor vehicle accidents.

Factors that contribute to falls among elderly patients include lengthy convalescent periods, a greater risk of incomplete recovery, medications, increasing physical disability, and impaired vision, hearing, or mental status. For example, once impaired, equilibrium takes longer to be restored in elderly people than in younger adults. Naturally, loss of balance increases the risk of falling. Besides causing physical harm, injuries from falls can trigger psychological problems, leading to a loss of self-confidence and hastening dependence and a move to a long-term care facility or nursing home.

Falls may be caused by extrinsic or environmental factors, such as poor lighting, slippery throw rugs, highly waxed floors, unfamiliar surroundings, or misuse of assistive devices. However, they usually result from intrinsic or physiologic factors, such as temporary muscle paralysis, vertigo, orthostatic hypotension, central nervous system lesions, dementia, failing eyesight, and decreased strength or coordination.[1]

In a health care facility, an accidental fall can change a short stay for a minor problem into a prolonged stay for serious and possibly life-threatening problems. The risk of falling is highest during the first week of a stay in a health care facility or nursing home. (See *Who's at risk for a fall?* page 298.)

Equipment
For fall management

Stethoscope ■ sphygmomanometer ■ analgesics ■ cold and warm compresses ■ pillows ■ blankets ■ emergency resuscitation equipment (crash cart), if needed ■ electrocardiogram (ECG) monitor, if needed.

Preparation of equipment

If you're helping a fallen patient, send an assistant to collect the assessment or resuscitation equipment you need.

Implementation

■ Confirm the patient's identity using at least two patient identifiers according to your facility's policy.[3]

For fall prevention

■ Assess your patient's risk of falling at least once each shift and according to your facility policy.[4] Your facility may require more frequent assessments. Note any changes in the patient's condition (such as decreased mental status) that may increase his

Who's at risk for a fall?[2]

Preventing falls begins with identifying the patients at greatest risk. Consider a patient with one or more of the following characteristics to be at risk.
- Age 75 or older
- Poor general health with a chronic disease
- Specific comorbidities (dementia, hip fracture, type 2 diabetes, Parkinson's disease, arthritis, depression)
- A history of a recent fall
- Altered mental status
- Use of assistive devices
- Gait or balance impairment
- Improperly fitted shoes or slippers
- Inappropriate use of restraints
- Urge urinary incontinence
- Sensory deficits—particularly visual deficits
- Neurologic deficits
- Use of high-risk medications, such as diuretics, strong analgesics, antipsychotics, and hypnotics

chances of falling. If you decide that he's at risk, take steps to reduce the danger.
- Correct potential dangers in the patient's room. Position the call light so that he can reach it. Provide adequate nighttime lighting.
- Place the patient's personal belongings and assistive devices (purse, wallet, books, tissues, urinal, commode, and cane or walker) within easy reach.
- Instruct the patient to rise slowly from a supine position *to avoid possible dizziness and loss of balance.*
- Keep the bed in its lowest position *so the patient can easily reach the floor when he gets out of bed. This position also reduces the distance to the floor in case he falls.* Lock the bed's wheels. If side rails are to be raised, observe the patient frequently.
- Advise the patient to wear nonskid footwear.
- Respond promptly to the patient's call light *to help limit the number of times he gets out of bed without help.*
- Check the patient at least every 2 hours. Check a high-risk patient every 30 minutes or according to your facility's policy.
- Alert other caregivers to the patient's risk of falling and to the interventions you've implemented.[4]
- Consider other precautions, such as placing two high-risk patients in the same room and having someone with them at all times.
- Encourage the patient to perform active range-of-motion (ROM) exercises *to improve flexibility and coordination.*
- Review medications that may contribute to a fall. (See *Medications associated with falls.*)
- Document the procedure.[5]

For fall management
- If you're with a patient as he falls and you can do so without significant risk of injury to yourself, try to break his fall with your body.

- Support him and guide him to the floor, particularly his head and trunk. If possible, help him to a supine position.
- Concentrate on maintaining proper body alignment while guiding the patient to the floor *to keep the center of gravity within your support base.* Spread your feet *to widen your support base.* Remember, the wider the base, the better your balance will be. Bend your knees—rather than your back—*to support the patient and to avoid injuring yourself.*
- Remain calm and stay with the patient *to prevent any further injury.*
- Ask another nurse to collect any tools you may need, such as a stethoscope, a sphygmomanometer and, if necessary, an ECG monitor.
- Assess the patient's circulation, airway, and breathing *to be sure the fall wasn't caused by respiratory or cardiac arrest.* If the patient is unresponsive and his breathing is abnormal (such as gasping for air) or absent, call a code and have a coworker obtain a defibrillator. Check for a pulse; if you don't feel a pulse within 10 seconds, immediately begin chest compressions. Compress the adult chest at a rate of at least 100 compressions per minute, with a compression depth of at least 2″ (5 cm). After compressions are started, deliver rescue breaths (each over 1 second) using a compression ratio of 30 chest compressions to 2 ventilations. When the defibrillator arrives, check the patient's rhythm and defibrillate if the patient has a shockable rhythm; otherwise continue cardiopulmonary resuscitation.[6]
- *To determine the extent of the patient's injuries,* look for lacerations, abrasions, and obvious deformities. Note any deviations from the patient's baseline condition. Notify the doctor. Determine if there was head trauma, which requires further diagnostic evaluation to rule out subdural hematoma.

NURSING ALERT *Patients taking anticoagulants or on aspirin therapy who experience head trauma are at increased risk for subdural hematoma.*

- If you weren't present during the fall, ask the patient or a witness what happened. Ask if the patient experienced pain or a change in level of consciousness.
- Don't move the patient until you evaluate his status fully. Provide reassurance, as needed, and observe for such signs and symptoms as confusion, tremor, weakness, pain, and dizziness.
- Assess the patient's limb strength and motion. Don't perform ROM exercises if you suspect a fracture or if the patient complains of any odd sensations or limited movement. If you suspect a disorder, don't move the patient until a doctor examines him.
- While the patient lies on the floor until the doctor arrives, offer pillows and blankets *for comfort.* If you suspect a spinal cord injury, don't place a pillow under his head; position a hard neck collar instead.
- If you don't detect any problems, return the patient to his bed with the help of another staff member. Never try to lift a patient alone *because you may injure yourself or the patient.*
- Take steps to control bleeding (if indicated) and to obtain an X-ray if you suspect a fracture. Provide first aid for minor injuries, as needed. Then monitor the patient's status for the next 48 hours or according to your facility's policy.[1]

- Even if the patient shows no signs of distress or has sustained only minor injuries, monitor his vital signs and neurologic assessments according to your facility's policy and until the patient is stable. Notify the doctor if you note any change from the baseline.
- Perform necessary measures to relieve the patient's pain and discomfort. Give analgesics, as ordered, following safe medication administration practices. Apply cold compresses for the first 24 hours and warm compresses, or according to the doctor's orders.
- Reassess the patient's environment and his risk of falling. Talk to him about the fall. Discuss why it occurred and how he thinks it could have been prevented. Refer patients to physical therapy, as indicated by the doctor, for gait retraining. Review the events that preceded the fall. Did the patient change position abruptly? Does he wear corrective lenses, and was he wearing them when he fell? Review medications that may have contributed to the fall, such as tranquilizers and opioids. (See *Medications associated with falls.*)
- Assess the patient for gait disturbances or improper use of a cane, crutches, or a walker.
- Perform hand hygiene.[7,8,9]
- Complete an incident report based on your facility's policy. Document any assessments, injuries, or interventions performed.[5]

Special considerations

- If your facility doesn't already have one, consider beginning a fall-prevention program, including an interdisciplinary fall team.

NURSING ALERT *Perform a risk assessment for falls on all admitted patients.*[4]

- For patients assessed as high risk for falls, consider using a device such as a pressure-pad alarm that's used in chairs and beds to signal when a patient gets up.[4] Alternatively, the patient can wear an alarm device just above the knee that sounds when the patient moves his leg to a vertical position.
- *To promote patient safety,* add an appropriate notation (such as "Risk for falls") to the Kardex and chart.[4]
- Provide emotional support. Let the elderly patient know that you recognize his limitations and acknowledge his fears. Point out measures that you'll take to provide a safe environment.
- After a fall, review the patient's medical history *to determine whether he's at risk for other complications.* For example, if he hit his head, check his history to see whether he takes anticoagulants. If he does, he's at greater risk for intracranial bleeding, and you'll need to monitor him accordingly.

Patient teaching

Teach the patient how to fall safely. Show him how to protect his hands and face. If he uses a walker or a wheelchair, demonstrate how to cope with and recover from a fall. Instruct him to survey the room for a low, sturdy, supportive piece of furniture (such as a coffee table). Then review the proper procedure for lifting himself off the floor and either standing up with the walker or getting into the wheelchair.

Before discharge, teach the patient and his family how to prevent accidental falls at home by correcting common household

---

Medications associated with falls

This chart highlights some classes of drugs that are commonly prescribed for older patients and the possible adverse effects of each that may increase a patient's risk of falling.

DRUG CLASS	ADVERSE EFFECTS
Diuretics	Hypovolemia, orthostatic hypotension, electrolyte imbalance, urinary incontinence
Antihypertensives, beta-adrenergic blockers, nitrates, vasodilators	Hypotension, syncope
Tricyclic antidepressants	Orthostatic hypotension
Antipsychotics	Orthostatic hypotension, muscle rigidity, sedation
Benzodiazepines and antihistamines	Excessive sedation, confusion, paradoxical agitation, loss of balance
Opioids	Hypotension, sedation, motor incoordination, agitation
Hypnotics	Excessive sedation, ataxia, poor balance, confusion, paradoxical agitation
Antidiabetic drugs	Acute hypoglycemia

---

hazards. Encourage them to take steps to ensure safety. (See *Promoting safety in the home,* page 300.)

As needed, refer the patient to the local visiting nurse association so that nursing services can continue after discharge and during convalescence.

Complications

Complications from a fall may include injury to the patient or to the health care worker attempting to assist the patient who has fallen.

Documentation

Document any measures taken to help prevent a fall, including patient and family teaching and their understanding of the teaching.

After a fall, complete a detailed incident report according to your facility policy to help track frequent patient falls so that prevention measures can be used with high-risk patients. Generally,

PATIENT TEACHING

Promoting safety in the home

Before your patient leaves the health care facility, provide him with the following tips for ensuring a safe home environment:

■ Secure all carpets and floor coverings around the edges, and tack down worn spots. Never use lightweight, loose mats or rugs on bare floors.

■ Make sure potential hazards such as stairs are well lighted. White paint on either side of a staircase can enhance visibility.

■ Install strong banisters along all indoor and outdoor steps.

■ Use a bedside lamp or low-wattage night-light in the bedroom *to avoid the need to grope around in the dark when getting out of bed.*

■ Fit secure handrails in convenient places in the shower and bathtub and around the toilet. Use nonskid mats inside and alongside every tub or shower.

■ Minimize clutter. Store children's toys, especially those on wheels, when not in use.

■ Walk carefully if a pet, such as a dog or a cat, is present.

■ Secure wires from electrical appliances to walls or moldings.

■ Store frequently used clothing and other items in places where they can be reached without standing on a stool or chair.

■ Select well-fitting shoes with nonskid soles, avoid long robes, and wear glasses if needed *to reduce the risk of accidental slips and falls.*

■ Sit on the edge of a bed or chair for a few minutes before rising.

■ Use a walking stick, cane, or walker whenever an unsteady feeling arises—but always inspect the condition of assistive devices before use.

this report isn't considered part of the patient's record. A copy, however, will go to the facility's administrator, who will evaluate care given on the unit and propose new safety policies, as appropriate. It may also go to other patient care teams, such as fall prevention teams.

The incident report should note where and when the fall occurred, how the patient was found, and in what position. Include the events preceding the fall, the names of witnesses, the patient's reaction to the fall, and a detailed description of his condition based on assessment findings. The patient's statement of the event is also included. Note any interventions taken and the names of other staff members who helped care for him after the fall. Record the doctor's name and the date and time that he was notified as well as the patient's health care power of attorney's name and the date and time notified. Include a copy of the doctor's report. Also note whether the patient was sent for diagnostic tests or transferred to another unit.

Include all of the information about the fall in the patient's record. Also document his vital signs and whether you're monitoring the patient for a severe complication.

REFERENCES

1 Gray-Micelli, D. (2008). "Falls: Nursing Standard of Practice Protocol: Fall Prevention" [Online]. Accessed September 2011 via the Web at http://consultgerirn.org/topics/falls/want_to_know_more (Level VII)

2 American Geriatrics Society, British Geriatrics Society, and American Academy of Orthopaedic Surgeons Panel on Falls Prevention. (2001, updated 2008). Guideline for the prevention of falls in older persons. *Journal of the American Geriatrics Society, 49*(5), 664–672.

3 The Joint Commission. (2012). Standard NPSG.01.01.01. *Comprehensive accreditation manual for hospitals: The official handbook.* Oakbrook Terrace, IL: The Joint Commission. (Level I)

4 The Joint Commission. (2012). Standard PC.01.02.08. *Comprehensive accreditation manual for hospitals: The official handbook.* Oakbrook Terrace, IL: The Joint Commission. (Level I)

5 The Joint Commission. (2012). Standard RC.01.03.01. *Comprehensive accreditation manual for hospitals: The official handbook.* Oakbrook Terrace, IL: The Joint Commission. (Level I)

6 American Heart Association. (2010). 2010 American Heart Association guidelines for cardiopulmonary resuscitation and emergency cardiovascular care. *Circulation, 122*(Suppl. 3), S676–S684. (Level I)

7 The Joint Commission. (2012). Standard NPSG.07.01.01. *Comprehensive accreditation manual for hospitals: The official handbook.* Oakbrook Terrace, IL: The Joint Commission. (Level I)

8 Centers for Disease Control and Prevention. (October 2002). Guideline for hand hygiene in health-care settings. *Morbidity and Mortality Weekly Report, 51*(RR-16), 1–45. (Level 1)

9 World Health Organization. (2009). *WHO guidelines on hand hygiene in health care: First global patient safety challenge. Clean care is safer care.* Geneva, Switzerland: World Health Organization. (Level I)

ADDITIONAL REFERENCES

Boddice, S.D., & Kogan, P. (2009). Research on patient safety: Falls and medications. *Home Healthcare Nurse, 27*(9), 555–560.

Hughes, K., et al. (2008). Older persons' perception of risk of falling: Implications for fall-prevention campaigns. *American Journal of Public Health, 98*(2), 351–357.

Oliver, D. (2007). Preventing falls and fall injuries in hospital: A major risk management challenge. *Clinical Risk, 13*(5), 173–178.

FECAL IMPACTION REMOVAL, DIGITAL

Fecal impaction is a large, hard, dry mass of stool in the folds of the rectum and, at times, in the sigmoid colon that results from prolonged retention and accumulation of stool. Common causes include poor bowel habits, inactivity, dehydration, improper diet (especially inadequate fluid intake), constipation-inducing drugs, and incomplete bowel cleaning after a barium enema or barium swallow. Digital removal of fecal impaction is used when oil retention and cleansing enemas, suppositories, and laxatives fail to clear the impaction. It typically requires a doctor's order.

This procedure is contraindicated during pregnancy; after rectal, genitourinary, abdominal, perineal, or gynecologic reconstructive surgery; in patients with myocardial infarction, coronary insufficiency, pulmonary embolus, heart failure, heart block, and Stokes-Adams syndrome (without pacemaker treatment); and in patients with GI or vaginal bleeding, hemorrhoids, rectal polyps, or blood dyscrasias.

Equipment

Gloves (two pairs) ▪ linen-saver pad ▪ bedpan ▪ plastic disposal bag ▪ soap ▪ water-filled basin ▪ towel ▪ water-soluble lubricant ▪ washcloth ▪ bath blanket.

Implementation

▪ Gather the appropriate equipment.
▪ Verify the doctor's order.
▪ Perform hand hygiene and put on gloves.[1,2,3]
▪ Confirm the patient's identity using at least two patient identifiers according to your facility's policy.[4]
▪ Explain the procedure to the patient and provide privacy. Answer all questions *to decrease anxiety and increase cooperation.*
▪ Perform an abdominal assessment.
▪ Assess the patient's pulse rate before performing the procedure *because anal stimulation may cause a vagal response.*
▪ Position the patient on his left side and flex his knees *to allow easier access to the sigmoid colon and rectum.* (See *Side-lying position.*)
▪ Drape the patient with a bath blanket, and place a linen-saver pad beneath the buttocks *to prevent soiling the bed linens.*
▪ Moisten a gloved index finger with water-soluble lubricant *to reduce friction during insertion, thereby avoiding injury to sensitive tissue.*
▪ Instruct the patient to breathe deeply *to promote relaxation.* Then gently insert your lubricated index finger beyond the anal sphincter until you touch the impaction. Rotate the finger gently around the stool *to dislodge and break it into small fragments.* Then work the fragments downward to the end of the rectum, and remove each one separately.
▪ Before removing your finger, gently stimulate the anal sphincter with a circular motion two or three times *to increase peristalsis and encourage evacuation.*
▪ Remove your finger and remove and discard your gloves. Perform hand hygiene and put on gloves. Then clean the anal area with soap and water, and pat dry with a towel.
▪ Offer the patient the bedpan or commode *because digital manipulation stimulates the urge to defecate.*
▪ Place disposable items in the plastic bag, and discard properly. If necessary, clean the bedpan and return it to the bedside stand.
▪ Remove your gloves and perform hand hygiene.[1,2,3]
▪ Document the procedure.[5]

Special considerations

▪ If the patient experiences pain, nausea, rectal bleeding, changes in pulse rate or skin color, diaphoresis, or syncope, stop the procedure immediately and notify the doctor.

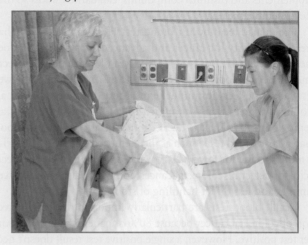

Side-lying position

Use a drawsheet or bath blanket to place the patient in a side-lying position.

Complications

Digital removal of fecal impaction can stimulate the vagus nerve and may decrease heart rate and cause syncope.

Documentation

Record the time and date of the procedure, the patient's response, and stool color, consistency, and odor.

REFERENCES

1 The Joint Commission. (2012). Standard NPSG.07.01.01. *Comprehensive accreditation manual for hospitals: The official handbook.* Oakbrook Terrace, IL: The Joint Commission. (Level I)
2 Centers for Disease Control and Prevention. (October 2002). Guideline for hand hygiene in health-care settings. *Morbidity and Mortality Weekly Report, 51*(RR-16), 1–45. (Level 1)
3 World Health Organization. (2009). *WHO guidelines on hand hygiene in health care: First global patient safety challenge. Clean care is safer care.* Geneva, Switzerland: World Health Organization. (Level I)
4 The Joint Commission. (2012). Standard NPSG.01.01.01. *Comprehensive accreditation manual for hospitals: The official handbook.* Oakbrook Terrace, IL: The Joint Commission. (Level I)
5 The Joint Commission. (2012). Standard RC.01.03.01. *Comprehensive accreditation manual for hospitals: The official handbook.* Oakbrook Terrace, IL: The Joint Commission. (Level I)

ADDITIONAL REFERENCES

Craven, R.F., & Hirnle, C.J. (2009). *Fundamentals of nursing: Human health and function* (6th ed.). Philadelphia, PA: Lippincott Williams & Wilkins.
Taylor, C., et al. (2011). *Fundamentals of nursing: The art and science of nursing care* (7th ed.). Philadelphia, PA: Lippincott Williams & Wilkins.

FECAL OCCULT BLOOD TESTS

Fecal occult blood tests help to determine the presence of occult blood (hidden GI bleeding) and to distinguish between true melena and melena-like stools. Certain medications, such as iron supplements and bismuth compounds, can darken stools so that they resemble melena.

The guaiac fecal occult blood test Hemoccult SENSA has greater sensitivity for cancer and advanced adenomas than does the Hemoccult II. Both tests produce a blue reaction in a fecal smear if occult blood loss exceeds 2 to 3 mL in 24 hours. A newer test called the fecal immunochemical test (FIT) detects human globin, a protein that—along with heme—constitutes human hemoglobin. This makes the FIT more specific for human blood than guaiac-based tests, such as the Hemoccult SENSA. The FIT is more specific for lower GI-type bleeding, improving its specificity for detecting colorectal cancer. Some FITs also require fewer samples and less direct handling of stool.

Occult blood tests are particularly important for early detection of colorectal cancer because 80% of patients with this disorder test positive. However, a single positive test result doesn't necessarily confirm GI bleeding or indicate colorectal cancer. To confirm a positive result, the test must be repeated at least three times while the patient follows a special diet, according to the manufacturer's recommendations for the particular occult blood test. Even then, a confirmed positive test doesn't necessarily indicate colorectal cancer. However, it does indicate the need for further diagnostic studies because GI bleeding can also result from noncancerous causes, such as ulcers, colon polyps, and diverticula.

These tests are easily performed on collected specimens or smears from digital rectal examination.

Equipment

Appropriate test kit ▪ laboratory biohazard transport bag ▪ wooden applicator ▪ gloves.

Implementation

- Verify the doctor's order.
- Gather the appropriate equipment.
- Perform hand hygiene and put on gloves.[1,2,3]
- Confirm the patient's identity using at least two patient identifiers according to your facility's policy.[4]
- Explain the procedure to the patient and check the patient's history for medications that may interfere with the test.
- Collect a stool specimen. (See "Stool specimen collection," page 674.)

Hemoccult slide test

- Open the flap on the slide packet, and use a wooden applicator to apply a thin smear of the stool specimen to the guaiac-impregnated filter paper exposed in box A. Or, after performing a digital rectal examination, wipe the finger you used for the examination on a square of the filter paper.
- Apply a second smear from another part of the specimen to the filter paper exposed in box B *because some parts of the specimen may not contain blood.*

- Allow the specimen to dry for 3 to 5 minutes.
- Open the flap on the reverse side of the slide package, and place two drops of Hemoccult developing solution on the paper over each smear. A blue reaction will appear in 30 to 60 seconds if the test is positive.
- Record the results and discard the slide package.

Fecal immunochemical test (FIT)

- Open the flap of the test card.
- Remove one of the long-handled brushes from the kit. Gently brush the surface of the stool with the brush; then rinse the brush in the toilet water surrounding the stool.
- Dab the brush onto the test card and close the flap.
- Place the test card in the laboratory biohazard transport bag and send it to the laboratory.

Completing the procedure

- Remove and discard your gloves and perform hand hygiene.[1,2,3]
- Document the procedure.[5]

Special considerations

- Test samples from several different portions of the same specimen *because occult blood from the upper GI tract isn't always evenly dispersed throughout the formed stool; likewise, blood from colorectal bleeding may occur mostly on the outer stool surface.*
- Check the expiration date on Hemoccult slides and developer, and protect unused slides from heat, moisture, light, and chemicals.
- Don't collect specimens during or until 3 days after a female patient's menstrual period *to avoid a false-positive test resulting from contamination of the specimen.*
- Keep in mind that ingestion of 2 to 5 mL of blood (from bleeding gums, for instance), active bleeding from hemorrhoids, or hematuria may also produce false-positive results.
- If repeated testing is necessary after a positive screening test, explain the test to the patient. Instruct him to maintain a high-fiber diet and to refrain from eating red meat, poultry, fish, turnips, and horseradish for 48 to 72 hours before the test as well as throughout the collection period *because these substances may alter test results.*
- As ordered, have the patient discontinue use of iron preparations, bromides, iodides, rauwolfia derivatives, indomethacin, colchicine, salicylates, potassium, bismuth compounds, steroids, and ascorbic acid for 48 to 72 hours before the test and during the test period *to ensure accurate test results and to avoid the possible bleeding that some of these compounds can cause.*

Patient teaching

If the patient will be using the Hemoccult slide packet or the FIT at home, advise him to complete the label on the slide packet before specimen collection. If he'll be using a ColoCARE test packet, inform him that this test is a preliminary screen for occult blood in his stool. Tell him he won't have to obtain a stool specimen to perform the test but that he should follow your instructions carefully. (See *Home tests for fecal occult blood.*)

Documentation

Record the time and date of the test, the result, and any unusual characteristics of the stool tested. Report positive results to the doctor. Document any patient teaching provided.

REFERENCES

1 The Joint Commission. (2012). Standard NPSG.07.01.01. *Comprehensive accreditation manual for hospitals: The official handbook.* Oakbrook Terrace, IL: The Joint Commission. (Level I)
2 Centers for Disease Control and Prevention. (October 2002). Guideline for hand hygiene in health-care settings. *Morbidity and Mortality Weekly Report, 51*(RR-16), 1–45. (Level 1)
3 World Health Organization. (2009). *WHO guidelines on hand hygiene in health care: First global patient safety challenge. Clean care is safer care.* Geneva, Switzerland: World Health Organization. (Level I)
4 The Joint Commission. (2012). Standard NPSG.01.01.01. *Comprehensive accreditation manual for hospitals: The official handbook.* Oakbrook Terrace, IL: The Joint Commission. (Level I)
5 The Joint Commission. (2012). Standard RC.01.03.01. *Comprehensive accreditation manual for hospitals: The official handbook.* Oakbrook Terrace, IL: The Joint Commission. (Level I)

ADDITIONAL REFERENCES

Allison, J.E. (2010). FIT: A valuable but underutilized screening test for colorectal cancer—It's time for a change. *American Journal of Gastroenterology, 105*(9), 2026–2028.
Brenner, H., et al. (2010). Low-dose aspirin use and performance of immunochemical fecal occult blood tests. *JAMA, 304*(22), 2513–2520.
Daly, J., et al. (2009). Colorectal cancer screening. *AJN, 109*(10), 60–62.
Deciphering diagnostics: What you need to know about FOBT (2008). *Nursing Made Incredibly Easy!, 6*(4), 32–34.
Fischbach, F., & Dunning, M.B. (2009). *A manual of laboratory and diagnostic tests* (8th ed.). Philadelphia, PA: Lippincott Williams & Wilkins.
Lippincott's visual encyclopedia of clinical skills. (2009). Philadelphia, PA: Lippincott Williams & Wilkins.
Nettina, S.M. (2010). *Lippincott manual of nursing practice* (9th ed.). Philadelphia, PA: Lippincott Williams & Wilkins.
Peters, D. (2008). Colon cancer screening: Recommendations and barriers to patient participation. *The Nurse Practitioner: The American Journal of Primary Health Care, 33*(12), 14–20.
Smeltzer, S.C., et al. (2010). *Brunner & Suddarth's textbook of medical-surgical nursing* (12th ed.). Philadelphia, PA: Lippincott Williams & Wilkins.

FEEDING

When confusion, arm or hand immobility, injury, weakness, or restrictions on activities or positions may prevent a patient from feeding himself, feeding the patient becomes a key nursing responsibility. Injured or debilitated patients may experience depression and subsequent anorexia. Meeting such patients' nutritional needs requires determining food preferences; conducting the feeding in a

Home tests for fecal occult blood

Most fecal occult blood tests require the patient to collect a specimen of his stool and smear some of it on a slide. In contrast, some tests don't require the patient to handle stool, making the procedure safer and simpler. One example is a test called ColoCARE.

If the patient is to perform the ColoCARE test at home, tell him to avoid red meat and vitamin C supplements for 2 days before the test. He should check with his doctor about discontinuing any medications before the test. Some drugs that may interfere with test results include aspirin, indomethacin, corticosteroids, reserpine, dietary supplements, anticancer drugs, and anticoagulants.

Tell the patient to flush the toilet twice just before performing the test *to remove any toilet-cleaning chemicals from the tank.* Tell him to defecate into the toilet but to throw no toilet paper into the bowl. Within 5 minutes, he should remove the test pad from its pouch and float it printed side up on the surface of the water. Tell him to watch the pad for 15 to 30 seconds for any evidence of blue or green color changes, and have him record the result on the reply card.

Emphasize that he should perform this test with three consecutive bowel movements and then send the completed card to his doctor. However, he should call his doctor immediately if he notes a positive color change in the first test.

friendly, unhurried manner; encouraging self-feeding to promote independence and dignity; and documenting intake and output. (See *Recording fluid intake and output,* page 304.)

Equipment

Meal tray ▪ overbed table ▪ linen-saver pad or towels ▪ clean linens ▪ disinfectant ▪ flexible straws ▪ basin of water ▪ soap ▪ washcloth ▪ hand towel ▪ spoon or feeding syringe ▪ Optional: assistive feeding devices.

Implementation

▪ Gather the appropriate equipment.
▪ Perform hand hygiene.[1,2,3]
▪ Confirm the patient's identity using at least two patient identifiers according to your facility's policy.[4]
▪ Explain the procedure to the patient *to decrease anxiety and increase cooperation.*
▪ *Because many adults consider being fed demeaning,* allow the patient some control over mealtime, such as letting her set the pace of the meal or decide the order in which she wants to eat various foods.

Recording fluid intake and output

Accurate intake and output records help evaluate a patient's fluid and electrolyte balance, suggest various diagnoses,
and influence the choice of fluid therapy. These records are mandatory for patients with burns, renal failure, electrolyte imbalance, recent surgical procedures, heart failure, or severe vomiting and diarrhea as well as for patients receiving diuretics or corticosteroids. Intake and output records are also significant in monitoring patients with nasogastric (NG) tubes or drainage collection devices and for those receiving IV therapy.

Fluid intake comprises all fluid entering the patient's body, including beverages, fluids contained in solid foods taken by mouth, and foods that aren't liquid at room temperature, such as flavored gelatin, custard, ice cream, and some beverages. Additional intake includes GI instillations, bladder irrigations, fluids ingested with medications, and IV fluids.

Fluid output consists of all fluid that leaves the patient's body, including urine, loose stools, vomitus, aspirated fluid loss, and drainage from surgical drains, NG tubes, and chest tubes.

When recording fluid intake and output, enlist the patient's help if possible. Record amount in milliliters (mL). Measure; don't estimate. For a small child, weigh diapers if appropriate. Monitor intake and output during each shift, and notify the doctor if amounts differ significantly over a 24-hour period. Document your findings in the appropriate location; describe any fluid restrictions and the patient's compliance.

■ Before the meal tray arrives, give the patient soap, a basin of water or a wet washcloth, and a hand towel *to clean her hands.* If necessary, wash her hands for her (as shown below).

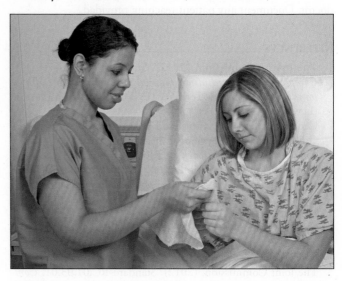

■ Wipe the overbed table with soap and water or disinfectant, especially if a urinal or bedpan was on it.
■ Confirm that the right tray has been delivered to the right patient.
■ Check the tray to make sure it contains foods and fluids appropriate for the patient's condition and prescribed diet.
■ Encourage the patient to feed herself if appropriate. If she's restricted to the prone or the supine position but can use her arms and hands, encourage her to try foods she can pick up, such as sandwiches. If she can assume Fowler's or semi-Fowler's position but has limited use of her arms or hands, teach her how to use assistive feeding devices. (See *Using assistive feeding devices.*)
■ If necessary, tuck a napkin or towel under her chin *to protect her gown from spills* (as shown below). Use a linen-saver pad or towel *to protect bed linens.*

■ Raise the head of the bed if allowed (as shown below). *Fowler's or semi-Fowler's position makes swallowing easier and reduces the risk of aspiration and choking.*

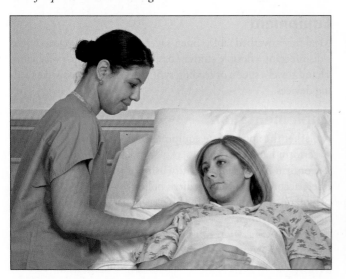

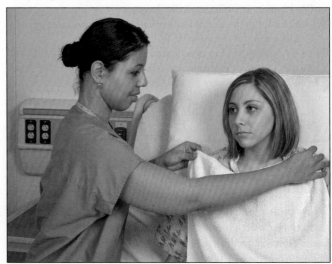

EQUIPMENT

Using assistive feeding devices

Various feeding devices can help the patient who has limited arm mobility, grasp, range of motion (ROM), or coordination. Before introducing your patient to an assistive feeding device, assess her ability to master it. Don't introduce a device she can't manage. If her condition is progressively disabling, encourage her to use the device only until her mastery of it falters.

Introduce the assistive device before mealtime, with the patient seated in a natural position. Explain its purpose, show the patient how to use it, and encourage her to practice. After meals, wash the device thoroughly and store it in the patient's bedside stand. Document the patient's progress and share it with staff and family members *to help reinforce the patient's independence*. Specific devices include the following:

Plate guard
This device blocks food from spilling off the plate. Attach the guard to the side of the plate opposite the hand the patient uses to feed herself. Guiding the patient's hand, show her how to push food against the guard *to secure it on the utensil*. Then have her try again with food of a different consistency. When the patient tires, feed her the rest of the meal. At subsequent meals, encourage the patient to feed herself for progressively longer periods until she can feed herself an entire meal.

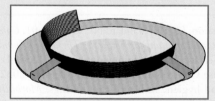

Swivel spoon
This utensil helps the patient with limited ROM in her forearm and will fit in universal cuffs.

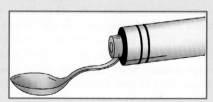

Universal cuffs
These flexible bands help the patient with flail hands or diminished grasp. Each cuff contains a slot that holds a fork or spoon. Attach the cuff to the hand the patient uses to feed herself. Then place the fork or spoon in the cuff slot. Bend the utensil to facilitate feeding.

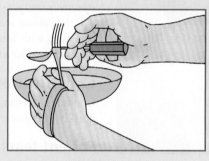

Long-handled utensils
These utensils have jointed stems to help the patient with limited ROM in her elbow and shoulder.

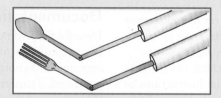

Utensils with built-up handles
These utensils can help the patient with diminished grasp. They can be purchased or can be improvised by wrapping tape around the handles.

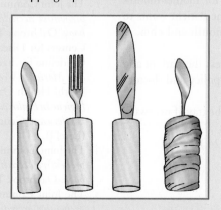

Spouted cups
These cups have a spout that can be used by patients experiencing tremors or who have unsteady arms and hands *to prevent spills and burns*.

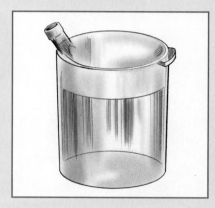

Slotted (nosey) cups
These cups have a cutout for the nose to allow the patient to drink without bending her neck or tilting her head. Some have handles on both sides to ensure a firm grasp.

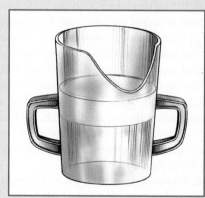

■ Position a chair next to the patient's bed *so you can sit comfortably if you need to feed her yourself.*

■ Set up the patient's tray, remove the plate from the tray warmer, and discard all plastic wrappings. Then cut the food into bite-sized pieces (as shown below). Season food according to the patient's request, as appropriate.

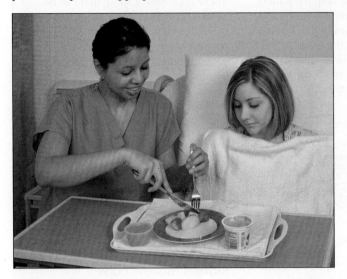

■ To help the blind or visually impaired patient feed herself, tell her that placement of various foods on her plate corresponds to the hours on a clock face. Maintain consistent placement for subsequent meals.

■ Ask the patient which food she prefers to eat first *to promote her sense of control over the meal. Some patients prefer to eat one food at a time, whereas others prefer to alternate foods.*

■ If the patient has difficulty swallowing, check the patient's medical record and care plan for any special instructions or swallowing techniques recommended by speech therapy. Offer liquids carefully with a spoon or feeding syringe *to help prevent aspiration.* Pureed or soft foods, such as custard or flavored gelatin, may be easier to swallow than liquids. If the patient doesn't have difficulty swallowing, use a flexible straw for liquids *to reduce the risk of spills.*

■ Ask the patient to indicate when she's ready for another mouthful. Pause between courses and whenever the patient wants to rest. During the meal, wipe the patient's mouth and chin, as needed.

■ If the patient is at risk for aspiration, assess the patient and obtain vital signs according to the facility's policy and doctor's order.

■ When the patient finishes eating, remove the tray. If necessary, clean up spills and change the bed linens.

■ Provide oral care. (See "Oral care", page 524.)

■ Perform hand hygiene.[1,2,3]

■ Document the procedure.[5]

Special considerations

■ Don't feed the patient too quickly *because this can cause anxiety and impair digestion.*

■ If the patient is restricted to the supine position, provide foods that can be chewed easily. Feed liquids carefully and only after the patient has swallowed any food in the mouth *to reduce the risk of aspiration.*

■ If the patient won't eat, try to find out why. For example, confirm food preferences. Also, make sure that the patient isn't in pain at mealtimes or hasn't received any treatments immediately before a meal that could be upsetting or cause nausea. Find out if any medications cause anorexia, nausea, or sedation. Clear the bedside of emesis basins, urinals, bedpans, and similar distractions at mealtimes.

■ Establish a pattern for feeding the patient, and share this information with the other staff members *so the patient doesn't need to repeatedly instruct staff members about preferred feeding techniques.*

■ If the patient and family are willing, suggest that family members assist with feeding. *Such assistance will make the patient feel more comfortable at mealtimes and may ease discharge planning.*

Complications

Choking and aspiration of food can occur if the patient is fed too quickly or is given excessively large mouthfuls.

Patient teaching

Teach the patient to use assistive devices as appropriate. Teach family members how to safely feed the patient if they're to assist with feeding at home. Review aspiration precautions as appropriate.

Documentation

Describe the feeding technique used in the nursing care plan to ensure continuity of care. Record the amount of food and fluid consumed; also note the fluids consumed on the intake and output record, if required. Note which foods the patient consistently fails to eat, and the reason, if known. Record the patient's level of independence. For the blind patient, record the pattern of feeding on the nursing care plan. Document any patient and family teaching and response to the teaching provided.

REFERENCES

1 The Joint Commission. (2012). Standard NPSG.07.01.01. *Comprehensive accreditation manual for hospitals: The official handbook.* Oakbrook Terrace, IL: The Joint Commission. (Level I)

2 Centers for Disease Control and Prevention. (October 2002). Guideline for hand hygiene in health-care settings. *Morbidity and Mortality Weekly Report, 51*(RR-16), 1–45. (Level 1)

3 World Health Organization. (2009). *WHO guidelines on hand hygiene in health care: First global patient safety challenge. Clean care is safer care.* Geneva, Switzerland: World Health Organization. (Level I)

4 The Joint Commission. (2012). Standard NPSG.01.01.01. *Comprehensive accreditation manual for hospitals: The official handbook.* Oakbrook Terrace, IL: The Joint Commission. (Level I)

5 The Joint Commission. (2012). Standard RC.01.03.01. *Comprehensive accreditation manual for hospitals: The official handbook.* Oakbrook Terrace, IL: The Joint Commission. (Level I)

FEEDING TUBE INSERTION AND REMOVAL

A feeding tube that's inserted nasally or orally into the stomach or duodenum allows a patient who can't or won't eat to receive nourishment. The feeding tube also permits supplemental feedings in a patient who has very high nutritional requirements, such as an unconscious patient or one with extensive burns. The preferred feeding tube route is nasal, but the oral route may be used for patients with such conditions as a head injury, deviated septum, or other nose injury.

The doctor may order duodenal feeding when the patient can't tolerate gastric feeding or when he expects gastric feeding to produce aspiration. Absence of bowel sounds or possible intestinal obstruction contraindicates using a feeding tube.

Feeding tubes differ somewhat from standard nasogastric tubes. Made of silicone, rubber, or polyurethane, feeding tubes have small diameters and great flexibility. These features reduce oropharyngeal irritation, necrosis from pressure on the tracheoesophageal wall, distal esophageal irritation, and discomfort from swallowing. To facilitate passage, some feeding tubes are weighted with tungsten, and some need a guide wire to keep them from curling in the back of the throat. These small-bore tubes usually have radiopaque markings and a water-activated coating, which provides a lubricated surface.

Feeding tubes should be removed when the patient no longer needs supplemental feedings.

Equipment
For feeding tube insertion
Feeding tube (#5 to #8 French, with or without guide) ▪ linen-saver pad ▪ gloves ▪ hypoallergenic tape ▪ water-soluble lubricant ▪ cotton-tipped applicators ▪ skin preparation product (such as compound benzoin tincture) ▪ facial tissues ▪ penlight ▪ small cup of water with straw or ice chips ▪ emesis basin ▪ 60-mL syringe ▪ pH test strip ▪ water ▪ permanent marker.

For feeding tube removal
Linen-saver pad ▪ gloves ▪ tube clamp ▪ 60-mL syringe.

Preparation of equipment
For feeding tube insertion
Perform hand hygiene.[1,2,3] Obtain the proper size tube. Usually, the doctor orders the smallest-bore tube that will allow free passage of the liquid feeding formula. Read the instructions on the tubing package carefully *because tube characteristics vary according to the manufacturer.* (For example, some tubes have marks at the appropriate lengths for gastric, duodenal, and jejunal insertion.) Examine the tube to make sure it's free from defects, such as cracks or rough or sharp edges. Run water through the tube *to check for patency, activate the coating, and facilitate removal of the guide.*

Determine the tube length needed to reach the stomach by first extending the distal end of the tube from the tip of the patient's nose to his earlobe. Coil this portion of the tube around your fingers *so the end stays curved until you insert it.* Then extend the uncoiled portion from the earlobe to the bottom of the xiphoid process.[4] Use a small piece of hypoallergenic tape to mark the total length of the two portions.

Implementation
▪ Verify the doctor's order.
▪ Confirm the patient's identity using at least two patient identifiers according to your facility's policy.[5]
▪ Explain the procedure to the patient *so he knows what to expect and can cooperate more fully.*
▪ Provide privacy.
▪ Perform hand hygiene and put on gloves.[1,2,3]
▪ Assist the patient into semi-Fowler's or high Fowler's position.[4]
▪ Place a linen-saver pad across the patient's chest *to protect him from spills.*

Inserting a feeding tube nasally
▪ Using the penlight, assess nasal patency. Inspect nasal passages for a deviated septum, polyps, or other obstructions. Occlude one nostril, then the other, *to determine which has the better airflow.* Assess the patient's history for nasal injury or surgery.
▪ Lubricate the curved tip of the tube (and the feeding tube guide, if appropriate) with a small amount of water-soluble lubricant *to ease insertion and prevent tissue injury.*
▪ Ask the patient to hold the emesis basin and facial tissues in case he needs them.
▪ To advance the tube, insert the curved, lubricated tip into the more patent nostril and direct it along the nasal passage. When it passes the nasopharyngeal junction, you'll feel some resistance. Unless contraindicated, instruct the patient to lower his chin to his chest *to close the trachea.* Then give him a small cup of water with a straw or ice chips. Direct him to sip the water or suck on the ice and swallow frequently *to ease the tube's passage.* Advance the tube as he swallows.

Inserting a feeding tube orally
▪ Have the patient lower his chin (unless contraindicated) *to close his trachea,* and ask him to open his mouth.
▪ Place the tip of the tube at the back of the patient's tongue, give water, and instruct the patient to swallow, as above. Remind him to avoid clamping his teeth down on the tube. Advance the tube as he swallows.

Positioning a tube
▪ Keep passing the tube until the tape marking the appropriate length reaches the patient's nostril or lips.
▪ If the tube has a guide wire, remove the guide wire with one hand while holding the tube in place at the nares.[4]
▪ Check the tube's placement and patency by attaching the syringe to the tube and gently aspirating stomach contents. Examine the aspirate and place a small amount on the pH test strip. Probability of gastric placement is increased if the aspirate has a typical gastric fluid appearance (grassy-green, clear and colorless with mucus shreds, or brown) and the pH is less than or equal to 5. If no gastric secretions return, the tube may be in the esophagus. You'll need to advance the tube or reinsert it and check placement again before proceeding.

NURSING ALERT *If using a postpyloric tube, gastric aspirate may not be a reliable indicator of tip position.*

■ To advance the tube to the duodenum, especially a tungsten-weighted tube, position the patient on his right side. *This position lets gravity assist tube passage through the pylorus.* Move the tube forward 2″ to 3″ (5 to 7.5 cm) hourly until X-ray studies confirm duodenal placement. (An X-ray must confirm placement before feeding begins *because duodenal feeding can cause nausea and vomiting if accidentally delivered to the stomach.*)

■ Ensure that tube placement is confirmed by X-ray before initial use. *X-ray confirmation is the only reliable method for confirming enteral tube placement.*

■ After confirming tube placement, remove the tape marking the tube length and mark the tube's exit point from the mouth or nostril with a marker. Check the mark regularly to see whether the length of the external portion of the tube has changed, indicating that the tube has moved.

■ Apply a skin preparation product to the patient's cheek *to help the tube adhere to the skin and prevent irritation.*

■ Tape the tube securely to the patient's cheek *to avoid excessive pressure on his nostrils or face.*

Removing a feeding tube

■ Flush the tube with air, then clamp or pinch the tube *to prevent fluid aspiration during withdrawal.*
■ Withdraw the tube gently but quickly.

Completing the procedure

■ Remove your gloves and perform hand hygiene.[1,2,3]
■ Document the procedure.[6]

Special considerations

■ Check gastric residual contents before each feeding or every 4 hours. Feeding should be held if residual volumes are greater than 200 mL on two successive assessments.

■ Flush the feeding tube according to your facility's policy (typically every 4 hours with from 20 to 30 mL of normal saline solution or warm water) *to maintain patency.* Retape the tube at least daily and as needed. Alternate taping the tube toward the inner and outer side of the nose *to avoid constant pressure on the same nasal area.* Inspect the skin for redness and breakdown.

■ Provide nasal hygiene daily using a cotton-tipped applicator and water-soluble lubricant *to remove crusted secretions.* Help the patient brush his teeth, gums, and tongue with mouthwash or saline solution at least twice daily.

■ Precise feeding-tube placement is especially important *because small-bore feeding tubes may slide into the trachea without causing immediate signs or symptoms of respiratory distress, such as coughing, choking, gasping, or cyanosis.* However, the patient will usually cough if the tube enters the larynx. *To make sure the tube clears the larynx,* ask the patient to speak. If he can't, the tube is in the larynx. Withdraw the tube immediately and reinsert it.

■ Check placement every 4 hours or according to your facility's policy.[7] When aspirating gastric contents to check tube placement, pull gently on the syringe plunger *to prevent trauma*

to the stomach lining or bowel. If you meet resistance during aspiration, stop the procedure *because resistance may result simply from the tube lying against the stomach wall.* If the tube coils above the stomach, you'll be unable to aspirate stomach contents. To rectify this, change the patient's position or withdraw the tube a few inches, readvance it, and try to aspirate again. If the tube was inserted with a guide wire, don't use the guide wire to reposition the tube. The doctor may do so, using fluoroscopic guidance.

Patient teaching

If your patient will use a feeding tube at home, make appropriate home care nursing referrals and teach the patient and caregivers how to use and care for a feeding tube. Teach them how to obtain equipment, insert and remove the tube, prepare and store feeding formula, and solve problems with tube position and patency.

Complications

Prolonged intubation may lead to skin erosion at the nostril, sinusitis, esophagitis, esophagotracheal fistula, gastric ulceration, and pulmonary and oral infection. (See *Managing tube feeding problems.*)

Documentation

For tube insertion, record the date, time, tube type and size, insertion site, area of placement, and confirmation of proper placement.

Record the date and time of tube removal and the patient's tolerance of the procedure.

REFERENCES

1 The Joint Commission. (2012). Standard NPSG.07.01.01. *Comprehensive accreditation manual for hospitals: The official handbook.* Oakbrook Terrace, IL: The Joint Commission. (Level I)
2 Centers for Disease Control and Prevention. (October 2002). Guideline for hand hygiene in health-care settings. *Morbidity and Mortality Weekly Report, 51*(RR-16), 1–45. (Level 1)
3 World Health Organization. (2009). *WHO guidelines on hand hygiene in health care: First global patient safety challenge. Clean care is safer care.* Geneva, Switzerland: World Health Organization. (Level I)
4 Lynn-McHale Wiegand, D. (Ed.). (2011). *AACN procedure manual for critical care* (6th ed.). Philadelphia, PA: Saunders.
5 The Joint Commission. (2012). Standard NPSG.01.01.01. *Comprehensive accreditation manual for hospitals: The official handbook.* Oakbrook Terrace, IL: The Joint Commission. (Level I)
6 The Joint Commission. (2012). Standard RC.01.03.01. *Comprehensive accreditation manual for hospitals: The official handbook.* Oakbrook Terrace, IL: The Joint Commission. (Level I)
7 American Association of Critical-Care Nurses (2009). "AACN Practice Alert: Verification of Feeding Tube Insertion (Blindly Inserted)" [Online]. Accessed August 2010 via the Web at http://www.aacn.org/WD/Practice/Docs/PracticeAlerts/Verification_of_Feeding_Tube_Placement_05-2005.pdf (Level I)

Managing tube feeding problems

COMPLICATIONS	NURSING INTERVENTIONS
Aspiration of gastric secretions	■ Discontinue feeding immediately. ■ Perform tracheal suction of aspirated contents if possible. ■ Notify the doctor. Prophylactic antibiotics and chest physiotherapy may be ordered. ■ Check tube placement before feeding *to prevent complications*.
Tube obstruction	■ Flush the tube with warm water. If necessary, replace the tube. ■ Flush the tube with 50 mL of water after each feeding *to remove excess sticky formula, which could occlude the tube*.
Oral, nasal, or pharyngeal irritation or necrosis	■ Provide frequent oral hygiene using mouthwash or swabs. Use petroleum jelly on cracked lips. ■ Change the tube's position. If necessary, replace the tube.
Vomiting, bloating, diarrhea, or cramps	■ Reduce the flow rate. ■ Administer metoclopramide as prescribed *to increase GI motility*. ■ Warm the formula to prevent GI distress. ■ For 30 minutes after feeding, position the patient on his right side with his head elevated *to facilitate gastric emptying*. ■ Notify the doctor. *He may want to reduce the amount of formula being given during each feeding.*
Constipation	■ Provide additional fluids if the patient can tolerate them. ■ Administer a bulk-forming laxative. ■ Increase fruit, vegetable, or sugar content of the feeding.
Electrolyte imbalance	■ Monitor blood glucose levels. ■ Notify the doctor. *He may want to adjust the formula content to correct the deficiency.*
Hyperglycemia	■ Monitor blood glucose levels. ■ Notify the doctor of elevated levels. ■ Administer insulin if ordered. ■ The doctor may adjust the sugar content of the formula.

ADDITIONAL REFERENCES

Gatt, M., & MacFie, J. (2009). Bedside postpyloric feeding tube placement: A pilot series to validate this novel technique. *Critical Care Medicine, 37*(2), 523–527.

Taylor, C., et al. (2011). *Fundamentals of nursing: The art and science of nursing care* (7th ed.). Philadelphia, PA: Lippincott Williams & Wilkins.

FEMORAL COMPRESSION

After a procedure involving an arterial access site (such as cardiac catheterization or angiography), femoral compression maintains hemostasis at the puncture site. A femoral compression device applies direct pressure to the arterial access site. A nylon strap is placed under the patient's buttocks and attached to the device with an inflatable plastic dome. Once the dome is positioned correctly over the puncture site, it's inflated to the set pressure. A doctor or specially trained nurses may apply the device.

Equipment

Femoral compression device strap ■ compression arch with dome and three-way stopcock ■ pressure inflation device ■ sterile transparent dressing ■ gloves ■ protective eyewear.

Implementation

After the arterial access procedure

■ Verify the doctor's order, including the amount of pressure to be applied and the length of time the device should remain in place.

- Confirm the patient's identity using at least two patient identifiers according to your facility's policy.[1]
- Explain the procedure to the patient and answer any questions *to decrease anxiety and increase cooperation.*
- Perform hand hygiene and put on gloves and protective eyewear.[2,3,4]
- Position the patient on the stretcher or bed; don't flex the involved extremity.
- Assess the condition of the puncture site, obtain vital signs, perform neurovascular checks, and assess pain, according to your facility's policy for arterial access procedures.

Applying the femoral compression device

- Place the device strap under the patient's hips before sheath removal (in cases that warrant the use of a sheath).
- With the assistance of another nurse, position the compression arch over the arterial puncture site, not the skin puncture site. Apply manual pressure over the dome area while the straps are secured to the arch.
- Once the dome is properly positioned over the arterial puncture site, connect the pressure inflation device to the stopcock that's attached to the device. Before inflation, verify the amplitude and location of the pedal pulse. Turn the stopcock to the open position and inflate the dome with the pressure inflation device to the ordered pressure. Typically, a venous sheath is removed at 20 to 30 mm Hg and an arterial sheath is removed at 60 to 80 mm Hg. Immediately after removal of the arterial sheath, inflate the device to 10 to 20 mm Hg over the systolic blood pressure. After 2 to 3 minutes, a reduction in pressure, usually a value between the patient's systolic and diastolic blood pressure, is ordered. Follow the doctor's specific orders for pressure changes.
- Assess the site for proper placement of the device and for signs of bleeding or hematoma. Assess distal pulses and perform neurovascular assessments according to your facility's policy. Confirm distal pulses after any adjustments of the device.

Maintaining the device

- When the patient is transferred to the nursing unit, assess the distal pulses, the puncture site, and placement of the device, and confirm the ordered amount of pressure.
- Check device placement, assess vital signs and the puncture site, and perform neurovascular checks every 2 hours or according to your facility's policy.
- Deflate the device hourly or as ordered and assess the puncture site for bleeding or hematoma. Assess for proper placement of the dome over the puncture site. Perform hand hygiene and put on gloves and protective eyewear to reposition the compression arch and dome as necessary. Re-inflate the device to the ordered pressure using the pressure inflation device.

Removing the device

- Explain the removal procedure to the patient.
- Perform hand hygiene[2,3,4] and put on gloves and protective eyewear. Remove the air from the dome. Leave the dome in place at 0 mm Hg pressure for at least 10 minutes; then loosen the straps and remove the device with a roll-off motion.

- Assess the puncture site for bleeding or hematoma. Apply a sterile transparent dressing according to your facility's policy.
- Check the puncture site and distal pulses, and perform neurovascular assessments every 15 minutes for the first half hour and every 30 minutes for the next 2 hours, or according to your facility's policy. Observe for signs of bleeding, hematoma, or infection.
- Dispose of the device according to your facility's policy.

Completing the procedure

- Remove and discard your protective wear and perform hand hygiene.[2,3,4]
- Document the procedure.[5]

Special considerations

- Advise the patient to use caution when moving in bed *to avoid malpositioning the device.* Instruct the patient not to bend the involved extremity.
- If you note external bleeding or signs of internal bleeding, remove the device, apply manual pressure, and notify the doctor.
- Change the dressing at the puncture site every 24 to 48 hours or according to your facility's policy. (The sterile transparent dressing permits inspection of the site for bleeding, drainage, or hematoma.)

Complications

Complications include bleeding, hematoma, retroperitoneal bleeding, and pseudoaneurysm. Other potential complications may include infection and deep vein thrombosis. Tissue damage may occur if prolonged pressure is maintained.

Documentation

Document sheath removal, initial application of the device, and the patient's tolerance of the procedure. Document vital signs, puncture site assessments, distal pulses, neurovascular assessments, periodic deflation, repositioning of the device, length of time the device was in place, and removal of the device. Document patient and family teaching, complications, and interventions.

REFERENCES

1 The Joint Commission. (2012). Standard NPSG.01.01.01. *Comprehensive accreditation manual for hospitals: The official handbook.* Oakbrook Terrace, IL: The Joint Commission. (Level I)

2 The Joint Commission. (2012). Standard NPSG.07.01.01. *Comprehensive accreditation manual for hospitals: The official handbook.* Oakbrook Terrace, IL: The Joint Commission. (Level I)

3 Centers for Disease Control and Prevention. (October 2002). Guideline for hand hygiene in health-care settings. *Morbidity and Mortality Weekly Report, 51*(RR-16), 1–45. (Level 1)

4 World Health Organization. (2009). *WHO guidelines on hand hygiene in health care: First global patient safety challenge. Clean care is safer care.* Geneva, Switzerland: World Health Organization. (Level I)

5 The Joint Commission. (2012). Standard RC.01.03.01. *Comprehensive accreditation manual for hospitals: The official handbook.* Oakbrook Terrace, IL: The Joint Commission. (Level I)

ADDITIONAL REFERENCES

Deuling, J.H., et al. (2008). Closure of the femoral artery after cardiac catheterization: A comparison of anglo-seal, starclose, and manual compression. *Catheterization and Cardiovascular Interventions, 71*(4), 518–523.

Dumont, C. (2007). Blood pressure and risks of vascular complications after percutaneous coronary interventions. *Dimensions in Critical Care Nursing, 26*(3), 121–127.

King, N.A., et al. (2008). A randomized controlled trial assessing the use of compression versus vasoconstriction in the treatment of femoral hematoma occurring after percutaneous coronary intervention. *Heart and Lung, 37*(3), 205–210.

Lynn-McHale Wiegand, D. (Ed.). (2011). *AACN procedure manual for critical care* (6th ed.). Philadelphia, PA: Saunders.

Schwarz, T., et al. (2009). Mechanical compression versus haemostatic wound dressing after femoral artery sheath removal: A prospective, randomized study. *Vasa, 38*(1), 53–59.

FOOT CARE

Daily bathing of feet and regular trimming of toenails promotes cleanliness, prevents infection, stimulates peripheral circulation, and controls odor by removing debris from between toes and under toenails. It's particularly important for bedridden patients and those especially vulnerable to foot infection. Increased susceptibility may be caused by peripheral vascular disease, diabetes mellitus, poor nutritional status, arthritis, or any condition that impairs peripheral circulation. In such patients, proper foot care should include meticulous cleanliness and regular observation for signs of skin breakdown. (See *Foot care for patients with diabetes.*) Patients should be taught proper foot care on at least a yearly basis.[1]

Toenail trimming is contraindicated in patients with toe infections, diabetes mellitus, neurologic disorders, renal failure, or peripheral vascular disease, unless performed by a doctor or podiatrist. Some facilities prohibit nurses from trimming toenails. Check your facility's policy before performing the procedure.

Equipment

Bath blanket ▪ large basin ▪ soap ▪ water ▪ towel ▪ linen-saver pad ▪ pillow ▪ washcloth ▪ toenail clippers ▪ orangewood stick ▪ emery board ▪ cotton-tipped applicator ▪ cotton ▪ lotion ▪ water-absorbent powder ▪ bath thermometer ▪ gloves (if the patient has open lesions) ▪ hospital-grade disinfectant.

Preparation of equipment

Fill the basin halfway with warm water. Test water temperature with a bath thermometer *because patients with diminished peripheral sensation could burn their feet in excessively hot water (over 105° F [40.6° C]) without feeling any warning pain.* The water temperature should feel comfortably warm.

Implementation

▪ Gather the equipment at the patient's bedside.
▪ Perform hand hygiene and put on gloves, if necessary.[3,4,5]

Foot care for patients with diabetes

Because diabetes mellitus can reduce blood supply to the feet, normally minor foot injuries can lead to dangerous infection. When caring for a patient with diabetes, keep these foot care guidelines in mind:

▪ Exercising the feet daily can help improve circulation. While the patient is sitting on the edge of the bed, ask him to point his toes upward, then downward, 10 times. Then have him make a circle with each foot 10 times.

▪ Shoes must fit properly. Instruct the patient to break in new shoes gradually by increasing wearing time by 30 minutes each day.[2] Also tell him to check his old shoes frequently *in case they develop rough spots in the lining.*

▪ Tell the patient to wear clean socks daily and to avoid socks with holes, darned spots, or rough, irritating seams.

▪ Advise the patient to see a doctor if he has corns or calluses.[2]

▪ Tell the patient to wear warm socks or slippers and to use extra blankets *to avoid cold feet.* He shouldn't use heating pads or hot-water bottles *because these items may cause burns.*

▪ Teach the patient to regularly inspect the skin on his feet for cuts, cracks, blisters, or red, swollen areas. Even slight cuts on the feet should receive a doctor's attention. As a first-aid measure, tell him to wash the cut thoroughly and apply a mild antiseptic. Urge him to avoid harsh antiseptics, such as iodine, *because they can damage tissue.*

▪ Advise the patient with diabetes to avoid tight-fitting garments or activities that can decrease circulation. The patient should especially avoid wearing elastic garters, sitting with knees crossed, picking at sores or rough spots on the feet, walking barefoot, or applying adhesive tape to the skin on his feet.

▪ Confirm the patient's identity using at least two patient identifiers according to your facility's policy.[6]
▪ Tell the patient that you'll wash his feet and provide foot and toenail care.
▪ Cover the patient with a bath blanket. Fanfold the top linen to the foot of the bed.
▪ Place a linen-saver pad and a towel under the patient's feet *to keep the bottom linen dry.* Then position the basin on the pad.
▪ Insert a pillow beneath the patient's knee *to provide support,* and cushion the rim of the basin with the edge of the towel *to prevent pressure on the patient's leg.*
▪ Immerse one foot in the basin. Allow it to soak for about 10 minutes and then wash it thoroughly with soap and water. *Soaking softens the skin and toenails, loosens debris under toenails, and comforts and refreshes the patient.*

■ After washing the foot, rinse it with a washcloth, remove it from the basin, and place it on the towel.

■ Dry the foot thoroughly, especially between the toes, *to avoid skin breakdown.* Blot gently to dry *because harsh rubbing may damage the skin.*

■ Empty the basin, refill it with warm water at the appropriate temperature, and soak and clean the other foot.

■ While the second foot is soaking, give the first one a pedicure. Using the cotton-tipped applicator, carefully clean the toenails. Using an orangewood stick, gently remove any dirt beneath the toenails; avoid injuring subungual skin.

■ Rinse the foot that has been soaking, dry it thoroughly, and give it a pedicure.

■ Apply lotion *to moisten dry skin,* or lightly dust water-absorbent powder between the toes *to absorb moisture.* Don't apply lotion between the toes *because lotion can cause skin maceration.*

■ Remove and clean all equipment and dispose of gloves, if used, and perform hand hygiene.[3,4,5]

■ Document the procedure.[7]

Special considerations

■ While providing foot care, observe the color, shape, and texture of the toenails. If you see redness, drying, cracking, blisters, discoloration, or other signs of traumatic injury, especially in patients with impaired peripheral circulation, notify the doctor. *Because such patients are vulnerable to infection and gangrene,* they need prompt treatment.[2]

■ When giving the bedridden patient foot care, perform range-of-motion exercises unless contraindicated *to stimulate circulation and prevent foot contractures or muscle atrophy.* Tuck folded 2″ × 2″ gauze pads between overlapping toes *to protect the skin from the toenails.* Apply heel protectors or protective boots *to prevent skin breakdown.*

■ If your facility's policy prevents you from trimming the patient's nails, consult a podiatrist if the nails need trimming.

Documentation

Record the date and time of foot care in your notes. Record and report any abnormal findings and any nursing actions you take. If toenail trimming was necessary, specify the name of the person who performed the trimming.

REFERENCES

1 American Diabetes Association. (2009). Standards of medical care in diabetes 2010. *Diabetes Care, 32*(Suppl.1), S13–S61.

2 American Diabetes Association. (2004). Preventive foot care in diabetes. *Diabetic Care, 27*(Suppl.1), S63–64.

3 The Joint Commission. (2012). Standard NPSG.07.01.01. *Comprehensive accreditation manual for hospitals: The official handbook.* Oakbrook Terrace, IL: The Joint Commission. (Level I)

4 Centers for Disease Control and Prevention. (October 2002). Guideline for hand hygiene in health-care settings. *Morbidity and Mortality Weekly Report, 51*(RR-16), 1–45. (Level 1)

5 World Health Organization. (2009). *WHO guidelines on hand hygiene in health care: First global patient safety challenge. Clean care is safer care.* Geneva, Switzerland: World Health Organization. (Level I)

6 The Joint Commission. (2012). Standard NPSG.01.01.01. *Comprehensive accreditation manual for hospitals: The official handbook.* Oakbrook Terrace, IL: The Joint Commission. (Level I)

7 The Joint Commission. (2012). Standard RC.01.03.01. *Comprehensive accreditation manual for hospitals: The official handbook.* Oakbrook Terrace, IL: The Joint Commission. (Level I)

FOREIGN BODY OBSTRUCTION AND MANAGEMENT

Most cases of foreign-body airway obstruction in adults occur while they're eating. In children, foreign-body airway obstruction occurs most often when they're eating or playing and typically involves such items as balloons, small objects, or such foods as hot dogs, rounded candies, nuts, or grapes. In infants, airway obstruction typically results from a liquid.

Foreign bodies can cause mild or severe airway obstruction. If the obstruction is mild and the patient is coughing forcefully, there's no reason to intervene; spontaneous coughing and breathing typically relieve the obstruction.[1]

If severe obstruction develops, you must intervene quickly to relieve the obstruction[1] because anoxia resulting from the obstruction may cause brain damage and death within 4 to 6 minutes. Intervene by administering abdominal thrusts, also called the *Heimlich maneuver,* which uses a subdiaphragmatic abdominal thrust to create diaphragmatic pressure in the static lung below the foreign body sufficient to expel the obstruction. Abdominal thrusts are used in conscious adult patients who can't speak, cough, or breathe.

If abdominal thrusts are ineffective, you may consider administering chest thrusts; this maneuver forces air out of the lungs, creating an artificial cough. Use chest thrusts for an obese patient, if you're unable to encircle the patient's abdomen, and for a patient who's in the late stages of pregnancy.[1] When administered to obese or pregnant patients who can't speak, cough, or breathe, chest thrusts work by forcing air out of the lungs, creating an artificial cough.[1]

For infants, deliver repeated cycles of five back blows followed by five chest compressions until the foreign body is expelled or the infant becomes unresponsive. Abdominal thrusts aren't recommended for infants because they may damage the infant's liver.

If a patient is unconscious or becomes unconscious despite your efforts, start cardiopulmonary resuscitation (CPR) immediately.

Equipment

No special equipment is required.

Implementation

■ Determine whether the patient is choking by asking, "Are you choking?" If the victim indicates "yes" by nodding her head without speaking, she has a severe airway obstruction.[1]

■ Activate the emergency response system quickly if the patient is having difficulty breathing. If another person is present, have him activate the system.

■ Talk to the patient to keep her calm, and explain what you're doing. Tell the patient that you'll try to dislodge the foreign body.[1]

For a conscious adult or child

■ Standing behind the patient, wrap your arms around her waist. Make a fist with one hand, and place the thumb side against her abdomen, slightly above the umbilicus and well below the xiphoid process. Then grasp your fist with the other hand (as shown below).

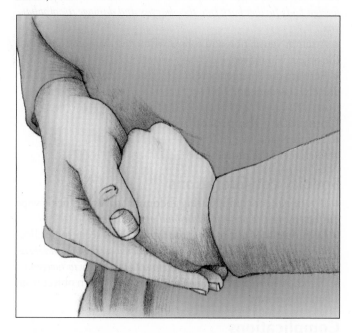

■ Squeeze the patient's abdomen using quick inward and upward thrusts. Each thrust should be a separate and distinct movement; each should be forceful enough to create an artificial cough that will dislodge an obstruction. Continue the abdominal thrust in rapid sequence until the obstruction is relieved or the patient becomes unresponsive.

■ Make sure you have a firm grasp on the patient *because the patient may lose consciousness and need to be lowered to the floor.*[1] Support the head and neck *to prevent injury.* If the patient becomes unconscious, start CPR and follow the steps for an unconscious adult or child.

■ Examine the patient for injuries, such as ruptured or lacerated abdominal or thoracic viscera, resulting from the procedure.

For an obese or pregnant adult

■ If the patient is conscious, stand behind her and place your arms under her armpits and around her chest.

■ Place the thumb side of your clenched fist against the middle of the sternum, avoiding the margins of the ribs and the xiphoid process (as shown at top of next column).

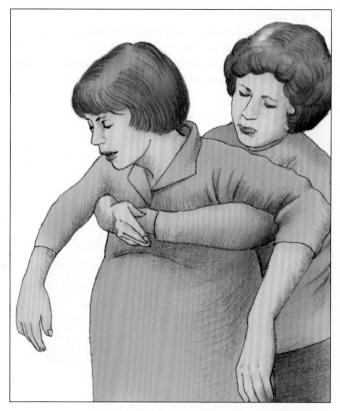

■ Grasp your fist with your other hand and perform a chest thrust with enough force to expel the foreign body. Continue until the patient expels the obstruction or loses consciousness. If the patient loses consciousness, carefully lower her to the floor and follow the steps outlined below for an unconscious adult or child.

■ Examine the patient for injuries, such as ruptured or lacerated abdominal or thoracic viscera, resulting from the procedure.

■ Notify the doctor of the patient's status, especially with loss of consciousness.

For an unconscious adult or child

■ For a patient who becomes unresponsive while trying to remove a foreign object, or if you come upon an unconscious patient, establish unresponsiveness by tapping the patient and shouting, "Are you alright?" Check to see if the patient is apneic or only gasping. If the patient is unresponsive and apneic or only gasping, call for help or activate the emergency response system.[1]

■ Begin CPR immediately, starting with chest compressions.[1]

■ Each time the airway is opened using a head-tilt, chin-lift maneuver, look for an object in the patient's mouth.[1]

■ Remove the object, if seen.[1]

NURSING ALERT *Never perform a blind finger-sweep to retrieve an object from a patient's airway. Remove visible objects.*[1]

■ Attempt to ventilate the patient and follow with 30 chest compressions.

■ Examine the patient for injuries, such as ruptured or lacerated abdominal or thoracic viscera, resulting from the procedure.

For an infant

■ Place the infant face down so that he's straddling your arm with his head lower than his trunk.[1]

■ Rest your forearm on your thigh and deliver five back blows with the heel of your hand between the infant's shoulder blades (as shown below).[1]

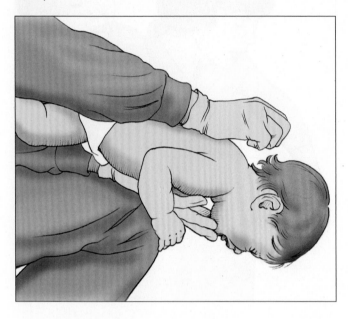

■ If you haven't removed the obstruction, place your free hand on the infant's back.

■ Supporting his neck, jaw, and chest with your other hand, turn him over onto your thigh.

■ Keep his head lower than his trunk.

■ Imagine a line between the infant's nipples and place the index finger of your free hand on his sternum, just below this imaginary line. Then place your middle and ring fingers next to your index finger and lift the index finger off his chest (as shown below).[1]

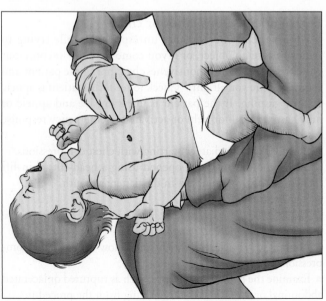

■ Deliver five chest thrusts as you would for chest compression, but at a slower rate.[1] *Don't perform abdominal thrust on an infant because it may damage the infant's liver.*[1]

■ Repeat the above steps until you've relieved the obstruction or the infant becomes unconscious.

■ If the infant becomes unconscious, call for help, and start to perform CPR beginning with chest compressions.[1] (See "Cardiopulmonary resuscitation, infant," page 125.)

■ After 30 chest compressions, open the airway.[1]

■ Before performing rescue breaths you should look in the infant's mouth for the foreign body. If you see the object, remove it. Never perform a blind finger-sweep on an infant *because it may push the foreign body further back into the pharynx and damage the oropharynx.*[1]

■ Attempt ventilation and follow with chest compressions until the object is removed.

■ Activate the emergency response system after 2 minutes if no one else has done so.[1]

Completing the procedure

■ Perform hand hygiene.[2,3,4]

■ Document the procedure.[5]

Special considerations

■ If your patient vomits during abdominal thrusts, quickly wipe out her mouth *to prevent additional obstruction.*

■ Even if your efforts to clear the airway don't seem to be effective, keep trying. *As oxygen deprivation increases, smooth and skeletal muscles relax, making your maneuvers more likely to succeed.*

■ Never perform a blind finger-sweep to retrieve an object from a patient's airway.[1]

Complications

Nausea, regurgitation, bruising, and achiness may develop after the patient can breathe independently. She may also be injured, possibly from incorrect placement of the rescuer's hands or because of osteoporosis or metastatic lesions that increase the risk of fracture.

Documentation

Record the date and time of the procedure, the patient's actions before the obstruction, the approximate length of time it took to clear the airway, and the type and size of the object removed. Also, note her vital signs after the procedure, any complications that occurred and nursing actions taken, and her tolerance of the procedure.

REFERENCES

1 American Heart Association. (2010). 2010 American Heart Association guidelines for cardiopulmonary resuscitation and emergency cardiovascular care. *Circulation, 122*(Suppl. 3), S685–S705. (Level I)

2 The Joint Commission. (2012). Standard NPSG.07.01.01. *Comprehensive accreditation manual for hospitals: The official handbook.* Oakbrook Terrace, IL: The Joint Commission. (Level I)

3 Centers for Disease Control and Prevention. (October 2002). Guideline for hand hygiene in health-care settings. *Morbidity and Mortality Weekly Report, 51*(RR-16), 1–45. (Level 1)
4 World Health Organization. (2009). *WHO guidelines on hand hygiene in health care: First global patient safety challenge. Clean care is safer care.* Geneva, Switzerland: World Health Organization. (Level I)
5 The Joint Commission. (2012). Standard RC.01.03.01. *Comprehensive accreditation manual for hospitals: The official handbook.* Oakbrook Terrace, IL: The Joint Commission. (Level I)

ADDITIONAL REFERENCE

Nettina, S.M. (2010). *Lippincott manual of nursing practice* (9th ed.). Philadelphia, PA: Lippincott Williams & Wilkins.

FUNCTIONAL ASSESSMENT

A functional assessment is used to evaluate the older adult's overall well-being and self-care abilities. It helps identify individual needs and care deficits, provide a basis for developing a care plan that enhances the abilities of the older adult with coexisting disease and chronic illness, and provide feedback about treatment and rehabilitation. You can use the information to identify and match the older adult's needs with such services as housekeeping, home health care, and day care to help the patient maintain independence. Any of several methods can help you perform a methodical functional assessment.

The *Katz Index of Independence in Activities of Daily Living* is a widely used tool for evaluating a person's ability to perform six daily personal care activities: bathing, dressing, toileting, transfer, continence, and feeding. It describes the patient's functional level at a specific point in time and objectively scores his performance on a three-point scale.

The *Lawton Instrumental Activities of Daily Living Scale* evaluates the ability of the patient to perform more complex personal care activities. It addresses the activities needed to support independent living, such as the ability to use the telephone, cook, shop, do laundry, manage finances, take medications, and prepare meals. The activities are rated on a three-point scale, ranging from independence, to needing some help, to complete disability. (See *Lawton Instrumental Activities of Daily Living Scale*, page 316.)

The *Barthel index* evaluates the following 10 self-care functions: feeding, moving from wheelchair to bed and returning, performing personal toilet, getting on and off the toilet, bathing, walking on a level surface or propelling a wheelchair, going up and down stairs, dressing and undressing, maintaining bowel continence, and controlling the bladder. Each item is scored according to the degree of assistance needed; over time, results reveal improvement or decline.

A similar scale, called the *Barthel Self-Care Rating Scale,* is a more detailed evaluation of function. Both tools provide information to help you determine the type of assistance needed.

In an attempt to improve the quality of care in extended care facilities, the federal government instituted major reforms through the Omnibus Budget Reconciliation Act of 1981 and its amendments. A standardized assessment tool called the *Minimum Data Set* was developed to make patient assessments more consistent and reliable throughout the country. All extended care facilities that receive federal funding are required to use this method.

The *Outcome and Assessment Information Set (OASIS),* now known *as OASIS-B,* is a standardized form required by the Health Care Financing Administration for Medicare-certified agencies. This form is a comprehensive assessment of home care patients. The OASIS-B was developed specifically to measure outcomes for adults who receive home care. The instrument allows the collection of data to measure changes in a patient's health status over time. Typically, you'll collect OASIS-B data when a patient starts home care, at the 60-day recertification point, and when the patient is discharged or transferred to another health care facility, such as a hospital or subacute care facility.

Equipment
- Facility-approved functional assessment tool.

Implementation
- Perform hand hygiene.[1,2,3]
- Confirm the patient's identity using at least two patient identifiers according to your facility's policy.[4]
- Explain the test to the patient, and tell him where it will take place.
- Review the patient's health history *to obtain subjective data about the patient and insight into problem areas and subtle physical changes.*
- If you don't already have it, obtain biographical data, including such information as the patient's name, age, and birth date.
- Using the functional assessment tool, ask the patient to answer the questions. If the patient is unable to answer, have his caregiver provide the answers.
- Perform hand hygiene.[1,2,3]
- Document the procedure.[5]

Special considerations
- In a long-term care facility, the physical assessment and care plan should be completed by a licensed nurse within 24 hours of a patient's admission. Functional assessment should be completed after a 7- to 14-day assessment period. A comprehensive care plan should be developed within 21 days.
- When using the Lawton scale, make sure you also evaluate the patient's safety. For example, even though a person may be able to cook a small meal for himself, he may leave the stove burner on after cooking.
- Both the Barthel index and the Barthel Self-Care Rating Scale are more likely to be used in rehabilitation and long-term care settings as tools to document improvement in a patient's abilities.

Documentation
Document all assessment findings according to your facility's policy.

Lawton Instrumental Activities of Daily Living Scale

The Lawton scale evaluates more sophisticated functions than the Katz index. Patients or caregivers can complete the form in a few minutes. The first answer in each case—except for 8a—indicates independence; the second, capability with assistance; and the third, dependence. In this version, the maximum score is 29, although scores have meaning only for a particular patient; for instance, declining scores over time that reveal deterioration. Questions 4 to 7 tend to be gender specific; modify them as necessary.

Name: _____

Rated by: _____ Date: _____

1. Can you use the telephone?
   without help   3
   with some help   2
   completely unable   1

2. Can you get to places beyond walking distance?
   without help   3
   with some help   2
   not without special arrangements   1

3. Can you go shopping for groceries?
   without help   3
   with some help   2
   completely unable   1

4. Can you prepare your own meals?
   without help   3
   with some help   2
   completely unable   1

5. Can you do your own housework?
   without help   3
   with some help   2
   completely unable   1

6. Can you do your own handyman work?
   without help   3
   with some help   2
   completely unable   1

7. Can you do your own laundry?
   without help   3
   with some help   2
   completely unable   1

8a. Do you take medicines or use any medications?
    Yes (If yes, answer Question 8b.)   1
    No (If no, answer Question 8c.)   2

8b. Do you take your own medicine?
    without help (in the right doses at the right times) 3
    with some help (if someone prepares it
    for you and/or reminds you to take it)   2
    completely unable   1

8c. If you had to take medicine, could you do it?
    without help (in the right doses at the right time) 3
    with some help (if someone prepared it for
    you and reminded you to take it)   2
    completely unable   1

9. Can you manage your own money?
   without help   3
   with some help   2
   completely unable   1

Adapted with permission from Lawton, M.P., & Brody, E.M. (1969). Assessment of older people: Self-maintaining and instrumental activities of daily living. *The Gerontologist, 9*(3), 179–186.

REFERENCES

1 The Joint Commission. (2012). Standard NPSG.07.01.01. *Comprehensive accreditation manual for hospitals: The official handbook.* Oakbrook Terrace, IL: The Joint Commission. (Level I)

2 Centers for Disease Control and Prevention. (October 2002). Guideline for hand hygiene in health-care settings. *Morbidity and Mortality Weekly Report, 51*(RR-16), 1–45. (Level 1)

3 World Health Organization. (2009). *WHO guidelines on hand hygiene in health care: First global patient safety challenge. Clean care is safer care.* Geneva, Switzerland: World Health Organization. (Level I)

4 The Joint Commission. (2012). Standard NPSG.01.01.01. *Comprehensive accreditation manual for hospitals: The official handbook.* Oakbrook Terrace, IL: The Joint Commission. (Level I)

5 The Joint Commission. (2012). Standard RC.01.03.01. *Comprehensive accreditation manual for hospitals: The official handbook.* Oakbrook Terrace, IL: The Joint Commission. (Level I)

ADDITIONAL REFERENCES

Moore, D.J., et al. (2008). The clinical usefulness of performance-based assessments of daily functioning for older adults. *Geriatrics, 6*(9), 16–20.

Wallace, M., & Shelkey, M. (2008). Monitoring functional status in hospitalized older adults. *AJN, 108*(4), 64–71; quiz 71–72.

GASTRIC LAVAGE

Gastric lavage flushes the stomach and removes ingested substances through a gastric lavage tube. The procedure may be used to empty the stomach in preparation for endoscopic examination or after poisoning or a drug overdose, especially in patients who have central nervous system depression or an inadequate gag reflex. However, the American Academy of Clinical Toxicology recommends using gastric lavage for managing instances of poisoning only when the patient has ingested a life-threatening amount of the poison and lavage can occur within 60 minutes of ingestion.[1]

Gastric lavage is typically done in the emergency department or on the intensive care unit by a doctor, gastroenterologist, or nurse; a wide-bore lavage tube is almost always inserted by a gastroenterologist.

This procedure is contraindicated after ingestion of a corrosive substance (such as lye, petroleum distillates, ammonia, alkalis, or mineral acids) because the lavage tube may perforate the already compromised esophagus.[1] Gastric lavage is also no longer recommended for routine management of hemorrhage. If it's used for hemorrhage, the risks should be weighed against the benefits.

Correct lavage tube placement is essential for patient safety because accidental misplacement (in the lungs, for example) followed by lavage can be fatal.

Equipment

2 to 3 L of normal saline solution, tap water, or appropriate antidote as ordered ▪ graduated container ▪ Ewald tube or any large-lumen gastric tube, typically #36 to #40 French (see *Using wide-bore gastric tubes,* page 318)[1] ▪ connection tubing ▪ intermittent suction setup ▪ water-soluble lubricant ▪ emesis basin ▪ ½" hypoallergenic tape ▪ 60-mL bulb or catheter-tip syringe or prepackaged syringe irrigation kit ▪ gloves ▪ face shield ▪ gown ▪ linen-saver pad or towel ▪ tonsillar or tonsil-tip suction device attached to suction ▪ Optional: anesthetic ointment, charcoal tablets or solution.

Preparation of equipment

Set up the lavage and suction equipment. Lubricate the end of the lavage tube with the water-soluble lubricant or anesthetic ointment.

Implementation

▪ Verify the doctor's order.
▪ Confirm the patient's identity using at least two patient identifiers according to your facility's policy.[2]
▪ Explain the procedure to the patient and provide privacy. Answer all questions *to decrease anxiety and increase cooperation.*
▪ Perform hand hygiene and put on a gown, gloves, and a face shield.[3,4,5]
▪ Drape the towel or linen-saver pad over the patient's chest *to protect him from soiling.*[6]

▪ Place the bed in semi-Fowler's position, ensuring the head of the bed is elevated 10 to 20 degrees, creating a slight reverse-Trendelenburg's position.[6]
▪ Place the patient in the left lateral decubitus position.
▪ The doctor or nurse inserts the lavage tube nasally or orally and advances it slowly and gently *because forceful insertion may injure tissues.* The tube's placement is checked by aspirating stomach contents with a 60-mL syringe and obtaining X-ray confirmation of placement.[6]
▪ *Because the patient may vomit when the lavage tube reaches the posterior pharynx during insertion,* be prepared to suction the airway immediately with either a tonsillar or a tonsil-tip suction device.
▪ After placement is confirmed, secure the lavage tube nasally or orally with tape.
▪ Aspirate stomach contents using a 60-mL syringe.
▪ Begin gastric lavage by slowly instilling 200 to 300 mL of fluid (for adults) using the 60-mL syringe.
▪ Aspirate the irrigant with the syringe and empty it into a graduated container or connect the lavage tube to the intermittent suction. Measure the outflow amount to make sure that it equals at least the amount of irrigant you instilled *to prevent accidental stomach distention and vomiting.* If the drainage amount falls significantly short of the instilled amount, reposition the tube until sufficient solution flows out.
▪ If the procedure is being performed for hemorrhage, repeat lavage intermittently until returned fluids appear clear, *signaling that bleeding has stopped.*
▪ If the procedure is being performed for an overdose, repeat lavage intermittently until the aspirated fluid is clear of toxic substances.
▪ Assess the patient's vital signs, urine output, and level of consciousness (LOC) every 15 minutes. Notify the doctor of any changes.
▪ If ordered, remove the lavage tube by clamping the tube and then pulling it out slowly and steadily.
▪ Dispose of soiled items in the appropriate receptacle.
▪ Remove your gloves, gown, and face shield and perform hand hygiene.[3,4,5]
▪ Document the procedure.[7]

Special considerations

▪ Never leave a patient alone during gastric lavage.
▪ Remember to keep tracheal suctioning equipment nearby, and watch closely for airway obstruction caused by vomiting or excess oral secretions. Throughout gastric lavage, you may need to suction the oral cavity frequently *to ensure an open airway and prevent aspiration.* For the same reasons, and if he doesn't exhibit an adequate gag reflex or is comatose, the patient may require an endotracheal tube before the procedure.[6]
▪ If ordered, after lavage to remove poisons or drugs, mix charcoal tablets or solution with the irrigant (water or normal saline solution) and administer the mixture through the gastric tube. The charcoal will absorb remaining toxic substances. The tube may be clamped temporarily, allowed to drain via gravity, attached to intermittent suction, or removed.
▪ When performing gastric lavage to stop bleeding, keep precise intake and output records *to determine the amount of*

EQUIPMENT

Using wide-bore gastric tubes

If you need to deliver a large volume of fluid rapidly through a gastric tube (when irrigating the stomach of a patient with profuse gastric bleeding or poisoning, for example), a wide-bore gastric tube usually serves best. Typically inserted orally, these tubes remain in place only long enough to complete the lavage and evacuate stomach contents.

Ewald tube
In an emergency, using this single-lumen tube with several openings at the distal end allows you to aspirate large amounts of gastric contents quickly.

Levacuator tube
This tube has two lumens. Use the larger lumen for evacuating gastric contents; the smaller, for instilling an irrigant.

Edlich tube
This single-lumen tube has four openings near the closed distal tip. A funnel or syringe may be connected at the proximal end. Like the Ewald tube, the Edlich tube lets you withdraw large quantities of gastric contents quickly.

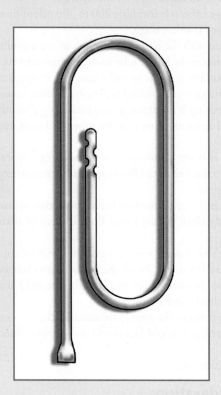
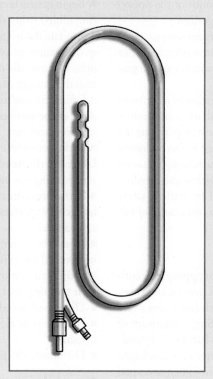
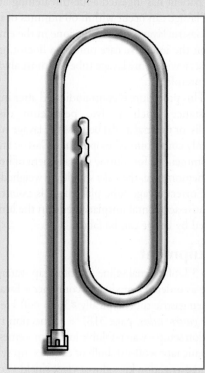

bleeding. When large volumes of fluid are instilled and withdrawn, serum electrolyte and arterial blood gas levels may be measured during or after lavage.

Complications
Vomiting and subsequent aspiration, the most common complications of gastric lavage, occur more often in a groggy patient. Bradyarrhythmias, laryngospasm, and hypoxia may occur.

Documentation
Record the date and time of lavage, the size and type of gastric tube used, the volume and type of irrigant, and the amount of drained gastric contents. Record this information on the intake-and-output record sheet, and include your observations, includ-

ing the color and consistency of drainage. Also keep precise records of the patient's vital signs and LOC, any drugs instilled through the tube, the time the tube was removed, and how well the patient tolerated the procedure.

REFERENCES

1   American Academy of Clinical Toxicology and European Association of Poison Centres and Clinical Toxicologists. (2004). "Position Paper: Gastric Lavage," *Journal of Toxicology. Clinical Toxicology, 42*(7), 933–43 [Online]. Accessed September 2011 via the Web at http://www.clintox.org/documents/positionpapers/GastricLavage.pdf (Level I)

2   The Joint Commission. (2012). Standard NPSG.01.01.01. *Comprehensive accreditation manual for hospitals: The official handbook.* Oakbrook Terrace, IL: The Joint Commission. (Level I)

3 The Joint Commission. (2012). Standard NPSG.07.01.01. *Comprehensive accreditation manual for hospitals: The official handbook*. Oakbrook Terrace, IL: The Joint Commission. (Level I)

4 Centers for Disease Control and Prevention. (October 2002). Guideline for hand hygiene in health-care settings. *Morbidity and Mortality Weekly Report, 51*(RR-16), 1–45. (Level 1)

5 World Health Organization. (2009). *WHO guidelines on hand hygiene in health care: First global patient safety challenge. Clean care is safer care*. Geneva, Switzerland: World Health Organization. (Level I)

6 Lynn-McHale Wiegand, D. (Ed.). (2011). *AACN procedure manual for critical care* (6th ed.). Philadelphia, PA: Saunders.

7 The Joint Commission. (2012). Standard RC.01.03.01. *Comprehensive accreditation manual for hospitals: The official handbook*. Oakbrook Terrace, IL: The Joint Commission. (Level I)

ADDITIONAL REFERENCES

Li, Y., et al. (2009). Systematic review of controlled clinical trials of gastric lavage in acute organophosphorus pesticide poisoning. *Clinical Toxicology, 47*(3), 179–192.

Pitera, A., & Sarko, J. (2010). Just say no: Gastric aspiration and lavage rarely provide benefit. *Annals of Emergency Medicine, 55*(4), 365–366.

GASTROSTOMY FEEDING BUTTON CARE AND REINSERTION

A gastrostomy feeding button serves as an alternative feeding device for an ambulatory patient who is receiving long-term enteral feedings. Approved by the Food and Drug Administration for 6-month implantation, feeding buttons can be used to replace gastrostomy tubes, if necessary.

The button has a mushroom dome at one end and two wing tabs and a flexible safety plug at the other. When inserted into an established stoma, the button lies almost flush with the skin, with only the wings and the top of the safety plug visible.

The button can usually be inserted into a stoma in less than 15 minutes. Besides its cosmetic appeal, the device is easily maintained, reduces skin irritation and breakdown, and is less likely to become dislodged or migrate than an ordinary feeding tube. A one-way, antireflux valve mounted just inside the mushroom dome prevents accidental leakage of gastric contents. The device usually requires replacement after 3 to 4 months, typically because the antireflux valve wears out.

Equipment

For care

Gloves ▪ feeding accessories, including adapter, feeding catheter, food syringe or bag, and formula ▪ catheter clamp ▪ cleaning equipment, including water, a syringe, cotton-tipped applicator, pipe cleaner, and mild soap or antiseptic solution ▪ Optional: IV pole, pump to provide continuous infusion over several hours.

For reinsertion

Gastrostomy feeding button of the correct size (or all three sizes, if the correct one isn't known) ▪ obturator ▪ antiseptic solution ▪ water-soluble lubricant ▪ gloves.

Preparation of equipment

Obtain the prescribed formula, frequency, amount, and rate of feeding. Gather the appropriate equipment. If using a feeding bag, fill the bag with formula and prime the tubing *to prevent air from entering the stomach and distending the abdomen*.

Make sure formula is at room temperature *because cold formula may cause cramping and discomfort*. Shake the formula container before opening it.

Implementation

▪ Verify the doctor's order.
▪ Confirm the patient's identify using at least two patient identifiers according to your facility's policy.[1]
▪ Explain the procedure to the patient and answer any questions *to decrease anxiety and increase cooperation*.
▪ Perform hand hygiene and put on gloves.[2,3,4]

For gastrostomy feeding button care

▪ Position the patient with the head of the bed raised 30 to 45 degrees.
▪ Attach the adapter and feeding catheter to the syringe or feeding bag tubing and prime the catheter.
▪ Open the safety plug and attach the adapter and feeding catheter to the button (as shown below). Elevate the syringe or feeding bag above stomach level, and gravity-feed the formula for 15 to 30 minutes, varying the height as needed *to alter the flow rate*. Refill the syringe before it's empty to *prevent air from entering the stomach and distending the abdomen*. Use a pump for continuous infusion or for feedings lasting several hours.

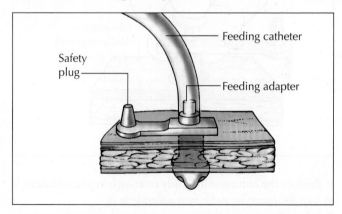

▪ After the feeding, lower the syringe or bag below stomach level *to allow burping* and flush the button with 10 mL of water.
▪ Remove the adapter and feeding catheter. The antireflux valve should prevent gastric reflux.
▪ Snap the safety plug in place *to keep the lumen clean and prevent leakage if the antireflux valve fails*.
▪ If the patient feels nauseated or vomits after the feeding, vent the button with the adapter and feeding catheter *to control emesis*.
▪ Maintain the head of the bed at 30 to 45 degrees for at least 1 hour after feedings.[5]
▪ Rinse the inside of the feeding catheter with water, and use a cotton-tipped applicator, if necessary, *to preserve patency and to dislodge formula or food particles*. Wash the catheter and syringe

or feeding bag in warm, soapy water and rinse thoroughly. Clean the catheter and adapter with a pipe cleaner. Rinse well before using for the next feeding. Soak the equipment once a week according to manufacturer's recommendations.

For gastrostomy feeding button reinsertion

■ Check your facility's policy *to be sure the procedure is approved for nursing personnel.*
■ Gather the appropriate equipment. If the old button will be reinserted, wash it with soap and water and rinse it thoroughly.
■ Position the patient *to easily access the stoma.*
■ Check the depth of the patient's stoma to make sure you have a feeding button of the correct size.
■ Clean around the stoma with mild soap and water or antiseptic solution.
■ Lubricate the obturator with a water-soluble lubricant, and distend the button several times *to ensure patency and function of the antireflux valve within the button.*
■ Lubricate the mushroom dome and the stoma.
■ Gently push the button through the stoma into the stomach (as shown below).

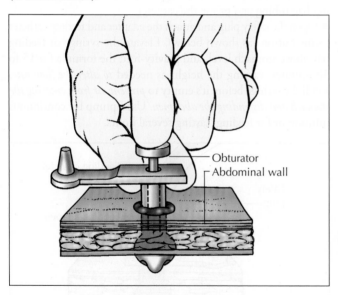

■ Remove the obturator by gently rotating it as you withdraw it *to keep the antireflux valve from adhering to it.*
■ After removing the obturator, make sure the antireflux valve is closed. Then close the flexible safety plug (as shown below), which should be relatively flush with the skin surface.

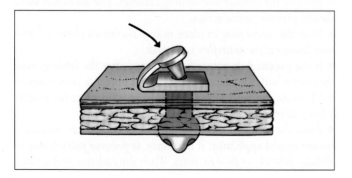

Completing the procedure

■ Remove and discard your gloves and perform hand hygiene.[2,3,4]
■ Document the procedure.[6]

Special considerations

■ If the button pops out while feeding, reinsert it, estimate the formula already delivered, and resume feeding.
■ Once daily, clean the peristomal skin with mild soap and water or povidone-iodine solution, and let the skin air-dry for 20 minutes *to avoid skin irritation.* Also clean the site whenever spillage from the feeding bag occurs.
■ If residual stomach content needs to be evaluated, the adapter and feeding catheter can be attached to the syringe to allow aspiration past the antireflux valve.
■ Medications to be administered through the gastrostomy button should be liquid preparations if at all possible or thoroughly crushed tablets mixed with water *to prevent blocking the button.* Discuss alternatives to enteric-coated tablets or capsules with the doctor or pharmacist.

Patient teaching

Before discharge, make sure the patient can insert and care for the gastrostomy feeding button. If possible, teach him or a family member how to reinsert the button by first practicing on a model. Offer written instructions and answer his questions on obtaining replacement supplies.

Complications

Frequent or large-volume feedings can cause bloating and retention. Dehydration, diarrhea, and vomiting can cause metabolic disturbances. Glycosuria, cramping, and abdominal distention usually indicate intolerance.

Complications from gastrostomy button reinsertion are rare and include irritation of the surrounding skin from the cleaning solutions.

Documentation

Record the feeding time, duration, amount and type of feeding formula used, and the patient's tolerance for the procedure. Record the patency and functioning of the button device. Maintain intake and output records as necessary. Note the appearance of the stoma and surrounding skin. Record the reason for reinsertion, the size of the button used, and the patient's tolerance of the procedure. Document any complications and nursing actions taken, and note the appearance of the stoma and surrounding skin. Document any patient teaching provided and the response to the teaching.

REFERENCES

1 The Joint Commission. (2012). Standard NPSG.01.01.01. *Comprehensive accreditation manual for hospitals: The official handbook.* Oakbrook Terrace, IL: The Joint Commission. (Level I)
2 The Joint Commission. (2012). Standard NPSG.07.01.01. *Comprehensive accreditation manual for hospitals: The official handbook.* Oakbrook Terrace, IL: The Joint Commission. (Level I)

3   Centers for Disease Control and Prevention. (October 2002). Guideline for hand hygiene in health-care settings. *Morbidity and Mortality Weekly Report, 51*(RR-16), 1–45. (Level 1)

4   World Health Organization. (2009). *WHO guidelines on hand hygiene in health care: First global patient safety challenge. Clean care is safer care.* Geneva, Switzerland: World Health Organization. (Level I)

5   Bankhead, R., et al. (2009). Enteral nutrition practice recommendations. *Journal of Parenteral and Enteral Nutrition, 33*(2), 122–167. (Level I)

6   The Joint Commission. (2012). Standard RC.01.03.01. *Comprehensive accreditation manual for hospitals: The official handbook.* Oakbrook Terrace, IL: The Joint Commission. (Level I)

ADDITIONAL REFERENCES

American Association of Critical-Care Nurses. (2009). "AACN Practice Alert: Verification of Feeding Tube Placement" [Online]. Accessed September 2011 via the Web at http://www.aacn.org/WD/Practice/Docs/PracticeAlerts/Verification_of_Feeding_Tube_Placement_05-2005.pdf

Lynn-McHale Wiegand, D. (Ed.). (2011). *AACN procedure manual for critical care* (6th ed.). Philadelphia, PA: Saunders.

Nettina, S.M. (2010). *Lippincott manual of nursing practice* (9th ed.). Philadelphia, PA: Lippincott Williams & Wilkins.

Taylor, C., et al. (2011). *Fundamentals of nursing: The art and science of nursing care* (7th ed.). Philadelphia, PA: Lippincott Williams & Wilkins.

HAIR CARE

Hair care involves combing and brushing the hair to stimulate scalp circulation, remove dead cells and debris, and distribute hair oils to produce a healthy sheen. Frequency of hair care depends on the length and texture of the patient's hair, the duration of hospitalization, and the patient's condition. Usually, hair should be combed and brushed daily.

Equipment

Comb ▪ brush ▪ bath towel ▪ gloves, as necessary ▪ alcohol or oil, as necessary.

Preparation of equipment

The comb and brush should be clean. If necessary, wash them in hot, soapy water. The comb should have dull, even teeth *to prevent scratching the scalp.* The brush should have stiff bristles *to enhance vigorous brushing and stimulation of circulation.*

Implementation

▪ Gather the equipment on the patient's bedside stand.
▪ Confirm the patient's identity using at least two patient identifiers according to your facility's policy.[1]
▪ Perform hand hygiene and, if necessary, put on gloves.[2,3,4]
▪ Tell the patient you're going to comb and brush his hair. If possible, encourage him to do this himself, assisting him as necessary.
▪ Adjust the bed to a comfortable working height *to prevent back strain.* If the patient's condition allows, help him to a sitting position by raising the head of the bed.
▪ Provide privacy, and drape a bath towel over the patient's pillow and shoulders *to catch loose hair and dirt.*
▪ For short hair, comb and brush one side at a time. For long or curly hair, turn the patient's head away from you, and then part his hair down the middle from front to back. Comb and brush the hair on the side facing you. Then turn the patient's head and comb and brush the opposite side. Part hair into small sections for easier handling. Comb one section at a time, working from the ends toward the scalp to remove tangles. Anchor each section of hair above the area being combed *to avoid hurting the patient.*
▪ If the hair is tangled, rub alcohol or oil on the hair strands to loosen them.
▪ After combing, brush the hair, making sure to get all the tangles out.
▪ Style the hair as the patient prefers. Braiding long or curly hair helps prevent snarling. To braid, part hair down the middle of the scalp and begin braiding near the face. Don't braid too tightly *to avoid patient discomfort.* Fasten the ends of the braids with hair ties. Pin the braids across the top of the patient's head or let them hang, as the patient desires, *so the finished braids don't press against the patient's scalp.*
▪ After styling the hair, carefully remove the towel by folding it inward. *This technique prevents loose hairs and debris from falling onto the pillow or into the patient's bed.*
▪ Remove and discard your gloves, and perform hand hygiene.[2,3,4]
▪ Document the procedure.[5]

Special considerations

▪ When giving hair care, check the patient's scalp carefully for signs of scalp disorders or skin breakdown, particularly if the patient is bedridden. Make sure each patient has his own comb and brush *to avoid cross-contamination.*

Documentation

Describe any scalp abnormalities in your notes.

REFERENCES

1   The Joint Commission. (2012). Standard NPSG.01.01.01. *Comprehensive accreditation manual for hospitals: The official handbook.* Oakbrook Terrace, IL: The Joint Commission. (Level I)

2   The Joint Commission. (2012). Standard NPSG.07.01.01. *Comprehensive accreditation manual for hospitals: The official handbook.* Oakbrook Terrace, IL: The Joint Commission. (Level I)

3   World Health Organization. (2009). *WHO guidelines on hand hygiene in health care: First global patient safety challenge. Clean care is safer care.* Geneva, Switzerland: World Health Organization. (Level I)

4   Centers for Disease Control and Prevention. (October 2002). Guideline for hand hygiene in health-care settings. *Morbidity and Mortality Weekly Report, 51*(RR-16), 1–45. (Level I)

5 The Joint Commission. (2012). Standard RC.01.03.01. *Comprehensive accreditation manual for hospitals: The official handbook.* Oakbrook Terrace, IL: The Joint Commission. (Level I)

ADDITIONAL REFERENCE

Craven, R.F., & Hirnle, C.J. (2012). *Fundamentals of nursing: Human health and function* (7th ed.). Philadelphia, PA: Lippincott Williams & Wilkins.

HALO-VEST TRACTION MANAGEMENT

Halo-vest traction immobilizes a patient's head and neck after traumatic injury to the cervical vertebrae as well as helping to prevent further injury to the spinal cord. It also can be used postoperatively to allow for bone healing. An orthopedic surgeon or neurosurgeon applies halo-vest traction, with assistance from a nurse. The procedure typically occurs in the emergency department, a specially equipped room, or the operating room after surgical reduction of vertebral injuries.

The halo-vest traction device consists of a metal ring that fits over the patient's head and metal bars that connect the ring to a plastic vest that distributes the weight of the entire apparatus around the chest. When in place, halo-vest traction allows the patient greater mobility than other forms of cervical traction. (See *Halo-vest traction device.*)

Equipment

Halo-vest traction unit ▪ halo ring ▪ gowns ▪ masks ▪ eye shields ▪ cervical collar or sandbags ▪ plastic vest ▪ board or padded headrest ▪ tape measure ▪ halo ring conversion chart ▪ clippers ▪ 4″ × 4″ sterile gauze pads ▪ antiseptic solution ▪ gloves ▪ sterile gloves ▪ Allen wrench ▪ four positioning pins ▪ multiple-dose vial of 1% lidocaine (with or without epinephrine) ▪ alcohol pads ▪ 3-mL syringe ▪ 25G needles ▪ five sterile skull pins (one more than needed) ▪ torque screwdriver ▪ sheepskin vest liners ▪ cotton-tipped applicators ▪ medicated powder or cornstarch ▪ sterile water or normal saline solution ▪ soap ▪ basin of warm water ▪ washcloth ▪ towel ▪ Optional: hair dryer, analgesics.

Most facilities supply packaged halo-vest traction units that include software (jacket and sheepskin liners), hardware (halo, head pins, upright bars, and screws), and tools (torque screwdriver, two conventional wrenches, Allen wrench, and screws and bolts).

Preparation of equipment

Obtain a halo-vest traction unit with halo rings and plastic vests in several sizes. Vest sizes are based on the patient's chest and head measurements. Check the expiration date of the prepackaged tray, and check the outside covering for damage *to ensure the sterility of the contents.* Then gather the equipment at the patient's bedside.

Implementation

▪ Verify the doctor's order.
▪ Gather the necessary equipment

▪ Conduct a preprocedure verification *to make sure that all relevant documentation, related information, and equipment are available and correctly identified to the patient's identifiers.*[1]
▪ Verify that the laboratory and imaging studies have been completed as ordered and that the results are in the patient's medical record. Notify the doctor of any unexpected results.[1]
▪ Perform hand hygiene.[2,3,4]
▪ Confirm the patient's identity using at least two patient identifiers according to your facility's policy.[5]
▪ Provide privacy.

Assisting with halo application

▪ Confirm that the doctor has obtained informed consent and make sure that the form is in the patient's medical record.[6,7]
▪ Obtain baseline vital signs and perform neurologic and pulmonary assessments.
▪ Check the support that was applied to the patient's neck on the way to the health care facility. If necessary, apply the cervical collar immediately or immobilize the head and neck with sandbags. Keep the cervical collar or sandbags in place until the halo is applied.[8] This support will then be carefully removed *to facilitate application of the vest.* Reassure the patient.
▪ Remove the headboard and any furniture at the head of the bed *to provide ample working space.* Then carefully place the patient's head on a board or on a padded headrest that extends beyond the edge of the bed.

NURSING ALERT To prevent further injury to the spinal cord, *never put the patient's head on a pillow before applying the halo.*

▪ Elevate the bed to a working level that gives the doctor easy access to the front and back of the halo unit.
▪ Stand at the head of the bed and see if the patient's chin lines up with his midsternum, *indicating proper alignment.* If ordered, support the patient's head in your hands and gently rotate the neck into alignment without flexing or extending it. Ask another nurse to help you with the procedure.
▪ Have the assisting nurse hold the patient's head and neck stable while the doctor removes the cervical collar or sandbags. This support should be maintained until the halo is secure while you assist with pin insertion.
▪ Conduct a time-out immediately before starting the procedure to perform a final assessment that the correct patient, site, positioning, and procedure are identified and, as applicable, that all relevant information and necessary equipment are available.[9] The doctor measures the patient's head with a tape measure and refers to the halo ring conversion chart to determine the correct ring size. (The ring should clear the head by ⅝″ [1.6 cm] and fit ½″ [1.3 cm] above the bridge of the nose.)
▪ The doctor selects four pin sites: ½″ above the lateral one-third of each eyebrow and ½″ above the top of each ear in the occipital area. He also takes into account the degree and type of correction needed to provide proper cervical alignment.
▪ Trim the hair at the pin sites with clippers *to facilitate subsequent care and help prevent infection.*
▪ Perform hand hygiene and put on sterile gloves, a gown, and eyewear.[2,3,4]

- Use 4″ × 4″ sterile gauze pads soaked in antiseptic solution to clean the sites and allow them to dry.
- Open the halo-vest unit using sterile technique *to avoid contamination*. The doctor puts on the sterile gloves and removes the halo and the Allen wrench. He then places the halo over the patient's head and inserts the four positioning pins *to hold the halo in place temporarily*.
- Help the doctor prepare the anesthetic. First, clean the injection port of the multiple-dose vial of lidocaine with the alcohol sponge. Then, invert the vial so the doctor can insert a 25G needle attached to the 3-mL syringe and withdraw the anesthetic.
- The doctor injects the anesthetic at the four pin sites. Change the needle on the syringe after each injection.
- The doctor removes four of the five skull pins from the sterile setup and firmly screws in each pin at a 90-degree angle to the skull. When the pins are in place, he removes the positioning pins. He then tightens the skull pins with the torque screwdriver.

Applying the vest
- After the doctor measures the patient's chest and abdomen, he selects a vest of appropriate size.
- Place the sheepskin liners inside the front and back of the vest *to make it more comfortable to wear and to help prevent pressure ulcers*.
- Help the doctor carefully raise the patient while the other nurse supports the patient's head and neck. Slide the back of the vest under the patient and gently lay him down. The doctor then fastens the front of the vest on the patient's chest using Velcro straps.
- The doctor attaches the metal bars to the halo and vest and tightens each bolt in turn *to avoid tightening any single bolt completely, causing maladjusted tension*.
- When halo-vest traction is in place, X-rays should be taken immediately *to check the depth of the skull pins and verify proper alignment*.

Caring for the patient
- Explain the procedure to the patient and his family.
- Obtain routine and neurologic vital signs as ordered.
NURSING ALERT *Notify the doctor immediately if you observe any loss of motor function or any decreased sensation from baseline;* these findings could indicate spinal cord trauma.
- *Because the vest limits chest expansion,* routinely assess pulmonary function, especially in a patient with pulmonary disease.
- Perform hand hygiene and put on gloves.[2,3,4]
- Visually assess the pin sites for drainage or signs of infection.
- Gently clean the pin sites with cleaning solution or chlorhexidine every 8 hours (or in accordance with your facility's policy) with cotton-tipped applicators. Use a clean cotton-tipped applicator for each individual site. Rinse the sites with normal saline solution *to remove any excess cleaning solution.*[10] *Meticulous pin-site care prevents infection and removes debris that might block drainage and lead to abscess formation.* Observe for signs of infection—a loose pin, swelling or redness, purulent drainage, or pain at the site—and notify the doctor if these signs develop.
- The doctor retightens the skull pins with the torque screwdriver 24 and 48 hours after the halo is applied. If the patient complains of a headache after the pins are tightened, obtain an

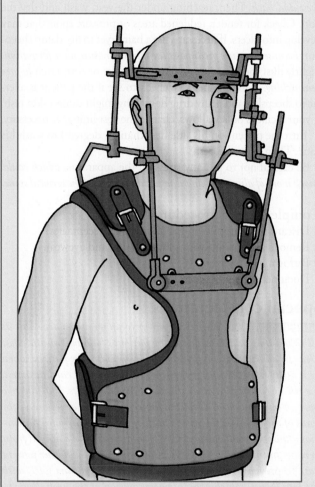

Halo-vest traction device

With the standard low-profile halo-vest traction device, traction and compression are produced by threaded support rods on either side of the halo ring. Flexion and extension are obtained by moving the swivel arm to an anterior or posterior position, depending on the location of the skull pins.

Advantages of this type of device include:
- immobilizing cervical spine fractures while allowing patient mobility
- facilitating surgery of the cervical spine and permitting flexion and extension
- allowing airway intubation without losing skeletal traction
- allowing necessary alignment through adjustments at the junction of the threaded support rods and horizontal frame.

order for an analgesic. If pain occurs with jaw movement or any movement of the head or neck, notify the doctor immediately *because this symptom may indicate that pins have slipped.*

■ Examine the halo-vest unit every shift *to make sure that the unit is secure and that the patient's head is centered within the halo.* If the vest fits correctly, you should be able to insert one or two fingers under the jacket at the shoulder and chest when the patient is lying supine.

■ Wash the patient's chest and back daily. First, place the patient on his back. Loosen the bottom Velcro straps *so you can get to the chest and back.* Then, reaching under the vest, wash and dry the skin. Check for tender, reddened areas or pressure spots that may develop into ulcers. If necessary, use a hair dryer to dry damp sheepskin *because moisture predisposes the skin to pressure ulcer formation.* Lightly dust the skin with medicated powder or cornstarch *to prevent itching.* If itching persists, check to see if the patient is allergic to sheepskin and if any drug he's taking might cause a skin rash. If your facility's policy allows, change the vest lining, as necessary.

■ Turn the patient on his side (less than 45 degrees) to wash his back. Then close the vest.

■ Be careful not to put any stress on the apparatus, *which could knock it out of alignment and lead to subluxation of the cervical spine.*

Completing the procedure
■ Discard used supplies in the appropriate receptacles.[10]
■ Remove and discard your gloves, gown, and eyewear.
■ Perform hand hygiene.[2,3,4]
■ Document the procedure.[11]

Special considerations

NURSING ALERT *Keep two conventional wrenches available at all times; they may be taped to the patient's halo vest on the chest area. In addition, a wrench should accompany the patient when he is away from the unit for testing. In the event of cardiac arrest, use the wrenches to remove the distal anterior bolts. Pull the two upright bars outward. Unfasten the Velcro straps, and remove the front of the vest. Use the sturdy back of the vest as a board for cardiopulmonary resuscitation (CPR). Some vests have a hinged front to raise the breastplate for CPR. Know the type of vest your patient has. To prevent subluxating the cervical injury, start CPR with the jaw thrust, which avoids hyperextension of the neck. Pull the patient's mandible forward while maintaining proper head and neck alignment.* This positioning pulls the tongue forward to open the airway.

■ Never lift the patient up by the vertical bars. *Doing so could strain or tear the skin at the pin sites or misalign the traction.*

■ *To prevent falls,* walk with the ambulatory patient. Remember, he'll have trouble seeing objects at or near his feet, and the weight of the halo-vest unit (about 10 lb [4.5 kg]) may throw him off balance. If the patient is in a wheelchair, lower the leg rests *to prevent the chair from tipping backward.*

■ *Because the vest limits chest expansion,* routinely assess pulmonary function, especially in a patient with pulmonary disease.

■ Skin breakdown can occur if the vest fits improperly or has inadequate padding. Prevent skin breakdown by ensuring adequate padding, turning, and repositioning of the patient.

Patient teaching
Teach the patient to turn slowly, in small increments, *to avoid losing his balance.* Remind him to avoid bending forward *because the extra weight of the halo apparatus could cause him to fall.* Teach him to bend at the knees rather than the waist.

Have a physical therapist teach the patient how to use assistive devices *to extend his reach and to help him put on socks and shoes.* Suggest that he wear shirts that button in front and that are larger than usual *to accommodate the halo vest.*

Most importantly, teach the patient about pin-site care and about shampooing and hair care. Instruct the patient and his family not to adjust the pins.

Complications
Manipulating the patient's neck during application of halo-vest traction may cause subluxation of the spinal cord, or it could push a bone fragment into the spinal cord, possibly compressing the cord and causing paralysis below the break.

Inaccurate positioning of the skull pins can lead to a puncture of the dura mater, causing a loss of cerebrospinal fluid and a serious central nervous system infection. Multiple retorquing of the pins increases the potential for a dural puncture.

Nonsterile technique during application of the halo or inadequate pin-site care can lead to infection at the pin sites and other complications, including pin-site loosening or dislodgement, swallowing problems, and ring migration.

Pressure ulcers can develop if the vest fits poorly or chafes the skin.

Documentation
Record the date and time that the halo-vest traction was applied. Also note the length of the procedure and the patient's response. Record the patient's vital signs and neurologic, pain, and pulmonary assessments. Document that a preprocedure verification and time-out were performed. Document the appearance of pin insertion sites, analgesics provided, and patient education performed.

When providing care to the patient with halo-vest traction, record routine vital signs as well as your pain, pulmonary, and neurologic assessments. Document pin-site care. Note any signs of infection or loose pins. Document patient teaching and the patient's response to the procedure.

References
1 The Joint Commission. (2012). Standard UP.01.01.01. *Comprehensive accreditation manual for hospitals: The official handbook.* Oakbrook Terrace, IL: The Joint Commission. (Level I)
2 The Joint Commission. (2012). Standard NPSG.07.01.01. *Comprehensive accreditation manual for hospitals: The official handbook.* Oakbrook Terrace, IL: The Joint Commission. (Level I)
3 Centers for Disease Control and Prevention. (October 2002). Guideline for hand hygiene in health-care settings. *Morbidity and Mortality Weekly Report, 51*(RR-16), 1–45. (Level I)
4 World Health Organization. (2009). *WHO guidelines on hand hygiene in health care: First global patient safety challenge. Clean care is safer care.* Geneva, Switzerland: World Health Organization. (Level I)

5 The Joint Commission. (2012). Standard NPSG.01.01.01. *Comprehensive accreditation manual for hospitals: The official handbook.* Oakbrook Terrace, IL: The Joint Commission. (Level I)

6 The Joint Commission. (2012). Standard RI.01.03.01. *Comprehensive accreditation manual for hospitals: The official handbook.* Oakbrook Terrace, IL: The Joint Commission. (Level I)

7 Centers for Medicare & Medicaid Services, Department of Health and Human Services. (2006). "Conditions of Participation: Patients' Rights," 42 CFR part 482.13 [Online]. Accessed November 2011 via the Web at https://www.cms.gov/CFCsAndCoPs/downloads/finalpatientrightsrule.pdf

8 American Association of Neuroscience Nurses. (2010). *Core curriculum for neuroscience nursing* (5th ed.). Philadelphia, PA: Saunders.

9 The Joint Commission. (2012). Standard UP.01.03.01. *Comprehensive accreditation manual for hospitals: The official handbook.* Oakbrook Terrace, IL: The Joint Commission. (Level I)

10 Lynn-McHale Wiegand, D. (Ed.). (2011). *AACN procedure manual for critical care* (6th ed.). Philadelphia, PA: Saunders.

11 The Joint Commission. (2012). Standard RC.01.03.01. *Comprehensive accreditation manual for hospitals: The official handbook.* Oakbrook Terrace, IL: The Joint Commission. (Level I)

ADDITIONAL REFERENCES

Holmes, S.B., & Brown, S.J. (2005). Skeletal pin site care: National Association of Orthopaedic Nurses guidelines for orthopaedic nursing. *Orthopaedic Nursing, 24*(2), 99–107.

Ivanic, P.C., et al. (2009). Effect of halo-vest components on stabilizing the injured cervical spine. *Spine, 34*(2), 167–175.

Lauweryns, P. (2010). Role of conservative treatment of cervical spine injury. *European Spine Journal, 19*(Suppl.), S23–S26.

Sarro, A., et al. (2010). Developing a standard of care for halo vest and pin site care including patient and family education: A collaborative approach among three greater Toronto-area teaching hospitals. *Journal of Neuroscience Nursing, 42*(3), 169–173.

Van Middendorp, J.J., et al. (2009). Incidence of and risk factors for complications associated with halo-vest immobilization: A prospective, descriptive cohort study of 239 patients. *Journal of Bone and Joint Surgery, 91*(1), 71–79.

HAND HYGIENE

The hands are the conduits for almost every transfer of potential pathogens from one patient to another, from a contaminated object to the patient, or from a staff member to the patient. Because of this, hand hygiene is the single most important procedure in preventing infection.[1,2,3,4] To protect patients from health care–associated infections, hand hygiene must be performed routinely and thoroughly. In effect, clean and healthy hands with intact skin, short fingernails, and no rings minimize the risk of contamination. Artificial nails may serve as a reservoir for microorganisms, and microorganisms are more difficult to remove from rough or chapped hands.[1,2,3,4]

Hand hygiene is a general term that's used by the Centers for Disease Control and Prevention (CDC) and the World Health Organization (WHO) to refer to hand washing, antiseptic hand wash, antiseptic hand rub, or surgical hand asepsis.

Washing with soap and water is appropriate when hands are visibly soiled or contaminated with blood or other body fluids, when exposure to potential spore-forming pathogens (*Clostridium difficile, Bacillus anthracis*) is strongly suspected or proven, and after using the restroom. Using an alcohol-based hand rub is appropriate for decontaminating the hands before direct patient contact; after removing gloves; before inserting an invasive device; after contact with the patient; when moving from a contaminated-body site to a clean-body site during patient care; after contact with body fluids or excretions, mucous membranes, nonintact skin, and wound dressings (if hands aren't visibly soiled); after removing gloves; and after contact with inanimate objects in the patient's environment.[1,2,4] (See *Your 5 moments for hand hygiene,* page 326.)

The CDC recommends performing hand hygiene with soap and water before eating;[1] the WHO recommends using either an alcohol-based hand rub or washing with soap and water before preparing food or handling medication.[2]

Equipment
Hand washing
Soap ▪ warm running water ▪ paper towels.

Hand sanitizing
Alcohol-based hand rub.

Implementation
Hand washing
▪ Remove rings according to your facility's policy *because they harbor dirt and skin microorganisms.* Remove your watch or wear it well above the wrist. If you wear nail polish, it must be kept in good repair to minimize its potential to harbor microorganisms; refer to your facility's policy pertaining to nail polish. Natural nails should be short (less than ¼" [0.6 cm]).[1,6,7]

▪ Wet your hands and wrists with warm (not hot) water and apply soap from a dispenser. Don't use bar soap *because it allows cross-contamination.* Hold your hands below elbow level *to prevent water from running up your arms and back down, thus contaminating clean areas.* (See *Proper hand-washing technique,* page 327.)

▪ Work up a generous lather by rubbing your hands together vigorously for about 15 seconds.[1] *Soap and warm water reduce surface tension and this, aided by friction, loosens surface microorganisms, which wash away in the lather.*

▪ Pay special attention to the area under fingernails and around cuticles as well as to the thumbs, knuckles, and sides of the fingers and hands *because microorganisms thrive in these protected or overlooked areas.* If you don't remove your wedding band, move it up and down your finger to clean beneath it.[1]

▪ Avoid splashing water on yourself or the floor *because microorganisms spread more easily on wet surfaces and because slippery floors are dangerous.* Avoid touching the sink or faucets *because they're considered contaminated.*

▪ Rinse hands and wrists well *because running water flushes suds, soil, and microorganisms away.*

Your 5 moments for hand hygiene

According to the World Health Organization (WHO), there are 5 key moments during patient care when health care workers should perform hand hygiene.[5]

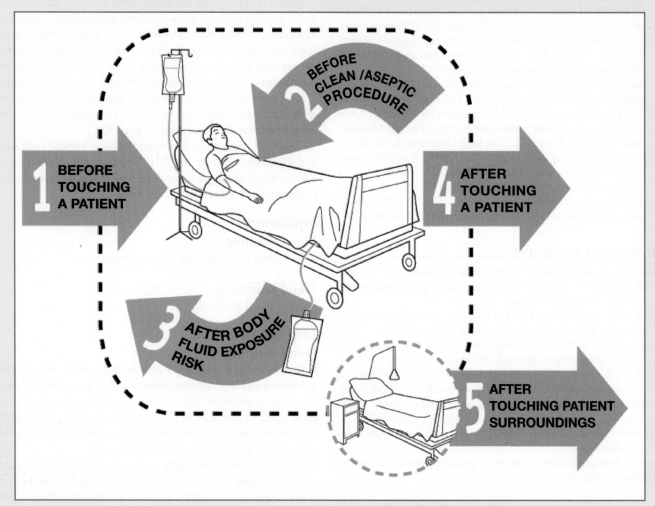

World Health Organization. (2009). "My 5 Moments for Hand Hygiene" [Online]. Accessed November 2011 via the Web at http://www.who.int/gpsc/5may/background/5moments/en/index.html

■ Pat hands and wrists dry with a paper towel. *Avoid rubbing, which can cause abrasion and chapping.*
■ If the sink isn't equipped with knee or foot controls, turn off the faucets by gripping them with a dry paper towel *to avoid recontaminating your hands.*

Hand sanitizing

■ Apply alcohol-based hand rub to the palm of one hand and then rub your hands together to cover all surfaces of the hands.[1,2]
■ Rub your hands together until all of the product has dried (usually 30 seconds).

Special considerations

■ Before participating in any sterile procedure or whenever your hands are grossly contaminated, wash your forearms also, and clean under the fingernails and in and around the cuticles. *Brushes, metal files, or other hard objects may injure your skin and, if reused, may be a source of contamination.*
■ The CDC hand hygiene guideline recommends that artificial nails or extenders not be worn when having direct contact with patients at high risk for acquiring infections, such as patients on intensive care or transplant units.[1] The WHO guidelines on hand hygiene in health care recommend that artificial nails or extenders not be worn when having direct contact with all patients.[2]
■ Don't use an alcohol-based hand rub if contact with items contaminated with *C. difficile* or *B. anthracis* occurs. *These organisms*

can form spores, and alcohol won't kill the spores. Instead, wash hands with soap and water.[1]

- If your hands aren't visibly soiled, an alcohol-based hand rub can be used for routine decontamination.
- If you're providing care in the patient's home, bring your own supply of soap and disposable paper towels. If there's no running water, disinfect your hands with an alcohol-based hand rub.
- Keep in mind that glove use doesn't eliminate the need for hand hygiene.
- Teach patients and their families about the importance of hand hygiene in preventing the spread of infection, and encourage them to remind health care workers to perform hand hygiene when necessary.[1,2]

Complications

Because frequent hand washing strips the skin of natural oils, this simple procedure can result in dryness, cracking, and irritation. However, these effects are probably more common after repeated use of antiseptic cleaning agents, especially in people with sensitive skin. *To help minimize irritation,* rinse your hands thoroughly, making sure they're free from residue.

To prevent your hands from becoming dry or chapped, apply an emollient hand cream after each washing or switch to a different cleaning agent. Make sure that the hand cream or lotion you use won't cause the material in your gloves to deteriorate. If you develop dermatitis, you may need to be evaluated by your employee health care provider *to determine whether you should continue to work until the condition resolves. Hands with dermatitis are more susceptible to becoming colonized with transient bacteria.*

REFERENCES

1   Centers for Disease Control and Prevention. (October 2002). Guideline for hand hygiene in health-care settings. *Morbidity and Mortality Weekly Report, 51*(RR-16), 1–45. (Level I)
2   World Health Organization. (2009). *WHO guidelines on hand hygiene in health care: First global patient safety challenge. Clean care is safer care.* Geneva, Switzerland: World Health Organization. (Level I)
3   Institute for Healthcare Improvement. "How-to Guide: Improving Hand Hygiene" [Online]. Accessed November 2011 via the Web at http://www.ihi.org/IHI/Topics/CriticalCare/IntensiveCare/Tools/HowtoGuideImprovingHandHygiene.htm (Level I)
4   The Joint Commission. (2012). Standard NPSG.07.01.01. *Comprehensive accreditation manual for hospitals: The official handbook.* Oakbrook Terrace, IL: The Joint Commission. (Level I)
5   World Health Organization. (2009). "My 5 Moments for Hand Hygiene" [Online]. Accessed November 2011 via the Web at http://www.who.int/gpsc/5may/background/5moments/en/index.html
6   Parry, M.F., et al. (2001). Candida osteomyelitis and diskitis after spinal surgery: An outbreak that implicates artificial nail use. *Clinical Infection Control, 32*(3), 352–357.
7   Salisbury, D.M., et al. (1997). The effect of rings on microbial load of health care workers hands. *American Journal of Infection Control, 25*(1), 24–27.

Proper hand-washing technique

To minimize the spread of infection, follow these basic hand-washing instructions.

With your hands angled downward under the faucet, adjust the water temperature until it's comfortably warm.

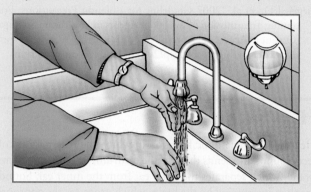

Work up a generous lather by scrubbing vigorously for 15 seconds. Be sure to clean beneath your fingernails, around your knuckles, and along the sides of your fingers and hands.

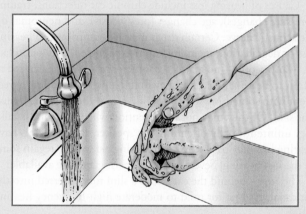

Rinse your hands completely *to wash away suds and microorganisms.* Pat dry with a paper towel. *To prevent recontaminating your hands on the faucet handles,* cover each one with a dry paper towel when turning off the water.

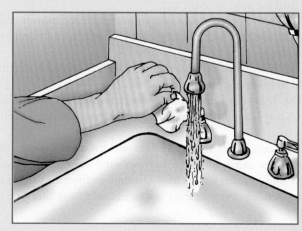

ADDITIONAL REFERENCES

Carrico, R. (Ed.). (2009). *APIC text of infection control and epidemiology* (3rd ed.). Washington, DC: Association for Professionals in Infection Control and Epidemiology, Inc.

The Joint Commission: Consensus Measurement in Hand Hygiene Project Expert Advisory Panel. (2009). *Measuring hand hygiene adherence: Overcoming the challenges.* Oakbrook Terrace, IL: The Joint Commission.

Siegel, J.D., et al. "2007 Guideline for Isolation Precautions: Preventing Transmission of Infectious Agents in Healthcare Settings" [Online]. Accessed September 2011 via the Web at http://www.cdc.gov/hicpac/2007ip/2007isolationprecautions.html

HEARING AID CARE

Hearing is an anatomic function in which the external ear collects sounds and sends them to the eardrum, or tympanic membrane, which separates the outer ear from the inner ear. Sounds are then interpreted by the brain, which processes the appropriate response. The three primary bones involved in sound transmission are the malleus (hammer), incus (anvil), and stapes (stirrup).

Causes of hearing loss include chronic ear infections, trauma (pressure changes), age changes (presbycusis), and neuromas on the acoustic nerve. Certain drugs may also contribute to hearing loss or degradation, including aspirin, naproxen, and ketorolac.

Many people—no matter what their age—are embarrassed to admit to hearing loss. They may find themselves nodding agreement with something someone said, even if they're unsure what was said. Or they may not pay attention when someone is talking, unintentionally offending the speaker. Patients who have hearing loss may be able to use a hearing aid to help regain some of the lost hearing. Several types of hearing aids are available:

■ The "open behind the ear" aid is a slim tube inserted into the ear canal. It's best for mild to moderate high-frequency hearing losses.

■ The "behind the ear" aid amplifies the sound from a customized ear mold that's placed in the ear canal. These aids are used for mild to moderate hearing loss.

■ The "full shell" aid is custom-made and fits on the outer ear. It's used for mild to severe loss.

■ The "half shell" models are also custom-made and provide optimal performance with greater comfort. They're used for mild to severe losses.

■ The "canal" aid fits inside the external ear canal and is used for mild to moderately severe loss.

■ The "mini-canal" fits almost completely inside the external ear canal and is appropriate for mild to moderately severe hearing loss.

■ The "completely in the canal" model fits deeply within the external ear canal. This type decreases wind noise, has less feedback, and provides a more natural sound. Individuals with mild to moderately severe hearing loss can benefit from this type of aid.

Patients generally wear hearing aids during the day only. At night and at times of rest, the hearing aid is usually removed. Because of the fragile nature of the hearing aid, it's important to clean it properly and carefully to avoid damage.

Equipment

Bath towel ■ facial tissue ■ cleaning brush, wire loop, or soft toothbrush ■ storage case ■ washcloth ■ water ■ soap ■ Optional: spare battery, dryer for hearing aids, gloves.

Implementation

■ Gather the appropriate equipment.
■ Perform hand hygiene.[1,2,3]
■ Confirm the patient's identity using at least two patient identifiers according to your facility's policy.[4]

Removing a hearing aid

■ Assess the patient's ear. If drainage is present, put on gloves.
■ Gently turn the hearing aid off *to prevent feedback during removal.*
■ Grasp the hearing aid and remove it from the ear.
■ Hold the hearing aid over a towel *to prevent damaging it if dropped.* Wipe the outside of the hearing aid with a tissue.

NURSING ALERT *Don't use alcohol or other solvents on the hearing aid because they may cause breakdown of the material.*

■ Carefully inspect the hearing aid and look for accumulated cerumen (earwax). Remove the cerumen using the cleaning brush or wire loop that was supplied with the hearing aid. If these items aren't available, use a soft toothbrush to gently remove the cerumen. Be careful not to push the cerumen into any openings.
■ Feel along the hearing aid for any rough areas that may irritate the ear canal.
■ Open the battery *to allow internal components exposure to air to dry.*
■ Place the hearing aid and battery in a storage container labeled with the patient's name, identification number, and room number.
■ Place a towel under the patient's ear and gently wash the ear and ear canal with a washcloth and soap and warm water.

Inserting a hearing aid

■ Remove the hearing aid from the storage case and close the battery door.
■ Check the battery by slowing turning the volume up to high. Place your hand over the hearing aid and listen for feedback. Turn the volume off *to prevent feedback while inserting the hearing aid.*
■ Look on the hearing aid and determine whether it's for the right or left ear. Right ear hearing aids will be marked with an R or have a red dot. Left ear hearing aids will be marked with an L or have a blue dot.
■ Hold the hearing aid gently and insert the shaped end into the ear canal. Avoid pulling on the ear, *which may alter the shape of the ear canal and cause the hearing aid to be improperly placed.*
■ Turn the volume up slowly to a comfortable level.

Completing the procedure

- Perform hand hygiene.[1,2,3]
- Document the procedure.[5]

Special considerations

- Many individuals with severe hearing loss have learned to read lips. Although this skill improves reception of the words, it doesn't improve the ability to hear. Face the patient when you speak to him and speak slowly.
- Keep background noise to a minimum if possible. *White noise can cause distractions, especially at higher frequencies.*
- Higher voices may be more difficult to hear, especially if the hearing loss is in the higher frequency, which more typically occurs in elderly patients. Patients with hearing loss may also have difficulty hearing such consonants as "p," "k," "f," "th," and "s."
- Avoid placing the hearing aid in direct sunlight or direct heat.

Patient teaching

Teach the patient how to properly remove, clean, and insert the hearing aid.

ELDER ALERT *Some elderly patients may have difficulty manipulating the hearing aids to correctly insert and clean them. If this is the case, refer them to an audiologist, who can recommend a hearing aid that will better fit their lifestyle.*

Tell the patient to keep the hearing aid in the storage case when not in use *to avoid damage.* Also, tell the patient to keep the hearing aid out of reach of animals. *Dogs are attracted to the smell of hearing aids and may damage them if they can reach them.* Instruct the patient to keep the batteries away from pets and children *to avoid accidental ingestion.* Tell the patient to keep the hearing aid dry and to remove it before showering, swimming, or participating in an activity with water. The patient should also avoid getting hairspray or cologne on the hearing aid.

Complications

Dropping the hearing aid may damage it. If there's moisture that gets into the hearing aid, either during wear or during cleaning, it may not transmit sound.

Documentation

Document the removal and cleaning of hearing aids. Document where the hearing aids were stored. If patient teaching was done, record the teaching performed and the patient's response to the teaching.[5]

REFERENCES

1 The Joint Commission. (2012). Standard NPSG.07.01.01. *Comprehensive accreditation manual for hospitals: The official handbook.* Oakbrook Terrace, IL: The Joint Commission. (Level I)
2 Centers for Disease Control and Prevention. (October 2002). Guideline for hand hygiene in health-care settings. *Morbidity and Mortality Weekly Report, 51*(RR-16), 1–45. (Level I)
3 World Health Organization. (2009). *WHO guidelines on hand hygiene in health care: First global patient safety challenge. Clean care is safer care.* Geneva, Switzerland: World Health Organization. (Level I)
4 The Joint Commission. (2012). Standard NPSG.01.01.01. *Comprehensive accreditation manual for hospitals: The official handbook.* Oakbrook Terrace, IL: The Joint Commission. (Level I)
5 The Joint Commission. (2012). Standard RC.01.03.01. *Comprehensive accreditation manual for hospitals: The official handbook.* Oakbrook Terrace, IL: The Joint Commission. (Level I)

ADDITIONAL REFERENCE

Desjardins, J.L., & Doherty, K.A. (2009). Do experienced hearing aid users know how to use their hearing aids correctly? *American Journal of Audiology, 18*(1), 69–76.

HEAT APPLICATION

Heat applied directly to the patient's body raises tissue temperature and enhances the inflammatory process by causing vasodilation and increasing local circulation, which promotes leukocytosis, suppuration, drainage, and healing. Heat also increases tissue metabolism, reduces pain caused by muscle spasm, and decreases congestion in deep visceral organs.

Direct heat may be dry or moist. Dry heat can be delivered at a higher temperature and for a longer time than moist heat. Devices for applying dry heat include the hot-water bottle, electric heating pad, K pad, and chemical hot pack.

Moist heat softens crusts and exudates, penetrates deeper than dry heat, is less drying to the skin, produces less perspiration, and is usually more comfortable for the patient. Devices for applying moist heat include warm compresses for small body areas and warm packs for large areas.

Direct heat treatment can't be used on a patient at risk for hemorrhage. It's also contraindicated if the patient has a sprained limb in the acute stage (because vasodilation would increase pain and swelling) or if he has a condition associated with acute inflammation such as appendicitis. Direct heat should be applied cautiously to pediatric and elderly patients as well as to patients with impaired renal, cardiac, or respiratory function; arteriosclerosis or atherosclerosis; or impaired sensation. It should be applied with extreme caution to heat-sensitive areas, such as scar tissue and stomas.

Equipment

For all methods

Patient thermometer ■ towel ■ adhesive tape or roller gauze ■ absorbent, protective cloth covering ■ Optional: sterile gloves.

For a hot-water bottle

Hot tap water ■ pitcher ■ bath (utility) thermometer.

For a K pad

Distilled water ■ temperature-adjustment key.

For a warm compress or pack (sterile or nonsterile)

Basin of hot tap water or container of sterile water, normal saline, or other solution, as ordered ■ hot-water bottle, K pad, or chemical hot pack ■ linen-saver pad ■ bath (utility) thermometer ■ Optional: forceps.

Sterile or nonsterile items, as appropriate, include compress material (flannel or 4″ × 4″ gauze pads) or pack material (absorbent towels or large absorbent pads), cotton-tipped applicators, forceps, a bowl or basin, a bath (utility) thermometer, waterproof covering, a towel, and dressings.

Preparation of equipment

Hot-water bottle

Fill the bottle with hot tap water *to detect leaks and warm the bottle;* then empty it. Run hot tap water into a pitcher and measure the water temperature with the bath thermometer. Adjust the temperature as ordered, usually to 115° to 125° F (46.1° to 51.7° C) for adults.

PEDIATRIC ALERT *Adjust water temperature to between 105° and 115° F (40.6° to 46.1° C) for children younger than age 2.*

ELDER ALERT *Adjust water temperature to between 105° and 115° F for elderly patients.*

Next, pour hot water into the bottle, filling it one-half to two-thirds full. *Partially filling the bottle keeps it lightweight and flexible to mold to the treatment area.* Squeeze the bottle until the water reaches the neck *to expel any air that would make the bottle inflexible and reduce heat conduction.* Fasten the top and cover the bag with an absorbent cloth. Secure the cover with tape or roller gauze.

Electric heating pad

Check the cord for frayed or damaged insulation. Then plug in the pad and adjust the control switch to the desired setting. Wrap the pad in a protective cloth covering, and secure the cover with tape or roller gauze.

K pad

Check the cord for frayed or damaged insulation, and fill the control unit two-thirds full with distilled water according to the manufacturer's directions. Don't use tap water *because it leaves mineral deposits in the unit.* Check for leaks, and then tilt the unit in several directions *to clear the pad's tubing of air.* Tighten the cap, and then loosen it a quarter turn *to allow heat expansion within the unit.* After making sure the hoses between the control unit and the pad are free of tangles, place the unit on the bedside table, slightly above the patient *so that gravity can assist water flow.* If the central supply department hasn't preset the temperature, use the temperature-adjustment key provided to set the temperature on the control unit (the usual temperature is 105° F [40.6° C]). Then place the pad in a protective cloth covering and secure the cover with tape or roller gauze. Plug in the unit, turn it on, and allow the pad to warm for 2 minutes.

Chemical hot pack

Select a pack of the correct size. Then follow the manufacturer's directions (strike, squeeze, or knead) *to activate the heat-producing chemicals.* Place the pack in a protective cloth covering and secure the cover with tape or roller gauze.

Sterile warm compress or pack

Warm the container of sterile water or solution by setting it in a sink or basin of hot water. Measure its temperature with a sterile bath thermometer. If a sterile thermometer is unavailable, pour some heated sterile solution into a clean container, check the temperature with a regular bath thermometer, and then discard the tested solution. Adjust the temperature by adding hot or cold water to the sink or basin until the solution reaches 131° F (55° C) for adults. Adjust the water to 105° F (40.6° C) for an eye compress.

PEDIATRIC ALERT *Adjust the water temperature to 105° F (40.6° C) for children.*

ELDER ALERT *Adjust the water temperature to 105° F for elderly patients.*

Pour the heated solution into a sterile bowl or basin. Then, using sterile technique, soak the compress or pack in the heated solution. If necessary, prepare a hot-water bottle, K pad, or chemical hot pack *to keep the compress or pack warm.*

Nonsterile warm compress or pack

Fill a bowl or basin with hot tap water or other solution, and measure the temperature of the fluid with a bath thermometer. Adjust the temperature as ordered, typically to 131° F (55° C) for adults or 105° F (40.6° C) for an eye compress.

PEDIATRIC ALERT *Adjust the water temperature to 105° F (40.6° C) for children.*

ELDER ALERT *Adjust the water temperature to 105° F (40.6° C) for elderly patients.*

Soak the compress or pack in the hot liquid. If necessary, prepare a hot-water bottle, K pad, or chemical hot pack *to keep the compress or pack warm.*

Implementation

- Verify the doctor's order and assess the patient's condition.
- Perform hand hygiene.[1,2,3]
- Confirm the patient's identity using at least two patient identifiers according to your facility's policy.[4]
- Explain the procedure to the patient, and tell him not to lean or lie directly on the heating device *because direct contact reduces air space and increases the risk of burns.* Warn him against adjusting the temperature of the heating device or adding hot water to a hot-water bottle. Advise him to report pain immediately and to remove the device if necessary.
- Provide privacy and make sure the room is warm and free of drafts. Perform hand hygiene.[1,2,3]
- Obtain the patient's temperature, pulse, and respirations *to serve as a baseline.* If heat treatment is being applied to raise the patient's body temperature, monitor temperature, pulse, and respirations throughout the application.
- Expose only the treatment area *because vasodilation will make the patient feel chilly.*

To apply a hot-water bottle, an electric heating pad, a K pad, or a chemical hot pack

■ Before applying the heating device, press it against your inner forearm *to test its temperature and heat distribution.* If it heats unevenly, obtain a new device.

■ Apply the device to the treatment area and, if necessary, secure it with tape or roller gauze. Begin timing the application.

■ Assess the patient's skin condition frequently; remove the device if you observe increased swelling or excessive redness, blistering, maceration, or pallor, or if the patient reports discomfort. Refill the hot-water bottle as necessary *to maintain the correct temperature.*

■ Remove the device after 20 to 30 minutes, or as ordered.

■ Dry the patient's skin with a towel and redress the site, if necessary. Take the patient's temperature, pulse, and respirations *for comparison with the baseline.* Position him comfortably in bed.

■ If the treatment is to be repeated, store the equipment in the patient's room, out of his reach; otherwise, return it to its proper place.

To apply a warm compress or pack

■ Place a linen-saver pad under the site.

■ Remove the warm compress or pack from the bowl or basin. (Use sterile forceps throughout the procedure if needed.)

■ Wring excess solution from the compress or pack. *Excess moisture increases the risk of burns.*

■ Apply the heating device gently to the affected site. After a few seconds, lift the device and check the skin for excessive redness, maceration, or blistering. When you're sure the device isn't causing a burn, mold it firmly to the skin *to keep out air, which reduces the temperature and effectiveness of the device.* Work quickly *so the device retains its heat.*

■ Apply a waterproof covering (sterile, if necessary) to the device. Secure it with tape or roller gauze *to prevent it from slipping.*

■ Place a hot-water bottle, K pad, or chemical hot pack over the device and waterproof covering *to maintain the correct temperature.* Begin timing the application.

■ Check the patient's skin every 5 minutes. Remove the device if the skin shows excessive redness, maceration, or blistering or if the patient experiences pain or discomfort. Change the device as needed to maintain the correct temperature.

■ After 15 or 20 minutes or as ordered, remove the device. Discard it into a waterproof trash bag.

■ Dry the patient's skin with a towel (sterile, if necessary). Note the condition of the skin and redress the area, if necessary. Take the patient's temperature, pulse, and respiration *for comparison with baseline.* Then make sure the patient is comfortable.

Completing the procedure

■ Perform hand hygiene.[1,2,3]

■ Document the procedure.[5]

Special considerations

■ Make sure the closure device isn't in direct contact with the patient's skin *because the closure device can cause burns.*

Using moist heat to relieve muscle spasm

Tell patients to choose moist heat rather than dry heat when attempting to ease muscle tension or spasm. *Moist heat is less drying to the skin, less apt to cause burns, less likely to cause excessive fluid and salt loss through sweating, and more likely to penetrate deeper tissues.* Instruct the patient to apply heat for 20 to 30 minutes, as follows:

■ Place a moist towel over the painful area.

■ Cover the towel with a hot-water bottle properly filled and at the correct temperature.

■ Remove the hot-water bottle and towel after 20 to 30 minutes. Don't continue the application for longer than 30 minutes *because therapeutic value decreases after that time.*

■ If the patient is unconscious, anesthetized, cognitively or neurologically impaired, or insensitive to heat, stay with him throughout the treatment.

■ When direct heat is ordered to decrease congestion within internal organs, the application must cover a large enough area *to increase blood volume at the skin's surface.* For relief of pelvic organ congestion, for example, apply heat over the patient's lower abdomen, hips, and thighs. *To achieve local relief,* you may concentrate heat only over the specified area. (See *Using moist heat to relieve muscle spasm.*)

■ As an alternative method to apply a sterile moist compress, use a bedside sterilizer to sterilize the compress. Saturate the compress with tap water or another solution and wring it dry. Then place it in the bedside sterilizer at 275° F (135° C) for 15 minutes. Remove the compress with sterile forceps or sterile gloves, and wring out the excess solution. Then place the compress in a sterile bowl and measure its temperature with a sterile thermometer.

■ Follow the manufacturer's instructions for heating compresses, and avoid overheating.

Complications

Because tissue damage may result from direct heat application, monitor the temperature of the compress carefully. Frequently assess the condition of the patient's skin under the heat application device.

Documentation

Record the time and date of heat application; the type, temperature or heat setting, duration, and site of application; the patient's temperature, pulse, respirations, and skin condition before, during, and after treatment; signs of complications; and the patient's tolerance for the treatment.

EQUIPMENT

Types of scales

Scale selection varies and is influenced by the status of the patient.

For ambulatory patients

For acutely ill or debilitated patients

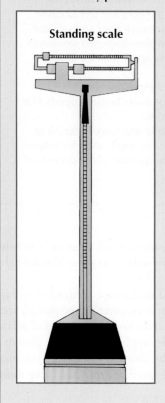

Standing scale

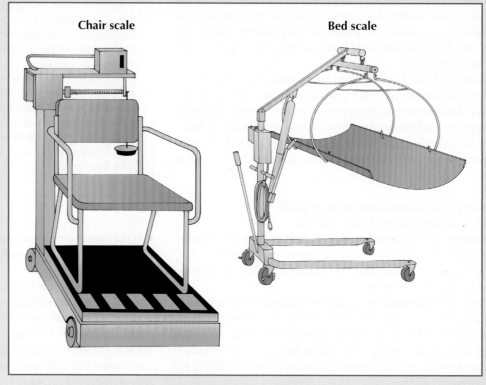

Chair scale

Bed scale

REFERENCES

1   The Joint Commission. (2012). Standard NPSG.07.01.01. *Comprehensive accreditation manual for hospitals: The official handbook.* Oakbrook Terrace, IL: The Joint Commission. (Level I)

2   Centers for Disease Control and Prevention. (October 2002). Guideline for hand hygiene in health-care settings. *Morbidity and Mortality Weekly Report*, *51*(RR-16), 1–45. (Level I)

3   World Health Organization. (2009). *WHO guidelines on hand hygiene in health care: First global patient safety challenge. Clean care is safer care.* Geneva, Switzerland: World Health Organization. (Level I)

4   The Joint Commission. (2012). Standard NPSG.01.01.01. *Comprehensive accreditation manual for hospitals: The official handbook.* Oakbrook Terrace, IL: The Joint Commission. (Level I)

5   The Joint Commission. (2012). Standard RC.01.03.01. *Comprehensive accreditation manual for hospitals: The official handbook.* Oakbrook Terrace, IL: The Joint Commission. (Level I)

ADDITIONAL REFERENCES

Craven, R.F., & Hirnle, C.J. (2012). *Fundamentals of nursing: Human health and function* (7th ed.). Philadelphia, PA: Lippincott Williams & Wilkins.

Taylor, C., et al. (2011). *Fundamentals of nursing: The art and science of nursing care* (7th ed.). Philadelphia, PA: Lippincott Williams & Wilkins.

HEIGHT AND WEIGHT MEASUREMENT

Most patients have their height and weight routinely measured during admission to a health care facility. An accurate record of the patient's height and weight is essential for calculating dosages of drugs, anesthetics, and contrast agents; assessing nutritional status; and determining the height-weight ratio. And because body weight provides the best overall picture of fluid status, monitoring weight daily proves important for patients receiving sodium-retaining or diuretic medications. Rapid weight gain may signal fluid retention; rapid weight loss may indicate diuresis.

Weight can be measured with a standing scale, chair scale, or bed scale. (See *Types of scales*.)

Equipment

Standing scale with measurement bar or chair or bed scale ■ wheelchair (if needed to transport patient) ■ drawsheet (for bed scale)

■ paper towel ■ Optional: Gloves, ruler (if scale doesn't have measuring bar), tape measure (to measure the height of a patient who is unable to stand), hospital-grade disinfectant.

Preparation of equipment

Select the appropriate scale, typically a standing scale for an ambulatory patient or a chair or bed scale for an acutely ill or debilitated patient. Then check to make sure the scale is balanced. Standing scales and, to a lesser extent, bed scales may become unbalanced when transported.

Implementation

■ Perform hand hygiene.[1,2,3]
■ Confirm the patient's identity using at least two patient identifiers according to your facility's policy.[4]
■ Explain the procedure to the patient. Refer to a chart of suggested healthy weight ranges *to determine norms for your patient's height and weight.* (See *Suggested weights for adults.*)

Using a standing scale

■ Place a paper towel on the scale's platform.
■ Zero the scale. If the scale has wheels, lock them before the patient steps on.
■ If you're using a digital scale, make sure the display reads 0 before use.
■ Tell the patient to remove his robe and slippers or shoes.
■ Assist the patient onto the scale and remain close to him *to prevent falls.*
■ If you're using an upright balance (gravity) scale, slide the lower rider to the groove representing the largest increment below the patient's estimated weight. Grooves represent 50, 100, 150, and 200 lb. Then slide the small upper rider until the beam balances. Add the upper and lower rider figures *to determine the weight.* (The upper rider is calibrated to eighths of a pound.)
■ Return the weight holder to its proper place.
■ If the scale is digital, read the display with the patient standing as still as possible.
■ While the patient is still on the scale, tell the patient to stand erect. Then raise the measuring bar until it touches the top of the patient's head. Extend the horizontal bar, and lower the bar until it touches the top of the patient's head. Read the patient's height.
■ Help the patient off the scale, and give him his robe and slippers or shoes.

Using a chair scale

■ Transport the patient to the weighing area or the scale to the patient's bedside.
■ Lock the scale in place *to prevent it from moving accidentally.*
■ If you're using a scale with a swing-away chair arm, unlock the arm. *When unlocked, the arm swings back 180 degrees to permit easy access.*
■ Position the scale beside the patient's bed or wheelchair with the chair arm open. Transfer the patient onto the scale, swing the chair arm to the front of the scale, and lock it in place.
■ If the chair scale is digital, make sure the display reads 0 before use. Press the button and record the patient's weight. If using a

---

Suggested weights for adults

This chart provides a guideline for determining healthy weights. Higher weights in each category typically apply to men, who average more muscle and bone; lower weights typically apply to women, who average less muscle and bone. Height is measured without shoes; weight is measured without clothes. The health risks of excess weight seem to apply to older and younger adults alike.

HEIGHT	WEIGHT (IN POUNDS)
4' 10"	91 to 119
4' 11"	92 to 124
5' 0"	97 to 138
5' 1"	101 to 143
5' 2"	104 to 148
5' 3"	107 to 152
5' 4"	111 to 157
5' 5"	114 to 162
5' 6"	118 to 167
5' 7"	121 to 172
5' 8"	125 to 178
5' 9"	129 to 183
5' 10"	132 to 188
5' 11"	136 to 194
6' 0"	140 to 199
6' 1"	144 to 205
6' 2"	148 to 210
6' 3"	152 to 216
6' 4"	156 to 222
6' 5"	160 to 228
6' 6"	164 to 234

---

multiple-weight scale, use the same process as a standing scale to determine the weight.
■ Help the patient off the scale.
■ Lock the main beam *to avoid damaging the scale during transport.* Then unlock the wheels and remove the scale from the patient's room.

Using a digital bed scale

■ Perform hand hygiene and follow standard precautions.[1,2,3]
■ Provide privacy, and tell the patient that you're going to weigh him on a special bed scale. Demonstrate its operation if appropriate.
■ Before using a bed scale, cover its stretcher with a drawsheet. Balance the scale with the drawsheet in place *to ensure accurate weighing.*
■ Release the stretcher to the horizontal position; then lock it in place.
■ Turn the patient on his side, facing away from the scale.
■ Roll the base of the scale under the patient's bed. Adjust the lever *to widen the base of the scale, providing stability.* Then lock the scale's wheels.

- Center the stretcher above the bed, lower it onto the mattress, and roll the patient onto the stretcher. Then position the circular weighing arms of the scale over the patient, and attach them securely to the stretcher bars.
- Pump the handle with long, slow strokes *to raise the patient a few inches off the bed.* Ensure that the patient doesn't lean on or touch the headboard, side rails, or other bed equipment *because this will affect weight measurement.*
- Press the operate button, and read the patient's weight on the digital display panel. Then press in the scale's handle *to lower the patient.*
- Detach the circular weighing arms from the stretcher bars, roll the patient off the stretcher and remove it, and position the patient comfortably in bed.
- Release the wheel lock and withdraw the scale. Return the stretcher to its vertical position.

Completing the procedure
- Perform hand hygiene.[1,2,3]
- Put on gloves and clean and disinfect the scale according to your facility's policy.
- Remove and discard gloves and perform hand hygiene.[1,2,3]
- Document the procedure.[5]

Measuring height without a scale
- Perform hand hygiene.[1,2,3]
- Confirm the patient's identity using at least two patient identifiers according to your facility's policy.[4]
- Explain the procedure to the patient.
- Have the patient remove his shoes and stand against a wall with his back and heels touching the wall. Use a straight, level object (such as a ruler) and place it on top of the patient' head parallel to the floor. Mark the location of the ruler on the wall. Measure the distance between the mark and the floor.
- If the patient is unable to stand, place him supine in bed with the head of the bed flat. Using a tape measure, measure from the top of the patient's head to his heels.
- Perform hand hygiene.[1,2,3]
- Document the procedure.[5]

Special considerations
- Some hospital beds contain a built-in scale. Make sure to zero the patient's bed with a sheet and patient gown on the bed before the patient is admitted *to ensure accurate weighing.* Then, with the patient in the bed, weigh him following manufacturer's instructions.
- Reassure and steady patients who are at risk for losing their balance on a scale.
- Weigh the patient at the same time each day (usually before breakfast), in similar clothing, and using the same scale. If the patient uses crutches, weigh him with the crutches. Then weigh the crutches and any heavy clothing and subtract their weight from the total to determine the patient's weight.
- When rolling the patient onto the stretcher, be careful not to dislodge IV catheters, indwelling catheters, and other supportive equipment.

- Report any change in weight of more than 2.2 lb (1 kg) per day.

Documentation
Record the patient's weight on the nursing assessment form and other medical records, as required by your facility.[5]

REFERENCES
1 The Joint Commission. (2012). Standard NPSG.07.01.01. *Comprehensive accreditation manual for hospitals: The official handbook.* Oakbrook Terrace, IL: The Joint Commission. (Level I)
2 Centers for Disease Control and Prevention. (October 2002). Guideline for hand hygiene in health-care settings. *Morbidity and Mortality Weekly Report, 51*(RR-16), 1–45. (Level I)
3 World Health Organization. (2009). *WHO guidelines on hand hygiene in health care: First global patient safety challenge. Clean care is safer care.* Geneva, Switzerland: World Health Organization. (Level I)
4 The Joint Commission. (2012). Standard NPSG.01.01.01. *Comprehensive accreditation manual for hospitals: The official handbook.* Oakbrook Terrace, IL: The Joint Commission. (Level I)
5 The Joint Commission. (2012). Standard RC.01.03.01. *Comprehensive accreditation manual for hospitals: The official handbook.* Oakbrook Terrace, IL: The Joint Commission. (Level I)

ADDITIONAL REFERENCES
Craven, R.F., & Hirnle, C.J. (2012). *Fundamentals of nursing: Human health and function* (7th ed.). Philadelphia, PA: Lippincott Williams & Wilkins.
Jensen, S. (2011). *Nursing health assessment: A best practice approach.* Philadelphia, PA: Lippincott Williams & Wilkins.
Rutala, W.A., et al. (2008). "Guideline for Disinfection and Sterilization in Healthcare Facilities, 2008" [Online]. Accessed November 2011 via the Web at http://www.cdc.gov/ncidod/dhqp/pdf/guidelines/Disinfection_Nov_2008.pdf

HEMODIALYSIS

Hemodialysis is a potentially lifesaving procedure that removes blood from the body, circulates it through a purifying dialyzer, and then returns it to the body. Various access sites can be used for this procedure, and access can be temporary or long term depending on the patient's requirements. Catheters are used for short-term access; for long-term access, arteriovenous (AV) fistulas are the preferred access because they last longer and are associated with fewer complications than other hemodialysis access sites.

The underlying mechanism in hemodialysis is differential diffusion across a semipermeable membrane, which extracts the by-products of protein metabolism (urea and uric acid) as well as creatinine and excess water. The membrane doesn't permit diffusion of large molecules, such as blood cells and plasma proteins. This process restores or maintains the balance of the body's buffer system and electrolytes, promoting a rapid return to normal serum values and helping to prevent complications associated with uremia. (See *How hemodialysis works.*)

How hemodialysis works

In hemodialysis, blood flows from the patient to an external dialyzer (or artificial kidney) through an access site. Inside the dialyzer, blood and dialysate flow countercurrently, divided by a semipermeable membrane. The composition of the dialysate resembles normal extracellular fluid. The blood contains an excess of specific solutes (metabolic waste products and some electrolytes), and the dialysate contains electrolytes that may be at abnormal levels in the patient's bloodstream. The dialysate's electrolyte composition can be modified to raise or lower electrolyte levels, depending on need.

Excretory function and electrolyte homeostasis are achieved by *diffusion*, the movement of a molecule across the dialyzer's semipermeable membrane from an area of higher solute concentration to an area of lower concentration. Water (solvent) crosses the membrane from the blood into the dialysate by *ultrafiltration*. This process removes excess water, waste products, and other metabolites through *osmotic pressure* and *hydrostatic pressure*. Osmotic pressure is the movement of water across the semipermeable membrane from an area of lesser solute concentration to one of greater solute concentration. Hydrostatic pressure forces water from the blood compartment into the dialysate compartment. Cleaned of impurities and excess water, the blood returns to the body through a venous site.

Types of dialyzers

There are two types of dialyzers: the hollow-fiber and the flat-plate or parallel flow-plate. The hollow-fiber and flat-plate dialyzers may be used several times on each patient. Heparin is used to prevent clot formation during hemodialysis.

The *hollow-fiber dialyzer,* the most common type, contains fine capillaries, with a semipermeable membrane enclosed in a plastic cylinder. Blood flows through these capillaries as the system pumps dialysate in the opposite direction on the outside of the capillaries.

The *flat-plate* or *parallel flow-plate dialyzer* has two or more layers of semipermeable membrane, bound by a semirigid or rigid structure. Blood ports are located at both ends, between the membranes. Blood flows between the membranes, and dialysate flows in the opposite direction along the outside of the membranes.

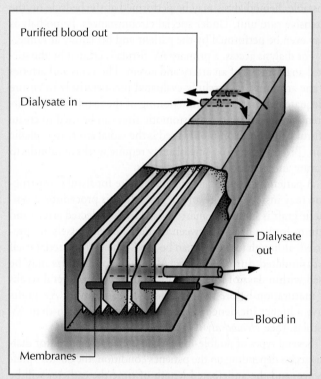

Dialysate delivery systems

Three system types can be used to deliver dialysate. The *batch system* uses a reservoir for recirculating dialysate. The *regenerative system* uses sorbents to purify and regenerate recirculating dialysate. The *proportioning system* (the most common) mixes concentrate with water to form dialysate, which then circulates through the dialyzer and goes down a drain after a single pass, followed by fresh dialysate.

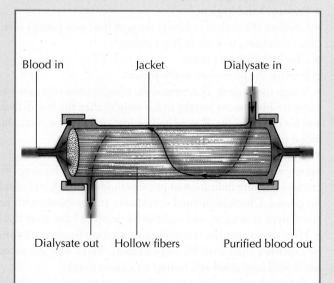

Hemodialysis provides temporary support for patients with acute, reversible renal failure as well as regular long-term treatment of patients with chronic end-stage renal disease. It may also be needed to remove toxic substances from the blood in cases of acute poisoning or barbiturate or analgesia overdose.

The patient's condition, along with such variables as the rate of creatinine accumulation and weight gain, determines the number and duration of hemodialysis treatments. To determine the patient's ultrafiltration requirements, the patient's present weight is compared with his weight after his last dialysis treatment and his target weight.

Specially trained personnel typically perform this procedure in a hemodialysis unit. However, if the patient is acutely ill and unstable, hemodialysis may be performed at the bedside on the intensive care unit. Under special circumstances, hemodialysis may even be performed by the patient and his family at home.

For dialysis access, a primary AV fistula is created by the surgical anastomosis of an artery and a vein. The veins and arteries of the arm must be carefully evaluated preoperatively to ensure adequate maturation and functioning of the fistula. Several different arterial-to-venous anastomotic sites can be used to create a fistula; the most commonly used is the radial artery to cephalic vein (Brescia-Cimino). A fistula may require weeks or months to mature and be usable for hemodialysis.

A patient whose vessels are inadequate for fistula construction may instead require an AV graft. In this procedure, a synthetic graft is surgically anastomosed to the selected artery and vein to form a bridge between them. The arm vessels are preferred, although leg vessels can be used. The graft material itself is cannulated during dialysis. Although some grafts may be used within days of their creation, most require several weeks of maturation before they can be used for dialysis. AV grafts have a higher incidence of thrombosis and infection than AV fistulas. (See *Hemodialysis access sites.*)

Several types of double-lumen catheters can be used for dialysis access depending on the patient's condition, the doctor's preference, and the anticipated length of time the catheter will be needed. The internal diameter of each lumen is approximately 12G to allow for high flow rates. The catheters have two ports—one colored red and one colored blue. The red port is used for withdrawing the patient's blood and sending it to the dialyzer; the blue port is used for returning the dialyzed blood to the patient.

Typically, double-lumen catheters are placed in the internal jugular or subclavian veins. The femoral vein is used only when other sites are unavailable. The internal jugular site is preferable to the subclavian site in patients who already have or will have permanent dialysis accesses placed in their arms because venous thrombosis is a common complication of venous catheters. In a patient with a permanent arm access, such as a bridge graft or fistula, a subclavian vein thrombosis on the contralateral side may impede the venous outflow from the permanent dialysis access, rendering it unusable.

Most double-lumen catheters are considered temporary dialysis accesses. However, a double-lumen, tunneled catheter with a Dacron cuff may be used for months.[3] This catheter is tunneled from the skin insertion site to the selected vein, and the Dacron cuff on the catheter under the skin acts as a barrier to infection.

Equipment
For general dialysis and initiating AV access
Hemodialysis machine with appropriate dialyzer and dialysate ▪ two 16G winged fistula needles ▪ two 10-mL syringes ▪ prescribed flush solution ▪ linen-saver pad ▪ antiseptic swabs ▪ antiseptic solution ▪ sterile 4″ × 4″ gauze pads ▪ sterile 2″ × 2″ gauze pads ▪ sterile drape ▪ sterile and clean gloves, a gown, and a face shield ▪ stethoscope ▪ adhesive tape ▪ Optional: tourniquet.

For initiating dialysis with a double-lumen catheter
Sphygmomanometer ▪ two 3-mL syringes ▪ two 5-mL syringes with prescribed anticoagulant flush ▪ syringe with prescribed anticoagulant.

For discontinuing dialysis with a double-lumen catheter
Two 10-mL syringes with normal saline for injection ▪ two 5-mL syringes with prescribed anticoagulant flush ▪ two sterile luer-lock caps ▪ stethoscope ▪ sphygmomanometer ▪ antiseptic swabs and solution ▪ sterile drape ▪ sterile 4″ × 4″ sterile gauze pads ▪ two 5-mL syringes with prescribed anticoagulant flush.

Preparation of equipment
Prepare the hemodialysis equipment following the manufacturer's instructions and your facility's protocol. *To maintain catheter patency,* carefully follow the manufacturer's instructions for specific catheter care and flushing procedures. Maintain strict sterile technique *to prevent introducing pathogens into the patient's bloodstream during dialysis.* Test the dialyzer and dialysis machine for residual disinfectant after rinsing and test all of the alarms.

Implementation
Initiating hemodialysis
▪ Gather and prepare the equipment.
▪ Perform hand hygiene.[4,5,6,7]
▪ Confirm the patient's identity using at least two patient identifiers according to your facility's policy.[8]
▪ Check the doctor's order.
▪ Explain the procedure to the patient.
▪ Weigh the patient. *To determine his ultrafiltration requirements,* compare his present weight to his weight after the last dialysis and his target weight. Record his baseline vital signs, and take his blood pressure while he's sitting and standing.
▪ Auscultate his heart for rate, rhythm, and abnormalities. Observe his respiratory rate, rhythm, and quality. Auscultate his lungs for crackles and any indication of possible fluid overload, and check for edema. Check his mental status, note any problems with his last dialysis treatment, and evaluate his previous laboratory data.
▪ Help the patient into a comfortable position (supine or sitting in a recliner chair with his feet elevated). Make sure the access site is well supported and resting on a clean drape.
▪ Perform hand hygiene; put on gloves, a gown, and a face shield; and follow standard precautions.[4,5,6,7]

Hemodialysis access sites

Hemodialysis requires vascular access. The site and type of access may vary, depending on the expected duration of dialysis, the surgeon's preference, and the patient's condition.

Subclavian vein catheterization

Using the Seldinger technique, the doctor inserts an introducer needle into the subclavian vein. He then inserts a guide wire through the introducer needle and removes the needle. Using the guide wire, he then threads a 5″ to 12″ (13- to 30-cm) plastic or Teflon catheter with a Y hub into the patient's vein.

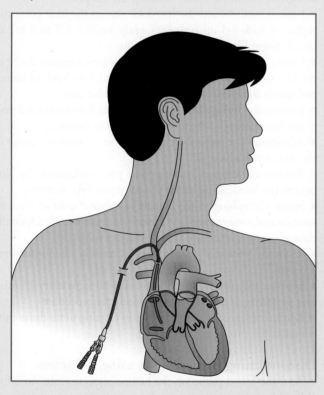

Use of the subclavian vein for catheter placement isn't recommended for patients who require permanent arteriovenous (AV) fistulas *because the risk of thrombosis may compromise AV fistula creation.*[1]

Femoral vein catheterization

Using the Seldinger technique, the doctor inserts an introducer needle into the left or right femoral vein. He then inserts a guide wire through the introducer needle and removes the needle.

Using the guide wire, he then threads either a 5″ to 12″ plastic or Teflon catheter with a Y hub, or two catheters, one for inflow and another placed about ½″ (1 cm) distal to the first for outflow. This catheter type should be used only when no other access site is available *because it's associated with an increased risk of infection and deep vein thrombosis.*[2]

AV fistula

To create a fistula, the surgeon makes an incision into the patient's wrist or lower forearm, followed by a small incision in the side of an artery, and then another in the side of a vein. He sutures the edges of the incisions together to make a common opening ⅛″ to ¼″ (0.3 to 0.6 cm) long. Because an AV fistula requires a 4- to 6-week healing time before it can be used as a dialysis access site, it's recommended that the fistula be created before hemodialysis is needed *so that the fistula is healed and ready for use when needed.*

AV graft

To create an AV graft, the surgeon makes an incision in the patient's forearm, upper arm, or thigh. He then tunnels a natural or synthetic graft under the skin and sutures the distal end to an artery and the proximal end to a vein.

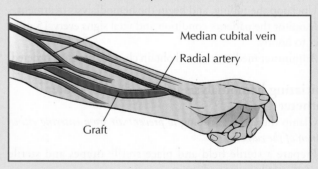

Median cubital vein
Radial artery
Graft

Initiating hemodialysis using AV access

■ Assess the AV access for patency. Check for the quality of the thrill and auscultate the bruit. Check for the presence of swelling, edema, erythema, or drainage.
■ Draw up the prescribed flush solution into each 10-mL syringe, and prime and clamp the tubing and needle just before cannulation.[1]
■ Wash the patient's access site using an antiseptic solution or antibacterial soap and water.[9]
■ Place the patient's access limb on a sterile drape.

■ Clean the skin over the AV access with antiseptic swabs according to the manufacturer's instructions using a chlorhexidine-based solution, alcohol, or a povidone-iodine solution. Apply a chlorhexidine-based solution using a back-and-forth friction scrub for 30 seconds and then allow it to dry. Apply alcohol using a rubbing motion for 1 minute immediately before accessing the fistula. Apply povidone-iodine solution for 2 to 3 minutes and allow it to dry.[9]
■ Remove and discard your gloves.
■ Perform hand hygiene.[4,5,6,7]
■ Put on another pair of clean gloves.

- Apply a tourniquet to the upper portion of the arm containing the fistula.
- Remove the needle guard from the first fistula needle (arterial), and squeeze the wings together.
- Insert the arterial needle into the fistula at a 25-degree angle (45-degree angle for a graft). Make sure the needle insertion site is at least 1″ (2.5 cm) from the arterial-venous anastomotic site. Be careful not to puncture the posterior wall of the access. Remove the tourniquet.[9]
- For a fistula, advance the needle, with the bevel up, to the hub of the needle. For a graft, after the tip of the needle penetrates the graft, rotate the needle 180 degrees and advance the needle to the hub with the bevel down.[9,10]
- Flush the needle *to prevent clotting*. Normal saline solution is the preferred flush solution, but some doctors may order an anticoagulant solution. Clamp the arterial needle tubing and secure the wing tips of the needle to the skin with adhesive tape *to prevent accidental dislodgement of the needle*.
- Perform the second access (venous) puncture with the other fistula needle, a few inches beyond the arterial needle (farther from the arterial-venous anastomosis). Be careful not to puncture the posterior wall of the access. Flush the needle with the appropriate solution. Clamp the venous needle tubing, and secure the wing tips of the venous needle to the patient's skin with adhesive tape.
- Remove the syringe from the end of the arterial needle tubing, uncap the arterial dialyzer tubing, and connect the two lines. Tape the connection securely *to prevent accidental separation of the tubing*.
- Remove the syringe from the end of the venous needle tubing, uncap the venous dialyzer tubing, and connect the two lines. Tape the connection securely *to prevent accidental separation of the tubing*.
- Unclamp the tubing, and begin the hemodialysis treatment.
- Monitor the patient's condition and vital signs every 15 minutes to hourly.
- Administer medications and obtain clotting times, as ordered.

Initiating hemodialysis using a double-lumen catheter

- Clamp the catheter tubing *to prevent air from entering either lumen of the catheter*.
- Prepare a sterile field and place sterile drapes and sterile 4″ × 4″ sterile gauze pads on it.
- Identify the red (arterial) and the blue (venous) ports, and place them near the sterile field. Place the dialyzer arterial and venous blood lines near the field.
- Open the sterile syringes and place them on the sterile field.
- Prepare the anticoagulant flush solution in the 5-mL syringes according to your facility's policy.
- Remove the dressing from the catheter exit site, making sure you don't dislodge the catheter.
- Discard the soiled dressing and your gloves in the appropriate receptacle.[10]
- Perform hand hygiene and put on sterile gloves.[4,5,6,7,9]
- Place a sterile drape beneath the catheter.
- Saturate 4″ × 4″ sterile gauze pads with antiseptic solution.

- Use a saturated gauze pad to scrub the red port for 1 minute. Then, wrap a saturated gauze pad around the red port and leave it in place for 3 to 5 minutes. Remove the gauze pad and discard it in the appropriate receptacle. Repeat these steps for the blue port.[10]
- Remove and discard the luer-lock cap on the red port and replace it with a 3-mL syringe. Unclamp the red port, aspirate 1.5 to 3 mL of blood, and reclamp the port.
- Soak 2″ × 2″ sterile gauze pads in antiseptic solution and then clean the connection site with them.
- Connect one of the 5-mL syringes with anticoagulant flush to the red port, unclamp the port, aspirate 1.5 to 3 mL of blood, and gently instill the flush. Reclamp the red port.
- Remove and discard the luer-lock cap on the blue port, and replace it with a 3-ml syringe. Gently aspirate 1.5 to 3 mL of blood, discard it, and reclamp the port.
- Connect the other 5-mL syringe (with anticoagulant flush) to the blue port, unclamp the port, aspirate 1.5 to 3 mL of blood, and gently instill the flush. Reclamp the blue port.
- Remove the syringe from the red port, and attach the red port to the line leading to the arterial port of the dialyzer.
- Administer the prescribed anticoagulant *to prevent clotting in the extracorporeal circuit*.
- Remove the syringe from the blue port, and attach the blue port to the line leading to the venous port of the dialyzer.
- Secure the tubing to the patient *to reduce tension on the connections and prevent trauma to the catheter insertion site*. Open the clamps to the arterial and venous dialyzer tubing.
- Begin the hemodialysis treatment according to your facility's protocol.
- Monitor the patient's condition and vital signs every 15 minutes to hourly, as necessary, throughout the procedure.
- Administer medications, and obtain clotting times during the hemodialysis procedure, as ordered.

Discontinuing hemodialysis using AV access

- Turn the blood pump on the hemodialysis machine to 50 to 100 mL/minute.
- Perform hand hygiene.[4,5,6,7]
- Put on gloves.
- Remove the tape from the connection site of the arterial lines. Clamp the needle tubing and disconnect the lines. The blood in the arterial line will continue to flow toward the dialyzer, followed by normal saline solution. Clamp the blood line just before the blood reaches the point where the saline enters the line.
- Unclamp the saline solution to allow a small amount of saline to flow through the line. Unclamp the dialyzer line to allow all blood to flow into the dialyzer, where it passes through the filter and back to the patient through the venous line.
- After the blood is retransfused, clamp the venous needle tubing and the dialyzer's venous line and turn off the blood pump.
- Remove the tape from the connection site of the venous lines and disconnect the lines.
- Remove the venipuncture needle completely, and then apply pressure to the site with a folded 4″ × 4″ sterile gauze pad using two fingers. You should be able to continue to feel a thrill both

above and below the compression site while holding pressure. *If inadequate pressure is used, a hematoma may develop; if excessive pressure is used, the access may thrombose.* Bleeding usually stops within 10 minutes.

■ Apply a dry sterile dressing to the site. Avoid circumferential taping of the dressing.

■ Repeat the procedure on the arterial needle and site.

■ When dialysis is complete, weigh the patient, obtain vital signs (including blood pressure while the patient is sitting and standing), and assess his mental status. Compare these findings with the predialysis assessment data.

■ Remove and discard your gloves and perform hand hygiene.[4,5,6,7]

■ Put on clean gloves and rinse and disinfect the delivery system according to the manufacturer's instructions.

Discontinuing hemodialysis with a double-lumen catheter

■ Perform hand hygiene; put on a gown, gloves, and a face shield; and follow standard precautions.[4,5,6,7]

■ Open the syringes, luer-lock caps, and gauze pads and place them on a sterile field.

■ Fill the two 5-mL syringes with the prescribed amount of anticoagulant flush.

■ Fill the two 10-mL syringes with normal saline for injection according to facility policy.

■ Clamp the tubing to the red and the blue catheter ports and the blood lines to the dialyzer.

■ Place a sterile drape beneath the ports.

■ Clean the connection points on the catheter, the clamps, and the blood lines with antiseptic solution.

■ Place a sterile drape under the catheter, and place two sterile 4″ × 4″ sterile gauze pads beneath the catheter ports.

■ Soak the 4″ × 4″ sterile gauze pads with antiseptic solution.

■ Remove and discard your gloves.

■ Perform hand hygiene and put on sterile gloves.[4,5,6,7]

■ Grasp the red port connection with the sterile gauze pad and disconnect it from the arterial dialyzer tubing.

■ Attach the 10-mL syringe (with normal saline) to the red port on the catheter and slowly flush the tubing.

■ Replace the 10-mL syringe on the red port with the 5-mL syringe filled with the prescribed anticoagulant flush and instill it. Remove the syringe, and cap the port with a sterile luer-lock cap.

■ Grasp the blue port connection with the sterile gauze pad and disconnect it from the venous dialyzer tubing

■ Attach the 10-mL syringe (with normal saline) to the blue catheter port and slowly flush the tubing.

■ Replace the 10-mL syringe on the blue port with the 5-mL syringe filled with the prescribed anticoagulant flush and instill it. Remove the syringe, and cap the port with a sterile luer-lock cap. Clamp both ports.

■ Position the patient supine with his head facing away from the catheter. Perform catheter insertion site care, and obtain a drainage specimen for culture, if necessary. (See "Central venous access catheter," page 133.)

■ Obtain the patient's postdialysis weight, vital signs, and neurologic, respiratory and hemodynamic parameters, and compare them to his predialysis baseline.

■ Remove and discard your gloves, remove other personal protective equipment, and perform hand hygiene.[4,5,6,7]

■ Put on gloves and rinse and disinfect the delivery system.

Completing the procedure
■ Remove and discard your gloves and perform hand hygiene.[4,5,6,7]
■ Document the procedure.[11]

Special considerations
NURSING ALERT To avoid pyrogenic reaction and bacteremia with septicemia resulting from contamination, *use strict sterile technique during the preparation of the machine. Discard equipment that has been disconnected and exposed to the air.*[1]

■ Immediately report any suspected machine malfunction or equipment defect.

■ Don't inject IV fluids or medications into either port of the double-lumen catheter.

■ If, while instilling the anticoagulant flush into either port, you meet resistance, stop flushing immediately. Clamp the port, replace the sterile luer-lock cap, and notify the doctor. Place a "do not use" message on the port until its patency is verified.

NURSING ALERT *Make sure you complete each step in the hemodialysis procedure correctly. Overlooking a single step or performing it incorrectly can cause unnecessary blood loss or inefficient treatment from poor clearances or inadequate fluid removal. For example, when preparing the equipment, never allow a saline solution bag to run dry while priming and soaking the dialyzer* because that could cause air to enter the patient portion of the dialysate system. *Failure to perform accurate hemodialysis therapy can lead to patient injury or death.*

■ If the patient receives meals during dialysis, make sure they're light.

■ Continue necessary drug administration during the hemodialysis treatment unless the drug would be removed in the dialysate; if so, administer the drug after dialysis.

Patient teaching
After surgery to create an AV access site
In the postoperative period, teach the patient to care for his AV access site. Teach him to keep the incision clean and dry *to prevent infection* and to clean it daily until it heals completely and the sutures are removed (usually 10 to 14 days after surgery). Teach him how to use a stethoscope to auscultate for his access bruit and how to palpate a thrill. He should check the access several times a day. He should notify the doctor of pain, swelling, redness, drainage, and any decrease in the access thrill or bruit.

Explain that after the access site heals, he may use the arm freely. Exercise is beneficial *because it stimulates vein enlargement.* He may start by squeezing a small rubber ball or other soft object for 15 minutes as advised by his doctor.

Teach the patient to avoid putting excessive pressure on the arm. He should not sleep on it, wear constricting clothing, or lift heavy objects with it. Also teach the patient that he should not allow anyone to take his blood pressure or draw blood from his access arm.

If the patient will be performing hemodialysis at home, thoroughly review all aspects of the procedure with the patient and his family. Give them the phone number of the dialysis center. Emphasize that training for home hemodialysis is a complex process requiring 2 to 3 months to ensure that the patient or family member performs it safely and competently. Keep in mind that this procedure is stressful.

After hemodialysis

Teach the patient to keep the dressings on the access site for several hours after his treatment. Teach him not to loosen the scabs on the needle insertion sites *because they may bleed or become infected.* If bleeding should occur, teach the patient to apply pressure to the needle sites with a clean towel or gauze for 10 to 15 minutes without lifting the pressure. *Prematurely releasing the pressure may disturb the clot formation.* Tell him to use enough pressure to stop the bleeding but not enough to occlude the pulse in his access. When the bleeding stops, have him tape the dressing in place. Instruct him never to wrap the tape all the way around his arm. If he can't stop the bleeding, he should go to the emergency department.

Complications

Bacterial endotoxins in the dialysate may cause fever. Improper access care and needle site asepsis or improper catheter and site asepsis may introduce bacteria into the bloodstream and cause sepsis. Rapid fluid removal and electrolyte changes during dialysis can cause early dialysis disequilibrium syndrome; signs and symptoms include headache, nausea, vomiting, restlessness, hypertension, muscle cramps, backache, and seizures.

Excessive removal of fluid during ultrafiltration can cause hypovolemia and hypotension. Diffusion of the sugar and sodium content of the dialysate solution into the blood can cause hyperglycemia and hypernatremia and subsequent hyperosmolarity.

Cardiac arrhythmias can occur from electrolyte and pH changes in the blood. They may also develop if the patient is taking antiarrhythmics *because the drugs may be removed during the treatment.* Angina may develop in patients with anemia or who have preexisting arteriosclerotic disease. Patients with reduced oxygen levels resulting from extracorporeal blood flow or membrane sensitivity may require oxygen administration during hemodialysis.

Some complications of hemodialysis can be fatal. An air embolus can result from tubing disconnection, if the dialyzer contains air, or if the saline solution container empties. Signs and symptoms may include dyspnea, chest pain, coughing, and cyanosis.

Hemolysis of the blood cells can result from obstructed flow of the dialysate concentrate or from incorrect setting of the conductivity alarm limits. Signs and symptoms include cherry red blood, chest pain, dyspnea, arrhythmias, hyperkalemia, and an abrupt decrease in hematocrit.

Hyperthermia, which can result from overheating of the dialysate, is potentially fatal.

Exsanguination can occur if the connections on the blood lines become separated or ruptured or the dialyzer membrane ruptures.

Improper access site cannulation or needle site care may cause hematoma, pseudoaneurysm formation, or even rupture of the graft and excessive bleeding.

Documentation

Record the time the treatment began along with the predialysis assessment and vital signs. Note any complications and nursing actions taken. Note any blood samples sent and the laboratory results obtained.

Record the time the treatment was completed and the patient's response to it. Record the condition of the AV access site or catheter insertion site with the date and time of the dressing change, how long it took to obtain hemostasis, and any culture specimens obtained.[11]

REFERENCES

1 National Kidney Foundation/KDOQI. (2006). "Clinical Practice Guidelines for Peritoneal Dialysis Adequacy, Update 2006" [Online]. Accessed November 2011 via the Web at http://www.kidney.org/professionals/KDOQI/guideline_upHD_PD_VA/index.htm (Level I).
2 Marschall, J., et al. (2008). Strategies to prevent central line-associated bloodstream infections in acute care hospitals. *Infection Control and Hospital Epidemiology, 29*(S1):S22–S30. (Level I)
3 O'Grady, N.P., et al. (2011, April). "Guidelines for the Prevention of Intravascular Catheter-Related Infections" [Online]. Accessed November 2011 via the Web at *http://www.cdc.gov/hicpac/pdf/guidelines/bsi-guidelines-2011.pdf*
4 The Joint Commission. (2012). Standard NPSG.07.01.01. *Comprehensive accreditation manual for hospitals: The official handbook.* Oakbrook Terrace, IL: The Joint Commission. (Level I)
5 World Health Organization. (2009). *WHO guidelines on hand hygiene in health care: First global patient safety challenge. Clean care is safer care.* Geneva, Switzerland: World Health Organization. (Level I)
6 Centers for Disease Control and Prevention. (2001). Recommendations for preventing transmission of infections among chronic hemodialysis patients. *Morbidity and Mortality Weekly Report, 50*(RR-05), 1–43. (Level I)
7 Centers for Disease Control and Prevention. (October 2002). Guideline for hand hygiene in health-care settings. *Morbidity and Mortality Weekly Report, 51*(RR-16), 1–45. (Level I)
8 The Joint Commission. (2012). Standard NPSG.01.01.01. *Comprehensive accreditation manual for hospitals: The official handbook.* Oakbrook Terrace, IL: The Joint Commission. (Level I)
9 National Kidney Foundation/KDOQI (2006). "Clinical Practice Guidelines for Vascular Access, Update 2006" [Online]. Accessed November 2011 via the Web at http://www.kidney.org/professionals/kdoqi/guideline_uphd_pd_va/va_guide3.htm
10 Lynn-McHale Wiegand, D. (Ed.). (2011). *AACN procedure manual for critical care* (6th ed.). Philadelphia, PA: Saunders.
11 The Joint Commission. (2012). Standard RC.01.03.01. *Comprehensive accreditation manual for hospitals: The official handbook.* Oakbrook Terrace, IL: The Joint Commission. (Level I)

ADDITIONAL REFERENCES

Burrow-Johnson, S., et al. (2006). *Nephrology nursing standards of practice and guidelines for care* (6th ed.). Pitman, NJ: Thomson Gale.

McCann, M., et al. (2008). Vascular access management I: An overview. *Journal of Renal Care, 34*(2), 77–84.

McCann, M., et al. (2009). Vascular access management II: AVF/AVG cannulation techniques and complications. *Journal of Renal Care, 35*(2), 90–98.

Nettina, S.M. (2010). *Lippincott manual of nursing practice* (9th ed.). Philadelphia, PA: Lippincott Williams & Wilkins.

Smeltzer, S.C., et al. (2010). *Brunner & Suddarth's textbook of medical-surgical nursing* (12th ed.). Philadelphia, PA: Lippincott Williams & Wilkins.

Standard 46. Vascular access device site care and dressing changes. Infusion nursing standards of practice. (2011). *Journal of Infusion Nursing, 34*(1S), S63–S64.

HEMOGLOBIN TESTING, BEDSIDE

Monitoring hemoglobin levels at the patient's bedside provides fast, accurate results that allow for immediate intervention, if necessary. In contrast, traditional monitoring methods take longer because they require sending blood samples to the laboratory for interpretation.

Several testing systems are available for bedside monitoring. Such systems are also convenient for the patient to use at home.

Normal hemoglobin values range from 12.5 to 15 g/dL. A below-normal hemoglobin value may indicate anemia, recent hemorrhage, or fluid retention, causing hemodilution. An elevated hemoglobin value suggests hemoconcentration from polycythemia or dehydration.

Equipment

Lancet ▪ microcuvette ▪ photometer ▪ gloves ▪ alcohol pads ▪ gauze pads.

Preparation of equipment

Turn on the photometer. If it hasn't been used recently, insert the control cuvette *to make sure that the photometer is working properly.*

Implementation

▪ Verify the doctor's order.
▪ Gather the appropriate equipment.
▪ Perform hand hygiene and put on gloves.[1,2,3]
▪ Confirm the patient's identity using at least two patient identifiers according to your facility's policy.[4]
▪ Explain the procedure to the patient.
▪ Tell him that he'll feel a pinprick in his finger during blood sampling.
▪ If needed, plug the photometer into the wall.
▪ Select an appropriate puncture site. For an adult, the middle and fourth fingers are the best choices. *The second finger is usually the most sensitive, and the thumb may have thickened skin or calluses.* Blood should circulate freely in the finger from which you're drawing blood, so avoid using a ring-bearing finger. *To ensure an adequate blood sample,* don't use a cold, cyanotic, or swollen area as the puncture site.

PEDIATRIC ALERT *For an infant, use the heel or great toe.*

▪ Keep the patient's finger straight and ask him to relax it. Holding his finger between the thumb and index finger of your nondominant hand, gently rock the patient's finger as you move your fingers from his top knuckle to his fingertip. *This action causes blood to flow to the sampling point.*
▪ Use an alcohol pad to clean the puncture site, wiping in a circular motion from the center of the site outward. Dry the site thoroughly with a gauze pad.
▪ Pierce the skin quickly and sharply with the lancet and apply the microcuvette, which automatically collects a precise amount of blood (approximately 5 μL).
▪ Place the microcuvette into the photometer. Results appear on the photometer screen in 40 seconds to 4 minutes.
▪ Place a gauze pad over the puncture site until the bleeding stops.
▪ Dispose of the lancet and microcuvette according to your facility's policy.
▪ Remove and discard your gloves and perform hand hygiene.[1,2,3]
▪ Put on gloves and clean and disinfect the photometer according to your facility's policy *so it's ready to use for another patient.*[5]
▪ Remove and discard your gloves and perform hand hygiene.[1,2,3]
▪ Notify the doctor if the test result is outside the expected parameters.[6]
▪ Document the procedure.[7]

Special considerations

▪ Before using a microcuvette, note its expiration date. Microcuvettes can be stored for up to 2 years; however, after the microcuvette vial is opened, the shelf life is 90 days.

Documentation

Document the values obtained from the photometer as well as the date and time of the test. Record the date and time the doctor was notified of abnormal results, any interventions performed, and the patient's response to these interventions.[7]

REFERENCES

1 The Joint Commission. (2012). Standard NPSG.07.01.01. *Comprehensive accreditation manual for hospitals: The official handbook.* Oakbrook Terrace, IL: The Joint Commission. (Level I)
2 Centers for Disease Control and Prevention. (October 2002). Guideline for hand hygiene in health-care settings. *Morbidity and Mortality Weekly Report, 51*(RR-16), 1–45. (Level I)
3 World Health Organization. (2009). *WHO guidelines on hand hygiene in health care: First global patient safety challenge. Clean care is safer care.* Geneva, Switzerland: World Health Organization. (Level I)
4 The Joint Commission. (2012). Standard NPSG.01.01.01. *Comprehensive accreditation manual for hospitals: The official handbook.* Oakbrook Terrace, IL: The Joint Commission. (Level I)
5 Rutala, W.A., et al. (2008). "Guideline for Disinfection and Sterilization in Healthcare Facilities, 2008" [Online]. Accessed November 2011 via the Web at http://www.cdc.gov/ncidod/dhqp/pdf/guidelines/Disinfection_Nov_2008.pdf (Level I)

Total hip replacement

To form a totally artificial hip, the surgeon cements a femoral head prosthesis in place to articulate with a cup, which he then cements into the deepened acetabulum. He may avoid using cement by implanting a prosthesis with a porous coating that promotes bony ingrowth.

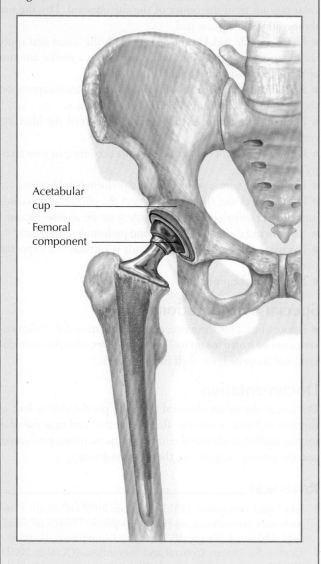

Acetabular cup

Femoral component

6 The Joint Commission. (2012). Standard NPSG.02.03.01. *Comprehensive accreditation manual for hospitals: The official handbook.* Oakbrook Terrace, IL: The Joint Commission. (Level I)

7 The Joint Commission. (2012). Standard RC.01.03.01. *Comprehensive accreditation manual for hospitals: The official handbook.* Oakbrook Terrace, IL: The Joint Commission. (Level I)

ADDITIONAL REFERENCE

Bubner, T.K., et al. (2009). Effectiveness of point-of-care testing for therapeutic control of chronic conditions: Results from the PoCT in general practice trial," *Medical Journal of Australia, 190*(11), 624–626.

Hip arthroplasty care

Hip arthroplasty involves surgical replacement of all or part of the hip joint. Hip replacement may be total, replacing the femoral head and acetabulum, or partial, replacing only one joint component. (See *Total hip replacement*.)

Hip replacement is done to decrease or eliminate pain and improve functional status. It's most commonly used to treat osteoarthritis. Other indications include rheumatoid arthritis, avascular necrosis, traumatic arthritis, hip fractures, benign and malignant bone tumors, ankylosing spondylitis, and juvenile rheumatoid arthritis.

Arthroplasty care includes maintaining alignment of the affected joint, assisting with exercises, and providing routine postoperative care. Nursing responsibility includes teaching, safe mobility, home care, and exercises that may continue for several years.

Equipment

Incentive spirometer ▪ compression stocking or sequential compression device ▪ sterile dressings ▪ hypoallergenic tape ▪ ice bag ▪ skin lotion ▪ warm water ▪ crutches or walker ▪ pain medications ▪ closed-wound drainage system ▪ pillow ▪ abduction splint ▪ anticoagulants.

Implementation

▪ Verify the doctor's orders.
▪ Confirm the patient's identity using at least two patient identifiers according to your facility's policy.[1]
▪ Explain all procedures to the patient.
▪ Perform hand hygiene.[2,3,4]
▪ Check vital signs every ten minutes until stable, every 30 minutes twice, then every 2 to 4 hours, and then routinely thereafter, according to facility policy. Report any changes in vital signs *because they may indicate infection, hemorrhage, or postoperative complications.*
▪ Encourage the patient to perform deep-breathing and coughing exercises. Assist with incentive spirometry to prevent postprocedure pneumonia.
▪ Perform bilateral neurovascular assessments every 2 hours for the first 48 hours and then every 4 hours *for signs of complications.* Check the affected leg for color, temperature, toe movement, sensation, edema, capillary filling, and pedal pulse. Investigate any complaints of pain, burning, numbness, or tingling.
▪ Apply the compression stocking or sequential compression device, if ordered, *to promote venous return and prevent venous thromboembolism.* Once every 8 hours, remove the stockings or compression device; inspect the legs, especially the heel, for pressure ulcers; and then reapply the stocking or device.

■ Assess the patient's pain and then administer pain medications, as ordered, following safe medication administration practices. Perform a follow-up assessment and notify the doctor if pain isn't adequately controlled.[5]

■ Administer anticoagulant therapy, as ordered, *to minimize the risk of venous thromboembolism.*

■ Make sure baseline coagulation studies have been obtained and are documented in the patient's medical record. (International Normalized Ratio [INR] should be monitored if the patient is receiving warfarin [Coumadin].) If a continuous infusion of heparin is prescribed, administer it using a programmable pump (preferably a smart pump with dose-range alerts) *to provide consistent and accurate dosing.*[6]

■ Observe for bleeding and for signs and symptoms of phlebitis, such as warmth, swelling, tenderness, and redness. Monitor laboratory results, including complete blood count, prothrombin time, partial thromboplastin time, and INR.

■ Check the dressings for excessive bleeding. Circle any drainage on the dressing and mark it with your initials, the date, and the time. As needed, apply more sterile dressings, using hypoallergenic tape. Report excessive bleeding to the doctor.

■ Observe the closed-wound drainage system for discharge color. (See "Closed-wound drain management," page 179.) *Proper drainage prevents hematoma. Purulent discharge and fever may indicate infection.* Empty and measure drainage, as ordered, using clean technique *to prevent infection.*

■ Monitor fluid intake and output daily; include wound drainage in the output measurement.

■ If the patient has an indwelling urinary catheter that was inserted for surgery, remove the catheter on postoperative day 1 or 2 (with the day of surgery considered day 0), according to facility policy or the doctor's order, to reduce the risk for catheter-associated urinary tract infection.[7,8] (See "Indwelling urinary catheter care and removal," page 374.)

■ Make sure prophylactic antibiotics are discontinued within 24 hours after surgery.[7,9]

■ Apply an ice bag, as ordered, to the affected site for the first 48 hours *to reduce swelling, relieve pain, and control bleeding.*

■ Help the patient use the trapeze to reposition himself every 2 hours. *These position changes enhance comfort, prevent pressure ulcers, and help prevent respiratory complications.* Then provide skin care for the back and buttocks, using warm water and lotion, as indicated.

■ Positioning varies based on the surgical approach used and the surgeon's preference. For the anterior approach, there should be no adduction past midline, no flexion greater than 90 degrees, and no external rotation past midline. For the posterior approach, there should be no adduction past midline, no flexion greater than 60 to 90 degrees, no internal rotation past midline, and no extension past neutral.

■ Keep the affected leg in abduction and in the neutral position *to stabilize the hip and keep the cup and femur head in the acetabulum.* Place a pillow between the patient's legs *to maintain hip abduction.*

■ Keep the patient in a supine position, with the affected hip in full extension, for 1 hour three times per day and at night *to prevent excessive hip flexion.*

■ On the day after surgery, have the patient begin plantar flexion and dorsiflexion exercises of the foot on the affected leg. When ordered, instruct him to begin quadriceps exercises. Collaborate with physical therapy professionals, as appropriate.

■ Instruct the patient to perform other muscle-strengthening exercises for affected and unaffected extremities, as ordered, *to help maintain muscle strength and range of motion and to help prevent phlebitis.*

■ Before ambulation, assess the patient's pain and give pain medication, as ordered, 30 minutes before activity *because movement is very painful.* Encourage the patient during exercise.[5]

■ Help the patient with progressive ambulation, using adjustable crutches or a walker when needed.

■ Perform hand hygiene.[2,3,4]

■ Document the procedure.[10]

Special considerations

■ Progressive ambulation protocols vary. Most patients are permitted to begin transfer and progressive ambulation with assistive devices on the first day. Collaborate with physical therapy professionals, as appropriate.

■ Educate the patient and family about measures to prevent surgical site infection.[11]

Complications

Immobility after arthroplasty may result in such complications as shock, pulmonary embolism, pneumonia, phlebitis, paralytic ileus, urine retention, and bowel impaction. A deep wound or infection at the prosthesis site is a serious complication that may force removal of the prosthesis. Although these are the most common complications, incidence has been significantly reduced because of the use of prophylactic antibiotics and anticoagulants and early mobilization. Dislocation of a total hip prosthesis may occur after violent hip flexion or adduction or during internal rotation. Signs of dislocation include inability to rotate the hip or bear weight, shortening of the leg, and increased pain.

Fat embolism, a potentially fatal complication resulting from release of fat molecules in response to increased intramedullary canal pressure from the prosthesis, may develop within 72 hours of surgery. Watch for such signs and symptoms as apprehension, diaphoresis, fever, dyspnea, pulmonary effusion, tachycardia, cyanosis, seizures, decreased level of consciousness, and a petechial rash on the chest and shoulders.

Documentation

Document any signs or symptoms of infection. Record the patient's neurovascular status. Document the patient's pain and response to pain medication.[5] Describe the patient's position (especially the position of the affected leg), skin care and condition, respiratory care and condition, and the use of elastic stockings. Document all exercises performed and their effect; also record ambulatory efforts, the type of support used, and the amount of traction weight.[10]

On the appropriate flowchart, record vital signs and fluid intake and output. Note the turning and skin care schedule and the current exercise and ambulation program. Record discharge instructions and how well the patient seems to understand them.

REFERENCES

1   The Joint Commission. (2012). Standard NPSG.01.01.01. *Comprehensive accreditation manual for hospitals: The official handbook.* Oakbrook Terrace, IL: The Joint Commission. (Level I)

2   The Joint Commission. (2012). Standard NPSG.07.01.01. *Comprehensive accreditation manual for hospitals: The official handbook.* Oakbrook Terrace, IL: The Joint Commission. (Level I)

3   World Health Organization. (2009). *WHO guidelines on hand hygiene in health care: First global patient safety challenge. Clean care is safer care.* Geneva, Switzerland: World Health Organization. (Level I)

4   Centers for Disease Control and Prevention. (October 2002). Guideline for hand hygiene in health-care settings. *Morbidity and Mortality Weekly Report, 51*(RR-16), 1–45. (Level I)

5   The Joint Commission. (2012). Standard PC.01.02.01. *Comprehensive accreditation manual for hospitals: The official handbook.* Oakbrook Terrace, IL: The Joint Commission. (Level I)

6   The Joint Commission. (2012). Standard NPSG.03.05.01. *Comprehensive accreditation manual for hospitals: The official handbook.* Oakbrook Terrace, IL: The Joint Commission. (Level I)

7   The Joint Commission. (2010). Surgical care improvement project national hospital inpatient quality measures. In *Specification manual for national hospital quality measures.* Oakbrook Terrace, IL: The Joint Commission. (Level I)

8   Gould, C.V., et al. (2009). "Guideline for Prevention of Catheter-associated Urinary Tract Infections, 2009" [Online]. Accessed November 2011 via the Web at http://www.cdc.gov/hicpac/cauti/001_cauti.html (Level I)

9   Anderson, D.J., et al. (2008). Compendium of strategies to prevent healthcare-associated infections in acute care hospitals: Strategies to prevent surgical site infections in acute care hospitals. *Infection Control and Hospital Epidemiology, 29*(Suppl. 1), 12–21.

10 The Joint Commission. (2012). Standard RC.01.03.01. *Comprehensive accreditation manual for hospitals: The official handbook.* Oakbrook Terrace, IL: The Joint Commission. (Level I)

11 The Joint Commission. (2012). Standard NPSG.07.05.01. *Comprehensive accreditation manual for hospitals: The official handbook.* Oakbrook Terrace, IL: The Joint Commission. (Level I)

ADDITIONAL REFERENCES

Colwell, C.W. (2009). The ACCP guidelines for thromboprophylaxis in total hip and knee arthroplasty. *Orthopedics, 32*(12 Suppl.), 67–73.

Smith-Miller, C.A., et al. (2009). A comparison of patient pain responses and medication regimens after hip/knee replacement. *Orthopedic Nursing, 28*(5), 242–249.

HOUR-OF-SLEEP CARE

Hour-of-sleep care meets the patient's physical and psychological needs in preparation for sleep. It includes providing for the patient's hygiene, making the bed clean and comfortable, and ensuring safety. For example, raising the bed's side rails can prevent the drowsy or sedated patient from falling out. This type of care also provides an opportunity to answer the patient's questions about the next day's tests and procedures and to discuss his worries and concerns.

Effective hour-of-sleep care prepares the patient for a good night's sleep. Ineffective care may contribute to sleeplessness, which can intensify patient anxiety and interfere with treatment and recuperation.

Equipment

Bedpan, urinal, or commode ■ basin ■ skin cleaner ■ towel ■ washcloth ■ toothbrush and toothpaste ■ denture cup and commercial denture cleaner, if necessary ■ lotion ■ clean linens, if necessary ■ blanket ■ facial tissues ■ gloves, if necessary ■ Optional: earplugs, gloves.

Preparation of equipment

Gather the equipment at the patient's bedside. For the ambulatory patient who is capable of self-care, gather skin cleaner, a washcloth, a towel, and oral hygiene items at the sink.

Implementation

■ Perform hand hygiene. Put on gloves, if necessary.[1,2,3]

■ Confirm the patient's identity using at least two patient identifiers according to your facility's policy.[4]

■ Tell the patient you will help him prepare for sleep, and provide privacy.

■ Offer the patient on bed rest a bedpan or urinal. Otherwise, assist the ambulatory patient to the bathroom or commode.

■ Fill the basin with warm water and bring it to the patient's bedside. Wash the patient's face and hands and dry them well. Encourage the patient to wash himself, if possible, *to promote independence.*

■ Provide toothpaste or a properly labeled denture cup and commercial denture cleaner. Assist the patient with oral hygiene, as necessary. (See "Oral care," page 524.) If the patient prefers to wear dentures until bedtime, leave denture-care items within easy reach.

■ After providing oral care, turn the patient on his side or stomach. Wash, rinse, and dry the patient's back and buttocks. Massage the back with lotion *to help relax the patient.* (For complete information on massage, see "Back care," page 48.)

■ While providing back care, observe the skin for redness, cracking, or other signs of breakdown. If the patient's gown is soiled or damp, provide a clean one and help him put it on, if necessary.

■ Check dressings, binders, antiembolism stockings, or other aids, changing or readjusting them as needed.

■ Refill the water container, and place it and a box of facial tissues within the patient's easy reach *to prevent falls if the patient needs to reach for these items.*

■ Straighten or change bed linens, as necessary, and fluff the patient's pillow. Clean linens are only needed if the linen is soiled. Cover the patient with a blanket or place one within easy reach *to prevent chills during the night.* Then position him comfortably.
■ Offer the patient ear plugs, if appropriate, *to help block noise from the unit.*
■ If the patient appears distressed, restless, or in pain, administer medications as needed following safe medication administration practices.[5]
■ After making the patient comfortable, evaluate his mental and physical condition.
■ Place the bed in a low position and, if appropriate, raise the side rails. Place the call bell within the patient's easy reach, and instruct him to call you whenever necessary.
■ Tidy the patient's environment: Move all breakables from the overbed table out of his reach, and remove any equipment and supplies that could cause falls should the patient get up during the night.
■ Turn off the overhead light and put on the night-light.
■ Remove and discard your gloves, if worn.
■ Perform hand hygiene.[1,2,3]
■ Document the procedure.[6]

Special considerations
■ Ask the patient about his sleep routine at home and, whenever possible, let him follow it.
■ Try to observe certain rituals, such as a bedtime snack, *which can aid sleep.* A back massage, a tub bath, or a shower can also help relax the patient and promote a restful night. If the patient normally bathes or showers before bedtime, let him do so if his condition and doctor's orders permit it.
■ Some patients may benefit from guided imagery and music therapy to help them sleep.

Documentation
Record the time and type of hour-of-sleep care in your notes. Include use of any special procedures such as relaxation techniques.[6]

REFERENCES
1 The Joint Commission. (2012). Standard NPSG.07.01.01. *Comprehensive accreditation manual for hospitals: The official handbook.* Oakbrook Terrace, IL: The Joint Commission. (Level I)
2 Centers for Disease Control and Prevention. (October 2002). Guideline for hand hygiene in health-care settings. *Morbidity and Mortality Weekly Report, 51*(RR-16), 1–45. (Level I)
3 World Health Organization. (2009). *WHO guidelines on hand hygiene in health care: First global patient safety challenge. Clean care is safer care.* Geneva, Switzerland: World Health Organization. (Level I)
4 The Joint Commission. (2012). Standard NPSG.01.01.01. *Comprehensive accreditation manual for hospitals: The official handbook.* Oakbrook Terrace, IL: The Joint Commission. (Level I)
5 The Joint Commission. (2012). Standard MM.06.01.01. *Comprehensive accreditation manual for hospitals: The official handbook.* Oakbrook Terrace, IL: The Joint Commission. (Level I)
6 The Joint Commission. (2012). Standard RC.01.03.01. *Comprehensive accreditation manual for hospitals: The official handbook.* Oakbrook Terrace, IL: The Joint Commission. (Level I)

ADDITIONAL REFERENCES
Craven, R.F., & Hirnle, C.J. (2012). *Fundamentals of nursing: Human health and function* (7th ed.). Philadelphia, PA: Lippincott Williams & Wilkins.
Taylor, C., et al. (2011). *Fundamentals of nursing: The art and science of nursing care* (7th ed.). Philadelphia, PA: Lippincott Williams & Wilkins.

HUMIDIFIER THERAPY

Humidifiers deliver a maximum amount of water vapor without producing particulate water. They're used to prevent drying and irritation of the upper airway in such conditions as croup, in which the upper airway is inflamed, or in a patient who has particularly thick and tenacious secretions.

Several types of humidifiers are available. (See *Types of humidifiers,* page 346.) Diffusion humidifiers (also known as *in-line humidifiers*) are added to oxygen delivery systems to humidify only the air being delivered to the patient. One type of diffusion humidifier—the *cascade bubble diffusion humidifier*—heats water vapor, which raises the moisture-carrying capacity of gas and increases the amount of humidity delivered to the patient. A *diffusion head humidifier* can be added to a low-flow oxygen delivery system to humidify the air being delivered to the patient, but it doesn't heat the water vapor. A *heated vaporizer* heats water vapor to raise the moisture-carrying capacity of gas, adding humidity to an entire room.

Equipment
Appropriate humidifier ■ sterile, distilled water (for all types) or tap water (for a heated vaporizer with a demineralizing capability) ■ container for waste water.

Bedside humidifier and heated vaporizer
Hospital-grade disinfectant.

Diffusion head humidifier
Flowmeter ■ oxygen source.

Preparation of equipment
For a bedside humidifier
Open the reservoir of the bedside humidifier and add sterile, distilled water to the fill line; then close the reservoir. Keep all room windows and doors closed tightly *to maintain adequate humidification.*

For a cascade bubble diffusion humidifier
The cascade bubble diffuser should be installed into the ventilator circuit according to the manufacturer's instructions. Unscrew the cascade reservoir and add sterile, distilled water to the fill line. Screw the top back onto the reservoir. Plug in the heater unit and set the temperature between 95° F (35° C) and 100.4° F (38° C).

EQUIPMENT

Types of humidifiers

	DESCRIPTION AND USES	ADVANTAGES	DISADVANTAGES
Bedside humidifier 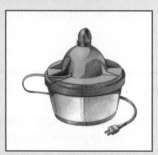	■ Spinning disk splashes water against a baffle, creating small drops and increasing evaporation; motor disperses mist to directly humidify room air.	■ May be used with all oxygen masks and nasal cannulas ■ Easy to operate ■ Inexpensive	■ Produces humidity inefficiently ■ Can't be used for a patient with a bypassed upper airway ■ May harbor bacteria and molds
Cascade bubble diffusion humidifier 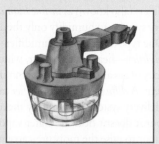	■ Gas is forced through a plastic grid in a reservoir of warmed water to create fine bubbles. It's commonly used in patients receiving mechanical ventilation or continuous positive airway pressure therapy.	■ Delivers 100% humidity at body temperature ■ Most effective of all evaporative humidifiers	■ If correct water level isn't maintained, mucosa may become irritated
Diffusion head humidifier 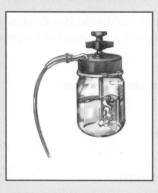	■ The diffusion head humidifier is most commonly used with low-flow oxygen delivery systems. Gas flows through the porous diffuser in the reservoir to increase gas-liquid interface, providing humidification to patients using a nasal cannula or oxygen mask (except the Venturi mask).	■ Easy to operate ■ Inexpensive	■ Provides only 20% to 30% humidity at body temperature ■ Can't be used for a patient with a bypassed upper airway
Heated vaporizer 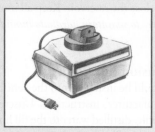	■ Water heated in the reservoir provides direct humidification to room air.	■ May be used with all oxygen masks and nasal cannulas ■ Easy to operate ■ Inexpensive	■ Can't guarantee the amount of humidity delivered ■ Risk of burn injury occurring if machine knocks over

For a diffusion head humidifier
Unscrew the humidifier reservoir and add sterile, distilled water to the appropriate level. (If using a disposable unit, screw the cap with the extension onto the top of the unit.) Then screw the reservoir back onto the humidifier, and attach the flowmeter to the oxygen source. Screw the diffusion head humidifier onto the flowmeter until the seal is tight. Then set the flowmeter at a rate of 2 L/minute and check for gentle bubbling. Next, check the positive-pressure release valve by occluding the end valve on the humidifier. The pressure should back up into the humidifier, signaled by a high-pitched whistle. If this whistle doesn't occur, tighten all connections and try again.

For a heated vaporizer
Remove the top of the vaporizer and fill the reservoir to the fill line with tap water. Replace the top securely.

Implementation
- Verify the doctor's order.
- Confirm the patient's identity using at least two patient identifiers according to your facility's policy.[1]
- Explain the procedure to the patient.
- Perform hand hygiene.[2,3,4]
- Make sure the humidifier has been prepared properly.

Bedside humidifier
- Plug the unit into the electrical outlet.
- Direct the humidifier unit's nozzle toward the patient but away from the patient's face for effective treatment. Check for a fine mist emission from the nozzle, *which indicates proper operation.*
- Check the unit every 4 hours for proper operation and water level. When refilling, unplug the unit, discard any old water, clean and disinfect it with a hospital-grade disinfectant, rinse the reservoir container, and refill with sterile, distilled water.
- Keep the unit cleaned and refilled with sterile water *to reduce the risk of bacterial growth.*

Cascade bubble diffusion humidifier
- Assess the temperature of the inspired gas near the patient's airway, every 2 hours for critical care and every 4 hours for general patient care. If the cascade becomes too hot, check the heater unit and reset or replace the unit, as necessary. *Overheated water vapor can cause respiratory tract burns.*
- Check the reservoir's water level every 2 to 4 hours, and fill it as necessary. *If the water level falls below the minimum water level mark, humidity will decrease to that of room air.*
- Be alert for condensation buildup in the tubing, which can result from the high humidification produced by the cascade.
- Check the tubing frequently and empty the condensate, as necessary, *so it can't drain into the patient's respiratory tract, encourage the growth of microorganisms, or obstruct dependent sections of tubing.* To do so, disconnect the tubing, drain the condensate into a container, and dispose of it properly. Never drain the condensate into the humidification system.

Diffusion head humidifier
- Attach the oxygen delivery device to the humidifier and then to the patient. Adjust the flowmeter to the appropriate oxygen flow rate.
- Check the reservoir every 4 hours. If the water level drops too low, empty the remaining water, rinse the jar, and refill it with sterile, distilled water. Alternately, replace a commercially prepared disposable unit at its low water mark. (As the reservoir water level decreases, the evaporation of water in the gas decreases, reducing humidification of the delivered gas.)
- Periodically assess the patient's sputum; *sputum that's too thick can hinder mobilization and expectoration.* If thick sputum occurs, the patient requires a device that can provide higher humidity.

Heated vaporizer
- Place the vaporizer about 4′ (1.2 m) from the patient, directing the steam toward but not directly onto the patient. Place the unit in a spot where it can't be overturned *to avoid hot-water burns.* This step is especially important if children will be in the room.
- Plug the unit into an electrical outlet. Steam should soon rise from the unit into the air. Close all windows and doors *to maintain adequate humidification.*
- Check the unit every 4 hours for proper functioning. If steam production seems insufficient, unplug the unit, discard the water, and refill with tap water, or clean the unit well.
- Also check the water level in the unit every 4 hours. To refill, unplug the unit, discard any old water, clean and disinfect with a hospital-grade disinfectant,[5] rinse the reservoir container, and refill with tap water as necessary.

Completing the procedure
- Perform hand hygiene.[2,3,4]
- Document the procedure.[6]

Special considerations
- Replace a bedside humidifier unit every 7 days, and send used units for proper decontamination.
- *Because the bedside humidifier or vaporizer doesn't deliver a precise amount of humidification,* assess the patient regularly *to determine the effectiveness of therapy.* Ask him if he's noticed any improvement, and evaluate his sputum.
- Change the cascade bubble diffusion humidifier regularly according to your facility's policy; change the diffusion head humidifier system regularly to prevent bacterial growth and invasion.
- Because the diffusion head humidifier creates a level of humidity comparable to that of ambient air, the diffusion head humidifier is use only for oxygen flow rates greater than 4 L/minute.
- Keep in mind that a humidifier that's not kept clean can cause or aggravate respiratory problems, especially for people allergic to molds. Refer to your facility's policy for changing and disposing of humidification equipment.

Patient teaching

Make sure the patient and his family understand the reason for using a humidifier and know how to use the equipment. Give them specific written guidelines concerning all aspects of home care.

Instruct the patient using a bedside humidifier at home to fill it with plain tap water but to periodically use sterile, distilled water *to prevent mineral buildup.*

Tell the patient using a bedside humidifier or heated vaporizer unit to rinse it with bleach and water every 5 days. Also tell him to run white vinegar through it *to help clean it, prevent bacterial buildup, and dissolve deposits.*

Complications

If contaminated, humidifiers can cause infection. Cascade bubble diffusion humidifiers can cause aspiration of tubal condensation, pulmonary burns if the air is heated, and infection if contaminated.

Documentation

Record the date and time when humidification began and was discontinued, the type of humidifier used, the patient's response to humidification, and any patient teaching provided.[6]

REFERENCES

1 The Joint Commission. (2012). Standard NPSG.01.01.01. *Comprehensive accreditation manual for hospitals: The official handbook.* Oakbrook Terrace, IL: The Joint Commission. (Level I)
2 The Joint Commission. (2012). Standard NPSG.07.01.01. *Comprehensive accreditation manual for hospitals: The official handbook.* Oakbrook Terrace, IL: The Joint Commission. (Level I)
3 Centers for Disease Control and Prevention. (October 2002). Guideline for hand hygiene in health-care settings. *Morbidity and Mortality Weekly Report, 51*(RR-16), 1–45. (Level I)
4 World Health Organization. (2009). *WHO guidelines on hand hygiene in health care: First global patient safety challenge. Clean care is safer care.* Geneva, Switzerland: World Health Organization. (Level I)
5 Rutala, W.A., et al. (2008). "Guideline for Disinfection and Sterilization in Healthcare Facilities, 2008" [Online]. Accessed November 2011 via the Web at http://www.cdc.gov/ncidod/dhqp/pdf/guidelines/Disinfection_Nov_2008.pdf (Level I)
6 The Joint Commission. (2012). Standard RC.01.03.01. *Comprehensive accreditation manual for hospitals: The official handbook.* Oakbrook Terrace, IL: The Joint Commission. (Level I)

ADDITIONAL REFERENCES

Coffin, S.E., et al. (2008). Supplement article: SHEA/IDSA practice recommendation: Strategies to prevent ventilator-associated pneumonia in acute care hospitals. *Infection Control and Hospital Epidemiology, 31*(S1).
Craven, R.F., & Hirnle, C.J. (2012). *Fundamentals of nursing: Human health and function* (7th ed.). Philadelphia, PA: Lippincott Williams & Wilkins.
Niel-Weise, B.S., et al. (2007). Humidification policies for mechanically ventilated intensive care patients and prevention of ventilator-associated pneumonia: A systematic review of randomized controlled trials. *Journal of Hospital Infection, 65*(4), 285–291.
Selvaraj, N. (2010). Artificial humidification for the mechanically ventilated patient. *Nursing Standard, 25*(8), 41–46.

HYPERTHERMIA-HYPOTHERMIA BLANKET USE

A blanket-sized aquamatic K pad, the hyperthermia-hypothermia blanket raises, lowers, or maintains body temperature through conductive heat or cold transfer between the blanket and the patient. It can be operated manually or automatically.

In manual operation, the nurse or doctor sets the temperature on the unit. The blanket reaches and maintains this temperature regardless of the patient's temperature. The temperature setting must be adjusted manually to reach a different setting. The nurse monitors the patient's body temperature with a conventional thermometer.

In automatic operation, the unit directly and continually monitors the patient's temperature by means of a thermistor probe (rectal, skin, or esophageal) and alternates heating and cooling cycles as necessary to achieve and maintain the desired body temperature. The thermistor probe also may be used in conjunction with manual operation but isn't essential. The unit is equipped with an alarm to warn of abnormal temperature fluctuations and a circuit breaker that protects against current overload.

The blanket is used most commonly to reduce high fever when more conservative measures—such as baths, ice packs, and antipyretics—are unsuccessful. Its other uses include maintaining normal temperature during surgery or shock; inducing hypothermia during surgery to decrease metabolic activity and thereby reduce oxygen requirements; reducing intracranial pressure; controlling bleeding and intractable pain in patients with amputations, burns, or cancer; and providing warmth in cases of mild to moderate hypothermia.

Equipment

Hyperthermia-hypothermia control unit ▪ fluid for the control unit (distilled water or distilled water and 20% ethyl alcohol) ▪ thermistor probe (rectal, skin, or esophageal) ▪ patient thermometer ▪ one or two hyperthermia-hypothermia blankets ▪ one or two disposable blanket covers (or one or two sheets or bath blankets) ▪ lanolin or a mixture of lanolin and cold cream ▪ adhesive tape ▪ towel ▪ sphygmomanometer ▪ gloves and gowns, if necessary ▪ Optional: protective wraps for the patient's hands and feet.

Disposable hyperthermia-hypothermia blankets are available for single-patient use.

Preparation of equipment

First, read the operation manual. Inspect the control unit and each blanket for leaks and the plugs and connecting wires for broken prongs, kinks, and fraying. If you detect or suspect malfunction, don't use the equipment.

Review the doctor's order, and prepare one or two blankets by covering them with disposable covers (or use a sheet or bath blanket when positioning the blanket on the patient). *The cover absorbs perspiration and condensation, which could cause tissue breakdown if left on the skin.* Connect the blanket to the control unit, and set the controls for manual or automatic operation and for the desired blanket or body temperature. Make sure the machine is properly grounded before plugging it in. Turn on the machine and add liquid to the unit reservoir, if necessary, as fluid fills the blanket. Allow the blanket to preheat or precool *so that the patient receives immediate thermal benefit.*

Implementation

■ Perform hand hygiene.[1,2,3]
■ Confirm the patient's identity using at least two patient identifiers according to your facility's policy.[4]
■ If the patient isn't already wearing a hospital gown, ask him to put one on. Use a gown with cloth ties rather than metal snaps or pins *to prevent heat or cold injury.*
■ Assess the patient's condition and explain the procedure to him. Provide privacy and make sure the room is warm and free from drafts.
■ Take the patient's temperature, pulse, respirations, and blood pressure *to serve as a baseline,* and assess his level of consciousness, pupil reaction, limb strength, and skin condition.
■ Keeping the bottom sheet in place and the patient recumbent, roll the patient to one side and slide the blanket halfway underneath him, so its top edge aligns with his neck. Then roll the patient back, and pull and flatten the blanket across the bed. Place a pillow under the patient's head. Make sure the patient's head doesn't lie directly on the blanket *because the blanket's rigid surface may be uncomfortable and the heat or cold may lead to tissue breakdown.* Use a sheet or bath blanket as insulation between the patient and the blanket. (See *Using a cooling system.*)
■ Apply lanolin or a mixture of lanolin and cold cream to the patient's skin where it touches the blanket *to help protect the skin from heat or cold sensation.*
■ In automatic operation, insert the thermistor probe in the patient's rectum and tape it in place *to prevent accidental dislodgment.* If rectal insertion is contraindicated, tuck a skin probe deep into the axilla, and secure it with tape. If the patient is comatose or anesthetized, you may want to insert an esophageal probe. Plug the other end of the probe into the correct jack on the unit's control panel.
■ Place a sheet or, if ordered, the second hyperthermia-hypothermia blanket over the patient *to increase the thermal benefit by trapping cooled or heated air.*
■ Wrap the patient's hands and feet if he wishes *to minimize chilling and promote comfort.* Monitor vital signs and perform a neurologic assessment every 5 minutes until the desired body temperature is reached and then every 15 minutes until the temperature is stable or as ordered.
■ Check fluid intake and output hourly or as ordered. Observe the patient regularly for color changes in skin, lips, and nail beds, and for edema, induration, inflammation, pain, or sensory impairment. If these complications occur, discontinue the procedure and notify the doctor.

EQUIPMENT

Using a cooling system

A hypothermia or cooling blanket is used to lower a patient's body temperature. The pad contains coils that circulate a chilled solution. While the blanket is in use, you must monitor the patient's temperature. The blanket's temperature can be adjusted to help keep the patient's temperature in the ordered range.

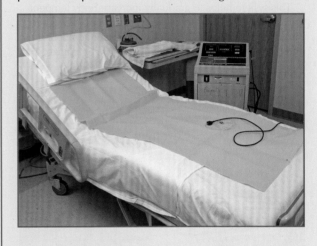

■ Reposition the patient every 30 minutes to 1 hour, unless contraindicated, *to prevent skin breakdown.* Keep the patient's skin, bedclothes, and blanket cover free of perspiration and condensation, and reapply cream to exposed body parts as needed.
■ After turning off the machine, follow the manufacturer's directions. *Some units must remain plugged in for at least 30 minutes to allow the condenser fan to remove water vapor from the mechanism.* Continue to monitor the patient's temperature until it stabilizes *because body temperature can fall as much as 5° F (2.8° C) after this procedure.*
■ Remove all equipment from the bed. Dry the patient and make him comfortable. Supply a fresh hospital gown, if necessary. Cover him lightly.
■ Continue to perform neurologic assessments and monitor vital signs, fluid intake and output, and general condition every 30 minutes for 2 hours and then hourly or as ordered.
■ Return the equipment to the central supply department for cleaning, servicing, and storage.
■ Perform hand hygiene.[1,2,3]
■ Document the procedure.[5]

Special considerations

■ If the patient shivers excessively during hypothermia treatment, discontinue the procedure and notify the doctor immediately. *By increasing metabolism, shivering elevates body temperature.*
■ Avoid lowering the temperature more than 1° F (0.6° C) every 15 minutes *to prevent premature ventricular contractions.*

EQUIPMENT

Using a warming system

Shivering, the compensatory response to falling body temperature, may use more oxygen than the body can supply—especially in a surgical patient. In the past, you would cover the patient with blankets to warm his body. Now, health care facilities may supply a warming system, such as the Bair Hugger patient-warming system.

This system helps to gradually increase body temperature. Like a large hair dryer, the warming unit draws air through a filter, warms the air to the desired temperature, and circulates it through a hose to a warming blanket placed over the patient.

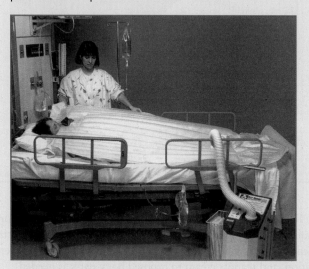

When using the warming system, be sure to:
- use a bath blanket in a single layer over the warming blanket *to minimize heat loss*
- place the warming blanket directly over the patient with the paper side facing down and the clear tubular side facing up
- make sure the connection hose is at the foot of the bed
- take the patient's temperature during the first 15 to 30 minutes and at least every 30 minutes while the warming blanket is in use
- obtain guidelines from the patient's doctor for discontinuing use of the warming blanket.

■ Don't use pins to secure catheters, tubes, or blanket covers *because an accidental puncture can result in fluid leakage and burns.*
■ With hyperthermia or hypothermia therapy, the patient may experience a secondary defense reaction (vasoconstriction or vasodilation, respectively) that causes body temperature to rebound, defeating the treatment's purpose.
■ If the patient requires isolation, place the blanket, blanket cover, and probe in a plastic bag clearly marked with the type of isola-

tion *so that the central supply department can give it special handling.* If the blanket is disposable, discard it, using appropriate precautions.
■ *To avoid bacterial growth in the reservoir or blankets,* always use sterile, distilled water and change it monthly. Check to see if facility policy calls for adding a bacteriostatic agent to the water. Avoid using deionized water *because it may corrode the system.*
■ *To gradually increase body temperature, especially in postoperative patients,* the doctor may order a disposable blanket warming system. (See *Using a warming system.*)

Complications

Use of a hyperthermia-hypothermia blanket can cause shivering, marked changes in vital signs, increased intracranial pressure, respiratory distress or arrest, cardiac arrest, oliguria, and anuria.

Documentation

Record the patient's pulse, respirations, blood pressure, neurologic signs, fluid intake and output, skin condition, and position changes. Record the patient's temperature and that of the blanket every 30 minutes while the blanket is in use. Also document the type of hyperthermia-hypothermia unit used; control settings (manual or automatic and temperature settings); date, time, duration, and patient's tolerance of treatment; and signs of complications.

REFERENCES

1 The Joint Commission. (2012). Standard NPSG.07.01.01. *Comprehensive accreditation manual for hospitals: The official handbook.* Oakbrook Terrace, IL: The Joint Commission. (Level I)
2 Centers for Disease Control and Prevention. (October 2002). Guideline for hand hygiene in health-care settings. *Morbidity and Mortality Weekly Report, 51*(RR-16), 1–45. (Level I)
3 World Health Organization. (2009). *WHO guidelines on hand hygiene in health care: First global patient safety challenge. Clean care is safer care.* Geneva, Switzerland: World Health Organization. (Level I)
4 The Joint Commission. (2012). Standard NPSG.01.01.01. *Comprehensive accreditation manual for hospitals: The official handbook.* Oakbrook Terrace, IL: The Joint Commission. (Level I)
5 The Joint Commission. (2012). Standard RC.01.03.01. *Comprehensive accreditation manual for hospitals: The official handbook.* Oakbrook Terrace, IL: The Joint Commission. (Level I)

ADDITIONAL REFERENCES

Arrich, J., et al. (2007). Clinical application of mild therapeutic hypothermia after cardiac arrest. *Critical Care Medicine, 35*(4), 1041–1047.
Cushman, L., et al. (2007). Bringing research to the bedside: The role of induced hypothermia in cardiac arrest. *Critical Care Nursing Quarterly, 30*(2), 143–153.
Ihn, C.H., et al. (2008). Comparison of three warming devices for the prevention of core hypothermia and post-anaesthesia shivering. *Journal of International Medical Research, 36*(5), 923–931.
Loke, A.Y., et al. (2005). Comparing the effectiveness of two types of cooling blankets for febrile patients. *Nursing Critical Care, 10*(5), 247–254.

IM INJECTION

IM injections deposit medication deep into muscle tissue. This route of administration provides rapid systemic action and absorption of relatively large doses (up to 4 mL in appropriate sites). IM injections are recommended for patients who can't take medication orally, when IV administration is inappropriate, and for drugs that are altered by digestive juices. Because muscle tissue has few sensory nerves, IM injections allow for less painful administration of irritating drugs.

The site for an IM injection must be chosen carefully, taking into account the patient's general physical status and the purpose of the injection. IM injections shouldn't be administered at inflamed, edematous, or irritated sites or at sites that contain moles, birthmarks, scar tissue, or other lesions. IM injections may also be contraindicated in patients with impaired coagulation mechanisms, occlusive peripheral vascular disease, edema, and shock; after thrombolytic therapy; and during an acute myocardial infarction (MI) because these conditions impair peripheral absorption. IM injections require sterile technique to maintain the integrity of muscle tissue.

Equipment

Patient's medication administration record ▪ prescribed medication ▪ sterile syringe and needle of appropriate size and gauge ▪ gloves ▪ alcohol pads ▪ Optional: gauze pad, 1″ tape, ice, filter needle.

The prescribed medication must be sterile. The needle may be packaged separately or already attached to the syringe. (See *Selecting the appropriate syringe and needle.*)

Preparation of equipment

Verify the order on the patient's medication record by checking it against the doctor's order.[1] Also note whether the patient has any allergies, especially before the first dose. Perform hand hygiene.[2,3,4] Avoid distractions and interruptions when preparing and administering medications *to prevent medication errors.*[5]

Check the prescribed medication for color and clarity. Also note the expiration date.[6] Never use medication that is cloudy or discolored or that contains a precipitate unless the manufacturer's instructions allow it. Remember that for some drugs (such as suspensions), the presence of drug particles is normal. Observe for abnormal changes. If in doubt, check with the pharmacist.

Choose equipment appropriate to the prescribed medication and injection site, and make sure it works properly. The needle should be straight, smooth, and free of burrs.

For single-dose ampules

Wrap an alcohol pad around the ampule's neck and snap off the top, directing the force away from your body. Attach a filter nee-

---

Selecting the appropriate syringe and needle

For an IM injection, the size of the syringe and the gauge and length of the needle are determined by several factors, including the amount and viscosity of the medication, the injection site chosen, and the patient's weight and amount of adipose tissue. Needles used for IM injections are longer than subcutaneous needles *because they must reach deep into the muscle.*

The volume of medication administered IM is usually 1 to 4 mL, so a 3- or 5-mL syringe is usually appropriate. The appropriate gauge of the needle is determined by the medication being administered. Biologic agents and medications in aqueous solutions should be administered with a 20G to 25G needle. Medications in oil-based solutions should be administered with an 18G to 25G needle.

Needle length depends on the injection site, the patient's size, and the amount of subcutaneous fat covering the muscle. Patients who are obese may require a longer needle (1½″ or longer) and thin or emaciated patients may require a shorter needle (½″ to 1″).[9] Needle lengths are based on the injection site chosen for an adult patient:

- Vastus lateralis: ½″ to 1″·
- Deltoid: ½″ to 1½″
- Ventrogluteal: ½″ to 1½″

---

dle to the syringe and withdraw the medication, keeping the needle's bevel tip below the level of the solution. Tap the syringe *to clear air from it.* Cover the needle with the needle sheath.

Before discarding the ampule, check the medication label against the patient's medication record.[1] Discard the filter needle and the ampule. Attach the appropriate needle to the syringe.

For single-dose or multidose vials

Reconstitute powdered drugs according to instructions. Make sure all crystals have dissolved in the solution. Warm the vial by rolling it between your palms *to help the drug dissolve faster.*

Wipe the stopper of the medication vial with an alcohol pad, and then draw up the prescribed amount of medication. Read the medication label as you select the medication, as you draw it up, and after you have drawn it up *to verify the correct dosage.*[1]

Don't use an air bubble in the syringe. Modern disposable syringes are calibrated to give the correct dose without an air bubble.

Gather all necessary equipment and proceed to the patient's room.

Implementation

- Perform hand hygiene.[2,3,4]
- Confirm the patient's identity using at least two patient identifiers according to your facility's policy.[7]

Locating IM injection sites

Deltoid

Have the patient sit or stand. Find the lower edge of the acromial process and the point on the lateral arm in line with the axilla. Insert the needle 1″ to 2″ (2.5 to 5 cm) below the acromial process, usually two or three finger-breadths, at a 90-degree angle or angled slightly toward the process. Typical injection: 0.5 mL (range: 0.5 to 2.0 mL).

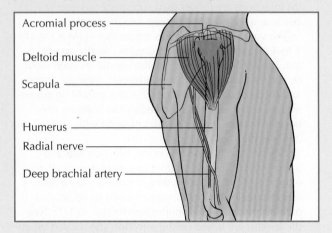

Acromial process
Deltoid muscle
Scapula
Humerus
Radial nerve
Deep brachial artery

Ventrogluteal

Have the patient sit, stand, lie laterally, or lie supine. Locate the greater trochanter of the femur with the heel of your hand. Then spread your index and middle fingers from the anterior superior iliac spine to as far along the iliac crest as you can reach. Insert the needle between the two fingers at a 90-degree angle to the muscle. (Remove your fingers before inserting the needle.) Typical injection: 1 to 4 mL.

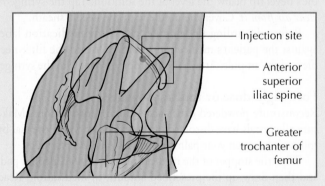

Injection site
Anterior superior iliac spine
Greater trochanter of femur

Vastus lateralis

Have the patient sit or lie supine. The knee may be slightly flexed and the foot may be externally rotated *to help relax the muscle.* Use the lateral muscle of the quadriceps group, from a handbreadth below the greater trochanter to a hand-breadth above the knee. Insert the needle into the middle third of the muscle parallel to the surface on which the patient is lying. Typical injection: 1 to 4 mL.

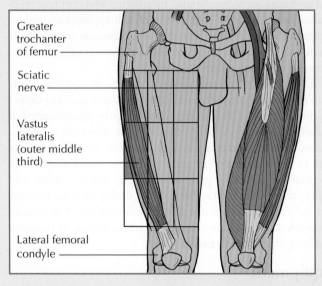

Greater trochanter of femur
Sciatic nerve
Vastus lateralis (outer middle third)
Lateral femoral condyle

- If your facility uses a bar code scanning system, scan your identification badge, the patient's identification bracelet, and the medication's bar code or follow the procedure for your facility's bar code system.
- Provide privacy and explain the procedure to the patient.
- Perform hand hygiene and put on gloves.[2,3,4]
- Select an appropriate injection site. The ventrogluteal site is used most commonly for healthy adults, although the deltoid

muscle may be used for a small-volume injection (2 mL or less). (See *Locating IM injection sites.*) Remember to always rotate injection sites for patients who require repeated injections.

PEDIATRIC ALERT *For infants and children, the vastus lateralis muscle of the thigh is used most commonly* because it's usually the best developed and contains no large nerves or blood vessels, minimizing the risk of serious injury.

■ Position and drape the patient appropriately using his bed linens, making sure the site is well exposed and that lighting is adequate (as shown below).

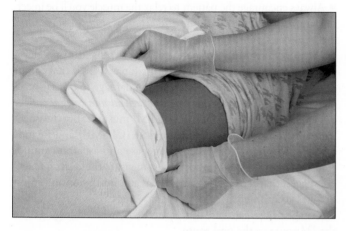

■ Loosen the protective needle sheath, but don't remove it (as shown below).

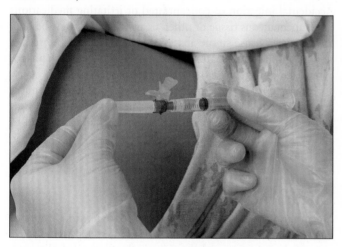

■ After selecting the injection site, gently tap it *to stimulate the nerve endings and minimize pain when the needle is inserted.* Clean the skin at the site with an alcohol pad (as shown below). Move the pad outward in a circular motion to a circumference of about 2″ (5 cm) from the injection site, and allow the skin to dry. Keep the alcohol pad for later use.

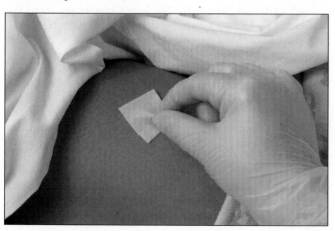

■ With the thumb and index finger of your nondominant hand, gently displace the skin and subcutaneous tissue of the injection site by pulling the skin laterally for the Z-track technique. (See "Z-track injection," page 797.)

■ While you hold the syringe in your dominant hand, remove the needle sheath by slipping it between the free fingers of your nondominant hand and then drawing back the syringe.

■ Position the syringe at a 90-degree angle to the skin surface, with the needle a couple of inches from the skin. Tell the patient that he'll feel a prick as you insert the needle. Then quickly and firmly thrust the needle through the skin and subcutaneous tissue, deep into the muscle.

■ Support the syringe with your nondominant hand, if desired. Pull back slightly on the plunger with your dominant hand to aspirate for blood if appropriate. Aspiration for blood isn't recommended for administration of immunizations and vaccines. If no blood appears, *slowly* inject the medication into the muscle. *A slow, steady injection rate allows the muscle to distend gradually and accept the medication under minimal pressure.* You should feel little or no resistance against the force of the injection.

NURSING ALERT *If blood appears in the syringe on aspiration, the needle is in a blood vessel. If this occurs, stop the injection, withdraw the needle, prepare another injection with new equipment, and inject another site. Don't inject the bloody solution.*

■ After the injection, gently but quickly remove the needle at a 90-degree angle. If present, activate the needle's safety mechanism *to prevent accidental needle-stick injury.*[8]

■ Release the displaced skin and subcutaneous tissue to seal the needle tract.

■ Using a gloved hand, cover the injection site immediately with the used alcohol pad and apply gentle pressure (as shown below).

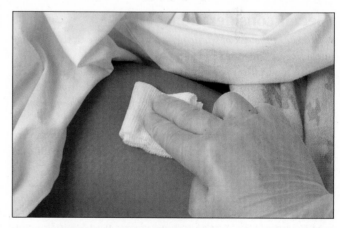

■ Remove the alcohol pad, and inspect the injection site for signs of active bleeding or bruising. If bleeding continues, apply pressure to the site; if bruising occurs, you may apply ice.

■ Watch for any adverse reactions at the site for 10 to 30 minutes after the injection.

ELDER ALERT *An elderly patient may bleed or ooze from the site after the injection because of decreased tissue elasticity. Applying a small pressure bandage may be helpful.*

Documenting administration of controlled substances

Regulations require controlled substances to be counted to ensure an accurate drug count, usually after each nursing shift. Some facilities use a computerized system that confirms the opioid count for each drug as it's used or removed from the system via a secure identification code; such a system eliminates the need for opioid counts during the day. Another regulation requires that a second nurse document your activity and observe you if part of a controlled substance dose must be wasted.

Before administering a controlled substance, regardless of the system being used, always verify the amount of drug in the container and follow your facility's policy for signing out the medication.

What to report

If you discover a discrepancy in the controlled substance count, follow your facility's reporting policy; you'll need to file an occurrence report as well. An investigation will follow.

- Discard all equipment according to standard precautions and your facility's policy. Don't recap needles; dispose of them in an appropriate sharps container *to avoid needle-stick injuries.*
- Remove your gloves and perform hand hygiene.[2,3,4]
- Document the procedure.[10]

Special considerations

- *Because of the risk of sciatic nerve injury,* the use of the dorsogluteal site isn't recommended for IM injections.
- If the medication isn't going to be administered immediately to the patient without a break in the process, clearly label the medication according to your facility's policy *to prevent a medication error.*[11]
- *To slow their absorption,* some drugs for IM administration are dissolved in oil or other special solutions. Mix these preparations well before drawing them into the syringe.

PEDIATRIC ALERT *The ventrogluteal muscles can be used as the injection site only after a toddler has been walking for about 1 year.*

- Never inject into sensitive muscles, especially those that twitch or tremble when you assess site landmarks and tissue depth. *Injections into these trigger areas may cause sharp or referred pain, such as the pain caused by nerve trauma.*
- Keep a rotation record that lists all available injection sites, divided into various body areas, for patients who require repeated injections. Rotate from a site in the first area to a site in each of the other areas. Then return to a site in the first area that is at least 1″ (2.5 cm) away from the previous injection site in that area.
- If the patient has experienced pain or emotional trauma from repeated injections, consider numbing the area before cleaning

it by holding ice on it for several seconds. If you must inject more than 4 mL of solution, divide the solution and inject it at two separate sites.

- Always encourage the patient to relax the muscle you'll be injecting *because injections into tense muscles are typically more painful and may bleed more readily.*
- IM injections can damage local muscle cells, causing elevations in serum enzyme levels (creatine kinase [CK]) that can be confused with elevations resulting from damage to cardiac muscle, as in MI. *To distinguish between skeletal and cardiac muscle damage,* diagnostic tests for suspected MI must identify the isoenzyme of CK specific to cardiac muscle (CK-MB) and include tests to determine lactate dehydrogenase and aspartate aminotransferase levels. If it's important to measure these enzyme levels, suggest that the doctor switch to IV administration and adjust dosages accordingly.
- Dosage adjustments are usually necessary when changing from the IM route to the oral route.

Complications

Accidental injection of concentrated or irritating medications into subcutaneous tissue or other areas where they can't be fully absorbed can cause sterile abscesses to develop. Such abscesses result from the body's natural immune response in which phagocytes attempt to remove the foreign matter.

Failure to rotate sites in patients who require repeated injections can lead to deposits of unabsorbed medications. Such deposits can reduce the desired pharmacologic effect and may lead to abscess formation or tissue fibrosis.

ELDER ALERT *Because elderly patients have decreased muscle mass, IM medications can be absorbed more quickly than expected.*

Documentation

Document the drug administered, dose, date, time, route of administration, and injection site. Also, note the patient's tolerance of the injection and the injection's effects, including any adverse effects. (See *Documenting administration of controlled substances.*)

REFERENCES

1 The Joint Commission. (2012). Standard MM.04.01.01. *Comprehensive accreditation manual for hospitals: The official handbook.* Oakbrook Terrace, IL: The Joint Commission. (Level I)
2 Centers for Disease Control and Prevention. (October 2002). Guideline for hand hygiene in health-care settings. *Morbidity and Mortality Weekly Report, 51*(RR-16), 1–45. (Level I)
3 The Joint Commission. (2012). Standard NPSG.07.01.01. *Comprehensive accreditation manual for hospitals: The official handbook.* Oakbrook Terrace, IL: The Joint Commission. (Level I)
4 World Health Organization. (2009). *WHO guidelines on hand hygiene in health care: First global patient safety challenge. Clean care is safer care.* Geneva, Switzerland: World Health Organization. (Level I)
5 Westbrook, J., et al. (2010). Association of interruptions with an increased risk and severity of medication administration errors. *Archives of Internal Medicine, 170*(8), 683–690.

6 The Joint Commission. (2012). Standard MM.06.01.01. *Comprehensive accreditation manual for hospitals: The official handbook.* Oakbrook Terrace, IL: The Joint Commission. (Level I)

7 The Joint Commission. (2012). Standard NPSG.01.01.01. *Comprehensive accreditation manual for hospitals: The official handbook.* Oakbrook Terrace, IL: The Joint Commission. (Level I)

8 Occupational Safety and Health Administration. "Bloodborne Pathogens, Standard Number 1910.1030" [Online]. Accessed November 2011 via the Web at http://www.osha.gov/pls/oshaweb/owadisp.show_document?p_table=STANDARDS&p_id=10051

9 Zaybak, A., et al. (2007). Does obesity prevent the needle from reaching muscle in intramuscular injections? *Journal of Advanced Nursing, 58*(6), 552–556.

10 The Joint Commission. (2012). Standard RC.01.03.01. *Comprehensive accreditation manual for hospitals: The official handbook.* Oakbrook Terrace, IL: The Joint Commission. (Level I)

11 The Joint Commission. (2012). Standard NPSG.03.04.01. *Comprehensive accreditation manual for hospitals: The official handbook.* Oakbrook Terrace, IL: The Joint Commission. (Level I)

ADDITIONAL REFERENCES

Carter-Templeton, H., & McCoy, T. (2008). Are we on the same page?: A comparison of intramuscular injection explanations in nursing fundamental texts. *MedSurg Nursing, 17*(4), 237–240.

Craven, R.F., & Hirnle, C.J. (2012). *Fundamentals of nursing: Human health and function* (7th ed.). Philadelphia, PA: Lippincott Williams & Wilkins.

Gittens, G., & Bunnell, T. (2009). Skin disinfection and its efficacy before administering injections. *Nursing Standard, 23*(39), 42–44.

Hughes, R., & Blegen, M. (2008). "Medication Administration Safety." In R. Hughes (Ed.), *Patient Safety and Quality: An Evidence-based Handbook for Nurses.* Rockville, MD: Agency for Healthcare Research and Quality [Online]. Accessed November 2011 via the Web at http://www.ahrq.gov/qual/nurseshdbk/docs/HughesR_MAS.pdf

Hunt, C.W. (2008). Which site is best for an IM injection? *Nursing, 38*(11), 62.

Hunter, J. (2008). Intramuscular injection techniques. *Nursing Standard, 22*(24), 35–40.

Lynn, P. (2011). *Taylor's clinical nursing skills* (3rd ed.). Philadelphia, PA: Lippincott Williams & Wilkins.

Malkin B. (2009). Are techniques used for intramuscular injection based on research evidence? *Nursing Times, 104*(50–51), 48–51.

Nettina, S.M. (2010). *Lippincott manual of nursing practice* (9th ed.). Philadelphia, PA: Lippincott Williams & Wilkins.

Occupational Safety and Health Administration. "Safety and Health Topics: Bloodborne Pathogens and Needlestick Prevention" [Online]. Accessed November 2011 via the Web at http://www.osha.gov/ SLTC/bloodbornepathogens

Petousis-Harris, H. (2008). Vaccine injection technique and reactogenicity—Evidence for practice. *Vaccine, 26*(50), 6299–6304.

Taylor, C., et al. (2011). *Fundamentals of nursing: The art and science of nursing care* (7th ed.). Philadelphia, PA: Lippincott Williams & Wilkins.

World Health Organization. "Guiding Principles to Ensure Injection Device Security" [Online]. Accessed November 2011 via the Web at http://www.who.int/injection_safety/WHOGuidPrinciplesInjEquipFinal.pdf

Zimmermann, P. (2010). Revisiting IM injections. *AJN, 110*(2), 60–61.

IMPAIRED SWALLOWING AND ASPIRATION PRECAUTIONS

Patients may experience impaired swallowing as a result of several specific problems. The first of these—oropharyngeal dysphagia—is impaired swallowing associated with deficits in oral and pharyngeal structure or function. Such patients are at especially high risk for aspiration, and many of them have silent aspiration. Patients at risk for oropharyngeal dysphagia include those with nervous system damage, such as that caused by stroke, head injury, or spinal cord injury; neuromuscular diseases, such as muscular dystrophy or cerebral palsy; progressive neurologic diseases, such as Parkinson's disease, multiple sclerosis, amyotrophic lateral sclerosis, or dementia; and head or neck cancer. Patients who have undergone facial, oral, or neck surgery; experienced neck trauma; or been intubated for longer than 3 days are also at risk.

The second type of impaired swallowing is associated with esophageal dysphagia and aspiration risk from gastroesophageal reflux disease, esophageal dysmotility or structural abnormality, delayed gastric emptying, or nasogastric tubes.

Finally, impaired swallowing can be associated with tracheostomy or ventilation support because of decreased sensation of the oral and pharyngeal cavities; decreased sensation of food or fluids penetrating the laryngeal vestibule and aspirating (dropping below the level of the vocal cords); decreased ability to cough aspirated material off the vocal cords; and decreased laryngeal elevation and airway closure.

Equipment

Meal tray ▪ call bell ▪ wall suction or portable suction apparatus ▪ suction kit ▪ gloves ▪ protective eyewear ▪ pulse oximeter.

Implementation

▪ Gather the appropriate equipment.
▪ Perform hand hygiene.[1,2,3]
▪ Confirm the patient's identity using at least two patient identifiers according to your facility's policy.[4]
▪ Explain the procedure to the patient and his family.
▪ Put on gloves and protective eyewear, if indicated, before suctioning the patient or providing oral care.
▪ Request a referral for and assist with a bedside swallow evaluation (usually conducted by a speech-language pathologist) as indicated.[5]

Managing impaired swallowing resulting from oropharyngeal dysphagia

▪ After completing the swallowing evaluation, develop a multidisciplinary management plan that includes common swallowing strategies, nutritional status, and supervision.[5]

Using common swallowing strategies
▪ Have suction equipment available at the bedside.
▪ Position the patient at a 90-degree angle during meals *to decrease the risk of aspiration.*

- Position the patient to sit up for 30 minutes after meals.
- Assist with or perform oral care before and after meals, and be sure to check for food residue.
- If applicable, ensure that dentures are in place, free from debris, and fit well.
- Crush medications, as appropriate, and mix in applesauce.
- Avoid mixed consistencies.
- Avoid straws.[6] Encourage small sips.
- If applicable, ensure that the temperature, consistency, and amount of foods and liquids are appropriate.[5] Water should be chilled; avoid tepid liquids or food.
- Minimize distractions when the patient is eating and drinking.
- Encourage slow intake with adequate chewing.
- If one side of the patient's face is paralyzed, place food on the unaffected side. Check the affected side of the mouth for food that may lodge in the cheek during and after meals. If appropriate, teach the patient to perform a finger sweep.
- If fatigue impairs swallowing, provide rest periods before and during meals as needed.
- Assess swallowing between bites by feeling the rise and fall of the larynx (Adam's apple).
- Use cold or sour foods and massage the cheeks or throat *to trigger swallowing.*
- Post swallowing precautions and feeding instructions in the patient's room.

Monitoring nutritional status
- Ask the dietitian to conduct a nutrition evaluation.
- Monitor the patient's hydration and nutrition.
- Implement calorie counts as ordered.
- Weigh the patient daily or as ordered.
- Consult with the patient and family regarding food and fluid preferences.
- Provide small, frequent meals and supplements.
- Praise the patient and family for achieving nutritional goals.

Using one-on-one supervision
- Ensure that someone remains with the patient throughout every meal.
- Provide feeding assistance or cueing for feeding and swallowing strategies during the entire meal, or ensure that a family member does so.[5]
- Encourage the patient to take 30 to 45 minutes to eat. *Patients with dysphagia typically need to eat slowly.*
- Monitor the patient for signs and symptoms of aspiration.

Using close supervision
- Check on the patient frequently during the meal; spend 3 to 5 minutes each time by re-cueing and reminding the patient to use swallowing strategies.[5]
- Monitor the patient for signs and symptoms of aspiration.
- Encourage the patient to increase intake, if needed, and provide other options *to maximize safety and nutritional intake.*
- Keep the call bell within reach.

Using distant supervision
- Provide initial cueing to initiate swallowing strategies.[5]
- Check on the patient by walking past his room frequently.
- Monitor the patient for signs and symptoms of aspiration.
- Assess the patient's progress at least two to three times during meals.
- Keep the call bell within reach.

Managing impaired swallowing resulting from esophageal dysphagia
- Monitor for reflux and aspiration risks related to esophageal dysphagia.
- Consult with a speech-language pathologist *to determine the need for alternative nutrition.*
- Monitor respiratory rate and depth; monitor breath sounds for crackles or wheezes, *which may indicate aspiration and airway obstruction.* Monitor for dyspnea and cyanosis.
- Monitor bowel sounds and assess for abdominal distention. *Absence of bowel sounds and increasing abdominal distention may indicate an ileus or bowel obstruction with resulting vomiting and risk for aspiration.*
- Monitor the patient's intake and output and daily weight. *Weight loss may indicate an esophageal problem.*
- Implement strategies for oral intake.
- Position the patient at a 90-degree angle during oral feeding, and maintain the patient in that position for 45 to 60 minutes after the meal *to decrease the risk for reflux, regurgitation, and aspiration.*
- If esophageal dysmotility exists, offer thickened liquids and pureed and moist foods that may be easier to swallow.[5]
- Feed the patient slowly; allow adequate time for esophageal emptying.
- If the patient feels full quickly, offer small, frequent meals of high-calorie foods.
- Alternate liquids and solids during feedings *to improve esophageal emptying of solids.*
- Avoid spicy and acidic foods, and decrease caffeine intake *to decrease reflux.*
- Tell the patient to avoid eating before bed, and keep the head of his bed elevated above a 30-degree angle at night.

Managing a patient with a feeding tube
- Initiate a dietary consult.
- Provide oral care for the patient who is on nothing-by-mouth status *to decrease colonization of bacteria in the mouth because he is at risk for secretion aspiration.*
- After feeding tube insertion, placement should be confirmed by X-ray. *X-ray confirmation of placement, especially of small-bore feeding tubes, is the gold standard for safe placement.*
- Trace the tubing from the patient to its point of origin before administering the feeding through the feeding tube *to make sure the feeding is administered through the proper port.*[7]
- Assess placement of the feeding tube before feeding and every 4 hours for a patient with a continuous feeding. Aspirate contents from the tube, note appearance and color (grassy-green, clear and colorless with mucus shreds, or brown), and determine

pH (less than or equal to 5). *Testing pH and noting aspirate characteristics are the most reliable means of determining tube placement.* Note that listening to stomach sounds as air is injected into the tube is no longer considered an accurate method for confirming placement.

■ If the assessment indicates the possibility of feeding solution in mucus coughed or suctioned from the trachea, test the mucus for glucose. A positive result may indicate tube displacement and aspiration of feeding solution.

■ Check gastric residuals every 4 hours during the first 48 hours of gastric feedings; after the enteral feeding goal rate is achieved, monitor residual every 6 to 8 hours in noncritically ill patients (every 4 hours in critically ill patients). Return residual to the stomach. Flush the feeding tube with 30 mL of water after measuring residual.

■ If residual volume is 250 mL or more, after a second residual check, a medication to improve gastric motility may be needed. Hold the feedings for residual greater than 500 mL (or according to your facility's policy) and assesses GI status.[8]

■ Maintain the patient in semi-Fowler's position (at least 30 degrees) during feedings and for 30 to 45 minutes after feeding *to promote movement of feeding solution through the stomach and into the small intestine, decreasing the risk of regurgitation and aspiration.*

Managing impaired swallowing resulting from tracheostomies or endotracheal tubes

■ Suction the patient as needed *to maintain a patent airway.*

■ Obtain a doctor's order for speaking valve trials as appropriate.

■ Follow speech therapy and doctor recommendations on cuff inflation versus deflation for oral intake. The patient may still be able to aspirate around an inflated cuff.

Managing impaired swallowing resulting from speaking valve trials

■ Have the speech-language pathologist assess the patient's tolerance for the speaking valve. *The speaking valve permits hands-free speech and can return oropharyngeal sensation and taste.*

■ Deflate the cuff before placing the valve. Monitor oxygen saturation at baseline, with the valve in place, and with valve removal.

■ Follow speaking valve recommendations for cleaning and wearing schedules.

■ Ensure the speaking valve is in place during meals (according to the speech-language pathologist's recommendations) *because it's usually safer to eat with the valve in place. The patient's ability to cough material off the vocal cords is increased.*

Completing the procedure

■ Perform hand hygiene.[1,2,3]

■ Document your actions.[9]

Special considerations

■ Monitor the patient for signs and symptoms of swallowing problems and aspiration. These include coughing before, during, or after eating; wet or "gurgling" voice; increased chest conges-

tion after eating; multiple swallows on one mouthful or washing down food with liquids; complaints of food getting "stuck" or painful swallowing; unexplained changes in the amount or rate of eating; drooling or spitting food out of the mouth; difficulty breathing during meals; weight loss and poor oral intake; recurrent pneumonias; low-grade temperatures shortly after meals; increased white blood cell counts; and leakage from the tracheostomy site.

■ Train and supervise the family to feed the patient as needed. Teach family members how to perform the abdominal thrust and how to use suction equipment as needed.

■ Angiotensin-converting enzyme inhibitors may improve the swallowing reflex in older patients with aspiration pneumonia.

Complications

Patients with impaired swallowing are more prone to airway obstruction and aspiration during meals. Aspiration may result in pneumonitis or pneumonia. Difficulty swallowing may result in decreased oral intake and eventually lead to dehydration and malnutrition.

Documentation

Record the amount of intake, the patient's food preference, his progress with meals, and any techniques effective in helping the swallowing process. Document the effectiveness of family teaching, complications that arose, and interventions taken to remedy the problem.

REFERENCES

1 The Joint Commission. (2012). Standard NPSG.07.01.01. *Comprehensive accreditation manual for hospitals: The official handbook.* Oakbrook Terrace, IL: The Joint Commission. (Level I)

2 Centers for Disease Control and Prevention. (October 2002). Guideline for hand hygiene in health-care settings. *Morbidity and Mortality Weekly Report, 51*(RR-16), 1–45. (Level I)

3 World Health Organization. (2009). *WHO guidelines on hand hygiene in health care: First global patient safety challenge. Clean care is safer care.* Geneva, Switzerland: World Health Organization. (Level I)

4 The Joint Commission. (2012). Standard NPSG.01.01.01. *Comprehensive accreditation manual for hospitals: The official handbook.* Oakbrook Terrace, IL: The Joint Commission. (Level I)

5 Smith Hammond, C.A., & Goldstein, L.B. (2006). Cough and aspiration of food and liquids due to oral-pharyngeal dysphagia: ACCP evidence-based clinical practice guidelines. *Chest, 129*(Suppl.1), 154S–168S.

6 Daniels, S.K., et al. (2004). Mechanism of sequential swallowing during straw drinking in healthy young and older adults. *Journal of Speech, Language, and Hearing Research, 47*(1), 33–45.

7 U.S. Food and Drug Administration. (2009). "Look. Check. Connect.: Safe Medical Device Connections Save Lives" [Online]. Accessed November 2011 via the Web at http://www.fda.gov/downloads/MedicalDevices/Safety/AlertsandNotices/UCM134873.pdf

8 Bankhead, R., et al. (2009). Enteral nutrition practice recommendations. *The American Society for Parenteral and Enteral Nutrition, 2*(33), 122–167.

9 The Joint Commission. (2012). Standard RC.01.03.01. *Comprehensive accreditation manual for hospitals: The official handbook.* Oakbrook Terrace, IL: The Joint Commission. (Level I)

ADDITIONAL REFERENCES

Eisenstadt, E. (2010). Dysphagia and aspiration pneumonia in older adults. *Journal of the American Academy of Nurse Practitioners, 22*(1), 17–22.

Serna, E.D., & McCarthy, M.S. (2006). Doing it better: Heads up to prevent aspiration during enteral feeding. *Nursing, 36*(1), 76–77.

Yoshikawa, M., et al. (2006). Influence of aging and denture use on liquid swallowing in healthy dentulous and edentulous older people. *Journal of the American Geriatrics Society, 54*(3), 444–449.

IMPLANTED PORT USE

Surgically implanted under local anesthesia by a surgeon or interventional radiologist, an implanted port, also known as a *vascular access device* or a *vascular access port,* is a type of central venous access device. It consists of a silicone or polyurethane catheter attached to a reservoir, which is covered with a self-sealing silicone septum. The catheter is placed in the central venous system with the reservoir typically implanted in a subcutaneous pocket in the upper anterior chest wall. Alternatively, the reservoir may be placed in the upper arm, abdomen, side, or back.

An implanted port is used most commonly when some type of long-term IV therapy is required and an external central venous device isn't appropriate or desirable. It can also be used to obtain blood samples for laboratory testing in these patients because they typically have limited vascular access. If the port isn't adequately flushed after blood withdrawal, a thrombotic catheter occlusion can occur.

NURSING ALERT *Limit blood sampling through the implanted port, when possible,* to reduce the risk for central line–associated bloodstream infections.

An implanted port also may be used to administer a bolus injection or a continuous infusion of IV fluids, if necessary. Bolus injection requires only the time it takes to push the plunger of the syringe. Note, however, that many drugs have minimum and maximum injection rates, which must be timed.

Depending on patient needs, the type of port selected may have one or two lumens. A port can be used immediately after placement, although some edema and tenderness may persist for about 72 hours, making the device initially difficult to palpate and slightly uncomfortable for the patient. (See *Understanding implanted ports.*)

Once implanted, the port is accessed using a noncoring needle when IV therapy, catheter flushing, or blood withdrawal is required. This type of needle has a deflected point, which slices the port's septum.

Only nurses who have been properly trained and validated may access and maintain implanted ports.[1]

Patients who require repeated computerized axial tomography scans with contrast may have a port implanted that has been specially developed to withstand the high pressures of power injectors. When using a power injector, a specialized access needle and tubing approved for power injection are required to ensure that the tubing and connections won't rupture or separate.

Equipment
Assisting with insertion
Noncoring needles (a noncoring needle has a deflected point, which slices the port's septum) of appropriate type and gauge ■ implanted port ■ sterile gloves and gown ■ mask ■ cap ■ antiseptic pads (alcohol, tincture of iodine, or chlorhexidine-based) ■ chlorhexidine sponges ■ extension tubing set, if needed ■ local anesthetic (lidocaine without epinephrine) ■ ice pack ■ syringes prefilled with heparin and preservative-free normal saline flush solutions ■ IV solution ■ sterile dressings ■ luer-lock injection cap ■ clamp ■ adhesive skin closures ■ suture removal set ■ insertion checklist.

Accessing a top-entry port
Noncoring needle of appropriate type and gauge and attached extension set tubing ■ gloves ■ sterile gloves ■ masks ■ sterile drape ■ 2% chlorhexidine applicator ■ 10-mL syringes prefilled with preservative-free normal saline solution ■ transparent semipermeable dressing ■ injection or access cap ■ catheter securement device, sterile tape, or sterile adhesive strips ■ Optional: antiseptic soap, water, local anesthetic, ice pack, syringe prefilled with heparin flush solution (100 units/mL), ordered IV fluid, IV administration set, clippers, 2″ × 2″ sterile gauze dressing.

Some facilities use an implantable port access kit.

Obtaining a blood sample
Gloves ■ appropriate antiseptic (alcohol, tincture of iodine, or chlorhexidine-based) ■ prefilled flush syringes of preservative-free normal saline solution ■ blood collection tubes ■ laboratory request forms and labels ■ laboratory biohazard transport bag ■ Optional: protective eyewear or face mask, sterile injection cap, syringe prefilled with heparin flush solution.

For Vacutainer method
Vacutainer with needleless adapter.

For syringe method
Blood transfer unit.

Administering a bolus injection
Patient's medication administration record ■ ordered medication in a syringe ■ 10-mL syringes filled with preservative-free normal saline solution ■ antiseptic pad (alcohol, tincture of iodine, or chlorhexidine-based) ■ heparin flush (100 units/mL) ■ Optional: port access equipment.

Administering a continuous infusion
Prescribed IV solution ■ IV administration set ■ gloves ■ antiseptic pads (alcohol, tincture of iodine, or chlorhexidine-based)

■ 10-mL syringe prefilled with preservative-free normal saline solution ■ Optional: infusion pump, filter.

Preparation of equipment

Assisting with insertion

Confirm the size and type of the device and the insertion site with the doctor. Attach the tubing to the solution container and prime the tubing with fluid. Prime the noncoring needle with the extension set. All priming must be done using strict sterile technique, and all tubing must be free of air.[2] After you've primed the tubing, recheck all connections for tightness. Make sure all open ends are covered with sealed caps.

Administering a bolus injection

Verify the order on the patient's medication record by checking it against the doctor's order.[3,4] Know the actions, adverse effects, and administration rate of the medication to be injected.[3]

Perform hand hygiene and put on gloves.[2,5,6,7] Avoid distractions and interruptions when preparing and administering medications *to prevent medication errors.*[8] Visually inspect the solution for particulates, discoloration, or other loss of integrity and check the expiration date. If the integrity is compromised or the medication is expired, obtain a replacement from the pharmacy.[4] If needed, draw up the prescribed medication in the syringe and dilute it, if necessary. Check the medication label three times while preparing it.[4] Many medications come in unit-dose syringes.

Administering a continuous infusion

Review the patient's medical record to determine the location of the implanted port and whether it's currently accessed with a noncoring needle. If needed, access the port using the appropriate noncoring needle.

Implementation

Assisting with insertion

■ Conduct a preprocedure verification *to make sure that all relevant documentation, related information, and equipment are available and correctly identified to the patient's identifiers.*[9]
■ Check the patient's history for hypersensitivity to local anesthetics or chlorhexidine.
■ Although the doctor is responsible for obtaining consent for the procedure, make sure the written document is signed, witnessed, and in the patient's medical record.[10,11]
■ Use an insertion checklist to adhere to infection prevention and safety practices during insertion. Stop the procedure immediately if you observe any breaks in sterile technique.
■ Perform hand hygiene *to prevent spreading microorganisms.*[5,6,7,8,12]
■ Confirm the patient's identity using at least two patient identifiers according to your facility's policy.[13]
■ Reinforce to the patient the doctor's explanation of the procedure, its benefit and risks, and what's expected of the patient during and after implantation.
■ Allay the patient's fears and answer questions about movement restrictions, cosmetic concerns, and management regimens.
■ Put on the mask, cap, sterile gloves, and gown.[2]

Understanding implanted ports

Typically, an implanted port is used to deliver intermittent infusions of medication, parenteral nutrition, chemotherapy, and blood products.[17] Because the device is completely covered by the patient's skin, the risk of extrinsic contamination is reduced. Patients may prefer this type of central line because it doesn't alter the body image and requires less routine catheter care. The implanted port consists of a catheter connected to a small reservoir. A septum designed to withstand multiple punctures seals the reservoir. To access the port, a special noncoring needle is inserted perpendicular to the reservoir.

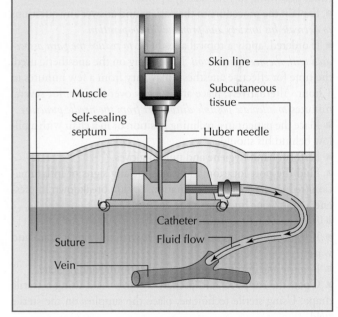

■ Conduct a time-out immediately before starting the procedure to determine that the correct patient, site, positioning, and procedure are identified, and confirm, as applicable, that relevant information and necessary equipment are available.[14] The doctor will surgically implant the port, most likely using a local anesthetic. Occasionally, however, a patient may receive a general anesthetic.
■ The insertion site is prepared using a chlorhexidine-based antiseptic and allowed to dry.
■ During the procedure, you may be responsible for handing equipment and supplies to the doctor.
■ After draping the patient from head to toe to comply with maximal barrier precautions,[2] the doctor makes a small incision and introduces the catheter, typically into the superior vena cava through the subclavian, jugular, or cephalic vein. After fluoroscopy verifies correct placement of the catheter tip, the doctor creates a subcutaneous pocket over a bony prominence in the chest wall. Then he tunnels the catheter to the pocket. Next, he connects

the catheter to the reservoir, places the reservoir in the pocket, and flushes it with heparin solution. Lastly, he sutures the reservoir to the underlying fascia and closes the incision.

■ Apply a sterile occlusive dressing.

■ Dispose of used equipment and discard of waste in the appropriate receptacle.

■ Remove and discard your personal protective equipment and perform hand hygiene.[5,6,,7,12]

■ Document the procedure.[15,16]

Accessing a top-entry port

■ Verify the doctor's order for obtaining access.

■ Check the patient's record for allergies.

■ Gather the necessary supplies.

■ Perform hand hygiene.[5,6,7,12]

■ Confirm the patient's identity using at least two patient identifiers according to your facility's policy.[13]

■ Explain the procedure to the patient and answer any questions *to decrease his anxiety and promote his cooperation.*

■ If ordered, apply a topical anesthetic *to reduce the pain associated with the needle insertion.* Depending on the anesthetic used, the time for effective anesthesia may vary from a few minutes to 1 hour. Alternatively, place an ice pack over the area for several minutes *to alleviate possible discomfort from the needle puncture.*

■ Place the patient in a reclining position or in a chair with a pillow behind his shoulder.

■ Perform hand hygiene and put on gloves.[5,6,7,12]

■ Find the port location and assess for any signs of inflammation (redness, swelling, or induration) or skin breakdown. If present, report your findings to the doctor.

■ If excessive hair is present, clip it.[18]

■ If the site is visibly soiled, wash it with antiseptic soap and water.

■ Remove and discard your gloves and perform hand hygiene.[5,6,7,12]

■ Open the supplies, and prepare a sterile field using a sterile drape. Using sterile technique, place the supplies on the sterile field.

■ Put on a mask (according to your facility's policy) and sterile gloves and wear them throughout the procedure.[1]

■ Prepare the noncoring needle by attaching a 10-mL syringe of sterile preservative-free normal saline solution and priming the extension set and needle.

■ Clean the area with the 2% chlorhexidine applicator, using a back-and-forth scrubbing motion, and allow the area to dry.[2,18]

■ Remove and discard your gloves and perform hand hygiene.[5,6,7,12] Put on a new pair of sterile gloves.

■ Palpate the area over the port *to find the port septum.*

■ Anchor the port with your nondominant hand. Then, using your dominant hand, aim the needle at the center of the device.

■ Insert the needle perpendicularly to the port septum. Push the needle through the skin and septum until you reach the bottom of the reservoir.

■ Check needle placement by aspirating for blood return.[1]

■ If you can't obtain blood, remove the needle and repeat the procedure. Ask the patient to raise his arms and perform Valsalva's maneuver. If you still don't get blood return, notify the

doctor; *a fibrin sleeve on the distal end of the catheter may be occluding the opening.* (See *Managing implanted port problems.*)

■ Flush the device with preservative-free normal saline solution. If you detect swelling or if the patient reports pain at the site, remove the needle and notify the doctor.

■ Secure the needle using a catheter securement device, sterile tape, or sterile adhesive strips. If necessary, place a folded 2″ × 2″ sterile gauze pad underneath the wings of the access needle without obscuring the insertion site *to prevent the needle from rocking within the septum.*

■ Cover the site with a transparent semipermeable dressing or gauze dressing.

■ Attach the end of the extension tubing to an IV infusion. If a continuous infusion isn't ordered, instill 3 mL of heparin (100 units/mL) *to heparin-lock the device.*[19] You may also attach an injection or access cap to the tubing if no infusion is being administered at this time.

■ Dispose of equipment and waste in an appropriate receptacle.[20,21]

■ Remove and discard your gloves and mask and perform hand hygiene.[5,6,7,12]

■ Document the procedure.[15,16]

Obtaining a blood sample

■ Verify the doctor's order for blood sampling.

■ Perform hand hygiene.[5,6,7,12]

■ Confirm the patient's identity using at least two patient identifiers according to your facility's policy.[13]

■ Explain the procedure to the patient *to allay the patient's anxiety and promote cooperation.*

■ Place the patient in a supine position with his head slightly elevated.

■ Label the discard blood collection tube *to prevent confusing it with the actual specimen.* If not already clearly marked, label the preservative-free normal saline flush syringe.[22]

■ Perform hand hygiene and put on gloves and protective eyewear or a face mask if splashing is likely.[5,6,7,12]

■ Locate the noncoring needle extension tubing.[1]

■ Stop any infusions that are infusing through the port *to prevent inaccurate blood test results.*[23]

■ Assess the skin overlying the port, the tissue surrounding the port, and the site of needle entry. Observe for signs of infection, thrombosis, device rotation, and skin erosion. Hold the procedure and call the doctor if you observe any complications.[2,24]

■ Close the clamp on the extension tubing and thoroughly disinfect the injection cap or access hub with an alcohol pad (or other appropriate disinfectant) using friction. Allow it to dry.[2,25,26]

■ Attach a prefilled syringe containing preservative-free normal saline solution and open the clamp. Aspirate for blood return and then instill the normal saline solution *to check the patency of the catheter.*[23] The minimum volume of normal saline solution instilled should be twice the internal volume of the catheter system. Reclamp the tubing and remove the syringe.[27]

■ Thoroughly disinfect the injection cap or access hub with an alcohol pad (or other appropriate disinfectant) using friction. Allow it to dry.[2,25]

TROUBLESHOOTING

Managing implanted port problems

This chart outlines common problems with implanted ports along with possible causes and nursing interventions.

PROBLEMS AND POSSIBLE CAUSES	NURSING INTERVENTIONS
INABILITY TO FLUSH THE DEVICE OR DRAW BLOOD	
Catheter lodged against the vessel wall	Reposition the patient.
	Teach the patient to change his position to free the catheter from the vessel wall.
	Raise the arm that's on the same side as the catheter.
	Roll the patient to his opposite side.
	Have the patient cough, sit up, or take a deep breath.
	Infuse 10 mL of preservative-free normal saline solution into the catheter.
	Regain access to the implanted port using a new needle.
Clot formation	Assess patency by trying to flush the port while the patient changes position.
	Notify the doctor; obtain an order for fibrinolytic agent instillation.
	Teach the patient to recognize clot formation, notify the doctor if it occurs, and avoid forcibly flushing the implanted port.
Incorrect needle placement or needle not advanced through septum	Regain access to the device.
	Teach the home care patient to push down firmly on the noncoring needle device in the septum and verify needle placement by aspirating for blood return.
Kinked catheter, catheter migration, or port rotation	Notify the doctor immediately.
	Tell the home care patient to notify the doctor if he has trouble using the implanted port.
Kinked tubing or closed clamp	Check the tubing or clamp.
INABILITY TO PALPATE THE DEVICE	
Deeply implanted port	Note the portal chamber scar.
	Use a deep palpation technique.
	Ask another nurse to try locating the port.
	Use a 1½″ or 2″ noncoring needle to access the implanted port.

Vacutainer method
■ Attach the needleless connector to the injection cap or the access hub, release the clamp, and engage the labeled discard blood collection tube *to aspirate the discard volume to clear the catheter's dead space volume and remove blood diluted by flush solution.* Limit the discard amount to 1.5 to 2 times the fill volume of the catheter.[25]
■ Clamp the extension tubing and remove the labeled discard blood collection tube from the Vacutainer.
■ Insert another blood collection tube, unclamp the catheter, and obtain a sample. Repeat as necessary until you've obtained all blood samples. Draw only the volume of blood needed for accurate testing *to prevent complications associated with blood loss.*[23]
■ Clamp the extension tubing and remove the Vacutainer and needleless connector from the injection cap or access hub.

■ Thoroughly disinfect the injection cap or access hub with an appropriate disinfectant using friction. Allow it to dry.[2,25,26] Connect a syringe containing preservative-free normal saline solution.
■ Open the clamp and flush the catheter system with preservative-free normal saline solution. Close the clamp.
■ Repeat the flushing procedure with a heparin flush solution according to your facility's policy, if the patient doesn't have a continuous infusion prescribed.[26,27,28]
■ Apply a new injection cap using strict sterile technique.[26]

Syringe method
■ Connect an empty labeled discard syringe to the catheter, release the clamp, and aspirate the discard volume. Limit the discard volume to 1.5 to 2 times the full volume of the catheter.

- Clamp the catheter and remove the labeled discard blood syringe and dispose of it appropriately.
- Thoroughly disinfect the injection cap with an antiseptic using friction. Allow it to dry.
- Connect an empty syringe to the catheter, release the clamp, and slowly withdraw the blood sample. If necessary, obtain multiple syringes of samples; draw only the volume of blood needed for accurate testing *to prevent complications associated with blood loss.*[23]
- Clamp the extension tubing and remove the syringe.
- Thoroughly disinfect the injection cap or access hub with an appropriate disinfectant using friction. Allow it to dry.[2,25,26]
- Connect the syringe containing preservative-free normal saline solution.
- Open the clamp and flush the catheter system with the normal saline solution. Close the clamp.
- Repeat the flushing procedure with a heparin flush solution according to your facility's policy, if the patient doesn't have a continuous infusion prescribed.[25,28]
- If needed, apply a new injection cap using strict sterile technique.[26]
- Use the blood transfer unit to transfer the blood into the appropriate blood collection tube.

Completing the procedure
- Label the samples in the presence of the patient *to prevent mislabeling.*[23]
- Place all blood collection tubes in a laboratory biohazard transport bag and send them to the laboratory with a completed laboratory request form.[21]
- Dispose of the equipment in the appropriate receptacle.[20,21]
- Remove and discard your gloves and protective eyewear and perform hand hygiene.[5,6,7,12]
- Document the procedure.[15,16]

Administering a bolus injection
- Review the patient's medical record to determine the location of the implanted port, whether it's currently accessed with a noncoring needle, and the patient's response to previous procedures.
- Ensure that a chest X-ray was obtained to confirm the placement of the catheter tip.
- Determine whether the patient has a history of allergies or other contraindications to the medication. Don't give the medication and notify the doctor if contraindications exist.[3]
- Review the patient's baseline vital signs and observe for changes that may indicate a local or systemic infection.
- Perform hand hygiene.[5,6,7,12]
- Confirm the patient's identity using at least two patient identifiers according to your facility's policy.[3,13]
- Verify the medication order, confirming that you have the right patient, medication, route, dose, and time of administration.[4]
- If your facility uses a bar code scanning system, be sure to scan your identification badge, the patient's identification bracelet, and the medication's bar code, or follow the procedure for your facility's bar code system.

- Discuss with the patient the medication to be administered, including potential adverse effects, and answer his questions.[3]
- Perform hand hygiene and put on gloves.[5,6,7,12]
- Thoroughly disinfect the injection port of the access tubing with an antiseptic pad using friction and allow it to dry.
- Connect a syringe filled with preservative-free saline solution to the access port.[27]
- Release the clamp and aspirate slowly to verify blood return.[27]
- Flush the tubing with preservative-free normal saline solution to clear the blood from the catheter.[25,27]
- Examine the skin surrounding the needle for signs of infiltration, such as swelling and tenderness. If you note these signs, stop the injection and intervene appropriately.

NURSING ALERT *Don't force the flush solution into the tubing.* If there is resistance, the catheter may be occluded.

- Remove and discard the saline syringe.
- Thoroughly disinfect the injection port with an antiseptic pad again using friction and allow the port to dry.[29]
- Attach the syringe with the medication for the IV bolus injection into the injection port of the tubing.
- Inject the medication at the required rate. Then remove the syringe from the injection port.
- Thoroughly disinfect the injection port with an antiseptic pad using friction and allow it to dry.
- Attach a second syringe filled with preservative-free saline solution and flush the tubing. (Remember to flush with preservative-free normal saline solution between infusions of incompatible drugs or fluids.) Remove the syringe.[25,27]
- Thoroughly disinfect the injection port with an antiseptic pad using friction and allow it to dry.
- Attach the syringe containing heparin flush solution and inject the heparin flush solution[25] according to your facility's policy. *Locking the device with heparin flush prevents clotting in the device.*[25,27]
- Close the clamp on the access tubing according to the type of needleless connector *to reduce blood reflux.*[25]

Administering a continuous infusion
- Make sure that a chest X-ray to confirm the placement of the catheter tip has been obtained.
- Verify the doctor's order for the type of infusion to be administered.
- Review the patient's baseline vital signs and observe for changes that may indicate a local or systemic infection.
- Compare the IV fluid label to the order in the patient's medical record.
- Visually inspect the IV solution for particulates, discoloration, or other loss of integrity, and check the expiration date. Replace the solution if the integrity is compromised or it's expired.
- Determine whether the patient has a history of allergies.
- Gather the necessary equipment.
- Perform hand hygiene.[5,6,7,12]
- Confirm the patient's identity using at least two patient identifiers according to your facility's policy.[13]
- Explain the procedure to the patient.

- Locate the noncoring needle extension tubing under the patient's gown.
- Assess the skin overlying the port, the tissue surrounding the port, and the site of needle entry. Observe for signs of infection, thrombosis, device rotation, and skin erosion. Hold the procedure and notify the doctor if any complications are observed.
- If your facility uses a bar code scanning system, scan your identification badge, the parent's identification band, and the solution's bar code according to your facility's policy.
- Put on gloves.
- Attach an infusion set and tubing to the bag of prescribed IV fluid.
- Prime the tubing of the IV infusion set so that no air remains in the tubing.
- If using an infusion pump, prime the appropriate tubing, and set the correct infusion parameters according to the doctor's orders and the manufacturer's instructions.
- Thoroughly disinfect the needleless injection or access cap on the extension tubing with an antiseptic pad using friction and allow it to dry.[2,29]
- Attach the syringe filled with sterile preservative-free normal saline solution to the injection cap.
- Release the clamp on the extension tubing.
- Pull back on the plunger of the syringe *to check for blood return.*[3]
- If you're unable to aspirate blood return to confirm needle placement, have the patient change positions, raise his arms over his head, take a deep breath and hold it, or cough *to increase intrathoracic pressure and increase yield for blood return.*[25] If you're still unable to obtain blood return and confirm noncoring needle placement, troubleshoot according to facility policy.

NURSING ALERT *If no blood return is obtained and needle placement is correct, don't proceed with fluid administration. Clamp the tubing and notify the doctor immediately* to ensure prompt intervention.

- Flush the port with the preservative-free normal saline solution.
- Clamp the extension set and remove the saline solution syringe.
- Thoroughly disinfect the needleless injection cap on the extension tubing with an antiseptic pad using friction and allow it to dry.[2,29]
- Connect and secure the prescribed IV fluid by connecting the infusion set tubing directly to the needleless injection cap of the extension tubing. Trace the tubing from the patient to its point of origin to make sure it's connected to the proper port.[3,30]
- Open the clamp and begin the infusion as prescribed.
- Examine the skin surrounding the needle for signs of extravasation or infiltration, such as swelling and tenderness. If you note these signs or if the patient complains of stinging, burning, or pain at the site, stop the infusion and intervene appropriately.
- Label the solution container with the date and time it was started and your initials.
- Label the IV tubing with the date and time of its first use and your initials. *Doing so helps identify proper change times.*

Completing the procedure

- Dispose of the used equipment and waste in the appropriate receptacle.[20,21]
- Remove and discard your gloves and perform hand hygiene.[5,6,7,12]
- Document the procedure.[15,16]

Special considerations

- After implantation, monitor the site for signs of hematoma and bleeding. Edema and tenderness may persist for about 72 hours. The incision site requires routine postoperative care for 7 to 10 days. You'll also need to assess the implantation site for signs of infection, device rotation, and skin erosion. You don't need to apply a dressing to the wound site except during infusions or to maintain an intermittent infusion device.
- Always use the smallest noncoring size needle necessary to accommodate the infusion *to prolong the life of the port and lessen the amount of pain experienced by the patient.*[1]
- Change the transparent semipermeable dressing at least every 7 days; change it sooner if its integrity is compromised.[1]
- As long as the gauze used to support the wings of the needle doesn't obscure or cover the catheter insertion site, it isn't considered a gauze dressing and doesn't require routine changing.[31]
- Alternative pain management strategies, such as distraction or relaxation techniques, may be helpful.
- Assess the implantation site for signs of infection, device rotation, and skin erosion.[31]
- Change the tubing and solution as you would for a long-term central venous infusion.
- If clotting threatens to occlude the implanted port, the doctor may order a fibrinolytic agent *to clear the catheter. Because such agents increase the risk of bleeding,* this intervention may be contraindicated in patients who have had surgery within the past 10 days, those who have active internal bleeding such as GI bleeding, and those who have experienced central nervous system damage, such as infarction, hemorrhage, traumatic injury, surgery, or primary or metastatic disease, within the past 2 months.
- Besides performing routine care measures, you must be prepared to handle several common problems that may arise during an infusion with an implanted port. Such problems include an inability to flush the port, withdraw blood from it, or palpate it.
- When obtaining a blood sample, use the minimal amount of discard blood *to help prevent anemia.*
- Try to consolidate all daily tests into one sampling *to reduce the risk for central line–associated bloodstream infections.*
- *Because there are different types of injection and access caps or needleless connectors,* always follow the manufacturer's guidelines for flush technique and when to clamp.[26]
- *If you're having difficulty aspirating blood, the catheter tip may be poorly positioned.* Ask the patient to cough, reposition him, turn his head, raise his arms above his head, or have him take a deep breath and hold it.
- If using a heparin flush, be aware of any effects it may have on specimens and flush the catheter before drawing a discard sample, if necessary.

■ When preparing to administer a bolus injection, always check drug compatibilities *because a drug may be incompatible with normal saline or heparin.*

■ Assess the implantation site for signs of infection, device rotation, and skin erosion.

■ While the patient is hospitalized, a needleless injection or access cap may be attached to the end of the extension set to provide ready access for intermittent infusions. *A cap reduces the discomfort of accessing the port and prolongs the life of the port septum by decreasing the number of needle punctures.*

■ With a continuous infusion, when the solution container is almost empty, obtain a new IV solution container, as ordered, and prepare it for administration.

■ Change the transparent dressing and needle every 7 days with a continuous infusion. Gauze dressings should be changed every 48 hours. However, any dressing should be changed immediately if its integrity is compromised. If gauze is used to support the wings of an access needle and if doesn't obscure the insertion site under the transparent semipermeable dressing, it can be changed every 7 days.[1]

■ Change the continuous infusion tubing no more frequently than every 96 hours; however, change it immediately upon suspected contamination or when the integrity of the product or system has been compromised.

Patient teaching

If your patient is going home, he'll need thorough teaching about procedures as well as follow-up visits from a home care nurse *to ensure safety and successful treatment.*[1] Tell the patient the type of port that he has in place and explain the importance of carrying a port identification card. If he'll be accessing the port himself, explain that the most uncomfortable part of the procedure is the actual insertion of the needle into the skin.

When the needle has penetrated the skin, the patient will feel mostly pressure. Eventually, the skin over the port will become desensitized from frequent needle punctures. Until then, the patient may want to use a topical anesthetic.

Stress the importance of pushing the needle into the port until the patient feels the needle bevel touch the back of the port. *Many patients tend to stop short of the back of the port, leaving the needle bevel in the rubber septum.*

Also stress the importance of monthly flushes when no more infusions are scheduled. If possible, instruct a family member in all aspects of care.[1]

If the patient is receiving an infusion at home, teach the patient and family member about checking the dressing daily. Also instruct the patient how to dress and undress to avoid pulling at the needle site; how to protect the site during bathing; immediately reporting pain, burning, stinging, or soreness at the site; and stopping the infusion and reporting wetness, leaking, or swelling at the site.[1]

Complications

A patient who has an implanted port faces risks similar to those associated with central venous access devices. (See *Risks of implanted port therapy.*)

Documentation

Document the site of the implanted port and the date and time of insertion. Document assessment findings, including the location and appearance of the site. When accessing the port, record the needle gauge and length used, appearance of any blood return and any unexpected outcomes, and your interventions. If an infusion is initiated, include the type, amount, and rate of the infusion.[31] When obtaining a blood sample, document the time and type of sample drawn, the volume of blood withdrawn, the amount and types of flushes used, the patency of the catheter, and the patient's tolerance of the procedure. When administering a bolus injection, document the drug, route, dose, time, and rate of administration; the type and amount of flush solution used; the presence of blood return; and the condition of the site. When administering a continuous infusion, include the type, amount, rate, and duration of the infusion; the appearance of the site; and any adverse reactions. Record the date and time you notified the doctor as well as the doctor's name and any orders received from him. Note the type and amount of flush solution used, the presence or absence of blood return, any resistance to flushing, and, if resistance was encountered, what interventions were implemented.

Also keep a record of all needle and dressing changes for continuous infusions; blood samples obtained, including the type and amount; and patient-teaching topics covered. Finally, document the removal of the infusion needle, status of the site, use of heparin flush, and any problems you found and resolved.[15,16]

REFERENCES

1 Standard 39. Implanted vascular access ports. Infusion nursing standards of practice. (2011). *Journal of Infusion Nursing, 34*(1S), S50–51. (Level I)

2 O'Grady, N.P., et al. (2011). "Guidelines for the Prevention of Intravascular Catheter-Related Infections" [Online]. Accessed November 2011 via the Web at http://www.cdc.gov/hicpac/pdf/guidelines/bsi-guidelines-2011.pdf (Level I)

3 Standard 61. Parenteral medication and solution administration. Infusion nursing standards of practice. (2011). *Journal of Infusion Nursing, 34*(1S), S86. (Level I)

4 The Joint Commission. (2012). Standard MM.06.01.01. *Comprehensive accreditation manual for hospitals: The official handbook.* Oakbrook Terrace, IL: The Joint Commission. (Level I)

5 The Joint Commission. (2012). Standard NPSG.07.01.01. *Comprehensive accreditation manual for hospitals: The official handbook.* Oakbrook Terrace, IL: The Joint Commission. (Level I)

6 Standard 19. Hand hygiene. Infusion nursing standards of practice. (2011). *Journal of Infusion Nursing, 34*(1S), S26–27. (Level I)

7 Centers for Disease Control and Prevention. (October 2002). Guideline for hand hygiene in health-care settings. *Morbidity and Mortality Weekly Report, 51*(RR-16), 1–45. (Level I)

8 Westbrook, J. et al. (2010). Association of interruptions with an increased risk and severity of medication administration errors. *Archives of Internal Medicine, 170*(8), 683–690. (Level VII)

9 The Joint Commission. (2012). Standard UP.01.01.01. *Comprehensive accreditation manual for hospitals: The official handbook.* Oakbrook Terrace, IL: The Joint Commission. (Level I)

10 Standard 12. Informed consent. Infusion nursing standards of practice. (2011). *Journal of Infusion Nursing, 34*(1S), S17. (Level I)

Risks of implanted port therapy

This chart shows possible complications of implanted port therapy and outlines signs and symptoms, possible causes, and nursing interventions.

COMPLICATION	SIGNS AND SYMPTOMS	POSSIBLE CAUSES	NURSING INTERVENTIONS
Extravasation	■ Burning sensation or swelling in subcutaneous tissue	■ Needle dislodged into subcutaneous tissue ■ Needle incorrectly placed in the port ■ Needle position not confirmed; needle pulled out of the septum ■ Rupture of the catheter along the tunnel route	■ Stop the infusion; remove the administration set but don't remove the needle. Aspirate fluid from the catheter using a small syringe and then remove the needle.[18] Assess the extent of extravasation using a standardized tool.[18] ■ Notify the doctor; prepare to administer an antidote, if ordered. ***Prevention*** ■ Teach the patient how to gain access to the device, verify its placement, and secure the needle before initiating an infusion.
Fibrin sheath formation	■ Blocked port and catheter lumen ■ Inability to flush the port or administer the infusion ■ Possible swelling, tenderness, and erythema in the neck, chest, and shoulder	■ Adherence of platelets to the catheter	■ Notify the doctor; prepare to administer a thrombolytic agent. ***Prevention*** ■ Use the port only to infuse fluids and medications; don't use it to obtain blood samples. ■ Administer only compatible substances through the port.
Site infection or skin breakdown	■ Erythema and warmth at the port site ■ Oozing or purulent drainage at the port site or pocket ■ Fever	■ Infected incision or pocket ■ Poor postoperative healing	■ Assess the site daily for redness; note drainage. ■ Notify the doctor. ■ Administer antibiotics, as prescribed. ■ Apply warm soaks for 20 minutes four times per day. ***Prevention*** ■ Teach the patient to inspect for and report redness, swelling, drainage, or skin breakdown at the port site.
Thrombosis	■ Inability to flush the port or administer the infusion	■ Frequent blood sampling ■ Infusion of packed red blood cells (RBCs)	■ Notify the doctor; obtain an order to administer a fibrinolytic agent. ***Prevention*** ■ Flush the implanted port thoroughly right after obtaining a blood sample. ■ Administer packed RBCs as a piggyback with normal saline solution and use an infusion pump; flush with normal saline solution between units.

(continued)

Risks of implanted port therapy *(continued)*

COMPLICATION	SIGNS AND SYMPTOMS	POSSIBLE CAUSES	NURSING INTERVENTIONS
Air embolism	■ Sudden onset of dyspnea ■ Breathlessness ■ Weak pulse; tachyarrhythmia ■ Increased central venous pressure ■ Loss of consciousness; altered mental status ■ Chest pain ■ Jugular venous distention ■ Wheezing, coughing ■ Numbness, paralysis ■ Altered speech	■ Entrance of air into the central line	■ Place patient in the left lateral decubitus position.[32] ■ Notify the doctor.

11 The Joint Commission. (2012). Standard RI.01.03.01. *Comprehensive accreditation manual for hospitals: The official handbook*. Oakbrook Terrace, IL: The Joint Commission. (Level I)

12 World Health Organization. (2009). *WHO guidelines on hand hygiene in health care: First global patient safety challenge. Clean care is safer care*. Geneva, Switzerland: World Health Organization. (Level I)

13 The Joint Commission. (2012). Standard NPSG.01.01.01. *Comprehensive accreditation manual for hospitals: The official handbook*. Oakbrook Terrace, IL: The Joint Commission. (Level I)

14 The Joint Commission. (2012). Standard UP.01.03.01. *Comprehensive accreditation manual for hospitals: The official handbook*. Oakbrook Terrace, IL: The Joint Commission. (Level I)

15 The Joint Commission. (2012). Standard RC.01.03.01. *Comprehensive accreditation manual for hospitals: The official handbook*. Oakbrook Terrace, IL: The Joint Commission. (Level I)

16 The Joint Commission. (2012). Standard RC.02.01.01. *Comprehensive accreditation manual for hospitals: The official handbook*. Oakbrook Terrace, IL: The Joint Commission. (Level I)

17 Standard 14. Documentation. Infusion nursing standards of practice. (2011). *Journal of Infusion Nursing, 34*(1S), S20–21. (Level I)

18 Standard 35. Vascular access site preparation and device placement. Infusion nursing standards of practice. (2011). *Journal of Infusion Nursing, 34*(1S), S44. (Level I)

19 Infusion Nurses Society. (2008). *Flushing protocols*. Boston, MA: Infusion Nurses Society.

20 Standard 22. Safe handling and disposal of sharps, hazardous material, and hazardous waste: Infusion nursing standards of practice. (2011). *Journal of Infusion Nursing, 34*(1S), S28. (Level I)

21 Occupational Safety and Health Administration. "Bloodborne Pathogens, Standard Number 1910.1030" [Online]. Accessed November 2011 via the Web at http://www.osha.gov/pls/oshaweb/owadisp.show_document?p_table=STANDARDS&p_id=10051 (Level I)

22 The Joint Commission. (2012). Standard NPSG.03.04.01. *Comprehensive accreditation manual for hospitals: The official handbook*. Oakbrook Terrace, IL: The Joint Commission. (Level I)

23 Standard 57. Phlebotomy. Infusion nursing standards of practice. (2011). *Journal of Infusion Nursing, 34*(1S), S77–80. (Level I)

24 Standard 18. Infection prevention. Infusion nursing standards of practice. (2011). *Journal of Infusion Nursing, 34*(1S), S25–26. (Level I)

25 Alexander, M., et al. (Eds.). (2010). *Infusion nursing: An evidence-based approach* (3rd ed.). Philadelphia, PA: Elsevier.

26 Standard 26. Add-on devices. Infusion nursing standards of practice. (2011). *Journal of Infusion Nursing, 34*(1S), S31. (Level I)

27 Standard 45. Flushing and locking. Infusion nursing standards of practice. (2011). *Journal of Infusion Nursing, 34*(1S), S59–63. (Level I)

28 Perry, A.G., et al. (2010). *Clinical nursing skills & techniques* (7th ed.). St. Louis, MO: Mosby Elsevier. (Level VII)

29 Standard 27. Needleless connectors. Infusion nursing standards of practice. (2011). *Journal of Infusion Nursing, 34*(1S), S32–33. (Level I)

30 U.S. Food and Drug Administration. (2009). "Look. Check. Connect.: Safe Medical Device Connections Save Lives" [Online]. Accessed November 2011 via the Web at http://www.fda.gov/downloads/MedicalDevices/Safety/AlertsandNotices/UCM134873.pdf (Level I)

31 Standard 46. Vascular access device site care and dressing changes. Infusion nursing standards of practice. (2011). *Journal of Infusion Nursing, 34*(1S), S63–64. (Level I)

32 Standard 50. Air embolism. Infusion nursing standards of practice. (2011). *Journal of Infusion Nursing, 34*(1S), S69–70. (Level I)

INCENTIVE SPIROMETRY

Incentive spirometry involves using a device to help the patient achieve maximal ventilation by providing feedback on respiratory effort. The device measures respiratory flow or respiratory volume and induces the patient to take a deep breath and hold it for several seconds. This deep breath increases lung volume, boosts alveolar inflation, and promotes venous return. Incentive spirometry is designed to replicate the natural mechanisms of sighing or yawning, thus preventing and reversing the alveolar collapse that causes atelectasis and pneumonitis. It's suggested that the patient do 5 to 10 breaths per session every hour while awake (approximately 100 breaths per day).[1]

Devices used for incentive spirometry provide a visual incentive to breathe deeply. Some are activated when the patient inhales a certain volume of air; the device then estimates the amount of air inhaled. Others contain plastic floats, which rise according to the amount of air the patient pulls through the device when he inhales.

Patients at low risk for developing atelectasis may use a flow incentive spirometer. Patients at high risk may need a volume incentive spirometer, which measures lung inflation more precisely.

Incentive spirometry benefits the patient on prolonged bed rest, especially the postoperative patient who may regain his normal respiratory pattern slowly due to such predisposing factors as abdominal or thoracic surgery, advanced age, inactivity, obesity, smoking, or decreased ability to cough effectively and expel lung secretions.

Equipment

Flow or volume incentive spirometer, as indicated, with sterile disposable tube and mouthpiece (the tube and mouthpiece are sterile on first use and clean on subsequent uses) ▪ stethoscope ▪ gloves ▪ watch ▪ pencil and paper ▪ hospital-grade disinfectant ▪ Optional: pillow.

Preparation of equipment

Gather the ordered equipment at the patient's bedside. Read the manufacturer's instructions for spirometer setup and operation. Remove the sterile flow tube and mouthpiece from the package, and attach them to the device. Set the flow rate or volume goal as determined by the doctor or respiratory therapist and based on the patient's preoperative performance. Turn on the machine if applicable.

Implementation

▪ Perform hand hygiene.[1,2,3,4,5]
▪ Confirm the patient's identity using at least two patient identifiers according to your facility's policy.[6]
▪ Assess the patient's condition.
▪ Explain the procedure to the patient, making sure he understands the importance of performing this exercise regularly *to maintain alveolar inflation.*
▪ Help the patient into a comfortable sitting or semi-Fowler's position *to promote optimal lung expansion.* If you're using a flow incentive spirometer and the patient is unable to assume or maintain this position, he can perform the procedure in any position as long as the device remains upright. *Tilting a flow incentive spirometer decreases the required patient effort and reduces the exercise's effectiveness.*
▪ Auscultate the patient's lungs *to provide a baseline for comparison with posttreatment auscultation.* Instruct the patient to exhale normally, insert the mouthpiece, close the lips tightly around it *because a weak seal may alter flow or volume readings,* and then

inhale as slowly and as deeply as possible (as shown below). If the patient has difficulty with this step, suggest sucking as one would through a straw but more slowly. Ask the patient to retain the entire volume of inhaled air for 3 seconds or, if you're using a device with a light indicator, until the light turns off. This deep breath creates sustained transpulmonary pressure near the end of inspiration and is sometimes called a sustained maximal inspiration.

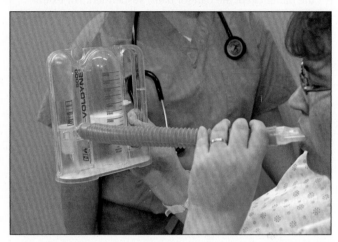

▪ Tell the patient to remove the mouthpiece and exhale normally. Let the patient relax and take several normal breaths before attempting another breath with the spirometer. Repeat this sequence 5 to 10 times during every waking hour. Note tidal volumes.
▪ Evaluate the patient's ability to cough effectively, encouraging coughing during and after each exercise session *because deep lung inflation may loosen secretions and facilitate their removal.* Observe any expectorated secretions.
▪ Auscultate the patient's lungs, and compare findings with the first auscultation.
▪ Perform hand hygiene and put on gloves.[1,2,3,4,5]
▪ Instruct the patient to remove the mouthpiece. Wash the mouthpiece in warm water and dry it. Avoid immersing the spirometer itself in water *because water enhances bacterial growth and impairs the internal filter's effectiveness in preventing inhalation of extraneous material.*
▪ Place the mouthpiece in a plastic storage bag between exercises, and label it and the spirometer, if applicable, with the patient's name *to avoid inadvertent use by another patient.* Keep the incentive spirometer within the patient's reach.
▪ Remove and discard your gloves and perform hand hygiene.[1,2,3,4,5]
▪ Disinfect your stethoscope using a disinfectant according to your facility's policy.
▪ Perform hand hygiene again.[1,2,3,4,5]
▪ Document the procedure.[7,8]

Special considerations

▪ If the patient is scheduled for surgery, make a preoperative assessment of his respiratory pattern and capability *to ensure the development of appropriate postoperative goals.* Teach the patient how to use the spirometer before surgery *so that he can concentrate on your instructions and practice the exercise.* A preoperative evaluation will also help in establishing a postoperative therapeutic goal.

Documenting flow and volume levels

If you've used a flow incentive spirometer, compute the volume by multiplying the setting by the duration that the patient kept the ball (or balls) suspended. For example, if the patient suspended the ball for 3 seconds at a setting of 500 mL during each of 10 breaths, multiply 500 mL by 3 seconds and then record this total (1,500 mL) and the number of breaths, as follows: 1,500 mL × 10 breaths.

If you've used a volume incentive spirometer, take the volume reading directly from the spirometer. For example, record 1,000 mL × 5 breaths.

■ Avoid exercise at mealtime *to prevent nausea*.
■ Provide paper and a pencil *so the patient can note exercise times*. Exercise frequency varies with condition and ability.
■ Immediately after surgery, monitor the exercise frequently *to ensure compliance and assess achievement*.
■ Premedicate for pain[9] as needed, following safe medication administration practices[10] *to improve comfort and effort*.
■ Some spirometers can be adapted for use by patients who have a tracheal stoma.
■ Remove the patient's dentures, if the fit is poor, *to create a better seal*.

Documentation

Record any teaching you provided. Document the baseline flow or volume levels, date and time of the procedure, type of spirometer, flow or volume levels achieved, and number of breaths taken. Also record the patient's condition before and after the procedure, his tolerance of the procedure, and the results of both auscultations.[7,8] (See *Documenting flow and volume levels*.)

REFERENCES

1 American Association for Respiratory Care. (1991). AARC clinical practice guideline: Incentive spirometry. *Respiratory Care, 36*(12), 1402–1405. (Level II)
2 The Joint Commission. (2012). Standard NPSG.07.01.01. *Comprehensive accreditation manual for hospitals: The official handbook*. Oakbrook Terrace, IL: The Joint Commission. (Level I)
3 Centers for Disease Control and Prevention. (October 2002). Guideline for hand hygiene in health-care settings. *Morbidity and Mortality Weekly Report, 51*(RR-16), 1–45. (Level I)
4 Siegel, J.D., et al. "2007 Guideline for Isolation Precautions: Preventing Transmission of Infectious Agents in Healthcare Settings" [Online]. Accessed September 2011 via the Web at http://www.cdc.gov/hicpac/2007ip/2007isolationprecautions.html (Level I)
5 World Health Organization. (2009). *WHO guidelines on hand hygiene in health care: First global patient safety challenge. Clean care is safer care*. Geneva, Switzerland: World Health Organization. (Level I)
6 The Joint Commission. (2012). Standard NPSG.01.01.01. *Comprehensive accreditation manual for hospitals: The official handbook*. Oakbrook Terrace, IL: The Joint Commission. (Level I)
7 The Joint Commission. (2012). Standard RC.01.03.01. *Comprehensive accreditation manual for hospitals: The official handbook*. Oakbrook Terrace, IL: The Joint Commission. (Level I)
8 The Joint Commission. (2012). Standard RC.02.01.01. *Comprehensive accreditation manual for hospitals: The official handbook*. Oakbrook Terrace, IL: The Joint Commission. (Level I)
9 The Joint Commission. (2012). Standard PC.01.02.01. *Comprehensive accreditation manual for hospitals: The official handbook*. Oakbrook Terrace, IL: The Joint Commission. (Level I)
10 The Joint Commission. (2012). Standard MM.06.01.01. *Comprehensive accreditation manual for hospitals: The official handbook*. Oakbrook Terrace, IL: The Joint Commission. (Level I)

ADDITIONAL REFERENCES

Guimarães, M.M., et al. (2009). Incentive spirometry for prevention of postoperative pulmonary complications in upper abdominal surgery. *Cochrane Database of Systematic Reviews*, (3), CD006058.
Nettina, S.M. (2010). *Lippincott manual of nursing practice* (9th ed.). Philadelphia, PA: Lippincott Williams & Wilkins.
Taylor, C., et al. (2011). *Fundamentals of nursing: The art and science of nursing care* (7th ed.). Philadelphia, PA: Lippincott Williams & Wilkins.
Westwood, K., et al. (2007). Incentive spirometry decreases respiratory complications following major abdominal surgery. *Surgeon, 5*(6), 339–342.

INCONTINENCE DEVICE APPLICATION, MALE

Many patients don't require an indwelling urinary catheter to manage their incontinence. For male patients, a male incontinence device, also known as a *condom catheter* or *penile sheath*, reduces the risk of urinary tract infection from catheterization, promotes bladder retraining when possible, helps prevent skin breakdown, and improves the patient's self-image. The device consists of a condom catheter secured to the shaft of the penis and connected to a leg bag or drainage bag. It has no contraindications but can cause skin irritation and edema.

Equipment

Condom catheter ■ drainage bag ■ extension tubing ■ hypoallergenic tape or incontinence sheath holder ■ commercial adhesive strip or skin-bond cement ■ plastic adhesive or Velcro, if needed ■ gloves ■ electric clippers, if needed ■ basin ■ soap ■ washcloth ■ towel.

Preparation of equipment

Fill the basin with lukewarm water. Then, bring the basin and the remaining equipment to the patient's bedside.

Implementation

- Perform hand hygiene and put on gloves.[1,2,3,4]
- Confirm the patient's identity using at least two patient identifiers according to your facility's policy.[5]
- Provide privacy and explain the procedure to the patient.
- Put on gloves.

Applying the device

- If the patient is circumcised, wash the penis with soap and water, rinse well, and pat dry with a towel. If the patient is uncircumcised, gently retract the foreskin and clean beneath it. Rinse well but don't dry *because moisture provides lubrication and prevents friction during foreskin replacement.* Replace the foreskin *to avoid penile constriction.* Then, if necessary, clip hair from the base and shaft of the penis *to prevent the adhesive strip or skin-bond cement from pulling pubic hair.*
- If you're using a precut commercial adhesive strip, insert the glans penis through its opening, and position the strip 1″ (2.5 cm) from the scrotal area. If you're using uncut adhesive, cut a strip to fit around the shaft of the penis. Remove the protective covering from one side of the adhesive strip and press this side firmly to the penis *to enhance adhesion.* Then remove the covering from the other side of the strip. If a commercial adhesive strip isn't available, apply skin-bond cement and let it dry for a few minutes.
- Position the rolled condom catheter at the tip of the penis, leaving ½″ (1.3 cm) between the condom end and the tip of the penis, with the drainage opening at the urinary meatus.
- Unroll the catheter upward, past the adhesive strip on the shaft of the penis. Then gently press the sheath against the strip until it adheres. (See *How to apply a condom catheter.*)
- After the condom catheter is in place, secure it with hypoallergenic tape or an incontinence sheath holder.
- Using extension tubing, connect the condom catheter to the leg bag or drainage bag.
- Remove and discard your gloves and perform hand hygiene.[1,2,3,4]
- Document the procedure.[6,7]

Removing the device

- Perform hand hygiene and put on gloves.[1,2,3,4]
- Confirm the patient's identity using at least two patient identifiers according to your facility's policy.[5]
- Explain the procedure to the patient and provide privacy.
- Simultaneously roll the condom catheter and adhesive strip off the penis and discard them. If you've used skin-bond cement rather than an adhesive strip, remove it with solvent. Also remove and discard the hypoallergenic tape or incontinence sheath holder.
- Clean the penis with lukewarm water, rinse thoroughly, and dry. Check for swelling or signs of skin breakdown.
- Remove the leg bag by closing the drain clamp, unlatching the leg straps, and disconnecting the extension tubing at the top of the bag.
- Remove and discard your gloves and perform hand hygiene.[1,2,3,4]
- Document the procedure.[6,7]

How to apply a condom catheter

Apply an adhesive strip to the shaft of the penis about 1″ (2.5 cm) from the scrotal area.

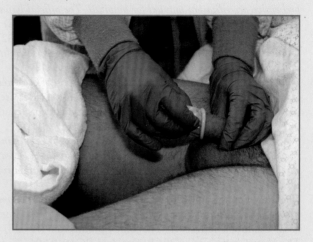

Then roll the condom catheter on to the penis past the adhesive strip. Leave about ½″ (1.3 cm) clearance at the end.

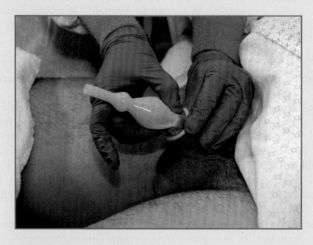

Press the sheath gently against the strip until it adheres.

Special considerations

- If hypoallergenic tape or an incontinence sheath holder isn't available, secure the condom with a strip of elastic adhesive or Velcro. Apply the strip snugly, but not too tightly *to prevent circulatory constriction.*
- Inspect the condom catheter for twists and the extension tubing for kinks *to prevent obstruction of urine flow, which could cause the condom to balloon, eventually dislodging it.*

Documentation

Record the date and time of application and removal of the incontinence device. Also note skin condition and the patient's response to the device, including voiding pattern, to assist with bladder retraining.[6,7]

REFERENCES

1   The Joint Commission. (2012). Standard NPSG.07.01.01. *Comprehensive accreditation manual for hospitals: The official handbook.* Oakbrook Terrace, IL: The Joint Commission. (Level I)

2   Centers for Disease Control and Prevention. (October 2002). Guideline for hand hygiene in health-care settings. *Morbidity and Mortality Weekly Report, 51*(RR-16), 1–45. (Level I)

3   Gould, C.V., et al. (2009). "Guideline for Prevention of Catheter-associated Urinary Tract Infections, 2009" [Online]. Accessed November 2011 via the Web at http://www.cdc.gov/hicpac/cauti/001_cauti.html (Level I)

4   World Health Organization. (2009). *WHO guidelines on hand hygiene in health care: First global patient safety challenge. Clean care is safer care.* Geneva, Switzerland: World Health Organization. (Level I)

5   The Joint Commission. (2012). Standard NPSG.01.01.01. *Comprehensive accreditation manual for hospitals: The official handbook.* Oakbrook Terrace, IL: The Joint Commission. (Level I)

6   The Joint Commission. (2012). Standard RC.01.03.01. *Comprehensive accreditation manual for hospitals: The official handbook.* Oakbrook Terrace, IL: The Joint Commission. (Level I)

7   The Joint Commission. (2012). Standard RC.02.01.01. *Comprehensive accreditation manual for hospitals: The official handbook.* Oakbrook Terrace, IL: The Joint Commission. (Level I)

ADDITIONAL REFERENCES

Brodie, A. (2006). A guide to the management of one-piece urinary sheaths. *Nursing Times, 102*(9), 49, 51.

de Zeeuw, S., and van Mastrigt, R. (2007). Increased postvoid residual after measuring the isovolumetric bladder pressure using the noninvasive condom catheter method. *BJU International, 100*(6), 1293–1297.

Milne, J.I., & Moore, K.N. (2006). Factors impacting self-care for urinary incontinence. *Urologic Nursing, 26*(1), 41–51.

Robinson, J. (2006). Continence: Sizing and fitting a penile sheath. *British Journal of Community Nursing, 11*(10), 420–427.

Saint, S., et al. (2006). Condom versus indwelling urinary catheters: A randomized trial. *Journal of the American Geriatric Society, 54*(7), 1055–1061.

INCONTINENCE MANAGEMENT, FECAL

Fecal incontinence is the involuntary passage of feces, which may occur gradually (as in dementia) or suddenly (as in spinal cord injury). It usually results from fecal stasis and impaction secondary to reduced activity, inappropriate diet, or untreated painful anal conditions. It can also result from chronic laxative use; reduced fluid intake; neurologic deficit; pelvic, prostatic, or rectal surgery; and the use of certain medications, including antihistamines, psychotropics, and iron preparations.

In elderly patients, fecal incontinence commonly follows any loss or impairment of anal sphincter control. The incontinence may be transient or permanent and affects up to 10% of patients in assisted living or extended care facilities. Not usually a sign of serious illness, fecal incontinence can seriously impair an elderly patient's physical and psychological well-being.

Patients with fecal incontinence should be carefully assessed for underlying disorders. Most can be treated; some can even be cured. Treatment aims to control the condition through bowel retraining or other behavioral management techniques, diet modification, drug therapy, pessaries, and, possibly, surgery.

Equipment

Gloves ▪ stethoscope ▪ lubricant ▪ skin protectant ▪ skin cleaner ▪ incontinence pads ▪ bedpan ▪ specimen container ▪ label ▪ laboratory request form ▪ Optional: stool collection kit.

Implementation

▪ Perform hand hygiene and put on gloves.[1,2,3]

▪ Confirm the patient's identity using at least two patient identifiers according to your facility's policy.[4]

▪ Ask the patient with fecal incontinence to identify its onset, duration, severity, and pattern (for instance, determine whether it occurs at night or with diarrhea). Focus the history on GI, neurologic, and psychological disorders.

▪ Note the frequency, consistency, and volume of stools passed in the past 24 hours.

▪ Protect the patient's bed with an incontinence pad.

▪ Obtain a stool specimen, if ordered. (See "Stool specimen collection," page 674.)

▪ Assess for chronic constipation, GI and neurologic disorders, and laxative abuse.[5] Inspect the abdomen for distention, and auscultate for bowel sounds. If not contraindicated, check for fecal impaction (a factor in overflow incontinence).

▪ Maintain effective hygienic care *to increase the patient's comfort and prevent skin breakdown and infection.* Clean the perineal area frequently with a skin cleaner, and apply a skin protectant cream after every incontinence episode.[6] Take steps to control foul odors as well.

▪ Assess the patient's medication regimen. Check for drugs that affect bowel activity, such as antibiotics, aspirin, some anticholinergic antiparkinsonian agents, aluminum hydroxide, calcium carbonate antacids, diuretics, iron preparations, opiates, tranquilizers, tricyclic antidepressants, and phenothiazines.

▪ For the neurologically capable patient with chronic incontinence, provide bowel retraining.

▪ Advise the patient to consume a fiber-rich diet that includes lots of raw, leafy vegetables (such as carrots and lettuce), unpeeled fruits (such as apples), and whole grains (such as wheat or rye breads and cereals). If the patient has a lactase deficiency, suggest that he take calcium supplements to replace calcium lost by eliminating dairy products from the diet.

▪ Encourage adequate fluid intake.

▪ Advise the patient to avoid caffeine, a gastrocolonic stimulant, after meals.

▪ Teach the elderly patient to gradually eliminate laxative use. Point out that using laxatives to promote regular bowel movement may have the opposite effect, producing either constipation or incontinence over time. Suggest natural laxatives, such as prunes and prune juice, instead.

- Promote regular exercise by explaining how it helps to regulate bowel motility. Even a nonambulatory patient can perform some exercises while sitting or lying in bed.
- Advise the patient to avoid brisk physical activity immediately after meals *to decrease urgency and diarrhea.*
- Remove and discard your gloves and perform hand hygiene.[1,2,3]
- Document the procedure.[7,8]

Special considerations

- Schedule extra time to provide encouragement and support for the patient, who may feel shame, embarrassment, and powerlessness from loss of control.

Complications

Skin breakdown and infection may result from incontinence. Psychological problems resulting from incontinence include social isolation, loss of independence, lowered self-esteem, and depression.

Documentation

Record all bladder and bowel retraining efforts, noting scheduled bathroom times, food and fluid intake, and elimination amounts, as appropriate. Document the duration of continent periods. Note any complications, including emotional problems and signs of skin breakdown and infection as well as the treatments given for them.[7,8]

REFERENCES

1 Centers for Disease Control and Prevention. (October 2002). Guideline for hand hygiene in health-care settings. *Morbidity and Mortality Weekly Report, 51*(RR-16), 1–45. (Level I)
2 World Health Organization. (2009). *WHO guidelines on hand hygiene in health care: First global patient safety challenge. Clean care is safer care.* Geneva, Switzerland: World Health Organization. (Level I)
3 The Joint Commission. (2012). Standard NPSG.07.01.01. *Comprehensive accreditation manual for hospitals: The official handbook.* Oakbrook Terrace, IL: The Joint Commission. (Level I)
4 The Joint Commission. (2012). Standard NPSG.01.01.01. *Comprehensive accreditation manual for hospitals: The official handbook.* Oakbrook Terrace, IL: The Joint Commission. (Level I)
5 Whitehead, W.E., et al. (2009). Fecal incontinence in US adults: Epidemiology and risk factors. *Gastroenterology, 137*(2), 512–517.
6 Beeckman D., et al. (2009). Prevention and treatment of incontinence-associated dermatitis: Literature review. *Journal of Advanced Nursing, 65*(6), 1141–1154.
7 The Joint Commission. (2012). Standard RC.01.03.01. *Comprehensive accreditation manual for hospitals: The official handbook.* Oakbrook Terrace, IL: The Joint Commission. (Level I)
8 The Joint Commission. (2012). Standard RC.02.01.01. *Comprehensive accreditation manual for hospitals: The official handbook.* Oakbrook Terrace, IL: The Joint Commission. (Level I)

ADDITIONAL REFERENCES

Abrams, P., et al. (2010). Fourth International Consultation on Incontinence Recommendations of the International Scientific Committee: Evaluation and treatment of urinary incontinence, pelvic organ prolapse, and fecal incontinence. *Neurology and Urodynamics, 29*(1), 213–240.

Beitz, J.M. (2006). Fecal incontinence in acutely and critically ill patients: Options in management. *Ostomy/Wound Management, 52*(12), 56–58, 60, 62–66.
Markland, A.D., et al. (2008). Correlates of urinary, fecal, and dual incontinence in older African-American and white men and women. *Journal of the American Geriatrics Society, 56*(2), 285–290.
Nix, D. (2006). Prevention and treatment of perineal skin breakdown due to incontinence. *Ostomy/Wound Management, 52*(4), 26–28.
Norton, C., et al. (2010). Management of fecal incontinence in adults. *Neurology and Urodynamics, 29*(1), 199–206.
Shamliyan, T., et al. (2007). Prevention of urinary and fecal incontinence in adults. *Evidence Report/Technology Assessment,* (161):1–379.

INCONTINENCE MANAGEMENT, URINARY

In elderly patients, urinary incontinence commonly follows any loss or impairment of urinary sphincter control. The incontinence may be transient or permanent. In all, about 10 million adults experience some form of urinary incontinence; this includes about 50% of the 1.5 million people in extended-care facilities.

Contrary to popular opinion, urinary incontinence is neither a disease nor a part of normal aging. It isn't inevitable and can be avoided or reversed with support and interventions. Incontinence may be caused by childbirth, confusion, dehydration, fecal impaction, or restricted mobility. It's also a sign of various disorders, such as prostatic hyperplasia, bladder calculus, bladder cancer, urinary tract infection (UTI), stroke, diabetic neuropathy, Guillain-Barré syndrome, multiple sclerosis, prostatic cancer, prostatitis, spinal cord injury, and urethral stricture. It may also result from urethral sphincter damage after prostatectomy. In addition, certain drugs, including diuretics, hypnotics, sedatives, anticholinergics, antihypertensives, and alpha antagonists, may trigger urinary incontinence.

Urinary incontinence is classified as acute or chronic. Acute urinary incontinence results from disorders that are potentially reversible, such as delirium, dehydration, urine retention, restricted mobility, fecal impaction, infection or inflammation, drug reactions, and polyuria. Chronic urinary incontinence occurs as four distinct types: stress, overflow, urge, and functional (total) incontinence.

With *stress incontinence,* leakage results from a sudden physical strain, such as a sneeze, cough, or quick movement. With *overflow incontinence,* urine retention causes dribbling because the distended bladder can't contract strongly enough to force a urine stream. With *urge incontinence,* the patient can't control the impulse to urinate. Finally, with *functional incontinence,* urine leakage occurs despite the fact that the bladder and urethra are functioning normally and is usually related to cognitive or mobility factors.

Patients with urinary incontinence should be carefully assessed for underlying disorders. Most can be treated; some can even be cured. Treatment aims to control the condition through bladder retraining or other behavioral management techniques, diet modification, drug therapy, pessaries and, possibly, surgery.

Artificial urinary sphincter implant

An artificial urinary sphincter implant can help restore continence to a patient with a neurogenic bladder. Criteria for inserting an implant include:
■ incontinence associated with a weak urinary sphincter
■ incoordination between the detrusor muscle and the urinary sphincter (if drug therapy fails)
■ inadequate bladder storage (if intermittent catheterization and drug therapy are unsuccessful).

Configuration and placement
An implant consists of a control pump, an inflatable cuff, and a pressure-regulating reservoir. The cuff is placed around the bladder neck, and the reservoir is placed under the rectus muscle in the abdomen. The reservoir holds fluid that inflates the cuff. In men, the surgeon places the control pump in the scrotum; in women, the surgeon places the pump in the labium.

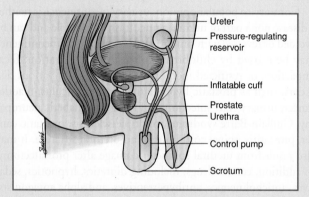

- Ureter
- Pressure-regulating reservoir
- Inflatable cuff
- Prostate
- Urethra
- Control pump
- Scrotum

Using the implant
To void, the patient squeezes the bulb to deflate the cuff, which opens the urethra by returning fluid to the balloon. After voiding, the cuff reinflates automatically, sealing the urethra until the patient needs to void again.

Complications and care
If complications develop, the implant may need to be repaired or removed. Possible complications include cuff leakage (uncommon), trapped blood or other fluid contaminants (which can cause control pump problems), skin erosion around the bulb or erosion in the bladder neck or the urethra, infection, inadequate occlusion pressures, and kinked tubing. If the bladder holds residual urine, intermittent self-catheterization may be needed.

Care includes avoiding strenuous activity for about 6 months after surgery and having regular checkups.

Corrective surgery for urinary incontinence includes transurethral resection of the prostate in men, urethral collagen injections for men or women, repair of the anterior vaginal wall or retropelvic suspension of the bladder in women, urethral sling, and bladder augmentation. (See *Artificial urinary sphincter implant*.)

Equipment
Bladder retraining record sheet ■ gloves ■ moisture barrier cream ■ incontinence pads ■ bedpan ■ specimen container ■ label ■ laboratory request form ■ Optional: urinary catheter.

Implementation
■ Perform hand hygiene.[1,2,3]
■ Confirm the patient's identity using at least two patient identifiers according to your facility's policy.[4]
■ Ask when the patient first noticed urine leakage and whether it began suddenly or gradually. Have him describe his typical urinary pattern: Does he usually experience incontinence during the day or at night? Does he get the urge to go again immediately after emptying the bladder? Does he get strong urges to go? Ask him to rate his urinary control: Does he have moderate control, or is he completely incontinent? If he sometimes urinates with control, ask him to identify when and how much he usually urinates.
■ Evaluate related problems, such as urinary hesitancy, frequency, urgency, nocturia, and decreased force or interruption of the urine stream. Ask the patient to describe any previous treatment received for incontinence or measures the patient has performed. Ask about medications, including nonprescription drugs.[5]
■ Assess the patient's environment. Is a toilet or commode readily available, and how long does the patient take to reach it? After the patient is in the bathroom, assess his manual dexterity; for example, how easily does he manipulate his clothes?
■ Evaluate the patient's mental status and cognitive function.
■ Quantify the patient's normal daily fluid intake.
■ Review the patient's medication and diet history for drugs and foods that affect digestion and elimination.
■ Review or obtain the patient's medical history, noting especially any incidence of UTI, diabetes, spinal injury or tumor, stroke, and bladder or pelvic surgery. For a female patient, also note the number and route of births and whether she's had a hysterectomy; for a male, note any prostate surgery. Assess for such disorders as delirium, dehydration, urine retention, restricted mobility, fecal impaction, infection, inflammation, and polyuria.[5]
■ Perform hand hygiene and put on gloves.[1,2,3]
■ Inspect the urethral meatus for obvious inflammation or anatomic defects. Have the female patient bear down while you note any urine leakage.
■ Gently palpate the abdomen for bladder distention, which signals urine retention.
■ Assess for costovertebral angle tenderness. If possible, have the patient examined by a urologist.
■ Obtain specimens for appropriate laboratory tests, as ordered. (See "Urine specimen collection," page 776.)
■ Begin incontinence management by implementing an appropriate bladder retraining program. (See *Correcting urinary incontinence with bladder retraining*.)

PATIENT TEACHING

Correcting urinary incontinence with bladder retraining

The incontinent patient typically feels frustrated, embarrassed, and hopeless. Fortunately, his problem can usually be corrected by bladder retraining—a program that aims to establish a regular voiding pattern. Follow these guidelines.

Assess elimination patterns

First, assess the patient's intake and voiding patterns and reason for each accidental voiding (such as a coughing spell). Use an incontinence monitoring record.

Establish a voiding schedule

Encourage the patient to void regularly, for example, every 2 hours. When he can stay dry for 2 hours, increase the interval by 30 minutes every day until he achieves a 3- to 4-hour voiding schedule. Teach the patient to practice relaxation techniques such as deep breathing, which help decrease the sense of urgency.

Record results and remain positive

Keep a record of continence and incontinence for about 5 days *to help reinforce the patient's efforts to remain continent*. Remember, both your own and your patient's positive attitudes are crucial to his successful bladder retraining.

Take steps for success

Here are some additional tips to boost the patient's success:
- Be sure to locate the patient's bed near a bathroom or portable toilet. Leave a light on at night. If the patient needs assistance getting out of bed or a chair, promptly answer the call for help.
- Teach the patient measures to prevent urinary tract infections, such as adequate fluid intake (at least 2,000 mL/day unless contraindicated), drinking cranberry juice to help acidify urine, wearing cotton underpants, and bathing with nonirritating soaps. If the patient has urge incontinence, cranberry juice is contraindicated.
- Encourage the patient to empty his bladder completely before and after meals and at bedtime.
- Advise him to urinate whenever the urge arises and never to ignore it.
- Instruct the patient to take prescribed diuretics upon rising in the morning.
- Advise him to limit the use of sleeping aids, sedatives, and alcohol; *they decrease the urge to urinate and can increase incontinence, especially at night.*
- If the patient is overweight, encourage weight loss.
- Suggest exercises to strengthen pelvic muscles.
- Instruct the patient to increase dietary fiber *to decrease constipation and incontinence.*
- Monitor the patient for signs of anxiety and depression.
- Reassure the patient that periodic incontinent episodes don't mean that the program has failed. Encourage persistence, tolerance, and a positive attitude.

NURSING ALERT *Obtain a 3- to 7-day bladder diary before implementing bladder retraining.*[5]
- *To ensure healthful hydration and to prevent UTIs,* make sure the patient maintains an adequate daily intake of fluids (six to eight 8-oz glasses). Restrict fluid intake after 6 p.m.
- *To manage stress incontinence,* begin an exercise program to help strengthen the pelvic floor muscles. (See *Strengthening pelvic floor muscles,* page 374.)
- *To manage functional incontinence,* frequently assess the patient's mental and functional status. Regularly remind him to void. Respond to his calls promptly, and help him get to the bathroom quickly. Provide positive reinforcement.
- Clean the perineal area frequently, and apply a moisture barrier cream. Also take steps to control foul odors.
- Remove and discard your gloves and perform hand hygiene.[1,2,3]
- Document the procedure.[6,7]

Special considerations

- Schedule extra time to provide encouragement and support for the patient, who may feel shame, embarrassment, and powerlessness from loss of control.

Complications

Skin breakdown and infection may result from incontinence. Psychological problems resulting from incontinence include social isolation, loss of independence, lowered self-esteem, and depression.

Documentation

Record all bladder retraining efforts, noting scheduled bathroom times, food and fluid intake, and elimination amounts, as appropriate. Document the duration of continent periods. Note any complications, including emotional problems and signs of skin breakdown and infection as well as the treatments given for them.[6,7]

REFERENCES

1 Centers for Disease Control and Prevention. (October 2002). Guideline for hand hygiene in health-care settings. *Morbidity and Mortality Weekly Report, 51*(RR-16), 1–45. (Level I)
2 World Health Organization. (2009). *WHO guidelines on hand hygiene in health care: First global patient safety challenge. Clean care is safer care.* Geneva, Switzerland: World Health Organization. (Level I)

PATIENT TEACHING

Strengthening pelvic floor muscles

Stress incontinence, the most common kind of urinary incontinence in women, usually results from weakening of the urethral sphincter. In men, it may sometimes occur after a radical prostatectomy.

You can help male and female patients prevent or minimize stress incontinence by teaching pelvic floor (Kegel) exercises to strengthen the pubococcygeal muscles.[5] Here's how.

Learning Kegel exercises

First, explain how to locate the muscles of the pelvic floor. Instruct the patient to tense the muscles around the anus, as if to retain stools.

To identify this area initially, teach the patient to tighten the muscles of the pelvic floor to stop the flow of urine while urinating and then to release the muscles to restart the flow. Once learned, these exercises can be done anywhere. Although Kegel exercises shouldn't be done while urinating, they can be done at any other time.

Establishing a regimen

Explain to the patient that contraction and relaxation exercises are essential to muscle retraining. Suggest that the patient start out by contracting the pelvic floor muscles for 5 seconds, relax for 5 seconds, and then repeat the procedure as often as needed. Typically, the patient starts with 10 contractions in the morning and 10 at night, gradually increasing the relaxation and contraction time.

Advise the patient not to use stomach, leg, or buttock muscles. Also discourage leg crossing or breath holding during these exercises.

3   The Joint Commission. (2012). Standard NPSG.07.01.01. *Comprehensive accreditation manual for hospitals: The official handbook.* Oakbrook Terrace, IL: The Joint Commission. (Level I)

4   The Joint Commission. (2012). Standard NPSG.01.01.01. *Comprehensive accreditation manual for hospitals: The official handbook.* Oakbrook Terrace, IL: The Joint Commission. (Level I)

5   Ghoniem, G., et al. (2008). Evaluation and outcome measures in the treatment of female urinary stress incontinence: International Urogynecological Association (IUGA) guidelines for research and clinical practice. *International Urogynecology Journal and Pelvic Floor Dysfunction, 19*(1), 5–33.

6   The Joint Commission. (2012). Standard RC.01.03.01. *Comprehensive accreditation manual for hospitals: The official handbook.* Oakbrook Terrace, IL: The Joint Commission. (Level I)

7   The Joint Commission. (2012). Standard RC.02.01.01. *Comprehensive accreditation manual for hospitals: The official handbook.* Oakbrook Terrace, IL: The Joint Commission. (Level I)

ADDITIONAL REFERENCES

Bradway, C. (2010). Urinary incontinence and co-morbid conditions: Opportunities for urologic nurses. *Urology Nursing, 30*(2), 109–110.

Bradway, C., & Cacchione, P. (2010). Teaching strategies for assessing and managing urinary incontinence in older adults. *Journal of Gerontology Nursing, 36*(7), 18–26.

Dingwall, L., & McLafferty, E. (2006). Do Nurses promote urinary continence in hospitalized older people? An exploratory study. *Journal of Clinical Nursing, 15*(10), 1276–1286.

Markland, A.D., et al. (2008). Correlates of urinary, fecal, and dual incontinence in older African-American and white men and women. *Journal of the American Geriatrics Society, 56*(2), 285–290.

Price, N., & Currie, I. (2010). Urinary incontinence in women: Diagnosis and management. *The Practitioner, 254*(1727), 27–32, 2–3.

Shamliyan, T., et al. (2007). Prevention of urinary and fecal incontinence in adults. *Evidence Report/Technology Assessment, (161):* 1–379.

Zarowitz, B.J., & Ouslander, J.G. (2006). Management of urinary incontinence in older persons. *Geriatric Nursing, 27*(5), 265–270.

INDWELLING URINARY CATHETER CARE AND REMOVAL

Intended to prevent infection and other complications by keeping an indwelling or Foley catheter insertion site clean, routine catheter care typically is performed after the patient's morning bath and immediately after perineal care. (Bedtime catheter care may have to be performed before perineal care.)

Because some studies suggest that catheter care increases the risk of infection and other complications rather than lowers it, many health care facilities don't recommend daily catheter care.[1] Because of this, individual facility policy dictates whether or not a patient receives such care. Regardless of the catheter care policy, the equipment and the patient's genitalia require inspection twice daily.

An indwelling urinary catheter should be removed when bladder decompression is no longer necessary, when the patient can resume voiding, or when the catheter is obstructed.[2] Depending on the length of the catheterization, the doctor may order bladder retraining before catheter removal. To prevent catheter-associated urinary tract infections, the catheter should be removed as soon as it's no longer needed.

Equipment

Gloves ▪ eight sterile 4″ × 4″ gauze pads ▪ basin ▪ washcloth ▪ soap and water ▪ leg bag ▪ drainage bag ▪ adhesive tape or leg band ▪ waste receptacle ▪ Optional: safety pin, rubber band, gooseneck lamp or flashlight, adhesive remover, antibiotic ointment, specimen container.

Commercially prepared catheter care kits containing all necessary supplies are available.

For catheter removal
Absorbent cotton ■ gloves ■ alcohol pad ■ 10-mL syringe with luer lock ■ bedpan.

Implementation
Catheter care
■ Perform hand hygiene, and put on gloves and a gown as needed.[3,4,5,6]
■ Confirm the patient's identity using at least two patient identifiers according to your facility's policy.[7]
■ Assemble the equipment and supplies at the bedside.
■ Explain the procedure and its purpose to the patient.
■ Provide the patient with the necessary equipment for self-cleaning, if possible.
■ Provide privacy.
■ Make sure the lighting is adequate *so that you can see the perineum and catheter tubing clearly.* Place a gooseneck lamp at the bedside, if needed.
■ Inspect the catheter for any problems, and check the urine drainage for mucus, blood clots, sediment, and turbidity. Then pinch the catheter between two fingers *to determine if the lumen contains any material.* If you notice any of these conditions (or if your facility's policy requires it), using sterile technique,[3,4] obtain a urine specimen from the specimen collection port. Collect at least 3 mL of urine, but don't fill the specimen cup more than halfway. Notify the doctor about your findings.
■ Inspect the outside of the catheter where it enters the urinary meatus *for encrusted material and suppurative drainage.* Also inspect the tissue around the meatus *for irritation or swelling.*
■ Remove the adhesive tape or leg band securing the catheter to the patient's thigh or abdomen. Inspect the area for signs of adhesive burns—redness, tenderness, or blisters.
■ Clean the outside of the catheter and the tissue around the meatus using soap and water. *To avoid contaminating the urinary tract,* always clean by wiping away from—never toward—the urinary meatus. Use a dry gauze pad to remove encrusted material.
NURSING ALERT *Don't pull on the catheter while you're cleaning it.* Pulling can injure the urethra and the bladder wall. It can also expose a section of the catheter that was inside the urethra, so that when you release the catheter, the newly contaminated section will reenter the urethra, introducing potentially infectious organisms.
■ Remove and discard your gloves and perform hand hygiene. Reapply the leg band, and reattach the catheter to the leg band. If a leg band isn't available, use a piece of adhesive tape to tape the catheter to the patient's leg or abdomen; retape the catheter on the opposite side of where it was before *to prevent skin hypersensitivity or irritation.*
NURSING ALERT *Provide enough slack before securing the catheter to prevent tension on the tubing, which could injure the urethral lumen or bladder wall.*[2]

■ Most drainage bags have a plastic clamp on the tubing to attach them to the sheet. Attach the drainage bag below bladder level to the bed frame.[2,3]
■ If necessary, clean residue from the previous tape site with an adhesive remover. Then dispose of all used supplies in a waste receptacle.
■ Perform hand hygiene.[3,4,5,6]
■ Document the procedure.[8,9]

Catheter removal
■ Gather the equipment at the patient's bedside.
■ Perform hand hygiene.
■ Confirm the patient's identity using at least two patient identifiers according to your facility's policy.[7]
■ Verify the doctor's order.
■ Explain the procedure and its purpose to the patient and tell him that he may feel slight discomfort.
■ Provide the patient with the necessary equipment for self-cleaning, if possible.
■ Provide privacy.
■ Perform hand hygiene, and put on gloves.[3,4,5,6]
■ Explain to the patient that you'll check him periodically during the first 6 to 24 hours after catheter removal *to make sure he resumes voiding.*
■ Attach the syringe to the luer-lock mechanism on the catheter.
■ Pull back on the plunger of the syringe *to deflate the balloon by aspirating the injected fluid.* The amount of fluid injected is usually indicated on the tip of the catheter's balloon lumen and in the patient's chart.
■ Grasp the catheter with the absorbent cotton, and gently withdraw it from the urethra.
■ Offer the patient a bedpan.
■ Measure and record the amount of urine in the collection bag before discarding it.
■ Dispose of used equipment in the appropriate receptacles.
■ Remove and discard your gloves. Perform hand hygiene.[3,4,5,6]
■ Document the procedure.[8,9]

Special considerations
■ The catheter should be removed as soon as it is no longer needed to prevent catheter-associated urinary tract infections.[2,3]
■ Some facilities require the use of specific cleaning agents for catheter care; check your facility's policy manual before beginning this procedure. A doctor's order will also be needed to apply antibiotic ointments to the urinary meatus after cleaning.
■ *To prevent reflux of urine, which may contain bacteria,* avoid raising the drainage bag above bladder level.[2] *To avoid damaging the urethral lumen or bladder wall,* always disconnect the drainage bag and tubing from the bed linen and bed frame before helping the patient out of bed.
■ When possible, attach a leg bag to allow the patient greater mobility.
■ Encourage patients with unrestricted fluid intake to increase intake to at least 30 mL/kg/day *to help flush the urinary system and reduce sediment formation.*

Teaching about leg bags

A urine drainage bag attached to the leg provides the catheterized patient with greater mobility. Because the bag is hidden under clothing, it may also help him feel more comfortable about catheterization. Leg bags are usually worn during the day and are replaced at night with a standard drainage bag.

If the patient will be discharged with an indwelling catheter, teach him how to attach and remove a leg bag. To demonstrate, you'll need a bag with a short drainage tube, two straps, an alcohol pad, adhesive tape, and a screw clamp or hemostat.

Attaching the leg bag
■ Provide privacy, and explain the procedure. Describe the advantages of a leg bag, but caution the patient that a leg bag is smaller than a standard drainage bag and may have to be emptied more frequently.
■ Remove the protective covering from the tip of the drainage tube. Then show the patient how to clean the tip with an alcohol pad, wiping away from the opening *to avoid contaminating the tube.* Show him how to attach the tube to the catheter.
■ Place the drainage bag on the patient's calf or thigh. Have him fasten the straps securely (as shown), and then show him how to tape the catheter to his leg. Emphasize that he must leave slack in the catheter to minimize pressure on the bladder, urethra, and related structures. *Excessive pressure or tension can lead to tissue breakdown.*
■ Also tell the patient not to fasten the straps too tightly *to avoid interfering with his circulation.*

Avoiding complications
■ Although most leg bags have a valve in the drainage tube that prevents urine reflux into the bladder, urge the patient to

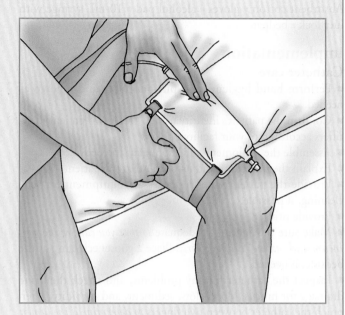

keep the drainage bag lower than his bladder at all times *because urine in the bag is a perfect growth medium for bacteria.* Caution him also not to go to bed or take long naps while wearing the leg bag.
■ *To prevent a full leg bag from damaging the bladder wall and urethra,* encourage the patient to empty the bag when it's half full or every 3 to 6 hours.[1] He should also inspect the catheter and drainage tube periodically for compression or kinking, *which could obstruct urine flow and result in bladder distention.*
■ Tell the patient to wash the leg bag with soap and water or a bacteriostatic solution before each use *to prevent infection.*

■ When changing a catheter after long-term use, you may need a larger-size catheter *because the meatus enlarges, causing urine to leak around the catheter.*
■ Don't clean the periurethral area with antiseptic; instead, clean the meatal surface during daily bathing *to reduce the risk of catheter-associated urinary tract infection.*[2,3]
■ After catheter removal, assess the patient for incontinence or dribbling, urgency, persistent dysuria or bladder spasms, fever, chills, or palpable bladder distention. Report these conditions to the doctor.

Patient teaching

If the patient will be discharged with an indwelling catheter, teach him how to use a leg bag. (See *Teaching about leg bags.*) Also instruct the patient to wash the urinary meatus and perineal area with soap and water twice daily and the anal area after each bowel movement.

Complications

Sediment buildup can occur anywhere in a catheterization system, especially in bedridden and dehydrated patients. Change the indwelling catheter as ordered or when malfunction, obstruction, or contamination occurs.

Acute renal failure may result from a catheter obstructed by sediment. Be alert for sharply reduced urine flow from the catheter. Assess for bladder discomfort or distention.

Urinary tract infection can result from catheter insertion or from intraluminal or extraluminal migration of bacteria up the catheter. Signs and symptoms may include cloudy or foul-smelling urine, hematuria, fever, malaise, tenderness over the bladder, and flank pain.

Major complications in removing an indwelling catheter include failure of the balloon to deflate and rupture of the balloon. If the balloon ruptures, cystoscopy is usually performed to ensure removal of any balloon fragments.

Documentation

Record the care you performed, any modifications, patient complaints, and the condition of the perineum and urinary meatus. Note the character of the urine in the drainage bag, any sediment buildup, and whether a specimen was sent for laboratory analysis. Also record fluid intake and output. An hourly record is usually necessary for critically ill patients and those with renal insufficiency who are hemodynamically unstable.[8,9]

Record the date and time of the catheter removal and the patient's tolerance of the procedure. Record when and how much he voided after catheter removal and any associated interventions.

REFERENCES

1 Clinical Practice Guidelines Task Force; Society of Urologic Nurses and Associates. (2006). Care of the patient with an indwelling catheter. *Urologic Nursing, 26*(1), 80–81. (Level I)
2 Gould, C.V., et al. (2009). "Guideline for Prevention of Catheter-associated Urinary Tract Infections, 2009" [Online]. Accessed November 2011 via the Web at http://www.cdc.gov/hicpac/cauti/001_cauti.html (Level I)
3 Lo, E. (2008). Strategies to prevent catheter-associated urinary tract infections in acute care hospitals. *Infection Control and Hospital Epidemiology 29*(Suppl. 1), S41–S50. (Level I)
4 The Joint Commission. (2012). Standard NPSG.07.06.01. *Comprehensive accreditation manual for hospitals: The official handbook.* Oakbrook Terrace, IL: The Joint Commission. (Level I)
5 The Joint Commission. (2012). Standard NPSG.07.01.01. *Comprehensive accreditation manual for hospitals: The official handbook.* Oakbrook Terrace, IL: The Joint Commission. (Level I)
6 Centers for Disease Control and Prevention. (October 2002). Guideline for hand hygiene in health-care settings. *Morbidity and Mortality Weekly Report, 51*(RR-16), 1–45. (Level I)
7 The Joint Commission. (2012). Standard NPSG.01.01.01. *Comprehensive accreditation manual for hospitals: The official handbook.* Oakbrook Terrace, IL: The Joint Commission. (Level I)
8 The Joint Commission. (2012). Standard RC.01.03.01. *Comprehensive accreditation manual for hospitals: The official handbook.* Oakbrook Terrace, IL: The Joint Commission. (Level I)
9 The Joint Commission. (2012). Standard RC.02.01.01. *Comprehensive accreditation manual for hospitals: The official handbook.* Oakbrook Terrace, IL: The Joint Commission. (Level I)

ADDITIONAL REFERENCES

Nettina, S.M. (2010). *Lippincott manual of nursing practice* (9th ed.). Philadelphia, PA: Lippincott Williams & Wilkins.
Reilly, L., et al. (2006). Reducing Foley catheter device days in an intensive care unit: Using the evidence to change practice. *AACN Advances in Critical Care, 17*(3), 272–283.
Ribby, K.J. (2006). Decreasing urinary tract infections through staff development, outcomes, and nursing process. *Journal of Nursing Care Quality, 21*(3), 272–276.
Willson, M., et al. (2009). Nursing interventions to reduce the risk of catheter-associated urinary tract infection: Part 2: Staff education, monitoring, and care techniques. *Journal of Wound, Ostomy, and Continence Nursing, 36*(2), 137–154.

INDWELLING URINARY CATHETER INSERTION

Also known as a *Foley* or *retention catheter,* an indwelling urinary catheter remains in the bladder to provide continuous urine drainage. A balloon inflated at the catheter's distal end prevents it from slipping out of the bladder after insertion.

Indwelling catheters are used most commonly to relieve bladder distention caused by urine retention and to allow continuous urine drainage when the urinary meatus is swollen from childbirth, surgery, or local trauma. Other indications for an indwelling catheter include urinary tract obstruction (by a tumor or enlarged prostate), urine retention or infection from neurogenic bladder paralysis caused by spinal cord injury or disease, and any illness in which the patient's urine output must be monitored closely. During bladder retraining for patients with neurologic disorders, such as stroke or spinal cord injury, bladder ultrasound scanning may be used to determine postvoid residual urine volume as well as the need for intermittent catheterization.

An indwelling catheter is inserted using sterile technique and only when absolutely necessary. Insertion should be performed with extreme care to prevent injury and infection. The catheter should be removed as soon as it is no longer needed to prevent catheter-associated urinary tract infections.[1,2,3]

Equipment

Sterile indwelling catheter (latex or silicone #10 to #22 French [average adult sizes are #16 to #18 French]) ▪ syringe filled with 5 to 8 mL of sterile water ▪ washcloth ▪ towel ▪ soap and water ▪ two linen-saver pads ▪ sterile gloves ▪ sterile drape ▪ sterile fenestrated drape ▪ sterile cotton-tipped applicators (or cotton balls and plastic forceps) ▪ antiseptic cleaning agent ▪ urine receptacle ▪ single-use packet of sterile, water-soluble lubricant ▪ sterile drainage collection bag ▪ intake and output sheet ▪ adhesive tape ▪ Optional: urine specimen container and laboratory request form, leg band with Velcro closure, gooseneck lamp or flashlight, pillows or rolled blankets or towels, ultrasound bladder scanner.

Prepackaged sterile disposable kits that usually contain all the necessary equipment are available. The syringes in these kits are prefilled with 10 mL of sterile water

Preparation of equipment

Verify the order on the patient's medical record to determine if a catheter size or type has been specified. Then perform hand hygiene, select the appropriate equipment, and assemble it at the patient's bedside.[1,4,5,6,7,8]

Implementation

▪ Confirm the patient's identity using at least two patient identifiers according to your facility's policy.[10]
▪ Explain the procedure to the patient and provide privacy. Check the chart and ask when the patient last voided.
▪ Percuss and palpate the bladder *to establish baseline data.* Ask if the patient feels the urge to void. If possible, measure the amount of urine in the bladder using ultrasonography.[1]

■ Have a coworker hold a flashlight or place a gooseneck lamp next to the patient's bed *so that you can see the urinary meatus clearly in poor lighting.*

■ You may need the assistant to help the patient stay in position or to direct the light.

For a female patient

■ Place the patient in the supine position, with her knees flexed and separated and her feet flat on the bed, about 2' (61 cm) apart. If she finds this position uncomfortable, have her flex one knee and keep the other leg flat on the bed. Or have the patient lie on her side with her knees drawn up to her chest during the catheterization procedure (as shown below). *This position may be especially helpful for elderly or disabled patients, such as those with severe contractures.*

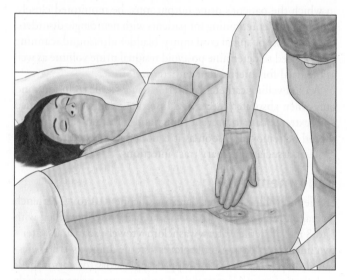

ELDER ALERT *The elderly patient may need pillows or rolled towels or blankets* to provide support with positioning.

■ You may need an assistant to help the patient stay in position or to direct the light. Ask the patient to hold the position *to give you a clear view of the urinary meatus and to prevent contamination of the sterile field.*

■ Perform hand hygiene and put on gloves.[1,4,5,6,7]

■ Use the washcloth to clean the patient's genital area and perineum thoroughly with soap and water. Dry the area with the towel. Then remove your gloves and perform hand hygiene again.[1,4,5,6,7]

■ Place the linen-saver pads on the bed between the patient's legs and under the hips. *To create the sterile field,* open the prepackaged kit or equipment tray and place it between the patient's legs. If the sterile gloves are the first item on the top of the tray, put them on. Place the sterile drape under the patient's hips. Then drape the patient's lower abdomen with the sterile fenestrated drape so that only the genital area remains exposed (as shown in next column).[7] Take care not to contaminate your gloves if you have them on already.

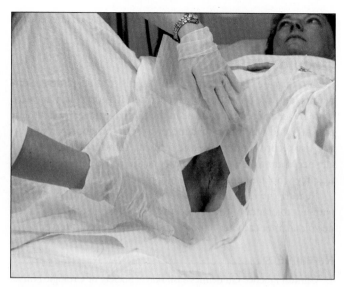

■ Open the rest of the kit or tray. Put on the sterile gloves if you haven't already done so.

■ Make sure the patient isn't allergic to iodine solution; if she is allergic, another antiseptic cleaning agent must be used.

■ Tear open the packet of antiseptic cleaning solution, and use it to saturate the sterile cotton balls or applicators. Be careful not to spill the solution on the equipment.

■ Open the packet of water-soluble lubricant, and apply it to the catheter tip; attach the drainage bag to the other end of the catheter. (If you're using a commercial kit, the drainage bag may already be attached.) Make sure all tubing ends remain sterile, and be sure the clamp at the emptying port of the drainage bag is closed *to prevent urine leakage from the bag.* Some drainage systems have an air-lock chamber *to prevent bacteria from traveling to the bladder from urine in the drainage bag.*

Note: Some urologists and nurses use a syringe prefilled with water-soluble lubricant and instill the lubricant directly into the female urethra, instead of on the catheter tip. *This method helps prevent trauma to the urethral lining as well as possible urinary tract infection.* Check your facility's policy.

■ Before inserting the catheter, inflate the balloon, as appropriate, with sterile water *to inspect it for leaks.* Be aware that some manufacturers recommend not inflating the balloon before insertion *because of the risk of microtears that may cause infection.* If you're unsure whether a balloon should be pretested, check the manufacturer's instructions included with the kit.

NURSING ALERT *Don't pretest balloons on silicone catheters.* Pretesting can cause a crease at the base of the balloon that can traumatize the urethra on insertion.

■ If you're pretesting the balloon, attach the water-filled syringe to the luer-lock; then push the plunger and check for seepage as the balloon expands (as shown on next page top). Aspirate the water to deflate the balloon. Also inspect the catheter for resiliency. *Rough, cracked catheters can injure the urethral mucosa during insertion, which can predispose the patient to infection.*

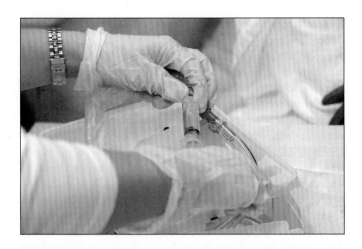

■ Separate the labia majora and labia minora as widely as possible with the thumb, middle, and index fingers of your nondominant hand so you have a full view of the urinary meatus. Keep the labia well separated throughout the procedure (as shown below), *so they don't obscure the urinary meatus or contaminate the area when it's cleaned.*

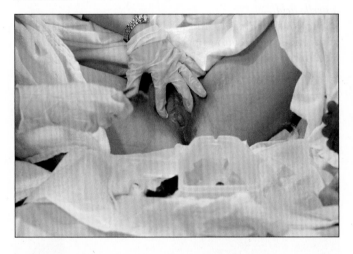

■ With your dominant hand, use a sterile, antiseptic-soaked, cotton-tipped applicator (or pick up a sterile cotton ball with the plastic forceps) and wipe one side of the urinary meatus with a downward motion (as shown below).[7]

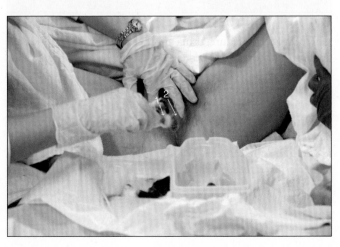

■ Wipe the other side with another sterile applicator or cotton ball in the same way. Then wipe directly over the meatus with still another sterile applicator or cotton ball. Take care not to contaminate your sterile glove.

■ Repeat the procedure, using another sterile applicator or cotton ball and taking care not to contaminate your sterile glove.

■ Pick up the catheter with your dominant hand, holding it 2″ to 3″ (5.1 to 7.6 cm) from the tip, and prepare to insert the lubricated tip into the urinary meatus.[7] *To facilitate insertion by relaxing the sphincter,* ask the patient to cough as you insert the catheter. Tell her to breathe deeply and slowly *to further relax the sphincter and reduce spasms.*

NURSING ALERT *Never force a catheter during insertion. Maneuver it gently as the patient bears down or coughs. If you still meet resistance, stop and notify the doctor. Sphincter spasms, strictures, or misplacement in the vagina may cause resistance.*

■ Advance the catheter 2″ to 3″ while continuing to hold the labia apart (as shown below)—until urine begins to flow.[7] If the catheter is inadvertently inserted into the vagina, leave it there as a landmark. Then begin the procedure over again using new supplies.

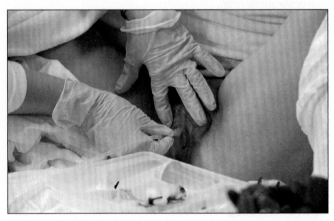

■ When urine stops flowing, attach the water-filled syringe to the luer lock.

■ Push the plunger and inflate the balloon (as shown below) *to keep the catheter in place in the bladder.*[7]

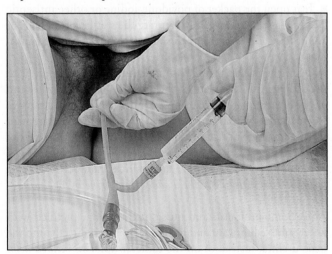

NURSING ALERT *Never inflate a balloon without first establishing urine flow, which assures you that the catheter is in the bladder.*

■ Hang the collection bag below bladder level *to prevent urine reflux into the bladder, which can cause infection, and to facilitate gravity drainage of the bladder.* Make sure the tubing doesn't get tangled in the bed's side rails.[1,2,3]

■ Tape the catheter to the patient's thigh *to prevent possible tension on the urogenital trigone.*[1,7]

■ As an alternative, secure the catheter to the patient's thigh using a leg band with a Velcro closure. *This method decreases skin irritation, especially in patients with long-term indwelling catheters.*

■ Dispose of all used supplies in the appropriate receptacles.

■ Remove your gloves and discard. Perform hand hygiene.[1,4,5,6,7]

■ Document the procedure.[11,12]

For a male patient

■ Place the patient in the supine position with his legs extended and flat on the bed. Ask the patient to hold the position *to give you a clear view of the urinary meatus and to prevent contamination of the sterile field.*

■ Perform hand hygiene and put on gloves.[1,4,5,6,7]

■ Use the washcloth to clean the patient's genital area and perineum thoroughly with soap and water. Dry the area with the towel.

■ Remove your gloves and perform hand hygiene again.[1,4,5,6,7]

■ Place the linen-saver pads on the bed between the patient's legs and under the hips.

■ *To create the sterile field,* open the prepackaged kit or equipment tray and place it next to the patient's hip. If the sterile gloves are the first item on the top of the tray, put them on. Place the sterile drape under the patient's hips. Then drape the patient's lower abdomen with the sterile fenestrated drape so that only the genital area remains exposed.[8] Take care not to contaminate your gloves if you have them on already.

■ Open the rest of the kit or tray. Put on the sterile gloves if you haven't already done so.

■ Make sure the patient isn't allergic to iodine solution; if he is allergic, another antiseptic cleaning agent must be used.

■ Tear open the packet of povidone-iodine or other antiseptic cleaning agent, and use it to saturate the sterile cotton balls or applicators. Be careful not to spill the solution on the equipment.

■ Open the packet of water-soluble lubricant and apply it to the catheter tip.[8] Then attach the drainage bag to the other end of the catheter. (If you're using a commercial kit, the drainage bag may already be attached.) Make sure all tubing ends remain sterile, and be sure the clamp at the emptying port of the drainage bag is closed *to prevent urine leakage from the bag.* Some drainage systems have an air-lock chamber *to prevent bacteria from traveling to the bladder from urine in the drainage bag.*

Note: Some urologists and nurses use a syringe prefilled with water-soluble lubricant and instill the lubricant directly into the male urethra, instead of on the catheter tip. *This method helps*

prevent trauma to the urethral lining as well as possible urinary tract infection. Check your facility's policy.

■ Before inserting the catheter, inflate the balloon, as appropriate, with sterile water *to inspect it for leaks.* Be aware that some manufacturers recommend not inflating the balloon before insertion *because of the risk of microtears that may cause infection.* If you're unsure whether a balloon should be pretested, check the manufacturer's instructions included with the kit.

NURSING ALERT *Don't pretest balloons on silicone catheters.* Pretesting can cause a crease at the base of the balloon that can traumatize the urethra on insertion.

■ If you're pretesting the balloon, attach the water-filled syringe to the luer lock; then push the plunger and check for seepage as the balloon expands. Aspirate the water to deflate the balloon. Also inspect the catheter for resiliency. *Rough, cracked catheters can injure the urethral mucosa during insertion, which can predispose the patient to infection.*

■ Hold the penis with your nondominant hand. If the patient is uncircumcised, retract the foreskin. Then gently lift and stretch the penis to a 60- to 90-degree angle.[8] Hold the penis this way throughout the procedure *to straighten the urethra and maintain a sterile field.*

■ Use your dominant hand to clean the glans with a sterile, antiseptic-soaked, cotton-tipped applicator or sterile cotton ball held in the forceps. Clean in a circular motion, starting at the urinary meatus and working outward (as shown below).[8]

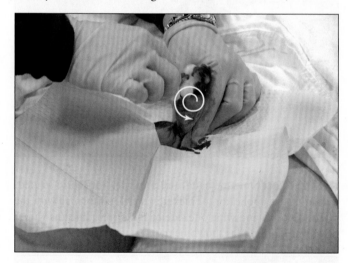

■ Repeat the procedure, using another sterile, antiseptic-soaked applicator or cotton ball and taking care not to contaminate your sterile glove.

■ Pick up the catheter with your dominant hand, holding it 2″ to 3″ (5.1 to 7.6 cm) from the tip, and prepare to insert the lubricated tip into the urinary meatus (as shown on next page). *To facilitate insertion by relaxing the sphincter,* ask the patient to cough as you insert the catheter. Tell him to breathe deeply and slowly *to further relax the sphincter and help prevent spasms.*[8]

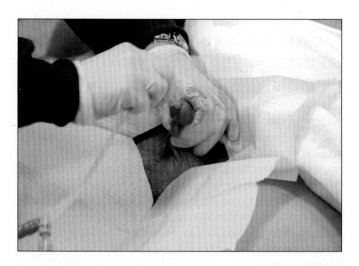

NURSING ALERT *Never force a catheter during insertion. Maneuver it gently as the patient bears down or coughs. If you still meet resistance, stop and notify the doctor.*[8] Sphincter spasms, strictures, or an enlarged prostate may cause resistance.

■ Advance the catheter to the bifurcation and check for urine flow.[8] If the foreskin was retracted, replace it *to prevent compromised circulation and painful swelling.*

■ When urine stops flowing, attach the water-filled syringe to the luer lock.

■ Push the plunger and inflate the balloon *to keep the catheter in place in the bladder.*[8]

NURSING ALERT *Never inflate a balloon without first establishing urine flow, which assures you that the catheter is in the bladder.*

■ Hang the collection bag below bladder level *to prevent urine reflux into the bladder, which can cause infection, and to facilitate gravity drainage of the bladder.*[1,2,3] Make sure the tubing doesn't get tangled in the bed's side rails.

■ Tape the catheter to the patient's abdomen or thigh *to prevent pressure on the urethra at the penoscrotal junction, which can lead to formation of urethrocutaneous fistulas. Taping this way also prevents traction on the bladder and alteration in the normal direction of urine flow in males.*

■ As an alternative, secure the catheter to the patient's thigh using a leg band with a Velcro closure. *This method decreases skin irritation, especially in patients with long-term indwelling catheters.*

■ Dispose of all used supplies in an appropriate receptacle.

■ Remove and discard your gloves. Perform hand hygiene.[1,4,5,6,7]

■ Document the procedure.[10,11]

Special considerations

■ Several types of catheters are available with balloons of various sizes. Each type has its own method of inflation and closure. For example, in one type of catheter, sterile solution or air is injected through the inflation lumen, and then the end of the injection port is folded over itself and fastened with a clamp or rubber band.

Note: Injecting a catheter with air makes identifying leaks difficult and doesn't guarantee deflation of the balloon for removal.

■ A similar catheter is inflated when a seal in the end of the inflation lumen is penetrated with a needle or the tip of the solution-filled syringe. Another type of balloon catheter self-inflates when a prepositioned clamp is loosened. The balloon size determines the amount of solution needed for inflation, and the exact amount is usually printed on the distal extension of the catheter used for inflating the balloon.

■ If the doctor orders a urine specimen for laboratory analysis, using sterile technique,[2,3] obtain it from the urine receptacle with a specimen collection container at the time of catheterization, and send it to the laboratory with the appropriate laboratory request form. Connect the drainage bag when urine stops flowing.

■ Inspect the catheter and tubing periodically while they're in place *to detect compression or kinking that could obstruct urine flow.* Explain the basic principles of gravity drainage *so that the patient realizes the importance of keeping the drainage tubing and collection bag lower than the bladder at all times.* If necessary, provide the patient with detailed instructions for performing clean intermittent self-catheterization.[1,2,3] (See "Self-catheterization," page 644.)

■ For monitoring purposes, empty the collection bag when one-half full, or every 3 to 6 hours. Excessive fluid volume may require more frequent emptying *to prevent traction on the catheter, which would cause the patient discomfort, and to prevent injury to the urethra and bladder wall.*

NURSING ALERT *Observe the patient carefully for adverse reactions caused by removing excessive volumes of residual urine, such as hypovolemic shock. Check your facility's policy beforehand to determine the maximum amount of urine that may be drained at one time (some facilities limit the amount, with upper limits ranging from 700 to 1,000 mL). Whether to limit the amount of urine drained is currently controversial. Clamp the catheter at the first sign of an adverse reaction, and notify the doctor.*

Patient teaching

If the patient will be discharged with a long-term indwelling catheter, teach the patient or family all aspects of daily catheter maintenance, including care of the skin and urinary meatus, signs and symptoms of urinary tract infection or obstruction, how to irrigate the catheter (if appropriate), and the importance of adequate fluid intake to maintain patency.

Complications

Urinary tract infection can result from the introduction of bacteria into the bladder. Improper insertion can cause traumatic injury to the urethral and bladder mucosa. Bladder atony or spasms can result from rapid decompression of a severely distended bladder.

Documentation

Record the date and time as well as the size and type of indwelling catheter used. Describe the amount, color, and other characteristics of urine emptied from the bladder. Your health care facility may require only the intake-and-output sheet for fluid-balance data. If large volumes of urine have been emptied, describe the patient's tolerance of the procedure. Note whether a urine specimen was sent for laboratory analysis.[10,11]

REFERENCES

1 Gould, C.V., et al. (2009). "Guideline for Prevention of Catheter-associated Urinary Tract Infections, 2009" [Online]. Accessed November 2011 via the Web at http://www.cdc.gov/hicpac/cauti/001_cauti.html (Level I)

2 Lo, E. (2008). Strategies to prevent catheter-associated urinary tract infections in acute care hospitals. *Infection Control and Hospital Epidemiology 29*(Suppl. 1), S41–S50. (Level I)

3 The Joint Commission. (2012). Standard NPSG.07.06.01. *Comprehensive accreditation manual for hospitals: The official handbook.* Oakbrook Terrace, IL: The Joint Commission. (Level I)

4 The Joint Commission. (2012). Standard NPSG.07.01.01. *Comprehensive accreditation manual for hospitals: The official handbook.* Oakbrook Terrace, IL: The Joint Commission. (Level I)

5 Centers for Disease Control and Prevention. (October 2002). Guideline for hand hygiene in health-care settings. *Morbidity and Mortality Weekly Report, 51*(RR-16), 1–45. (Level I)

6 World Health Organization. (2009). *WHO guidelines on hand hygiene in health care: First global patient safety challenge. Clean care is safer care.* Geneva, Switzerland: World Health Organization. (Level I)

7 Society of Urologic Nurses and Associates. (2005). "Clinical Practice Guidelines: Female Urethral Catheterization" [Online]. Accessed November 2011 via the Web at http://www.suna.org/resources/ femaleCatheterization.pdf

8 Society of Urologic Nurses and Associates. (2005). "Clinical Practice Guidelines: Male Urethral Catheterization" [Online]. Accessed November 2011 via the Web at http://www.suna.org/resources/maleCatheterization.pdf

9 The Joint Commission. (2012). Standard NPSG.01.01.01. *Comprehensive accreditation manual for hospitals: The official handbook.* Oakbrook Terrace, IL: The Joint Commission. (Level I)

10 The Joint Commission. (2012). Standard RC.01.03.01. *Comprehensive accreditation manual for hospitals: The official handbook.* Oakbrook Terrace, IL: The Joint Commission. (Level I)

11 The Joint Commission. (2012). Standard RC.02.01.01. *Comprehensive accreditation manual for hospitals: The official handbook.* Oakbrook Terrace, IL: The Joint Commission. (Level I)

ADDITIONAL REFERENCES

Godfrey, H., & Fraczyk, L. (2005). Preventing and managing catheter-associated urinary tract infections. *British Journal of Community Nursing, 105*(5), 205–206, 208–212.

Nasiriani, K., et al. (2009). Comparison of the effect of water vs. povidone-iodine solution for periurethral cleaning in women requiring an indwelling catheter prior to gynecologic surgery. *Urology Nursing, 29*(2), 118–121, 131.

Nettina, S.M. (2010). *Lippincott manual of nursing practice* (9th ed.). Philadelphia, PA: Lippincott Williams & Wilkins.

Niël-Weise, B.S., & Van den Broek, P.J. (2005). Urinary catheter policies for long-term bladder drainage. *Cochrane Database of Systemic Reviews,* (1), CD004201.

INDWELLING URINARY CATHETER IRRIGATION

Irrigation of the bladder shouldn't be done routinely. If an obstruction is anticipated, closed continuous irrigation may be used to prevent it. (See "Continuous bladder irrigation," page 207.) To relieve an obstruction resulting from clots, mucus, or other causes, an intermittent method of irrigation may be used.[1] Whenever possible, the catheter should be irrigated through a closed system to decrease the risk for infection.[2,3]

Before initiating catheter irrigation, a bladder scanner may be used to confirm whether a decrease in urine output results from a blockage or reduced urine in the bladder, reducing the number of unnecessary irrigations and minimizing breaks in the closed drainage system.[4]

If obstruction occurs and it's likely that the catheter material is contributing to obstruction, change the catheter.[2] To help prevent catheter-associated urinary tract infections, the catheter should be removed as soon as it's no longer needed.[1,2,3,4,5]

Equipment

Ordered irrigating solution (such as normal saline solution) ▪ sterile basin ▪ 30- to 60-mL syringe ▪ 18G blunt-end needle (if system isn't needleless) ▪ sterile alcohol pads ▪ gloves ▪ linen-saver pad ▪ intake-output sheet ▪ clamp.

Commercially packaged kits containing sterile irrigating solution, a graduated receptacle, and a 50-mL catheter tip syringe may be available.

Preparation of equipment

Check the expiration date on the irrigating solution. *To prevent vesical spasms during instillation of solution,* warm it to room temperature. Never heat the solution on a burner or in a microwave oven. *Hot irrigating solution can injure the patient's bladder.*

Implementation

▪ Verify the doctor's order.
▪ Perform hand hygiene.[6,7,8]
▪ Confirm the patient's identity using at least two patient identifiers according to your facility's policy.[9]
▪ Gather the equipment and supplies at the bedside.
▪ Perform hand hygiene and put on gloves.[6,7,8]
▪ Explain the procedure to the patient, and provide privacy.
▪ Empty the catheter drainage bag. Measure the amount of urine, noting the color and characteristics of the urine.
▪ Expose the catheter's aspiration port and place a linen-saver pad under it *to protect the bed linens.*
▪ Create a sterile field at the patient's bedside. Using sterile technique, pour the prescribed amount of solution into the basin.
▪ Place the tip of the syringe into the solution and fill the syringe with the appropriate amount (as shown on next page top).

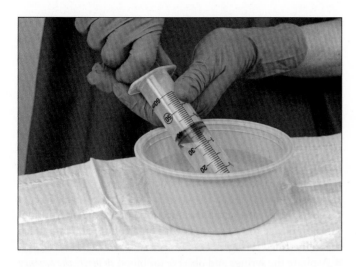

■ Clean the aspiration port with an alcohol pad (as shown below) *to remove as many bacterial contaminants as possible.*

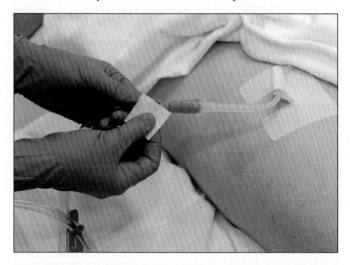

■ Clamp the catheter tubing below the aspiration port (as shown below).

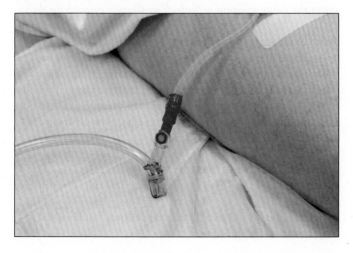

■ Attach the syringe to the port, or insert the blunt-tip needle into the port if a needleless system isn't in place.

■ Instill the irrigating solution into the catheter. If necessary, refill the syringe and repeat this step until you've instilled the prescribed amount of irrigating solution.

■ Remove the syringe and unclamp the drainage tube *to allow the irrigant and urine to flow into the drainage bags.*

■ Make sure the catheter tubing is secured to the patient's leg and that the drainage bag is below the level of the bladder.[1,2,3,5]

■ Dispose of all used supplies in the appropriate receptacle.

■ Remove your gloves and perform hand hygiene.[6,7,8]

■ Document the procedure.[10,11]

Special considerations

■ If you encounter any resistance during instillation of the irrigating solution, don't try to force the solution into the bladder. Instead, stop the procedure and notify the doctor. If an indwelling catheter becomes totally obstructed, obtain an order to remove it and replace it with a new one *to prevent bladder distention, acute renal failure, urinary stasis, and subsequent infection.*

■ Encourage catheterized patients not on restricted fluid intake to increase intake to 30 mL/kg/day *to help flush the urinary system and reduce sediment formation.*[3]

Documentation

Note the amount, color, and consistency of return urine flow, and document the patient's tolerance for the procedure. Also note any resistance during instillation of the solution. If the return flow volume is less than the amount of solution instilled, note this on the intake-and-output balance sheets and in your notes.[10,11]

REFERENCES

1 Lo, E. (2008). Strategies to prevent catheter-associated urinary tract infections in acute care hospitals. *Infection Control and Hospital Epidemiology 29*(Suppl. 1), S41–S50.

2 Gould, C.V., et al. (2009). "Guideline for Prevention of Catheter-associated Urinary Tract Infections, 2009" [Online]. Accessed November 2011 via the Web at http://www.cdc.gov/hicpac/cauti/001_cauti.html (Level I)

3 Clinical Practice Guidelines Task Force; Society of Urologic Nurses and Associates. (2006). Care of the patient with an indwelling catheter. *Urologic Nursing, 26*(1), 80–81. (Level I)

4 Association for Professionals in Infection Control and Epidemiology. (2008). "Guide to the Elimination of Catheter-Associated Urinary Tract Infections (CAUTIs)" [Online]. Accessed November 2011 via the Web at http://www.apic.org/Content/NavigationMenu/PracticeGuidance/APICEliminationGuides/CAUTI_Guide.pdf

5 The Joint Commission. (2012). Standard NPSG.07.06.01. *Comprehensive accreditation manual for hospitals: The official handbook.* Oakbrook Terrace, IL: The Joint Commission. (Level I)

6 The Joint Commission. (2012). Standard NPSG.07.01.01. *Comprehensive accreditation manual for hospitals: The official handbook.* Oakbrook Terrace, IL: The Joint Commission. (Level I)

7 Centers for Disease Control and Prevention. (October 2002). Guideline for hand hygiene in health-care settings. *Morbidity and Mortality Weekly Report, 51*(RR-16), 1–45. (Level I)

8 World Health Organization. (2009). *WHO guidelines on hand hygiene in health care: First global patient safety challenge. Clean care is safer care.* Geneva, Switzerland: World Health Organization. (Level I)

9 The Joint Commission. (2012). Standard NPSG.01.01.01. *Comprehensive accreditation manual for hospitals: The official handbook.* Oakbrook Terrace, IL: The Joint Commission. (Level I)

10 The Joint Commission. (2012). Standard RC.01.03.01. *Comprehensive accreditation manual for hospitals: The official handbook.* Oakbrook Terrace, IL: The Joint Commission. (Level I)

11 The Joint Commission. (2012). Standard RC.02.01.01. *Comprehensive accreditation manual for hospitals: The official handbook.* Oakbrook Terrace, IL: The Joint Commission. (Level I)

Additional references

Nettina, S.M. (2010). *Lippincott manual of nursing practice* (9th ed.). Philadelphia, PA: Lippincott Williams & Wilkins.

Taylor, C., et al. (2011). *Fundamentals of nursing: The art and science of nursing care* (7th ed.). Philadelphia, PA: Lippincott Williams & Wilkins.

Intermittent infusion device drug administration

An intermittent infusion injection device, or *saline lock,* eliminates the need for multiple venipunctures or for maintaining venous access with a continuous IV infusion. This device allows intermittent administration by infusion or by IV bolus injection.

Equipment

Patient's medical record, including medication record ■ gloves ■ antiseptic pads (alcohol, tincture of iodine, or chlorhexidine-based) ■ two prefilled preservative-free normal saline flush syringes ■ prescribed medication in an IV container with administration set (for infusion) or in a syringe (for IV bolus) ■ labels ■ Optional: extra intermittent infusion device.

Implementation

■ Avoid distractions and interruptions when preparing and administering medications *to prevent medication errors.*[1]

■ Verify the order on the patient's medication record by checking it against the doctor's order.[2,3]

■ Compare the medication label to the doctor's order to verify the correct medication, indication, dose, route, and time of administration.[3]

■ Check the expiration date; return the medication to the pharmacy if it's expired.[3]

■ Check the patient's medical record for any allergy or other contraindication to the prescribed medication. If an allergy or other contraindication is present, don't administer the medication and notify the doctor.[3]

■ Visually inspect the medication for discoloration or any other loss of integrity. Don't administer the medication if its integrity is compromised.[3]

■ Perform hand hygiene.[4,5,6,7]

■ If you'll be infusing medication, insert the administration set spike into the IV container, attach the needleless adapter, and prime the line. If you'll be giving an IV injection, fill a syringe with the prescribed drug and label it.[8]

■ Confirm the patient's identity using at least two patient identifiers according to your facility's policy.[9,10]

■ If your facility uses a bar code scanning system, be sure to scan your identification badge, the patient's identification bracelet, and the medication's bar code or follow the procedure for your facility's bar code system.

■ Explain the procedure to the patient.

■ Put on gloves.[11]

■ Assess the IV site. Scrub the injection port of the intermittent infusion device for 15 seconds with an alcohol pad, and attach the saline-filled syringe.[12]

■ Aspirate the syringe and observe for blood *to verify the patency of the device.*[10] Flush the catheter with the preservative-free normal saline solution.

NURSING ALERT *Stop the injection immediately if you feel any resistance* because resistance indicates that the device is occluded. *If resistance occurs, remove the device and insert a new intermittent infusion device.*

■ If you feel no resistance, watch for signs and symptoms of infiltration (puffiness or pain at the site) as you slowly inject the saline solution. If these occur, insert a new intermittent infusion device.

■ Remove the saline syringe.

Administering IV bolus injections

■ Thoroughly disinfect the injection port with an antiseptic pad using friction.[12]

■ Insert the syringe with the medication for the IV bolus injection into the injection port of the device.

■ Inject the medication at the required rate. Then remove the syringe from the injection port.

■ Thoroughly disinfect the injection port with an antiseptic pad using friction.[12]

■ Attach the saline-filled syringe into the injection port and slowly inject the saline solution *to flush all medication through the device.*

Administering an infusion

■ Insert the administration set attached to the infusion bag.

■ Open the infusion line, and adjust the flow rate as necessary.

■ Infuse medication for the prescribed length of time; then disinfect the port, and flush the device with preservative-free normal saline solution, as you would after a bolus or push injection, according to your facility's policy.

Completing the procedures

■ Dispose of the used equipment in the appropriate receptacle.[11,13]

■ Remove and discard your gloves, and perform hand hygiene.[4,5,6,7]

■ Document the procedure.[10,14,15]

Special considerations

■ Intermittent infusion devices should be changed regularly (usually every 96 hours), according to standard precautions guidelines and your facility's policy.[12]

■ Before administering an injectable drug, make sure you know the prescribed infusion rate and infusion time period.

Complications

Infiltration and a specific reaction to the infused medication are the most common complications.

Documentation

Record the type and amount of drug administered and times of administration. Include all IV solutions used to dilute the medication and flush the line on the intake record. Also document the use of saline solution.

REFERENCES

1 Westbrook, J. et al. (2010). Association of interruptions with an increased risk and severity of medication administration errors. *Archives of Internal Medicine, 170*(8), 683–690.

2 The Joint Commission. (2012). Standard MM.04.01.01. *Comprehensive accreditation manual for hospitals: The official handbook.* Oakbrook Terrace, IL: The Joint Commission. (Level I)

3 The Joint Commission. (2012). Standard MM.06.01.01. *Comprehensive accreditation manual for hospitals: The official handbook.* Oakbrook Terrace, IL: The Joint Commission. (Level I)

4 Centers for Disease Control and Prevention. (October 2002). Guideline for hand hygiene in health-care settings. *Morbidity and Mortality Weekly Report, 51*(RR-16), 1–45. (Level I)

5 The Joint Commission. (2012). Standard NPSG.07.01.01. *Comprehensive accreditation manual for hospitals: The official handbook.* Oakbrook Terrace, IL: The Joint Commission. (Level I)

6 Standard 19. Hand hygiene. Infusion nursing standards of practice. (2011). *Journal of Infusion Nursing, 34*(1S), S26–27. (Level I)

7 World Health Organization. (2009). *WHO guidelines on hand hygiene in health care: First global patient safety challenge. Clean care is safer care.* Geneva, Switzerland: World Health Organization. (Level I)

8 Standard 45. Flushing and locking. Infusion nursing standards of practice. (2011). *Journal of Infusion Nursing, 34*(1S), S59–63. (Level I)

9 The Joint Commission. (2012). Standard NPSG.01.01.01. *Comprehensive accreditation manual for hospitals: The official handbook.* Oakbrook Terrace, IL: The Joint Commission. (Level I)

10 Standard 61. Parenteral medication and solution administration. Infusion nursing standards of practice. (2011). *Journal of Infusion Nursing, 34*(1S), S86.

11 Occupational Safety and Health Administration. "Bloodborne Pathogens, Standard Number 1910.1030" [Online]. Accessed November 2011 via the Web at http://www.osha.gov/pls/oshaweb/owadisp.show_document?p_table=STANDARDS&p_id=10051

12 O'Grady, N.P., et al. (2011). "Guidelines for the Prevention of Intravascular Catheter-Related Infections" [Online]. Accessed November 2011 via the Web at http://www.cdc.gov/hicpac/pdf/guidelines/bsi-guidelines-2011.pdf

13 Standard 22. Safe handling and disposal of sharps, hazardous material, and hazardous waste: Infusion nursing standards of practice. (2011). *Journal of Infusion Nursing, 34*(1S), S28.

14 The Joint Commission. (2012). Standard RC.01.03.01. *Comprehensive accreditation manual for hospitals: The official handbook.* Oakbrook Terrace, IL: The Joint Commission. (Level I)

15 The Joint Commission. (2012). Standard RC.02.01.01. *Comprehensive accreditation manual for hospitals: The official handbook.* Oakbrook Terrace, IL: The Joint Commission. (Level I)

ADDITIONAL REFERENCES

Alexander, M., et al. (Eds.). (2010). *Infusion nursing: An evidence-based approach* (3rd ed.). Philadelphia, PA: Elsevier.

Infusion Nurses Society. (2011). *Policies and procedures for infusion nursing* (4th ed.). Boston, MA: Infusion Nurses Society.

Nettina, S.M. (2010). *Lippincott manual of nursing practice* (9th ed.). Philadelphia, PA: Lippincott Williams & Wilkins.

Scales, K. (2008). Intravenous therapy: A guide to good practice. *British Journal of Nursing, 17*(19), S4–S12.

Standard 19. Hand hygiene. Infusion nursing standards of practice. (2011). *Journal of Infusion Nursing, 34*(1S), S26–27. (Level I)

Standard 22. Safe handling and disposal of sharps, hazardous materials, and hazardous waste. Infusion nursing standards of practice. (2011). *Journal of Infusion Nursing, 34*(1S), S28. (Level I)

Standard 61. Parenteral medication and solution administration. Infusion nursing standards of practice. (2011). *Journal of Infusion Nursing, 34*(1S), S86. (Level I)

Taylor, C., et al. (2011). *Fundamentals of nursing: The art and science of nursing care* (7th ed.). Philadelphia, PA: Lippincott Williams & Wilkins.

INTERMITTENT INFUSION DEVICE INSERTION

Also called a *saline lock,* an intermittent infusion device consists of a catheter with an injection cap attached. Filled with saline solution to prevent blood clot formation, the device maintains venous access in patients who are receiving IV medication regularly or intermittently but who don't require continuous infusion. An intermittent infusion device is superior to an IV line that's maintained at a moderately slow infusion rate because it minimizes the risk of fluid overload and electrolyte imbalance. It also cuts costs, reduces the risk of contamination by eliminating IV solution containers and administration sets, increases patient comfort and mobility, reduces patient anxiety, and, if inserted in a large vein, allows collection of multiple blood samples without repeated venipuncture.

For intermittent infusion device insertion, choose a vein on the dorsal and ventral surfaces of the upper extremities, including the metacarpal, cephalic, basilic, and median veins. When choosing a site, avoid areas of flexion; areas where there is pain on palpation; veins that are compromised by bruising, infiltration, phlebitis, sclerosis, or cord formation; and areas where procedures are planned. Because of the risk of nerve damage, avoid the lateral surface of the wrist for about 4 to 5 inches. Also avoid the ventral surface of the wrist because of the associated pain on insertion and the risk of nerve damage. Avoid using veins of the lower extremities because of the increased risk of tissue damage, thrombophlebitis, and ulceration. In a patient who has had breast surgery with axillary node dissection, don't use veins in the upper extremity on the affected side; also don't choose veins on an extremity affected by radiation therapy, lymphedema, or stroke.

If the patient has stage 4 or 5 chronic kidney disease, avoid using upper arm veins or forearms that could be used for dialysis access. Collaborate with the patient and his doctor to discuss the risks and benefits of using a vein in an affected extremity if no other options exist.[1]

Equipment

IV access device with safety shield[2] ▪ needleless system device ▪ syringe prefilled with preservative-free normal saline solution ▪ single-use tourniquet (preferably latex-free) ▪ antiseptic pads (alcohol, tincture of iodine, or chlorhexidine-based) ▪ chlorhexidine solution (tincture of iodine, povidone iodine, or alcohol may be used if contraindication exists to chlorhexidine) ▪ transparent semipermeable dressing ▪ catheter securement device, sterile hypoallergenic tape, or sterile surgical strips ▪ gloves ▪ Optional: soap and water, arm board, warm packs, ultrasound device with sterile probe cover, sterile ultrasound gel, local anesthetic, scissors or clippers.

Implementation

▪ Perform hand hygiene.[3,4,5,6]
▪ Confirm the patient's identity using at least two patient identifiers according to your facility's policy.[7]
▪ Explain the procedure to the patient, and describe the purpose of the intermittent infusion device. Provide the patient with information about the insertion process, expected duration of therapy, care and maintenance of the device, and signs and symptoms of complications and when to report them.
▪ Remove the set from its packaging, disinfect the port with an antiseptic pad, and inject preservative-free normal saline solution to fill the tubing and needleless system. *This process removes air from the system, preventing formation of an air embolus.*
▪ Select the puncture site. If long-term therapy is anticipated, start with a vein at the most distal site *so that you can move proximally as needed for subsequent IV insertion sites.*[8] For infusion of an irritating medication, choose a large vein distal to any nearby joint. Make sure the intended vein can accommodate the cannula.
▪ Place the patient in a comfortable, reclining position, leaving his arm in a dependent position *to increase venous fill of the lower arms and hands.* If the patient's skin is cold, cover the entire arm with warm packs for 5 to 10 minutes.

Applying the tourniquet

▪ Apply a tourniquet about 4″ to 6″ (10 to 15 cm) above the intended puncture site to dilate the vein. Check for a radial pulse. If it isn't present, release the tourniquet and reapply it with less tension *to prevent arterial occlusion.*[9]
▪ Lightly palpate the vein with the index and middle fingers of your nondominant hand. Stretch the skin *to anchor the vein.* If the vein feels hard or ropelike, select another.
▪ If the vein is easily palpable but not sufficiently dilated, one or more of the following techniques may help raise the vein: Place the extremity in a dependent position for several seconds, or lightly

stroke the vessel downward; if you have selected a vein in the arm or hand, tell the patient to open and close his fist several times.
▪ Leave the tourniquet in place for no more than 3 minutes. If you can't find a suitable vein and prepare the site in that time, release the tourniquet for a few minutes. Then reapply it and continue the procedure.

Preparing the site

▪ If the intended insertion site is visibly soiled, clean it with soap and water before applying the antiseptic solution.[8]
▪ Clip the hair around the insertion site with scissors or electric clippers if needed.[3,8]
▪ Administer a local anesthetic if indicated and prescribed.[3]
▪ Disinfect the site with chlorhexidine using a back-and-forth scrubbing motion for 30 seconds *to remove flora that would otherwise be introduced into the vascular system with the venipuncture.* Allow the antiseptic to dry.[3,8]
▪ Reapply the tourniquet.
▪ Use the ultrasound device with a sterile probe cover to locate the vein if necessary.
▪ Using the thumb of your nondominant hand, stretch the skin taut below the puncture site to stabilize the vein.
▪ Grasp the access cannula with your dominant hand, remove the cover, and examine the cannula tip.[8] If the edge isn't smooth, discard and replace the device.

Inserting the device

▪ Tell the patient that you are about to insert the device.
▪ Hold the needle bevel up and enter the skin directly over the vein at a 0 to 15 degree angle.
▪ Aggressively push the needle directly through the skin and into the vein in one motion. Check the flashback chamber behind the hub for blood return, *signifying that the vein has been properly accessed.* (You may not see a blood return in a small vein.)
▪ Then level the insertion device slightly by lifting the tip of the device up *to prevent puncturing the back wall of the vein with the access device.*
▪ Advance the needle fully, if possible, and hold it in place.
▪ Release the tourniquet, open the administration set clamp slightly, and check for free flow or infiltration.
▪ Release the tourniquet and remove the inner needle. While stabilizing the vein with one hand, use the other to advance the catheter into the vein.
▪ After the venous access device has been inserted, clean the skin completely.
▪ Secure the catheter using a catheter securement device, sterile hypoallergenic tape, or sterile surgical strips. Apply a transparent semipermeable dressing.[3,10,11]
▪ Loop the tubing, if applicable, *so the injection port is free and easily accessible.*
▪ Thoroughly disinfect the needleless injection portion with an antiseptic pad using friction and allow it to dry.
▪ Attach a prefilled syringe of preservative-free normal saline solution to the needleless injection port. Slowly aspirate until a brisk blood return is obtained and then slowly flush the catheter with the preservative-free normal saline solution.[12,13]

■ Clamp the catheter to reduce blood reflux; the clamping sequence depends on the type of needleless port used. For a positive-pressure needleless port, clamp the catheter after removing the syringe; for a negative-pressure needleless port, maintain pressure on the syringe plunger while clamping the catheter; for a neutral needleless port, clamp the device before or after disconnecting the syringe.[12]

■ On the dressing label, write the time, date, and your initials and the gauge and length of the catheter; place the label on the dressing.[10]

■ Discard used supplies in the appropriate receptacle.

■ Remove and discard your gloves and perform hand hygiene.[3,4,5,6]

■ Document the procedure.[14,15]

Special considerations

■ According to the Centers for Disease Control and Prevention, there is no need to replace peripheral IV catheters more frequently than every 72 to 96 hours.[3]

■ If the patient feels a burning sensation during the injection of saline, stop the injection and check cannula placement. If the cannula is in the vein, inject the saline at a slower rate *to minimize irritation.* If the cannula isn't in the vein, remove and discard it. Then select a new venipuncture site and, using fresh equipment, restart the procedure.

■ If the doctor orders discontinuing an IV infusion and inserting an intermittent infusion device in its place, convert the existing line by disconnecting the IV tubing and inserting a male adapter plug into the device. (See *Converting an IV line to an intermittent infusion device.*)

Complications

Use of an intermittent infusion device has the same potential complications as the use of a peripheral IV catheter. (See "IV catheter insertion and removal," page 421.)

Documentation

Record the date and time of insertion; type, brand, and gauge and length of the vascular access device; anatomic location of the insertion site; the patient's tolerance of the procedure; the number and location of attempts; and functionality of the device. Record the local anesthetic, if used, site preparation, and whether an ultrasound device was used to guide the insertion.[14,15]

REFERENCES

1 Standard 33. Site selection. Infusion nursing standards of practice. (2011). *Journal of Infusion Nursing, 34*(1S), S40–43. (Level I)

2 Standard 32. Vascular access device selection. Infusion nursing standards of practice. (2011). *Journal of Infusion Nursing, 34*(1S), S37–40. (Level I)

3 O'Grady, N.P., et al. (2011). "Guidelines for the Prevention of Intravascular Catheter-Related Infections" [Online]. Accessed November 2011 via the Web at http://www.cdc.gov/hicpac/pdf/guidelines/bsi-guidelines-2011.pdf

4 The Joint Commission. (2012). Standard NPSG.07.01.01. *Comprehensive accreditation manual for hospitals: The official handbook.* Oakbrook Terrace, IL: The Joint Commission. (Level I)

Converting an IV line to an intermittent infusion device

Many types of adapter caps allow you to convert an existing IV line into an intermittent infusion device. To make the conversion, follow these steps:

■ Prime the male adapter plug with normal saline solution.

■ Clamp the IV tubing and remove the administration set from the cannula hub.

■ Insert the male adapter cap.

■ Flush the access with the remaining solution *to prevent clot formation.*

Short male adapter
This short luer-lock adapter cap twists into place.

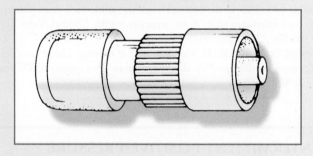

5 Standard 19. Hand hygiene. Infusion nursing standards of practice. (2011). *Journal of Infusion Nursing, 34*(1S), S26–27. (Level I)

6 World Health Organization. (2009). *WHO guidelines on hand hygiene in health care: First global patient safety challenge. Clean care is safer care.* Geneva, Switzerland: World Health Organization. (Level I)

7 The Joint Commission. (2012). Standard NPSG.01.01.01. *Comprehensive accreditation manual for hospitals: The official handbook.* Oakbrook Terrace, IL: The Joint Commission. (Level I)

8 Standard 35. Vascular access site preparation and device placement. Infusion nursing standards of practice. (2011). *Journal of Infusion Nursing, 34*(1S), S44. (Level I)

9 Standard 31. Tourniquets. Infusion nursing standards of practice. (2011). *Journal of Infusion Nursing, 34*(1S), S36. (Level I)

10 Standard 46. Vascular access device site care and dressing changes. Infusion nursing standards of practice. (2011). *Journal of Infusion Nursing, 34*(1S), S63–64. (Level I)

11 Standard 36. Vascular access device stabilization. Infusion nursing standards of practice. (2011). *Journal of Infusion Nursing, 34*(1S), S46. (Level I)

12 Infusion Nurses Society. (2011). *Policies and procedures for infusion nursing* (4th ed.). Boston, MA: Infusion Nurses Society.

13 Standard 45. Flushing and locking. Infusion nursing standards of practice. (2011). *Journal of Infusion Nursing, 34*(1S), S59–63. (Level I)

14 The Joint Commission. (2012). Standard RC.01.03.01. *Comprehensive accreditation manual for hospitals: The official handbook.* Oakbrook Terrace, IL: The Joint Commission. (Level I)

15 The Joint Commission. (2012). Standard RC.02.01.01. *Comprehensive accreditation manual for hospitals: The official handbook.* Oakbrook Terrace, IL: The Joint Commission. (Level I)

ADDITIONAL REFERENCES

Alexander, M., et al. (Eds.). (2010). *Infusion nursing: An evidence-based approach* (3rd ed.). Philadelphia, PA: Elsevier.

Aziz, A.M. (2009). Improving peripheral IV cannula care: Implementing high-impact interventions. *British Journal of Nursing, 18*(20), 1242–1246.

Infusion Nurses Society. (2008). *Flushing protocols.* Boston, MA: Infusion Nurses Society.

Lee, W.L., et al. (2009). Risk factors for peripheral intravenous catheter infection in hospitalized patients: A prospective study of 3165 patients. *American Journal of Infection Control, 37*(8), 683–686.

Mok, E., et al. (2007). A randomized controlled trial for maintaining peripheral intravenous lock in children. *International Journal of Nursing Practice, 13*(1), 33–45.

Nettina, S.M. (2010). *Lippincott manual of nursing practice* (9th ed.). Philadelphia, PA: Lippincott Williams & Wilkins.

Scales, K. (2008). Intravenous therapy: A guide to good practice. *British Journal of Nursing, 17*(19), S4–S12.

Szablewski, S.G., et al. (2009). Describing saline-lock usage patterns on a telemetry unit: A retrospective study. *Clinical Nurse Specialist, 23*(6), 296–304.

Taylor, C., et al. (2011). *Fundamentals of nursing: The art and science of nursing care* (7th ed.). Philadelphia, PA: Lippincott Williams & Wilkins.

INTERMITTENT POSITIVE-PRESSURE BREATHING

Intermittent positive-pressure breathing (IPPB) delivers room air or oxygen into the lungs at a pressure higher than atmospheric pressure. This delivery ceases when pressure in the mouth or in the breathing circuit tube increases to a predetermined airway pressure.

IPPB was formerly the mainstay of pulmonary therapy, with its proponents claiming that the device delivered aerosolized medications deeper into the lungs, decreased the work of breathing, and assisted in the mobilization of secretions. Studies now show that IPPB has no clinical benefit over handheld nebulizers. However, it continues to be used selectively to treat atelectasis not responsive to other procedures, such as incentive spirometry or chest physiotherapy.[1]

Equipment

IPPB machine with all necessary circuit tubing ▪ mouthpiece or mask ▪ noseclips, if necessary ▪ source of pressurized gas at 50 psi, if necessary ▪ oxygen, if desired ▪ prescribed medication and normal saline solution ▪ 3-mL syringe ▪ sphygmomanometer ▪ stethoscope ▪ specimen cup or facial tissues and waste bag ▪ warm, soapy water ▪ Optional: suction equipment.

Preparation of equipment

Follow the manufacturer's instructions to set up the equipment properly. Label all medications, medication containers, and other solutions.

Implementation

▪ Verify the doctor's orders.
▪ Perform hand hygiene and follow standard precautions.[2,3,4]
▪ Confirm the patient's identity using at least two patient identifiers according to your facility's policy.[5]
▪ Explain the procedure to the patient *to decrease anxiety and ensure his cooperation.*
▪ Tell the patient to sit erect in a chair, if possible, *to allow for optimal lung expansion.* Otherwise, place him in semi-Fowler's position.
▪ Take baseline blood pressure and heart rate measurements, especially if a bronchodilator will be administered, and listen to breath sounds *for posttreatment comparisons.*
▪ Instill the ordered medication or normal saline solution into the nebulizer cup. Turn on the IPPB machine at the appropriate settings as determined by the doctor or respiratory therapist.
▪ Instruct the patient to breathe deeply and slowly through his mouth as if sucking on a straw. Encourage the patient to let the machine do the work.
▪ During treatment, instruct the patient to hold his breath for a few seconds after full inspiration *to allow for greater distribution of gas and medication.* Then instruct him to exhale normally.
▪ During treatment, take the patient's blood pressure and heart rate. *IPPB treatment increases intrathoracic pressure and may temporarily decrease cardiac output and venous return, resulting in tachycardia, hypotension, or headache. Monitoring also detects reactions to the bronchodilator.* If you find a sudden change in blood pressure or increase in heart rate by 20 or more beats per minute, stop the treatment and notify the doctor.
▪ If the patient is tolerating the treatment, continue until the medication in the nebulizer is exhausted, usually about 10 minutes.
▪ After treatment, or as needed, have the patient either expectorate into tissues and discard them in a waste bag or expectorate in a specimen cup; alternatively, you can suction him as necessary. Listen to his breath sounds, and compare them with the pretreatment assessment.
▪ Shake excess moisture from the nebulizer and the mouthpiece or mask. After 24 hours of use, either discard the equipment or clean it with warm, soapy water. Then remove the equipment, rinse with sterile water, and air dry. When it's dry, store it in a clean plastic bag.
▪ Perform hand hygiene.[2,3,4]
▪ Document the procedure.[6,7]

Special considerations

▪ If possible, avoid administering IPPB treatment immediately before or after a meal *because the treatment may induce nausea and because a full stomach reduces lung expansion.*
▪ Never give IPPB treatment without medication or sterile saline in the nebulizer, *which could dry the patient's airways and make secretions more difficult to mobilize.*
▪ If the purpose of treatment is to mobilize secretions, use a specimen cup to measure the secretions obtained.
▪ If the patient wears dentures, leave them in place *to ensure a proper seal,* but remove them if they slide out of position.

■ If the patient has an artificial airway, use a special adapter, such as mechanical ventilation tubing, to give IPPB treatments.

■ When using a mask to administer treatments, allow the patient frequent rest periods, and observe for gastric distention *because this issue is more likely to occur with a mask.*

■ If the patient's blood pressure is stable during the initial treatment, you may not need to check it during subsequent treatments unless he has a history of cardiovascular disease, hypotension, or sensitivity to any drug delivered in the treatment.

Patient teaching

If the patient will be using IPPB at home, provide appropriate patient teaching. Have him demonstrate the proper setup, use, and cleaning of the equipment before discharge. Tell him that he shouldn't change the pressure settings without checking with his doctor. Suggest that the patient avoid using IPPB immediately before or after a meal because of possible nausea and reduced lung expansion. Instruct him to discontinue treatment and call his doctor if he experiences dizziness.

Complications

Gastric insufflation may result from swallowed air and occurs more commonly with a mask than with a mouthpiece. Dizziness can result from hyperventilation. The work of breathing can be increased, especially if the patient is uncomfortable with or frightened by the machine. Decreased blood pressure can result from decreased venous return, especially in the patient with hypovolemia or cardiovascular disease. Increased intracranial pressure can result from impeded venous return from the brain. Spontaneous pneumothorax may result from increased intrathoracic pressure; this complication is rare but is most likely to occur in patients with emphysematous blebs.

Documentation

Record the date, time, and duration of treatment; medication administered; pressure used; vital signs; breath sounds before and after treatment; amount of sputum produced; any complications and nursing actions taken; the patient's tolerance of the procedure; and any patient teaching provided.[6,7]

REFERENCES

1 American Association for Respiratory Care. (2003). AARC clinical practice guideline: Intermittent positive pressure breathing—2003 revision & update. *Respiratory Care, 48*(5), 540–546. (Level I)

2 The Joint Commission. (2012). Standard NPSG.07.01.01. *Comprehensive accreditation manual for hospitals: The official handbook.* Oakbrook Terrace, IL: The Joint Commission. (Level I)

3 Centers for Disease Control and Prevention. (1997). Guidelines for prevention of nosocomial pneumonia. *Morbidity and Mortality Weekly Report, 46*(RR-1), 1–79.

4 World Health Organization. (2009). *WHO guidelines on hand hygiene in health care: First global patient safety challenge. Clean care is safer care.* Geneva, Switzerland: World Health Organization. (Level I)

5 The Joint Commission. (2012). Standard NPSG.01.01.01. *Comprehensive accreditation manual for hospitals: The official handbook.* Oakbrook Terrace, IL: The Joint Commission. (Level I)

6 The Joint Commission. (2012). Standard RC.01.03.01. *Comprehensive accreditation manual for hospitals: The official handbook.* Oakbrook Terrace, IL: The Joint Commission. (Level I)

7 The Joint Commission. (2012). Standard RC.02.01.01. *Comprehensive accreditation manual for hospitals: The official handbook.* Oakbrook Terrace, IL: The Joint Commission. (Level I)

ADDITIONAL REFERENCES

Guérin, C., et al. (2010). The short-term effects of intermittent positive-pressure breathing treatments on ventilation in patients with neuromuscular disease. *Respiratory Care, 55*(7), 866–872.

Laffont, I., et al. (2008). Intermittent positive-pressure breathing effects in patients with high spinal cord injury. *Archives of Physical Medicine and Rehabilitation, 89*(8), 1575–1579.

Nettina, S.M. (2010). *Lippincott manual of nursing practice* (9th ed.). Philadelphia, PA: Lippincott Williams & Wilkins.

Taylor, C., et al. (2011). *Fundamentals of nursing: The art and science of nursing care* (7th ed.). Philadelphia, PA: Lippincott Williams & Wilkins.

INTERMITTENT URINARY CATHETERIZATION

Intermittent (straight) urinary catheter insertion involves inserting a temporary catheter into the bladder to drain urine. In contrast with an indwelling urinary catheter, an intermittent catheter is removed as soon as the urine is drained. It's a preferred alternative to indwelling urinary catheter insertion for managing patients with neurogenic bladder and urinary retention because it's associated with lower infection rates than indwelling urinary catheterization.[1,2,3,4]

Intermittent urinary catheterization has been used in patients with spinal cord injury, spinal tumors, diabetic neuropathy, multiple sclerosis, spina bifida, myelodysplasia, bladder outlet obstruction, and continent urinary diversion. It's also been used to manage incontinence and postoperative urinary retention as well as to collect urine samples for culture and sensitivity.

Intermittent urinary catheterization is used long-term or short-term, depending on the patient's condition. When used routinely, it should be performed at regular intervals throughout the day according to the patient's fluid intake to prevent bladder overdistention.[2]

In a health care facility, use sterile or clean technique for insertion, depending on your facility's policy. At home, the patient may use clean technique without increasing the risk for a urinary tract infection.[4]

Equipment

Sterile urethral catheter (latex or silicone #10 to #22 French) ■ washcloth ■ towel ■ soap and water ■ gloves ■ two linen-saver pads ■ sterile gloves ■ sterile drape ■ sterile fenestrated drape ■ sterile cotton-tipped applicators (or cotton balls and plastic forceps) ■ antiseptic cleaning agent ■ urine drainage receptacle ■ sterile water-soluble lubricant ■ intake and output record

■ Optional: urine specimen container, laboratory request form, gooseneck lamp or flashlight, pillows or rolled blankets or towels, bladder ultrasonography equipment, catheter storage container, specimen supplies.

Prepackaged sterile disposable kits that usually contain all the necessary equipment are available.

Implementation

■ Gather the appropriate equipment.
■ Verify the doctor's order.
■ Check the patient's medical record for a history of hypersensitivity to iodine or latex.
■ Perform hand hygiene and put on gloves.[5,6,7]
■ Provide privacy and explain the procedure to the patient *to allay anxiety and promote cooperation during the procedure.*
■ Confirm the patient's identity using at least two patient identifiers according to your facility's policy.[8]
■ Check the patient's intake and output record to see the time and amount of the most recent voiding and confirm the time with the patient.
■ Percuss and palpate the patient's bladder *to establish baseline data.* Ask if the patient feels the urge to void. If possible, measure the volume of urine in the bladder using bladder ultrasonography; *ultrasonography helps prevent unnecessary catheterization.*[2]
■ Have a coworker hold a flashlight or place a gooseneck lamp next to the patient's bed *so that you can visualize the urinary meatus in poor lighting.*

For a female patient

■ Place the patient in the supine position, with her knees flexed and separated and her feet flat on the bed, about 2″ (61 cm) apart. If she finds this position uncomfortable, have her flex one knee and keep the other leg flat on the bed. Or have the patient lie on her side with her knees drawn up to her chest during the catheterization procedure (as shown below). *This position may be especially helpful for elderly or disabled patients, such as those with severe contractures.*

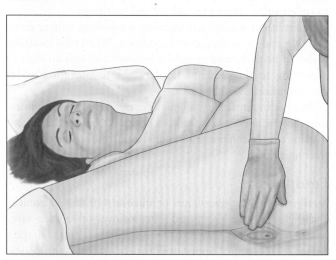

ELDER ALERT *An elderly patient may need pillows or rolled towels or blankets* to provide support with positioning.

■ You may need an assistant to help the patient stay in position or to direct the light. Ask the patient to hold her position *to give you a clear view of the urinary meatus and to prevent contamination of the sterile field.*
■ Place the linen-saver pads on the bed between the patient's legs and under her hips *to prevent inadvertent soiling of the patient's bed linens.* Use warm soapy water and a washcloth to clean the patient's genital area and perineum thoroughly. Dry the area with the towel. Then remove your gloves and perform hand hygiene.
■ *To create the sterile field,* open the prepackaged kit or equipment tray and place it between the patient's legs. If the sterile gloves are the first item on the top of the tray, put them on. Place the sterile drape under the patient's hips. Then drape the patient's lower abdomen with the sterile fenestrated drape so that only the genital area remains exposed (as shown below). Make sure you don't contaminate your gloves if you have them on already.[3,6,9]

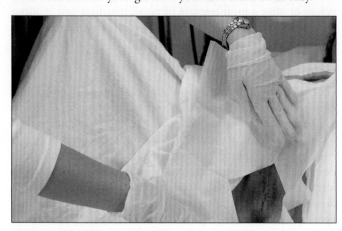

■ Open the rest of the kit or tray. Put on the sterile gloves if you haven't already done so.
■ Tear open the packet of antiseptic cleaning solution, and use it to saturate the sterile cotton balls or applicators.
■ Open the packet of water-soluble lubricant, and apply it to the catheter tip.[4]
■ Separate the labia majora and labia minora as widely as possible with the thumb, middle, and index fingers of your nondominant hand *so you have a full view of the urinary meatus.* Keep the labia well separated throughout the procedure (as shown below), *so they don't obscure the urinary meatus or contaminate the area when it's cleaned.*

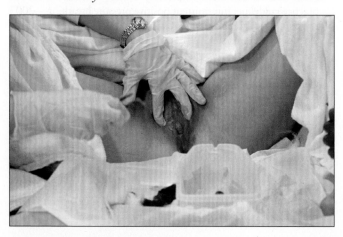

■ With your dominant hand, use a sterile, antiseptic-soaked, cotton-tipped applicator (or pick up a sterile cotton ball with the plastic forceps) and wipe one side of the urinary meatus with a downward motion (as shown below).

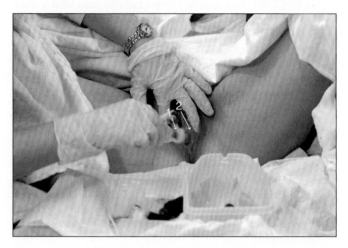

■ Wipe the other side with another sterile applicator or cotton ball in the same way. Then wipe directly over the meatus with still another sterile applicator or cotton ball. Take care not to contaminate your sterile glove.
■ Repeat the procedure, using another sterile applicator or cotton ball. Make sure that you don't contaminate your sterile glove.
■ Pick up the straight catheter with your dominant hand, holding it 2″ to 3″ (5.1 cm to 7.6 cm) from the tip, and prepare to insert the lubricated tip into the urinary meatus. *To facilitate insertion by relaxing the sphincter,* ask the patient to cough as you insert the catheter. Tell her to breathe deeply and slowly *to further relax the sphincter and reduce spasms.*[9]

NURSING ALERT *Never force a catheter during insertion. Maneuver it gently as the patient bears down or coughs. If you still meet resistance, stop and notify the doctor. Sphincter spasms, strictures, or misplacement in the vagina may cause resistance.*

■ Slowly and gently advance the catheter 2″ to 4″ while continuing to hold the labia apart until urine begins to flow.[4] If the catheter is inadvertently inserted into the vagina, leave it there as a landmark. Then begin the procedure over again using new supplies.
■ Drain the urine into the urine receptacle.
■ Hold the catheter in place until the urine flow stops and the bladder is empty.
■ When flow has stopped, slowly remove the catheter, allowing urine to drain from the lower half of the bladder. Completely remove the catheter when there's no further urine flow.[4]
■ If the catheter is disposable, discard it in the appropriate receptacle. If it's reusable, clean the catheter with mild soap and water and store it in a clean, dry container.[4]
■ Discard all used supplies in the appropriate receptacle.
■ Remove and discard your gloves and perform hand hygiene.[5,6,7]
■ Document the procedure.[10,11]

For a male patient
■ Place the patient in the supine position with his legs extended and flat on the bed. Ask the patient to remain in that position *to*

give you a clear view of the urinary meatus and to prevent contamination of the sterile field.
■ Place a linen-saver pad on the bed between the patient's legs and under his hips *to prevent inadvertent soiling of bed linens.*
■ Use warm soapy water and a washcloth to clean the patient's genital area and perineum thoroughly. Dry the area with the towel.
■ Replace the linen-saver pad if the existing one is wet or soiled.
■ Remove and discard your gloves and perform hand hygiene.[5,6,7]
■ *To create the sterile field,* open the prepackaged kit or equipment tray and place it next to the patient's hip. If the sterile gloves are the first item on the top of the tray, put them on. Place the sterile drape under the patient's hips. Then drape the patient's lower abdomen with the sterile fenestrated drape so that only the genital area remains exposed. Make sure you don't contaminate your gloves if you have them on already.[3,6,12,13]
■ Open the rest of the kit or tray. Put on the sterile gloves if you haven't already done so.
■ Tear open the packet of antiseptic cleaning agent, and use it to saturate the sterile cotton balls or applicators.
■ Open the packet of water-soluble lubricant and apply it to the catheter tip.[4]
■ Hold the penis with your nondominant hand. If the patient is uncircumcised, retract the foreskin. Then gently lift and stretch the penis to a 60- to 90-degree angle. Hold the penis this way throughout the procedure *to straighten the urethra and maintain a sterile field.*
■ Use your dominant hand to clean the glans with a sterile, antiseptic-soaked, cotton-tipped applicator or sterile cotton ball held in the forceps. Clean in a circular motion, starting at the urinary meatus and working outward (as shown below).

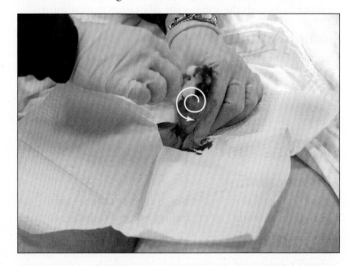

■ Repeat the procedure, using another sterile applicator or cotton ball. Make sure that you don't contaminate your sterile glove.
■ Pick up the catheter with your dominant hand, holding it 2″ to 3″ (5.1 cm to 7.6 cm) from the tip, and prepare to insert the lubricated tip into the urinary meatus. *To facilitate insertion by relaxing the sphincter,* ask the patient to cough as you insert the catheter. Tell him to breathe deeply and slowly *to further relax the sphincter and reduce spasms.*[13]

NURSING ALERT *Never force a catheter during insertion. Maneuver it gently as the patient bears down or coughs. If you still meet resistance, stop and notify the doctor.* Sphincter spasms, strictures, or an enlarged prostate may cause resistance.

■ Gently insert the catheter into the meatus, approximately 6″ to 8″ (15 to 20 cm) or until the urine begins to flow.[4]

■ As you reach the level of the prostate you'll meet some resistance; tell the patient to breathe deeply and slowly and continue to advance the catheter.

■ If the foreskin was retracted, replace it *to prevent compromised circulation and painful swelling.*

■ Drain the urine into the urine receptacle.

■ Hold the catheter in place until the urine flow stops and the bladder is empty.

■ When flow has stopped, slowly remove the catheter, allowing urine to drain from the lower half of the bladder. Completely remove the catheter when there's no further urine flow.[4]

■ If the catheter is disposable, discard it in the appropriate receptacle. If it is reusable, clean the catheter with mild soap and water and store it in a clean, dry container.[4]

■ Discard all the used supplies in the appropriate receptacle.

■ Remove and discard your gloves and perform hand hygiene.[5,6,7]

■ Document the procedure.[10,11]

Special considerations

■ Perform intermittent catheterization at regular *intervals to prevent bladder overdistention.*[6]

■ If the doctor orders a urine specimen for laboratory analysis, obtain it from the urine receptacle with a specimen collection container at the time of catheterization, label it in the presence of the patient to prevent mislabeling, and send it to the laboratory in a biohazard bag with the appropriate laboratory request form.

Complications

Complications include urethral false passages, urethral strictures, bladder perforation, and deterioration of the upper urinary tracts.[4] Urinary tract infection can result from the introduction of bacteria into the bladder. Improper insertion can cause traumatic injury to the urethral and bladder mucosa. Bladder atony or spasms can result from rapid decompression of a severely distended bladder.

Documentation

Record the date, time, and size and type of catheter used. Also describe the amount, color, and other characteristics of urine emptied from the bladder. Your facility may require only the intake and output record for fluid-balance data. Describe the patient's tolerance of the procedure. Note whether a urine specimen was sent for laboratory analysis.[10,11]

REFERENCES

1 Association for Professionals in Infection Control and Epidemiology. (2008). "Guide to the Elimination of Catheter-Associated Urinary Tract Infections (CAUTIs)" [Online]. Accessed November 2011 via the Web at http://www.apic.org/Content/NavigationMenu/PracticeGuidance/APICEliminationGuides/CAUTI_Guide.pdf

2 Gould, C.V., et al. (2009). "Guideline for Prevention of Catheter-associated Urinary Tract Infections, 2009" [Online]. Accessed November 2011 via the Web at http://www.cdc.gov/hicpac/cauti/001_cauti.html (Level I)

3 Lo, E. (2008). Strategies to prevent catheter-associated urinary tract infections in acute care hospitals. *Infection Control and Hospital Epidemiology 29*(Suppl. 1), S41–S50.

4 Society of Urologic Nurses and Associates. (2006). "Clinical Practice Guidelines: Adult Clean Intermittent Catheterization" [Online]. Accessed November 2011 via the Web at http://www.suna.org/resources/adultCICGuide.pdf (Level VII)

5 Centers for Disease Control and Prevention. (October 2002). Guideline for hand hygiene in health-care settings. *Morbidity and Mortality Weekly Report, 51*(RR-16), 1–45. (Level I)

6 The Joint Commission. (2012). Standard NPSG.07.01.01. *Comprehensive accreditation manual for hospitals: The official handbook.* Oakbrook Terrace, IL: The Joint Commission. (Level I)

7 World Health Organization. (2009). *WHO guidelines on hand hygiene in health care: First global patient safety challenge. Clean care is safer care.* Geneva, Switzerland: World Health Organization. (Level I)

8 The Joint Commission. (2012). Standard NPSG.01.01.01. *Comprehensive accreditation manual for hospitals: The official handbook.* Oakbrook Terrace, IL: The Joint Commission. (Level I)

9 Society of Urologic Nurses and Associates. (2005). "Clinical Practice Guidelines: Female Urethral Catheterization" [Online]. Accessed November 2011 via the Web at http://www.suna.org/resources/femaleCatheterization.pdf

10 The Joint Commission. (2012). Standard RC.01.03.01. *Comprehensive accreditation manual for hospitals: The official handbook.* Oakbrook Terrace, IL: The Joint Commission. (Level I)

11 The Joint Commission. (2012). Standard RC.02.01.01. *Comprehensive accreditation manual for hospitals: The official handbook.* Oakbrook Terrace, IL: The Joint Commission. (Level I)

12 The Joint Commission. (2012). Standard NPSG.07.06.01. *Comprehensive accreditation manual for hospitals: The official handbook.* Oakbrook Terrace, IL: The Joint Commission. (Level I)

13 Society of Urologic Nurses and Associates. (2005). "Clinical Practice Guidelines: Male Urethral Catheterization" [Online]. Accessed November 2011 via the Web at http://www.suna.org/resources/maleCatheterization.pdf

INTERNAL FIXATION MANAGEMENT

In internal fixation, also known as *surgical reduction* or *open reduction–internal fixation*, the doctor implants fixation devices to stabilize the fracture. Internal fixation devices include nails, screws, pins, wires, and rods, all of which may be used in combination with metal plates. These devices remain in the body indefinitely unless the patient experiences adverse reactions after the healing process is complete. (See *Reviewing internal fixation devices.*)

Typically, internal fixation is used to treat fractures of the face and jaw, spine, and arms and legs as well as fractures involving a joint (most commonly, the hip). Internal fixation permits earlier mobilization and can shorten hospitalization, particularly in elderly patients with hip fractures.

Nursing management for a patient who undergoes internal fixation involves monitoring neurovascular status, administering

EQUIPMENT

Reviewing internal fixation devices

In trochanteric or sub-trochanteric fractures, the surgeon may use a hip pin or nail, with or without a screw plate. A pin or plate with extra nails stabilizes the fracture by impacting the bone ends at the fracture site.

In an uncomplicated fracture of the femoral shaft, the surgeon may use an intramedullary rod. This device permits early ambulation with partial weight bearing.

Another choice for fixation of a long-bone fracture is a screw plate, shown here on the tibia.

In an arm fracture, the surgeon may fix the involved bones with a plate, rod, or nail. Most radial and ulnar fractures may be fixed with plates, whereas humeral fractures are commonly fixed with rods.

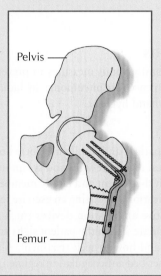
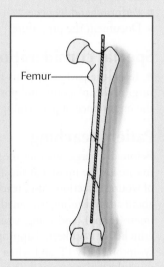
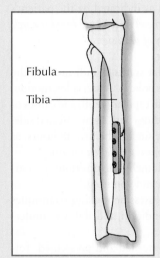
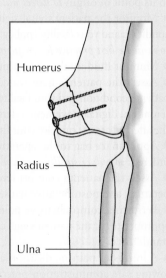

medications, managing the patient's pain, preventing infection, and assisting with ambulation and exercises.

Equipment

Ice bag ▪ pain medication ▪ incentive spirometer ▪ compression stockings ▪ sequential compression device.

For a patient with a leg fracture, you may also need an overhead frame with trapeze, pressure-relief mattress, crutches or walker, and pillow; hip fractures may require abductor pillows.

Implementation

Preoperative care
▪ Verify the doctor's orders.
▪ Perform hand hygiene.[1,2,3]
▪ Confirm the patient's identity using at least two patient identifiers according to your facility's policy.[4]
▪ Reinforce the doctor's explanation of the procedure, and answer the patient's questions. Ensure that the patient has signed a consent form, according to your facility's policy.[5]
▪ Perform a comprehensive pain assessment using techniques appropriate for the patient's age, condition, and ability to understand.[6]
▪ Assess the patient for pain and administer pain medication, as prescribed, using safe medication administration practices. Per-

form a follow-up pain assessment and notify the doctor if pain isn't adequately controlled.[6]
▪ Tell the patient what to expect during postoperative assessment and monitoring.
▪ Teach the patient how to cough, deep breathe, and use an incentive spirometer *to reduce the risk of postprocedure pneumonia.*[7]
▪ Prepare the patient for proposed exercise and progressive ambulation regimens, if necessary.
▪ Conduct a preprocedure verification to make sure that all relevant documentation and related information or equipment is available and correctly identified to the patient's identifiers.[8]
▪ Verify that the laboratory and imaging studies have been completed, as ordered, and that the results are in the patient's medical record. Notify the doctor of any unexpected results.[8]
▪ Ensure that the patient has had nothing by mouth for 6 to 8 hours before the procedure, except in emergency situations.
▪ Verify that the patient has patent IV access *to administer prophylactic antibiotics (commonly administered 1 hour before the incision or 2 hours before if vancomycin or fluoroquinolones are prescribed), IV fluids, and blood products, as prescribed.*[9,10]
▪ Perform hand hygiene.[1,2,3]
▪ Document the procedure.[11,12]

Postoperative care

- Perform hand hygiene.[1,2,3]
- Receive hand-off communication from the person who assumed care of the patient in the postanesthesia care unit; ask questions as needed.[13]
- Confirm the patient's identity using at least two patient identifiers according to your facility's policy.[4]
- Assess the patient's respiratory status and oxygen saturation level.[14]
- Assess patency of the patient's IV catheter; insert a new one if necessary.
- Trace each tubing that the patient has in place from the patient to its point of origin *to detect misconnections.*[15]
- Monitor the patient's vital signs as indicated by the patient's condition and your facility's policy; *there's no evidence-based research to indicate best practice for frequency of vital signs.*[14]
- Monitor fluid intake and output.
- Assess the patient's neurovascular status as indicated by the patient's condition and your facility's policy.[14] Assess color, motion, sensation, digital movement, edema, capillary refill, and pulses of the affected area. Compare your findings with the unaffected side.
- Apply an ice bag to the operative site for the first 48 hours, as ordered, *to reduce swelling, relieve pain, and lessen bleeding.*
- Assess the patient's comfort level, including positioning, temperature, and postoperative nausea and vomiting.[14]
- Perform a comprehensive pain assessment using techniques appropriate for the patient's age, condition, and ability to understand.[6,14]
- Administer pain medication as needed and prescribed, following safe administration practices, *to promote comfort.* If the patient is using patient-controlled analgesia, instruct him to administer a dose before exercising or mobilizing.[16]
- Assess the patient's safety needs including his risk for falling. Implement the appropriate measures *to ensure patient safety.*[14]
- Reassess the patient's pain[6,14] and ask about the presence of burning, tingling, or numbness, *which may indicate infection or impaired circulation.*
- Elevate the affected limb on a pillow, if appropriate, *to minimize edema.*
- Assess the condition and color of the patient's skin.[14]
- Check surgical dressings for excessive drainage or bleeding.[14]
- Assess the incision site for signs of infection, such as erythema, drainage, edema, and unusual pain.
- Assist and encourage the patient to perform range-of-motion and other muscle strengthening exercises, as ordered, *to promote circulation, improve muscle tone, and maintain joint function.*
- *To prevent postprocedure pneumonia,* have the patient cough, deep breathe, and use an incentive spirometer according to the doctor's order.[7] (See "Incentive spirometry," page 366.)
- Apply compression stockings or a sequential compression device, as appropriate, *to prevent venous thromboembolism (VTE).* The patient may also require a pressure-relief mattress. (See "Sequential compression therapy," page 645.)
- Teach the patient to perform early progressive ambulation and mobilization[7,17] using an overhead frame with a trapeze, crutches, or a walker, as appropriate.

- Continue anticoagulation therapy, as ordered by the doctor *to prevent VTE.* Make sure baseline coagulation studies have been obtained and are documented in the patient's medical record. (International Normalized Ratio should be monitored if the patient is receiving warfarin [Coumadin].)[17,18]
- Make sure prophylactic antibiotics are discontinued within 24 hours after surgery.[18]
- If the patient has an indwelling urinary catheter that was inserted for surgery, remove the catheter on postoperative day 1 or 2 (with the day of surgery considered day 0), according to facility policy or the doctor's order, *to reduce the risk for catheter-associated urinary tract infection.*[18] (See "Indwelling urinary catheter care and removal," page 374.)
- Perform hand hygiene.[1,2,3]
- Document the procedure.[11,12]

Special considerations

- Teach the patient and his family about measures to prevent surgical site infections and postprocedure pneumonia, including the importance of performing hand hygiene.[9,10]

Patient teaching

Before discharge, instruct the patient and family members how to care for the incisional site and recognize signs and symptoms of wound infection. Also, teach the patient and family members about administering pain medication, practicing an exercise regimen (if any), and using assistive ambulation devices (such as crutches or a walker), if appropriate. Teach the patient signs and symptoms of VTE and when and how to seek treatment. Also teach the patient about the prescribed anticoagulation regimen.[17]

Complications

Wound infection and, more critically, infection involving metal fixation devices may require reopening the incision, draining the suture line and, possibly, removing the fixation device. Any such infection would require wound dressings and antibiotic therapy. Other complications may include malunion, nonunion, fat or pulmonary embolism, neurovascular impairment, and chronic pain.

Documentation

In the patient record, document perioperative findings on cardiovascular, respiratory, and neurovascular status. Document pain medications administered, including the amount, route, and patient tolerance. Describe the wound appearance and alignment of the affected bone. Document the patient's response to teaching about appropriate exercise, care of the incision site, use of assistive devices (if appropriate), anticoagulant therapy, signs and symptoms that should be reported to the doctor, and where and when to seek treatment.[11,12]

REFERENCES

1 Centers for Disease Control and Prevention. (October 2002). Guideline for hand hygiene in health-care settings. *Morbidity and Mortality Weekly Report, 51*(RR-16), 1–45. (Level I)

2 World Health Organization. (2009). *WHO guidelines on hand hygiene in health care: First global patient safety challenge. Clean care is safer care.* Geneva, Switzerland: World Health Organization. (Level I)

3 The Joint Commission. (2012). Standard NPSG.07.01.01. *Comprehensive accreditation manual for hospitals: The official handbook.* Oakbrook Terrace, IL: The Joint Commission. (Level I)

4 The Joint Commission. (2012). Standard NPSG.01.01.01. *Comprehensive accreditation manual for hospitals: The official handbook.* Oakbrook Terrace, IL: The Joint Commission. (Level I)

5 The Joint Commission. (2012). Standard RI.01.03.01. *Comprehensive accreditation manual for hospitals: The official handbook.* Oakbrook Terrace, IL: The Joint Commission. (Level I)

6 The Joint Commission. (2012). Standard PC.01.02.07. *Comprehensive accreditation manual for hospitals: The official handbook.* Oakbrook Terrace, IL: The Joint Commission. (Level I)

7 Centers for Disease Control and Prevention. (2004). Guidelines for preventing health-care– associated pneumonia, 2003. *Morbidity and Mortality Weekly Report, 53*(RR-03), 1–36.

8 The Joint Commission. (2012). Standard UP.01.01.01. *Comprehensive accreditation manual for hospitals: The official handbook.* Oakbrook Terrace, IL: The Joint Commission. (Level I)

9 The Joint Commission. (2012). Standard NPSG.07.05.01. *Comprehensive accreditation manual for hospitals: The official handbook.* Oakbrook Terrace, IL: The Joint Commission. (Level I)

10 Anderson, D.J., et al. (2008). Compendium of strategies to prevent healthcare-associated infections in acute care hospitals: Strategies to prevent surgical site infections in acute care hospitals. *Infection Control and Hospital Epidemiology,* (29), S1. (Level 1)

11 The Joint Commission. (2012). Standard RC.01.03.01. *Comprehensive accreditation manual for hospitals: The official handbook.* Oakbrook Terrace, IL: The Joint Commission. (Level I)

12 The Joint Commission. (2012). Standard RC.02.01.01. *Comprehensive accreditation manual for hospitals: The official handbook.* Oakbrook Terrace, IL: The Joint Commission. (Level I)

13 Recommended practices for transfer of patient care information. (2010). In R. Conner, et al. (Eds.). *Perioperative standards and recommended practices.* Denver, CO: AORN. (Level I)

14 American Society of PeriAnesthesia Nurses. (2010). Practice recommendation 2: Components of initial, ongoing, and discharge assessment and management. In *Perianesthesia nursing standards and practice recommendations: 2010–2012.* Cherry Hill, NJ: American Society of PeriAnesthesia Nurses.

15 U.S. Food and Drug Administration. (2009). "Look. Check. Connect.: Safe Medical Device Connections Save Lives" [Online]. Accessed November 2011 via the Web at http://www.fda.gov/downloads/MedicalDevices/Safety/AlertsandNotices/UCM134873.pdf

16 The Joint Commission. (2012). Standard MM.06.01.01. *Comprehensive accreditation manual for hospitals: The official handbook.* Oakbrook Terrace, IL: The Joint Commission. (Level I)

17 Institute for Clinical Systems Improvement. (September 2011). "Health Care Guideline: Venous Thromboembolism Prophylaxis, Eighth Edition" [Online]. Accessed November 2011 via the Web at http:// www.icsi.org/venous_thromboembolism_prophylaxis__2__guideline_/venous_thromboembolism_prophylaxis__guideline__47057.html

18 The Joint Commission. (2010). Surgical Care Improvement Project national hospital inpatient quality measures. In *Specification manual for national hospital quality measures.* Oakbrook Terrace, IL: The Joint Commission. (Level I)

ADDITIONAL REFERENCES

American Society of PeriAnesthesia Nurses. "Clinical Guideline for Pain and Comfort" [Online]. Accessed November 2011 via the Web at http://www.aspan.org/Portals/6/docs/ClinicalPractice/Guidelines/ASPAN_ClinicalGuideline_PainComfort.pdf

Anderson, D.J., et al. (2008). Compendium of strategies to prevent healthcare-associated infections in acute care hospitals: Strategies to prevent surgical site infections in acute care hospitals. *Infection Control and Hospital Epidemiology,* (29), S1.

Institute for Healthcare Improvement. (2008). *5 million lives campaign getting started kit: Prevent surgical site infections.* Cambridge, MA: Institute for Healthcare Improvement.

INTRA-ABDOMINAL PRESSURE MONITORING

Intra-abdominal pressure monitoring measures the pressure in the abdominal compartment. It can be assessed indirectly in the patient with an indwelling urinary catheter by measuring the pressure in the bladder with a needle that connects a pressure transducer to the urinary catheter or by inserting an IV catheter into the sampling port. Pressure in the abdomen may rise from such conditions as intraperitoneal bleeding, third-space fluid resuscitation, peritonitis, ascites, gaseous bowel distention, abdominal surgery, and trauma.

If pressure in the abdominal cavity becomes greater than the pressure in the capillaries that perfuse the abdominal organs, ischemia and infarction may result. Increased intra-abdominal pressure can also lead to reduced cardiac output, increased systemic vascular resistance, increased vascular resistance, and reduced venous return. By measuring intra-abdominal pressure, the nurse can detect a rise in pressure and initiate life-saving measures.[1]

To help prevent catheter-associated urinary tract infections, the catheter should be removed as soon as it's no longer needed.[2,3]

Equipment

Indwelling urinary catheter with drainage bag ■ gloves ■ cardiac monitor ■ pressure cable for monitor interface ■ 500- or 1,000-mL bag of IV normal saline solution ■ appropriate-size pressure bag ■ IV tubing ■ pressure tubing, pressure transducer with flush device, and two stopcocks ■ 30-mL luer-lock syringe ■ clamp ■ antiseptic cleaning solution ■ tape ■ IV pole.

Several commercially prepared kits are available. Examples include the Bard and AbViser intra-abdominal pressure monitoring systems.

Preparation of equipment

Before setting up the monitoring system, perform hand hygiene.[4,5,6] Maintain asepsis throughout preparation and wear the appropriate personal protective equipment. (For instructions on setting up and priming the monitoring system, see "Transducer system setup," page 739.)

Verify the doctor's order. Assemble the equipment, taking care not to contaminate dead-end caps, stopcocks, and syringes.

Connect the IV tubing to the transducer, the transducer to two successive stopcocks, and then the second stopcock to the pressure tubing and monitor cable. Attach a 30-mL syringe to the side port of the first stopcock. Place the transducer in the transducer holder attached to the IV pole. Hang the 500-mL bag of normal saline solution from an IV pole, attach the IV tubing, and flush the entire line system of air. Use the pressure bag to pressurize the system to 300 mm Hg. Attach the cable from the transducer to the monitor and select a 30 mm Hg scale for monitoring pressure.

Implementation

■ Perform hand hygiene and put on gloves.[4,5,6]
■ Confirm the patient's identity using at least two patient identifiers according to your facility's policy.[7]
■ Explain the procedure to the patient, including the purpose of intra-abdominal pressure monitoring and anticipated duration of catheter placement, *to reduce anxiety and enhance cooperation.*
■ Insert an indwelling urinary catheter, if the patient doesn't already have one in place. (See "Indwelling urinary catheter care and removal," page 374.)
■ Place the IV pole with the monitoring system next to the patient.
■ With the patient supine and the head of the bed flat, level and zero the transducer to the iliac crest at the midaxillary line *to cancel out the effect of atmospheric pressure.*[1] *The supine position prevents the abdominal organs from exerting pressure down on the bladder, falsely elevating the readings.* If the patient can't tolerate the head of the bed being flat, place the transducer at the level of the bladder.
■ Clean the indwelling urinary catheter sampling port with antiseptic solution according to facility policy *to reduce the risk of infection* and attach the end of the pressure tubing to the sampling port.[2,3]
■ Clamp the urinary catheter just distal to the connection of the catheter and drainage bag *to keep saline from draining out of the bladder while filling the bladder.*
■ Open the stopcock from the flush line to the syringe and fill the syringe with 25 mL of fluid from the IV normal saline solution bag.[8]
■ Close the stopcock to the flush line and open it to the urinary catheter and instill 25 mL of normal saline solution into the bladder. *This volume won't overdistend the bladder and produce a falsely high reading.*[8]
■ Push out any air seen in between the clamp and the urinary catheter by opening the clamp and allowing the normal saline solution to flow past the clamp. Then reclamp the tubing.
■ Close the stopcock to the syringe, and open it to the pressure tubing and the transducer.
■ Wait 30 seconds after instilling the saline,[1] and then obtain the intra-abdominal pressure with the patient in the supine position and the point of leveling at the symphysis pubis.
■ Obtain the pressure reading at the end of expiration *to minimize the effects of respiration.*[1] Fluctuation should be evident in the waveform with the heartbeat or respiratory pattern.

■ After the reading is obtained, turn the stopcock off to the pressure tubing and catheter, release the clamp, and allow the instilled normal saline solution to drain.
■ Measure the urinary output after subtracting the 25 mL of instilled normal saline solution *to maintain accurate intake and output.*[8]
■ Remove the pressure tubing from the sampling port or leave it in place if subsequent monitoring is necessary. Tape the connections securely.
■ Dispose of used supplies in appropriate receptacles.
■ Perform hand hygiene.[4,5,6]
■ Document the procedure.[9,10]

Special considerations

■ Monitor intra-abdominal pressure at least every 4 hours or according to facility policy.[1] Report an increasing intra-abdominal pressure to the doctor. Intra-abdominal pressures 12 mm Hg or higher signal intra-abdominal hypertension, but a pressure greater than 20 mm Hg is considered abdominal compartment syndrome, possibly requiring decompression surgery.[8]
■ Patients at risk for intra-abdominal hypertension should be assessed for signs of reduced organ perfusion, such as reduced or absent urinary output, increasing serum creatinine levels, hypotension, reduced cardiac output, increased central venous and pulmonary artery pressures, increased intracerebral pressure, increased serum lactate levels, increased peak airway pressure, decreased tidal volume, hypoxemia, hypercarbia, GI bleeding, and impaired peripheral circulation.
■ If a patient can't lie in a supine position to obtain a reading, take the reading with the head of the bed elevated. Make sure the transducer is at the level of the bladder for all readings. Document the position the patient was in for the reading, and obtain all further readings from this position.

Complications

Intra-abdominal pressures that exceed 20 mm Hg are usually associated with irreversible organ damage, leading to abdominal compartment syndrome and multiple-organ-dysfunction syndrome. With increased pressure readings and signs of reduced organ perfusion, surgical intervention may be required to preserve organ function and decrease morbidity and mortality associated with intra-abdominal hypertension and abdominal compartment syndrome. The presence of an indwelling urinary catheter and entering the closed system for pressure monitoring increases the risk of infection.

Documentation

Describe any patient teaching performed. Record the date and time of the reading. Document if the system was leveled and zeroed and the patient's position during the reading. Note the amount of normal saline solution instilled. Record the intra-abdominal pressure reading. Frequent intra-abdominal pressure readings may be recorded on a frequent parameter assessment sheet. Indicate if anyone was notified of an abnormal reading, whether orders were given, what treatments were performed, and what response the patient had.[9,10]

Record any vital signs taken and assessments done at the time of the reading. Record urinary output after subtracting the amount of instilled normal saline solution. Urinary output may also be documented on the frequent parameter assessment sheet. Chart any urinary catheter care performed. Note the patient's tolerance of the procedure. If a strip of the waveform is available, place it in the medical record, noting the date, time, and patient's name on the strip.

REFERENCES

1 World Society of Abdominal Compartment Syndrome. (2006). "WSACS Consensus Definitions and Recommendations" [Online]. Accessed November 2011 via the Web at http://www.wsacs.org/consensus.php (Level I)
2 The Joint Commission. (2012). Standard NPSG.07.06.01. *Comprehensive accreditation manual for hospitals: The official handbook.* Oakbrook Terrace, IL: The Joint Commission. (Level I)
3 Lo, E. (2008). Strategies to prevent catheter-associated urinary tract infections in acute care hospitals. *Infection Control and Hospital Epidemiology 29*(Suppl. 1), S41–S50. (Level I)
4 The Joint Commission. (2012). Standard NPSG.07.01.01. *Comprehensive accreditation manual for hospitals: The official handbook.* Oakbrook Terrace, IL: The Joint Commission. (Level I)
5 World Health Organization. (2009). *WHO guidelines on hand hygiene in health care: First global patient safety challenge. Clean care is safer care.* Geneva, Switzerland: World Health Organization. (Level I)
6 Centers for Disease Control and Prevention. (October 2002). Guideline for hand hygiene in health-care settings. *Morbidity and Mortality Weekly Report, 51*(RR-16), 1–45. (Level I)
7 The Joint Commission. (2012). Standard NPSG.01.01.01. *Comprehensive accreditation manual for hospitals: The official handbook.* Oakbrook Terrace, IL: The Joint Commission. (Level I)
8 Lynn-McHale Wiegand, D. (Ed.). (2011). *AACN procedure manual for critical care* (6th ed.). Philadelphia, PA: Saunders.
9 The Joint Commission. (2012). Standard RC.01.03.01. *Comprehensive accreditation manual for hospitals: The official handbook.* Oakbrook Terrace, IL: The Joint Commission. (Level I)
10 The Joint Commission. (2012). Standard RC.02.01.01. *Comprehensive accreditation manual for hospitals: The official handbook.* Oakbrook Terrace, IL: The Joint Commission. (Level I)

ADDITIONAL REFERENCES

Cheatham, M.L., et al. (2007). Results from the International Conference of Experts on Intra-abdominal Hypertension and Abdominal Compartment Syndrome. II. Recommendations. *Intensive Care Medicine, 33*(6), 951–962.
De Keulenaer, B.L., et al. (2009). What is normal intra-abdominal pressure and how is it affected by positioning, body mass and positive end-expiratory pressure? *Intensive Care Medicine, 35*(6), 969–976.
Gallagher, J. (2010). Intra-abdominal hypertension: Detecting and managing a lethal complication of critical illness. *AACN Advanced Critical Care, 21*(2), 205–217.
Kimball, E.J., et al. (2009). A comparison of infusion volumes in the measurement of intra-abdominal pressure. *Journal of Intensive and Critical Care Medicine, 24*(4), 261–268.

INTRA-AORTIC BALLOON COUNTERPULSATION

Providing temporary support for the heart's left ventricle, intra-aortic balloon counterpulsation (IABC) mechanically displaces blood within the aorta by means of an intra-aortic balloon attached to an external pump console. The balloon is usually inserted through the common femoral artery and positioned with its tip just distal to the left subclavian artery. When used correctly, IABC improves two key aspects of myocardial physiology: it increases the supply of oxygen-rich blood to the myocardium, and it decreases myocardial oxygen demand and consumption.

IABC is recommended for patients with a wide range of low-cardiac-output disorders or cardiac instability, including refractory anginas, ventricular arrhythmias associated with ischemia, pump failure caused by cardiogenic shock, intraoperative myocardial infarction (MI), or low cardiac output after bypass surgery. IABC is also indicated for patients with low cardiac output secondary to acute mechanical defects after MI (such as ventricular septal defect, papillary muscle rupture, or left ventricular aneurysm).

Perioperatively, the technique is used to support and stabilize patients with a suspected high-grade lesion who are undergoing such procedures as angioplasty, thrombolytic therapy, cardiac surgery, and cardiac catheterization.

IABC is contraindicated in patients with end-stage renal disease, irreversible brain damage, severe aortic regurgitation, aortic aneurysm, or severe peripheral vascular disease.

The doctor removes the balloon when the patient's hemodynamic status remains stable after the frequency of balloon augmentation is decreased.

Equipment
For assisting with insertion
IABC console and balloon catheters ▪ insertion kit ▪ Dacron graft (for a surgically inserted balloon) ▪ electrocardiogram (ECG) monitor and electrodes ▪ IV solution and infusion set ▪ sedative ▪ arterial line catheter ▪ temporary pacemaker setup ▪ 18G angiography needle ▪ sterile drape ▪ sterile gloves ▪ gown ▪ mask ▪ sutures ▪ suction setup ▪ oxygen setup and ventilator, if necessary ▪ defibrillator and emergency medications ▪ fluoroscope ▪ indwelling urinary catheter ▪ urinometer ▪ arterial blood gas (ABG) kits and tubes for laboratory studies ▪ antiseptic solution ▪ clippers.

For maintaining the IABC
IABC console and balloon catheters ▪ ECG monitor and electrodes ▪ IV solution ▪ arterial line tubing, transducer, and pressure bag or device ▪ suction setup ▪ oxygen ▪ thermometer ▪ stethoscope ▪ emergency equipment and medications ▪ ABG kits and tubes for laboratory studies ▪ dressing materials ▪ gloves.

For assisting with removal
Dressing materials ▪ gloves ▪ suture removal kit.

EQUIPMENT

How the intra-aortic balloon pump works

Made of polyurethane, the intra-aortic balloon is attached to an external pump console by means of a large-lumen catheter. These illustrations show the direction of blood flow when the pump inflates and deflates the balloon.

Balloon inflation
The balloon inflates as the aortic valve closes and diastole begins. The balloon inflation displaces blood superiorly, which, in turn, augments coronary artery blood flow.

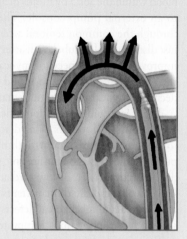

Balloon deflation
The balloon deflates before ventricular ejection, when the aortic valve opens. This deflation permits ejection of blood from the left ventricle against a lowered resistance. As a result, aortic end-diastolic pressure and afterload decrease and cardiac output rises.

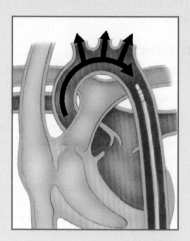

Preparation of equipment

When assisting with insertion, you or a perfusionist must zero and balance the pressure transducer in the external pump console and calibrate the oscilloscope monitor to ensure accuracy depending on your facility's policy.

When maintaining IABC, have the defibrillator, the suction setup, the temporary pacemaker setup, and emergency medications readily available *in case the patient develops severe complications.*

Implementation

- Perform hand hygiene.[1,2,3]
- Confirm the patient's identity using at least two patient identifiers according to your facility's policy.[4]

For assisting with insertion

- Reinforce the doctor's explanation of the procedure, explaining that the doctor will place a special balloon catheter in the patient's aorta *to help his heart pump more easily.* Briefly explain the insertion procedure, and mention that the catheter will be connected to a large console next to his bed. Tell him that the balloon will temporarily reduce his heart's workload *to promote rapid healing of the ventricular muscle.* Let him know that it will be removed after his heart can resume an adequate workload. (See *How the intra-aortic balloon pump works.*)
- Confirm that a written consent is obtained and that the consent is in the patient's medical record.[5,6]
- Conduct a pre-procedure verification process *to make sure that all relevant documentation, related information, or equipment is available and correctly identified to the patient's identifiers.*[7]
- Perform hand hygiene and put on sterile gloves.[1,2,3,8]
- Make sure the patient has an arterial line *for withdrawing blood samples, monitoring blood pressure, and assessing the timing and*

effectiveness of therapy; a pulmonary artery catheter *to allow measurement of pulmonary artery pressure (PAP), aspiration of blood samples, and cardiac output studies (increased PAP indicates increased myocardial workload and ineffective balloon pumping);* and a peripheral IV catheter or central venous access device in place *for administering fluids and medications.*

- Obtain the patient's baseline vital signs. Attach the patient to an ECG machine for continuous monitoring. Be sure to apply chest electrodes in a standard lead II position—or in whatever position produces the largest R wave—*because the R wave triggers balloon inflation and deflation.* Obtain a baseline ECG.
- Attach another set of ECG electrodes to the patient unless the ECG pattern is being transmitted from the patient's bedside monitor to the balloon pump monitor through another cable.
- Administer oxygen, as ordered and as necessary.
- Insert an indwelling catheter *so you can measure the patient's urine output and assess his fluid balance and renal function.*
- *To reduce the risk of infection,* clip hair bilaterally from the lower abdomen to the lower thigh, including the pubic area.
- Observe and record the patient's peripheral leg pulse and document sensation, movement, color, and temperature of the legs.
- Administer a sedative, as ordered, following safe medication administration practices.[9]
- Have the defibrillator, suction setup, temporary pacemaker setup, and emergency medications readily available in case the patient develops complications (such as arrhythmia) during insertion.
- Perform hand hygiene and then put on a cap, mask, gown, and sterile gloves to comply with maximal barrier precautions during insertion.[1,2,3,8]
- Before the doctor inserts the balloon, he puts on a surgical cap, sterile gloves, a gown, and a mask following maximal barrier precautions. He cleans the site with antiseptic solution and drapes

the patient using a sterile drape and observing maximal barrier precautions.

■ Conduct a time-out immediately before starting the procedure *to determine that the correct patient, site, positioning, and procedure are identified and to confirm, as applicable, that relevant information and necessary equipment are available.*[10]

Inserting the intra-aortic balloon percutaneously

■ The doctor may insert the balloon percutaneously through the femoral artery into the descending thoracic aorta using a modified Seldinger technique. First, he accesses the vessel with an 18G angiography needle and removes the inner stylet.

■ Then he passes the guide wire through the needle and removes the needle.

■ After passing a #8 French vessel dilator over the guide wire into the vessel, he removes the vessel dilator, leaving the guide wire in place.

■ Next, the doctor passes an introducer (dilator and sheath assembly) over the guide wire into the vessel until about 1″ (2.5 cm) remains above the insertion site. He then removes the inner dilator, leaving the introducer sheath and guide wire in place.

■ After passing the balloon over the guide wire into the introducer sheath, the doctor advances the catheter into position, ⅜″ to ¾″ (1 to 2 cm) distal to the left subclavian artery under fluoroscopic guidance.

■ The doctor attaches the balloon to the control system to initiate counterpulsation. The balloon catheter then unfurls.

Inserting the intra-aortic balloon surgically

■ If the doctor chooses not to insert the catheter percutaneously, he usually inserts it by femoral arteriotomy.

■ After making an incision and isolating the femoral artery, the doctor attaches a Dacron graft to a small opening in the arterial wall.

■ He then passes the catheter through this graft. Using fluoroscopic guidance as necessary, he advances the catheter up the descending thoracic aorta and places the catheter tip between the left subclavian artery and the renal arteries.

■ The doctor sews the Dacron graft around the catheter at the insertion point and connects the other end of the catheter to the pump console. (See *Surgical insertion sites for the intra-aortic balloon.*)

Completing the procedure

■ Discard used supplies, remove and discard your personal protective equipment, and perform hand hygiene.[1,2,3]

■ Document the procedure.[11,12]

For maintaining the IABC

■ Put on gloves if you will be assessing the insertion site.[8]

■ Interpret waveforms and monitor balloon function. (See *Interpreting intra-aortic balloon waveforms,* page 400.)

NURSING ALERT *If the pump console malfunctions or becomes inoperable, don't let the balloon catheter remain dormant for more than 15 minutes. Get another pump console, and attach it to the balloon; then resume pumping. In the meantime, inflate the balloon manually, using a 60-mL syringe and room air, a*

Surgical insertion sites for the intra-aortic balloon

If an intra-aortic balloon can't be inserted percutaneously, the doctor will insert it surgically, using a femoral or transthoracic approach.

Femoral approach
Insertion through the femoral artery requires a cutdown and an arteriotomy. The doctor passes the balloon through a Dacron graft that has been sewn to the artery.

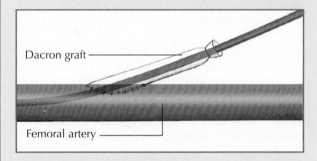

Transthoracic approach
If femoral insertion is unsuccessful, the doctor may use a transthoracic approach. He inserts the balloon in an antegrade direction through the subclavian artery and then positions it in the descending thoracic aorta.

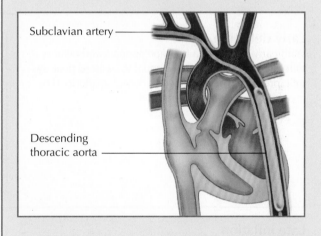

minimum of once every 5 minutes to prevent thrombus formation in the catheter. *The volume of inflation is equal to 10 mL less than the balloon size marked on the catheter. Never manually inflate the balloon if rupture is suspected.*

■ Monitor the patient's vital signs and level of conscious every 15 minutes for 1 hour and according to the patient's condition.[13]

■ Assess and record pedal and posterior tibial pulses as well as color, sensation, and temperature in the affected limb every 15 minutes for 1 hour, then hourly. Notify the doctor immediately if you detect circulatory changes; the balloon may need to be removed.

■ Observe and record the patient's baseline arm pulses, arm sensation and movement, and arm color and temperature every

Interpreting intra-aortic balloon waveforms

During intra-aortic balloon counterpulsation, you can use electrocardiogram (ECG) and arterial pressure waveforms to determine whether the balloon pump is functioning properly.

Normal inflation-deflation timing

Balloon inflation occurs after aortic valve closure; deflation, during isovolumetric contraction, just before the aortic valve opens. In a properly timed waveform, like the one shown, the inflation point lies at or slightly above the dicrotic notch. Both inflation and deflation cause a sharp V. Peak diastolic pressure exceeds peak systolic pressure; peak systolic pressure exceeds assisted peak systolic pressure.

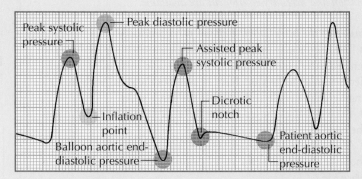

Early inflation

With *early inflation*, the inflation point lies before the dicrotic notch. Early inflation dangerously increases myocardial stress and decreases cardiac output.

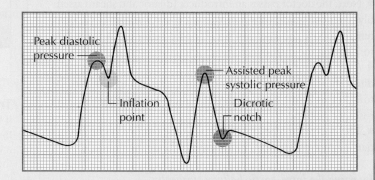

Early deflation

With *early deflation,* a U shape appears and peak systolic pressure is less than or equal to assisted peak systolic pressure. This event won't decrease afterload or myocardial oxygen consumption.

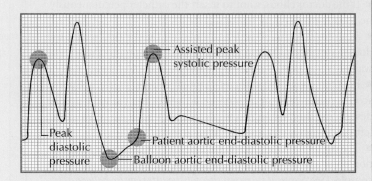

Late inflation

With *late inflation*, the dicrotic notch precedes the inflation point, and the notch and the inflation point create a W shape. Late inflation can lead to a reduction in peak diastolic pressure, coronary and systemic perfusion augmentation time, and augmented coronary perfusion pressure.

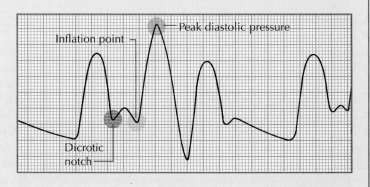

Interpreting intra-aortic balloon waveforms (continued)

Late deflation

With *late deflation,* peak systolic pressure exceeds assisted peak systolic pressure. This event threatens the patient by increasing afterload, myocardial oxygen consumption, cardiac workload, and preload. It occurs when the balloon has been inflated for too long or fails to receive the input signal from the ECG, indicating the start of systole (QRS complex).

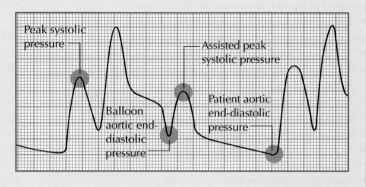

15 minutes for 1 hour after balloon insertion, then every 2 hours while the balloon is in place or according to your facility's policy. *Loss of left arm pulses may indicate upward balloon displacement.* Notify the doctor of any changes.
■ Monitor the patient's urine output every hour. Note baseline serum creatinine levels, and monitor these levels daily. *Changes in urine output and serum creatinine levels may signal reduced renal perfusion from downward balloon displacement.*
■ Auscultate for heart and breath sounds as needed or every 4 hours. If the patient's condition permits, put IABC on standby to auscultate the heart and lungs so IABC noises don't interfere with your assessment.[13]
■ Auscultate for and record bowel sounds every 4 hours. Check for abdominal distention and tenderness as well as changes in the patient's elimination patterns.
■ Measure the patient's temperature every 1 to 4 hours or according to your facility's policy. If it's elevated, obtain blood samples for a culture, send them to the laboratory immediately, and notify the doctor.
■ Maintain the head of the bed less than 45 degrees to prevent kinking and migration of the catheter.[13]
■ Monitor the patient's hematologic status. Observe for bleeding gums, blood in the urine or stools, petechiae, and bleeding at the insertion site. Monitor his platelet count, hemoglobin levels, and hematocrit daily.[13] Expect to administer blood products to maintain hematocrit at 30%. If the platelet count drops, expect to administer platelets.
■ If heparin is used for arterial lumen patency, monitor partial thromboplastin time (PTT) every 6 hours while the heparin dose is adjusted to maintain PTT at 1½ to 2 times the normal value, then every 12 to 24 hours while the balloon remains in place.
■ Measure pulmonary artery pressure and pulmonary artery wedge pressure (PAWP) every 1 to 2 hours, as ordered. *A rising PAWP reflects preload, signaling increased ventricular pressure and workload*; notify the doctor if this occurs.
■ Obtain samples for ABG analysis, as ordered.
■ Monitor serum electrolyte levels—especially sodium and potassium—*to assess the patient's fluid and electrolyte balance and help prevent arrhythmias.*

■ Watch for signs and symptoms of a dissecting aortic aneurysm: a blood pressure differential between the left and right arms, elevated blood pressure, syncope, pallor, diaphoresis, dyspnea, a throbbing abdominal mass, a reduced red blood cell count with an elevated white blood cell count, and pain in the chest, abdomen, or back. Notify the doctor immediately if you detect any of these complications.
■ Assess the cardiac index, systemic blood pressure, and PAWP *to help the doctor evaluate the patient's readiness for weaning*—usually about 24 hours after balloon insertion. The patient's hemodynamic status should be stable on minimal doses of inotropic agents, such as dopamine (Intropin) or dobutamine (Dobutrex).
■ Discard used supplies, remove and discard your gloves, and perform hand hygiene.[1,2,3]
■ Document the procedure.[11,12]

Weaning a patient from IABC

■ Perform hand hygiene.[1,2,3]
■ To begin weaning, gradually decrease the frequency of balloon augmentation to 1:2, as ordered. Although each facility has its own weaning protocol, be aware that assist frequency is usually maintained for an hour or longer. If the patient's hemodynamic indices remain stable during this time, weaning may continue by decreasing the frequency of balloon augmentation to 1:3, and so on.
■ Avoid leaving the patient on a low augmentation volume for more than 2 hours *to prevent embolus formation.*
■ If augmentation volume is reduced for weaning, return the pump to full augmentation volume at a ratio of 1:1 for 5 minutes each hour *to decrease the risk of platelet aggregation.*
■ Assess the patient's tolerance of weaning. Signs and symptoms of poor tolerance include hypotension, confusion, disorientation, urine output below 30 mL/hour, cold and clammy skin, chest pain, arrhythmias, ischemic ECG changes, and elevated pulmonary artery occlusion pressure. If the patient develops any of these problems, notify the doctor immediately.
■ Perform hand hygiene.[1,2,3]
■ Document the procedure.[11,12]

For assisting with removal

■ Perform hand hygiene and put on gloves.[1,2,3]
■ Make sure PTT is within normal limits before the balloon is removed *to prevent hemorrhage at the insertion site.*
■ The control system is turned off and the connective tubing is disconnected from the catheter *to ensure balloon deflation.*
■ The doctor removes the sutures securing the balloon and then withdraws the balloon until the proximal end of the catheter contacts the distal end of the introducer sheath.
■ The doctor then applies pressure below the puncture site and removes the balloon and introducer sheath as a unit, allowing a few seconds of free bleeding *to prevent thrombus formation.*
■ *To promote distal bleedback,* the doctor applies pressure above the puncture site.
■ Apply direct pressure to the site for 30 minutes or until bleeding stops.[13] (In some facilities, this is the doctor's responsibility.)
■ If the balloon was inserted surgically, the surgeon will close the Dacron graft and suture the insertion site. The cardiologist usually removes a percutaneous catheter.
■ After balloon removal, provide wound care according to your facility's policy. Apply a pressure dressing and keep it in place for 2 to 4 hours.[13]
■ Record the patient's pedal and posterior tibial pulses, and the color, temperature, and sensation of the affected limb.
■ Maintain the patient on bed rest, with the head of the patient's bed elevated 30 degrees or less, and keep the affected extremity straight for 8 hours according to your facility policy.[13]
■ Discard used supplies, remove and discard your gloves, and perform hand hygiene.[1,2,3]
■ Document the procedure.[11,12]

Special considerations

■ Before using the IABC control system, make sure you know what the alarms and messages mean and how to respond to them.
■ Inflation and deflation need to be timed to the patient's cardiac cycle *to achieve optimal counterpulsation.* Determine timing using the patient's ECG signal (inflation occurs in the middle of the T wave; deflation occurs just before the end of the QRS complex), his arterial waveform, or the intrinsic pump rate.

NURSING ALERT *You must respond immediately to alarms and messages.*

■ Don't use the arterial lumen of the IABC catheter for blood sampling.
■ Site care and frequency depend on the type of dressing used. Change a transparent semipermeable dressing at least every 7 days and a gauze dressing every 2 days.[14] Change the dressing sooner if drainage, site tenderness, signs of infection, or compromised dressing integrity occur.
■ Clean the catheter-site junction with an antiseptic pad (chlorhexidine-based is preferred), allow it to dry, replace the securement device (if used), and then apply a sterile occlusive dressing.[15] If povidone-iodine solution is used, don't allow it to come in contact with the catheter.
■ Watch for pump interruptions, which may result from loose ECG electrodes or leadwires, static or 60-cycle interference, catheter kinking, or improper body alignment.

■ After removal, assess the patient's vital signs and hemodynamic parameters every 15 minutes for 1 hour, every 30 minutes for the next hour, and then hourly as the patient's condition warrants.[13] Notify the doctor of any abnormalities.

Complications

IABC may cause several complications. The most common, arterial embolism, stems from clot formation on the balloon surface. Other potential complications include extension or rupture of an aortic aneurysm, femoral or iliac artery perforation, femoral artery occlusion, balloon rupture, sepsis, and limb ischemia. Bleeding at the insertion site may become aggravated by pump-induced thrombocytopenia caused by platelet aggregation around the balloon.

Removal of IABC may cause bleeding and hematoma formation at the insertion site. Bleeding at the insertion site may become aggravated by pump-induced thrombocytopenia caused by platelet aggregation around the balloon.

Documentation

Document all aspects of patient preparation and assessment, including any patient and family teaching provided. Also document the procedure, interventions, complications, and patient's response.[11,12]

When managing IABC, document all aspects of patient assessment and management, including the patient's response to therapy. If you're responsible for the IABC device, document all routine checks, problems, and troubleshooting measures. If a technician is responsible for the IABC device, record only when and why the technician was notified as well as the result of his actions on the patient, if any. Also document any teaching of the patient and family as well as their responses.[11,12]

Document all aspects of patient assessment and management related to removal, including the condition of the insertion site after removal, wound care performed, and the patient's tolerance of the procedure. Document any patient teaching and the patient's understanding of your teaching.[11,12]

REFERENCES

1 The Joint Commission. (2012). Standard NPSG.07.01.01. *Comprehensive accreditation manual for hospitals: The official handbook.* Oakbrook Terrace, IL: The Joint Commission. (Level I)
2 Centers for Disease Control and Prevention. (October 2002). Guideline for hand hygiene in health-care settings. *Morbidity and Mortality Weekly Report, 51*(RR-16), 1–45. (Level I)
3 World Health Organization. (2009). *WHO guidelines on hand hygiene in health care: First global patient safety challenge. Clean care is safer care.* Geneva, Switzerland: World Health Organization. (Level I)
4 The Joint Commission. (2012). Standard NPSG.01.01.01. *Comprehensive accreditation manual for hospitals: The official handbook.* Oakbrook Terrace, IL: The Joint Commission. (Level I)
5 The Joint Commission. (2012). Standard RI.01.03.01. *Comprehensive accreditation manual for hospitals: The official handbook.* Oakbrook Terrace, IL: The Joint Commission. (Level I)
6 Centers for Medicare & Medicaid Services, Department of Health and Human Services. (2006). "Conditions of Participation: Patients' Rights," 42 CFR part 482.13 [Online]. Accessed November 2011 via the Web at https://www.cms.gov/CFCsAndCoPs/downloads/finalpatientrightsrule.pdf

7 The Joint Commission. (2012). Standard UP.01.01.01. *Comprehensive accreditation manual for hospitals: The official handbook.* Oakbrook Terrace, IL: The Joint Commission. (Level I)

8 Siegel, J. D., et al. "2007 Guideline for Isolation Precautions: Preventing Transmission of Infectious Agents in Healthcare Settings" [Online]. Accessed September 2011 via the Web at http://www.cdc.gov/hicpac/2007ip/2007isolationprecautions.html

9 The Joint Commission. (2012). Standard MM.06.01.01. *Comprehensive accreditation manual for hospitals: The official handbook.* Oakbrook Terrace, IL: The Joint Commission. (Level I)

10 The Joint Commission. (2012). Standard UP.01.03.01. *Comprehensive accreditation manual for hospitals: The official handbook.* Oakbrook Terrace, IL: The Joint Commission. (Level I)

11 The Joint Commission. (2012). Standard RC.01.03.01. *Comprehensive accreditation manual for hospitals: The official handbook.* Oakbrook Terrace, IL: The Joint Commission. (Level I)

12 The Joint Commission. (2012). Standard RC.02.01.01. *Comprehensive accreditation manual for hospitals: The official handbook.* Oakbrook Terrace, IL: The Joint Commission. (Level I)

13 Lynn-McHale Wiegand, D. (Ed.). (2011). *AACN procedure manual for critical care* (6th ed.). Philadelphia, PA: Saunders.

14 O'Grady, N. P., et al. (2011). "Guidelines for the Prevention of Intravascular Catheter-Related Infections" [Online]. Accessed November 2011 via the Web at http://www.cdc.gov/hicpac/pdf/guidelines/bsi-guidelines-2011.pdf (Level I)

15 Standard 46. Vascular access device site care and dressing changes. Infusion nursing standards of practice. (2011). *Journal of Infusion Nursing, 34*(1S), S63–S64. (Level I)

ADDITIONAL REFERENCES

Dyub, A.M., et al. (2008). Preoperative intra-aortic balloon pump in patients undergoing coronary bypass surgery: A systematic review and meta-analysis. *Journal of Cardiac Surgery, 23*(1), 79–86.

Lewis, P.A., et al. (2009). The intra-aortic balloon pump in heart failure management: Implications for nursing practice. *Australian Critical Care, 22*(3), 125–131.

Santa-Cruz, R.A., et al. (2006). Aortic counterpulsation: A review of the hemodynamic effects and indications for use. *Catheterization and Cardiovascular Interventions, 67*(1), 68–77.

Sice, A. (2006). Intra-aortic balloon counterpulsation complicated by limb ischaemia: A reflective commentary. *Nursing in Critical Care, 11*(6), 297–304.

Theologou, T., et al. (2011). Preoperative intra aortic balloon pumps in patients undergoing coronary artery bypass grafting. *Cochrane Database of Systematic Reviews,* (1), CD004472.

Trost, J.C., & Hillis, L.D. (2006). Intra-aortic balloon counterpulsation. *American Journal of Cardiology, 97*(9), 1391–1398.

Woods, S.L., et al. (Eds.). (2010). *Cardiac nursing.* Philadelphia, PA: Lippincott Williams & Wilkins.

INTRACRANIAL PRESSURE MONITORING

Intracranial pressure (ICP) monitoring measures pressure exerted by the brain, blood, and cerebrospinal fluid (CSF) against the inside of the skull. Indications for monitoring ICP include head trauma with bleeding or edema, overproduction or insufficient absorption of CSF, cerebral hemorrhage, and space-occupying brain lesions. ICP monitoring can detect elevated ICP early, before clinical danger signs develop.[1] Prompt intervention can then help avert or diminish neurologic damage caused by cerebral hypoxia and shifts of brain mass.

The four basic ICP monitoring systems are intraventricular catheter, subarachnoid bolt, epidural or subdural sensor, and intraparenchymal pressure monitoring. (See *Understanding ICP monitoring,* pages 404 and 405.) Regardless of which system is used, the procedure is typically performed by a neurosurgeon in the operating room, emergency department, or intensive care unit. Insertion of an ICP monitoring device requires sterile technique to reduce the risk of central nervous system (CNS) infection. Setting up equipment for the monitoring systems also requires strict asepsis.[1]

Equipment

Monitoring unit and transducers as ordered ■ sterile 4″ × 4″ gauze pads ■ linen-saver pads ■ electric clippers ■ sterile drapes ■ povidone-iodine solution ■ sterile gown ■ surgical mask ■ gloves ■ sterile gloves ■ sterile marker ■ sterile labels ■ head dressing supplies (two rolls of 4″ elastic gauze dressing, one roll of 4″ roller gauze, adhesive tape) ■ Optional: suction apparatus, IV pole.

You may need to gather other equipment as instructed by the doctor, such as the drill and bits, scalp retractor, and a scalp staple.

Preparation of equipment

Various types of preassembled ICP monitoring units are available, each with its own setup protocols. These units are designed to reduce the risk of infection by eliminating the need for multiple stopcocks, manometers, and transducer dome assemblies. When preparing the equipment, label all medications, medication containers, and other solutions on and off the sterile field.[2] Some facilities use units that have miniaturized transducers rather than transducer domes.

Monitoring units and setup protocols are varied and complex and differ among health care facilities. Check your facility's guidelines for your particular unit.

Implementation

■ Perform hand hygiene.[3,4,5]
■ Confirm the patient's identity using at least two patient identifiers according to your facility's policy.[6]
■ Explain the procedure to the patient or his family.
■ Make sure that an informed consent has been obtained and documented in the medical record.[7]
■ Provide privacy if the procedure is being done in an open emergency department or intensive care unit.
■ Conduct a preprocedure verification process *to make sure that all relevant documentation, related information, and equipment are available and correctly identified to the patient identifiers.*[8]
■ Verify that the laboratory and imaging studies have been completed as ordered and that the results are in the patient's medical record. Notify the doctor of any unexpected results.[8]
■ Perform hand hygiene and put on gloves. Wear appropriate personal protective equipment.[3,4,5]
■ Obtain baseline routine and neurologic vital signs *to aid in prompt detection of decompensation during the procedure.*[1]

EQUIPMENT

Understanding ICP monitoring

Intracranial pressure (ICP) can be monitored using one of four systems.

Intraventricular catheter monitoring

In this procedure, which monitors ICP directly, the doctor inserts a small polyethylene or silicone rubber catheter into the lateral ventricle through a burr hole.

Although this method measures ICP most accurately, it carries the greatest risk of infection. This is the only type of ICP monitoring that allows evaluation of brain compliance and drainage of significant amounts of cerebrospinal fluid (CSF).

Contraindications usually include stenotic cerebral ventricles, cerebral aneurysms in the path of catheter placement, and suspected vascular lesions.

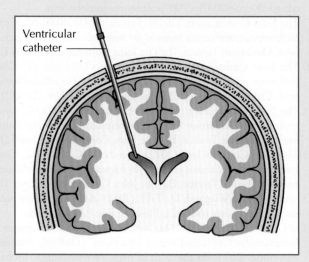

Ventricular catheter

Subarachnoid bolt monitoring

This procedure involves insertion of a special bolt into the subarachnoid space through a twist-drill burr hole that's positioned in the front of the skull behind the hairline.

Placing the bolt is easier than placing an intraventricular catheter, especially if a computed tomography scan reveals that the cerebrum has shifted or the ventricles have collapsed. This type of ICP monitoring also carries less risk of infection and parenchymal damage *because the bolt doesn't penetrate the cerebrum.*

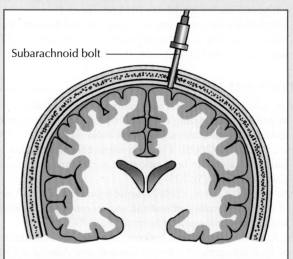

Subarachnoid bolt

■ Place the patient in the supine position, and elevate the head of the bed 30 degrees (or as ordered).[1]

■ Place linen-saver pads under the patient's head. Clip his hair at the insertion site, as indicated by the doctor, *to decrease the risk of infection.* Carefully fold and remove the linen-saver pads *to avoid spilling loose hair onto the bed.*

■ Drape the patient with sterile drapes.

■ Verify that the insertion site has been identified before preparing the site. *Doing so will minimize the risk of preparing the wrong area.*[9] Then scrub the insertion site for 2 minutes with antiseptic solution.

■ The doctor puts on the sterile gown, mask, and sterile gloves.

■ Make sure a time-out is conducted immediately before the doctor starts the procedure *to identify the correct patient, site, positioning,*

and procedure and to ensure that all relevant information and necessary equipment is available.[10]

■ The doctor opens the interior wrap of the sterile supply tray and proceeds with insertion of the catheter or bolt.

■ *To facilitate placement of the device,* hold the patient's head in your hands or attach a long strip of 4″ roller gauze to one side rail, and bring it across the patient's forehead to the opposite rail. Reassure the conscious patient *to help ease his anxiety.* Talk to him frequently *to assess his level of consciousness (LOC) and detect signs of deterioration.* Watch for cardiac arrhythmias and abnormal respiratory patterns.

■ After insertion, remove and discard your gloves. Perform hand hygiene,[3,4,5] put on sterile gloves, clean around the insertion site with antiseptic solution, and apply a sterile dressing to the site.[1]

Understanding ICP monitoring *(continued)*

Epidural or subdural sensor monitoring

ICP can also be monitored from the epidural or subdural space. For epidural monitoring, a fiber-optic sensor is inserted into the epidural space through a burr hole. This system's main drawback is its questionable accuracy *because ICP isn't being measured directly from a CSF-filled space.*

For subdural monitoring, a fiber-optic transducer-tipped catheter is tunneled through a burr hole, and its tip is placed on brain tissue under the dura mater. The main drawback to this method is its inability to drain CSF.

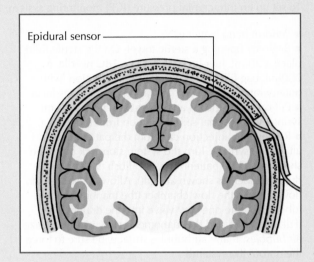

Intraparenchymal pressure monitoring

In this procedure, the doctor inserts a catheter through a small subarachnoid bolt and, after puncturing the dura mater, advances the catheter a few centimeters into the brain's white matter. There's no need to balance or calibrate the equipment after insertion.

Although this method doesn't provide direct access to CSF, measurements are accurate *because brain tissue pressures correlate well with ventricular pressures.* Intraparenchymal monitoring may be used to obtain ICP measurements in patients with compressed or dislocated ventricles.

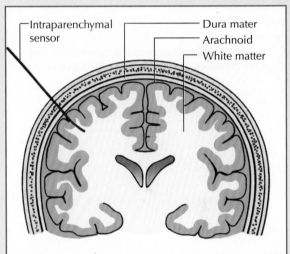

- If not done by the doctor, connect the catheter to the appropriate monitoring device, depending on the system used.[1] Make sure to trace the tubing from the patient to the point of origin before attaching it *to make sure that it's connected to the proper port.*[11] (See *Setting up an ICP monitoring system,* page 406.)
- If the doctor has set up a ventriculostomy drainage system, attach the drip chamber to the headboard or bedside IV pole as ordered.

NURSING ALERT *Positioning the drip chamber too high may raise ICP; positioning it too low may cause excessive CSF drainage.*

- Dispose of used supplies in the appropriate receptacle.
- Remove your personal protective equipment and perform hand hygiene.[3,4,5]
- Document the procedure.[12,13]

Special considerations

- Inspect the insertion site at least every 24 hours (or according to your facility's policy) for redness, swelling, and drainage. Clean the site and apply a dry sterile dressing when the dressing is loose or soiled, or according to your facility's policy.
- Assess the patient's clinical status, and take routine and neurologic vital signs every hour, or as ordered. Make sure you've obtained orders for pressure parameters from the doctor.[1]
- Calculate cerebral perfusion pressure (CPP) hourly; use the equation CPP = MAP − ICP (MAP refers to mean arterial pressure). If CPP isn't within the specified parameters, notify the doctor.[1]
- Observe digital ICP readings and waves. Remember, the trend of readings is more significant than any single reading. Remember that when measuring ICP using the intraventricular catheter or subarachnoid bolt, make sure the transducer is in the exact same position in relation to patient landmarks with each measurement. (See *Interpreting ICP waveforms,* page 407.) If you observe continually elevated ICP readings, note how long they're sustained. If they last several minutes, notify the doctor immediately. Finally, record and describe any CSF drainage.

(Text continues on page 408.)

Setting up an ICP monitoring system

To set up an intracranial pressure (ICP) monitoring system, follow these steps, using strict sterile technique.

■ Perform hand hygiene.[3,4,5]
■ Begin by opening a sterile towel. On the sterile field, place a 20-mL luer-lock syringe, an 18G needle, a 250-mL bag filled with normal saline solution (with outer wrapper removed), and a disposable transducer.
■ Put on sterile gloves and gown, and fill the 20-mL syringe with normal saline solution from the IV bag.
■ Remove the injection cap from the patient line and attach the syringe. Turn the system stopcock off to the short end of the patient line, and flush through to the drip chamber (as shown at right). Allow a few drops to flow through the flow chamber (the manometer), the tubing, and the one-way valve into the drainage bag. (Fill the tubing and the manometer slowly *to minimize air bubbles*. If any air bubbles surface, be sure to force them from the system.)

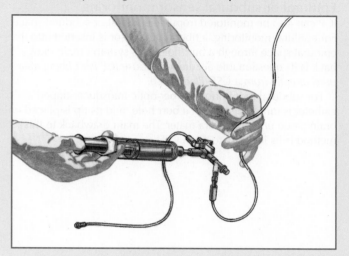

■ Attach the manometer to the IV pole at the head of the bed.
■ Slide the drip chamber onto the manometer, and align the chamber to the zero point (as shown at right).

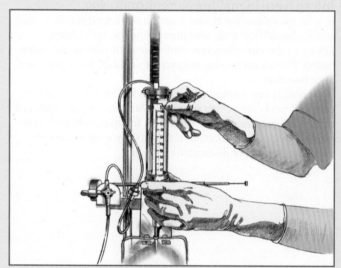

■ Next, connect the transducer to the monitor.
■ Remove and discard your gloves and perform hand hygiene.[3,4,5]
■ Put on a new pair of sterile gloves.
■ Keeping one hand sterile, turn the patient stopcock off to the patient.
■ Align the zero point with the center line of the patient's head, level with the middle of the ear.
■ Lower the flow chamber to zero, and turn the stopcock off to the dead-end cap. With a clean hand, balance the system according to monitor guidelines.
■ Turn the system stopcock off to drainage, and raise the flow chamber to the ordered height (as shown at right).
■ Return the stopcock to the ordered position, and observe the monitor for the return of ICP patterns.
■ Remove and discard your gloves and perform hand hygiene.[3,4,5]

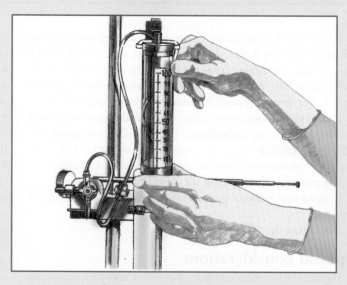

Interpreting ICP waveforms

Three waveforms—A, B, and C—are used to monitor intracranial pressure (ICP). A waves are an ominous sign of intracranial decompensation and poor compliance. B waves correlate with changes in respiration, and C waves correlate with changes in arterial pressure.

Normal waveform

A normal ICP waveform typically shows a steep upward systolic slope followed by a downward diastolic slope with a dicrotic notch. In most cases, this waveform occurs continuously and indicates an ICP between 0 and 15 mm Hg—normal pressure.

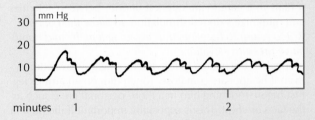

A waves

The most clinically significant ICP waveforms are A waves, which may reach elevations of 50 to 100 mm Hg, persist for 5 to 20 minutes, then drop sharply—signaling exhaustion of the brain's compliance mechanisms. A waves may come and go, spiking from temporary rises in thoracic pressure or from any condition that increases ICP beyond the brain's compliance limits. Activities such as sustained coughing or straining during defecation can cause temporary elevations in thoracic pressure.

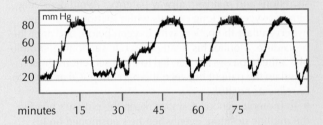

B waves

B waves, which appear sharp and rhythmic with a sawtooth pattern, occur every 1½ to 2 minutes and may reach elevations of 50 mm Hg. The clinical significance of B waves isn't clear, but the waves correlate with respiratory changes and may occur more frequently with decreasing compensation. Because B waves sometimes precede A waves, notify the doctor if B waves occur frequently.

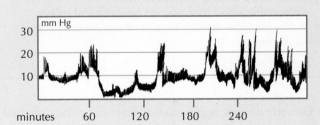

C waves

Like B waves, C waves are rapid and rhythmic, but they aren't as sharp. Clinically insignificant, they may fluctuate with respirations or systemic blood pressure changes.

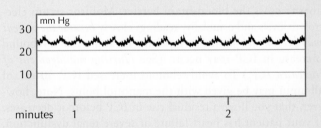

When equipment malfunctions

A waveform that looks like the one shown at right signals a problem with the transducer or monitor. Check for line obstruction, and determine if the transducer needs rebalancing.

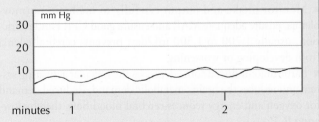

Nursing management of increased ICP

By performing nursing care gently, slowly, and cautiously, you can best help manage—or even significantly reduce—increased intracranial pressure (ICP). If possible, urge your patient to participate in his own care. Here are some steps you can take to manage increased ICP.

■ Plan your care to include rest periods between activities and minimize external stimulation *to allow the patient's ICP to return to baseline, thus avoiding lengthy and cumulative pressure elevations.*

■ Speak to the patient before attempting any procedures, even if he appears comatose. Touch him on an arm or leg first before touching him in a more personal area, such as the face or chest. This is especially important if the patient doesn't know you or if he's confused or sedated.

■ Suction the patient only when it's necessary to remove secretions and maintain airway patency. Avoid depriving him of oxygen for long periods while suctioning; always hyperventilate the patient with oxygen before and after the procedure. Monitor his heart rate while suctioning. If multiple catheter passes are needed to clear secretions, hyperventilate the patient between them *to bring ICP as close to baseline as possible.*

■ To promote venous drainage, keep the patient's head in the midline position, even when he's positioned on his side.[1] Avoid flexing the neck or hip more than 90 degrees, and keep the head of the bed elevated 30 to 45 degrees. Keep endotracheal tube ties and rigid cervical collars secure but loose enough *to prevent compression of the jugular veins.*

■ Avoid the prone position.

■ *To avoid increasing intrathoracic pressure, which raises ICP,* discourage Valsalva's maneuver and isometric muscle contractions. To avoid isometric contractions, distract the patient when giving him painful injections (by asking him to wiggle his toes and by massaging the area before injection to relax the muscle) and have him concentrate on breathing through difficult procedures such as bed-to-stretcher transfers. To keep the patient from holding his breath when moving around in bed, tell him to relax as much as possible during position changes. If necessary, administer a stool softener to help prevent constipation and unnecessary straining during defecation.

■ If the patient is heavily sedated, monitor his respiratory rate and blood gas levels. *Depressed respirations will compromise ventilations and oxygen exchange. Maintaining adequate respiratory rate and volume helps reduce ICP.*

■ If you're in a specialty unit, you may be able to hyperventilate the patient *to counter sustained ICP elevations.* This procedure is one of the best ways to reduce high ICP at bedside for short periods. Consult your facility's protocol.

■ Osmotic diuretic agents such as mannitol reduce cerebral edema by shrinking intracranial contents. Given by IV drip or bolus, mannitol draws water from tissues into plasma; it doesn't cross the blood-brain barrier. Monitor serum electrolyte levels and osmolality readings closely *because the patient may become dehydrated very quickly.* Be aware that a rebound increase in ICP may occur. (See *Nursing management of increased ICP.*) To avoid rebound increased ICP, 50-mL of albumin may be given with the mannitol bolus. Note, however, that you'll see a residual rise in ICP before it decreases. If your patient has heart failure or severe renal dysfunction, monitor for problems in adapting to the increased intravascular volumes.

■ Monitor intake and output carefully to maintain normovolemia, ensure adequate MAP, and ensure good CPP. Fluid restriction, usually 1,200 to 1,500 mL/day, prevents cerebral edema from developing or worsening.

■ Barbiturate-induced coma depresses the reticular activating system and reduces the brain's metabolic demand. Reduced demand for oxygen and energy reduces cerebral blood flow, thereby lowering ICP.

■ Hyperventilation with oxygen from a handheld resuscitation bag or ventilator helps rid the patient of excess carbon dioxide, constricting cerebral vessels and reducing cerebral blood volume and ICP. However, only normal brain tissues respond because blood vessels in damaged areas have reduced vasoconstrictive ability. Hyperventilation should only be done in an acute situation to decrease ICP until other measures can be instituted.[1]

NURSING ALERT *Hyperventilation with a handheld resuscitation bag or a ventilator should be performed with care because hyperventilation can cause ischemia.*[1]

■ Before tracheal suctioning, hyperventilate the patient with 100% oxygen as ordered. Apply suction for a maximum of 15 seconds. Avoid inducing hypoxia *because this condition greatly increases cerebral blood flow.*

■ Because fever raises brain metabolism, which increases cerebral blood flow, fever reduction (achieved by administering acetaminophen, sponge baths, or a hypothermia blanket) also helps to reduce ICP. However, rebound increases in ICP and brain edema may occur if rapid rewarming takes place after hypothermia or if cooling measures induce shivering.

■ Withdrawal of CSF through the drainage system reduces CSF volume and thus reduces ICP. Although less commonly used, surgical removal of a skull-bone flap provides room for the swollen brain to expand. If this procedure is performed, keep the site clean and dry *to prevent infection* and maintain sterile technique when changing the dressing.

Complications

CNS infection, the most common hazard of ICP monitoring, can result from contamination of the equipment setup or of the insertion site.

NURSING ALERT *Excessive loss of CSF can result from faulty stopcock placement or a drip chamber that's positioned too low. Such loss can rapidly decompress the cranial contents and damage bridging cortical veins, leading to hematoma formation. Decompression can also lead to rupture of existing hematomas or aneurysms, causing hemorrhage.*

Watch for signs of impending or overt decompensation: pupillary dilation (unilateral or bilateral); decreased pupillary response to light; decreasing LOC; rising systolic blood pressure and widening pulse pressure; bradycardia; slowed, irregular respirations; and, in late decompensation, decerebrate posturing.

Documentation

Record the time and date of the insertion procedure and the patient's response. Note the insertion site and the type of monitoring system used. Record ICP digital readings and waveforms and CPP hourly in your notes, on a flowchart, or directly on readout strips, depending on your facility's policy. Document any factors that may affect ICP (for example, drug therapy, stressful procedures, or sleep).[12,13]

Record routine and neurologic vital signs hourly, and describe the patient's clinical status. Note the amount, character, and frequency of any CSF drainage (for example, "between 6 p.m. and 7 p.m., 15 mL of blood-tinged CSF"). Also record the ICP reading in response to drainage.[12,13]

REFERENCES

1 American Association of Neuroscience Nursing. (2011). *Guide to the care of the patient with intracranial pressure monitoring/extraventricular drainage or lumbar drain: AANN reference series for clinical practice.* Glenview, IL: American Association of Neuroscience Nurses.

2 The Joint Commission. (2012). Standard NPSG.03.04.01. *Comprehensive accreditation manual for hospitals: The official handbook.* Oakbrook Terrace, IL: The Joint Commission. (Level I)

3 The Joint Commission. (2012). Standard NPSG.07.01.01. *Comprehensive accreditation manual for hospitals: The official handbook.* Oakbrook Terrace, IL: The Joint Commission. (Level I)

4 Centers for Disease Control and Prevention. (October 2002). Guideline for hand hygiene in health-care settings. *Morbidity and Mortality Weekly Report, 51*(RR-16), 1–45. (Level I)

5 World Health Organization. (2009). *WHO guidelines on hand hygiene in health care: First global patient safety challenge. Clean care is safer care.* Geneva, Switzerland: World Health Organization. (Level I)

6 The Joint Commission. (2012). Standard NPSG.01.01.01. *Comprehensive accreditation manual for hospitals: The official handbook.* Oakbrook Terrace, IL: The Joint Commission. (Level I)

7 The Joint Commission. (2012). Standard RI.01.03.01. *Comprehensive accreditation manual for hospitals: The official handbook.* Oakbrook Terrace, IL: The Joint Commission. (Level I)

8 The Joint Commission. (2012). Standard UP.01.01.01. *Comprehensive accreditation manual for hospitals: The official handbook.* Oakbrook Terrace, IL: The Joint Commission. (Level I)

9 The Joint Commission. (2012). Standard UP.01.02.01. *Comprehensive accreditation manual for hospitals: The official handbook.* Oakbrook Terrace, IL: The Joint Commission. (Level I)

10 The Joint Commission. (2012). Standard UP.01.03.01. *Comprehensive accreditation manual for hospitals: The official handbook.* Oakbrook Terrace, IL: The Joint Commission. (Level I)

11 U.S. Food and Drug Administration. (2009). "Look. Check. Connect.: Safe Medical Device Connections Save Lives" [Online]. Accessed November 2011 via the Web at http://www.fda.gov/downloads/MedicalDevices/Safety/AlertsandNotices/UCM134873.pdf

12 The Joint Commission. (2012). Standard RC.01.03.01. *Comprehensive accreditation manual for hospitals: The official handbook.* Oakbrook Terrace, IL: The Joint Commission. (Level I)

13 The Joint Commission. (2012). Standard RC.02.01.01. *Comprehensive accreditation manual for hospitals: The official handbook.* Oakbrook Terrace, IL: The Joint Commission. (Level I)

ADDITIONAL REFERENCES

Forsyth, R.J., et al. (2010). Routine intracranial pressure monitoring in acute coma. *Cochrane Database of Systematic Reviews*, (2), CD002043.

Hickey, J.V. (2009). *The clinical practice of neurological and neurosurgical nursing* (6th ed.). Philadelphia, PA: Lippincott Williams & Wilkins.

Lynn-McHale Wiegand, D. (Ed.). (2011). *AACN procedure manual for critical care* (6th ed.). Philadelphia, PA: Saunders.

May, K. (2009). The pathophysiology and causes of raised intracranial pressure. *British Journal of Nursing, 18*(15), 911–914.

Wolfe, T.J., & Torbey, M.T. (2009). Management of intracranial pressure. *Current Neurology and Neuroscience Reports, 9*(6), 477–485.

INTRADERMAL INJECTION

Because little systemic absorption of intradermally injected agents takes place, this type of injection is used primarily to produce a local effect, as in allergy or tuberculin testing. Intradermal injections are administered in small volumes—usually 0.1 mL or less—into the outer layers of the skin.

The ventral forearm is the most commonly used site for intradermal injection because of its easy accessibility and lack of hair. In extensive allergy testing, the outer aspect of the upper arms may be used, as well as the area of the back located between the scapulae. (See *Intradermal injection sites,* page 410.)

Equipment

Patient's medication record and chart ■ tuberculin syringe with a 26G or 27G ½″ to ⅜″ needle ■ prescribed medication ■ gloves ■ alcohol pads ■ gauze pads ■ pen, if needed.

Implementation

■ Verify the doctor's order for the prescribed drug, dosage, and route.[1] Compare the order with the drug label.

Intradermal injection sites

The most common intradermal injection site is the ventral forearm. Other sites (indicated by dotted areas) include the upper chest, upper arm, and shoulder blades. Skin in these areas is usually lightly pigmented, thinly keratinized, and relatively hairless, facilitating detection of adverse reactions.

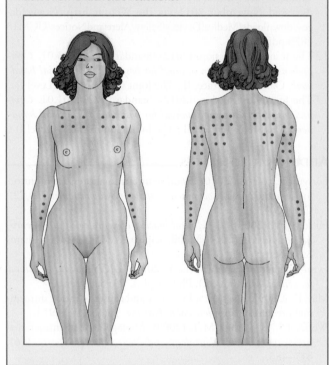

■ Review the patient's medical record for drug allergies.[1]

■ Avoid distractions and interruptions when preparing and administering the medication to prevent medication errors.[2]

■ Check the prescribed medication for color and clarity, observe for abnormal changes, and note the medication's expiration date.[3] If the medication has expired, return it to the pharmacy and obtain a new vial.

■ Select the appropriately sized needle.

■ Perform hand hygiene.[4,5,6]

■ Confirm the patient's identity using at least two patient identifiers according to your facility's policy.[7]

■ Explain the procedure to the patient.

■ Tell the patient where you'll be giving the injection.

■ Provide privacy.

■ If your facility uses a bar code scanning system, scan your identification badge, the patient's identification bracelet, and the medication's bar code.

■ Instruct the patient to sit up and to extend her arm and support it on a flat surface, with the ventral forearm exposed (as shown below).

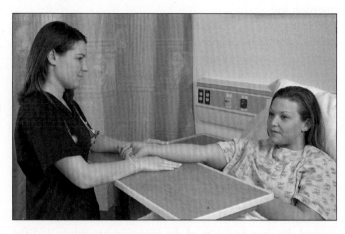

■ Put on gloves.

■ With an alcohol pad, clean the surface of the ventral forearm about two or three fingerbreadths distal to the antecubital space (as shown below). Be sure the test site you have chosen is free of hair or blemishes. Allow the skin to dry completely before administering the injection.

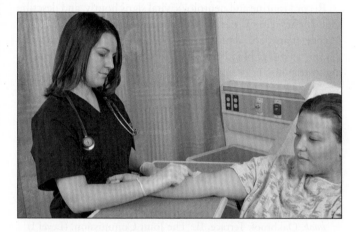

■ While holding the patient's forearm in your hand, stretch the skin taut with your thumb (as shown below).

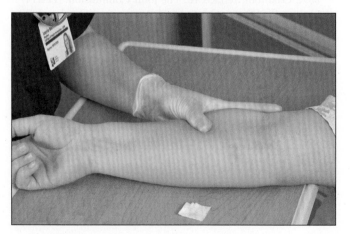

Giving an intradermal injection

Secure the forearm. Insert the needle at a 10- to 15-degree angle so that it just punctures the skin's surface. The antigen should raise a small wheal as it's injected.

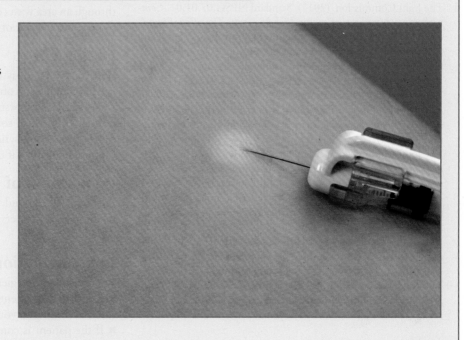

■ With your free hand, hold the needle at a 10- to 15-degree angle to the patient's arm, with its bevel up (as shown below).[8]

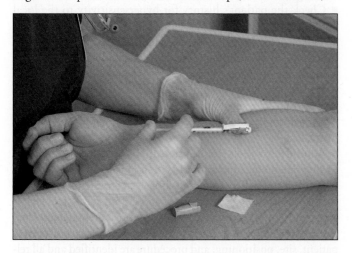

■ Insert the needle about ⅛″ (0.3 cm) below the epidermis. Stop when the needle's bevel tip is under the skin, and inject the antigen slowly. You should feel some resistance as you do this, and a wheal should form as you inject the antigen. (See *Giving an intradermal injection.*) If no wheal forms, you have injected the antigen too deeply; withdraw the needle, and administer another test dose at least 2″ (5 cm) from the first site.

■ Withdraw the needle at the same angle at which it was inserted. Don't rub the site. *Rubbing could irritate the underlying tissue, which may affect test results.*

■ If you're administering multiple antigens, inject them at sites at least 2″ apart.

■ Circle each test site with a marking pen, and label each site according to the recall antigen given. Instruct the patient to refrain from washing off the circles until the test is completed.

■ Don't recap the needle. Dispose of needles and syringes according to your facility's policy.

■ Remove and discard your gloves in the appropriate container and perform hand hygiene.[4,5,6]

■ Assess the patient's response to the skin testing in 24 to 48 hours.

■ Document the procedure.[9,10]

Special considerations

■ In patients who are hypersensitive to the test antigens, a severe anaphylactic response can result. This reaction requires immediate epinephrine injection and other emergency resuscitation procedures. Be especially alert after giving a test dose of penicillin or tetanus antitoxin.

Documentation

On the patient's medical record, document the type and amount of medication given, the time it was given, and the injection site. Note skin reactions and other adverse reactions.[9,10]

REFERENCES

1 The Joint Commission. (2012). Standard MM.04.01.01. *Comprehensive accreditation manual for hospitals: The official handbook.* Oakbrook Terrace, IL: The Joint Commission. (Level I)

2 Westbrook, J. et al. (2010). Association of interruptions with an increased risk and severity of medication administration errors. *Archives of Internal Medicine, 170*(8), 683–690.

3 The Joint Commission. (2012). Standard MM.06.01.01. *Comprehensive accreditation manual for hospitals: The official handbook*. Oakbrook Terrace, IL: The Joint Commission. (Level I)

4 The Joint Commission. (2012). Standard NPSG.07.01.01. *Comprehensive accreditation manual for hospitals: The official handbook*. Oakbrook Terrace, IL: The Joint Commission. (Level I)

5 Centers for Disease Control and Prevention. (October 2002). Guideline for hand hygiene in health-care settings. *Morbidity and Mortality Weekly Report, 51*(RR-16), 1–45. (Level I)

6 World Health Organization. (2009). *WHO guidelines on hand hygiene in health care: First global patient safety challenge. Clean care is safer care*. Geneva, Switzerland: World Health Organization. (Level I)

7 The Joint Commission. (2012). Standard NPSG.01.01.01. *Comprehensive accreditation manual for hospitals: The official handbook*. Oakbrook Terrace, IL: The Joint Commission. (Level I)

8 Tarnow, K., & King, N. (2004). Intradermal injections: Traditional bevel up versus bevel down. *Applied Nursing Research, 17*(4), 275–282. (Level VI)

9 The Joint Commission. (2012). Standard RC.01.03.01. *Comprehensive accreditation manual for hospitals: The official handbook*. Oakbrook Terrace, IL: The Joint Commission. (Level I)

10 The Joint Commission. (2012). Standard RC.02.01.01. *Comprehensive accreditation manual for hospitals: The official handbook*. Oakbrook Terrace, IL: The Joint Commission. (Level I)

ADDITIONAL REFERENCES

Craven, R.F., & Hirnle, C.J. (2012). *Fundamentals of nursing: Human health and function* (7th ed.). Philadelphia, PA: Lippincott Williams & Wilkins.

Nettina, S.M. (2010). *Lippincott manual of nursing practice* (9th ed.). Philadelphia, PA: Lippincott Williams & Wilkins.

Taylor, C., et al. (2011). *Fundamentals of nursing: The art and science of nursing care* (7th ed.). Philadelphia, PA: Lippincott Williams & Wilkins.

INTRAOSSEOUS INFUSION

When rapid venous access is difficult or impossible, intraosseous infusion (IO) allows short-term delivery of fluids, medications, or blood into the bone marrow. Most commonly performed on infants and children, this technique is used in such emergencies as cardiopulmonary arrest or circulatory collapse, hypovolemia from traumatic injury or dehydration, status epilepticus, status asthmaticus, burns, near drowning, and overwhelming sepsis. It can also be used in adults in emergency situations when IV access can't be established.[1] If needed during cardiac arrest, don't interrupt cardiopulmonary resuscitation (CPR) for cannula insertion.[2]

Any drug that can be given IV can be given by IO infusion with comparable absorption and effectiveness. IO infusion is commonly undertaken at the anterior surface of the tibia. Alternative sites include the iliac crest, spinous process and, rarely, the upper anterior portion of the sternum. Only personnel trained in this procedure should perform it. Usually, a nurse assists with the procedure, unless specially trained to perform it. (See *Understanding IO infusion*.)

This procedure is contraindicated in osteogenesis imperfecta, osteoporosis, and ipsilateral fracture because of the potential for subcutaneous extravasation. IO infusion is also contraindicated through an area with cellulitis or an infected burn because doing so increases the risk of infection.

Equipment

Bone marrow biopsy needle or specially designed IO infusion needle (cannula and obturator) ■ antiseptic solution ■ sterile gauze pads ■ sterile gloves ■ sterile drape ■ syringe with preservative-free normal saline flush solution ■ IV fluids and tubing ■ 1% lidocaine ■ 3- to 5-mL syringe ■ tape ■ sterile marker ■ sterile labels ■ Optional: sedative, if ordered.

Preparation of equipment

Prepare IV fluids and tubing as ordered. Label all medications, medication containers, and other solutions on and off the sterile field.[3]

Implementation

■ Perform hand hygiene.[4,5,6]

■ Confirm the patient's identity using at least two patient identifiers according to your facility's policy.[7]

■ If the patient is conscious, explain the procedure *to allay his fears and promote his cooperation*.

■ If time permits, ensure that the patient or a responsible family member understands the procedure and a consent form has been signed.[8,9]

■ Check the patient's history for hypersensitivity to the local anesthetic.

■ Tell the patient which bone site will receive the infusion. Inform him that he will receive a local anesthetic and will feel pressure from needle insertion.

■ If time permits, perform a preprocedure verification to make sure that all relevant documentation, related information, and equipment are available and correctly identified to the patient's identifiers.[10]

■ Administer a sedative, if ordered, before the procedure following safe medication administration practices.[11]

■ Position the patient based on the selected puncture site.

■ Perform hand hygiene again[4,5,6] and put on sterile gloves.[12]

■ If time allows, conduct a time-out immediately before starting the procedure to perform a final assessment that the correct patient, site, positioning, and procedure are identified and all relevant information and necessary equipment are available.[10]

■ Using sterile technique, the doctor cleans the puncture site with an antiseptic pad and allows it to dry. He then covers the area with a sterile drape.

■ Using sterile technique, hand the doctor the 3- or 5-mL syringe with 1% lidocaine *so that he can anesthetize the infusion site*.[1]

■ The doctor inserts the infusion needle through the skin and into the bone at an angle of 10 to 15 degrees from vertical. He advances it with a forward and backward rotary motion through the periosteum until the needle penetrates the marrow cavity. The needle should "give" suddenly as it enters the marrow and should stand erect when released.

- Then the doctor removes the obturator from the needle and attaches a 5-mL syringe. He aspirates some bone marrow *to confirm needle placement.*
- The doctor replaces this syringe with the syringe containing the flush solution and flushes the cannula *to confirm needle placement and clear the cannula of clots or bone particles.*
- Next, the doctor removes the syringe of flush solution and attaches IV tubing to the cannula *to allow infusion of medications and IV f luids.*
- Clean the infusion site with antiseptic solution and allow it to dry; then secure the site with tape and a sterile gauze dressing.[1]
- Label the dressing with the date, the time, and your initials.[13]
- Monitor the patient's vital signs and check the infusion site for bleeding and extravasation.
- Remove and discard your gloves and perform hand hygiene.[4,5,6]
- Document the procedure.[14,15]

Special considerations

- The doctor should discontinue IO infusion as soon as conventional vascular access is established (preferably within 2 to 4 hours). IO infusion should remain in place no longer than 24 hours.[1] *Prolonged infusion significantly increases the risk of infection.*
- After you (if you're specially trained) or the doctor removes the needle, apply firm pressure to the site for 5 minutes and place antiseptic ointment and a sterile occlusive dressing over the injection site.
- IO flow rates are determined by needle size and flow through the bone marrow. Fluids should flow freely if needle placement is correct.

Complications

Common complications include extravasation of fluid into subcutaneous tissue, resulting from incorrect needle placement; subperiosteal effusion, resulting from failure of fluid to enter the marrow space; and clotting in the needle, resulting from delayed infusion or failure to flush the needle after placement. Other complications include subcutaneous abscess, osteomyelitis, and epiphyseal injury.

Documentation

Record the time, date, location, and patient's tolerance of the procedure. Document the amount of fluid infused on the intake-and-output record. Document patient teaching and the patient's understanding of your teaching.[14,15]

REFERENCES

1 Standard 59. Intraosseous access devices. Infusion nursing standards of practice. (2011). *Journal of Infusion Nursing, 34*(1S), S82–S83. (Level I)

2 American Heart Association. (2010). 2010 American Heart Association guidelines for cardiopulmonary resuscitation and emergency cardiovascular care. *Circulation, 122*(Suppl. 3), S729–S767. (Level I)

Understanding IO infusion

During intraosseous (IO) infusion, the bone marrow serves as a noncollapsible vein; thus, fluid infused into the marrow cavity rapidly enters the circulation by way of an extensive network of venous sinusoids. Here, the needle is shown positioned in the patient's tibia.

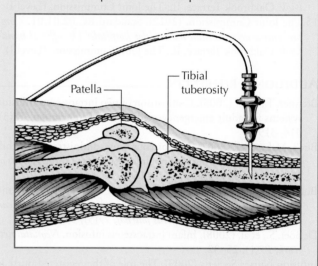

3 The Joint Commission. (2012). Standard NPSG.03.04.01. *Comprehensive accreditation manual for hospitals: The official handbook.* Oakbrook Terrace, IL: The Joint Commission. (Level I)

4 The Joint Commission. (2012). Standard NPSG.07.01.01. *Comprehensive accreditation manual for hospitals: The official handbook.* Oakbrook Terrace, IL: The Joint Commission. (Level I)

5 Centers for Disease Control and Prevention. (October 2002). Guideline for hand hygiene in health-care settings. *Morbidity and Mortality Weekly Report, 51*(RR-16), 1–45. (Level I)

6 World Health Organization. (2009). *WHO guidelines on hand hygiene in health care: First global patient safety challenge. Clean care is safer care.* Geneva, Switzerland: World Health Organization. (Level I)

7 The Joint Commission. (2012). Standard NPSG.01.01.01. *Comprehensive accreditation manual for hospitals: The official handbook.* Oakbrook Terrace, IL: The Joint Commission. (Level I)

8 The Joint Commission. (2012). Standard RI.01.03.01. *Comprehensive accreditation manual for hospitals: The official handbook.* Oakbrook Terrace, IL: The Joint Commission. (Level I)

9 Centers for Medicare & Medicaid Services, Department of Health and Human Services. (2006). "Conditions of Participation: Patients' Rights," 42 CFR part 482.13 [Online]. Accessed November 2011 via the Web at https://www.cms.gov/CFCsAndCoPs/downloads/finalpatientrightsrule.pdf

10 The Joint Commission. (2012). Standard UP.01.01.01. *Comprehensive accreditation manual for hospitals: The official handbook.* Oakbrook Terrace, IL: The Joint Commission. (Level I)

11 The Joint Commission. (2012). Standard MM.06.01.01. *Comprehensive accreditation manual for hospitals: The official handbook.* Oakbrook Terrace, IL: The Joint Commission. (Level I)

12 Siegel, J.D., et al. "2007 Guideline for Isolation Precautions: Preventing Transmission of Infectious Agents in Healthcare Settings" [Online]. Accessed September 2011 via the Web at http://www.cdc.gov/hicpac/2007ip/2007isolationprecautions.html

13 Standard 46. Vascular access device site care and dressing changes. Infusion nursing standards of practice. (2011). *Journal of Infusion Nursing, 34*(1S), S63–64. (Level I)

14 The Joint Commission. (2012). Standard RC.01.03.01. *Comprehensive accreditation manual for hospitals: The official handbook.* Oakbrook Terrace, IL: The Joint Commission. (Level I)

15 The Joint Commission. (2012). Standard RC.02.01.01. *Comprehensive accreditation manual for hospitals: The official handbook.* Oakbrook Terrace, IL: The Joint Commission. (Level I)

ADDITIONAL REFERENCES

Brenner, T., et al. (2008). Comparison of two intraosseous infusion systems for adult emergency medical use. *Resuscitation, 78*(3), 314–319.

Buck, M.L., et al. (2007). Intraosseous drug administration in children and adults during cardiopulmonary resuscitation. *Annals of Pharmacotherapy, 41*(10), 1679–1686.

Burgert, J.M. (2009). Intraosseous infusion of blood products and epinephrine in an adult patient in hemorrhagic shock. *American Association of Nurse Anesthetists Journal, 77*(5), 359–363.

DeBoer, S., et al. (2008). Infant intraosseous infusion. *Neonatal network, 27*(1), 25–32.

Infusion Nurses Society. (2009). The role of the registered nurse in the insertion of intraosseous access devices. *Journal of Infusion Nursing, 32*(4), 187–188.

Langley, D.M., & Moran, M. (2008). Intraosseous needles: They're not just for kids anymore. *Journal of Emergency Nursing, 34*(4), 318–319.

Nettina, S.M. (2010). *Lippincott manual of nursing practice* (9th ed.). Philadelphia, PA: Lippincott Williams & Wilkins.

Verger, J.T., & Lebet, R.M. (Eds.). (2008). *AACN procedure manual for pediatric acute and critical care.* St. Louis, MO: Saunders.

INTRAPLEURAL DRUG ADMINISTRATION

An intrapleural drug is injected through the chest wall into the pleural space or instilled through a chest tube placed intrapleurally for drainage. Doctors use intrapleural administration to promote analgesia, treat spontaneous pneumothorax, resolve pleural effusions, and administer chemotherapy.

Intrapleurally administered drugs diffuse across the parietal pleura and innermost intercostal muscles to affect the intercostal nerves. During intrapleural injection of a drug, the needle passes through the intercostal muscles and parietal pleura on its way to the pleural space.

Drugs commonly given by intrapleural injection include tetracycline, streptokinase, anesthetics, and chemotherapeutic agents (to treat malignant pleural effusion or lung adenocarcinoma).

Contraindications for this route include pleural fibrosis or adhesions, which interfere with diffusion of the drug to the intended site; pleural inflammation; sepsis; and infection at the puncture site. Patients with bullous emphysema and those receiving respiratory therapy using positive end-expiratory pressure also shouldn't have intrapleural injections because the injections may exacerbate an already compromised pulmonary condition.

Equipment

If a patient has emphysema, pleural effusion, or pneumothorax, an intrapleural drug is given through either a #16 to #20 or a #28 to #40 chest tube. Otherwise, it's given through a 16G to 18G blunt-tipped intrapleural (epidural) needle and catheter. Accessory equipment depends on the type of access device the doctor uses. All equipment must be sterile.

For intrapleural catheter insertion

Sterile gloves ■ sterile cap ■ sterile mask ■ sterile gown ■ sterile gauze ■ antiseptic solution ■ sterile drape ■ local anesthetic, such as 1% lidocaine ■ 3- to 5-mL syringe with 22G 1″ and 25G ⅝″ needles ■ 18G needle or scalpel ■ saline-lubricated glass syringe ■ sterile dressings ■ sutures ■ tape ■ blunt-tipped intrapleural needle ■ intrapleural catheter.

For chest tube insertion

Sterile towels ■ sterile gloves ■ sterile cap ■ sterile mask ■ sterile gown ■ sterile gauze ■ antiseptic solution ■ 3- to 5-mL syringe ■ local anesthetic, such as 1% lidocaine ■ 18G needle or scalpel ■ chest tube with or without trocar (#16 to #20 catheter for air or serous fluid; #28 to #40 for blood, pus, or thick fluid) ■ two rubber-tipped clamps, if necessary ■ sutures ■ sterile drain dressings ■ tape ■ thoracic drainage system and tubing.

For drug administration

Sterile gloves ■ sterile gauze pads ■ antiseptic solution ■ prescribed medication ■ appropriate-sized needles and syringes ■ 1% lidocaine, if necessary ■ infusion pump ■ sterile dressings ■ tape ■ two rubber-tipped clamps, if necessary.

For chemotherapy administration

Nonlinting, nonabsorbent disposable gown ■ sterile powder-free chemotherapy gloves ■ face shield ■ National Institute for Occupational Safety and Health–approved respirator mask (if aerosolization is likely) ■ antiseptic solution ■ prescribed chemotherapeutic medication ■ sterile gauze pads ■ infusion pump with programmable dosing limits ■ syringe with a luer-lock connector ■ administration set ■ spill kit ■ hazardous waste receptacle.

Preparation of equipment

When administering chemotherapy, make sure a spill kit is readily available to clean up spills immediately should they occur.

Implementation

■ Perform hand hygiene.[1,2,3]
■ Confirm the patient's identity using at least two patient identifiers according to your facility's policy.[4]
■ Explain the procedure to the patient *to allay his fears.* Encourage him to follow instructions.
■ Ensure that a consent form has been properly signed and witnessed.[5,6]

- Perform hand hygiene and put on sterile gloves and other protective equipment as appropriate.[1,2,3,7]
- Make sure that the insertion site is marked to prevent inserting the catheter in the incorrect location.
- Conduct a time-out immediately before starting the procedure *to perform a final assessment that the correct patient, site, positioning, and procedure are identified and, as applicable, all relevant information and necessary equipment are available.*[8]

Inserting an intrapleural catheter

- The doctor inserts the intrapleural catheter at the patient's bedside with the nurse assisting.
- Position the patient on his side with the affected side up. The doctor will insert the catheter into the fourth to eighth intercostal space, 3″ to 4″ (7.5 to 10 cm) from the posterior midline. (See *Inserting an intrapleural catheter.*)
- The doctor puts on a sterile cap, gown, and mask and sterile gloves, cleans around the puncture site with an antiseptic-soaked gauze pad and allows it to dry, and then covers the area with a sterile drape. Next, he fills the 3- to 5-mL syringe with local anesthetic and injects it into the skin and deep tissues.
- The doctor punctures the skin with the 18G needle or scalpel, which helps the blunt-tipped intrapleural needle penetrate the skin over the superior edge of the lower rib in the chosen interspace. Keeping the bevel tilted upward, he directs the needle medially at a 30- to 40-degree angle to the skin. When the needle tip punctures the posterior intercostal membrane, he removes the stylet and attaches a saline-lubricated glass syringe containing 2 to 4 mL of air to the needle hub.
- During puncture, tell the patient to hold his breath (or momentarily disconnect him from mechanical ventilation) until the needle is removed. *Doing so helps prevent the needle from injuring lung tissue.*
- The doctor advances the needle slowly. When the needle punctures the parietal pleura, negative intrapleural pressure moves the plunger outward. He then removes the syringe from the needle and threads the intrapleural catheter through the needle until he has advanced it about 2″ (5 cm) into the pleural space. Without removing the catheter, he carefully withdraws the needle.
- Tell the patient that he can breathe again (or reconnect mechanical ventilation).
- Blood in the needle means that the catheter probably is misplaced in a blood vessel, and aspirated air means that it's probably in a lung. The doctor will then order a chest X-ray *to verify placement and to detect such complications as pneumothorax.*
- Apply a sterile occlusive dressing over the insertion site *to prevent catheter dislodgment.* Label the dressing with the date, the time, and your initials. Obtain the patient's vital signs every 15 minutes for the first hour after the procedure and then as needed.
- Perform a comprehensive pain assessment using techniques appropriate for the patient's age, condition, and ability to understand and respond appropriately.[9]

Inserting a chest tube

- The doctor inserts the chest tube with the nurse assisting. (See "Chest tube insertion," page 173.)

Inserting an intrapleural catheter

In intrapleural administration, the doctor injects a drug into the pleural space using a catheter.

Help the patient lie on one side with the affected side up. The doctor inserts a needle into the fourth to eighth intercostal space, 3″ to 4″ (7.5 to 10 cm) from the posterior midline. He then advances the needle medially over the superior edge of the patient's rib through the intercostal muscles until it tangentially penetrates the parietal pleura (as shown). The catheter is advanced into the pleural space through the needle, which is then removed.

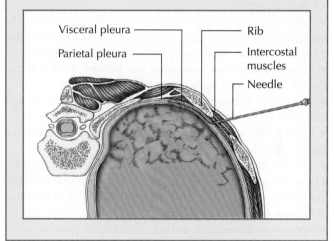

- First, position the patient with the affected side up, and drape him with sterile towels.
- The doctor puts on a sterile cap, gown, and mask and sterile gloves; disinfects the appropriate site with an antiseptic-soaked gauze pad; allows it to dry; and then drapes the insertion site using a sterile drape. If the patient has a pneumothorax, the doctor uses the second intercostal space as the access site *because air rises to the top of the pleural space.* If the patient has a hemothorax or pleural effusion, the doctor uses the sixth to eighth intercostal space *because fluid settles to the bottom of the pleural space.*
- The doctor fills the syringe with a local anesthetic and injects it into the site. He makes a small incision with the 18G needle or scalpel, inserts the appropriate-sized chest tube, and immediately connects it to the thoracic drainage system or clamps it close to the patient's chest. He then sutures the tube to the patient's skin.
- Tape the chest tube to the patient's chest distal to the insertion site *to help prevent accidental dislodgment.* Also tape the junction of the chest tube and drainage tube *to prevent their separation.* Apply a petroleum dressing at the junction between the skin and chest tube, apply sterile drain dressings, cover them with gauze, and tape them in place, creating an occlusive dressing. Label the dressing with the date, the time, and your initials.
- After insertion, the doctor verifies tube placement and monitors for complications with an X-ray.

■ Obtain the patient's vital signs every 15 minutes for 1 hour and then as needed or according to your facility's policy.

■ Perform a comprehensive pain assessment using techniques appropriate for the patient's age, condition, and ability to understand and respond appropriately.[9]

■ Auscultate the patient's lungs at least every 4 hours, according to your facility's policy, *to assess air exchange in the affected lung.* Diminished breath or absent breath sounds mean that the lung hasn't reexpanded.

Administering medication

■ The doctor injects medication through the intrapleural catheter or chest tube, with the nurse assisting.

■ Position the patient with the affected side up *to gain access to the injection port.*

■ Assist the doctor with removing the dressing from the intrapleural catheter or chest tube and clamp the drainage tube, if present. Discard the dressing in the appropriate receptacle.

■ Remove and discard your gloves and perform hand hygiene. Put on a new pair of sterile gloves.[1,2,3]

■ The doctor disinfects the access port of the catheter or chest tube with an antiseptic-soaked gauze pad and allows it to dry.

■ Draw up the appropriate medication dose and hand it to the doctor with the vial for verification.

■ The doctor injects the medication. If it's an anesthetic, he gives a bolus or loading dose initially and then a continuous infusion. For tetracycline, he mixes it with an anesthetic such as lidocaine *to alleviate pain during injection.*

■ Apply new dressings as needed. Monitor the patient closely during and after drug administration *to gauge the effectiveness of drug therapy and to check for complications and adverse effects.*

Administering chemotherapy

■ Verify the doctor's order for the chemotherapeutic agent. Make sure the order contains the patient's complete name and a second identifier, the date, the patient's diagnosis, any applicable allergies, the regimen name and number (if applicable), treatment criteria, dosage calculation method, the patient's height and weight, and any other variables used to calculate the dose, the dosage, the route and rate of administration, the administration schedule, duration of therapy, cumulative lifetime dose (if applicable), sequence of drug administration (if applicable), and any supportive care treatments appropriate for the regimen.[6,10]

■ Verify that the patient received written educational materials appropriate for his reading level and understanding and that the materials include information about his diagnosis, chemotherapy plan, possible long- and short-term adverse effects, risks associated with the regimen, reportable signs and symptoms, monitoring, and follow-up care.[10]

■ Make sure that written informed consent has been obtained and that the form is in the patient's medical record.[5,10]

■ Wash your hands and put on personal protective equipment (two pairs of gloves, a gown, a face shield, and a respirator if necessary). Make sure your inner glove cuff is worn under the gown cuff and the outer glove cuff extends over the gown cuff *to fully protect your skin.* Inspect your gloves to make sure they're physically intact.[11,12]

■ Perform an independent double-check with another practitioner approved to administer chemotherapy *to verify the medication name, dose, volume, rate of administration, route of administration, expiration date and time, and the appearance and physical integrity of the medication.* Document that the verification is in the patient's medical record.[10]

■ Confirm the treatment plan, drug route, and symptom management plan with the patient.[10]

■ Position the patient with the affected side up *to gain access to the injection port.*

■ Assist the doctor with removing the dressing from the intrapleural catheter or chest tube, and discard it in the appropriate receptacle. If a pleural effusion is present, it must be completely drained from the pleural cavity before the medication is instilled.[11] Clamp the drainage tube, if present.

■ Remove and discard your gloves and put on two new pairs of gloves.

■ Place a linen-saver pad underneath the work area *to absorb droplets of the medication that may spill.*[10]

■ Assist the doctor with preparing the access port. The doctor thoroughly disinfects the access port of the catheter or chest tube with an antiseptic-soaked gauze pad and then allows it to dry.

■ The doctor injects the medication or begins an infusion. Trace the tubing from the patient to its point of origin *to make sure the tubing is connected to the proper port before the infusion is started.*[13]

■ Apply new dressings, as needed. Label the dressings with the date, the time, and your initials.

■ Discard the linen-saver pad and other used equipment in the proper receptacle.

■ After instillation, clamp the tubing and reposition the patient every 10 to 15 minutes for 2 hours, or according to the doctor's order.[11]

■ Monitor the patient closely for signs of respiratory distress, allergic reaction, or other adverse reactions to the medication.

■ If the medication was administered by infusion, remove the medication container with the tubing attached, and dispose of it in the proper receptacle; don't remove the spike from the container *to prevent exposure to the hazardous medication.*[11] If the medication container will be used to collect drainage after the prescribed dwell time, leave it hanging on an IV pole at the patient's bedside. After the prescribed dwell time, lower the bag to a dependent position, unclamp the tubing, and allow fluid to drain by gravity. After the prescribed volume drains, disconnect the tubing from the injection port and discard it, the fluid, and the container in the proper receptacle.

Completing the procedure

■ Discard used supplies, remove your personal protective equipment, and perform hand hygiene.[1,2,3]

■ Document the procedure.[14,15]

Special considerations

■ If the patient is receiving a continuous infusion, label the solution bag clearly. Cover all injection ports so that other drugs aren't injected into the pleural space accidentally.

■ If the chest tube dislodges, cover the site at once with a sterile gauze pad and tape it in place. Stay with the patient, monitor his vital signs, and observe carefully for signs and symptoms of tension pneumothorax: hypotension, distended jugular veins, absent breath sounds, tracheal shift, hypoxemia, dyspnea, tachypnea, diaphoresis, chest pain, and a weak, rapid pulse. Have another nurse call the doctor and gather the equipment for reinsertion.

■ Keep rubber-tipped clamps at the bedside. If a commercial chest tube system cracks or a tube disconnects, use the clamps to clamp the chest tube close to the insertion site temporarily. Be sure to observe the patient closely for signs of tension pneumothorax *because no air can escape from the pleural space while the tube is clamped.*

■ Wrap a piece of petroleum gauze around the chest tube at the insertion site to make an airtight seal, apply sterile split dressings around the chest tube at the insertion site, and then apply sterile dressings and tape them in place, forming an occlusive dressing. Label the dressing with the date, the time, and your initials.

■ When handling chemotherapy agents, change your gloves regularly (every 30 to 60 minutes), whenever your gloves become damaged, and if contact with the drug is known or suspected.[12]

Complications

Pneumothorax or tension pneumothorax may occur if the doctor accidentally injects air into the pleural cavity. These complications are more likely to occur in a patient who is on mechanical ventilation.

Accidental catheter placement in the lung can lead to respiratory distress; catheter placement within a vessel can increase the medication's effects. With catheter fracture, lung puncture may occur. Laceration of intercostal vessels can cause bleeding.

Local anesthetic toxicity can lead to tinnitus, metallic taste, light-headedness, somnolence, visual and auditory disturbances, restlessness, delirium, slurred speech, nystagmus, muscle tremor, seizures, arrhythmias, and cardiovascular collapse. A local anesthetic containing epinephrine can cause tachycardia and hypertension.

Intrapleural chemotherapeutic drugs can irritate the pleura chemically and cause such systemic effects as neutropenia and thrombocytopenia. Administering intrapleural tetracycline without an anesthetic can cause pain.

The insertion site can become infected. However, meticulous skin preparation, strict sterile technique, and sterile dressings usually prevent infection.

Documentation

Document the date and time of catheter insertion, the doctor's name, and the site of the catheter. Document the patient's tolerance of the procedure. Record the date, time, drug administered, drug dosage, patient's response to the treatment, and condition of the catheter insertion site. Note any adverse reactions to the medication, that the doctor was notified, prescribed interventions, and the patient's response to such interventions.

REFERENCES

1 The Joint Commission. (2012). Standard NPSG.07.01.01. *Comprehensive accreditation manual for hospitals: The official handbook.* Oakbrook Terrace, IL: The Joint Commission. (Level I)
2 Centers for Disease Control and Prevention. (October 2002). Guideline for hand hygiene in health-care settings. *Morbidity and Mortality Weekly Report, 51*(RR-16), 1–45. (Level I)
3 World Health Organization. (2009). *WHO guidelines on hand hygiene in health care: First global patient safety challenge. Clean care is safer care.* Geneva, Switzerland: World Health Organization. (Level I)
4 The Joint Commission. (2012). Standard NPSG.01.01.01. *Comprehensive accreditation manual for hospitals: The official handbook.* Oakbrook Terrace, IL: The Joint Commission. (Level I)
5 The Joint Commission. (2012). Standard RI.01.03.01. *Comprehensive accreditation manual for hospitals: The official handbook.* Oakbrook Terrace, IL: The Joint Commission. (Level I)
6 Centers for Medicare & Medicaid Services, Department of Health and Human Services. (2006). "Conditions of Participation: Patients' Rights," 42 CFR part 482.13 [Online]. Accessed November 2011 via the Web at https://www.cms.gov/CFCsAndCoPs/downloads/finalpatientrightsrule.pdf
7 Siegel, J.D., et al. "2007 Guideline for Isolation Precautions: Preventing Transmission of Infectious Agents in Healthcare Settings" [Online]. Accessed September 2011 via the Web at http://www.cdc.gov/hicpac/2007ip/2007isolationprecautions.html
8 The Joint Commission. (2012). Standard UP.01.01.01. *Comprehensive accreditation manual for hospitals: The official handbook.* Oakbrook Terrace, IL: The Joint Commission. (Level I)
9 The Joint Commission. (2012). Standard PC.01.02.01. *Comprehensive accreditation manual for hospitals: The official handbook.* Oakbrook Terrace, IL: The Joint Commission. (Level I)
10 Jacobson, J., et al. (2009). American Society of Clinical Oncology/Oncology Nursing Society Chemotherapy Administration safety standards. *Journal of Clinical Oncology, 27*(32), 5469–5475.
11 Polovich, M., et al. (2009). *Chemotherapy and biotherapy guidelines and recommendations for practice* (3rd ed.). Pittsburgh, PA: Oncology Nursing Society.
12 National Institute for Occupational Safety and Health. (2008). "Workplace Solutions: Personal Protective Equipment for Health Care Workers Who Work with Hazardous Drugs" [Online]. Accessed November 2011 via the Web at http://www.cdc.gov/niosh/docs/wp-solutions/2009-106/pdfs/2009-106.pdf
13 U.S. Food and Drug Administration. (2009). "Look. Check. Connect.: Safe Medical Device Connections Save Lives" [Online]. Accessed November 2011 via the Web at http://www.fda.gov/downloads/MedicalDevices/Safety/AlertsandNotices/UCM134873.pdf
14 The Joint Commission. (2012). Standard RC.01.03.01. *Comprehensive accreditation manual for hospitals: The official handbook.* Oakbrook Terrace, IL: The Joint Commission. (Level I)
15 The Joint Commission. (2012). Standard RC.02.01.01. *Comprehensive accreditation manual for hospitals: The official handbook.* Oakbrook Terrace, IL: The Joint Commission. (Level I)

ADDITIONAL REFERENCES

Demmy, T.L., et al. (2009). Chest tube-delivered bupivacaine improves pain and decreases opioid use after thoracoscopy. *Annals of Thoracic Surgery, 87*(4), 1040–1046; discussion 1046–1047.

Levinson, G.M., & Pennington, D.W. (2007). Intrapleural fibrinolytics combined with image-guided chest tube drainage for pleural infection. *Mayo Clinic Proceedings, 82*(4), 407–413.

Maskell, N., et al. (2006). Intrapleural streptokinase for pleural infection. *British Medical Journal, 332*(7540), 552.

Tokuda, Y., et al. (2006). Intrapleural fibrinolytic agents for empyema and complicated parapneumonic effusions: A meta-analysis. *Chest, 129*(3), 783–790.

IONTOPHORESIS

Iontophoresis is a technique for delivering dermal analgesia quickly (in 10 to 20 minutes) with minimal discomfort and without distorting the tissue. The Numby 900 iontophoretic drug-delivery system is a handheld device with two electrodes that uses a mild electric current to deliver charged ions of lidocaine 2% and epinephrine 1:100,000 solution into the skin. The device is powered by a 9-volt battery.

Local anesthetic agents, such as those administered through iontophoresis, should be considered before IV insertion.[1] Because iontophoresis acts quickly, it's an excellent choice for numbing an IV insertion site, especially in children.

Equipment

Dose-control device with battery ■ drug-delivery electrode kit ■ lidocaine 2% with epinephrine 1:100,000 solution ■ alcohol pads ■ syringe with needle ■ gloves ■ tongue blade.

Implementation

■ Perform hand hygiene.[2,3,4]
■ Confirm the patient's identity using at least two patient identifiers according to your facility's policy.[5]
■ Ask the patient or, if the patient is a child, ask the parents if he has any allergies or sensitivity to medications. Avoid using iontophoresis in patients with implanted devices such as a pacemaker.
■ Explain the procedure to the patient and tell him that he may feel tingling or warmth under the electrode pads while they're on the skin.
■ Assess the patient for appropriate electrode placement. You'll place a medication-delivery electrode over the intended IV insertion site. The second electrode, which drives drug ions into the skin, must be applied over a muscle 4″ to 6″ (10 to 15 cm) away.
■ Put on gloves. Examine the patient's skin and select intact electrode placement sites, avoiding areas with pimples, unhealed wounds, or ingrown hairs. With alcohol pads, briskly rub an area slightly larger than the electrode at each site.
■ Remove the paper flap from the back of the drug-delivery electrode.
■ Draw up the lidocaine with epinephrine in a syringe. Remove the needle from the syringe and saturate the medication pad with the amount of lidocaine and epinephrine solution indicated on

the electrode pad (as shown below). The amount of lidocaine and epinephrine solution required to saturate the pad varies with pad size: for a standard-sized pad, use about 1 mL; for a large pad, use about 2.5 mL.

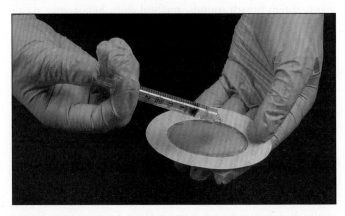

■ Remove the remaining backing from the drug-delivery pad and apply the pad to the selected site. Remove the backing from the grounding electrode and apply it to the second prepared site.
■ Connect the lead clips: red (positive charge) to the drug-delivery electrode and black (negative charge) to the grounding electrode.
■ Turn on the device (as shown below).

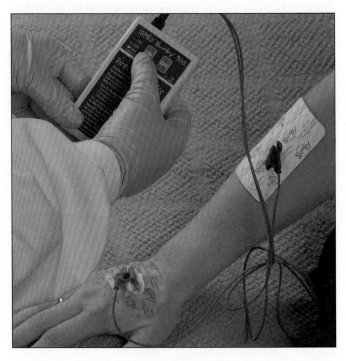

■ As indicated by the green light, the device will automatically operate at the lowest current, 2 milliamperes (mA), unless you increase the level to 3 or 4 mA by pressing the ON button. If your patient has discomfort at a higher setting, reduce the current by pushing the ON button until the appropriate light indicates the desired level. The device is calibrated to deliver a dose of 40 mA-minutes, after which it will automatically stop. If the setting remains at 4 mA, treatment is completed in 10 minutes. However, if you decrease the setting because the patient has discomfort, the device will automatically adjust to a longer treatment time to deliver the entire dose.

- After the dose has been delivered, remove the electrodes. Assess the skin at the drug-delivery site for numbness by touching it with a blunt object such as a tongue blade.
- Promptly prepare the site and perform the venipuncture *because the numbness may last only a few minutes.*
- Remove and discard your gloves and perform hand hygiene.[2,3,4]
- Document the procedure.[6,7]

Special considerations

- *To avoid interfering with energy emission,* don't tape or compress the electrodes.
- If you need to stop the treatment for any reason, press the OFF button and hold it. The lights will indicate decreasing current levels; then the device will beep and turn off. Don't disconnect the lead clips or the electrodes until all signals have stopped *because the device is still transmitting energy until it turns off.*

Complications

Allergic reaction may occur in patients sensitive to lidocaine or epinephrine.

Documentation

Document the treatment, the sites used, and whether analgesia was achieved. Also document an allergic response, if any. Record any patient teaching and the patient's understanding of your teaching.[6,7]

REFERENCES

1 Standard 34. Local anesthesia for vascular access device placement and access. Infusion nursing standards of practice. (2011). *Journal of Infusion Nursing, 34*(1S), S43–44. (Level I)
2 Centers for Disease Control and Prevention. (October 2002). Guideline for hand hygiene in health-care settings. *Morbidity and Mortality Weekly Report, 51*(RR-16), 1–45. (Level I)
3 World Health Organization. (2009). *WHO guidelines on hand hygiene in health care: First global patient safety challenge. Clean care is safer care.* Geneva, Switzerland: World Health Organization. (Level I)
4 The Joint Commission. (2012). Standard NPSG.07.01.01. *Comprehensive accreditation manual for hospitals: The official handbook.* Oakbrook Terrace, IL: The Joint Commission. (Level I)
5 The Joint Commission. (2012). Standard NPSG.01.01.01. *Comprehensive accreditation manual for hospitals: The official handbook.* Oakbrook Terrace, IL: The Joint Commission. (Level I)
6 The Joint Commission. (2012). Standard RC.01.03.01. *Comprehensive accreditation manual for hospitals: The official handbook.* Oakbrook Terrace, IL: The Joint Commission. (Level I)
7 The Joint Commission. (2012). Standard RC.02.01.01. *Comprehensive accreditation manual for hospitals: The official handbook.* Oakbrook Terrace, IL: The Joint Commission. (Level I)

ADDITIONAL REFERENCES

Becker, B., et al. (2005). Ultrasound with topical anesthetic rapidly decreases pain of intravenous cannulation. *Academic Emergency Medicine, 12*(4), 289–295.
Lindley, P., et al. (2009). Comparison of postoperative pain management using two patient-controlled analgesia methods: Nursing perspective. *Journal of Advanced Nursing, 65*(7), 1370–1380.
Pasero, C. (2006). Lidocaine iontophoresis for dermal procedure analgesia. *Journal of Perianesthesia Nursing, 21*(1), 48–52.
Viscusi, E.R., et al. (2006). An iontophoretic fentanyl patient-activated analgesic delivery system for postoperative pain: A double-blind, placebo-controlled trial. *Anesthesia and Analgesia, 102*(1), 188–194.

IV BOLUS INJECTION

The IV bolus injection method allows rapid drug administration. It can be used in an emergency to provide an immediate drug effect. It can also be used to administer drugs that can't be given IM, to achieve peak drug levels in the bloodstream, and to deliver drugs that can't be diluted, such as diazepam, digoxin, and phenytoin. The term *bolus* usually refers to the concentration or amount of a drug. *IV push* is a technique for rapid IV injection.

Bolus doses of medication may be injected directly through an existing venous access device or through an implanted port. The medication administered by these methods usually takes effect rapidly, so the patient must be monitored for an adverse reaction, such as cardiac arrhythmia and anaphylaxis. IV bolus injections are contraindicated when rapid drug administration could cause life-threatening complications. The safe rate of injection is specified by the drug's manufacturer.

Equipment

Patient's medication record ■ patient's medical records ■ gloves ■ antiseptic pads (alcohol, tincture of iodine, or chlorhexidine-based) ■ prescribed medication ■ prefilled-syringe containing preservative-free normal saline solution ■ syringe and needleless adapter ■ diluent, if needed ■ Optional: second syringe (and needleless adapter) filled with preservative-free normal saline solution.

A useful dosage form is the ready injectable. (See *Using a ready injectable,* page 420.)

Implementation

- Avoid distractions and interruptions when preparing and administering medications *to prevent medication administration errors.*[1]
- Verify the order on the patient's medication record by checking it against the doctor's order in his medical record.[2]
- Compare the medication label to the doctor's order to *verify the correct medication, indication, dose, route, and time of administration.*[2]
- Check the expiration date; return the medication to the pharmacy if it's expired.[2]
- Check the patient's medical record for an allergy or other contraindication to the prescribed medication. If an allergy or other contraindication is present, don't administer the medication and notify the doctor.[2]

EQUIPMENT

Using a ready injectable

A commercially premeasured medication packaged with a syringe and needle, the ready injectable allows for rapid drug administration in an emergency. Preparing a ready injectable usually takes only 15 to 20 seconds. Other advantages include the reduced risk of breaking sterile technique during administration and the easy identification of medication and dose.

When using a ready injectable, be sure to give the precise dose prescribed. For example, if a 50-mg/mL cartridge is supplied but the patient's prescribed dose is 25 mg, you must administer only 0.5 mL, half of the volume contained in the cartridge. Be alert for potential medication errors whenever dispensing medications in premeasured dosage forms.

- Visually inspect the medication for discoloration or any other loss of integrity. Don't administer the medication if its integrity is compromised.
- Check the compatibility of the medication with the IV solution and any medicated infusions that are infusing.
- Perform hand hygiene and put on gloves.[3,4,5,6]
- If the medication isn't in a prefilled syringe, dilute it and draw it up in a syringe using sterile technique. Check the medication label three times while preparing it *to prevent medication administration errors.*
- Confirm the patient's identity using at least two patient identifiers according to your facility's policy.[7,8]
- Explain the procedure to the patient.
- If the patient is receiving the medication for the first time, inform the patient or his family about possible significant adverse reactions or other concerns related to administering the medication.
- If your facility uses a bar code scanning system, scan your identification badge, the patient's identification bracelet, and the medication's bar code.
- Close the flow clamp; thoroughly disinfect the needleless injection port with an antiseptic pad using friction. Allow it to dry.[9]
- Attach a prefilled syringe containing preservative-free normal saline solution to the injection port; aspirate for blood return *to verify catheter patency* and then flush the catheter.[8]
- Remove and discard the syringe in a puncture-resistant sharps container.
- Thoroughly disinfect the injection port with an antiseptic pad using friction and allow it to dry.[9]
- Attach the medication syringe to the injection port and inject the medication, as prescribed.
- If the medication is compatible with the patient's prescribed IV solution, open the clamp and adjust the flow rate; if the medication is incompatible, flush the catheter with preservative-free normal saline solution, and then open the clamp and adjust the flow rate.
- Discard used supplies in the appropriate receptacle.
- Remove and discard your gloves and perform hand hygiene.[3,4,5,6]
- Document the procedure.[10,11]

Special considerations

- If you're giving a medication that's incompatible with preservative-free normal saline solution, flush the device with dextrose 5% in water followed by preservative-free normal saline solution.[8]

Complications

Because drugs administered by IV bolus injections are delivered directly into the circulatory system and can produce an immediate effect, an acute allergic reaction or anaphylaxis can develop rapidly. If signs of anaphylaxis (dyspnea, cyanosis, seizures, and increasing respiratory distress) occur, notify the doctor immediately and begin emergency procedures, as necessary. Also watch for signs and symptoms of extravasation, such as paint, redness, or swelling. If extravasation occurs, stop the injection, estimate the amount of infiltration, and notify the doctor. Excessively rapid drug administration may cause adverse effects, depending on the medication administered.

Documentation

Record the amount and type of drug administered, time of injection, appearance of the site, duration of administration, and patient's tolerance of the procedure. Also note the drug's effect and any adverse reactions. Document any patient teaching provided.

REFERENCES

1 Westbrook, J. et al. (2010). Association of interruptions with an increased risk and severity of medication administration errors. *Archives of Internal Medicine, 170*(8), 683–690.

2 The Joint Commission. (2012). Standard MM.06.01.01. *Comprehensive accreditation manual for hospitals: The official handbook.* Oakbrook Terrace, IL: The Joint Commission. (Level I)

3 Standard 19. Hand hygiene. Infusion nursing standards of practice. (2011). *Journal of Infusion Nursing, 34*(1S), S26–27. (Level I)

4 Centers for Disease Control and Prevention. (October 2002). Guideline for hand hygiene in health-care settings. *Morbidity and Mortality Weekly Report, 51*(RR-16), 1–45. (Level I)

5 World Health Organization. (2009). *WHO guidelines on hand hygiene in health care: First global patient safety challenge. Clean care is safer care.* Geneva, Switzerland: World Health Organization. (Level I)

6 The Joint Commission. (2012). Standard NPSG.07.01.01. *Comprehensive accreditation manual for hospitals: The official handbook.* Oakbrook Terrace, IL: The Joint Commission. (Level I)

7 The Joint Commission. (2012). Standard NPSG.01.01.01. *Comprehensive accreditation manual for hospitals: The official handbook.* Oakbrook Terrace, IL: The Joint Commission. (Level I)

8 Standard 61. Parenteral medication and solution administration. Infusion nursing standards of practice. (2011). *Journal of Infusion Nursing, 34*(1S), S86.

ng standards
), S32–S33.

)3.01. *Com-
official hand-
1. (Level I)*

11 The Joint Commission. (2012). Standard RC.02.01.01. *Comprehensive accreditation manual for hospitals: The official handbook.* Oakbrook Terrace, IL: The Joint Commission. (Level I)

ADDITIONAL REFERENCES

Dolan, S.A., et al. (2010). APIC position paper: Safe injection, infusion, and medication vial practices in health care. *American Journal of Infection Control, 38*(3), 167–172.

Nettina, S.M. (2010). *Lippincott manual of nursing practice* (9th ed.). Philadelphia, PA: Lippincott Williams & Wilkins.

O'Grady, N.P., et al. (2011). "Guidelines for the Prevention of Intravascular Catheter-Related Infections" [Online]. Accessed November 2011 via the Web at http://www.cdc.gov/hicpac/pdf/guidelines/bsi-guidelines-2011.pdf

Taylor, C., et al. (2011). *Fundamentals of nursing: The art and science of nursing care* (7th ed.). Philadelphia, PA: Lippincott Williams & Wilkins.

IV CATHETER INSERTION AND REMOVAL

Peripheral IV catheter insertion involves selection of a venipuncture device and an insertion site, application of a tourniquet, preparation of the site, and venipuncture. Selection of a venipuncture device and site depends on the type of solution to be used; frequency and duration of infusion; patency and location of accessible veins; the patient's age, size, and condition; and, when possible, the patient's preference.[1,2,3]

If possible, choose a vein in the nondominant arm or hand. Use veins on the dorsal and ventral surfaces of the upper extremities, including the metacarpal, cephalic, basilic, and median veins. When choosing a site, avoid areas of flexion; areas where there's pain on palpation; veins that are compromised by bruising, infiltration, phlebitis, sclerosis, or cord formation; and areas where procedures are planned. Avoid the lateral surface of the wrist for about 4″ to 5″ (10 to 12.5 cm) because of the risk for nerve damage; avoid the ventral surface of the wrist because of the associated pain on insertion and the risk for nerve damage.

Also avoid using veins of the lower extremities because of the increased risk for tissue damage, thrombophlebitis, and ulceration. In a patient who has had breast surgery with axillary node dissection, don't use veins in the upper extremity on the affected side; also don't choose veins on an extremity affected by radiation therapy, lymphedema, or stroke. If the patient has stage 4 or 5 chronic kidney disease, avoid using upper arm veins or forearms that could be used for dialysis access. Collaborate with the patient and his doctor to discuss the risks and benefits of using a vein in an affected extremity if no other options exist.[2]

A peripheral catheter allows administration of fluids, medication, blood, and blood components and maintains IV access to the patient. It's removed upon completion of therapy, for can-nula site changes, when contamination is suspected, and for suspected infection or infiltration.[4,5]

According to the Centers for Disease Control and Prevention, a peripheral IV catheter should be replaced no more frequently than every 72 to 96 hours to reduce the risk of infection and phlebitis in adults.[1] If an IV catheter is inserted in an emergency situation, it should be removed as soon as possible, within 48 hours.[1]

Equipment

Chlorhexidine solution (tincture of iodine, povidone iodine, or alcohol may be used if there's a contraindication to chlorhexidine) ▪ gloves ▪ single-use tourniquet (preferably latex-free) ▪ IV access devices with safety shields[3] ▪ IV solution with attached and primed administration set ▪ IV pole ▪ transparent semipermeable dressing ▪ catheter securement device, sterile hypoallergenic tape, or sterile surgical strips ▪ Optional: arm board, roller gauze, tube gauze, warm packs, scissors, clippers, ultrasound device with sterile probe cover, sterile ultrasound gel, local anesthetic, basin of water, soap.

Commercial venipuncture kits come with or without an IV access device. (See *Comparing venous access devices,* page 422.) In many facilities, venipuncture equipment is kept on a tray or cart, allowing more choice of access devices and easy replacement of contaminated items.

Preparation of equipment

Check the information on the label of the IV solution container, including the patient's name and identification number, the type of solution, the time and date of its preparation, the preparer's name, and the ordered infusion rate. Compare the doctor's orders with the solution label *to verify that the solution is the correct one.*[6]

Inspect the solution for discoloration or other loss of integrity and make sure that it hasn't expired.[7] Then select the gauge of catheter that's appropriate for the patient's diagnosis, prescribed type and duration of therapy (therapy that's required for less than 1 week), available access sites, and your experience with insertion. Also take into consideration complications that are associated with the particular type catheter. If blood transfusion is necessary, a 14G to 24G catheter may be used in adults.[3]

If you're using a winged infusion set, connect the adapter to the administration set, and unclamp the line until fluid flows from the open end of the needle cover. Then close the clamp and place the needle on a sterile surface, such as the inside of its packaging. If you're using a catheter device, open its package *to allow easy access.*

Implementation

▪ Perform hand hygiene.[1,8,9,10,11]
▪ Place the IV pole in the proper slot in the patient's bed frame. If you're using a portable IV pole, position it close to the patient.
▪ Hang the IV solution with attached primed administration set on the IV pole.
▪ Confirm the patient's identity using at least two patient identifiers according to your facility's policy.[12]

EQUIPMENT

Comparing venous access devices

Most IV infusions are delivered through one of two basic types of venous access devices: an over-the-needle cannula or a winged infusion set. To improve IV therapy and guard against accidental needle sticks, you should use a needle-free system and shielded or retracting peripheral IV catheters. Steel-winged devices should be limited to single-dose or short-term administration.[3]

Over-the-needle cannula

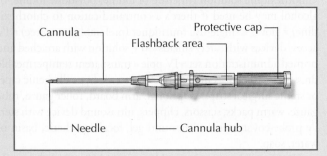

Cannula — Protective cap — Flashback area — Needle — Cannula hub

Purpose
Long-term therapy for an active or agitated patient

Advantages
More comfortable for the patient once it's in place; contains radio-paque thread for easy location. Activity-restricting device, such as arm board, rarely required.

Disadvantage
More difficult to insert than other devices

Winged infusion set

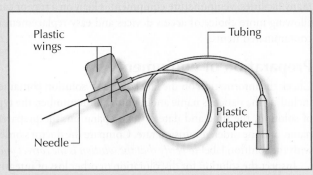

Plastic wings — Tubing — Plastic adapter — Needle

Purpose
Short-term therapy or single-dose administration.[3]

Advantages
Less painful to insert; ideal for nonirritating IV push drugs.

Disadvantage
May easily cause infiltration

■ Explain the procedure to the patient *to ensure his cooperation and reduce anxiety. Anxiety can cause a vasomotor response resulting in venous constriction.*

■ Provide the patient with information about the insertion process, expected duration of therapy, care and maintenance of the IV catheter, and the signs and symptoms of complications and when to report them.[13,14,15]

Selecting the site

■ Select the puncture site. If long-term therapy is anticipated, start with a vein at the most distal site *so that you can move proximally as needed for subsequent IV insertion sites.*[2] For infusion of an irritating medication, choose a large vein distal to any nearby joint. Make sure the intended vein can accommodate the cannula.

■ Place the patient in a comfortable, reclining position, leaving the arm in a dependent position *to increase venous fill of the lower arms and hands.* If the patient's skin is cold, cover his entire arm with warm pack for 5 to 10 minutes or submerge it in warm water.

Applying the tourniquet

■ Apply a tourniquet about 4″ to 6″ (10 to 15 cm) above the intended puncture site *to dilate the vein* (as shown below). Check for a radial pulse. If it isn't present, release the tourniquet and reapply it with less tension *to prevent arterial occlusion.*[14]

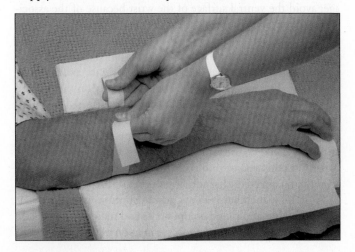

- Lightly palpate the vein with the index and middle fingers of your nondominant hand. Stretch the skin *to anchor the vein*. If the vein feels hard or ropelike, select another.
- If the vein is easily palpable but not sufficiently dilated, one or more of the following techniques may help raise the vein. Place the extremity in a dependent position for several seconds or lightly stroke the vessel downward. If you have selected a vein in the arm or hand, tell the patient to open and close his fist several times.[15]
- Leave the tourniquet in place for no more than 3 minutes while you locate a suitable vein. Release the tourniquet for a few minutes.

Preparing the site

- If the intended insertion site is visibly soiled, clean it with soap and water before applying the antiseptic solution.[5,15]
- Clip the hair around the insertion site, if needed, with a scissors or electric clippers.[15]
- Administer a local anesthetic if indicated and prescribed.[5,15]
- Perform hand hygiene and put on gloves.[1,8,9,10,11]
- Clean the site with chlorhexidine using a back-and-forth scrubbing motion for at least 30 seconds[5] to remove flora that would otherwise be introduced into the vascular system with the venipuncture. Allow the antiseptic to dry.
- Reapply the tourniquet.
- Use the handheld ultrasound device with a sterile probe cover to locate the vein, if necessary.
- Using the thumb of your nondominant hand, stretch the skin taut below the puncture site *to stabilize the vein*.[5]
- Grasp the access cannula. If you're using a winged infusion set, hold the short edges of the wings (with the needle's bevel facing upward) between the thumb and forefinger of your dominant hand. Then squeeze the wings together. If you're using an over-the-needle cannula, grasp the plastic hub with your dominant hand, remove the cover, and examine the cannula tip. If the edge isn't smooth, discard and replace the device.

Inserting the device

- Tell the patient that you are about to insert the device.
- Hold the needle bevel up and enter the skin directly over the vein at a 0- to 15-degree angle.
- Aggressively push the needle directly through the skin and into the vein in one motion. Check the flashback chamber behind the hub for blood return, *signifying that the vein has been properly accessed.* (You may not see a blood return in a small vein.)
- Then level the insertion device slightly by lifting the tip of the device up *to prevent puncturing the back wall of the vein with the access device.*
- If you're using a winged infusion set, advance the needle fully, if possible, and hold it in place. Release the tourniquet, open the administration set clamp slightly, and check for free flow or infiltration.
- If you're using an over-the-needle cannula, advance the device 2 to 3 mm *to ensure that the cannula itself, not just the introducer needle, has entered the vein.* Then remove the tourniquet. Grasp the cannula hub to hold it in the vein, and withdraw the needle.

As you withdraw it, press lightly on the catheter tip *to prevent bleeding* (as shown below).

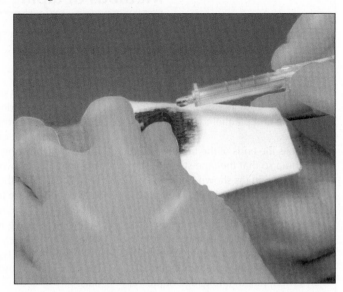

- To advance the cannula while infusing IV solution, release the tourniquet and remove the inner needle. Using sterile technique, attach the IV tubing and begin the infusion. While stabilizing the vein with one hand, use the other to advance the catheter into the vein. When the catheter is advanced, decrease the IV flow rate. *This method reduces the risk of puncturing the vein's opposite wall because the catheter is advanced without the needle and because the rapid flow dilates the vein.*
- To advance the cannula before starting the infusion, first release the tourniquet. While stabilizing the vein with one hand, use the other to advance the catheter up to the hub (as shown below). Next, remove the inner needle and, using sterile technique, quickly attach the IV tubing. *This method often results in less blood being spilled.*

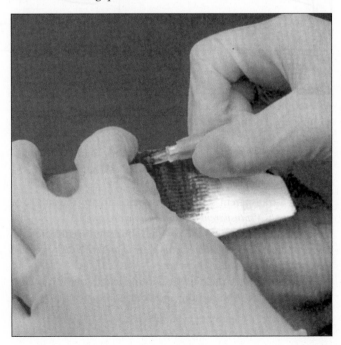

Methods of taping a venous access site

When using tape to secure the access device to the insertion site, use one of the basic methods described below. Use only sterile tape when securing a venous access site.[13]

Chevron method
■ Cut a long strip of ½" (1.3-cm) tape and place it sticky side up under the cannula and parallel to the short strip of tape.
■ Cross the ends of the tape over the cannula so that the tape sticks to the patient's skin (as shown below).
■ Apply a piece of 1" (2.5-cm) tape across the two wings of the chevron.
■ Loop the tubing and secure it with another piece of 1" tape. Once the dressing is secured, apply a label. On the label, write the date and time of insertion, length and gauge of the vascular access device, and your initials.[5,16]

U method
■ Cut a 2" (5-cm) strip of ½" tape. With the sticky side up, place it under the hub of the cannula.
■ Bring each side of the tape up, folding it over the wings of the cannula in a U shape (as shown below). Press it down parallel to the hub.
■ Now apply tape to stabilize the catheter.
■ Once a dressing is secured, apply a label. On the label, write the date and time of insertion, type and gauge of the needle or cannula, and your initials.[5,16]

H method
■ Cut three strips of 1" (2.5-cm) tape.
■ Place one strip of tape over each wing, keeping the tape parallel to the cannula (as shown below).
■ Now place the other strip of tape perpendicular to the first two. Put it either directly on top of the wings or just below the wings, directly on top of the tubing.
■ Make sure the cannula is secure, and then apply a dressing and a label. On the label, write the date and time of insertion, length and gauge of the vascular access device, and your initials.[5,16]

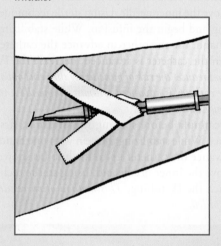 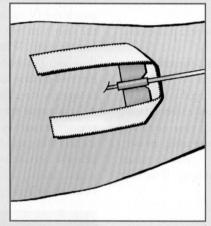 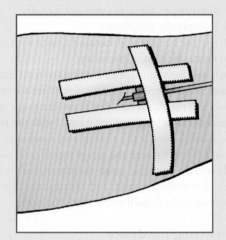

Dressing the site
■ After the venous access device has been inserted, clean the skin completely. Then regulate the flow rate.
■ Apply a catheter securement device *to secure the catheter.* If a catheter securement device isn't available, use sterile 1" hypoallergenic tape or sterile surgical strips *to secure the device.* (See *Methods of taping a venous access site.*)[13]
■ Apply a transparent semipermeable dressing to the site. (See *How to apply a transparent semipermeable dressing.*)[1,16]
■ Loop the IV tubing on the patient's limb, and secure the tubing with tape. *The loop allows some slack to prevent dislodgment of the cannula from tension on the line.*
■ Label the site with the type, gauge, and length of the catheter; the date and time of insertion; and your initials.[5,16]

■ Adjust the flow rate as ordered. Trace the tubing from the patient to its point of origin *to make sure you've attached the tubing to the correct port.*[7,17]
■ If the puncture site is near a movable joint, place a padded arm board under the joint and secure it with roller gauze or tape *to provide stability because excessive movement can dislodge the venous access device and increase the risk of thrombophlebitis and infection.*[18]
■ Check frequently for impaired circulation distal to the infusion site anytime an arm board is used.
■ Discard used supplies in an appropriate receptacle and perform hand hygiene.[1,5,8,9,10,11] Document the procedure.[19,20]

Removing an IV catheter
■ Verify the order to remove the peripheral IV catheter.[4]
■ Perform hand hygiene.[1,8,9,10,11]

- Confirm the patient's identity using at least two patient identifiers according to your facility's policy.[12]
- Using sterile technique, open the gauze pad and adhesive bandage and place them within reach on a clean barrier.
- Put on gloves.
- To remove the IV catheter, first clamp the IV tubing *to stop the flow of solution*. Then gently remove the transparent dressing, catheter securement device, and all tape from the skin (as shown below).

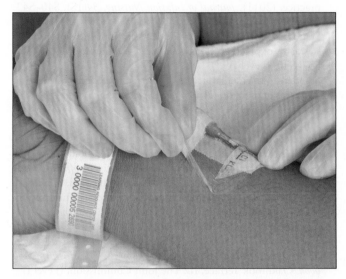

- Hold the sterile gauze pad over the puncture site with one hand, and use your other hand to withdraw the cannula slowly and smoothly, keeping it parallel to the skin (as shown below).

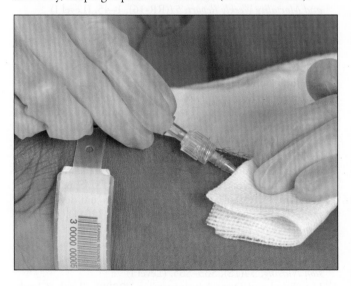

- Inspect the cannula tip; if it isn't smooth, assess the patient immediately, and notify the doctor.
- Using the gauze pad, apply firm pressure over the puncture site for 1 to 2 minutes after removal or until bleeding has stopped.[5,21]

How to apply a transparent semipermeable dressing

To secure the IV insertion site, you can apply a transparent semipermeable dressing as follows:
- Make sure the insertion site is clean and dry.
- Remove the dressing from the package and, using sterile technique, remove the protective seal. Avoid touching the sterile surface.
- Place the dressing directly over the insertion site and the hub (as shown). Don't cover the tubing. Also, don't stretch the dressing; *doing so may cause itching*.

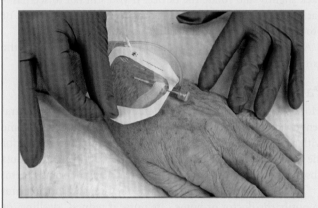

- Tuck the dressing around and under the cannula hub *to make the site impervious to microorganisms*.
- To remove the dressing, grasp one corner, and then lift and stretch it. If removal is difficult, try loosening the edges with alcohol or water.

- Clean the site and apply the adhesive bandage (as shown below). If blood oozes, apply a pressure bandage.

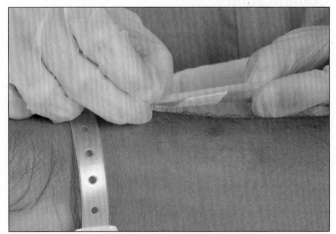

- If drainage appears at the puncture site, consider culturing the catheter according to your facility's policy; *a draining site may be infected*.[1,5,21]
- Discard used supplies in an appropriate receptacle.

■ Remove and discard your gloves and perform hand hygiene.[1,8,9,10,11]
■ Document the procedure.[19,20]

Special considerations

ELDER ALERT *Apply the tourniquet carefully to avoid pinching the skin. If necessary, apply it over the patient's gown. Make sure skin preparation materials are at room temperature to avoid vasoconstriction resulting from lower temperatures.*

■ No more than two attempts at insertion should be made by one nurse *because unsuccessful attempts limit future attempts and cause the patient unnecessary pain.*[15]
■ If you fail to see flashback after the needle enters the vein, pull back slightly and rotate the device. If you still fail to see flashback, remove the cannula and try again with a new cannula or proceed according to your facility's policy.[15]
■ After removal, change the dressing every 24 hours until the exit site heals.[5]

Patient teaching

Most patients who receive IV therapy at home have a central venous access device. But if you're caring for a patient going home with a peripheral catheter, you should teach him how to care for the IV site and identify certain complications. If the patient must observe movement restrictions, make sure he understands them.

Teach the patient how to examine the site, and instruct him to notify the doctor or home care nurse if redness, swelling, or discomfort develops or if the dressing becomes moist. Also tell the patient to report any problems with the IV line—for instance, if the solution stops infusing or if an alarm goes off on an infusion pump.

If the patient is using an intermittent infusion device, teach him how and when to flush it. Finally, teach the patient to document daily whether the IV site is free from pain, swelling, and redness.

Complications

Peripheral IV catheter complications can result from the catheter (infection and phlebitis) or from the solution (circulatory overload, infiltration, sepsis, and allergic reaction). (See *Risks of peripheral IV therapy.*)

Documentation

Document the date and time of insertion; the type, gauge, and length of the vascular access device; the anatomic location of the insertion site; the number and location of attempts; and the functionality of the device.

Record the local anesthetic, if used, site preparation, and whether an ultrasound device was used to guide insertion. Also document the type and flow rate of the IV solution, the name and dose of medication in the solution (if any), any adverse reactions and actions taken to correct them, patient teaching, and evidence of patient understanding.

Record the date and time of the catheter removal, the site from which the catheter was removed, the condition of the catheter site and catheter, the patient's tolerance of the procedure, and any patient teaching provided.

REFERENCES

1 O'Grady, N.P., et al. (2011). "Guidelines for the Prevention of Intravascular Catheter-Related Infections" [Online]. Accessed November 2011 via the Web at http://www.cdc.gov/hicpac/pdf/guidelines/bsi-guidelines-2011.pdf
2 Standard 33. Site selection. Infusion nursing standards of practice. (2011). *Journal of Infusion Nursing, 34*(1S), S40–S43. (Level I)
3 Standard 32. Vascular access device selection. Infusion nursing standards of practice. (2011). *Journal of Infusion Nursing, 34*(1S), S37–S40. (Level I)
4 Standard 44. Vascular access device removal. Infusion nursing standards of practice. (2011). *Journal of Infusion Nursing, 34*(1S), S57–S59. (Level I)
5 Infusion Nurses Society. (2011). *Policies and procedures for infusion nursing* (4th ed.). Boston, MA: Infusion Nurses Society.
6 The Joint Commission. (2012). Standard MM.06.01.01. *Comprehensive accreditation manual for hospitals: The official handbook.* Oakbrook Terrace, IL: The Joint Commission. (Level I)
7 Standard 61. Parenteral medication and solution administration. Infusion nursing standards of practice. (2011). *Journal of Infusion Nursing, 34*(1S), S86. (Level I)
8 The Joint Commission. (2012). Standard NPSG.07.01.01. *Comprehensive accreditation manual for hospitals: The official handbook.* Oakbrook Terrace, IL: The Joint Commission. (Level I)
9 Standard 19. Hand hygiene. Infusion nursing standards of practice. (2011). *Journal of Infusion Nursing, 34*(1S), S26–S27.
10 Centers for Disease Control and Prevention. (October 2002). Guideline for hand hygiene in health-care settings. *Morbidity and Mortality Weekly Report, 51*(RR-16), 1–45. (Level I)
11 World Health Organization. (2009). *WHO guidelines on hand hygiene in health care: First global patient safety challenge. Clean care is safer care.* Geneva, Switzerland: World Health Organization. (Level I)
12 The Joint Commission. (2012). Standard NPSG.01.01.01. *Comprehensive accreditation manual for hospitals: The official handbook.* Oakbrook Terrace, IL: The Joint Commission. (Level I)
13 Standard 36. Vascular access device stabilization. Infusion nursing standards of practice. (2011). *Journal of Infusion Nursing, 34*(1S), S46. (Level I)
14 Standard 31. Tourniquets. Infusion nursing standards of practice. (2011). *Journal of Infusion Nursing, 34*(1S), S36. (Level I)
15 Standard 35. Vascular access site preparation and device placement. Infusion nursing standards of practice. (2011). *Journal of Infusion Nursing, 34*(1S), S44–S46. (Level I)
16 Standard 46. Vascular access device site care and dressing changes. Infusion nursing standards of practice. (2011). *Journal of Infusion Nursing, 34*(1S), S63–S65. (Level I)
17 U.S. Food and Drug Administration. (2009). "Look. Check. Connect.: Safe Medical Device Connections Save Lives" [Online]. Accessed November 2011 via the Web at http://www.fda.gov/downloads/MedicalDevices/Safety/AlertsandNotices/UCM134873.pdf
18 Standard 37. Joint stabilization. Infusion nursing standards of practice. (2011). *Journal of Infusion Nursing, 34*(1S), S47. (Level I)

(*Text continues on page 431.*)

Risks of peripheral IV therapy

COMPLICATIONS	SIGNS AND SYMPTOMS	POSSIBLE CAUSES	NURSING INTERVENTIONS
LOCAL COMPLICATIONS			
Phlebitis[21]	■ Tenderness at tip of and proximal to venous access device ■ Redness at tip of cannula and along vein ■ Swelling and induration over vein ■ Palpable venous cord ■ Elevated temperature ■ Pain ■ Purulent drainage	■ Poor blood flow around venous access device ■ Friction from cannula movement in vein ■ Venous access device left in vein too long ■ Drug or solution with high or low pH or high osmolarity ■ Clotting at cannula tip	■ Use a standardized scale to assess the severity of phlebitis. ■ Discontinue the infusion and then remove venous access device. ■ Determine whether the cause was mechanical, chemical or bacterial. ■ Apply warm soaks for 20 minutes three to four times per day as ordered. ■ Notify the doctor. ■ Replace the device in the opposite extremity. Consult with the doctor about central venous access device placement if the probable cause is irritating fluid. ■ Document patient's condition and your interventions.[19,20] ***Prevention*** ■ Secure the device *to prevent motion*.
Infiltration	■ Swelling at and above IV site (may extend along entire limb) ■ Discomfort, burning, or pain at site (may be painless) ■ Tight feeling at site ■ Decreased skin temperature around site ■ Blanching at site ■ Fluid drainage from insertion site ■ Loss of blood return during aspiration ■ Slower infusion rate	■ Venous access device dislodged from vein ■ Perforated vein	■ Stop the infusion. ■ Remove the catheter.[22] ■ Apply warm soaks *to aid absorption* and elevate the limb. ■ Check for pulse and capillary refill periodically *to assess circulation*. ■ Restart the infusion in another limb. ■ Document the patient's condition and your interventions.[19,20] ■ Notify the doctor that infiltration has occurred, if severe. Treatment depends on the severity and type of solution infiltrated. ***Prevention*** ■ Check the IV site frequently. ■ Aspirate for blood return to ensure catheter patency before beginning the infusion.[22] ■ Teach the patient to observe the IV site and report pain, burning, or swelling. ■ Stabilize the catheter to minimize movement at the insertion site.[22]
Cannula dislodgment	■ Cannula partly backed out of vein ■ Solution infiltrating	■ Loosened tape, or tubing snagged in bed linens, resulting in partial retraction of cannula ■ Pulled out by confused patient	■ If no infiltration occurs, retape without pushing cannula back into vein. Never reinsert the cannula into the vein. If pulled out, apply pressure to IV site with sterile dressing.[13] ***Prevention*** ■ Secure the device on insertion.

(continued)

Risks of peripheral IV therapy *(continued)*

COMPLICATIONS	SIGNS AND SYMPTOMS	POSSIBLE CAUSES	NURSING INTERVENTIONS
LOCAL COMPLICATIONS *(continued)*			
Occlusion	▪ Infusion doesn't flow ▪ Infusion pump alarms "occlusion" ▪ Discomfort at insertion site	▪ IV flow interrupted ▪ Saline lock not flushed ▪ Blood backflow in line when patient walks ▪ Line clamped too long ▪ Hypercoagulable patient	▪ Use mild flush injection. Don't force it. If unsuccessful, remove the IV catheter and insert a new one. ***Prevention*** ▪ Maintain IV flow rate. ▪ Flush promptly after intermittent piggyback administration. ▪ Have the patient walk with his arm bent at the elbow *to reduce the risk of blood backflow.*
Vein irritation or pain at IV site	▪ Pain during infusion ▪ Possible blanching if vasospasm occurs ▪ Red skin over vein during infusion ▪ Rapidly developing signs of phlebitis	▪ Solution with high or low pH or high osmolarity, such as phenytoin and some antibiotics (vancomycin and nafcillin)	▪ Decrease the flow rate. ▪ Try using an electronic flow device *to achieve a steady flow.* ***Prevention*** ▪ Dilute solutions before administration. For example, give antibiotics in 250-mL solution rather than 100-mL solution. If the drug has a low pH, ask the pharmacist if the drug can be buffered with sodium bicarbonate. (Refer to your facility's policy.) ▪ If long-term therapy with an irritating drug is planned, ask the doctor to use a central venous access device.
Severed cannula	▪ Leakage from cannula shaft	▪ Cannula inadvertently cut by scissors ▪ Reinsertion of stylet into cannula	▪ If a broken part is visible, attempt to retrieve it. If unsuccessful, notify the doctor. ▪ If a portion of the cannula enters the bloodstream, place the tourniquet above the IV site *to prevent progression of the broken part.* ▪ Notify the doctor and radiology department. ▪ Document the patient's condition and your interventions.[19,20] ***Prevention*** ▪ Don't use scissors around the IV site. ▪ Never reinsert the stylet into cannula.[15] ▪ Remove unsuccessfully inserted cannula and stylet together.
Hematoma	▪ Tenderness at venipuncture site ▪ Bruised area around site ▪ Inability to advance or flush IV catheter	▪ Vein punctured through opposite wall at time of insertion ▪ Leakage of blood from stylet displacement	▪ Remove the venous access device. ▪ Apply direct pressure and elevate the extremity until bleeding has stopped. ▪ Recheck for bleeding. ▪ Document the patient's condition and your interventions. ***Prevention*** ▪ Choose a vein that can accommodate the size of the venous access device. ▪ Release the tourniquet as soon as successful insertion is achieved.

Risks of peripheral IV therapy *(continued)*

COMPLICATIONS	SIGNS AND SYMPTOMS	POSSIBLE CAUSES	NURSING INTERVENTIONS
LOCAL COMPLICATIONS *(continued)*			
Venous spasm	■ Pain along vein ■ Flow rate sluggish when clamp completely open ■ Blanched skin over vein	■ Severe vein irritation from irritating drugs or fluids ■ Administration of cold fluids or blood ■ Very rapid flow rate (with fluids at room temperature)	■ Apply warm soaks over the vein and surrounding area. ■ Decrease the flow rate. ***Prevention*** ■ Use a blood warmer for blood or packed red blood cells.
Thrombosis	■ Painful, reddened, and swollen vein ■ Sluggish or stopped IV flow	■ Injury to endothelial cells of vein wall, allowing platelets to adhere and thrombi to form	■ Remove the venous access device; restart the infusion in the opposite limb if possible. ■ Apply cold compresses. ■ Watch for IV therapy–related infection; thrombi provide an excellent environment for bacterial growth. ***Prevention*** ■ Use proper venipuncture technique *to reduce injury to the vein.* ■ Avoid starting an IV in the lower extremities.
Thrombophlebitis	■ Severe discomfort ■ Reddened, swollen, and hardened vein	■ Thrombosis and inflammation	■ Remove the venous access device; restart the infusion in the opposite limb if possible. ■ Apply cold compresses. ■ Watch for IV therapy–related infection. Thrombi provide an excellent environment for bacterial growth. ***Prevention*** ■ Check the site frequently. Remove the venous access device at the first sign of redness and tenderness.
Nerve, tendon, or ligament damage	■ Extreme pain (similar to electrical shock when nerve is punctured) ■ Numbness and muscle contraction ■ Delayed effects, including paralysis, numbness, and deformity	■ Improper venipuncture technique, resulting in injury to surrounding nerves, tendons, or ligaments ■ Tight taping or improper splinting with arm board	■ Stop the procedure and remove the device. ***Prevention*** ■ Don't repeatedly penetrate tissues with a venous access device. ■ Don't apply excessive pressure when taping; don't encircle the limb with tape. ■ Pad arm boards and tape securing arm boards if possible.
Vasovagal reaction	■ Sudden collapse of vein during venipuncture ■ Sudden pallor, sweating, faintness, dizziness, and nausea ■ Decreased blood pressure	■ Vasospasm from anxiety or pain	■ Lower the head of the bed. ■ Have the patient take deep breaths. ■ Check vital signs. ***Prevention*** ■ Prepare the patient for therapy *to relieve his anxiety.* ■ Use local anesthetic *to prevent pain.*

(continued)

Risks of peripheral IV therapy *(continued)*

COMPLICATIONS	SIGNS AND SYMPTOMS	POSSIBLE CAUSES	NURSING INTERVENTIONS
SYSTEMIC COMPLICATIONS			
Circulatory overload	■ Discomfort ■ Neck vein engorgement ■ Respiratory distress ■ Increased blood pressure ■ Crackles ■ Increased difference between fluid intake and output	■ Roller clamp loosened to allow run-on infusion ■ Flow rate too rapid ■ Miscalculation of fluid requirements	■ Raise the head of the bed. ■ Slow the infusion rate, but don't remove the IV catheter. ■ Administer oxygen as needed. ■ Notify the doctor. ■ Administer medications (probably furosemide) as prescribed. ***Prevention*** ■ Use a pump for elderly or compromised patients. ■ Recheck calculations of fluid requirements. ■ Monitor infusion frequently.
Systemic infection (septicemia or bacteremia)	■ Fever, chills, and malaise for no apparent reason ■ Contaminated IV site, usually with no visible signs of infection at site	■ Failure to maintain sterile technique during insertion or site care ■ Severe phlebitis, which can set up ideal conditions for organism growth ■ A poorly secured device that can move, which can introduce organisms into bloodstream ■ Prolonged indwelling time of device ■ Weak immune system	■ Notify the doctor. ■ Administer medications as prescribed. ■ Culture the site and device.[23] ■ Monitor vital signs. ***Prevention*** ■ Use scrupulous sterile technique when handling solutions and tubing, inserting venous access device, and discontinuing infusion. ■ Secure all connections and use only luer-lock–designed devices.[24] ■ Change IV solutions, tubing, and venous access devices at recommended times.
Air embolism[25]	■ Sudden onset of dyspnea ■ Breathlessness ■ Tachyarrhythmias ■ Weak pulse ■ Increased central venous pressure ■ Hypotension ■ Loss of consciousness ■ Continued coughing ■ Chest pain ■ Jugular venous distention ■ Wheezing ■ Altered mental status ■ Altered speech ■ Numbness ■ Paralysis	■ Solution container empty ■ Solution container empties, and added container pushes air down the line (if line not purged first) ■ Disconnected tubing from venous access device or IV bag	■ Clamp, fold, or close the existing catheter or occlude the insertion site.[25] ■ Place the patient in a left lateral decubitus position, if not contraindicated by other conditions.[25] ■ Administer oxygen. ■ Notify the doctor. ■ Document the patient's condition and your interventions.[19,20] ***Prevention*** ■ Purge administration sets and add-on devices of air completely before starting an infusion.[5] ■ Use an air-detection device on the pump or an air-eliminating filter proximal to the IV site. ■ Secure connections. ■ Use luer-lock connections on catheter-administration set junctions.[5] ■ Place the patient in a position with the insertion site at or below heart level when changing administration sets or needleless connectors.[5] ■ Trace the tubing from the patient to its point of origin to prevent misconnections.[5,17]

Risks of peripheral IV therapy *(continued)*

COMPLICATIONS	SIGNS AND SYMPTOMS	POSSIBLE CAUSES	NURSING INTERVENTIONS
SYSTEMIC COMPLICATIONS *(continued)*			
			■ Have the patient perform Valsalva's maneuver, if able, when you're changing administration tubing or the needleless connector if a clamp isn't present on the catheter's exterior. If it is present, clamp it.
Allergic reaction	■ Itching ■ Watery eyes and nose ■ Bronchospasm ■ Wheezing ■ Urticarial rash ■ Edema at IV site ■ Anaphylactic reaction, which may occur within minutes or up to 1 hour after exposure (flushing, chills, anxiety, agitation, itching, palpitations, paresthesia, throbbing in ears, wheezing, coughing, seizures, cardiac arrest)	■ Allergens, such as medications	■ If a reaction occurs, stop the infusion immediately and infuse normal saline solution. ■ Maintain a patent airway. ■ Notify the doctor. ■ Administer an antihistamine, a steroid, an anti-inflammatory, and antipyretic drugs, as prescribed. ■ Give epinephrine, as prescribed. Repeat as needed and prescribed. ■ Administer steroids if prescribed. ***Prevention*** ■ Obtain the patient's allergy history. Be aware of cross-allergies. ■ Assist with test dosing and document any new allergies. ■ Monitor the patient carefully during the first 15 minutes of administration of a new drug.

19 The Joint Commission. (2012). Standard RC.01.03.01. *Comprehensive accreditation manual for hospitals: The official handbook.* Oakbrook Terrace, IL: The Joint Commission. (Level I)

20 The Joint Commission. (2012). Standard RC.02.01.01. *Comprehensive accreditation manual for hospitals: The official handbook.* Oakbrook Terrace, IL: The Joint Commission. (Level I)

21 Standard 47. Phlebitis. Infusion nursing standards of practice. (2011). *Journal of Infusion Nursing, 34*(1S), S65. (Level I)

22 Standard 48. Infiltration and extravasation. Infusion nursing standards of practice. (2011). *Journal of Infusion Nursing, 34*(1S), S66–S68. (Level I)

23 Standard 49. Infection. Infusion nursing standards of practice. (2011). *Journal of Infusion Nursing, 34*(1S), S68. (Level I)

24 Standard 26. Add-on devices. Infusion nursing standards of practice. (2011). *Journal of Infusion Nursing, 34*(1S), S31. (Level I)

25 Standard 50. Air embolism. Infusion nursing standards of practice. (2011). *Journal of Infusion Nursing, 34*(1S), S69–S70. (Level I)

ADDITIONAL REFERENCES

Aziz, A.M. (2009). Improving peripheral IV cannula care: Implementing high-impact interventions. *British Journal of Nursing, 18*(20), 1242–1246.

Lee, W.L., et al. (2009). Risk factors for peripheral intravenous catheter infection in hospitalized patients: A prospective study of 3165 patients. *American Journal of Infection Control, 37*(8), 683–686.

Nettina, S.M. (2010). *Lippincott manual of nursing practice* (9th ed.). Philadelphia, PA: Lippincott Williams & Wilkins.

Scales, K. (2008). Intravenous therapy: A guide to good practice. *British Journal of Nursing, 17*(19), S4–S12.

Taylor, C., et al. (2011). *Fundamentals of nursing: The art and science of nursing care* (7th ed.). Philadelphia, PA: Lippincott Williams & Wilkins.

Weinstein, S.M. (2007). *Plumer's principles and practices of intravenous therapy* (8th ed.). Philadelphia, PA: Lippincott Williams & Wilkins.

IV CATHETER MAINTENANCE

Routine maintenance of an IV site includes regular assessment of the site and periodic changes of the dressing, along with solution changes, and regular tubing changes, which help prevent complications, such as thrombophlebitis and infection. They should be performed according to your facility's policy.

Routine site care and IV dressing changes aren't recommended for short peripheral IV catheters unless the dressing becomes soiled or damp or is no longer intact.[1,2] Dressings are also changed when the device is changed; the IV catheter should be changed when clinically indicated by the patient's condition, integrity of the vein and skin, length and type of prescribed therapy, integrity and patency of the existing catheter, and the patient's care location.[2] Peripheral IV catheters should be replaced no more frequently than every 72 to 96 hours to reduce the risk for infection and phlebitis in adults;[1] follow your facility's policy for IV maintenance. If an IV catheter is inserted during an emergency, it should be replaced as soon as possible, within 48 hours.[2]

The IV administration set should be changed no more frequently than every 96 hours, although it should be changed immediately upon suspected contamination, when the integrity of the product or system has been compromised, or whenever the peripheral IV site is rotated.[1,3]

Another aspect of IV catheter maintenance, ensuring an accurate flow rate helps prevent complications. Calculated from a doctor's order, flow rate is usually expressed as the total volume of IV solution infused over a prescribed interval or as the total volume given in milliliters per hour. Many devices can regulate the flow of IV solution, including clamps, the flow regulator (or rate minder), and the volumetric pump. With any device, flow rate can be easily monitored by using a time tape, which indicates the prescribed solution level at hourly intervals. IV time tapes are rarely used in acute care settings, but may be found in long-term or subacute care settings.

Equipment

For a dressing change

Gloves ■ antiseptic solution ■ transparent semipermeable dressing ■ catheter securement device, sterile tape, or sterile surgical strips ■ label ■ Optional: sterile 2″ × 2″ gauze pad and adhesive bandage, as needed.

For a solution change

Solution container ■ antiseptic pad (alcohol, tincture of iodine, or chlorhexidine-based) ■ gloves.

For an IV tubing change

IV administration set ■ new bag of prescribed IV fluids (as needed) ■ gloves ■ transparent semipermeable dressing ■ sterile 2″ × 2″ gauze pads ■ label.

For using a time tape

IV solution ■ IV administration set with clamp ■ 1″ paper or adhesive tape (or preprinted time tape) ■ pen.

Preparation of equipment

If your facility keeps IV equipment and dressings in a tray or cart, have it nearby, if possible, *because you may have to select a new venipuncture site, depending on the current site's condition.*

When possible, change the solution and tubing at the same time *to decrease the risk of contamination.*[3]

If you're changing both the solution and the tubing, attach and prime the IV administration set, including add-on devices, before entering the patient's room.

Implementation

■ Verify the doctor's order.

■ Perform hand hygiene *to prevent the spread of microorganisms.*[1,4,5,6,7]

■ Confirm the patient's identity using at least two patient identifiers according to your facility's policy.[8]

■ Explain the procedure to the patient *to allay his fears and ensure cooperation.*

Changing a dressing

■ Open all supply packages.
■ Put on gloves.
■ Remove the old dressing (as shown below).

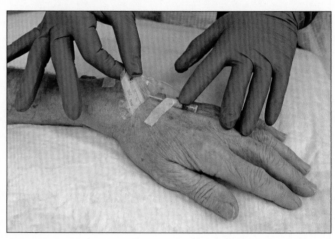

■ Hold the cannula in place with your nondominant hand *to prevent accidental movement or dislodgment, which could puncture the vein and cause infiltration* (as shown below).

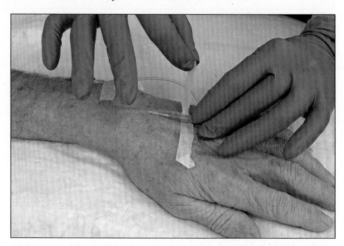

■ Assess the venipuncture site for signs of infection (redness and pain at the puncture site), infiltration (coolness, blanching, and edema at the site), and thrombophlebitis (redness, firmness, tenderness, warmth, palpable venous cord, and edema).[1] If any such signs are present, cover the area with a sterile 2″ × 2″ gauze pad and remove the catheter. Apply pressure to the area until the bleeding stops, and apply an adhesive bandage. Then, using fresh equipment and solution, start the IV in another appropriate site, preferably on the opposite extremity.

■ If the venipuncture site is intact, stabilize the cannula and carefully clean around the puncture site with antiseptic solution (as shown below). Cleaning methods vary with the type of antiseptic used. Apply chlorhexidine using a side-to-side motion for at least 30 seconds.[9] Allow the area to dry completely.

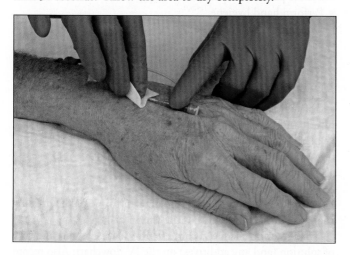

■ Secure the catheter with a catheter securement device, sterile tape, or sterile surgical strips.[9]
■ Cover the site with a transparent semipermeable dressing.[9] *The transparent dressing allows visualization of the insertion site and maintains sterility.* Place it over the insertion site to halfway up the cannula (as shown below).

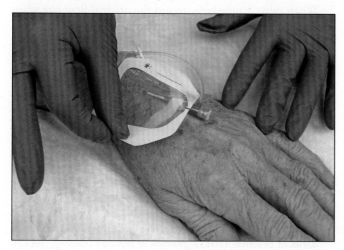

■ Label the dressing with the date and time of the procedure.[2]
■ Discard used supplies in the appropriate receptacle.
■ Remove and discard your gloves and perform hand hygiene.[1,4,5,6,7]
■ Document the procedure.[10,11]

Changing the solution

■ If your facility uses a bar code scanning system, scan your identification badge, the patient's identification band, and the IV fluid's bar code or follow your facility's policy.
■ Inspect the new solution container for cracks, leaks, and other damage. Check the solution for discoloration, turbidity, and par-

ticulates. Note the date and time the solution was mixed and its expiration date.[12]
■ Clamp the tubing when inverting it *to prevent air from entering the tubing.* Keep the drip chamber half full. Put the IV pump on standby or pause.
■ If you're replacing a bag, remove the seal or tab from the new bag and remove the old bag from the pole. Remove the spike, insert it into the new bag, and adjust the flow rate or restart the pump.[9]
■ If you're replacing a bottle, remove the cap and seal from the new bottle and disinfect the rubber port with an antiseptic pad. Clamp the line, pause the pump, remove the spike from the old bottle, and insert the spike into the new bottle. Then hang the new bottle and adjust the flow rate or restart the pump.
■ Label the solution container with the date and time and place a time strip on the solution.
■ Discard used supplies in an appropriate receptacle.
■ Perform hand hygiene.[1,4,5,6,7]
■ Document the procedure.[10,11]

Changing the tubing

■ Hang the IV container and primed set on the pole.
■ Put on gloves and assess the IV site for redness, swelling, or pain.
■ Remove the dressing over the IV cannula, if needed, *to access the hub.*
■ Place a sterile gauze pad under the needle or cannula hub *to create a sterile field.*
■ Clamp the existing administration set and then clamp the IV catheter *to prevent accidental exposure to blood and to reduce the risk of air embolism.*[9]
■ Gently disconnect the old tubing (as shown below), being careful not to dislodge or move the IV device. (If you have trouble disconnecting the old tubing, use a hemostat to hold the hub securely while twisting the tubing *to remove it.* Or, use one hemostat on the venipuncture device and another on the hard plastic end of the tubing. Then pull the hemostats in opposite directions. Don't clamp the hemostats shut *because this could crack the tubing adapter or the venipuncture device.*)

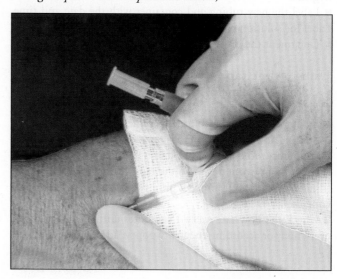

- Thoroughly disinfect the catheter hub with an antiseptic pad using friction and allow it to dry.[9]
- Remove the protective cap from the new tubing, and connect the new adapter to the cannula. Hold the hub securely *to prevent dislodging the needle or cannula tip.*
- Observe for blood backflow into the new tubing *to verify that the catheter is still in place.* (You may not be able to do this with a small-gauge catheter.)
- Trace the tubing from the patient to its point of origin *to make sure you've connected the administration tubing to the proper port.*[13]
- Unclamp the catheter *to resume infusion.*[9]
- Adjust the clamp to maintain the appropriate flow rate (as shown below).

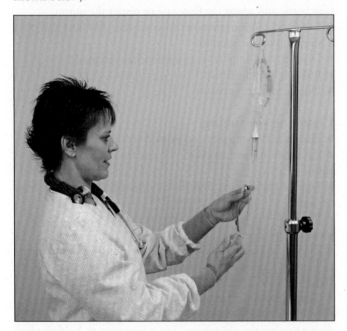

- Redress the catheter insertion site and IV tubing, and recheck the IV flow rate *because taping may alter it.*
- Discard used supplies in an appropriate receptacle.
- Remove and discard your gloves and perform hand hygiene.[1,4,5,6,7]
- Label the new tubing and container with the date and time. Label the solution container with a time strip.
- Document the procedure.[10,11]

Using a time tape

- Calculate the number of milliliters to be infused per hour.
- Place a piece of tape or preprinted time tape vertically on the container alongside the volume-increment markers.
- Starting at the current solution level, move down the number of milliliters to be infused in 1 hour, and mark the appropriate time and a horizontal line on the tape at this level. Then continue to mark 1-hour intervals until you reach the bottom of the container.
- Check the flow rate every 15 minutes until stable, and then every hour or according to facility policy; adjust, as needed.

- Compare the time to the appropriate infusion level on the tape and recheck the flow rate. Assess for deviations from recommended intake. (See *Managing IV flow rate deviations.*)
- With each check, inspect the IV site for complications, and assess the patient's response to therapy.
- Perform hand hygiene.[1,4,5,6,7]
- Document the procedure.[10,11]

Special considerations

- If you crack the adapter or hub (or if you accidentally dislodge the cannula from the vein), remove the cannula. Apply pressure and an adhesive bandage *to stop any bleeding.* Perform a venipuncture at another site, and reinsert a new IV catheter.
- Check the prescribed IV flow rate before and after each solution change *to prevent errors.*

Documentation

For a dressing change, record the date and time of the dressing change and the appearance of the site.

For a solution change, record the time, date, and rate and type of solution (and any additives) on the IV flowchart. Also record the appearance of the site.

For a tubing change, record the date and time of the tubing change, the appearance of the site, the type of dressing applied, and any patient teaching and the patient's understanding of your teaching. Document the patient's tolerance of the procedure as well as the type of IV fluid hung and the rate of infusion.

When using a time tape, record the original flow rate when beginning the infusion through the peripheral IV catheter. If you adjust the rate, record the change, the date and time, and your initials. Document any patient teaching provided and the patient's understanding of your teaching.

REFERENCES

1 O'Grady, N.P., et al. (2011). "Guidelines for the Prevention of Intravascular Catheter-Related Infections" [Online]. Accessed November 2011 via the Web at http://www.cdc.gov/hicpac/pdf/guidelines/bsi-guidelines-2011.pdf

2 Standard 46. Vascular access device site care and dressing changes. Infusion nursing standards of practice. (2011). *Journal of Infusion Nursing, 34*(1S), S63–S64. (Level I)

3 Standard 43. Administration set change. Infusion nursing standards of practice. (2011). *Journal of Infusion Nursing, 34*(1S), S55–S57. (Level I)

4 The Joint Commission. (2012). Standard NPSG.07.01.01. *Comprehensive accreditation manual for hospitals: The official handbook.* Oakbrook Terrace, IL: The Joint Commission. (Level I)

5 Standard 19. Hand hygiene. Infusion nursing standards of practice. (2011). *Journal of Infusion Nursing, 34*(1S), S26–S27. (Level I)

6 Centers for Disease Control and Prevention. (October 2002). Guideline for hand hygiene in health-care settings. *Morbidity and Mortality Weekly Report, 51*(RR-16), 1–45. (Level I)

7 World Health Organization. (2009). *WHO guidelines on hand hygiene in health care: First global patient safety challenge. Clean care is safer care.* Geneva, Switzerland: World Health Organization. (Level I)

TROUBLESHOOTING

Managing IV flow rate deviations

PROBLEM	POSSIBLE CAUSES	NURSING INTERVENTIONS
Flow rate too slow	■ Venous spasm after insertion	■ Apply warm soaks over site.
	■ Venous obstruction from bending arm	■ Secure with an arm board if necessary. ■ Change IV site.
	■ Pressure change (decreasing fluid in bottle causes solution to run slower because of decreasing pressure)	■ Readjust flow rate.
	■ Elevated blood pressure	■ Readjust flow rate. Use infusion pump to ensure correct flow rate.
	■ Cold solution	■ Allow solution to warm to room temperature before hanging.
	■ Change in solution viscosity from medication added	■ Readjust flow rate.
	■ IV container too low or patient's arm too high	■ Hang container higher or remind patient to keep his arm below heart level.
	■ Bevel against vein wall (positional cannulation)	■ Withdraw needle slightly, or place a folded 2″ × 2″ gauze pad over or under catheter hub to change angle.
	■ Excess tubing dangling below insertion site	■ Replace tubing with shorter piece, or tape excess tubing to IV pole, below flow clamp. (Make sure tubing isn't kinked.)
	■ Cannula too small	■ Remove cannula in use, and insert a larger-bore cannula, or use an infusion pump.
	■ Infiltration or clotted cannula	■ Remove cannula in use, and insert a new cannula.
	■ Kinked tubing	■ Check tubing over its entire length and unkink it. ■ Replace tubing if it remains kinked.
	■ Clogged filter	■ Remove filter and replace with a new one.
	■ Tubing memory (tubing compressed at clamped area)	■ Massage or milk tubing by pinching and wrapping it around a pencil four or five times. Quickly pull pencil out of coiled tubing. ■ Replace tubing if necessary.
Flow rate too fast	■ Patient or visitor manipulated clamp	■ Instruct patient not to touch clamp. Place tape over it. Administer IV solution with infusion pump.
	■ Tubing disconnected from catheter	■ Restart IV with new catheter with luer-lock connections.
	■ Change in patient position	■ Readjust flow rate.
	■ Flow clamp drifted because of patient movement	■ Place tape below clamp.

Using IV clamps

With a roller clamp, you can increase or decrease the flow through the IV line by turning a wheel.

With a slide clamp, you can open or close the line by moving the clamp horizontally. However, you can't make fine adjustments to the flow rate.

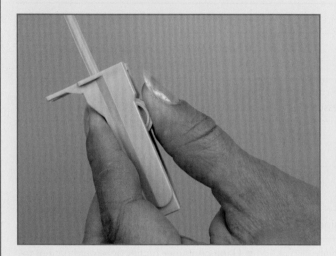
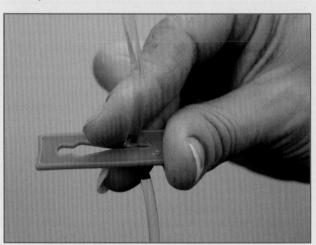

8 The Joint Commission. (2012). Standard NPSG.01.01.01. *Comprehensive accreditation manual for hospitals: The official handbook.* Oakbrook Terrace, IL: The Joint Commission. (Level I)

9 Infusion Nurses Society. (2011). *Policies and procedures for infusion nursing* (4th ed.). Boston, MA: Infusion Nurses Society.

10 The Joint Commission. (2012). Standard RC.01.03.01. *Comprehensive accreditation manual for hospitals: The official handbook.* Oakbrook Terrace, IL: The Joint Commission. (Level I)

11 The Joint Commission. (2012). Standard RC.02.01.01. *Comprehensive accreditation manual for hospitals: The official handbook.* Oakbrook Terrace, IL: The Joint Commission. (Level I)

12 Standard 61. Parenteral medication and solution administration. Infusion nursing standards of practice. (2011). *Journal of Infusion Nursing, 34*(1S), S86. (Level I)

13 U.S. Food and Drug Administration. (2009). "Look. Check. Connect.: Safe Medical Device Connections Save Lives" [Online]. Accessed November 2011 via the Web at http://www.fda.gov/downloads/MedicalDevices/Safety/AlertsandNotices/UCM134873.pdf

ADDITIONAL REFERENCES

Alexander, M., et al. (Eds.). (2010). *Infusion nursing: An evidence-based approach* (3rd ed.). Philadelphia, PA: Elsevier.

Nettina, S.M. (2010). *Lippincott manual of nursing practice* (9th ed.). Philadelphia, PA: Lippincott Williams & Wilkins.

IV INFUSION RATES AND MANUAL CONTROL

Calculated from a doctor's orders, infusion flow rate is usually expressed as the total volume of IV solution infused over a prescribed interval or as the total volume given in milliliters per hour. Many devices can regulate the flow of IV solution, including clamps, the flow regulator (or rate minder), and the volumetric pump. (See *Using IV clamps.*)

When regulated by a clamp, flow rate is usually measured in drops per minute; by a volumetric pump, in milliliters per hour. The flow regulator can be set to deliver the desired amount of solution, also in milliliters per hour. Less accurate than infusion pumps, flow regulators are most reliable when used with inactive adult patients. With any device, flow rate can be easily monitored by using a time tape, which indicates the prescribed solution level at hourly intervals. (See "IV catheter maintenance," page 431.)

Equipment

IV solution ▪ IV administration set with clamp ▪ watch with second hand ▪ drip rate chart, as necessary.

Standard macrodrip sets deliver from 10 to 20 drops/mL, depending on the manufacturer; microdrip sets, 60 drops/mL; and blood transfusion sets, 10 drops/mL. A commercially available adapter can convert a macrodrip set to a microdrip system.

Implementation

▪ Verify the doctor's order for the prescribed flow rate.[1]
▪ Gather the equipment.
▪ Perform hand hygiene.[2,3,4]

Calculating infusion rates

When calculating the infusion rate of IV solutions, remember that the number of drops required to deliver 1 mL varies with the type and manufacturer of the administration set used. The first illustration shows a standard (macrodrip) set, which delivers from 10 to 20 drops/mL. The second illustration shows a pediatric (microdrip) set, which delivers about 60 drops/mL. The third illustration shows a blood transfusion set, which delivers about 10 drops/mL.

To calculate the infusion rate, you must know the calibration of the drip rate for each manufacturer's product. Use this formula to calculate specific drip rates:

$$\frac{\text{volume of infusion (in mL)}}{\text{time of infusion (in minutes)}} \times \text{drip factor (in drops/mL)} = \text{drops/minute}$$

Macrodrip set

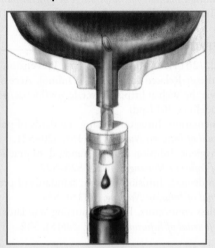

Microdrip set

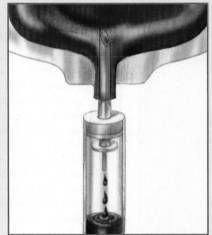

Blood transfusion set

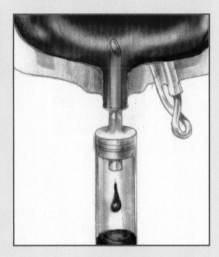

- Confirm the patient's identity using at least two patient identifiers according to your facility's policy.[5]
- Attach the administration set to the IV solution and prime the tubing. (See "IV therapy preparation," page 443.) Trace the tubing from the patient to its point of origin *to make sure you've connected it to the proper port before beginning the infusion.*[6]
- The flow rate requires close monitoring and correction *because such factors as venous spasm, venous pressure changes, patient movement or manipulation of the clamp, and bent or kinked tubing can cause the rate to vary markedly.*
- Determine the proper drip rate, or use your unit's drip rate chart. (See *Calculating infusion rates.*)
- After calculating the desired drip rate, remove your watch and hold it next to the drip chamber *so that you can observe the watch and drops simultaneously.*
- Release the clamp to the approximate drip rate. Then count drops for 1 minute *to account for flow irregularities.*
- Adjust the clamp as necessary, and count drops for 1 minute. Continue to adjust the clamp and count drops until the correct rate is achieved.
- Check the flow rate every 15 minutes until stable, and then every hour or according to your facility's policy; adjust as needed.
- With each check, inspect the IV site for complications, and assess the patient's response to therapy.

- Perform hand hygiene.[2,3,4]
- Document the procedure.[7,8]

Special considerations

- If the infusion rate slows significantly, a slight rate increase may be necessary. If the rate must be increased by more than 30% to achieve the infusion volume goal, consult the doctor. When infusing drugs, use an IV pump, if possible, *to avoid flow rate inaccuracies.* Always use a pump when infusing solutions by way of a central venous access device.
- Large-volume solution containers have about 10% more fluid than the amount indicated on the bag *to allow for tubing purges.* Thus, a 1,000-mL bag or bottle contains an additional 100 mL; similarly, a 500-mL container holds an extra 50 mL; and a 250-mL container holds an extra 25 mL.

Complications

An excessively slow flow rate may cause insufficient intake of fluids, drugs, and nutrients; an excessively rapid rate of fluid or drug infusion may cause circulatory overload—possibly leading to heart failure and pulmonary edema—as well as other adverse drug effects. (See "IV catheter maintenance," page 431.)

Infusion pumps

Infusion pumps (like the one shown here) electronically regulate the flow of IV solutions and drugs. You'll use them when a precise flow rate is require—for instance, when administering total parenteral nutrition solutions and chemotherapeutic or cardiovascular agents.

Infusion pump

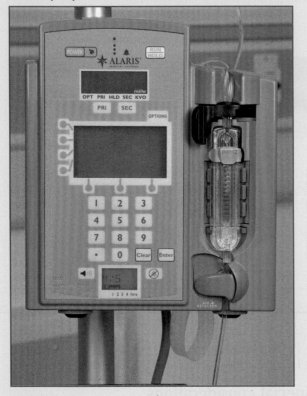

Documentation

Record the original flow rate when setting up a peripheral line. If you adjust the rate, record the change, the date and time, and your initials. Document the patient's response to therapy and any patient teaching provided.

REFERENCES

1 The Joint Commission. (2012). Standard MM.04.01.01. *Comprehensive accreditation manual for hospitals: The official handbook.* Oakbrook Terrace, IL: The Joint Commission. (Level I)

2 The Joint Commission. (2012). Standard NPSG.07.01.01. *Comprehensive accreditation manual for hospitals: The official handbook.* Oakbrook Terrace, IL: The Joint Commission. (Level I)

3 Centers for Disease Control and Prevention. (October 2002). Guideline for hand hygiene in health-care settings. *Morbidity and Mortality Weekly Report, 51*(RR-16), 1–45. (Level I)

4 World Health Organization. (2009). *WHO guidelines on hand hygiene in health care: First global patient safety challenge. Clean care is safer care.* Geneva, Switzerland: World Health Organization. (Level I)

5 The Joint Commission. (2012). Standard NPSG.01.01.01. *Comprehensive accreditation manual for hospitals: The official handbook.* Oakbrook Terrace, IL: The Joint Commission. (Level I)

6 Standard 61. Parenteral medication and solution administration. Infusion nursing standards of practice. (2011). *Journal of Infusion Nursing, 34*(1S), S86. (Level I)

7 The Joint Commission. (2012). Standard RC.01.03.01. *Comprehensive accreditation manual for hospitals: The official handbook.* Oakbrook Terrace, IL: The Joint Commission. (Level I)

8 The Joint Commission. (2012). Standard RC.02.01.01. *Comprehensive accreditation manual for hospitals: The official handbook.* Oakbrook Terrace, IL: The Joint Commission. (Level I)

ADDITIONAL REFERENCES

O'Grady, N.P., et al. (2011). "Guidelines for the Prevention of Intravascular Catheter-Related Infections" [Online]. Accessed November 2011 via the Web at http://www.cdc.gov/hicpac/pdf/guidelines/bsi-guidelines-2011.pdf

Standard 14. Documentation. Infusion nursing standards of practice. (2011). *Journal of Infusion Nursing, 34*(1S), S20–S21.

Standard 19. Hand hygiene. Infusion nursing standards of practice. (2011). *Journal of Infusion Nursing, 34*(1S), S26–S27.

Standard 26. Add-on devices. Infusion nursing standards of practice. (2011). *Journal of Infusion Nursing, 34*(1S), S31.

Standard 27. Needleless connectors. Infusion nursing standards of practice. (2011). *Journal of Infusion Nursing, 34*(1S), S32.

IV PUMP USE

Various types of pumps electronically regulate the flow of IV solutions or drugs with great accuracy. (See *Infusion pumps.*)

Volumetric pumps, used for high-pressure infusion of drugs or for highly accurate delivery of fluids or drugs, have mechanisms to propel the solution at the desired rate under pressure. (Pressure is brought to bear only when gravity flow rates are insufficient to maintain preset infusion rates.) The peristaltic pump applies pressure to the IV tubing to force the solution through it. (Not all peristaltic pumps are volumetric; some count drops.) The piston-cylinder pump pushes the solution through special disposable cassettes. Most of these pumps operate at high pressures (up to 45 psi), delivering from 1 to 999 mL/hour with about 98% accuracy; some pumps operate at 10 to 25 psi. The portable syringe pump delivers very small amounts of fluid over a long period of time. It's used for administering fluids to infants and for delivering intra-arterial drugs.

Other specialized devices include smart pumps (such as bar code automated programming devices), the controlled-release infusion system, the secondary syringe converter, and patient-controlled analgesia. (See *Understanding smart pumps.*)

Pumps have various detectors and alarms that automatically signal or respond to the completion of an infusion, air in the line,

Understanding smart pumps

Conventional, general-purpose infusion pumps allow nurses to program an hourly infusion rate and volume. A smart pump has software that allows the pump to be programmed with a facility's guidelines for specific drugs and patients, making it a customized drug library. These pumps can help you intercept and correct potentially serious infusion mistakes before they happen.

Before smart pumps are used at the bedside, a facility programs the pumps with its own specific information. These profiles specify the infusion requirements for different types of patients, such as adults and children, and care areas, such as pediatric, maternal, oncology, intensive care, and postanesthesia care units. Each profile includes a drug library that contains facility-defined drug infusion parameters, such as acceptable concentrations, infusion rates, dosing units, and maximum and minimum loading and maintenance dose bolus limits. The maximum rate and pressure at which the infusion will run can also be programmed into the software. A team that typically consist of pharmacists, doctors, and nurses within each facility sets up and manages these profiles based on the facility's own best-practice guidelines.

Smart pumps vary by manufacturer, with some pumps even incorporating bar code technology on each IV medication bag. The bar code automatically programs the pump according to a current drug order.

Programming the pump

When you turn on a typical smart pump, it asks you to designate the specific patient care area you're going to use it in. Then it automatically configures itself to provide you with the infusion parameters for that area. Because a pump may be used in different types of patient care units and departments throughout the facility, this feature adds an extra layer of safety.

You then program the pump by choosing the intended drug and concentration from the smart pump's list and entering the ordered dose and infusion rate. The pump checks this information against the drug library. If the parameters you've programmed match those in the pump's drug library for that patient care area, the pump allows the infusion to begin. However, if what you've programmed is outside of the specified limits, the pump alerts you with a visual and audible alarm and lets you know which parameter lies outside of the recommended range.

Depending on the pump's settings, it will sound a soft or hard alarm. If your facility's policy permits it, you can override a soft alarm to allow the infusion to begin at the current settings. However, a hard alarm requires you to reprogram the pump with settings that lie within your facility's specified limits before allowing the infusion to run.

A smart pump also logs and tracks all alerts, recording the time, date, drug, concentration, and infusion rate, as well as your action—including whether you overrode the alert or reprogrammed the pump with different settings. This provides your facility with data it can use to shape current practice guidelines and identify process improvements.

Guidelines for safe administration

Health care facilities provide safer, more effective care when they follow these guidelines from the Institute for Healthcare Improvement before deploying smart pumps:

- Standardize concentrations within the health care facility; asking a health care worker to choose from several concentrations increases the risk of selection error.
- Standardize dosing units for a given drug; for instance, always use either mcg/minute or mcg/kg/minute for nitroglycerin, but not both.
- Standardize drug nomenclature; for example, agree to use the abbreviation KCl for potassium chloride consistently rather than allowing a variety of terms, such as K, pot chloride, or potassium chloride (spelled out).
- Make sure that all concentrations, dose units, and nomenclature used in the smart pump are consistent with those used in the medication administration record, pharmacy computer system, and electronic medical record.
- Meet with all relevant clinicians to agree on the proper upper and lower hard and soft dose limits.
- Monitor the frequency and type of alert overrides to determine if alert settings have been properly configured or if they need adjustment.
- Make sure the pump's smart feature is used in all parts of the facility; for instance, if the operating room sets up the pump volumetrically without the smart feature, but the intensive care unit uses the smart feature, an error may occur if the pump isn't reprogrammed properly.
- Make sure to establish upper and lower dose limits for bolus doses, when applicable.
- Have a biomedical technician identify previously unidentified risks for failure when the pumps are deployed.
- Establish procedures that allow staff members, when necessary, to administer drugs in nonstandard concentrations as well as to administer drugs that aren't in the drug library.
- Deploy one type of smart pump throughout the health care facility; doing so helps prevent errors that may occur when different types of pumps are used on different units.

low battery power, and occlusion or inability to deliver at the set rate. Depending on the problem, these devices may sound or flash an alarm, shut off, or switch to a keep-vein-open rate.

Equipment

Infusion pump ■ IV pole ■ IV solution ■ sterile administration set ■ sterile tubing or cassette, if needed (tubing and cassettes vary among manufacturers) ■ alcohol pads ■ gloves ■ adhesive tape.

Preparation of equipment

Verify the doctor's order and gather the appropriate equipment. Inspect the IV solution to make sure that it's labeled properly, its integrity is intact, it contains the right solution in the right concentration, and it hasn't expired.[1] Perform hand hygiene.[2,3,4,5,6] Attach the pump to the IV pole (as shown below).

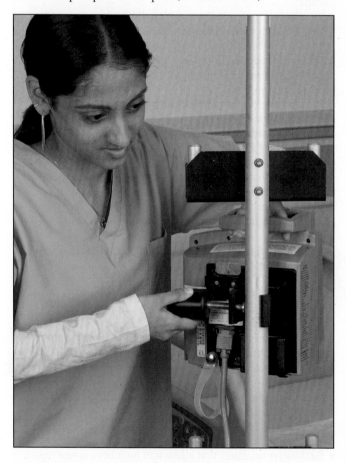

Access the port on the IV container and swab with alcohol, if appropriate. Insert the administration set spike, and fill the drip chamber to at least ⅓ full *to prevent air bubbles from entering the tubing.*[3] Next, prime the tubing and close the clamp. Follow the manufacturer's instructions for placement of tubing in the pump.

Implementation

■ Perform hand hygiene.[2,3,4,5,6]
■ Confirm the patient's identity using at least two patient identifiers according to your facility's policy.[7]
■ Explain the procedure to the patient *to ease his anxiety and ensure his cooperation.*

■ If your facility uses a bar code automated pump, scan your identification (ID) badge, the patient's ID bracelet, and the patient ID on the medication bag, or follow the procedure for your facility's bar code system *to ensure that the right patient is receiving the infusion.*
■ Position the pump on the same side of the bed as the IV or anticipated venipuncture site *to avoid crisscrossing IV lines over the patient.* Plug in the machine.
■ Put on gloves.
■ Assess the IV site and the patency of the IV catheter. If necessary, perform the venipuncture. (See "IV catheter insertion and removal," page 421.) If connecting to a venous access device, confirm placement and patency.
■ Attach the IV tubing to the catheter using sterile technique. Trace the tubing from the patient to its point of origin to make sure that you've attached it to the proper hub.[1,8]
■ Depending on the machine, turn it on and enter the desired infusion rate and volume. Always set the volume dial at 50 mL less than the prescribed volume or 50 mL less than the volume in the container *so that you can hang a new container before the old one empties.*
■ Confirm that the right information is displayed on the pump, open the tubing clamp, and then push the RUN or START button (as shown below).

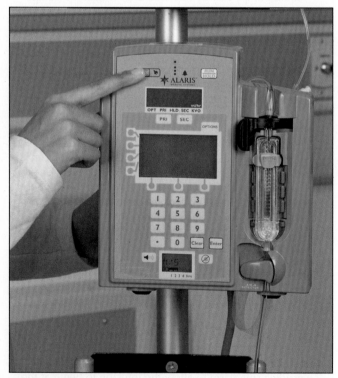

■ Recheck the patency of the IV catheter and watch for infiltration.
■ Check that all connections are secure *to prevent leaking, bleeding, and contamination.*[8]
■ Turn on the alarm switches, and explain the alarm system to the patient *to prevent anxiety when a change in the infusion activates an alarm.*

- Remove and discard your gloves and perform hand hygiene.[2,3,4,5,6]
- Document the procedure.[9,10]

Special considerations

- Monitor the pump and the patient frequently *to ensure the device's correct operation and flow rate and to detect infiltration and such complications as infection and air embolism.*
- If electrical power fails, the pumps automatically switch to battery power.
- Check the manufacturer's recommendations before administering opaque fluids, such as blood, *because some pumps fail to detect opaque fluids and others may cause hemolysis of infused blood.*
- Change the tubing and cassette no more frequently than every 96 hours; however, change it immediately upon suspected contamination or when the integrity of the product or system has been compromised.[3,11]
- If a catheter-associated infection is suspected or documented, follow your facility's policy regarding tubing changes.
- Remove IV solutions from the refrigerator 1 hour before infusing them to help release small gas bubbles from the solutions. *Small bubbles in the solution can join to form larger bubbles, which can activate the pump's air-in-line alarm.* Aspirate large air bubbles from the tubing before they reach the cassette.
- If the alarm sounds, mute the alarm and check the pump for a problem message, such as infusion complete, occlusion, air in line, or low battery. Address the problem, assess the IV and infusion components, restart the infusion, and reset the alarm.

Patient teaching

Make sure the patient and his family understand the purpose of using the pump. If necessary, demonstrate how the device works. Also demonstrate how to maintain the system (tubing, solution, and site assessment and care) until you're confident that the patient and family members can proceed safely. As time permits, have the patient repeat the demonstration. Discuss which complications to watch for, such as infiltration, and review measures to take if complications occur. Schedule a teaching session with the patient or family members *so you can answer questions they may have about the procedure before the patient's discharge.*

Explain the signs and symptoms of IV infiltration to the patient; instruct him to call for assistance if they occur. Discuss potential adverse effects of IV medication administration, if appropriate, and what signs and symptoms to report. If the patient is ambulatory, discuss his ability to unplug the pump and wheel the IV pole with him. Discourage the patient from touching the controls on the infusion pump, and instruct him to call for assistance if the pump sounds an alarm.

Complications

Complications associated with IV pumps are the same as those associated with peripheral lines. (See "IV catheter insertion and removal," page 421.) Keep in mind that infiltration can develop rapidly with infusion by a volumetric pump *because the increased subcutaneous pressure won't slow the infusion rate until significant edema occurs.*

Documentation

In addition to routine documentation of the IV infusion, record the use of a pump on the IV record and in your notes. Also document any patient teaching provided and the patient's understanding of your teaching.[9,10]

REFERENCES

1 Standard 61. Parenteral medication and solution administration. Infusion nursing standards of practice. (2011). *Journal of Infusion Nursing, 34*(1S), S86. (Level I)

2 Centers for Disease Control and Prevention. (October 2002). Guideline for hand hygiene in health-care settings. *Morbidity and Mortality Weekly Report, 51*(RR-16), 1–45. (Level I)

3 O'Grady, N.P., et al. (2011). "Guidelines for the Prevention of Intravascular Catheter-Related Infections" [Online]. Accessed November 2011 via the Web at http://www.cdc.gov/hicpac/pdf/guidelines/bsi-guidelines-2011.pdf

4 Standard 19. Hand hygiene. Infusion nursing standards of practice. (2011). *Journal of Infusion Nursing, 34*(1S), S26–S27. (Level I)

5 The Joint Commission. (2012). Standard NPSG.07.01.01. *Comprehensive accreditation manual for hospitals: The official handbook.* Oakbrook Terrace, IL: The Joint Commission. (Level I)

6 World Health Organization. (2009). *WHO guidelines on hand hygiene in health care: First global patient safety challenge. Clean care is safer care.* Geneva, Switzerland: World Health Organization. (Level I)

7 The Joint Commission. (2012). Standard NPSG.01.01.01. *Comprehensive accreditation manual for hospitals: The official handbook.* Oakbrook Terrace, IL: The Joint Commission. (Level I)

8 U.S. Food and Drug Administration. (2009). "Look. Check. Connect.: Safe Medical Device Connections Save Lives" [Online]. Accessed November 2011 via the Web at http://www.fda.gov/downloads/MedicalDevices/Safety/AlertsandNotices/UCM134873.pdf

9 The Joint Commission. (2012). Standard RC.01.03.01. *Comprehensive accreditation manual for hospitals: The official handbook.* Oakbrook Terrace, IL: The Joint Commission. (Level I)

10 The Joint Commission. (2012). Standard RC.02.01.01. *Comprehensive accreditation manual for hospitals: The official handbook.* Oakbrook Terrace, IL: The Joint Commission. (Level I)

11 Standard 43. Administration set change. Infusion nursing standards of practice. (2011). *Journal of Infusion Nursing, 34*(1S), S55–S57. (Level I)

ADDITIONAL REFERENCES

Alexander, M., et al. (Eds.). (2010). *Infusion nursing: An evidence-based approach* (3rd ed.). Philadelphia, PA: Elsevier.

Infusion Nurses Society. (2011). *Policies and procedures for infusion nursing* (4th ed.). Boston, MA: Infusion Nurses Society.

Institute for Healthcare Improvement. "Reduce Adverse Drug Events (ADEs) Involving Intravenous Medications: Implement Smart Infusion Pumps" [Online]. Accessed November 2011 via the Web at http://www.ihi.org/IHI/Topics/PatientSafety/MedicationSystems/Changes/IndividualChanges/ImplementSmartInfusionPumps.htm

Kaufman, M. "New IV smart pump technologies prevent medication errors, ADRs" [Online]. Accessed November 2011 via the Web at http://formularyjournal.modernmedicine.com/formulary/Technology+News/New-IV-smart-pump-technologies-prevent-medication-/ArticleStandard/Article/detail/611706

Standard 29. Flow-control devices. Infusion nursing standards of practice. (2011). *Journal of Infusion Nursing, 34*(1S), S34. (Level I)

IV SECONDARY LINE INFUSION

A secondary IV line is a complete IV set, container, tubing, and microdrip or macrodrip system, connected to the lower Y port (secondary port) of a primary line instead of to the IV catheter. It can be used for continuous or intermittent drug infusion. When used continuously, a secondary IV line permits drug infusion and titration while the primary line maintains a constant total infusion rate.

When used intermittently, a secondary IV line is commonly called a *piggyback set.* In this case, the primary line maintains venous access between drug doses. Typically, a piggyback set includes a small IV container, short tubing, and a macrodrip system. This set connects to the primary line's upper Y port, also called a *piggyback port.* Antibiotics are most commonly administered by intermittent (piggyback) infusion. To make this set work, the primary IV container must be positioned below the piggyback container. (The manufacturer provides an extension hook for that purpose.)

IV pumps should be used to maintain constant infusion rates, especially with a drug such as lidocaine. A pump allows more accurate titration of drug dosage and helps maintain venous access.

Equipment

Patient's medication record ▪ patient's medication administration record ▪ prescribed IV medication ▪ prescribed IV solution ▪ administration set with secondary injection port ▪ needleless adapter ▪ antiseptic pads (alcohol, tincture of iodine, or chlorhexidine-based) ▪ 1″ adhesive tape ▪ time tape ▪ labels ▪ infusion pump ▪ extension hook and appropriate solution for intermittent piggyback infusion ▪ Optional: normal saline solution for infusion with incompatible solutions.

For intermittent infusion, the primary line typically has a piggyback port with a backcheck valve that stops the flow from the primary line during drug infusion and returns to the primary flow after infusion. A volume-control set can also be used with an intermittent infusion line.

Preparation of equipment

Verify the order on the patient's medication record by checking it against the doctor's order.[1] Perform hand hygiene.[2,3,4,5] Inspect the IV container for cracks, leaks, and contamination, and check drug compatibility with the primary solution. Verify the expiration date. Check to see whether the primary line has a secondary injection port. If it doesn't and the medication is to be given regularly, replace the IV set with a new one that has a secondary injection port.

If necessary, add the drug to the secondary IV solution. To do so, remove any seals from the secondary container, and wipe the main port with an alcohol pad. Inject the prescribed medication, and gently agitate the solution to mix the medication thoroughly. Properly label the IV mixture. Insert the administration set spike and attach the needleless system. Open the flow clamp and prime the line. Then close the flow clamp.

Some medications are available in vials that are suitable for hanging directly on an IV pole. Instead of preparing medication and injecting it into a container, you can inject diluent directly into the medication vial. Then you can spike the vial, prime the tubing, and hang the set, as directed.

Implementation

▪ Perform hand hygiene.[2,3,4,5]
▪ Confirm the patient's identity by checking at least two patient identifiers according to your facility's policy.[6,7]
▪ If your facility uses a bar code scanning system, scan your identification (ID) badge, the patient's ID bracelet, and the medication's bar code.
▪ Assess the patient's IV site for pain, redness, or swelling and ensure patency.
▪ If the drug is incompatible with the primary IV solution, replace the primary solution with a fluid that's compatible with both solutions, such as normal saline solution, and flush the line before starting the drug infusion. Many facility protocols require that the primary IV solution be removed and that a sterile IV plug be inserted into the container until it's ready to be rehung. *This protocol maintains the sterility of the solution and prevents someone else from inadvertently restarting the incompatible solution before the line is flushed with normal saline solution.*
▪ Hang the secondary set's container, and thoroughly disinfect the injection port of the primary line with an antiseptic pad using friction. Allow it to dry.[8]
▪ Trace the tubing from the patient to its point of origin *to make sure that it's attached to the proper port.*[7]
▪ Insert the needleless adapter from the secondary line into the injection port, and secure it to the primary line.
▪ To run the secondary set's container by itself, lower the primary set's container with an extension hook. To run both containers simultaneously, place them at the same height. (See *Assembling a piggyback set.*)
▪ Open the clamp and adjust the drip rate. For continuous infusion, set the secondary solution to the desired drip rate; then adjust the primary solution *to achieve the desired total infusion rate.*
▪ For intermittent infusion, adjust the primary drip rate, as required, on completion of the secondary solution. If the secondary solution tubing is being reused, close the clamp on the tubing and remove the needless adapter and replace it with a new sterile one.[9] Don't attach the exposed end of the administration set to a port on the same set.[9] If the tubing won't be reused, discard it appropriately with the IV container.
▪ Perform hand hygiene.[2,3,4,5]
▪ Document the procedure.[10,11]

Special considerations

■ Whenever possible, use a pump for drug infusion.
■ When reusing secondary tubing, change it according to your facility's policy, usually every 24 hours.[9] Similarly, inspect the injection port for leakage with each use, and change it more often if needed.
■ Unless you're piggybacking lipids, don't piggyback a secondary IV line to a total parenteral nutrition line *because of the risk of contamination.* Check your facility's policy for possible exceptions.

Complications

The patient may experience an adverse reaction to the infused drug. In addition, repeated punctures of the secondary injection port can damage the seal, possibly allowing leakage or contamination.

Documentation

Record the amount and type of drug and the amount of IV solution on the intake and output and medication records. Note the date, duration and rate of infusion, and the patient's response, where applicable.[10,11]

REFERENCES

1 The Joint Commission. (2012). Standard MM.04.01.01. *Comprehensive accreditation manual for hospitals: The official handbook.* Oakbrook Terrace, IL: The Joint Commission. (Level I)
2 The Joint Commission. (2012). Standard NPSG.07.01.01. *Comprehensive accreditation manual for hospitals: The official handbook.* Oakbrook Terrace, IL: The Joint Commission. (Level I)
3 Centers for Disease Control and Prevention. (October 2002). Guideline for hand hygiene in health-care settings. *Morbidity and Mortality Weekly Report, 51*(RR-16), 1–45. (Level I)
4 World Health Organization. (2009). *WHO guidelines on hand hygiene in health care: First global patient safety challenge. Clean care is safer care.* Geneva, Switzerland: World Health Organization. (Level I)
5 Standard 19. Hand hygiene. Infusion nursing standards of practice. (2011). *Journal of Infusion Nursing, 34*(1S), S26–S27. (Level I)
6 The Joint Commission. (2012). Standard NPSG.01.01.01. *Comprehensive accreditation manual for hospitals: The official handbook.* Oakbrook Terrace, IL: The Joint Commission. (Level I)
7 Standard 61. Parenteral medication and solution administration. Infusion nursing standards of practice. (2011). *Journal of Infusion Nursing, 34*(1S), S86. (Level I)
8 O'Grady, N.P., et al. (2011). "Guidelines for the Prevention of Intravascular Catheter-Related Infections" [Online]. Accessed November 2011 via the Web at http://www.cdc.gov/hicpac/pdf/guidelines/bsi-guidelines-2011.pdf
9 Standard 43. Administration set change. Infusion nursing standards of practice. (2011). *Journal of Infusion Nursing, 34*(1S), S55–S57. (Level I)
10 The Joint Commission. (2012). Standard RC.01.03.01. *Comprehensive accreditation manual for hospitals: The official handbook.* Oakbrook Terrace, IL: The Joint Commission. (Level I)
11 The Joint Commission. (2012). Standard RC.02.01.01. *Comprehensive accreditation manual for hospitals: The official handbook.* Oakbrook Terrace, IL: The Joint Commission. (Level I)

Assembling a piggyback set

A piggyback set is useful for intermittent drug infusion. To work properly, the secondary set's container must be positioned higher than the primary set's container.

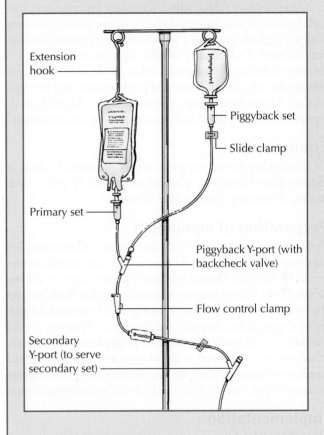

Extension hook

Piggyback set

Slide clamp

Primary set

Piggyback Y-port (with backcheck valve)

Flow control clamp

Secondary Y-port (to serve secondary set)

ADDITIONAL REFERENCES

Infusion Nurses Society. (2011). *Policies and procedures for infusion nursing* (4th ed.). Boston, MA: Infusion Nurses Society.
Nettina, S.M. (2010). *Lippincott manual of nursing practice* (9th ed.). Philadelphia, PA: Lippincott Williams & Wilkins.
Scales, K. (2008). Intravenous therapy: A guide to good practice. *British Journal of Nursing, 17*(19), S4–S12.

IV THERAPY PREPARATION

Selection and preparation of appropriate equipment are essential for accurate delivery of an IV solution. The type of IV administration set used depends on the rate and type of infusion desired and the type of IV solution container used. Two types of drip sets are available: the macrodrip and the microdrip. The macrodrip set can deliver a solution in large quantities at rapid rates because it delivers a larger amount with each drop. The microdrip set, used for pediatric patients and certain adult patients who require small or closely regulated amounts of IV solution, delivers a smaller quantity with each drop.

Although plastic bags are often used to hold IV fluids, there may be times when you'll use a bottle as a container. Glass bottles are usually used to hold medications that are unstable in a plastic bag, such as nitroglycerin. The bottle may be vented or nonvented.

Administration tubing with a secondary injection port permits separate or simultaneous infusion of two solutions; tubing with a piggyback port and a backcheck valve permits intermittent infusion of a secondary solution and, on its completion, a return to infusion of the primary solution. Vented IV tubing is selected for solutions in nonvented bottles; nonvented tubing is selected for solutions in bags or vented bottles.[1] Assembly of IV equipment requires sterile technique to prevent contamination.[1]

Equipment

IV solution bag ▪ antiseptic pads (alcohol, tincture of iodine, or chlorhexidine-based) ▪ IV administration set ▪ IV pole ▪ medication, if necessary ▪ in-line filter, if needed.

Preparation of equipment

Perform hand hygiene *to prevent introducing contaminants during preparation.*[2,3,4,5,6] Verify the type, volume, and expiration date of the IV solution. Discard outdated solution. Squeeze the bag *to detect leaks.* If the solution is contained in a glass bottle, inspect the bottle for chips or cracks. Examine the IV solution for particles, abnormal discoloration, and cloudiness. If present, discard the solution and notify the pharmacy or dispensing department. If ordered, add medication to the solution, and place a completed medication-added label on the bag. Remove the administration set from its box, and check for cracks, holes, and missing clamps.

Implementation

Preparing the bag

▪ Slide the flow clamp of the administration set tubing down to the drip chamber or injection port, and close the clamp.
▪ Place the bag on a flat, stable surface or hang it on an IV pole.
▪ Remove the protective cap or tear the tab from the tubing insertion port (as shown below).

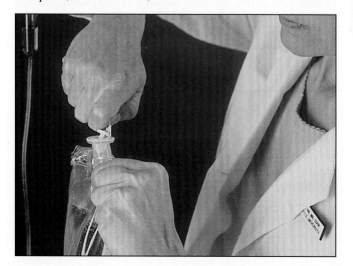

▪ Remove the protective cap from the administration set spike.
▪ Hold the port firmly with one hand, and insert the spike with your other hand (as shown below). Be careful not to contaminate the IV bag insertion port or the IV tubing spike.

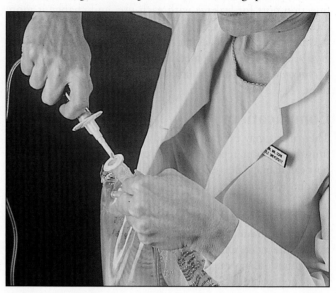

▪ Hang the bag on the IV pole, if you haven't already, and squeeze the drip chamber until it's half full (as shown below).

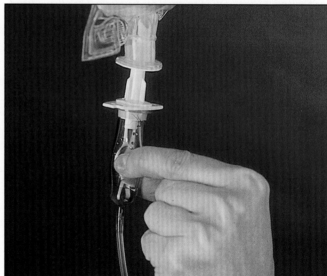

▪ Label the bag with the patient's name and identification number, date and time, the bag number, ordered rate and duration of infusion, and your initials.
▪ Perform hand hygiene.[2,3,4,5,6]
▪ Document the procedure.[7,8]

Preparing a bottle

- Slide the flow clamp of the administration set tubing down to the drip chamber or injection port, and close the clamp.
- For a nonvented bottle, remove the bottle's metal cap and inner disk, if present. For a vented bottle, remove the bottle's metal cap and latex diaphragm to release the vacuum. If the vacuum isn't intact, discard the bottle and begin again.
- Place the bottle on a stable surface and disinfect the rubber stopper with an antiseptic pad.[3]
- Remove the protective cap from the administration set spike, and push the spike through the center of the nonvented bottle's rubber stopper. Avoid twisting or angling the spike *to prevent pieces of the stopper from breaking off and falling into the solution.* If using a vented bottle, push the spike through the insertion port next to the air vent tube opening.
- Invert the nonvented bottle. If its vacuum is intact, you'll hear a hissing sound and see air bubbles rise (this may not occur if you've already added medication). If the vacuum isn't intact, discard the bottle and begin again.
- Hang the bottle on the IV pole, and squeeze the drip chamber until it's half full.
- Perform hand hygiene.[2,3,4,5,6]
- Document the procedure.[7,8]

Priming the tubing

- Once you have spiked the solution container and squeezed the drip chamber to be half full, hang the solution on the IV pole.
- Leave the protective cover on the end of the tubing, aim the distal end of the tubing over a wastebasket or sink, and slowly open the flow clamp.
- If a filter is necessary, purge the tubing before attaching it *to avoid forcing air into the filter and, possibly, clogging some filter channels.* Attach a filter to the end of the IV tubing, and follow the manufacturer's instructions for filling and priming it. Most filters are positioned with the distal end of the tubing facing upward so that the solution will completely wet the filter membrane and all air bubbles will be eliminated from the line. (See *Indications for in-line filters.*)
- Leave the clamp open until the IV solution flows through the entire length of tubing *to release trapped air bubbles and force out all the air.*
- Invert all Y-ports and backcheck valves and tap them, if necessary, *to fill them with solution.*
- Close the clamp. Then loop the tubing over the IV pole.
- Label the IV container with the patient's name and room number, date and time, container number, ordered rate and duration of infusion, and your initials.
- Perform hand hygiene.[2,3,4,5,6]
- Document the procedure.[7,8]

Special considerations

- Always use sterile technique when preparing IV solutions.[1] If you contaminate the administration set or container, replace it with a new one *to prevent introducing contaminants into the system.*

Indications for in-line filters

An in-line filter removes pathogens and particles from IV solutions, *helping to reduce the risk of infusion phlebitis.* Because an in-line filter is expensive and its installation is awkward and time-consuming, these filters aren't used routinely. Many health care facilities require that a filter be used only when administering an admixture. If you're unsure of whether to use a filter, check your facility's policy and the manufacturer's specific recommendations. Use this list of do's and don'ts as a guide.

Do's
Do use an in-line filter:
- when administering solutions to an immunodeficient patient
- when administering total parenteral nutrition
- when using additives comprising many separate particles, such as antibiotics requiring reconstitution, or when administering several additives
- when using rubber injection ports or plastic diaphragms repeatedly
- when phlebitis is likely to occur.

Change the in-line filter according to the manufacturer's recommendations (and with administration set change). *If you don't, bacteria trapped in the filter releases endotoxin, a pyrogen small enough to pass through the filter into the bloodstream.*

Use an add-on filter of larger pore size (1.2 microns) when infusing lipid emulsions or total nutrient admixtures that require filtration.

If a positive-pressure electronic infusion device is used, consider the psi rating of the filter. If the psi from the infusion device exceeds that of the filter, the filter will crack or break under the pressure.

Don'ts
Don't use an in-line filter:
- when administering solutions with large particles, such as blood and its components, suspensions, lipid emulsions, and high-molecular-volume plasma expanders, *because the particle will clog the filter and stop IV flow*
- when administering a small-volume IV push medication *because the filter may absorb it.*

- Change the IV tubing no more frequently than 96 hours; however, change it immediately upon suspected contamination or when the integrity of the product or system has been compromised.[1,3] Change the filter according to the manufacturer's recommendations or sooner if it becomes clogged.
- If necessary, you can use vented tubing with a vented bottle. To do this, don't remove the latex diaphragm. Instead, insert the spike into the larger indentation in the diaphragm.

Teaching your patient about IV therapy

Many patients are apprehensive about peripheral IV therapy. So before you begin therapy, tell your patient what to expect before, during, and after the procedure. *Thorough patient teaching can reduce anxiety, making therapy easier.* Follow these guidelines.

Before insertion
■ Describe the procedure to the patient. Tell him that "intravenous" means inside the vein and that a plastic catheter will be placed in his vein. Explain that fluids containing nutrients or medications will flow from a bag or bottle through a length of tubing and then through the plastic catheter into his vein.
■ Tell him about how long the catheter will stay in place. Explain that the doctor will decide how much and what type of fluid the patient needs.
■ If the patient will receive a local anesthetic at the insertion site, ask him if he's allergic to lidocaine. If in doubt, use another anesthetic. Tell him that this injection will numb the site to reduce the pain of IV device insertion.
■ If no anesthetic will be used, tell the patient that he may feel transient pain at the insertion site but that the discomfort will stop when the catheter is in place.

■ Tell him that IV fluid may feel cold at first but that this sensation should last only a few minutes.

During therapy
■ Instruct the patient to report any discomfort after the catheter has been inserted and the fluid has begun to flow.
■ Explain any restrictions as ordered. As appropriate, tell the patient that he may be able to walk and, depending on the insertion site and the device, to shower or take a tub bath during therapy.
■ Teach him how to care for the IV line. Tell him not to pull at the insertion site or tubing, not to remove the container from the IV pole, and not to kink the tubing or lie on it. Instruct him to call a nurse if the flow rate suddenly slows or speeds up.

At removal
■ Explain that removing a peripheral IV catheter is a simple procedure. Tell the patient that pressure will be applied to the site until bleeding stops. Reassure him that when the device is out and bleeding stops, he'll be able to use the affected arm or leg as before therapy.

■ If a catheter-associated infection is suspected or documented, follow your facility's policy regarding tubing changes.

Patient teaching
Before initiation of IV therapy, the patient should be told what to expect. (See *Teaching your patient about IV therapy.*)

Documentation
Document the type and amount of solution, the rate used, and any additives added to the solution.[7,8]

REFERENCES
1 Standard 43. Administration set change. Infusion nursing standards of practice. (2011). *Journal of Infusion Nursing, 34*(1S), S55–S57. (Level I)
2 The Joint Commission. (2012). Standard NPSG.07.01.01. *Comprehensive accreditation manual for hospitals: The official handbook.* Oakbrook Terrace, IL: The Joint Commission. (Level I)
3 O'Grady, N.P., et al. (2011). "Guidelines for the Prevention of Intravascular Catheter-Related Infections" [Online]. Accessed November 2011 via the Web at http://www.cdc.gov/hicpac/pdf/guidelines/bsi-guidelines-2011.pdf
4 Standard 19. Hand hygiene. Infusion nursing standards of practice. (2011). *Journal of Infusion Nursing, 34*(1S), S26–S27. (Level I)
5 Centers for Disease Control and Prevention. (October 2002). Guideline for hand hygiene in health-care settings. *Morbidity and Mortality Weekly Report, 51*(RR-16), 1–45. (Level I)
6 World Health Organization. (2009). *WHO guidelines on hand hygiene in health care: First global patient safety challenge. Clean care is safer care.* Geneva, Switzerland: World Health Organization. (Level I)
7 The Joint Commission. (2012). Standard RC.01.03.01. *Comprehensive accreditation manual for hospitals: The official handbook.* Oakbrook Terrace, IL: The Joint Commission. (Level I)
8 The Joint Commission. (2012). Standard RC.02.01.01. *Comprehensive accreditation manual for hospitals: The official handbook.* Oakbrook Terrace, IL: The Joint Commission. (Level I)

ADDITIONAL REFERENCES
Alexander, M., et al. (Eds.). (2010). *Infusion nursing: An evidence-based approach* (3rd ed.). Philadelphia, PA: Elsevier.
Infusion Nurses Society. (2011). *Policies and procedures for infusion nursing* (4th ed.). Boston, MA: Infusion Nurses Society.
Nettina, S.M. (2010). *Lippincott manual of nursing practice* (9th ed.). Philadelphia, PA: Lippincott Williams & Wilkins.
Taylor, C., et al. (2011). *Fundamentals of nursing: The art and science of nursing care* (7th ed.). Philadelphia, PA: Lippincott Williams & Wilkins.

JUGULAR VENOUS OXYGEN SATURATION MONITORING

Jugular venous oxygen saturation ($SjvO_2$) monitoring measures the venous oxygenation saturation of blood as it leaves the brain, reflecting the oxygen saturation of blood after cerebral perfusion has taken place. After comparing $SjvO_2$ with the arterial venous oxygenation, you can determine whether blood flow to the brain matches the brain's metabolic demand.

$SjvO_2$ monitoring is often used with other types of cerebral hemodynamic monitoring—such as intracranial pressure (ICP) monitoring—to provide detailed information regarding pressure and perfusion states during treatment. Treatment regimens can be titrated to enhance pressure and perfusion.

$SjvO_2$ normally ranges from 55% to 70%. Values higher than 70% indicate hyperperfusion; values between 40% and 54% indicate relative hypoperfusion. Values lower than 40% indicate ischemia.

Data from monitoring can also be used to calculate:
- cerebral extraction of oxygen ($CeO_2 = SaO_2 - SjvO_2$)
- cerebral arterial oxygen content ($CaO_2 = 1.34 \times Hgb \times SaO_2 - 0.0031 \times PaO_2$)
- global cerebral oxygen extraction ratio ($O_2ER = SaO_2 - SjvO_2/Sa_2$) and jugular venous oxygen content saturation ($CjvO_2 = 1.34 \times Hgb \times SjvO_2 + 0.0031 \times PjvO_2$)
- arteriovenous jugular oxygen content ($AVjDO_2 = CaO_2 - CjvO_2$), which helps determine cerebral oxygen use, metabolic demand, and adequacy of oxygen delivery.

Monitoring of $SjvO_2$ allows the nurse to maximize the balance between cerebral perfusion, oxygenation, and metabolism. Criteria for $SjvO_2$ monitoring include any neurologic injury in which ischemia is a threat, including intraoperative monitoring, subarachnoid hemorrhage, and postacute head injury with increased ICP.

Equipment

Sterile towels ▪ sterile drapes ▪ surgical caps ▪ gowns ▪ sterile gloves ▪ masks ▪ antiseptic scrub ▪ antiseptic solution ▪ central venous catheter insertion kit ▪ 1% or 2% lidocaine without epinephrine ▪ 5- or 10-mL syringe with an 18G or 23G needle ▪ #5 French percutaneous introducer ▪ #4 French fiber-optic $SjvO_2$ catheter ▪ oximetric monitor with cable ▪ 500 mL of normal saline solution (heparinized or nonheparinized, according to your facility's policy) ▪ pressure tubing with continuous flush device ▪ pressure bag or device ▪ sterile occlusive dressing ▪ sterile labels.

Implementation

- Perform hand hygiene.[1,2,3]
- Confirm the patient's identity using at least two patient identifiers according to your facility's policy.[4]

- Explain the procedure to the patient and provide privacy.

Inserting the catheter

- Conduct a preprocedure verification process *to make sure that all relevant documentation, related information, and equipment are available and correctly identified to the patient identifiers.*[5]
- Prime the pressure tubing system, removing all air bubbles and maintaining sterility of system for insertion.
- Follow the manufacturer's instructions for in vitro calibration of the catheter before insertion.
- Conduct a time-out *to make sure that the correct patient, site, and procedure are verified.*[6]
- Position the patient with his head elevated 30 to 45 degrees and his neck in a neutral position. Document baseline ICP.[7]
- Turn the patient's head laterally, away from the site chosen for catheter insertion. Note and document any change in ICP.
- Perform hand hygiene.[1,2,3]
- Put on a cap, mask, gown, and sterile gloves.
- Using sterile technique, open and prepare the central venous catheter insertion tray, and add a #5 French sterile introducer and a #4 French fiber-optic $SjvO_2$ catheter.
- Label all medications, medication containers, and other solutions on and off the sterile field.[8]
- After the doctor puts on a cap, mask, gown, and sterile gloves, he will scrub the insertion site with a chlorhexidine-based antiseptic solution for 30 seconds, using a vigorous side-to-side motion. He will then position the sterile drapes, using maximum barrier precautions and exposing only the insertion site.
- Assist the doctor during insertion as needed, making sure sterile technique is maintained.
- Monitor the patient's neurologic status, vital signs, ICP, and pain during insertion and immediately after insertion.

NURSING ALERT *Because the catheter in the jugular bulb can inhibit venous outflow, a sustained ICP of more than 5 mm Hg over preinsertion baseline may be an indication for catheter removal.*

- After the line is in place, carefully trace the pressure tubing from the point of origin and attach it to the line.[9] Confirm the patency of both jugular catheter lumens by aspirating and flushing.
- Apply the sterile occlusive dressing.
- Obtain a lateral cervical spine or lateral skull X-ray *to confirm catheter placement at the level of the jugular bulb.*
- Draw an initial jugular venous blood gas sample and perform in vivo calibration according to the manufacturer's instructions. *In vivo calibration is necessary to ensure reliability of the data.*
- Discard used supplies in an appropriate receptacle.
- Remove and discard your gloves, gown, mask, and cap.
- Perform hand hygiene.[1,2,3]

Ongoing monitoring

- Record baseline parameters for $SjvO_2$. Calculate $AVjDO_2$, CeO_2, and O_2ER as a baseline.
- Continuously monitor $SjvO_2$.
- Record $SjvO_2$ and ICP values and note trends. Assess ICP in relation to $SjvO_2$. Notify the doctor of any deviation from the

Common causes of desaturation

You may encounter periods of desaturation and need to be prepared to take action. This table lists common causes of desaturation and appropriate interventions.

CAUSE	NURSING INTERVENTIONS
Systemic hypoxemia (one of the most common causes of cerebral hypoxia)	If the oxygen saturation is less than 90%, increase the oxygen percentage or fraction of inspired oxygen and adjust the ventilator settings as ordered.
Anemia (hemoglobin less than 9 g/L)	Report abnormal results to the doctor, and administer a blood transfusion if ordered.
Systemic hypotension (mean blood pressure less than 70 mm Hg)	Report abnormal results to the doctor, and administer a fluid challenge or vasopressors if ordered.
Increased intracranial pressure (greater than 20 mm Hg)	Elevate the head of the bed 30 degrees, decrease external stimuli, administer osmotic diuretics such as mannitol, and adjust the ventilator settings to produce mild hyperventilation (partial pressure of arterial carbon dioxide of 30 to 35 mm Hg). Other measures may include drainage of cerebrospinal fluid and methods to reduce cerebral oxygen demand, such as sedation, neuromuscular blockade, or barbiturate coma.

trend. *Increased ICP is a frequent cause of desaturation in patients with brain injury.*
- Calculate CeO_2 and O_2ER, as indicated.
- Identify $SjvO_2$ desaturations and notify the doctor. (See *Common causes of desaturation.*)

NURSING ALERT *Repeated patterns of desaturation have been shown to be predictors of poor outcomes in patients with severe head injury. Desaturations are emergent events requiring immediate interventions to restore cerebral blood flow and oxygen delivery.*

- Perform in vivo calibration with a jugular blood gas sample, as recommended by the monitor manufacturer (usually performed

every 24 hours, with $SjvO_2$ desaturations, and when data reliability is in question).

NURSING ALERT *A significant change in readings following sampling can signify errors related to aspiration of blood. Avoid errors by aspirating blood slowly during sampling procedure (1 mL/minute).*

- Document the procedure.[10,11]

Special considerations

- Maintain a safe environment during monitoring *to prevent accidental dislodgement of the catheter.*
- Use sedation or analgesia, as indicated, *to maintain, monitor, and enhance cerebral perfusion pressure (CPP).*
- Change the dressing using sterile technique if it becomes soiled or loosened and as indicated by your facility's policy for central venous access device redressing.
- Change the IV solution and tubing for the catheter according to your facility's policy for central lines.
- Replace an $SjvO_2$ catheter with low light intensity. Check the fiber-optic catheter for obstruction, occlusion, or damage to the fiber-optics. Aspirate the catheter until blood can be freely sampled and normal light intensity is displayed. If you can't aspirate a blood sample, the catheter needs to be replaced.
- For an $SjvO_2$ catheter with high light intensity, adjust the patient's head to ensure a neutral neck position. High light intensity indicates a vessel-wall artifact and is usually encountered during repositioning of the patient.
- *To prevent catheter coiling,* identify rhythmic fluctuations in $SjvO_2$ trends. Those unrelated to changes in ICP, CPP, or systemic blood pressure signify coiling of the catheter. Obtain a lateral cervical spine or lateral skull X-ray *to assess position of the catheter in the external jugular vein* (compare to the X-ray done on insertion). If coiling is confirmed, consider replacing the catheter.
- Assess line necessity daily, and make sure the line is removed when no longer needed *to reduce the risk of a health care facility–associated bloodstream infection.*

Complications

Complications associated with $SvjO_2$ monitoring are similar to complications that can occur with any central line, the most common being line sepsis. Other risks include pneumothorax, carotid artery puncture, internal jugular thrombosis, and excessive bleeding.

In rare instances, the catheter can also cause impaired cerebral venous drainage and increase ICP.

Documentation

Document difficulties encountered during insertion, depth (in centimeters) of the catheter, patient tolerance of the procedure, and the ICP reading during insertion. Record the baseline $SjvO_2$ reading and initial CeO_2 and $AVjDO_2$ calculations. Record $SjvO_2$ and ICP hourly. Record CeO_2, $AVjDO_2$, and O_2ER, when indicated. Document your assessment of the insertion site, expected and unexpected outcomes, nursing actions taken, and patient and family education provided.

REFERENCES

1 The Joint Commission. (2010). Standard NPSG.07.01.01. *Comprehensive accreditation manual for hospitals: The official handbook.* Oakbrook Terrace, IL: The Joint Commission. (Level I)

2 Centers for Disease Control and Prevention. (October 2002). Guideline for hand hygiene in health-care settings. *Morbidity and Mortality Weekly Report, 51*(RR-16), 1–45. (Level I)

3 World Health Organization. (2009). *WHO guidelines on hand hygiene in health care: First global patient safety challenge. Clean care is safer care.* Geneva, Switzerland: World Health Organization. (Level I)

4 The Joint Commission. (2012). Standard NPSG.01.01.01. *Comprehensive accreditation manual for hospitals: The official handbook.* Oakbrook Terrace, IL: The Joint Commission. (Level I)

5 The Joint Commission. (2012). Standard UP.01.01.01. *Comprehensive accreditation manual for hospitals: The official handbook.* Oakbrook Terrace, IL: The Joint Commission. (Level I)

6 The Joint Commission. (2012). Standard UP.01.03.01. *Comprehensive accreditation manual for hospitals: The official handbook.* Oakbrook Terrace, IL: The Joint Commission. (Level I)

7 Ng, I., et al. (2004). Effects of head posture on cerebral hemodynamics: its influences on intracranial pressure, cerebral perfusion pressure, and cerebral oxygenations. *Neurosurgery, 54*(3), 593–597. (Level VI)

8 The Joint Commission. (2012). Standard NPSG.03.04.01. *Comprehensive accreditation manual for hospitals: The official handbook.* Oakbrook Terrace, IL: The Joint Commission. (Level I)

9 U.S. Food and Drug Administration. (2009). "Look. Check. Connect. Safe Medical Device Connections Save Lives" [Online]. Accessed August 2011 via the Web at http://www.fda.gov/downloads/MedicalDevices/Safety/AlertsandNotices/UCM134873.pdf

10 The Joint Commission. (2012). Standard RC.01.03.01. *Comprehensive accreditation manual for hospitals: The official handbook.* Oakbrook Terrace, IL: The Joint Commission. (Level I)

11 The Joint Commission. (2012). Standard RC.02.01.01. *Comprehensive accreditation manual for hospitals: The official handbook.* Oakbrook Terrace, IL: The Joint Commission. (Level I)

ADDITIONAL REFERENCES

American Association of Neuroscience Nurses. (2004). *Core curriculum for neuroscience nursing* (4th ed.). Philadelphia, PA: Saunders.

Dunn, I.F., et al. (2006). Neuromonitoring in neurological critical care. *Neurocritical Care, 4*(1), 83–92.

Lynn-McHale Wiegand, D. (Ed.). (2011). *AACN procedure manual for critical care* (6th ed.). Philadelphia, PA: Saunders.

Tobias, J.D. (2006). Cerebral oxygenation monitoring: Near-infrared spectroscopy. *Expert Review of Medical Devices, 3*(2), 235–243.

KNEE ARTHROPLASTY POSTPROCEDURE CARE

Knee arthroplasty involves surgical replacement of all or part of the knee joint. In partial knee replacement, either the medial or lateral compartment of the knee joint is replaced. Total knee replacement is commonly used to treat severe pain, joint contractures, and deterioration of joint surfaces, conditions that prohibit full extension or flexion.

Arthroplasty postprocedure care includes maintaining alignment of the affected joint, assisting with exercises, and providing routine postoperative care. Nursing responsibilities include teaching, safe mobility, home care, and exercises that may continue for several years.

Equipment

Incentive spirometer ▪ continuous passive motion (CPM) machine ▪ compression stockings or sequential compression device ▪ sterile gloves ▪ gloves ▪ sterile dressings ▪ hypoallergenic tape ▪ ice bag ▪ skin lotion ▪ warm water ▪ crutches or walker ▪ pain medications ▪ closed-wound drainage system ▪ IV antibiotics ▪ pillow.

After total knee replacement, a knee immobilizer may be applied in the operating room, or the leg may be placed in CPM.

Implementation

▪ Confirm the doctor's orders.
▪ Confirm the patient's identity using at least two patient identifiers according to your facility's policy.[1]
▪ Explain all the procedures.
▪ Perform hand hygiene and follow standard precautions.[2,3,4]
▪ Check vital signs every 15 minutes until stable, then every 30 minutes twice, then every 2 to 4 hours, and then routinely thereafter, according to facility policy. Report any changes in vital signs *because they may indicate infection, hemorrhage, or postoperative complications.*
▪ Encourage the patient to perform deep-breathing and coughing exercises. Assist with incentive spirometry *to prevent postprocedure pneumonia.*
▪ Perform a bilateral neurovascular assessment every 2 hours for the first 48 hours and then every 4 hours or according to your facility's policy *for signs of complications.* Check the affected leg for color, temperature, toe movement, sensation, edema, capillary filling, and pedal pulse. Investigate any complaints of pain, burning, numbness, or tingling.
▪ Apply the compression stockings or sequential compression device, as ordered, *to promote venous return and prevent venous thromboembolism.* Once every 8 hours, remove the stockings or compression device, inspect the legs—especially the heels—for pressure ulcers, and reapply the stockings or device.

■ Assess the patient's pain and administer pain medications, as ordered, following safe medication administration practices.[5,6]

■ Make sure prophylactic antibiotics are discontinued within 24 hours after surgery.[7,8]

■ Administer anticoagulant therapy, as ordered, *to minimize the risk of venous thromboembolism*. If a continuous infusion of heparin is prescribed, administer it using a programmable pump (preferably a smart pump with dose-range alerts) *to provide consistent and accurate dosing*.[9] Observe for bleeding and for signs and symptoms of phlebitis, such as warmth, swelling, tenderness, and redness. Monitor laboratory results, such as complete blood count, prothrombin time, International Normalized Ratio, and partial thromboplastin time.[7]

■ Check dressings for excessive bleeding. Circle any drainage on the dressing and mark it with your initials, the date, and the time. As needed, apply more sterile dressings, using hypoallergenic tape.[10] Report excessive bleeding to the doctor.

■ Observe the closed-wound drainage system for discharge color. (See "Closed-wound drainage management," page 179.) *Proper drainage prevents hematoma. Purulent discharge and fever may indicate infection.* Empty and measure drainage, as ordered, using clean technique *to prevent infection*.

■ Monitor the patient's fluid intake and output daily; include wound drainage in the output measurement.

■ If the patient has an indwelling urinary catheter that was inserted for surgery, remove the catheter on postoperative day 1 or 2 (with the day of surgery considered day 0), according to your facility policy or the doctor's order, *to reduce the risk for catheter-associated urinary tract infection*.[7] (See "Indwelling urinary catheter care and removal," page 374.)

■ Apply an ice bag, as ordered, to the affected site for the first 48 hours *to reduce swelling, relieve pain, and control bleeding*.

■ Help the patient use the trapeze to reposition himself every 2 hours. *These position changes enhance comfort, prevent pressure ulcers, and help prevent respiratory complications.* Then provide skin care for the back and buttocks, using warm water and lotion, as indicated.

■ Instruct the patient to perform muscle-strengthening exercises for extremities, as ordered, *to help maintain muscle strength and range of motion and to help prevent phlebitis*. Collaborate with physical therapy professionals, as appropriate.

■ Elevate the affected leg, as ordered, *to reduce swelling*.

■ Instruct the patient to begin quadriceps exercises and straight-leg raising, when ordered (usually on the second postoperative day). Encourage flexion-extension exercises, when ordered (usually after the first dressing change). Collaborate with physical therapy professionals, as appropriate.

■ If the doctor orders use of the CPM machine, he will adjust the machine daily *to gradually increase the degree of flexion of the affected leg*. Typically, patients can dangle their feet on the first day after surgery and begin ambulation with partial weight-bearing, as tolerated (cemented knee) or toe-touch ambulation only (uncemented knee) by the second day. The patient may need to wear a knee immobilizer for support when walking; otherwise, he should be in CPM for most of the day and night or during waking hours only. (See "Continuous passive motion device use," page 209.)

■ The degree of flexion, extension, and weight-bearing status will depend on the doctor's specific orders, the surgical approach used, and the surgeon's preference.

■ Before ambulation, give an analgesic, as ordered, 30 minutes before activity *because movement is very painful*. Encourage the patient during exercise.[5]

■ Help the patient with progressive ambulation, using adjustable crutches or a walker when needed.

■ Educate the patient and his family about measures to prevent surgical site infection.

■ Perform hand hygiene.[2,3,4]

■ Document the procedure.[11,12]

Complications

Immobility after arthroplasty may result in such complications as shock, pulmonary embolism, pneumonia, phlebitis, paralytic ileus, urine retention, and bowel impaction. A deep wound or infection at the prosthesis site is a serious complication that may force removal of the prosthesis.

Fat embolism, a potentially fatal complication resulting from release of fat molecules in response to increased intramedullary canal pressure from the prosthesis, may develop within 72 hours after surgery. Watch for such signs and symptoms as apprehension, diaphoresis, fever, dyspnea, pulmonary effusion, tachycardia, cyanosis, seizures, decreased level of consciousness, and a petechial rash on the chest and shoulders.

Documentation

Record the patient's neurovascular status and maintenance and settings of the CPM device. Describe the patient's position (especially the position of the affected leg), skin care and condition, respiratory care and condition, and the use of compression stockings. Document all exercises performed and their effect; also record ambulatory efforts, the type of support used, and the amount of traction weight. On the appropriate flowchart, record vital signs and fluid intake and output. Note the turning and skin care schedule and the current exercise and ambulation program. Record discharge instructions and how well the patient seems to understand them.

REFERENCES

1 The Joint Commission. (2012). Standard NPSG.01.01.01. *Comprehensive accreditation manual for hospitals: The official handbook.* Oakbrook Terrace, IL: The Joint Commission. (Level I)

2 The Joint Commission. (2012). Standard NPSG.07.01.01. *Comprehensive accreditation manual for hospitals: The official handbook.* Oakbrook Terrace, IL: The Joint Commission. (Level I)

3 Centers for Disease Control and Prevention. (October 2002). Guideline for hand hygiene in health-care settings. *Morbidity and Mortality Weekly Report, 51*(RR-16), 1–45. (Level I)

4 World Health Organization. (2009). *WHO guidelines on hand hygiene in health care: First global patient safety challenge. Clean care is safer care.* Geneva, Switzerland: World Health Organization. (Level I)

5 The Joint Commission. (2012). Standard PC.01.02.01. *Comprehensive accreditation manual for hospitals: The official handbook.* Oakbrook Terrace, IL: The Joint Commission. (Level I)

6 The Joint Commission. (2012). Standard MM.06.01.01. *Comprehensive accreditation manual for hospitals: The official handbook.* Oakbrook Terrace, IL: The Joint Commission. (Level I)

7 The Joint Commission. (2010). Surgical Care Improvement Project national hospital inpatient quality measures. In *Specification manual for national hospital quality measures.* Oakbrook Terrace, IL: The Joint Commission. (Level I)

8 Anderson, D.J., et al. (2008). Compendium of strategies to prevent healthcare-associated infections in acute care hospitals: Strategies to prevent surgical site infections in acute care hospitals. *Infection Control and Hospital Epidemiology,* (29), S1. (Level 1)

9 The Joint Commission. (2012). Standard NPSG.03.05.01. *Comprehensive accreditation manual for hospitals: The official handbook.* Oakbrook Terrace, IL: The Joint Commission. (Level I)

10 The Joint Commission. (2012). Standard NPSG.07.05.01. *Comprehensive accreditation manual for hospitals: The official handbook.* Oakbrook Terrace, IL: The Joint Commission. (Level I)

11 The Joint Commission. (2012). Standard RC.01.03.01. *Comprehensive accreditation manual for hospitals: The official handbook.* Oakbrook Terrace, IL: The Joint Commission. (Level I)

12 The Joint Commission. (2012). Standard RC.02.01.01. *Comprehensive accreditation manual for hospitals: The official handbook.* Oakbrook Terrace, IL: The Joint Commission. (Level I)

ADDITIONAL REFERENCES

Berger, R.A., & Walsh, S.M. (2009). Outpatient total knee arthroplasty: Pathways and protocols. *Techniques in Knee Surgery, 8*(2), 115–118.

Burge, D.M. (2009). Relationship between patient trust of nursing staff, postoperative pain, and discharge functional outcomes following a total knee arthroplasty. *Orthopedic Nursing, 28*(6), 295–301.

Colwell, C.W. (2009). The ACCP guidelines for thromboprophylaxis in total hip and knee arthroplasty. *Orthopedics, 32*(12 Suppl.), 67–73.

Jacobson, A.F., et al. (2008). "Patients' perspectives on total knee replacement," *AJN, 108*(5), 54–63.

Roman, M. (2009). Total knee arthroplasty. *MedSurg Nursing, 18*(5), 317–318.

Smith-Miller, C.A., et al. (2009). A comparison of patient pain responses and medication regimens after hip/knee replacement. *Orthopedic Nursing, 28*(5), 242–249.

LARYNGEAL MASK AIRWAY INSERTION

The laryngeal mask airway (LMA) is used to establish and maintain a patent airway in the unconscious patient. It's used extensively in the operating room by anesthesia personnel and is also appropriate for emergency airway and ventilatory support when endotracheal (ET) intubation isn't immediately possible. The LMA may also be used in place of a face mask during adult, pediatric, and neonatal resuscitation.[1,2,3]

The LMA consists of a semirigid tube attached to a silicone mask. The mask is placed into the patient's mouth and advanced blindly until it rests above the larynx. The patient may then breathe spontaneously or be assisted with moderate positive-pressure ventilation.

The LMA doesn't always protect the patient from regurgitation and aspiration, so it should be used in patients with full stomachs only in emergency situations in which intubation isn't possible, or if ventilation by face mask is ineffective. However, regurgitation is less likely and aspiration uncommon with the LMA when compared with the bag-mask device.[1] In addition, the LMA should only be inserted into the patient who has lost protective cough and gag reflexes. The LMA should be used cautiously in patients with delayed gastric emptying because of the risk of regurgitation.

Types of LMAs used outside of the operating room include reusable (requiring cleaning and sterilization between uses) and disposable (for single-patient use). An intubating LMA is also available; it's used to provide a patent airway, which facilitates ET intubation.

Occasionally, patients can't be adequately ventilated with the LMA, even after successful insertion; ET intubation supplies should be readily available, if needed.[1]

Equipment

Appropriately sized LMA based on patient's weight (reusable, disposable, or intubating) (see *LMA specifications,* page 452) ▪ syringe of appropriate size for inflating cuff ▪ water-soluble lubricant ▪ gloves and other personal protective equipment ▪ oxygen equipment ▪ tape or device to secure the tube ▪ bag-valve mask device ▪ bite block ▪ stethoscope ▪ suction equipment ▪ pulse oximeter, if available ▪ capnometer.

Preparation of equipment

Perform hand hygiene thoroughly *to reduce the transmission of microorganisms.*[4,5,6] While the equipment is being prepared, ventilate and oxygenate the patient with a bag-valve or mouth-to-mouth mask device, if necessary. Remove the LMA from its package and visually inspect it for discoloration, cracks, or kinks in the tube; also make sure it's the right size. Inspect the airway opening and check that the aperture bars are intact. Manually tighten the connector, if needed.

Test the patency of the cuff by first withdrawing all air and then overinflating it with air injected through the pilot balloon. While inflated, visually inspect the cuff for symmetry; then deflate the cuff. Don't use the LMA if it's leaking air or if you note that the cuff is asymmetrical when you inflate it. Assemble suction equipment and check that it's working properly.

Implementation

▪ If this is a planned procedure, verify the order in the patient's medical record *to ensure that the right procedure is being performed on the right patient at the right time.*[7]

▪ Perform hand hygiene.[4,5,6]

▪ Confirm the patient's identity using at least two patient identifiers according to your facility's policy.[8]

LMA specifications

The following chart will help you choose the right size laryngeal mask airway (LMA) for your patient.

LMA SIZE	PATIENT SIZE	MAXIMAL CUFF INFLATION VOLUME	OVERINFLATION VOLUME FOR CUFF TEST
1	Up to 5 kg (11 lb)	4 mL	8 mL
1½	5–10 kg (11–22 lb)	7 mL	10 mL
2	10–20 kg (22–44 lb)	10 mL	15 mL
2½	20–30 kg (44–66 lb)	14 mL	21 mL
3	30–50 kg (66–110 lb)	20 mL	30 mL
4	50–70 kg (110–154 lb)	30 mL	45 mL
5	70–100 kg (154–220 lb)	40 mL	60 mL
6	Greater than 100 kg (220 lb)	50 mL	75 mL

■ Assess the patient's level of consciousness. The patient should be unconscious and unresponsive *because the LMA shouldn't be inserted into a patient who may resist insertion.*

■ Put on gloves and personal protective equipment *to reduce contact with body secretions and the transmission of microorganisms.*

■ Teach the family about the procedure, as the patient's condition allows, *to provide them with information and reduce anxiety.*

■ Lubricate the posterior surface of the LMA, using a water-soluble lubricant, *to ease insertion.*[9] Avoid getting the lubricant on the anterior surface of the cuff *because the lubricant may be aspirated.*

■ Place the patient in the supine position with a folded towel or blanket under the head to flex the neck and extend the head (the "sniffing position") *to ease insertion of the LMA.*

■ Stand behind the patient's head and place your nondominant hand under the patient's head, lifting the head slightly and keeping upward pressure.[9]

■ Hold the LMA in your dominant hand like a pencil, with your index finger placed at the junction of the mask and the tube (as shown below). The lumen of the LMA should be facing up, with the lubricated posterior surface facing the floor.

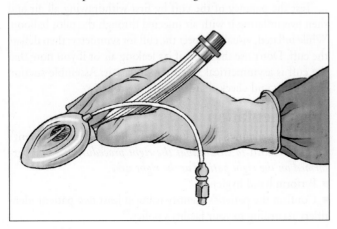

■ Extend the patient's head while flexing the neck and flatten the LMA against the patient's hard palate.[9] Use your middle finger to gently press down on the patient's jaw.

■ Flex your wrist fully so that the tip of the LMA points toward the patient's head and down, and use your index finger to insert the tip of the LMA into the patient's mouth (as shown below).

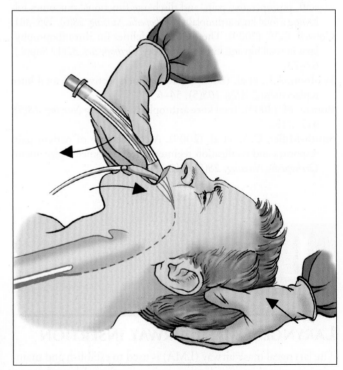

■ Press the posterior surface of the LMA against the hard palate and advance it into the oropharynx (as shown below).[9] *By applying pressure up against the hard palate, the LMA will advance to the proper position.*

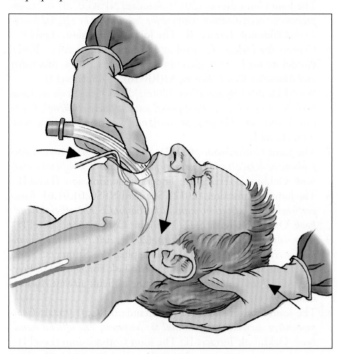

■ Use your middle finger to open the patient's jaw and check that the cuff is compressed against the hard palate. If the cuff isn't flattened against the hard palate, remove the LMA and insert it again.

■ While maintaining pressure on the LMA so that it stays pressed against the hard palate, extend your index finger fully while continuing to advance the LMA until you meet resistance at the hypopharynx (as shown below). The LMA should now be in the correct position.

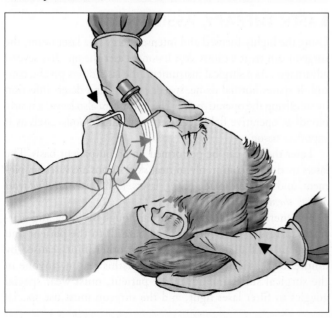

■ Remove your nondominant hand from under the patient's head, and use it to hold the LMA in place while removing your index finger (as shown below).[9]

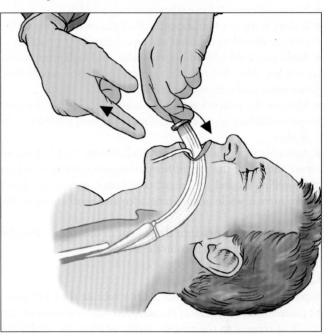

■ Without holding the LMA, use the syringe to inflate the cuff to an intracuff pressure of about 60 cm H_2O.[9] *Inflating the cuff without holding the tube allows it to settle itself into the correct position during cuff inflation.* Only one-half the maximum inflation volume is required to make a seal. Don't overinflate the cuff.

■ Check the patient's mouth to make sure the cuff isn't visible, and observe for minor outward movement of the tube and minor neck bulging in the area of the cricothyroid, *indicating proper tube placement and cuff inflation.*

■ Verify correct placement by auscultating for bilateral breath sounds with a stethoscope, and by capnography and pulse oximetry, if available.[10]

■ Use a bag-valve device connected to an oxygen source, if indicated, to gently deliver ventilations using a peak airway pressure less than 20 cm H_2O and a tidal volume of 8 mL/kg of body weight or less. *Using low pressure ventilations avoids exceeding cuff pressure and reduces the risk of forcing air into the stomach.*

■ Insert a bite block *to keep the patient from biting on the tube, which may cause it to become occluded or move out of proper position.*[9]

■ Tape the LMA and bite block securely to the patient's face or use a commercial device to secure the tube.

■ Remove and discard your gloves and other personal protective equipment and perform hand hygiene.[4,5,6]

■ Document the procedure.[11,12]

Special considerations

■ If there is a risk that the patient may have neck trauma, insert the LMA with the patient's neck in a neutral position.

■ Introducers, which are used in place of your index finger, may be available from the manufacturer to assist with insertion. The introducer maintains contact between the posterior aspect of the tube and the patient's hard palate and should be used according to the manufacturer's instructions.

■ Never use extreme force when inserting a LMA.

■ If there is any concern about the final placement of the LMA, the device should be removed and repositioned.

■ Avoid use of the LMA in patients who need high pressures for ventilation. *The LMA has a low-pressure seal, which may be ineffective when used with high pressures.*

■ Monitor the patient's respiratory status continually *to ensure proper ventilation, oxygenation, and tube placement while the LMA is in place.*

■ Assess for an air leak, *which may indicate that the LMA isn't in correct position.* If the patient has prolonged expirations and no oval swelling around the cricoid membrane, remove the LMA and reinsert it while maintaining adequate ventilations to the patient.

■ If the patient vomits, turn the patient to the side *to allow for drainage of contents* and suction the airway.

Complications

Aspiration of stomach contents is a risk because the LMA doesn't protect the airway. Use of excessive force during insertion can result in trauma to the mouth, teeth, or pharynx, including lacerations, bleeding, and edema. Use of excessive air to inflate the cuff can result in edema or nerve damage. Other complications include hoarseness, dysphagia, stridor, dysarthria, and dysphonia.

Documentation

Document why LMA insertion was needed. Record the method of ventilating and oxygenating used while preparing for LMA insertion. Note that the cuff was tested for patency and that the device was visually inspected, with no irregularities observed. Record the date, time, and name of the person performing the procedure. Include the size of the LMA, volume of air used to inflate the cuff, and number of attempts to achieve proper placement. Record the methods used to determine proper tube placement. Include placement of the bite block and how the bite block and tube were secured. Document whether the patient was breathing spontaneously or receiving assisted or controlled ventilations. Include the amount of oxygen delivered as well as any evidence of trauma to the airway from insertion of the LMA. Record frequent assessments of tube placement and respiratory status on a frequent patient assessment sheet. Include any teaching and support given to the family.[10,11]

References

1 American Heart Association. (2010). 2010 American Heart Association guidelines for cardiopulmonary resuscitation and emergency cardiovascular care. *Circulation, 122*(Suppl. 3), S729–767. (Level I)

2 American Heart Association. (2010). Pediatric advanced life support: 2010 American Heart Association guidelines for cardiopulmonary resuscitation and emergency cardiovascular care. *Circulation, 122*(Suppl. 3), S876–908. (Level I)

3 American Heart Association. (2010). Neonatal resuscitation: 2010 American Heart Association Guidelines for cardiopulmonary resuscitation and emergency cardiovascular care. *Circulation, 122*(Suppl. 3), S909–919. (Level I)

4 The Joint Commission. (2012). Standard NPSG.07.01.01. *Comprehensive accreditation manual for hospitals: The official handbook.* Oakbrook Terrace, IL: The Joint Commission. (Level I)

5 Centers for Disease Control and Prevention. (October 2002). Guideline for hand hygiene in health-care settings. *Morbidity and Mortality Weekly Report, 51*(RR-16), 1–45. (Level I)

6 World Health Organization. (2009). *WHO guidelines on hand hygiene in health care: First global patient safety challenge. Clean care is safer care.* Geneva, Switzerland: World Health Organization. (Level I)

7 The Joint Commission. (2012). Standard UP.01.01.01. *Comprehensive accreditation manual for hospitals: The official handbook.* Oakbrook Terrace, IL: The Joint Commission. (Level I)

8 The Joint Commission. (2012). Standard NPSG.01.01.01. *Comprehensive accreditation manual for hospitals: The official handbook.* Oakbrook Terrace, IL: The Joint Commission. (Level I)

9 Lynn-McHale Wiegand, D. (Ed.). (2011). *AACN procedure manual for critical care* (6th ed.). Philadelphia, PA: Saunders.

10 American Society of Anesthesiologists Task Force. (2003). Practice guidelines for management of the difficult airway. *Anesthesiology, 98*(5), 1269–1277. (Level I)

11 The Joint Commission. (2012). Standard RC.01.03.01. *Comprehensive accreditation manual for hospitals: The official handbook.* Oakbrook Terrace, IL: The Joint Commission. (Level I)

12 The Joint Commission. (2012). Standard RC.02.01.01. *Comprehensive accreditation manual for hospitals: The official handbook.* Oakbrook Terrace, IL: The Joint Commission. (Level I)

Additional reference

Middleton P. (2009). Insertion techniques of the laryngeal mask airway: A literature review. *Journal of Perioperative Practice, 19*(1), 31–35.

Laser therapy, assisting

Using the highly focused and intense energy of a laser beam, the surgeon can treat various skin lesions. Laser therapy has several advantages. As a surgical instrument, the laser offers precise control. It spares normal tissue, speeds healing, and deters infection by sterilizing the operative site. The laser beam also leaves a nearly bloodless operative field because it seals tiny blood vessels as it vaporizes tissue.

Laser therapy can be performed on an outpatient basis. The lasers used most commonly to treat skin lesions are vascular, pigment, and carbon dioxide (CO_2) lasers. (See *Understanding types of laser therapy.*)

In general, laser surgery is safe, although bleeding and scarring can result. One pronounced hazard, to the patient and treatment staff alike, is eye damage or other injury caused by unintended laser beam reflection. For this reason, anyone in the surgical suite, including the patient, must wear special goggles to filter laser light, and the surgeon must use special nonreflective instruments. Access to the room must be strictly controlled, and all windows must be covered.

Equipment

Laser ▪ filtration face masks ▪ protective eyewear (approved by the laser safety officer [LSO])[1] ▪ laser vacuum ▪ extra vacuum filters ▪ surgical drape ▪ prescribed cleaning solution ▪ sterile gauze ▪ non-adherent dressings ▪ surgical tape ▪ cotton-tipped applicators ▪ nonreflective surgical instruments ▪ gown ▪ sterile gloves.

Preparation of equipment

Perform hand hygiene[2,3,4] and gather the equipment. Prepare the tray. It should include a local anesthetic, as ordered, and dry and wet gauze. *The gauze will be used to control bleeding, protect healthy tissue, and abrade and remove any eschar, which would otherwise inhibit laser absorption.* Prepare nonreflective surgical instruments as needed.

Cover all the windows and door windows in the treatment room to prevent the laser from being seen through the windows, creating a potential for exposure.[1]

Fire is a significant hazard during laser use. Make sure that water, saline, and a fire extinguisher are readily available for use during the procedure.[1]

Implementation

▪ Make sure the doctor has obtained informed consent and that it's documented in the patient's medical record.[5,6]
▪ Conduct a preprocedure verification *to make sure that all relevant documentation, related information, and equipment are available and correctly identified to the patient identifiers.*[7]
▪ Perform hand hygiene.[2,3,4]
▪ Confirm the patient's identity using at least two patient identifiers according to your facility's policy.[8]
▪ Tell the patient how the laser works and name its benefits. Point out the equipment and outline the procedure *to help allay the patient's concerns.*
▪ Put on a cap, a gown, a filtration face mask, and protective eyewear.
▪ If appropriate, make sure the surgical site is marked according to facility policy.[9]
▪ Position the patient comfortably, drape him, and place normal saline solution–saturated gauze, if needed, over exposed tissue around the operative site. *To avoid thermal injuries,* make sure that all surgical drapes at the site are moist.[1]
▪ Place protective eyewear on the patient: goggles or glasses designed for the type of laser if the patient will remain awake during the procedure; wet eye pads, laser-specific eyeshields, or specific protection designated by the LSO if the patient will undergo general anesthesia; or metal corneal eye shields if the patient is undergoing laser on or around the eyelids.[1]
▪ Confirm that everyone in the room, including the patient, is wearing protective eyewear *to filter the laser light.*[1]
▪ Keep the door to the surgical suite closed and post warning signs regarding the type of laser used at all entrances to the laser treatment area *to keep unprotected people from inadvertently entering the room.*[1]

Understanding types of laser therapy

Laser therapy is now an essential tool for treating many types of skin lesions. The number of lasers used in dermatology continues to grow, and each type is used for specific conditions.

The term *laser* is an acronym for Light Amplification by the Stimulated Emission of Radiation. When directed toward the skin, most of this light energy is absorbed by chromophores, substances that absorb specific wavelengths of light. This is the basis of selective photothermolysis, which has revolutionized cutaneous laser surgery. Melanin is the target chromophore in pigmented lesions, and oxyhemoglobin within microvessels is the target chromophore in vascular lesions.

Each type of laser has a different use.

Lasers for vascular lesions
The laser most commonly used for vascular lesions is the pulsed dye laser (PDL). Other lasers used to treat vascular lesions include the copper vapor, argon, argon-pumped tunable dye, potassium-titanyl-phosphate (KTP), krypton, and neodymium:yttrium-aluminum-garnet (Nd:YAG). Vascular lesions appropriate for laser therapy include port-wine stains, hemangiomas, venous lake, rosacea, telangiectasia, and Kaposi's sarcoma.

Lasers for pigmented lesions
Lasers that effectively treat tattoos and dermal and epidermal pigmented lesions include Q-switched ruby, Q-switched Nd:YAG, Q-switched alexandrite, and PDL. Pigmented lesions appropriate for laser treatment include tattoos, nevi of Ota, melasma, solar lentigo, café au lait spots, Becker's nevi, and epidermal nevi.

Lasers for hair removal
Lasers used to eliminate unwanted hair include ruby, alexandrite, and Nd:YAG. Laser treatment is only effective in removing dark-colored hair; it doesn't effectively remove blonde, red, white, or gray hair.

▪ Make sure that the surgical team conducts a time-out immediately before the surgeon begins the procedure *to perform a final assessment that the correct patient, site, positioning, and procedure are identified and, as applicable, all relevant information and necessary equipment are available.*[9]
▪ Make sure that the skin preparation product and hand antiseptic agents are completely dry before the laser is turned on *to prevent surgical fires. Use of nonflammable preparation agents minimize the risk.*[1]
▪ Keep sponges and drapes near the surgical site moist to reduce the risk of fire. Ensure that wet towels and normal saline solution are available on the sterile field *to extinguish a fire if one occurs.*[1]

■ After the surgeon administers the anesthetic and it takes effect, activate the laser vacuum. The CO_2 laser has a vacuum hose attached to a separate apparatus. Use this apparatus *to clear the surgical site.* The vacuum has a filter that traps and collects most of the vaporized tissue. Change the filter whenever suction decreases, and follow facility guidelines for filter disposal.

■ When the surgeon finishes the procedure, perform hand hygiene,[2,3,4] put on sterile gloves, and apply direct pressure with a sterile gauze pad to any bleeding wound for 20 minutes. If a wound continues to bleed, notify the doctor.

■ When the bleeding is controlled, use sterile technique to clean the area with a cotton-tipped applicator dipped in the prescribed cleaning solution. Then size and cut a nonadherent dressing. Secure the dressing with surgical tape.

■ Discard equipment and supplies according to your facility's policy.

■ Remove and discard your personal protective equipment and perform hand hygiene.[2,3,4]

■ Document the procedure.[10,11]

Special considerations

■ Vascular and pigment lasers won't result in a wound; only superficial skin changes will occur.

■ The nurse must have thorough knowledge of how each laser operates and of laser safety considerations for both the patient and the health care providers.[1]

Patient teaching

Before the procedure, tell the patient that the surgeon uses the laser beam much as he would a scalpel to excise the lesion. Explain that the laser causes a burnlike wound that can be deep. Inform the patient that the wound will appear charred. Also, tell the patient that some of the eschar will be removed during the initial postoperative cleaning and that more will gradually dislodge at home. Warn the patient to expect a burning odor and smoke during the procedure. A machine called a smoke evacuator, which sounds like a vacuum cleaner, will clear it away. Advise the patient that he may sense heat from the laser. Urge him to tell the doctor at once if pain develops.

Teach the patient how to dress his wound or care for his skin daily as ordered by the surgeon. Tell him that he can take showers, but he shouldn't immerse the wound in water *to promote wound healing and prevent infection.* If the wound bleeds at home, demonstrate how to apply direct pressure on the site with clean gauze or a washcloth for 20 minutes. If pressure doesn't control the bleeding, tell the patient to call his doctor.

If the patient's foot or leg was operated on, urge him to keep the extremity elevated and to use it as little as possible *because pressure can inhibit healing.* Warn the patient to protect the treated area from exposure to the sun *to avoid changes in pigmentation.* Tell him to call the doctor if he develops a temperature of 100° F (37.8° C) or higher that persists longer than 1 day.

Complications

Pain, bruising, redness, and blistering may occur after laser surgery. Scarring, pigment changes, and infection are rare complications of laser surgery.

Documentation

Most patients who have laser surgery for skin lesions are treated as outpatients. Note the patient's skin condition before and after the procedure. Also document any bleeding, record the type of dressing applied, and list the patient's complaints of pain. Note whether the patient comprehends home care instructions.[10,11]

REFERENCES

1 Recommended practices for laser safety. (2010). In R. Conner, et al (Eds.). *Perioperative standards and recommended practices.* Denver, CO: AORN. (Level I)

2 Centers for Disease Control and Prevention. (October 2002). Guideline for hand hygiene in health-care settings. *Morbidity and Mortality Weekly Report, 51*(RR-16), 1–45. (Level I)

3 World Health Organization. (2009). *WHO guidelines on hand hygiene in health care: First global patient safety challenge. Clean care is safer care.* Geneva, Switzerland: World Health Organization. (Level I)

4 The Joint Commission. (2012). Standard NPSG.07.01.01. *Comprehensive accreditation manual for hospitals: The official handbook.* Oakbrook Terrace, IL: The Joint Commission. (Level I)

5 The Joint Commission. (2012). Standard RI.01.03.01. *Comprehensive accreditation manual for hospitals: The official handbook.* Oakbrook Terrace, IL: The Joint Commission. (Level I)

6 Centers for Medicare & Medicaid Services, Department of Health and Human Services. (2006). "Conditions of Participation: Patients' Rights," 42 CFR part 482.13 [Online]. Accessed November 2011 via the Web at https://www.cms.gov/CFCsAndCoPs/downloads/finalpatientrightsrule.pdf

7 The Joint Commission. (2012). Standard UP.01.01.01. *Comprehensive accreditation manual for hospitals: The official handbook.* Oakbrook Terrace, IL: The Joint Commission. (Level I)

8 The Joint Commission. (2012). Standard NPSG.01.01.01. *Comprehensive accreditation manual for hospitals: The official handbook.* Oakbrook Terrace, IL: The Joint Commission. (Level I)

9 The Joint Commission. (2012). Standard UP.01.03.01. *Comprehensive accreditation manual for hospitals: The official handbook.* Oakbrook Terrace, IL: The Joint Commission. (Level I)

10 The Joint Commission. (2012). Standard RC.01.03.01. *Comprehensive accreditation manual for hospitals: The official handbook.* Oakbrook Terrace, IL: The Joint Commission. (Level I)

11 The Joint Commission. (2012). Standard RC.02.01.01. *Comprehensive accreditation manual for hospitals: The official handbook.* Oakbrook Terrace, IL: The Joint Commission. (Level I)

ADDITIONAL REFERENCES

Battle, E.F., Jr., & Soden, C.E., Jr. (2009). The use of lasers in darker skin types. *Seminars in Cutaneous Medicine and Surgery, 28*(2), 130–140.

Huikeshoven, M., et al. (2007). Redarkening of port-wine stains 10 years after pulsed-dye-laser treatment. *New England Journal of Medicine, 356*(12), 1235–1240.

Wiper, A., et al. (2007). Amiodarone-induced skin pigmentation: Q-switched laser therapy, an effective treatment option. *Heart, 93*(1), 15.

LATEX ALLERGY PROTOCOL

Latex is a natural product of the rubber tree and is used in many products in the health care field. With the increased use of latex in barrier protection and medical equipment, more and more nurses and patients are becoming hypersensitive to it.

Certain groups of people are at increased risk for developing latex allergy. These include people who have had or will undergo multiple surgical procedures (such as those with a history of spina bifida), health care workers (especially those who work in the emergency department or operating room), workers who manufacture latex and latex-containing products, and people with a genetic predisposition to latex allergy. Some studies also suggest that pregnant patients may have a higher risk of latex allergy than nonpregnant patients.[1]

People allergic to certain cross-reactive foods—including bananas, avocados, chestnuts, cherries, grapes, kiwis, passion fruit, tomatoes, and peaches—may also be allergic to latex. Exposure to latex elicits an allergic response similar to the one elicited by these foods.

For those with latex allergy, latex becomes a hazard when the protein in latex comes in direct contact with mucous membranes or is inhaled, which happens when powdered latex surgical gloves are used. People with asthma are at greater risk for developing worsening signs and symptoms from airborne latex.

The diagnosis of latex allergy is based on the patient's history and physical examination. Laboratory testing should be performed to confirm or eliminate the diagnosis. Skin testing, such as the skin-prick or patch test, may be performed. The radioallergosorbent test (RAST) measures the serum level of latex-specific immunoglobulin E in the blood. Other serum blood tests include Pharmacia CAP, AlaSTAT, and HYTEC.

Latex allergy can produce a myriad of signs and symptoms, including generalized itching (on the hands and arms, for example); itchy, watery, or burning eyes; sneezing and coughing (hay fever–type symptoms); rash; hives; bronchial asthma, scratchy throat, or difficulty breathing; edema of the face, hands, or neck; and anaphylaxis.

To help identify the patient at risk for latex allergy, ask latex allergy–specific questions during the health history. (See *Latex allergy screening.*) If the patient's history reveals a latex sensitivity, the doctor assigns him to one of three categories based on the extent of his sensitization:

■ Group 1 patients have a history of anaphylaxis or a systemic reaction when exposed to a natural latex product.
■ Group 2 patients have a clear history of an allergic reaction of a nonsystemic type.
■ Group 3 patients don't have a previous history of latex hypersensitivity but are designated as high risk because of an associated medical condition, occupation, or crossover allergy.

If you determine that your patient has a sensitivity to latex, make sure that he doesn't come in contact with latex because such contact could result in a life-threatening hypersensitivity reaction. Creating a latex-safe environment is the only way to safeguard your patient. Many facilities now designate nonlatex equipment, which is usually kept on a cart that can be moved into the patient's room.

Latex allergy screening

To determine if your patient has a latex sensitivity or allergy, ask the following screening questions:
■ What is your occupation?
■ Have you experienced an allergic reaction, local sensitivity, or itching following exposure to any latex products, such as balloons, dishwashing gloves, or condoms?
■ Do you have shortness of breath or wheezing after blowing up balloons or after a dental visit?
■ Do you have itching in or around your mouth after eating a banana?
If your patient answers yes to any of these questions, proceed with the following questions:
■ Do you have a history of allergies, dermatitis, or asthma? If so, what type of reaction do you have?
■ Do you have any congenital abnormalities? If yes, explain.
■ Do you have any food allergies? If so, what specific allergies do you have? Describe your reaction.
■ If you experience shortness of breath or wheezing when blowing up latex balloons, describe your reaction.
■ Have you had any previous surgical procedures? Did you experience associated complications? If so, describe them.
■ Have you had previous dental procedures? Did complications result? If so, describe them.
■ Are you exposed to latex in your occupation? Do you experience a reaction to latex products at work? If so, describe your reaction.

Equipment

Latex allergy patient identification wristband ■ nonlatex equipment, including room contents ■ anaphylaxis kit ■ Optional: latex allergy sign.

Preparation of equipment

After you've determined that the patient has a latex allergy or is sensitive to latex, arrange for him to be placed in a private room. If that isn't possible, make the room latex-safe, even if the roommate hasn't been designated as hypersensitive to latex. *This intervention prevents the spread of airborne particles from latex products used on the other patient.*

Implementation
For all patients
■ Assess for possible latex allergy in all patients being admitted.

Anesthesia induction and latex allergy

Latex allergy can cause signs and symptoms in both conscious and anesthetized patients.

CAUSES OF INTRAOPERATIVE REACTION	SIGNS AND SYMPTOMS IN A CONSCIOUS PATIENT	SIGNS AND SYMPTOMS IN AN ANESTHETIZED PATIENT
■ Latex contact with mucous membrane ■ Latex contact with intraperitoneal serosal lining ■ Inhalation of airborne latex particles during anesthesia ■ Injection of antibiotics and anesthetic agents through latex ports	■ Abdominal cramping ■ Anxiety ■ Bronchoconstriction ■ Diarrhea ■ Feeling of faintness ■ Generalized pruritus ■ Itchy eyes ■ Nausea ■ Shortness of breath ■ Swelling of soft tissue (hands, face, tongue) ■ Vomiting ■ Wheezing	■ Bronchospasm ■ Cardiopulmonary arrest ■ Facial edema ■ Flushing ■ Hypotension ■ Laryngeal edema ■ Tachycardia ■ Urticaria ■ Wheezing

For patients in groups 1 and 2

■ If the patient has a confirmed latex allergy, bring a cart with nonlatex supplies into his room.

■ Document on the patient's chart and in the facility database (according to facility policy) that the patient has a latex allergy. If policy requires that the patient wear a latex allergy identification bracelet, place it on the patient.

■ Post a latex allergy sign in the patient's room.

■ If the patient will be receiving anesthesia, make sure that "latex allergy" is clearly visible on the front of his chart. (See *Anesthesia induction and latex allergy*.) Notify the circulating nurse on the surgical unit, the postanesthesia care unit nurses, and any other team members that the patient has a latex allergy.

■ If the patient must be transported to another area of the health care facility, make certain that the nonlatex cart accompanies him and that all health care workers who come in contact with him wear nonlatex gloves. The patient may need to wear a mask with cloth ties when leaving his room *to protect him from inhaling airborne latex particles.*

■ Check adhesives and tapes, including electrocardiogram (ECG), electrodes, and dressing supplies, for latex content.

■ Notify central supply, the dietary department, and the pharmacy about the patient's allergy.

■ If the patient will have an IV line, make sure that IV access is accomplished using all nonlatex products. Post a latex allergy sign on the IV tubing *to prevent access of the line using latex products.*

■ If latex tubing must be used, flush the IV tubing with 50 mL of IV solution to rinse it out *because of latex ports in the IV tubing.*

■ Place a warning label on IV bags that reads "Do not use latex injection ports."

■ Use a nonlatex tourniquet. If none are available, use a latex tourniquet over clothing.

■ Remove the vial stopper to mix and draw up medications.

■ Use nonlatex oxygen administration equipment. Remove the elastic, and tie equipment on with gauze.

■ Wrap your stethoscope, blood pressure cuff and tubing, and ECG wires with a nonlatex product *to protect the patient from latex contact.*

■ Apply transparent dressing over the patient's finger before using pulse oximetry to create a barrier.

■ Use nonlatex syringes when administering medication through a syringe.

■ Make sure that an anaphylaxis kit is readily available. *If your patient has an allergic reaction to latex, you must act immediately.*

■ Have a special latex-free crash cart outside the patient's room during his hospitalization.

■ Document your actions.[2,3]

Special considerations

■ Remember that signs and symptoms of latex allergy usually occur within 30 minutes of anesthesia induction. However, the time of onset can range from 10 minutes to several hours.

■ Don't forget that, as a health care worker, you're in a position to develop a latex hypersensitivity. If you suspect that you're sensitive to latex, contact the employee health services department concerning facility protocol for latex-sensitive employees. Use nonlatex products as often as possible *to help reduce your exposure to latex.* If latex gloves must be worn, powder-free latex gloves are recommended. *When powdered gloves are used, the natural rubber latex (NRL) proteins attach to the cornstarch powder particles and become airborne with glove donning and removal.*

■ Don't assume that if something doesn't look like rubber it isn't latex. Latex can be found in a wide variety of equipment, including ECG leads, oral and nasal airway tubing, tourniquets, nerve stimulation pads, temperature strips, and blood pressure cuffs.

Patient teaching

Teach the patient that the best prevention of an allergic reaction is to avoid latex exposure. Encourage the patient to obtain and wear a medical alert bracelet. Instruct the patient to tell all health care providers, including dentists, about his latex allergy. Instruct the patient to read labels on household rubber items for latex content.

Documentation

Document the results of latex allergy screening, the date and time of screening, and notification of staff of the patient's status. Document placement of signs and warning labels and any patient teaching provided.[2,3]

REFERENCES

1 Draisci, G., et al. (2011). Latex sensitization: A special risk for the obstetric population? *Anesthesiology, 114*(3), 565–569.
2 The Joint Commission. (2012). Standard RC.01.03.01. *Comprehensive accreditation manual for hospitals: The official handbook.* Oakbrook Terrace, IL: The Joint Commission. (Level I)
3 The Joint Commission. (2012). Standard RC.02.01.01. *Comprehensive accreditation manual for hospitals: The official handbook.* Oakbrook Terrace, IL: The Joint Commission. (Level I)

ADDITIONAL REFERENCES

National Institute for Occupational Safety and Health. "Latex Allergy: A Prevention Guide," Publication No. 98-113 [Online]. Accessed January 2012 via the Web at http://www.cdc.gov/niosh/docs/98-113/
Noble, K.A. (2005). The patient with latex allergy. *Journal of Perioperative Nursing, 20*(4), 285–288.
Pontén, A., & Dubnika, I. (2009). Delayed reactions to reusable protective gloves. *Contact Dermatitis, 60*(4), 227–229.
Reines, H.D., & Seifert, P. C. (2005). Patient safety: Latex allergy. *Surgical Clinics of North America, 85*(6), 1329–1340.
Society of Gastroenterology Nurses and Associates, Inc. (2007). "Guidelines for Preventing Sensitivity and Allergic Reactions to Natural Rubber Latex in the Workplace" [Online]. Accessed January 2012 via the Web at http://www.sgna.org/Portals/0/Education/Practice%20Guidelines/LatexAllergyGuideline.pdf

LIPID EMULSION ADMINISTRATION

Given as a separate solution in conjunction with parenteral nutrition or as a component of a total nutrient admixture or three-in-one solution, lipid emulsions are a source of calories and essential fatty acids. A deficiency in essential fatty acids can hinder wound healing, adversely affect production of red blood cells, and impair prostaglandin synthesis.

Lipid emulsions given alone can be administered through either a peripheral or a central venous line. Central venous access is preferred if lipid infusion is ordered for more than 48 hours and is required if it accompanies hypertonic parenteral nutrition solution.[1]

Lipid emulsions are contraindicated in patients who have a condition that disrupts normal fat metabolism, such as patho-logic hyperlipidemia, lipid nephrosis, or acute pancreatitis. They also can't be given to patients with severe egg allergies. They must be used cautiously in patients who have liver or pulmonary disease, anemia, or coagulation disorders as well as in those who are at risk for developing a fat embolism.

Equipment

Lipid emulsion ■ IV administration set with vented spike ■ tape ■ time tape ■ antiseptic pads (alcohol, tincture of iodine, or chlorhexidine-based) ■ IV pump ■ gloves.

If administering the lipid emulsion as part of a 3-in-1 solution, also obtain a filter that's 1.2 microns or greater *because lipids will clog a smaller filter.*[1,2]

Preparation of equipment

Inspect the lipid emulsion for opacity and consistency of color and texture. If the emulsion looks frothy or oily or contains particles, or if you think its stability or sterility is questionable, return the bottle to the pharmacy. *To prevent aggregation of fat globules,* don't shake the lipid container excessively. Protect the emulsion from freezing, and never add anything to it. Make sure you have the correct lipid emulsion.

Implementation

■ Verify the doctor's order.[3]
■ Perform hand hygiene and put on gloves.[4,5,6]
■ Confirm the patient's identity using at least two patient identifiers according to your facility's policy.[7]
■ Explain the procedure to the patient *to promote his cooperation.*
■ Connect the IV administration set tubing to a needleless connector; the needleless connector connects piggyback tubing to primary tubing.
■ Close the flow clamp on the administration set tubing. Check that luer-lock connections are secure *to prevent accidental separation, which can lead to air embolism, exsanguination, or sepsis.*
■ Using aseptic technique, remove the protective cap from the lipid emulsion bottle, and clean the rubber stopper with an antiseptic pad.
■ Hold the bottle upright and, using strict aseptic technique, insert the vented spike through the inner circle of the rubber stopper.
■ Invert the bottle, and squeeze the drip chamber until it fills to the level indicated in the tubing package instructions.
■ Open the flow clamp and prime the tubing and filter. Gently tap the tubing *to dislodge air bubbles trapped in the Y-ports.* If necessary, attach a time tape to the lipid emulsion container *to monitor fluid intake.*
■ Label the tubing, noting the date and time the tubing was hung.
■ Thoroughly disinfect the access port on the primary tubing with an antiseptic pad and allow it to dry.[8]
■ Trace the tubing from the patient to its point of origin and then connect the lipid emulsion tubing to the primary tubing below the in-line filter.[9]
■ If this is the patient's first lipid infusion, administer a test dose at the rate of 1 mL/minute for 30 minutes.

■ Monitor the patient's vital signs, and watch for signs and symptoms of an adverse reaction, such as fever; flushing, sweating, or chills; a pressure sensation over the eyes; nausea; vomiting; headache; chest and back pain; tachycardia; dyspnea; and cyanosis. An allergic reaction usually stems from either the source of lipids or from eggs, which occur in the emulsion as egg phospholipids, an emulsifying agent.

■ If the patient has no adverse reactions to the test dose, begin the infusion at the prescribed rate. The maximum infusion rate is 125 mL/hour for a 10% lipid emulsion and 60 mL/hour for a 20% lipid emulsion.

■ Remove and discard your gloves and perform hand hygiene.[4,5,6]

■ Document the procedure.[10]

Special considerations

■ Always maintain strict aseptic technique while preparing and handling equipment.[1,11]

■ Observe the patient's reaction to the lipid emulsion. Most patients report a feeling of satiety; some complain of an unpleasant metallic taste.

■ Change the administration set and the lipid emulsion container every 24 hours when given continuously.[1] If lipids are given intermittently, change the administration set with each new container. Change immediately upon suspected contamination, or when the integrity of the system has been compromised.[11]

■ Monitor the patient for hair or skin changes. Also, closely monitor his lipid tolerance rate. Cloudy plasma in a centrifuged sample of citrated blood indicates that the lipids haven't been cleared from the patient's bloodstream.

■ A lipid emulsion may clear from the blood at an accelerated rate in patients with full-thickness burns, multiple traumatic injuries, or a metabolic imbalance. *This is because catecholamines, adrenocortical hormones, thyroxine, and growth hormone enhance lipolysis and embolization of fatty acids.*

■ Obtain weekly laboratory tests, as ordered. Usual tests include liver function studies, prothrombin time, platelet count, and serum triglyceride levels. Whenever possible, draw blood for triglyceride levels at least 6 hours after the completion of the lipid emulsion infusion *to avoid falsely elevated results.*

■ *A lipid emulsion is an excellent medium for bacterial growth.* Therefore, never rehang a partially empty bottle of emulsion.

■ Complete the infusion of lipid emulsions within 12 to 24 hours.[1]

Complications

Immediate or early adverse reactions to lipid emulsion therapy, which occur in fewer than 1% of patients, include fever, dyspnea, cyanosis, nausea and vomiting, headache, flushing, diaphoresis, lethargy, syncope, chest and back pain, slight pressure over the eyes, irritation at the infusion site, hyperlipidemia, hypercoagulability, and thrombocytopenia.

PEDIATRIC ALERT *Thrombocytopenia has been reported in infants receiving a 20% IV lipid emulsion. In premature or low-birth-weight infants, peripheral parenteral nutrition with a lipid emulsion may cause lipids to accumulate in an infant's lungs.*

Delayed but uncommon complications associated with prolonged administration of lipid emulsion include hepatomegaly, splenomegaly, jaundice secondary to central lobular cholestasis, and blood dyscrasias (such as thrombocytopenia, leukopenia, and transient increases in liver function studies). Dry or scaly skin, thinning hair, abnormal liver function studies, and thrombocytopenia may indicate a deficiency of essential fatty acids. For unknown reasons, some patients develop brown pigmentation in the reticuloendothelial system.

Report any adverse reactions to the patient's doctor *so that he can change the parenteral nutrition regimen as needed.*

Documentation

Record the times of all dressing changes and solution changes, the condition of the catheter insertion site, your asssessments of the patient's condition, and any complications and resulting interventions. Document patient and family teaching.

REFERENCES

1 Standard 43. Administration set change. Infusion nursing standards of practice. (2011). *Journal of Infusion Nursing, 34*(1S), S55–S57. (Level I)

2 Standard 28. Filters. Infusion nursing standards of practice. (2011). *Journal of Infusion Nursing, 34*(1S), S33–S34. (Level I)

3 The Joint Commission. (2012). Standard MM.04.01.01. *Comprehensive accreditation manual for hospitals: The official handbook.* Oakbrook Terrace, IL: The Joint Commission. (Level I)

4 The Joint Commission. (2012). Standard NPSG.07.01.01. *Comprehensive accreditation manual for hospitals: The official handbook.* Oakbrook Terrace, IL: The Joint Commission. (Level I)

5 Centers for Disease Control and Prevention. (October 2002). Guideline for hand hygiene in health-care settings. *Morbidity and Mortality Weekly Report, 51*(RR-16), 1–45. (Level I)

6 World Health Organization. (2009). *WHO guidelines on hand hygiene in health care: First global patient safety challenge. Clean care is safer care.* Geneva, Switzerland: World Health Organization. (Level I)

7 The Joint Commission. (2012). Standard NPSG.01.01.01. *Comprehensive accreditation manual for hospitals: The official handbook.* Oakbrook Terrace, IL: The Joint Commission. (Level I)

8 Standard 65. Parenteral nutrition. Infusion nursing standards of practice. (2011). *Journal of Infusion Nursing, 34*(1S), S91–S93. (Level I)

9 U.S. Food and Drug Administration. (2009). "Look. Check. Connect.: Safe Medical Device Connections Save Lives" [Online]. Accessed November 2011 via the Web at http://www.fda.gov/downloads/MedicalDevices/Safety/AlertsandNotices/UCM134873.pdf

10 The Joint Commission. (2012). Standard RC.01.03.01. *Comprehensive accreditation manual for hospitals: The official handbook.* Oakbrook Terrace, IL: The Joint Commission. (Level I)

11 O'Grady, N.P., et al. (2011). "Guidelines for the Prevention of Intravascular Catheter-Related Infections" [Online]. Accessed November 2011 via the Web at http://www.cdc.gov/hicpac/pdf/guidelines/bsi-guidelines-2011.pdf (Level I)

ADDITIONAL REFERENCES

Standard 14. Documentation. Infusion nursing standards of practice. (2011). *Journal of Infusion Nursing, 34*(1S), S20–S21.

Standard 65. Parenteral nutrition. Infusion nursing standards of practice. (2011). *Journal of Infusion Nursing, 34*(1S), S91–93. (Level I)

Weinstein, S.M. (2007). *Plumer's principles and practices of intravenous therapy* (8th ed.). Philadelphia, PA: Lippincott Williams & Wilkins.

LOW-AIR-LOSS THERAPY BED USE

Low-air-loss therapy beds, composed of segmented cushions that provide surface area for pressure relief, help prevent and treat skin breakdown as well as minimize pain. These beds are indicated for patients with skin grafts and surgical flaps, pressure ulcers, edema, and malnutrition as well as for oncology, orthopedic, and transplant patients. Studies have also shown that low-air-loss beds are effective in preventing pressure ulcers in obese patients.[1]

The segmented air cushions, covered by a low-friction fabric, inflate and rest on a bed frame (similar to a standard bed frame), reducing pressure on skin surfaces and diminishing shearing forces when repositioning the patient.

Note: A maximum-inflate feature allows the entire surface to become firm for patient repositioning. The system is also capable of deflating quickly in emergencies.

As with a standard bed frame, the head and foot of the bed can be adjusted. Low-air-loss therapy beds circulate cool air, which helps to evaporate moisture and reduce temperature, thereby reducing excess skin moisture and preventing maceration. (See *Low-air-loss therapy bed.*)

Some models are equipped with pulsation or rotational capability. Pulsation promotes circulation, which improves healing; the rotational capability makes turning easier, helping to mobilize secretions and prevent pulmonary complications. Larger beds are available for patients who weigh more than 300 lb (136 kg). Pressure zones may also be adjusted, and adjustable lumbar supports are available in some models.

A low-air-loss therapy bed is contraindicated for patients with an unstable cervical, thoracic, or lumbar fracture. Patients with uncontrolled diarrhea, hemodynamic instability, severe agitation, or uncontrolled claustrophobia may not benefit from this bed.

Equipment

Low-air-loss therapy bed ▪ turning sheet ▪ Optional: gloves.

Preparation of equipment

The manufacturer's representative or a trained staff member usually prepares the bed for use. The unit is plugged in and turned on to inflate the bed. Make sure the bed inflates properly and the equipment is in working order. The settings are adjusted as appropriate (such as degrees of rotation). Fully inflate until the patient is moved onto it.

Implementation

▪ Perform hand hygiene and, if necessary, put on gloves.[2,3,4]
▪ Confirm the patient's identity using at least two patient identifiers according to your facility's policy.[5]

EQUIPMENT

Low-air-loss therapy bed

The low-air-loss therapy bed reduces pressure on skin surfaces and may be used for patients such with conditions as immobility, malnutrition, incontinence, contractures, fractures, or amputations. Some models come with special features, such as rotational or percussion options.

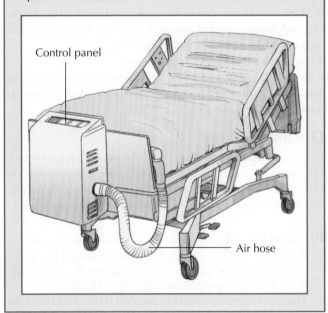

▪ Explain and, if possible, demonstrate the operation of the low-air-loss therapy bed. Tell the patient the reason for its use. Explain any special features of the bed (such as lumbar supports and rotation).
▪ With the help of four or more coworkers, transfer the patient to the bed using a lift sheet. (See "Transfer within a facility," page 741.)
▪ Start with the settings as set by the representative, monitor the patient for comfort, and ensure proper functioning of the bed.
▪ Adjust the inflation settings on the control panel according to the patient's comfort and therapeutic use.
▪ Remove and discard your gloves if worn, and perform hand hygiene.[2,3,4]
▪ Document the procedure.[6,7]

Special considerations

▪ Encourage coughing and deep breathing every 2 hours.
▪ If the bed doesn't rotate, turn the patient at least every 2 hours and reposition using an approved turning sheet. Some beds come with special foam wedges that are used for repositioning.
▪ To turn and reposition the patient, use the maximum-inflate feature to fully inflate the bed. Use the turning sheet to position

the patient and place the pillows or foam wedges. Then return the bed to the correct patient settings.

■ If the bed is rotational, verify that invasive lines and tubes are secured at the correct angle *to minimize the risk for binding, disconnecting, or dislodging.*

■ To position a bedpan, deflate the seat portion of the bed, roll the patient away from you, and place the bedpan on the turning sheet. Then reposition the patient. To remove the bedpan, hold it steady, roll the patient away from you, and remove the bedpan. Then reinflate the seat portion of the bed.

■ Don't use pins or clamps to secure sheets or tubing, *because they may puncture the bed and result in air loss.* Take care to avoid puncturing the bed when giving injections.

■ Assess the patient's skin every 2 hours.

■ Engage the emergency or cardiopulmonary resuscitation button during cardiac arrest *to help ensure adequate chest compressions.*

Documentation

Record the duration of therapy and the patient's response to it. Document the condition of the patient's skin, including the presence of pressure ulcers and other wounds. Document the patient's comfort level and tolerance of rotational angles, as applicable.[6,7]

REFERENCES

1 Pemberton, V., et al. (2009). The effect of using a low-air-loss surface on the skin integrity of obese patients: Results of a pilot study. *Ostomy/Wound Management, 55*(2), 44–48.

2 The Joint Commission. (2012). Standard NPSG.07.01.01. *Comprehensive accreditation manual for hospitals: The official handbook.* Oakbrook Terrace, IL: The Joint Commission. (Level I)

3 Centers for Disease Control and Prevention. (October 2002). Guideline for hand hygiene in health-care settings. *Morbidity and Mortality Weekly Report, 51*(RR-16), 1–45. (Level I)

4 World Health Organization. (2009). *WHO guidelines on hand hygiene in health care: First global patient safety challenge. Clean care is safer care.* Geneva, Switzerland: World Health Organization. (Level I)

5 The Joint Commission. (2012). Standard NPSG.01.01.01. *Comprehensive accreditation manual for hospitals: The official handbook.* Oakbrook Terrace, IL: The Joint Commission. (Level I)

6 The Joint Commission. (2012). Standard RC.01.03.01. *Comprehensive accreditation manual for hospitals: The official handbook.* Oakbrook Terrace, IL: The Joint Commission. (Level I)

7 The Joint Commission. (2012). Standard RC.02.01.01. *Comprehensive accreditation manual for hospitals: The official handbook.* Oakbrook Terrace, IL: The Joint Commission. (Level I)

ADDITIONAL REFERENCES

Ahrens, T., et al. (2004). Effect of kinetic therapy on pulmonary complications. *American Journal of Critical Care, 13*(5), 376–383.

Brienza, D.M., & Geyer, M.J. (2005). Using support surfaces to manage tissue integrity. *Advances in Skin and Wound Care, 18*(3), 151–157.

Collins, F. (2004). Russka pressure-relieving low air-loss mattress system," *British Journal of Nursing, 13*(6 Suppl.), S50–54.

McInnes, E., et al. (2011). Support surfaces for pressure ulcer prevention. *Cochrane Database of Systemic Reviews,* (4), CD001735.

Ochs, R.F., et al. (2005). Comparison of air-fluidized therapy with other support surfaces used to treat pressure ulcers in nursing home residents. *Ostomy Wound Management, 51*(2), 38–68.

LUMBAR PUNCTURE, ASSISTING

Lumbar puncture involves the insertion of a sterile needle into the subarachnoid space of the spinal canal, usually between the third and fourth lumbar vertebrae. This procedure is used to determine the presence of blood in cerebrospinal fluid (CSF), to obtain CSF specimens for laboratory analysis, and to inject dyes for contrast in radiologic studies. The pressure of CSF, which flows freely between the brain and the spinal column, may be measured during the procedure. It's also used to administer drugs or anesthetics.

Performed by a doctor with a nurse assisting, lumbar puncture requires sterile technique and careful patient positioning. This procedure is contraindicated in patients with increased intracranial pressure (ICP) with mass effect, with a lumbar deformity, with a platelet count of less than $50,000/mm^3$, who have an International Normalized Ratio greater than 1.5, who are receiving anticoagulants,[1] or who have an infection at the puncture site.

Equipment

Overbed table ■ one or two pairs of sterile gloves for the doctor ■ sterile gloves for the nurse ■ face masks[1] ■ antiseptic solution ■ sterile gauze pads ■ antiseptic pads ■ sterile fenestrated drape ■ 3-mL syringe for local anesthetic ■ 25G ¾" sterile needle for injecting anesthetic ■ local anesthetic (usually 1% lidocaine) ■ 22G 3½" spinal needle with stylet[2] ■ three-way stopcock ■ manometer ■ small adhesive bandage ■ three sterile collection tubes with stoppers ■ laboratory request forms ■ labels ■ light source such as a gooseneck lamp ■ sterile marker ■ sterile labels ■ laboratory transport bag ■ Optional: patient-care reminder.

Disposable lumbar puncture trays contain most of the needed sterile equipment.

Implementation

■ Perform a preprocedure verification *to make sure that all relevant documentation, related information, and equipment are available and correctly identified to the patient's identifiers.*[3]

■ Perform hand hygiene.[4,5,6]

■ Gather the equipment and take it to the patient's bedside.

■ Confirm the patient's identity using at least two patient identifiers according to your facility's policy.[7]

■ Explain the procedure to the patient *to ease his anxiety and ensure his cooperation.*

■ Make sure an informed consent form has been obtained and documented in the patient's medication record.[8,9]

■ Inform the patient that he may experience headache after lumbar puncture, but reassure him that his cooperation during the procedure minimizes such an effect.

■ Check the patient's history for hypersensitivity to local anesthetic.

■ Immediately before the procedure, provide privacy and instruct the patient to void.

Positioning for lumbar puncture

Have the patient lie on his side at the edge of the bed, with his chin tucked to his chest and his knees drawn up to his abdomen. Make sure the patient's spine is curved and his back is at the edge of the bed (as shown below). *This position widens the spaces between the vertebrae, easing insertion of the needle.*

To help the patient maintain this position, place one of your hands behind his neck and the other hand behind his knees, and pull gently. Hold the patient firmly in this position throughout the procedure *to prevent accidental needle displacement.* Typically, the doctor inserts the needle between the third and fourth lumbar vertebrae (as shown below).

Patient positioning

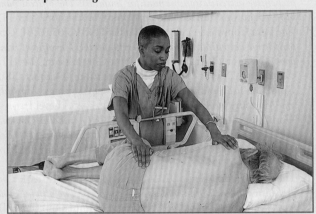

Needle insertion

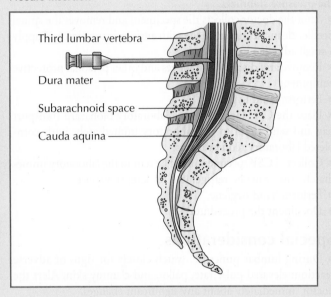

Third lumbar vertebra

Dura mater

Subarachnoid space

Cauda aquina

■ Perform hand hygiene.[4,5,6]

■ Open the equipment tray on an overbed table, being careful not to contaminate the sterile field when you open the wrapper. Label all medications, medication containers, and other solutions on and off the sterile field.[10]

■ Provide adequate lighting at the puncture site, and adjust the height of the patient's bed *to allow the doctor to perform the procedure comfortably.*

■ Position the patient and reemphasize the importance of remaining as still as possible *to minimize discomfort and trauma.* (See *Positioning for lumbar puncture.*)

■ Perform hand hygiene.[4,5,6]

■ Put on a cap, mask with face shield, sterile gown, and sterile gloves.[1]

■ Conduct a time-out before starting the procedure *to determine that the correct patient, site, positioning, and procedure are identified and confirmed as applicable.*[11]

■ The doctor cleans the puncture site with sterile gauze pads soaked in antiseptic solution, wiping in a circular motion away from the puncture site; he uses three different pads *to prevent contamination of spinal tissues by the body's normal skin flora.* Next, he drapes the area with the fenestrated drape *to provide a sterile field.* (If the doctor uses antiseptic sponges instead of sterile gauze pads, he may remove his sterile gloves and put on another pair *to avoid introducing antiseptic solution into the subarachnoid space with the lumbar puncture needle.*)

NURSING ALERT *Chlorhexidine is neurotoxic and shouldn't be used to prepare the skin for lumbar puncture.*[12]

■ If no ampule of anesthetic is included on the equipment tray, disinfect the injection port of a multidose vial of anesthetic with an antiseptic pad. Then invert the vial 45 degrees so that the doctor can insert a 25G needle and syringe and withdraw the anesthetic for injection.

■ Before the doctor injects the anesthetic, tell the patient he'll experience a transient burning sensation and local pain. Ask him to report any other persistent pain or sensations *because they may indicate irritation or puncture of a nerve root, requiring repositioning of the needle.*

■ When the doctor inserts the sterile spinal needle into the subarachnoid space between the third and fourth lumbar vertebrae, instruct the patient to remain still and breathe normally. If necessary, hold the patient firmly in position *to prevent sudden movement that may displace the needle.*

■ If the lumbar puncture is being performed to administer contrast media for radiologic studies or spinal anesthetic, the doctor injects the dye or anesthetic at this time.

■ When the needle is in place, the doctor attaches a manometer with a three-way stopcock to the needle hub *to read CSF pressure.* If ordered, help the patient extend his legs *to provide a more accurate pressure reading.*

■ The doctor then detaches the manometer and allows CSF to drain from the needle hub into the collection tubes. When he has collected 2 to 3 mL in each tube, mark the tubes in sequence and insert a stopper to secure them. Label the specimens in the presence of the patient to prevent mislabeling.[7]

■ If the doctor suspects an obstruction in the spinal subarachnoid space, he may check for Queckenstedt's sign. After he takes an initial CSF pressure reading, compress the patient's jugular vein for 10 seconds, as ordered. *This increases ICP and, if no subarachnoid block exists, causes CSF pressure to rise as well.* The doctor then takes pressure readings every 10 seconds until the pressure stabilizes.

■ After the doctor collects the specimens and removes the spinal needle, clean the puncture site with antiseptic solution and apply a small adhesive bandage.

■ Remove and discard your gloves and other personal protective equipment.

■ Perform hand hygiene.[4,5,6]

■ Place the CSF specimens in a laboratory biohazard transport bag and send them to the laboratory immediately, with completed laboratory request forms.

■ Collected CSF specimens must be sent to the laboratory immediately; they can't be refrigerated for later transport.

■ Perform hand hygiene.[4,5,6]

■ Document the procedure.[13,14]

Special considerations

■ During lumbar puncture, watch closely for signs of adverse reaction: elevated pulse rate, pallor, and clammy skin. Alert the doctor immediately about any significant changes.

■ The doctor may order for the patient to remain flat or at a 30-degree angle for 30 minutes to several hours. Check the doctor's orders for the specific position and duration.

■ Encourage the patient to drink fluids after the procedure *to restore spinal fluid volume and reduce the risk of headache.*

■ Check the puncture site for redness, swelling, and drainage every hour for the first 4 hours, and then every 4 hours for the first 24 hours.

■ If CSF pressure is elevated, assess the patient's neurologic status every 15 minutes for 4 hours or according to your facility's policy. If he's stable, assess him every hour for 2 hours and then every 4 hours or according to the pretest schedule.

■ In obese patients, the doctor may use an ultrasound *to help determine accurate needle placement.*[15]

Complications

Headache is the most common adverse effect of lumbar puncture. Others may include a reaction to the anesthetic, meningitis, epidural or subdural abscess, bleeding into the spinal canal, CSF leakage through the dural defect remaining after needle withdrawal, local pain caused by nerve root irritation, edema or hematoma at the puncture site, transient difficulty voiding, and fever. The most serious complications of lumbar puncture, although rare, are tonsillar herniation and medullary compression.

Documentation

Record the initiation and completion times of the procedure, the patient's response, administration of drugs, number of specimen tubes collected, time of transport to the laboratory, and color, consistency, and any other characteristics of the collected specimens. Document patient teaching.[13,14]

REFERENCES

1 Siegel, J.D., et al. "2007 Guideline for Isolation Precautions: Preventing Transmission of Infectious Agents in Healthcare Settings" [Online]. Accessed September 2011 via the Web at http://www.cdc.gov/hicpac/2007ip/2007isolationprecautions.html

2 Armon, C., et al. (2005). Addendum to assessment: Prevention of post-lumbar puncture headaches: Report of the Therapeutics and Technology Assessment Subcommittee of the American Academy of Neurology. *Neurology, 65*(4), 510–512.

3 The Joint Commission. (2012). Standard UP.01.01.01. *Comprehensive accreditation manual for hospitals: The official handbook.* Oakbrook Terrace, IL: The Joint Commission. (Level I)

4 The Joint Commission. (2012). Standard NPSG.07.01.01. *Comprehensive accreditation manual for hospitals: The official handbook.* Oakbrook Terrace, IL: The Joint Commission. (Level I)

5 Centers for Disease Control and Prevention. (October 2002). Guideline for hand hygiene in health-care settings. *Morbidity and Mortality Weekly Report, 51*(RR-16), 1–45. (Level I)

6 World Health Organization. (2009). *WHO guidelines on hand hygiene in health care: First global patient safety challenge. Clean care is safer care.* Geneva, Switzerland: World Health Organization. (Level I)

7 The Joint Commission. (2012). Standard NPSG.01.01.01. *Comprehensive accreditation manual for hospitals: The official handbook.* Oakbrook Terrace, IL: The Joint Commission. (Level I)

8 The Joint Commission. (2012). Standard RI.01.03.01. *Comprehensive accreditation manual for hospitals: The official handbook.* Oakbrook Terrace, IL: The Joint Commission. (Level I)

9 Centers for Medicare & Medicaid Services, Department of Health and Human Services. (2006). "Conditions of Participation: Patients' Rights," 42 CFR part 482.13 [Online]. Accessed November 2011 via the Web at https://www.cms.gov/CFCsAndCoPs/downloads/finalpatientrightsrule.pdf

10 The Joint Commission. (2012). Standard NPSG.03.04.01. *Comprehensive accreditation manual for hospitals: The official handbook.* Oakbrook Terrace, IL: The Joint Commission. (Level I)

11 The Joint Commission. (2012). Standard UP.01.03.01. *Comprehensive accreditation manual for hospitals: The official handbook.* Oakbrook Terrace, IL: The Joint Commission. (Level I)

12 Recommended practices for preoperative patient skin antisepsis. (2010). In R. Conner, et al. (Eds.). *Perioperative standards and recommended practices.* Denver, CO: AORN.

13 The Joint Commission. (2012). Standard RC.01.03.01. *Comprehensive accreditation manual for hospitals: The official handbook.* Oakbrook Terrace, IL: The Joint Commission. (Level I)

14 The Joint Commission. (2012). Standard RC.02.01.01. *Comprehensive accreditation manual for hospitals: The official handbook.* Oakbrook Terrace, IL: The Joint Commission. (Level I)

15 Strony, R. (2010). Ultrasound-assisted lumbar puncture in obese patients. *Critical Care Clinics, 26*(4), 661–664.

ADDITIONAL REFERENCES

Lynn-McHale Wiegand, D. (Ed.). (2011). *AACN procedure manual for critical care* (6th ed.). Philadelphia, PA: Saunders.

Nettina, S.M. (2010). *Lippincott manual of nursing practice* (9th ed.). Philadelphia, PA: Lippincott Williams & Wilkins.

MANUAL VENTILATION

A handheld resuscitation bag is an inflatable device that can be attached to a face mask or directly to an endotracheal (ET) or tracheostomy tube, allowing manual delivery of oxygen or room air to the lungs of a patient who can't breathe by himself. Typically used in emergencies, manual ventilation also can be performed while the patient is temporarily disconnected from a mechanical ventilator, such as during a tubing change, during transport, or before suctioning. In such instances, use of the handheld resuscitation bag maintains ventilation.

During cardiopulmonary resuscitation (CPR), however, using a handheld resuscitation bag to administer rescue breaths is less important than providing high-quality chest compressions. Lone rescuers should begin chest compressions first. After 30 compressions, the rescuer should then administer two breaths. When a second person arrives, a handheld resuscitation bag can be used to administer two breaths after every 30 compressions.

Equipment

Handheld resuscitation bag ▪ mask, if needed ▪ oxygen source (wall unit or tank) ▪ oxygen tubing ▪ nipple adapter attached to oxygen flowmeter ▪ gloves ▪ gown, goggles, or face shield, if needed ▪ oropharyngeal or nasopharyngeal airway ▪ Optional: oxygen accumulator (oxygen reservoir), positive end-expiratory pressure (PEEP) valve, suction source, tubing, catheters. (See *Using a PEEP valve*.)

Preparation of equipment

Unless the patient is intubated or has a tracheostomy, select a mask that fits snugly over the mouth and nose. Attach the mask to the resuscitation bag.

If oxygen is readily available, connect the handheld resuscitation bag to the oxygen source. Attach one end of the tubing to the bottom of the bag and the other end to the nipple adapter on the flowmeter of the oxygen source.

Turn on the oxygen, and adjust the flow rate to 15 L. If the patient has a low partial pressure of arterial oxygen, he'll need a higher fraction of inspired oxygen (FIO_2). *To increase the concentration of inspired oxygen,* you can add an oxygen accumulator (also called an oxygen reservoir). This device, which attaches to an adapter on the bottom of the bag, permits an FIO_2 of up to 100%. If time allows, set up suction equipment.

Implementation

▪ Perform hand hygiene,[1,2,3] put on gloves and other personal protective equipment, and follow standard precautions.[4]
▪ Explain the procedure to the patient. Answer any questions *to decrease anxiety and increase cooperation.*

Using a PEEP valve

To add positive end-expiratory pressure (PEEP) to manual ventilation, attach a PEEP valve to the resuscitation bag. *This addition may improve oxygenation if the patient hasn't responded to increased fraction of inspired oxygen levels.* Always use a PEEP valve to manually ventilate a patient who has been receiving PEEP on the ventilator.

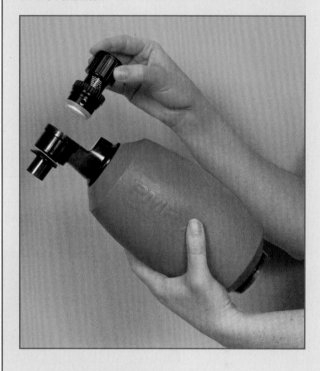

▪ Before using the handheld resuscitation bag, check the patient's upper airway for foreign objects. If present, remove them *because this alone may restore spontaneous respirations in some instances. Also, foreign matter or secretions can obstruct the airway and impede resuscitation efforts.*
▪ Suction the patient *to remove any secretions that may obstruct the airway.* If necessary, insert an oropharyngeal or nasopharyngeal airway *to maintain airway patency.* If the patient has a tracheostomy or ET tube in place, suction the tube.
▪ If appropriate, remove the bed's headboard and stand at the head of the bed *to help keep the patient's neck extended and to free space at the side of the bed for other activities such as CPR.*
▪ Unless the patient has evidence of head or neck trauma, use the head-tilt, chin-lift maneuver to open the patient's airway *to move the tongue away from the base of the pharynx and prevent obstruction of the airway.*[5]
▪ Apply the mask. (See *How to apply a handheld resuscitation bag and mask,* page 466.)
▪ Keeping your nondominant hand on the patient's mask, exert downward pressure *to seal the mask against his face.* For

EQUIPMENT

How to apply a handheld resuscitation bag and mask

1. Place the mask over the patient's face so that the apex of the triangle covers the bridge of his nose and the base lies between his lower lip and chin, creating a tight seal.

2. Make sure that the patient's mouth remains open underneath the mask. Attach the bag to the mask and to the tubing leading to the oxygen source.

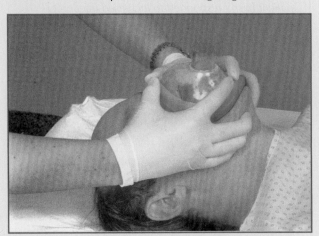

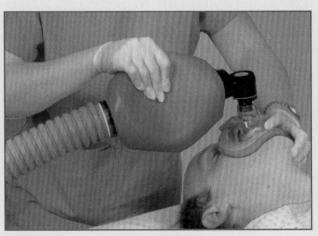

3. Or, if the patient has a tracheostomy or endotracheal tube in place, remove the mask from the bag and attach the handheld resuscitation bag directly to the tube.

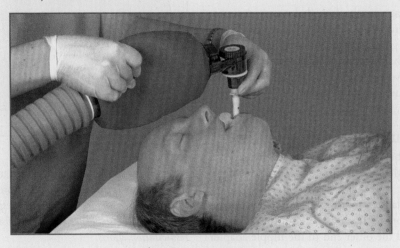

the adult patient, use your dominant hand to compress the bag to deliver 600 mL of air over 1 second *to produce a rise in the patient's chest.*[5]

PEDIATRIC ALERT *For infants and children, use a pediatric handheld resuscitation bag. With infants and children, use only enough force and tidal volume to make the chest rise visibly with each bag compression. Each breath should be given over 1 second.*[5]

■ Deliver breaths with the patient's own inspiratory effort, if any is present. Don't attempt to deliver a breath as the patient exhales.

■ Observe the patient's chest *to ensure that it rises and falls with each compression.*[5] If ventilation fails to occur, check the fit of the mask and the patency of the patient's airway; if necessary, reposition his head and ensure patency with an oral airway.

■ Assist with ET intubation if necessary.

■ Remove and discard your gloves, remove other personal protective equipment, and perform hand hygiene.[1,2,3]

■ Document the procedure.[6]

Special considerations

■ Avoid neck hyperextension if the patient has a possible cervical injury; instead, use the jaw-thrust technique to open the airway. If you need both hands to keep the patient's mask in place with a good seal and maintain hyperextension, use the lower part of your arm to compress the bag against your side.

■ Observe for vomiting through the clear part of the mask. If vomiting occurs, stop the procedure immediately, lift the mask, wipe and suction vomitus, and resume resuscitation.

■ Underventilation commonly occurs because the handheld resuscitation bag is difficult to keep positioned tightly on the patient's face while ensuring an open airway. What's more, the volume of air delivered to the patient varies with the type of bag used and the hand size of the person compressing the bag. For these reasons, have someone assist with the procedure, if possible.

■ It isn't possible to deliver an accurate or exact tidal volume while using a handheld resuscitation bag and mask.[7]

■ If a second rescuer relieves you in performing chest compressions during CPR and you're using the handheld resuscitation bag and mask to deliver breaths, make sure the use of the bag doesn't interfere with the performance of chest compressions.[5]

Complications

Aspiration of vomitus can result in pneumonia, and gastric distention may result from air forced into the patient's stomach. In an emergency, hyperventilation of the patient may cause increased intrathoracic pressure with a subsequent decrease in coronary and cerebral perfusion pressures.

Documentation

In an emergency, record the date and time of the procedure; the reason for initiating the procedure; any complications and the nursing action taken; and the patient's response to treatment, according to your facility's protocol for respiratory arrest.

In a nonemergency situation, record the date and time of the procedure as well as the reason and length of time the patient was disconnected from mechanical ventilation and received manual ventilation. Note the patient's tolerance of the procedure along with any complications and nursing actions taken.

REFERENCES

1 The Joint Commission. (2012). Standard NPSG.07.01.01. *Comprehensive accreditation manual for hospitals: The official handbook.* Oakbrook Terrace, IL: The Joint Commission. (Level I)

2 Centers for Disease Control and Prevention. (October 2002). Guideline for hand hygiene in health-care settings. *Morbidity and Mortality Weekly Report, 51*(RR-16), 1–45. (Level 1)

3 World Health Organization. (2009). *WHO guidelines on hand hygiene in health care: First global patient safety challenge. Clean care is safer care.* Geneva, Switzerland: World Health Organization. (Level I)

4 Siegel, J.D., et al. "2007 Guideline for Isolation Precautions: Preventing Transmission of Infectious Agents in Healthcare Settings" [Online]. Accessed September 2011 via the Web at http://www.cdc.gov/hicpac/2007ip/2007isolationprecautions.html

5 American Heart Association. (2010). 2010 American Heart Association guidelines for cardiopulmonary resuscitation and emergency cardiovascular care. *Circulation, 122*(Suppl. 3), S729–S767, S876–S908. (Level I)

6 The Joint Commission. (2012). Standard RC.01.03.01. *Comprehensive accreditation manual for hospitals: The official handbook.* Oakbrook Terrace, IL: The Joint Commission. (Level I)

7 Lee, H.M., et al. (2008). Can you deliver accurate tidal volume by manual resuscitator? *Emergency Medicine Journal, 25*(10), 632–634. (Level VI)

ADDITIONAL REFERENCES

Lynn-McHale Wiegand, D. (Ed.). (2011). *AACN procedure manual for critical care* (6th ed.). Philadelphia, PA: Saunders.

Nettina, S.M. (2010). *Lippincott manual of nursing practice* (9th ed.). Philadelphia, PA: Lippincott Williams & Wilkins.

MASSIVE INFUSION DEVICE USE

A massive infusion device is a mechanical device that's used in patients who need rapid fluid replacement with blood products and IV fluids. Patients with life-threatening conditions, such as severe trauma, gastrointestinal hemorrhage, postoperative hemorrhage, septic shock, or burns may need the use of a rapid infusion device to deliver large volumes of fluid within a short period.[1]

A massive infusion device can warm IV fluid or blood to room temperature, and then administer the fluid rapidly at rates up to 30,000 mL/hour. Remember that the device requires specialized IV tubing that expands under pressure.[1]

Equipment

IV fluids or blood products ■ specialized infusion set ■ replaceable filter or vent ■ blood administration set ■ IV pole ■ gown and face protection ■ gloves ■ large-bore needle ■ massive infusion device ■ antiseptic solution ■ male luer-lock cap ■ blankets.

Implementation

■ Verify the doctor's order.

■ Confirm that written informed consent was obtained and that the consent is in the patient's medical record.[3]

■ Verify that baseline hemoglobin, hematocrit, electrolyte levels, and coagulation studies have been obtained *to serve as a comparison and help guide fluid replacement.*[2]

■ Perform hand hygiene.[3,4,5]

■ Confirm the patient's identity using with at least two patient identifiers according to your facility's policy.[6]

■ Make sure that the patient and his family understand the procedure. Answer any questions *to evaluate their understanding of the information provided.*

■ Insert an indwelling urinary catheter, as ordered, if the patient doesn't already have one in place, *to help monitor fluid resuscitation efforts.* (See "Indwelling urinary catheter insertion," page 377.)

■ Perform hand hygiene and put on sterile gloves and other personal protective equipment as needed.[3,4,5]

■ Make sure that the patient has patent IV access. If he doesn't, insert an IV catheter *to administer IV fluid and medications, as needed, until a central venous catheter can be inserted.* (See "IV catheter insertion and removal," page 421.)

Changing the infusion bag

Follow these steps when an infusion is empty and you need to replace it with another infusion bag:

■ Close the clamp on the side of the Y-connector with the empty bag, and then open the clamp on the side of the Y-connector with the remaining full infusion bag.

■ Turn the switch at the top of the pressure chamber to OFF.

■ Open the pressure chamber door, remove the empty bag from the Y-connector, and replace it with a new one.

■ Close and latch the pressure chamber door, and turn the switch at the top of the pressure chamber to ON. Always have a new infusion bag ready to infuse *because any interruption in fluid or blood administration may cause a sudden drop in the patient's blood pressure, which may harm the patient's vital organs.*

■ Assist the doctor with central venous catheter or pulmonary artery catheter insertion *to facilitate administration of large fluid volumes and to help monitor the patient's fluid status.* (See "Central venous access catheter," page 133.)[1]

■ Assist the doctor with arterial catheter insertion *for continuous blood pressure assessment.* (See "Arterial pressure monitoring," page 29.)[1]

■ Turn on the infusion device *to allow the system to warm up.*

■ If infusing blood products, follow your facility's policy for pretransfusion blood verification with two qualified health care providers.[7]

■ Remove the administration set from its packaging and close all of the clamps on the Y-set.

■ Connect fluid or blood, as ordered, to each side of the Y-set and hang the bags on the hooks provided within the rapid infuser pressure chambers. Leave the chamber doors open.[1]

■ Secure the heat exchanger and gas vent filter in their proper positions following the manufacturer's instructions.[1]

■ Fill the drip chambers on the administration set halfway (by squeezing them) *to prevent air from entering the tubing.*[1]

■ Open the clamp on one side of the Y-set, remove the cap from the end of the tubing, open the clamp on the lower end of the tubing, remove the filter from its holder, and invert it. Then, begin priming the tubing of the administration set. Tap the filter *to help remove air.* Inspect the tubing and filter when finished *to make sure there are no air bubbles.*[1]

■ Slowly begin the infusion to assess for air bubbles; if more than ¼" (0.6 cm) of air remains in the top of the filter, replace it.[1]

■ Put a new male luer-lock cap on the end of the tubing, close the clamps, and then close and latch the pressure chamber doors.

■ Perform function and alarm checks according to the manufacturer's instructions *to make sure that the machine is functioning properly.*

■ When the temperature readout on the infusion device reaches 106° F (41° C), turn the switch at the top of the pressure cham-

ber to ON. *Turning on the machine causes the chambers to pressurize to 300 mm Hg, allowing fluid to flow through the administration tubing at a faster rate than with gravity alone.*[1]

■ Clean the injection port with antiseptic solution according to your facility's policy. Trace the tubing from the patient to its point of origin *to make sure that you're attaching the tubing to the proper port,* and then connect the distal end of the tubing to the patient's IV catheter and begin the infusion.

■ Monitor the patient's vital signs every 5 to 15 minutes, as indicated. As the patient's condition stabilizes, monitor vital signs less frequently (every 30 minutes until the patient's blood pressure is stable for longer than 2 hours), according to your facility policy.

■ Monitor core temperature every 15 to 30 minutes and maintain a core temperature no lower than 97° F (36° C) *to prevent hypothermia-induced coagulopathies.*[1]

■ Assess the patient's hemodynamic parameters every 15 to 30 minutes and urine output every 30 to 60 minutes, as ordered, *to evaluate the patient's fluid volume status, which indicates the effectiveness of fluid resuscitation and guides therapy.*

■ Inspect the IV sites every 15 minutes; *rapid infusion increases the risk for infiltration.*

■ If the patient is receiving blood products, monitor him closely for signs of transfusion reaction, such as fever, chills, flushing, nausea, chest tightness, restlessness, apprehension, and back pain.

■ Obtain an arterial blood gas sample *to monitor oxygenation and acid-base balance.* (See "Arterial puncture for blood gas analysis," page 35.)

■ When the infusion is complete, change the IV fluid or blood bag. (See *Changing the infusion bag.*)

■ Discard the empty infusion bag in the proper receptacle or per your facility's policy. Some facilities require empty blood transfusion bags to be returned to the blood bank.

■ Obtain blood samples for hemoglobin, hematocrit, lactic acid, electrolytes, and coagulation studies, as ordered. (See "Venipuncture," page 781.)

■ Discard trash in the proper receptacles.

■ Cover the patient with blankets *to keep him warm and prevent hypothermia.*

■ Remove and discard your gloves and other personal protective equipment, as appropriate. Perform hand hygiene.[3,4,5]

■ Document the procedure.[8]

Special considerations

■ Rapid infusion devices are designed for use during rapid fluid infusion only; they aren't appropriate when a specific drip rate is required.

■ Most devices increase the flow rate gradually *to prevent damage to the vein;* adjust the roller clamp if the rate needs to be decreased.

Complications

Possible complications include electrolyte imbalance, fluid overload, acid-base imbalance, infiltration (extravasation), pulmonary edema, heart failure, interstitial edema, acute respiratory distress syndrome, and hypothermia.

Documentation

Document the transfusion of all blood products in the patient's record; include the product type, the date and time of the infusion, and the unique number or lot number for blood products. Obtain the patient's core temperature before the start of massive infusions, and monitor it during and afterwards. Carefully document the amounts and types of fluids given and correlating vital signs. Incorporate your documentation of massive fluid infusion into the existing required documentation protocol for resuscitation documentation.

REFERENCES

1 Lynn-McHale Wiegand, D. (Ed.). (2011). *AACN procedure manual for critical care* (6th ed.). Philadelphia, PA: Saunders.
2 The Joint Commission. (2012). Standard RI.01.03.01. *Comprehensive accreditation manual for hospitals: The official handbook.* Oakbrook Terrace, IL: The Joint Commission. (Level I)
3 The Joint Commission. (2012). Standard NPSG.07.01.01. *Comprehensive accreditation manual for hospitals: The official handbook.* Oakbrook Terrace, IL: The Joint Commission. (Level I)
4 Centers for Disease Control and Prevention. (October 2002). Guideline for hand hygiene in health-care settings. *Morbidity and Mortality Weekly Report, 51*(RR-16), 1–45. (Level 1)
5 World Health Organization. (2009). *WHO guidelines on hand hygiene in health care: First global patient safety challenge. Clean care is safer care.* Geneva, Switzerland: World Health Organization. (Level I)
6 The Joint Commission. (2012). Standard NPSG.01.01.01. *Comprehensive accreditation manual for hospitals: The official handbook.* Oakbrook Terrace, IL: The Joint Commission. (Level I)
7 The Joint Commission. (2012). Standard NPSG.01.03.01. *Comprehensive accreditation manual for hospitals: The official handbook.* Oakbrook Terrace, IL: The Joint Commission. (Level I)
8 The Joint Commission. (2012). Standard RC.01.03.01. *Comprehensive accreditation manual for hospitals: The official handbook.* Oakbrook Terrace, IL: The Joint Commission. (Level I)

ADDITIONAL REFERENCES

Kleinman, S. "Massive Blood Transfusion" [Online]. Accessed January 2012 via the Web at http://www.uptodate.com/contents/massive-blood-transfusion
Siegel, J.D., et al. "2007 Guideline for Isolation Precautions: Preventing Transmission of Infectious Agents in Healthcare Settings" [Online]. Accessed September 2011 via the Web at http://www.cdc.gov/hicpac/2007ip/2007isolationprecautions.html

MECHANICAL TRACTION MANAGEMENT

Mechanical traction exerts a pulling force on a part of the body—usually the spine, pelvis, or long bones of the arms and legs. It can be used to reduce fractures, treat dislocations, correct or prevent deformities, improve or correct contractures, or decrease muscle spasms. Depending on the injury or condition, an orthopedist may order either skin or skeletal traction.

Applied directly to the skin and thus indirectly to the bone, skin traction is ordered when a light, temporary, or noncontinuous pulling force is required. Contraindications for skin traction include a severe injury with open wounds, an allergy to tape or other skin traction equipment, circulatory disturbances, dermatitis, and varicose veins.

With skeletal traction, an orthopedist inserts a pin or wire through the bone and attaches the traction equipment to the pin or wire to exert a direct, constant, longitudinal pulling force. Indications for skeletal traction include fractures of the tibia, femur, and humerus. Infections such as osteomyelitis contraindicate skeletal traction.

The design of the patient's bed usually dictates the type of traction frame used.

Setup of the specific traction can be done by a nurse with special skills, an orthopedic technician, or the doctor. Instructions for setting up these traction units usually accompany the equipment.

After the patient is placed in the specific type of traction ordered by the orthopedist, the nurse is responsible for assessing and managing the patient's pain; preventing complications from immobility; routinely inspecting the equipment; adding traction weights, as ordered; and, in patients with skeletal traction, monitoring the pin insertion sites for signs of infection.

Equipment
IV-type basic frame
102″ (259 cm) plain bar ▪ 27″ (69 cm) double-clamp bar ▪ 48″ (122 cm) swivel-clamp bar ▪ two 36″ (91 cm) plain bars ▪ four 4″ (10 cm) IV posts with clamps ▪ cross clamp ▪ trapeze with clamp ▪ wall bumper or roller.

IV-type Balkan traction frame
Two 102″ plain bars ▪ two 27″ double-clamp bars ▪ two 48″ swivel-clamp bars ▪ five 36″ plain bars ▪ four 4″ IV posts with clamps ▪ eight cross clamps ▪ trapeze with clamp ▪ wall bumper or roller.

Claw-type basic frame
102″ plain bar ▪ two 66″ (168 cm) swivel-clamp bars ▪ two upper-panel clamps ▪ two lower-panel clamps ▪ trapeze with clamp ▪ wall bumper or roller.

Preparation of equipment

Arrange with central supply or the appropriate department to have the traction equipment transported to the patient's room on a traction cart.

Implementation
▪ Confirm the doctor's order.
▪ Confirm the patient's identity using at least two patient identifiers according to your facility's policy.[1]
▪ Explain the purpose of traction to the patient and answer all questions *to decrease anxiety and increase cooperation.* Emphasize the importance of maintaining proper body alignment after the traction equipment is set up.
▪ Perform hand hygiene.[2,3,4]

IV-type basic traction frame

With an IV-type basic frame, IV posts, placed in IV holders, support the horizontal bars across the foot and head of the bed. These horizontal bars then support the two uprights.

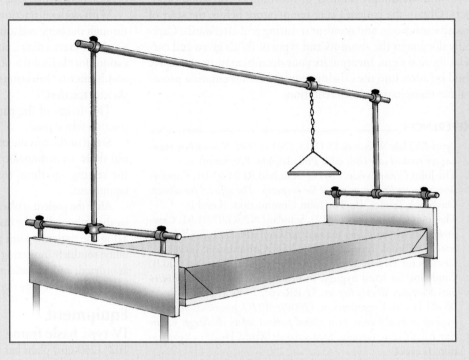

IV-type basic frame

■ Attach one 4″ IV post with clamp to each end of both 36″ horizontal plain bars.

■ Secure an IV post in each IV holder at the bed corners. Using a cross clamp, fasten the 48″ vertical swivel-clamp bar to the middle of the horizontal plain bar at the foot of the bed.

■ Fasten the 27″ vertical double-clamp bar to the middle of the horizontal plain bar at the head of the bed.

■ Attach the 102″ horizontal plain bar to the tops of the two vertical bars, making sure the clamp knobs point up.

■ Using the appropriate clamp, attach the trapeze to the horizontal bar about 2′ (60 cm) from the head of the bed. (See *IV-type basic traction frame*.)

■ Attach a wall bumper or roller to the vertical bar or bars at the head of the bed *to protect the walls from damage caused by the bed or equipment.*

■ Perform hand hygiene.[2,3,4]

■ Document the procedure.[4,5]

IV-type Balkan traction frame

■ Attach one 4″ IV post with clamp to each end of two 36″ horizontal plain bars.

■ Secure an IV post in each IV holder at the bed corners.

■ Attach a 48″ vertical swivel-clamp bar, using a cross clamp, to each IV post clamp on the horizontal plain bar at the foot of the bed.

■ Fasten one 36″ horizontal plain bar across the midpoints of the two 48″ swivel-clamp bars, using two cross clamps.

■ Attach a 27″ vertical double-clamp bar to each IV post clamp on the horizontal bar at the head of the bed.

■ Using two cross clamps, fasten a 36″ horizontal plain bar across the midpoints of two 27″ double-clamp bars.

■ Clamp a 102″ horizontal plain bar onto the vertical bars on each side of the bed; make sure the clamp knobs point up.

■ Use two cross clamps to attach a 36″ horizontal plain bar across the two overhead bars, about 2′ (60 cm) from the head of the bed.

■ Attach the trapeze to this 36″ horizontal bar. (See *IV-type Balkan traction frame.*)

■ Attach a wall bumper or roller to the vertical bar or bars at the head of the bed *to protect the walls from damage caused by the bed or equipment.*

■ Perform hand hygiene.[2,3,4]

■ Document the procedure.[5]

Claw-type basic frame

■ Attach one lower-panel and one upper-panel clamp to each 66″ swivel-clamp bar.

■ Fasten one bar to the footboard and one to the headboard by turning the clamp knobs clockwise until they're tight and then pulling back on the upper clamp's rubberized bar until it's tight.

EQUIPMENT

IV-type Balkan traction frame

The IV-type Balkan frame features IV posts and horizontal bars (secured in the same manner as those for the IV-type basic frame) that support four uprights.

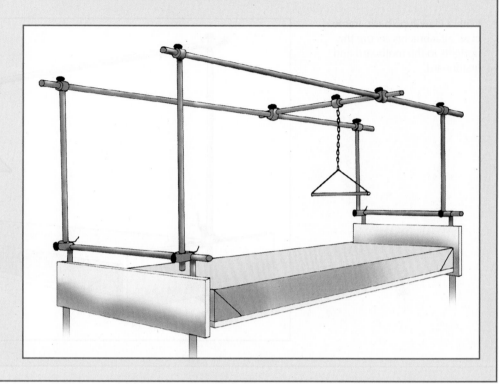

■ Secure the 102″ horizontal plain bar atop the two vertical bars, making sure that the clamp knobs point up.
■ Using the appropriate clamp, attach the trapeze to the horizontal bar about 2′ from the head of the bed. (See *Claw-type basic traction frame,* page 472.)
■ Attach a wall bumper or roller to the vertical bar or bars at the head of the bed *to protect the walls from damage caused by the bed or equipment.*
■ Perform hand hygiene.[2,3,4]
■ Document the procedure.[5]

Special considerations
■ Countertraction must always be provided by the patient's body weight, pull of weights in the opposite direction, or elevation of the bed.
■ The line of pull should be maintained at all times.
■ The weights should hang freely at all times.
■ Friction should be prevented on the traction apparatus.
■ When using skin traction, apply ordered weights slowly and carefully *to avoid jerking the affected extremity.* Arrange the weights so they don't hang over the patient *to avoid injury in case the ropes break.*
■ When applying Buck's traction, make sure the line of pull is always parallel to the bed and not angled downward *to prevent pressure on the heel.* Placing a flat pillow under the extremity may be helpful as long as it doesn't alter the line of pull.

Complications
Immobility during traction may result in pressure ulcers, osteoporosis, muscle atrophy, weakness, or contractures. Immobility can also cause GI disturbances such as constipation; urinary problems, including stasis and calculi; respiratory problems, such as stasis of secretions and hypostatic pneumonia; and circulatory disturbances, including stasis and thrombophlebitis.

Prolonged immobility, especially after traumatic injury, may promote depression or other emotional disturbances. Skeletal traction may cause osteomyelitis originating at the pin or wire sites.

Documentation
In the patient record, document the time the traction was set up and the amount of traction weight used; note that the weight is hanging freely. Record the patient's tolerance of traction. Also document the patent's neurovascular integrity, skin condition, and respiratory status. Note whether any pain medications were administered and their effectiveness.

REFERENCES
1 The Joint Commission. (2012). Standard NPSG.01.01.01. *Comprehensive accreditation manual for hospitals: The official handbook.* Oakbrook Terrace, IL: The Joint Commission. (Level I)

Claw-type basic traction frame

With a claw-type basic frame, claw attachments secure the uprights to the footboard and headboard.

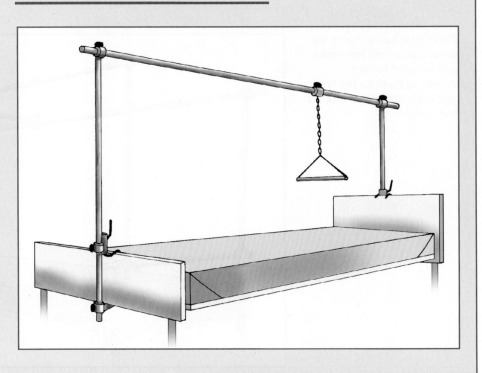

2 The Joint Commission. (2012). Standard NPSG.07.01.01. *Comprehensive accreditation manual for hospitals: The official handbook.* Oakbrook Terrace, IL: The Joint Commission. (Level I)

3 Centers for Disease Control and Prevention. (October 2002). Guideline for hand hygiene in health-care settings. *Morbidity and Mortality Weekly Report, 51*(RR-16), 1–45. (Level 1)

4 World Health Organization. (2009). *WHO guidelines on hand hygiene in health care: First global patient safety challenge. Clean care is safer care.* Geneva, Switzerland: World Health Organization. (Level I)

5 The Joint Commission. (2012). Standard RC.01.03.01. *Comprehensive accreditation manual for hospitals: The official handbook.* Oakbrook Terrace, IL: The Joint Commission. (Level I)

MECHANICAL VENTILATION, POSITIVE PRESSURE

A mechanical ventilator moves air in and out of a patient's lungs. Although the equipment serves to ventilate a patient, it doesn't ensure adequate gas exchange. Mechanical ventilators may use either positive or negative pressure to ventilate patients.

Positive-pressure ventilators cause inspiration while increasing tidal volume (V_T). The inspiratory cycles of these ventilators may vary in volume, pressure, time, or frequency. For example, a volume-cycled ventilator—the type most commonly used—delivers a preset volume of air each time, regardless of the amount of lung resistance. A pressure-cycled ventilator generates flow until the machine reaches a preset pressure regardless of the volume delivered or the time required to achieve the pressure. A time-cycled ventilator generates flow for a preset amount of time. A high-frequency ventilator uses high respiratory rates and low V_T to maintain alveolar ventilation.

Equipment

Oxygen source ▪ air source that can supply 50 psi ▪ mechanical ventilator ▪ humidifier ▪ ventilator circuit tubing, connectors, and adapters ▪ condensation collection trap ▪ spirometer, respirometer, or electronic device to measure flow and volume ▪ in-line thermometer ▪ gloves and other personal protective equipment ▪ handheld resuscitation bag with reservoir ▪ suction equipment ▪ sterile distilled water ▪ equipment for arterial blood gas (ABG) analysis ▪ soft restraints, if indicated ▪ oximeter or capnography device ▪ oral care products ▪ Optional: chlorhexidine oral care product, as prescribed.

Mechanical ventilation glossary

Although a respiratory therapist usually monitors ventilator settings based on the doctor's order, you should understand all of the following terms.

Assist-control mode: The ventilator delivers a preset tidal volume (V_T) at a preset rate; however, the patient can initiate additional breaths, which trigger the ventilator to deliver the preset V_T at positive pressure.

Continuous positive airway pressure (CPAP): This setting prompts the ventilator to deliver positive pressure to the airway throughout the respiratory cycle. It works only on patients who can breathe spontaneously.

Control mode: The ventilator delivers a preset V_T at a fixed rate regardless of whether the patient is breathing spontaneously.

Fraction of inspired oxygen (FIO_2): This is the amount of oxygen delivered to the patient by the ventilator. The dial or digital display on the ventilator that sets this percentage is labeled by the term oxygen concentration or oxygen percentage.

Inspiratory-expiratory (I:E) ratio: This ratio compares the duration of inspiration to the duration of expiration. The I:E ratio of normal, spontaneous breathing is 1:2, meaning that expiration is twice as long as inspiration.

Inspiratory flow rate (IFR): The IFR denotes the V_T delivered within a certain time. Its value can range from 20 to 120 L/minute.

Minute ventilation or minute volume (VE): This measurement results from the multiplication of respiratory rate and V_T.

Peak inspiratory pressure (PIP): Measured by the pressure manometer on the ventilator, PIP reflects the amount of pressure required to deliver a preset V_T.

Plateau pressure: Airway pressure measured after a 0.5 second pause at the end of inspiration, plateau pressure indicates the stiffness of the lungs.

Positive end-expiratory pressure (PEEP): In PEEP mode, the ventilator is triggered to apply positive pressure at the end of each expiration to increase the area for oxygen exchange by helping to inflate and keep open collapsed alveoli.

Pressure support: A ventilator adjunct, pressure support delivers positive pressure, supplementing the spontaneous breath of a patient on the ventilator. It's used to reduce the work of breathing associated with the artificial airway or increase the volume of the patient's spontaneous breath.

Respiratory rate: The number of breaths per minute delivered by the ventilator; also called frequency.

Sensitivity setting: A setting that determines the amount of effort the patient must exert to trigger the inspiratory cycle.

Sigh volume: A ventilator-delivered breath that's $1\frac{1}{4}$ times as large as the patient's V_T.

Synchronized intermittent mandatory ventilation (SIMV): The ventilator delivers a preset number of breaths at a specific V_T. The patient may supplement these mechanical ventilations with his own breaths, in which case the V_T and rate are determined by his own inspiratory ability.

Tidal volume (V_T): This refers to the volume of air delivered to the patient with each cycle, usually 8 to 10 mL/kg.

Preparation of equipment

In most facilities, respiratory therapists assume responsibility for setting up the ventilator. If necessary, however, check the manufacturer's instructions for setting it up. In some cases, you'll need to add sterile distilled water to the humidifier and connect the ventilator to the appropriate gas source.

Plug the ventilator into the electrical outlet and turn it on. Adjust the settings on the ventilator, as ordered. (See *Mechanical ventilation glossary.*) Make sure the ventilator's alarms are set, as ordered, and that the humidifier is filled with the sterile distilled water. Attach a capnographic device to measure carbon dioxide levels *to confirm placement of the endotracheal (ET) tube and detect any disconnection from the ventilator and other complications.*

Implementation

■ Verify the doctor's order.
■ If the patient isn't already intubated, prepare him for intubation. (See "Endotracheal intubation," page 260.)
■ Gather and prepare the necessary equipment.
■ Confirm the patient's identity using with at least two patient identifiers according to your facility's policy.[1]

■ When possible, explain the procedure to the patient and his family *to help reduce anxiety and fear.* Assure the patient and his family that staff members are nearby to provide care.
■ Make sure the patient is being adequately oxygenated, using manual ventilation, if necessary.
■ Perform hand hygiene, and put on gloves and personal protective equipment.[2,3,4]
■ As the patient's condition allows, perform a complete physical assessment, and draw blood for ABG analysis *to establish a baseline.*
■ Assist with intubation (if necessary) and then connect the ET tube to the ventilator. Observe for chest expansion, and auscultate for bilateral breath sounds *to verify that the patient is being ventilated.* Monitor the patient's pulse oximetry.
■ Suction the patient using a closed-suction catheter, if necessary.
■ Monitor the patient's ABG values after the initial ventilator setup (usually 20 to 30 minutes), after changes in ventilator settings, and as the patient's clinical condition indicates *to determine whether the patient is being adequately ventilated and to avoid oxygen toxicity.* Be prepared to adjust ventilator settings based on ABG analysis.
■ Check the ventilator tubing frequently for condensation, *which can cause resistance to airflow and which may also be aspirated by*

the patient. As needed, drain the condensate into a collection trap. Keep the circuit closed during condensate drainage *to prevent bacterial contamination.*[5] Don't drain the condensate into the humidifier *because the condensate may be contaminated with the patient's secretions.* Also avoid accidental drainage of condensation into the patient's airway when moving the tubing or the patient.[5]

■ Inspect heat and moisture exchangers, and replace inserts or filters contaminated by secretions. Note humidifier settings. The heated humidifier should be set to deliver an inspired gas temperature of 91.4° F (33° C) plus or minus 3.6° F (2° C) and should provide a minimum of 30 mg/L of water vapor with routine use to an intubated patient.[6]

■ If you're using a heated humidifier, monitor the inspired air temperature as close to the patient's airway as possible. The inspiratory gas shouldn't be warmer than 98.6° F (37° C) at the opening of the airway. Check that the high temperature alarm is set no higher than 98.6° F and no lower than 86° F (30° C).[6] Observe the amount and consistency of the patient's secretions.

■ Check the in-line thermometer *to make sure the temperature of the air delivered to the patient is close to body temperature.*

■ When monitoring the patient's vital signs, count spontaneous breaths as well as ventilator-delivered breaths.

■ Change, clean, or dispose of the ventilator tubing and equipment when visibly soiled or malfunctioning and according to your facility's policy *to reduce the risk of bacterial contamination.*[5,6,7]

■ Provide emotional support to the patient during all phases of mechanical ventilation *to reduce his anxiety and promote successful treatment.* Even if the patient is unresponsive, continue to explain all procedures and treatments to him.

■ Make sure the ventilator alarms are on at all times. *These alarms alert nursing staff members to potentially hazardous conditions and changes in patient status.*

■ Unless contraindicated, turn the patient from side to side every 1 to 2 hours *to facilitate lung expansion and removal of secretions.* Perform active or passive range-of-motion exercises for all extremities *to reduce the hazards of immobility.* If the patient's condition permits, position him upright at regular intervals *to increase lung expansion.*

■ Elevate the head of the bed 30 to 45 degrees, unless contraindicated, *to promote air exchange and prevent ventilator-associated pneumonia.* If the patient is unable to bend at the hip, maintain the patient in reverse Trendelenburg's position.[5,8,9]

■ Assess the patient's peripheral circulation, and monitor his urine output for signs of decreased cardiac output. Monitor the patient for signs and symptoms of fluid volume excess or dehydration.

■ Perform routine oral care according to your facility's policy, and perform oral care daily using chlorhexidine solution, as prescribed, *to prevent ventilator-associated pneumonia.*[9]

■ The patient should be maintained on deep vein thrombosis and peptic ulcer prophylaxis *to decrease the risk of these common complications.*[5,8,9]

■ Place the call light within the patient's reach, and establish a method of communication, such as a communication board, *because intubation and mechanical ventilation impair the patient's ability to speak.* An artificial airway may help the patient to speak by allowing air to pass through his vocal cords.

■ Administer a sedative or neuromuscular blocking agent, as ordered, *to relax the patient or eliminate spontaneous breathing efforts that can interfere with the ventilator's action.* Remember that the patient receiving a neuromuscular blocking agent requires close observation *because of his inability to breathe or communicate.*

■ Take steps to ensure the patient's safety, such as raising the side rails of his bed while turning him and covering and lubricating his eyes.

■ Remove and discard gloves and personal protective equipment. Perform hand hygiene.[2,3,4]

■ Document the procedure.[10]

Special considerations

■ If an alarm sounds and the problem can't be identified easily, disconnect the patient from the ventilator and use a handheld resuscitation bag to ventilate him. (See *Responding to ventilator alarms.*)

■ If the patient is receiving a neuromuscular blocking agent, make sure he also receives a sedative. *Neuromuscular blocking agents cause paralysis without altering the patient's level of consciousness (LOC).* Reassure the patient and his family that the paralysis is temporary. Also make sure emergency equipment is readily available in case the ventilator malfunctions or the patient is extubated accidentally.

■ A sedation vacation strategy should be discussed with the doctor during multidisciplinary rounds *to assess for readiness for weaning.*[5,8,9]

■ Interrupt sedation daily, according to your facility's policy, and assess the patient's readiness to wean.

■ If the patient is ready to wean, begin to wean the patient from the ventilator, as ordered.

■ In the postoperative patient, assess for pain, and administer analgesics, as needed and ordered.

■ If the patient is receiving enteral feedings, avoid gastric overdistention *to reduce the risk of aspiration.*[8]

■ Make sure the patient gets adequate rest and sleep *because fatigue can delay weaning from the ventilator.* Provide subdued lighting, safely muffle equipment noises, and restrict staff access to the area *to promote quiet during rest periods.*

Patient teaching

Educate the patient and his family about measures to prevent ventilator-associated pneumonia, including maintaining the head of the bed at 30 to 45 degrees. Encourage them to alert staff members when the bed doesn't appear to be positioned correctly.[9]

If the patient will be discharged on a ventilator, evaluate ability and motivation of family members or other caregivers to provide such care. Well before discharge, develop a teaching plan that addresses the patient's needs. For example, teaching should include information about ventilator care and settings, artificial airway care, suctioning, respiratory therapy, communication, nutrition, therapeutic exercise, signs and symptoms of infection, and ways to troubleshoot minor equipment malfunctions.

TROUBLESHOOTING

Responding to ventilator alarms

SIGNAL	POSSIBLE CAUSE	NURSING INTERVENTIONS
Low-pressure alarm	■ Tube disconnected from ventilator	■ Reconnect the tube to the ventilator.
	■ Endotracheal (ET) tube displaced above vocal cords or tracheostomy tube extubated	■ Check tube placement and reposition if needed. If extubation or displacement has occurred, ventilate the patient manually and call the doctor immediately.
	■ Leaking tidal volume from low cuff pressure (from an underinflated or ruptured cuff or a leak in the cuff or one-way valve)	■ Listen for a whooshing sound around the tube, indicating an air leak. If you hear one, check cuff pressure. If you can't maintain pressure, call the doctor; he may need to insert a new tube.
	■ Ventilator malfunction	■ Disconnect the patient from the ventilator and ventilate him manually if necessary. Obtain another ventilator.
	■ Leak in ventilator circuitry (from loose connection or hole in tubing, loss of temperature-sensitive device, or cracked humidification jar)	■ Make sure all connections are intact. Check for holes or leaks in the tubing and replace if necessary. Check the humidification jar and replace if cracked.
High-pressure alarm	■ Increased airway pressure or decreased lung compliance caused by worsening disease	■ Auscultate the lungs for evidence of increasing lung consolidation, barotrauma, or wheezing. Call the doctor if indicated.
	■ Patient biting on oral ET tube	■ Insert a bite block if needed. ■ Consider pain medication or sedation if appropriate.
	■ Secretions in airway	■ Look for secretions in the airway. To remove them, suction the patient or have him cough.
	■ Condensate in large-bore tubing	■ Check tubing for condensate and remove any fluid.
	■ Intubation of right mainstem bronchus	■ Auscultate the lungs for evidence of diminished or absent breath sounds in the left lung fields.
	■ Patient coughing, gagging, or attempting to talk	■ Check tube position. If the tube has slipped, call the doctor; he may need to reposition it.
	■ Chest wall resistance	■ If the patient fights the ventilator, the doctor may order a sedative or neuromuscular blocking agent.
	■ Failure of high-pressure relief valve	■ Reposition the patient to see if doing so improves chest expansion. If repositioning doesn't help, administer the prescribed analgesic. ■ Have faulty equipment replaced.
	■ Bronchospasm	■ Assess the patient for the cause. Report to the doctor, and treat as ordered.

Also evaluate the patient's need for adaptive equipment, such as a hospital bed, wheelchair or walker with a ventilator tray, patient lift, and bedside commode. Determine whether the patient needs to travel; if so, select appropriate portable and backup equipment.

Before discharge, have the patient's caregiver demonstrate his ability to use the equipment. At discharge, contact a durable medical equipment vendor and a home health nurse to follow up with the patient. Also, refer the patient to community resources, if available.

Complications

Mechanical ventilation can cause tension pneumothorax, decreased cardiac output, oxygen toxicity, fluid volume excess (from humidification), infection, and such GI complications as distention or bleeding from stress ulcers.

Documentation

Document the date and time mechanical ventilation was initiated. Name the type of ventilator used for the patient, and note its settings. Describe the patient's subjective and objective response to mechanical ventilation, including vital signs, breath sounds, neurologic status, readiness to wean, use of accessory muscles, intake and output, and weight. List any complications and nursing actions taken. Record all pertinent laboratory data, including ABG analysis results and oxygen saturation levels. Describe the patient's LOC, respiratory effort, arrhythmias, skin color, and need for suctioning. Document interventions, such as elevating the head of bed, providing oral care, interrupting sedation, and weaning, and note the patient's response to these interventions.

If the patient was receiving pressure-support ventilation (PSV) or using a T-piece or tracheostomy collar, note the duration of spontaneous breathing and the patient's ability to maintain the weaning schedule. If using intermittent mandatory ventilation, with or without PSV, record the control breath rate, the time of each breath reduction, and the rate of spontaneous respirations.

Document any patient and family teaching provided.[10]

REFERENCES

1 The Joint Commission. (2012). Standard NPSG.01.01.01. *Comprehensive accreditation manual for hospitals: The official handbook.* Oakbrook Terrace, IL: The Joint Commission. (Level I)
2 The Joint Commission. (2012). Standard NPSG.07.01.01. *Comprehensive accreditation manual for hospitals: The official handbook.* Oakbrook Terrace, IL: The Joint Commission. (Level I)
3 Centers for Disease Control and Prevention. (October 2002). Guideline for hand hygiene in health-care settings. *Morbidity and Mortality Weekly Report, 51*(RR-16), 1–45. (Level 1)
4 World Health Organization. (2009). *WHO guidelines on hand hygiene in health care: First global patient safety challenge. Clean care is safer care.* Geneva, Switzerland: World Health Organization. (Level I)
5 Association for Professional in Infection Control and Epidemiology. (2009). "Guide to the Elimination of Ventilator-Associated Pneumonia" [Online]. Accessed January 2012 via the Web at http://www.apic.org/Resource_/EliminationGuideForm/18e326ad-b484-471c-9c35-6822a53ee4a2/File/VAP_09.pdf
6 American Association for Respiratory Care. (1992). AARC clinical practice guideline: Humidification during mechanical ventilation. *Respiratory Care, 36*(8), 887–890. (Level I)
7 American Association for Respiratory Care. (2003). AARC evidence-based clinical practice guideline: Care of the ventilator circuit and its relation to ventilator-associated pneumonia. *Respiratory Care, 48*(9), 869–879. (Level I)
8 Coffin, S.E., et al. (2008). Strategies to prevent ventilator-associated pneumonia in acute care hospitals. *Infection Control and Hospital Epidemiology, 29*(1), S31–S40.
9 Institute for Healthcare Improvement. (2010). *5 million lives campaign getting started kit: Prevent ventilator-associated pneumonia.* Cambridge, MA: Institute for Healthcare Improvement. (Level I)
10 The Joint Commission. (2012). Standard RC.01.03.01. *Comprehensive accreditation manual for hospitals: The official handbook.* Oakbrook Terrace, IL: The Joint Commission. (Level I)

ADDITIONAL REFERENCES

Lynn-McHale Wiegand, D. (Ed.). (2011). *AACN procedure manual for critical care* (6th ed.). Philadelphia, PA: Saunders.
Nettina, S.M. (2010). *Lippincott manual of nursing practice* (9th ed.). Philadelphia, PA: Lippincott Williams & Wilkins.

METERED-DOSE INHALER USE

A metered-dose inhaler delivers topical medications to the respiratory tract, producing local and systemic effects. The mucosal lining of the respiratory tract absorbs the inhalant almost immediately. Examples of common inhalants include bronchodilators, which improve airway patency and facilitate mucous drainage; mucolytics, which attain a high local concentration to liquefy tenacious bronchial secretions; and corticosteroids, which decrease inflammation.

The use of these inhalers may be contraindicated in patients who can't form an airtight seal around the device and in patients who lack the coordination or clear vision to assemble the inhaler. Some patients use a spacer to assist them with the airtight seal. Specific inhalants may also be contraindicated. For example, bronchodilators are contraindicated if the patient has tachycardia or a history of cardiac arrhythmias associated with tachycardia.

Equipment

Patient's medication record and chart ■ metered-dose inhaler and prescribed medication ■ normal saline solution (or another appropriate solution) for gargling ■ Optional: emesis basin.

Implementation

■ Verify the order on the patient's medication record by checking it against the doctor's order.[1]
■ Perform hand hygiene.[2,3,4]

- Check the label on the inhaler against the order on the medication record. Verify the expiration date.[1]
- Confirm the patient's identity using at least two patient identifiers according to your facility's policy.[5]
- If your facility uses a bar code scanning system, be sure to scan your identification badge, the patient's identification bracelet, and the medication's bar code.
- Explain the procedure to the patient. Answer any questions *to decrease anxiety and increase cooperation.*
- Shake the inhaler bottle *to mix the medication and aerosol propellant.*
- Remove the mouthpiece and cap. Keep in mind that some metered-dose inhalers have a spacer built into the inhaler. Pull the spacer away from the section holding the medication canister until it clicks into place.
- Insert the metal stem on the bottle into the small hole on the flattened portion of the mouthpiece. Then turn the bottle upside down.
- Have the patient exhale; then have him place the mouthpiece in his mouth and close his lips around it (as shown below).

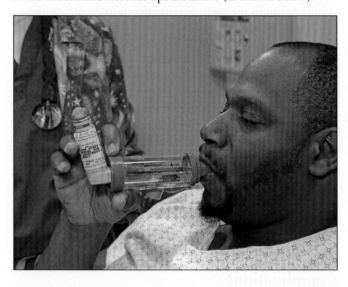

- As you firmly push the bottle down against the mouthpiece, ask the patient to inhale slowly and to continue inhaling until his lungs feel full. *This action draws the medication into his lungs.* Compress the bottle against the mouthpiece only once.
- Remove the mouthpiece from the patient's mouth and tell him to hold his breath for several seconds *to allow the medication to reach the alveoli.* Then, instruct him to exhale slowly through pursed lips *to keep the distal bronchioles open, allowing increased absorption and diffusion of the drug and better gas exchange.*
- Have the patient gargle with water, if desired, *to remove medication from the mouth and back of the throat.* (The lungs retain only about 10% of the inhalant; most of the remainder is exhaled, but substantial amounts may remain in the oropharynx.)
- Rinse the mouthpiece thoroughly with warm water *to prevent accumulation of residue.*
- Perform hand hygiene.[2,3,4]
- Document the procedure.[6]

Special considerations

Spacer inhalers may be recommended *to provide greater therapeutic benefit for children and for patients who have difficulty with coordination.* A spacer attachment is an extension to the inhaler's mouthpiece that provides more dead-air space for mixing the medication. Some inhalers have built-in spacers.

Patient teaching

Teach the patient how to use the inhaler *so that he can continue treatments himself after discharge, if necessary.* Explain that overdosage, which commonly occurs, can cause the medication to lose its effectiveness. Tell him to record the date and time of each inhalation as well as his response *to prevent overdosage and to help the doctor determine the drug's effectiveness.* Also, note whether the patient uses an unusual amount of medication—for example, more than one cartridge every 3 weeks. Inform the patient of possible adverse reactions.

If more than one inhalation is ordered, advise the patient to wait at least 2 minutes before repeating the procedure.

If the patient is also using a steroid inhaler, instruct him to use the bronchodilator first and then wait 5 minutes before using the steroid. *This process allows the bronchodilator to open the air passages for maximum effectiveness.*

Complications

Complications are related to the medication being administered.

Documentation

Record the inhalant administered as well as the dose and time. Note any significant change in the patient's heart rate and any other adverse reactions.

REFERENCES

1 The Joint Commission. (2012). Standard MM.06.01.01. *Comprehensive accreditation manual for hospitals: The official handbook.* Oakbrook Terrace, IL: The Joint Commission. (Level I)
2 The Joint Commission. (2012). Standard NPSG.07.01.01. *Comprehensive accreditation manual for hospitals: The official handbook.* Oakbrook Terrace, IL: The Joint Commission. (Level I)
3 Centers for Disease Control and Prevention. (October 2002). Guideline for hand hygiene in health-care settings. *Morbidity and Mortality Weekly Report, 51*(RR-16), 1–45. (Level 1)
4 World Health Organization. (2009). *WHO guidelines on hand hygiene in health care: First global patient safety challenge. Clean care is safer care.* Geneva, Switzerland: World Health Organization. (Level I)
5 The Joint Commission. (2012). Standard NPSG.01.01.01. *Comprehensive accreditation manual for hospitals: The official handbook.* Oakbrook Terrace, IL: The Joint Commission. (Level I)
6 The Joint Commission. (2012). Standard RC.01.03.01. *Comprehensive accreditation manual for hospitals: The official handbook.* Oakbrook Terrace, IL: The Joint Commission. (Level I)

ADDITIONAL REFERENCES

Leach, C.L. (2007). Inhalation aspects of therapeutic aerosols. *Toxicologic Pathology, 35*(1), 23–26.

Nettina, S.M. (2010). *Lippincott manual of nursing practice* (9th ed.). Philadelphia, PA: Lippincott Williams & Wilkins.

Taylor, C., et al. (2011). *Fundamentals of nursing: The art and science of nursing care* (7th ed.). Philadelphia, PA: Lippincott Williams & Wilkins.

MIXED VENOUS OXYGEN SATURATION MONITORING

This procedure uses a fiber-optic thermodilution pulmonary artery (PA) catheter to continuously monitor oxygen delivery to tissues and oxygen consumption by tissues. Monitoring of mixed venous oxygen saturation ($S\bar{v}O_2$) allows rapid detection of impaired oxygen delivery, such as from decreased cardiac output, hemoglobin level, or arterial oxygen saturation. It also helps evaluate a patient's response to drug therapy, endotracheal tube suctioning, ventilator setting changes, positive end-expiratory pressure, and fraction of inspired oxygen. $S\bar{v}O_2$ usually ranges from 60% to 80%.

Equipment

Fiber-optic PA catheter ▪ co-oximeter and monitor ▪ optical module and cable ▪ gloves.

Preparation of equipment

Review the manufacturer's instructions for assembly and use of the fiber-optic PA catheter. Connect the optical module and cable to the monitor. Next, peel back the wrapping covering the catheter just enough to uncover the fiber-optic connector. Attach the fiber-optic connector to the optical module while allowing the rest of the catheter to remain in its sterile wrapping. Calibrate the fiber-optic catheter by following the manufacturer's instructions.

To prepare for the rest of the procedure, follow the instructions for pulmonary catheter insertion, as described in "Pulmonary artery pressure and pulmonary artery wedge pressure monitoring," page 610. (See *$S\bar{v}O_2$ monitoring equipment*.)

Implementation

▪ Verify the doctor's order.
▪ Confirm the patient's identity using with at least two patient identifiers according to your facility's policy.[1]
▪ Perform hand hygiene and put on gloves.[2,3,4]
▪ Explain the procedure to the patient and answer any questions *to allay his fears and promote cooperation.*
▪ Assist with the insertion of the fiber-optic catheter just as you would for a PA catheter.
▪ After the catheter is inserted, confirm that the light intensity tracing on the graphic printout is within normal range *to ensure correct positioning and function of the catheter.*
▪ Observe the digital readout and record the $S\bar{v}O_2$ on graph paper. Repeat readings at least once each hour *to monitor and document trends.*

▪ Set the machine alarms 10% above and 10% below the patient's current $S\bar{v}O_2$ reading.

Recalibrating the monitor

▪ Draw a mixed venous blood sample from the distal port of the PA catheter. Label the sample in the presence of the patient *to prevent mislabeling.*[1] Send it to the laboratory for analysis *to compare the laboratory's $S\bar{v}O_2$ reading with that of the fiber-optic catheter.*
▪ If the catheter values and the laboratory values differ by more than 4%, follow the manufacturer's instructions to enter the $S\bar{v}O_2$ value obtained by the laboratory into the co-oximeter.
▪ Recalibrate the monitor every 24 hours or whenever the catheter has been disconnected from the optical module.
▪ Remove and discard your gloves and perform hand hygiene.[2,3,4]
▪ Document the procedure.[5]

Special considerations

▪ If the patient's $S\bar{v}O_2$ drops below 60% or varies by more than 10% for 3 minutes or longer, reassess the patient. If the $S\bar{v}O_2$ doesn't return to the baseline value after nursing interventions, notify the doctor. *A decreasing $S\bar{v}O_2$, or a value less than 60%,* indicates impaired oxygen delivery, as occurs in hemorrhage, hypoxia, shock, arrhythmias, or suctioning. $S\bar{v}O_2$ may also decrease as a result of increased oxygen demand from such causes as hyperthermia, shivering, or seizures.
▪ If the intensity of the tracing is low, ensure that all connections between the catheter and co-oximeter are secure and that the catheter is patent and not kinked.
▪ If the tracing is damped or erratic, try to aspirate blood from the catheter *to check for patency.* If you can't aspirate blood, notify the doctor *so that he can replace the catheter.* Also check the PA waveform *to determine whether the catheter has wedged.* If the catheter has wedged, turn the patient from side to side and instruct him to cough. If the catheter remains wedged, notify the doctor immediately.

Complications

Thrombosis can result from local irritation by the catheter; however, a heparinized flush helps prevent this complication. Thromboembolism also can occur if a thrombus breaks off and lodges in the circulatory system. Monitor the patient for signs of infection, such as redness or drainage at the catheter site.

Documentation

Record the $S\bar{v}O_2$ value on a flowchart and attach a tracing, as ordered. Note any significant changes in the patient's status and the results of any interventions. For comparison, note the $S\bar{v}O_2$ as measured by the fiber-optic catheter whenever a blood sample is obtained for laboratory analysis of $S\bar{v}O_2$.

REFERENCES

1 The Joint Commission. (2012). Standard NPSG.01.01.01. *Comprehensive accreditation manual for hospitals: The official handbook.* Oakbrook Terrace, IL: The Joint Commission. (Level I)

EQUIPMENT

S⊽O₂ monitoring equipment

The mixed venous oxygen saturation (S⊽O₂) monitoring system consists of a flow-directed pulmonary artery (PA) catheter with fiber-optic filaments, an optical module, and a co-oximeter. The co-oximeter displays a continuous digital S⊽O₂ value; the strip recorder prints a permanent record.

Catheter insertion follows the same technique as with any thermodilution flow-directed PA catheter. The distal lumen connects to an external PA pressure monitoring system, the proximal or central venous pressure lumen connects to another monitoring system or to a continuous flow administration unit, and the optical module connects to the co-oximeter unit.

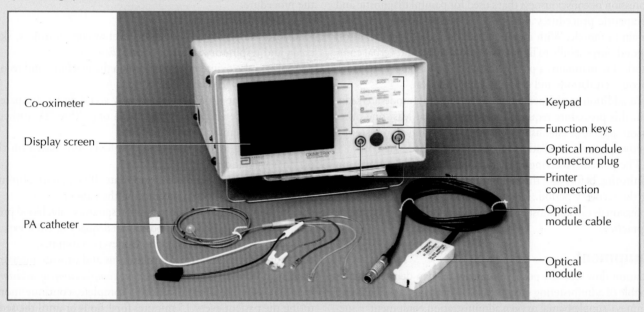

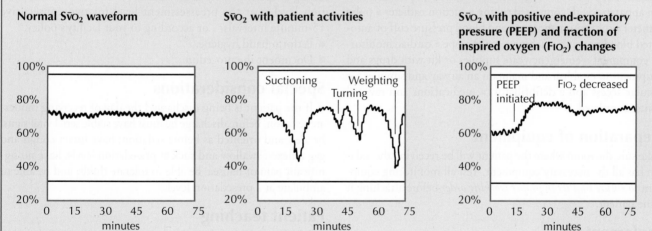

Normal S⊽O₂ waveform

S⊽O₂ with patient activities

S⊽O₂ with positive end-expiratory pressure (PEEP) and fraction of inspired oxygen (FIO₂) changes

2 The Joint Commission. (2012). Standard NPSG.07.01.01. *Comprehensive accreditation manual for hospitals: The official handbook.* Oakbrook Terrace, IL: The Joint Commission. (Level I)

3 Centers for Disease Control and Prevention. (October 2002). Guideline for hand hygiene in health-care settings. *Morbidity and Mortality Weekly Report, 51*(RR-16), 1–45. (Level 1)

4 World Health Organization. (2009). *WHO guidelines on hand hygiene in health care: First global patient safety challenge. Clean care is safer care.* Geneva, Switzerland: World Health Organization. (Level I)

5 The Joint Commission. (2012). Standard RC.01.03.01. *Comprehensive accreditation manual for hospitals: The official handbook.* Oakbrook Terrace, IL: The Joint Commission. (Level I)

ADDITIONAL REFERENCES

Lorentzen, A.G., et al. (2008). Central venous oxygen saturation cannot replace mixed venous saturation in patients undergoing cardiac surgery. *Journal of Cardiothoracic and Vascular Anesthesia, 22*(6), 853–857.

Lynn-McHale Wiegand, D. (Ed.). (2011). *AACN procedure manual for critical care* (6th ed.). Philadelphia, PA: Saunders.

Yazigi, A., et al. (2008). Comparison of central venous to mixed venous oxygen saturation in patients with low cardiac index and filling pressures after coronary artery surgery. *Journal of Cardiothoracic and Vascular Anesthesia, 22*(1), 77–83.

MODERATE SEDATION

Moderate sedation, also called *conscious sedation,* is a drug-induced depression of consciousness that's used for painful diagnostic and therapeutic procedures and those for which the patient must remain immobile. With moderate sedation, the patient can still respond purposefully to light tactile stimulation and verbal commands. He maintains a patent airway as well as adequate spontaneous ventilations and cardiovascular function.

In addition to the person administering the moderate sedation, this procedure requires the presence of at least one other person capable of establishing a patent airway and administering positive-pressure ventilation to the patient, if necessary.[1]

The patient receiving moderate sedation requires sedation monitoring before and throughout the procedure as well as during the recovery period. Doctors, nurses, and other health care professionals can administer moderate sedation within their scope of practice.

Equipment

Sedation flow record ▪ positive-pressure oxygen delivery system capable of administering greater than 90% oxygen for at least 60 minutes ▪ supplemental oxygen administration equipment[1] ▪ suction apparatus with connected tubing ▪ suction catheter ▪ pulse oximeter ▪ sphygmomanometer and blood pressure cuff or automated blood pressure machine ▪ stethoscope ▪ cardiac monitoring equipment ▪ emergency care supplies or kit with drugs and equipment to establish and maintain an airway and supplies for vascular access and a defibrillator[1] ▪ medications and reversal agents, as ordered.

Preparation of equipment

Make sure the room where the patient will be receiving the sedation has all the necessary equipment. Test all monitoring equipment *to ensure that it's in proper working order* before attaching it to the patient.

Implementation

▪ Verify the doctor's order for moderate sedation.[2]

▪ Review the patient's medical record and make sure the following information is documented: any preexisting medical conditions, previous anesthesia and sedation experiences, current medications, allergies, the last time the patient ate or had oral fluids, a recent height and weight, and physical examination findings, including evaluation of the airway and a cardiac and respiratory assessment.[1,3]

▪ Ensure that informed consent for the procedure to be performed has been obtained and is included in the patient's medical record.[4,5]

▪ Confirm the patient's identity using with at least two patient identifiers according to your facility's policy.[6]

▪ Explain the procedure to the patient and his family, and answer their questions *to decrease anxiety and increase cooperation.*

▪ If the patient is to be discharged less than 12 hours after receiving sedation, verify that arrangements have been made to transport the patient home and that an adult will be available in case complications arise.

▪ Ensure that the patient has had nothing by mouth except for clear liquids and prescribed medications for at least 8 hours before the procedure.

▪ Perform hand hygiene.[7,8,9]

▪ Record the patient's vital signs, level of consciousness, skin color, and respiratory status *to use as a baseline.*[3]

▪ Apply a pulse oximeter probe, turn on the machine, and record the patient's oxygen saturation.

▪ Ensure that the patient has a patent IV access device. If a patent IV access device isn't present, establish one.[1] (See "IV catheter insertion and removal," page 421.)

▪ Confirm the medication dosage calculations based on the patient's weight or body surface area.

▪ Administer the sedation as appropriate. If you aren't administering the sedation, begin monitoring the patient.

▪ Continuously monitor the patient's respiratory rate, blood pressure, oxygen saturation, head position, adequacy of chest expansion, and level of consciousness at least every 5 minutes.[1,5,10]

▪ Monitor the patient for complications and provide interventions as indicated.[11] (See *Responding to complications of sedation.*)

▪ When sedation administration is complete, continue monitoring the patient every 15 minutes for 1 hour or until the sedation level is at the preassessment level for two consecutive 15-minute intervals,[12] or according to your facility's policy.[1]

▪ Perform hand hygiene.[7,8,9]

▪ Document the procedure.[13]

Special considerations

▪ If the patient is being discharged the day of receiving moderate sedation, before discharge he must have stable serial vital signs; be alert and oriented as before sedation; have intact cough and gag reflexes; swallow and suck at presedation levels; have no significant pain or nausea; be able to tolerate fluids; and be able to ambulate at a presedation level.

Patient teaching

After completion of the procedure, reinforce patient education with written instructions for the patient and his family to take home. Explain when to seek immediate emergency care. Teach the patient and his family about pain management. Reinforce the importance of having someone available to assist the patient with care for 24 hours following the procedure.

Complications

It's possible for the patient to become oversedated during moderate sedation. Other complications of moderate sedation include aspiration of gastric contents, respiratory depression or failure, and adverse reactions to the medication. Observe the patient for airway obstruction, respiratory depression, hypotension, and drug-specific complications.

Preexisting respiratory conditions, such as chronic obstructive pulmonary disease or asthma, and hepatic or renal dysfunction can increase the risk of adverse reactions. Age and overall health can also increase the risk of adverse reactions. In general, children (because of their smaller body mass) and older adults (because of decreased renal and hepatic function and relative loss of muscle) are at greater risk. Drug interactions, such as those that occur with cimetidine and droperidol or when opioids and sedatives are used in combination, can have synergistic effects. (See *Responding to complications of sedation.*)

Documentation

Document the procedure and all of the patient's vital signs on your facility's sedation flow sheet. Also document how the patient tolerated the procedure and any complications or adverse effects. Record all medications administered, including any medications administered to manage the recovery of the patient. Document IV fluids administered, including the type and amount. Document any adverse effects experienced in response to medications administered. Note patient teaching provided.

REFERENCES

1 Practice guidelines for sedation and analgesia by non-anesthesiologists: An updated report by the American Society of Anesthesiologists Task Force on Sedation and Analgesia by Non-Anesthesiologists. (2002). *Anesthesiology, 96,* 1004–1017. (Level I)

2 The Joint Commission. (2012). Standard MM.06.01.01. *Comprehensive accreditation manual for hospitals: The official handbook.* Oakbrook Terrace, IL: The Joint Commission. (Level I)

3 The Joint Commission. (2012). Standard PC.03.01.01. *Comprehensive accreditation manual for hospitals: The official handbook.* Oakbrook Terrace, IL: The Joint Commission. (Level I)

4 The Joint Commission. (2012). Standard RI.01.03.01. *Comprehensive accreditation manual for hospitals: The official handbook.* Oakbrook Terrace, IL: The Joint Commission. (Level I)

5 Standard 67. Moderate sedation/analgesia using intravenous sedation. Infusion nursing standards of practice. (2011). *Journal of Infusion Nursing, 34*(1S), S95. (Level I)

6 The Joint Commission. (2012). Standard NPSG.01.01.01. *Comprehensive accreditation manual for hospitals: The official handbook.* Oakbrook Terrace, IL: The Joint Commission. (Level I)

7 The Joint Commission. (2012). Standard NPSG.07.01.01. *Comprehensive accreditation manual for hospitals: The official handbook.* Oakbrook Terrace, IL: The Joint Commission. (Level I)

8 Centers for Disease Control and Prevention. (October 2002). Guideline for hand hygiene in health-care settings. *Morbidity and Mortality Weekly Report, 51*(RR-16), 1–45. (Level 1)

9 World Health Organization. (2009). *WHO guidelines on hand hygiene in health care: First global patient safety challenge. Clean care is safer care.* Geneva, Switzerland: World Health Organization. (Level I)

10 The Joint Commission. (2012). Standard PC.03.01.05. *Comprehensive accreditation manual for hospitals: The official handbook.* Oakbrook Terrace, IL: The Joint Commission. (Level I)

11 The Joint Commission. (2012). Standard MM.07.01.01. *Comprehensive accreditation manual for hospitals: The official handbook.* Oakbrook Terrace, IL: The Joint Commission. (Level I)

TROUBLESHOOTING

Responding to complications of sedation

This table reviews nursing interventions for various complications of sedation.

COMPLICATION	NURSING INTERVENTIONS
Airway obstruction or respiratory depression	■ Reposition the head. ■ Suction. ■ Insert an oral airway. ■ Tell the patient to take a deep breath. ■ Stimulate the patient by rubbing his arms or legs. ■ Administer oxygen. ■ Manually ventilate with a bag-valve mask device.
Oversedation	■ Maintain airway, breathing, and circulation. ■ Have drugs to reverse sedation (such as naloxone for opiates or flumazenil for benzodiazepines) immediately available and administer, as ordered, if the patient is too deeply sedated. ■ Monitor respiratory status until stable.
Cardiac arrhythmias	■ Note baseline heart rate and rhythm. ■ Obtain an apical pulse for 1 minute. ■ Examine electrocardiogram patterns if indicated. ■ Ensure that the patient has a patent airway. ■ Monitor oxygen saturation levels. ■ Administer oxygen. ■ Administer fluids and antiarrhythmic drugs as ordered.
Hypotension	■ Investigate possible causes. ■ Support respiratory status. ■ Administer fluids and vasopressors as ordered.
Hypertension	■ Administer additional sedation or analgesia.

12 The Joint Commission. (2012). Standard PC.03.01.07. *Comprehensive accreditation manual for hospitals: The official handbook.* Oakbrook Terrace, IL: The Joint Commission. (Level I)

13 The Joint Commission. (2012). Standard RC.01.03.01. *Comprehensive accreditation manual for hospitals: The official handbook.* Oakbrook Terrace, IL: The Joint Commission. (Level I)

ADDITIONAL REFERENCE

McQuaid, K.R., & Laine, L. (2008). A systematic review and meta-analysis of randomized, controlled trials of moderate sedation for routine endoscopic procedures. *Gastrointestinal Endoscopy, 67*(6), 910–923.

MUCUS CLEARANCE DEVICE

Patients with chronic respiratory disorders, such as cystic fibrosis, bronchitis, or bronchiectasis, require therapy to mobilize and remove mucus secretions from the lungs. A handheld mucus clearance device, also known as the *flutter,* can help such patients cough up secretions more easily.

The device works by using a ball valve that vibrates as the patient exhales vigorously through it. The vibrations propagate throughout the airways during expiration, loosening the mucus. As the patient repeats this process, the mucus progressively moves up the airways until the patient can easily cough it out. A licensed practitioner should determine the frequency and duration of device use.

When used before bronchodilator therapy in patients with chronic obstructive pulmonary disease, the mucus clearance device has been shown to improve the patient's response to the bronchodilator.

Equipment

Mucus clearance device ▪ emesis basin ▪ tissues ▪ trash bag ▪ stethoscope ▪ oral care supplies (see "Oral care," page 524) ▪ Optional: gloves.

Implementation

▪ Verify the doctor's order.
▪ Confirm the patient's identity using with at least two patient identifiers according to your facility's policy.[1]
▪ Perform hand hygiene, put on gloves as needed, and follow standard precautions.[2,3,4]
▪ Explain the procedure to the patient and answer any questions *to decrease anxiety and increase cooperation.* Tell him that this device will help move the mucus through his airways so that he can eventually expectorate it.
▪ Auscultate the patient's lungs and perform a baseline assessment.
▪ Have the patient sit with his back straight and his head tilted backward slightly so that his throat and trachea are wide open. *This position allows exhaled air to flow smoothly from the lungs and out through the device.*
▪ If the patient prefers, he may place his elbows on a table at a height that prevents him from slouching, *which would interfere with smooth breathing.*

▪ Tell the patient to hold the device so that the stem is parallel to the floor. *This position places the interior cone of the device at a 30-degree tilt, which allows the ball inside the device to bounce and roll freely in the cone.*
▪ Have the patient draw a deep breath and hold it for 2 to 3 seconds. This inhalation step is very important; *the inspired air is evenly distributed throughout the lungs, especially in the small airways, where infection and airway damage can occur.*
▪ After 2 to 3 seconds, instruct the patient to place the device in his mouth and then exhale at a steady rate for as long as he can. *Explain that if he breathes out too quickly and forcefully, the ball won't vibrate or flutter properly, thereby defeating the purpose of the device.*
▪ Tell the patient to keep his cheeks as flat and hard as possible while exhaling *to direct the air out through the device most effectively.* Suggest that he hold his cheeks lightly with his other hand *to help learn the technique.*
▪ After the patient has completely exhaled, he can remove the device from his mouth, take in another full breath, and cough. The entire procedure can be repeated several times, as recommended by a licensed practitioner.
▪ Tell the patient to expectorate the mucus into an emesis basin or tissue.
▪ Observe the type, amount, color, and odor of expectorated secretions.
▪ Dispose of secretions appropriately.
▪ Auscultate for the patient's breath sounds *to determine the effectiveness of his coughing,* and compare your findings with the baseline assessment.
▪ Have the patient perform oral care.
▪ Remove and discard your gloves. Perform hand hygiene.[2,3,4]
▪ Document the procedure.[5]

Special considerations

▪ Alternatively, after completely exhaling, the patient can leave the device in his mouth, draw another big breath through his nose, hold it for 2 to 3 seconds, and repeat the exhalation maneuver. He can breathe through the device up to five times before taking the final breath and cough.
▪ *To help the patient achieve the best fluttering effect,* you may need to place one hand on his back and the other on his chest as he exhales through the device. If he's achieving the maximum effect, you'll feel the vibrations in his lungs as he exhales. If results are unsatisfactory at first, tell the patient to adjust the angle at which he's holding the device until optimal fluttering occurs.
▪ If the patient's final cough doesn't seem to work, he can try repeated, controlled, short, rapid exhalations (huffing), as though he were trying to cough a bread crumb out of his throat, *to aid mucus removal.*

Patient teaching

Tell the patient to clean the device after each use *to remove mucus from the internal components.* Instruct him to clean it more thoroughly every 2 days. All parts should be washed in a solution of mild soap or detergent. Tell him not to use bleach or other chlorine-containing products. After thorough cleaning, all parts should be rinsed under a stream of hot tap water, wiped with a clean towel, and reassembled and stored in a clean, dry place.

Documentation

Record your patient teaching as well as the patient's tolerance of the procedure. Record the amount, color, and odor of any secretions that the patient is able to expectorate. Document the patient's breath sounds before and after he's used the device and coughed. Also record the number of times the patient repeated the procedure and the success of his coughing efforts.

REFERENCES

1 The Joint Commission. (2012). Standard NPSG.01.01.01. *Comprehensive accreditation manual for hospitals: The official handbook.* Oakbrook Terrace, IL: The Joint Commission. (Level I)
2 The Joint Commission. (2012). Standard NPSG.07.01.01. *Comprehensive accreditation manual for hospitals: The official handbook.* Oakbrook Terrace, IL: The Joint Commission. (Level I)
3 Centers for Disease Control and Prevention. (October 2002). Guideline for hand hygiene in health-care settings. *Morbidity and Mortality Weekly Report, 51*(RR-16), 1–45. (Level 1)
4 World Health Organization. (2009). *WHO guidelines on hand hygiene in health care: First global patient safety challenge. Clean care is safer care.* Geneva, Switzerland: World Health Organization. (Level I)
5 The Joint Commission. (2012). Standard RC.01.03.01. *Comprehensive accreditation manual for hospitals: The official handbook.* Oakbrook Terrace, IL: The Joint Commission. (Level I)

ADDITIONAL REFERENCES

Morrison, L., & Agnew, J. (2009). Oscillating devices for airway clearance in people with cystic fibrosis. *Cochrane Database of Systematic Reviews* (1), CD006842.
Taylor, C., et al. (2011). *Fundamentals of nursing: The art and science of nursing care* (7th ed.). Philadelphia, PA: Lippincott Williams & Wilkins.

NASAL IRRIGATION

Irrigation of the nasal passages soothes irritated mucous membranes and washes away crusted mucus, secretions, and foreign matter. Left unattended, these deposits may impede sinus drainage and nasal airflow and cause headaches, infections, and unpleasant odors. Irrigation may be done with a bulb syringe or an electronic irrigating device.

Nasal irrigation benefits patients with acute or chronic nasal conditions, including sinusitis, rhinitis, Wegener's granulomatosis, and Sjögren's syndrome.[1] In addition, the procedure may help people who regularly inhale toxins or allergens-paint fumes, sawdust, pesticides, or coal dust, for example. Nasal irrigation is routinely recommended after some nasal surgeries to enhance healing by removing postoperative eschar and to aid remucosolization of the sinus cavities and ostia.

Contraindications for nasal irrigation may include advanced destruction of the sinuses, frequent nosebleeds, and foreign bodies in the nasal passages (which could be driven farther into the passages by the irrigant). However, some patients with these conditions may benefit from irrigation.

Equipment

Bulb syringe or an oral irrigating device (such as a Water Pik) ▪ rigid or flexible disposable irrigation tips (for one-patient use) ▪ hypertonic saline solution ▪ plastic sheet ▪ towels ▪ facial tissues ▪ bath basin ▪ gloves ▪ hospital-grade disinfectant.

Preparation of equipment

Warm the saline solution to about 105° F (40.6° C). If you'll be irrigating with a bulb syringe, draw some irrigant into the bulb and then expel it *to rinse any residual solution from the previous irrigation and warm the bulb.*

If you're using an oral irrigating device, plug the instrument into an electrical outlet in an area near the patient. Then, run about 1 cup (240 mL) of saline solution through the tubing *to rinse residual solution from the lines and warm the tubing.* Next, fill the reservoir of the device with warm saline solution.

Implementation

▪ Verify the doctor's order.[2]
▪ Confirm the patient's identity using at least two patient identifiers according to your facility's policy.[3]
▪ Perform hand hygiene and put on gloves.[4,5,6]
▪ Explain the procedure to the patient and answer any questions *to decrease anxiety and increase cooperation.*
▪ Place a towel on his upper body to protect his clothing from getting wet. Place a plastic sheet on the bed, if indicated.
▪ Have the patient sit comfortably near the equipment in a position that allows the bulb or catheter tip to enter his nose and the returning irrigant to flow into the bath basin or sink. (See *Positioning the patient for nasal irrigation,* page 484.)
▪ Remind the patient to keep his mouth open and to breathe rhythmically during irrigation. *This action causes the soft palate to seal the throat, allowing the irrigant to stream out the opposite nostril and carry discharge with it.*
▪ Instruct the patient not to speak or swallow during the irrigation *to avoid forcing infectious material into the sinuses or eustachian tubes.*
▪ Remove the irrigating tip from the patient's nostril if he reports the need to sneeze or cough *to avoid injuring the nasal mucosa.*

Using a bulb syringe

▪ Fill the bulb syringe with saline solution and insert the tip about ½″ (1.3 cm) into the patient's nostril.
▪ Squeeze the bulb until a gentle stream of warm irrigant washes through the nose. Avoid forceful squeezing, *which may drive debris from the nasal passages into the sinuses or eustachian tubes and introduce infection.* Alternate the nostrils until the return irrigant runs clear.

Positioning the patient for nasal irrigation

Whether you're teaching a patient to perform nasal irrigation with a bulb syringe or an oral irrigating device, the irrigation will progress more easily once the patient learns how to hold her head for optimal safety, comfort, and effectiveness.

Help the patient to sit upright with her head bent forward over the basin or sink and well-flexed on her chest. Her nose and ear should be on the same vertical plane.

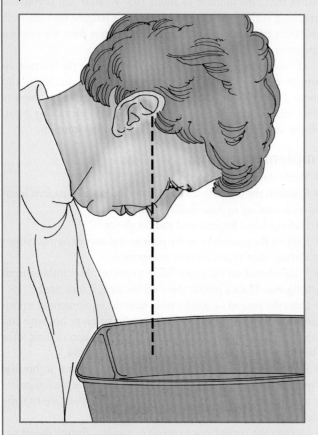

Explain that she's less likely to breathe in the irrigant when holding her head in this position. This position should also keep the irrigant from entering the eustachian tubes, which will now lie above the level of the irrigation stream.

Using an oral irrigating device

■ Insert the irrigation tip into the nostril about ½″ to 1″ (1.3 to 2.5 cm) and turn on the irrigating device. Begin with a low pressure setting (increasing the pressure as needed) *to obtain a gentle stream of irrigant.* Again, be careful not to drive material from the nose into the sinuses or eustachian tubes. Irrigate both nostrils.

■ Inspect returning irrigant. Changes in color, viscosity, or volume may signal an infection and should be reported to the doctor. Also report blood or necrotic material.

Completing the procedure

■ After irrigation, have the patient wait a few minutes before blowing excess fluid from both nostrils at once. *Gentle blowing through both nostrils prevents fluid or pressure buildup in the sinuses. This action also helps to loosen and expel crusted secretions and mucus.*
■ Clean the bulb syringe or irrigating device with soap and water and then disinfect as recommended. Rinse and dry the device.
■ Remove and discard your gloves. Perform hand hygiene.[4,5,6]
■ Document the procedure.[7]

Special considerations

■ Expect fluid to drain from the patient's nose for a brief time after the irrigation and before he blows his nose.
■ Be sure to insert the irrigation tip far enough to ensure that the irrigant cleans the nasal membranes before draining out. A typical amount of irrigant ranges from 500 to 1,000 mL.

Patient teaching

To continue nasal irrigations at home, teach the patient how to prepare saline solution. Tell him to fill a clean 1-L plastic bottle with bottled or distilled water (4 cups + 1 oz = 1 L), add 1 tsp of salt, and shake the solution until the salt dissolves. Teach him how to disinfect used irrigation devices.

Documentation

Write down the time and duration of the procedure and the amount of irrigant used. Describe the appearance of the returned solution. Record your assessment of the patient's comfort level and breathing ease before and after the procedure. Document patient teaching and the patient's understanding of the teaching.

REFERENCES

1 Rabago, D., et al. (2008). Nasal irrigation for chronic sinus symptoms in patients with allergic rhinitis, asthma, and nasal polyposis: A hypothesis generating study. *Wisconsin Medical Journal, 107*(2), 69–75.
2 The Joint Commission. (2012). Standard MM.04.01.01. *Comprehensive accreditation manual for hospitals: The official handbook.* Oakbrook Terrace, IL: The Joint Commission. (Level I)
3 The Joint Commission. (2012). Standard NPSG.01.01.01. *Comprehensive accreditation manual for hospitals: The official handbook.* Oakbrook Terrace, IL: The Joint Commission. (Level I)
4 The Joint Commission. (2012). Standard NPSG.07.01.01. *Comprehensive accreditation manual for hospitals: The official handbook.* Oakbrook Terrace, IL: The Joint Commission. (Level I)
5 Centers for Disease Control and Prevention. (October 2002). Guideline for hand hygiene in health-care settings. *Morbidity and Mortality Weekly Report, 51*(RR-16), 1–45. (Level I)
6 World Health Organization. (2009). *WHO guidelines on hand hygiene in health care: First global patient safety challenge. Clean care is safer care.* Geneva, Switzerland: World Health Organization. (Level I)
7 The Joint Commission. (2012). Standard RC.01.03.01. *Comprehensive accreditation manual for hospitals: The official handbook.* Oakbrook Terrace, IL: The Joint Commission. (Level I)

ADDITIONAL REFERENCES _____

Kassel, J.C., et al. (2010). Saline nasal irrigation for acute upper respiratory tract infections. *Cochrane Database of Systematic Reviews,* (3), CD006821.

Pynnonen, M.A., et al. (2007). Nasal saline for chronic sinonasal symptoms: A randomized controlled trial. *Archives of Otolaryngology-Head & Neck Surgery, 133*(11), 1115–1120.

Rabago, D., & Zgierska, A. (2009). Saline nasal irrigation for upper respiratory conditions. *American Family Physician, 80*(10), 1117–1119.

Smeltzer, S.C., et al. (2010). *Brunner & Suddarth's textbook of medical surgical-nursing* (12th ed.). Philadelphia, PA: Lippincott Williams & Wilkins.

Stankiewicz, J.A., et al. (2008). Nasal amphotericin irrigation in chronic rhinosinusitis. *Current Opinion in Otolaryngology & Head and Neck Surgery, 16*(1), 44–46.

Taylor, C., et al. (2011). *Fundamentals of nursing: The art and science of nursing care* (7th ed.). Philadelphia, PA: Lippincott Williams & Wilkins.

NASAL MEDICATION ADMINISTRATION

Medications can be instilled into the nostril by drops, which may be directed at a specific area of the nasal passage. This method results in increased local effects with minimal systemic effects.

Medication can also be administered using a nasal inhaler, which delivers topical medications to the respiratory tract, producing local and systemic effects. The mucosal lining of the respiratory tract absorbs the inhalant almost immediately. Examples of common inhalants include bronchodilators, which improve airway patency and facilitate mucous drainage; mucolytics, which attain a high local concentration to liquefy tenacious bronchial secretions; and corticosteroids, which decrease inflammation. Inhalants may be contraindicated in patients who lack the coordination or clear vision necessary to assemble a turbo-inhaler. Specific inhalants may also be contraindicated. For example, bronchodilators are contraindicated if the patient has tachycardia or a history of cardiac arrhythmias associated with tachycardia.

A third method, nasal aerosols diffuse medication throughout the nasal passages. This method results in increased local effects with minimal systemic effects.

Most nasal medications, such as phenylephrine, are vasoconstrictors, which relieve nasal congestion by coating and shrinking swollen mucous membranes. Because vasoconstrictors may be absorbed systemically, they're usually contraindicated in hypersensitive patients. Other types of nasal medications include antiseptics, anesthetics, and corticosteroids. Local anesthetics may be administered to promote patient comfort during rhinolaryngologic examination, laryngoscopy, bronchoscopy, and endotracheal intubation. Corticosteroids reduce inflammation in allergic or inflammatory conditions and nasal polyps.

Equipment

Patient's medication record and chart ▪ prescribed medication ▪ Optional: pillow, small piece of soft rubber or plastic tubing, gloves, emesis basin, normal saline solution (or another appropriate solution) for gargling.

Implementation

▪ Verify the order on the patient's medication record by checking it against the doctor's order.[1]
▪ Perform hand hygiene and put on gloves, as needed.[2,3,4]
▪ Check the label on the inhaler three times. Verify the expiration date.[1]
▪ Confirm the patient's identity using at least two patient identifiers according to your facility's policy.[5]
▪ If your facility uses a bar code scanning system, be sure to scan your identification badge, the patient's identification bracelet, and the medication's bar code.
▪ Explain the procedure to the patient. Answer any questions *to decrease anxiety and increase cooperation.*
▪ Have the patient blow his nose *to clear his nostrils.*

For nose drop instillation

▪ When possible, position the patient so that the drops flow back into the nostrils, toward the affected area. (See *Positioning the patient for nose drop instillation,* page 486.)
▪ Draw up medication into the dropper.
▪ Push up the tip of the patient's nose slightly. Position the dropper just above the nostril, and direct its tip toward the midline of the nose *so that the drops flow toward the back of the nasal cavity rather than down the throat.*
▪ Insert the dropper about ⅜″ (1 cm) into the nostril. Don't let the dropper touch the sides of the nostril *because this would contaminate the dropper or could cause the patient to sneeze.*
▪ Instill the prescribed number of drops, observing the patient carefully for signs of discomfort.
▪ *To prevent the drops from leaking out of the nostrils,* ask the patient to keep her head tilted back for at least 5 minutes and to breathe through her mouth. *This also allows sufficient time for the medication to constrict mucous membranes.*
▪ Keep an emesis basin handy *so that the patient can expectorate any medication that flows into the oropharynx and mouth.* Use a facial tissue to wipe any excess medication from the patient's nostrils and face.
▪ Clean the dropper by separating the plunger and pipette and flushing them with warm water. Allow them to air-dry.

For nasal inhaler and aerosol drug instillation

▪ Insert the medication cartridge according to the manufacturer's instructions. With some models, you'll fit the medication cartridge over a small hole in the adapter. When inserting a refill cartridge, first remove the protective cap from the stem. Spacer inhalers may be recommended.
▪ Shake the medication cartridge and then insert it in the adapter. (Before inserting a refill cartridge, remove the protective cap from the stem.)
▪ Remove the protective cap from the adapter tip.
▪ Hold the inhaler with your index finger on top of the cartridge and your thumb under the nasal adapter. The adapter tip should be pointing toward the patient.

Positioning the patient for nose drop instillation

To reach the ethmoid and sphenoid sinuses, have the patient lie on her back with her neck hyperextended and her head tilted back over the edge of the bed. Support her head with one hand *to prevent neck strain.*

To reach the maxillary and frontal sinuses, have the patient lie on her back with her head toward the affected side and hanging slightly over the edge of the bed. Ask her to rotate her head laterally after hyperextension, and support her head with one hand *to prevent neck strain.*

To administer drops for relief of ordinary nasal congestion, help the patient to a reclining or supine position with her head tilted slightly toward the affected side. Aim the dropper upward, toward the patient's eye, rather than downward, toward her ear.

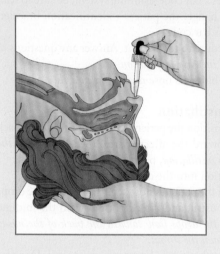

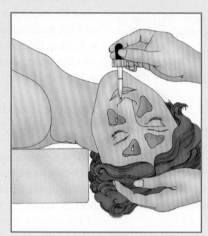

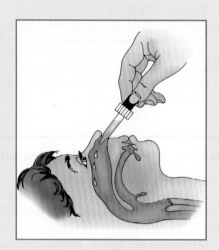

■ Have the patient tilt his head back. Then tell him to place the adapter tip into one nostril, pointing it slightly away from the nasal septum, while occluding the other nostril with his finger.

■ Instruct the patient to inhale gently as he presses the adapter and the cartridge together firmly *to release a measured dose of medication.* Be sure to follow the manufacturer's instructions. *With some medications, such as dexamethasone sodium phosphate (Turbinaire), drug administration by inhaler isn't desirable.*

■ Tell the patient to remove the inhaler from his nostril and to hold his breath for a few seconds.

■ Have the patient exhale through his mouth.

■ Shake the inhaler, and have the patient repeat the procedure in the other nostril.

■ Have the patient gargle with water or saline *to remove medication from his mouth and throat.*

■ Remove the medication cartridge from the nasal inhaler, and wash the nasal adapter in lukewarm water. Let the adapter dry thoroughly before reinserting the cartridge.

Completing the procedure
■ Remove and discard gloves.
■ Perform hand hygiene.[2,3,4]
■ Document the procedure.[6]

Special considerations
■ Instruct the patient not to blow his nose for 15 minutes after the medication is given.

PEDIATRIC ALERT *Before instilling nose drops in a young child, attach a small piece of tubing to the end of the dropper. Do the same for an uncooperative patient.*

■ When using an aerosol, be careful not to puncture or incinerate the pressurized cartridge. Store it at temperatures below 120° F (48.9° C).

■ *To prevent the spread of infection,* label the medication bottle so that it will be used only for that patient.

■ After using the nasal aerosol, the patient should wait at least 15 minutes before blowing his nose *to allow the medication time to be absorbed.*

Patient teaching
Teach the patient how to instill nasal medications correctly *so that he can continue treatment after discharge, if necessary.* Caution him against using nasal medications longer than prescribed *because they may cause a rebound effect that worsens the condition.* A rebound effect occurs when the medication loses its effectiveness and relaxes the vessels in the nasal turbinates, producing a stuffiness that can be relieved only by discontinuing the medication.

Inform the patient of possible adverse reactions. In addition, explain that when corticosteroids are given by nasal aerosol, therapeutic effects may not appear for 2 days to 2 weeks. Teach the patient good oral and nasal hygiene.

Explain that overdosage—which commonly occurs—can cause the medication to lose its effectiveness. Tell him to record the date and time of each inhalation or instillation as well as his response *to prevent overdosage and to help the doctor determine the drug's effectiveness.* Also, note whether the patient uses an unusual amount of medication. Inform the patient of possible adverse reactions.

If more than one inhalation is ordered, advise the patient to wait at least 2 minutes before repeating the procedure. If the patient is also using a steroid inhaler, instruct him to use the bronchodilator first and then wait 5 minutes before using the steroid. *This approach allows the bronchodilator to open the air passages for maximum effectiveness.*

Complications

Complications are related to the medication being administered. Use of nasal inhalers may also cause drying of the nasal membranes and epistaxis.

Some nasal medications may cause restlessness, palpitations, nervousness, and other systemic effects. For example, excessive use of corticosteroid aerosols may cause hyperadrenocorticism and adrenal suppression.

Documentation

Record the medication instilled and its concentration, the number of drops or instillations administered, and whether the medication was instilled in one or both nostrils. Also note the time and date of instillation and any resulting adverse effects.

REFERENCES

1 The Joint Commission. (2012). Standard MM.06.01.01. *Comprehensive accreditation manual for hospitals: The official handbook.* Oakbrook Terrace, IL: The Joint Commission. (Level I)
2 The Joint Commission. (2012). Standard NPSG.07.01.01. *Comprehensive accreditation manual for hospitals: The official handbook.* Oakbrook Terrace, IL: The Joint Commission. (Level I)
3 Centers for Disease Control and Prevention. (October 2002). Guideline for hand hygiene in health-care settings. *Morbidity and Mortality Weekly Report, 51*(RR-16), 1–45. (Level I)
4 World Health Organization. (2009). *WHO guidelines on hand hygiene in health care: First global patient safety challenge. Clean care is safer care.* Geneva, Switzerland: World Health Organization. (Level I)
5 The Joint Commission. (2012). Standard NPSG.01.01.01. *Comprehensive accreditation manual for hospitals: The official handbook.* Oakbrook Terrace, IL: The Joint Commission. (Level I)
6 The Joint Commission. (2012). Standard RC.01.03.01. *Comprehensive accreditation manual for hospitals: The official handbook.* Oakbrook Terrace, IL: The Joint Commission. (Level I)

ADDITIONAL REFERENCES

Leach, C.L. (2007). Inhalation aspects of therapeutic aerosols. *Toxicologic Pathology, 35*(1), 23–26.
Nettina, S.M. (2010). *Lippincott manual of nursing practice* (9th ed.). Philadelphia, PA: Lippincott Williams & Wilkins.
Taylor, C., et al. (2011). *Fundamentals of nursing: The art and science of nursing care* (7th ed.). Philadelphia, PA: Lippincott Williams & Wilkins.

NASAL PACKING, ASSISTING

In the highly vascular nasal mucosa, even seemingly minor injuries can cause major bleeding and blood loss. When routine therapeutic measures, such as direct pressure, cautery, and vasoconstrictive drugs, fail to control epistaxis (nosebleed), the patient's nose may have to be packed to stop anterior bleeding (which runs out of the nose) or posterior bleeding (which runs down the throat). If blood drains into the nasopharyngeal area or lacrimal ducts, the patient may also appear to bleed from the mouth and eyes.

Most nasal bleeding originates at a plexus of arterioles and venules in the anteroinferior septum. Only about 1 in 10 nosebleeds occurs in the posterior nose, which usually bleeds more heavily than the anterior location.

A nurse typically assists a doctor with anterior or posterior nasal packing. She may also assist with nasal balloon catheterization—a procedure that applies pressure to a posteior bleeding site.

Whichever procedure the patient undergoes, you should provide ongoing encouragement and support to reduce his discomfort and anxiety. You should also perform ongoing assessment to determine the procedure's success and to detect possible complications.

Equipment

Gowns ▪ goggles ▪ masks ▪ sterile gloves ▪ sedative, as ordered ▪ clamp ▪ patient drape (towels, incontinence pads, or gown) ▪ nasal speculum and tongue depressors (may be in preassembled head and neck examination kit) ▪ directed illumination source (such as headlamp or strong flashlight) or fiber-optic nasal endoscope, light cables, and light source ▪ suction apparatus with sterile suction-connecting tubing and sterile nasal aspirator tip ▪ sterile bowl and sterile saline solution for flushing out suction apparatus ▪ sterile tray or sterile towels ▪ local anesthetic spray (topical 4% lidocaine) or vial of local anesthetic solution (such as 2% lidocaine or 1% to 2% lidocaine with epinephrine 1:100,000) ▪ 10-mL syringe with 22G 1½″ needle ▪ silver nitrate sticks ▪ topical nasal vasoconstrictor decongestant (such as 0.5% phenylephrine) ▪ sterile normal saline solution (1-g container and 60-mL syringe with luer-lock tip, or 5-mL bullets for moistening nasal tampons) ▪ equipment for measuring vital signs ▪ packages of 1½″ petroleum strip gauze ▪ two #14 or #16 French catheters with 30-mL balloon ▪ alcohol pad ▪ cotton-tipped applicators ▪ petroleum jelly ▪ additional medications, as ordered.

Preparation of equipment

Gather all equipment at the patient's bedside. Make sure the headlamp works. Plug in the suction apparatus if necessary or turn on the suction regulator. Connect the tubing from the collection

Inserting anterior nasal packing

The doctor may treat an anterior nosebleed by packing the anterior nasal cavity with a 3″ to 4″ (7.5- to 10-cm) strip of antibiotic-impregnated petroleum gauze (as shown) or with a nasal tampon.

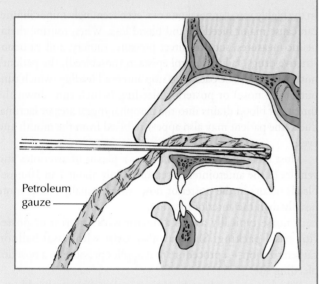

Petroleum gauze

A nasal tampon is made of tightly compressed absorbent material with or without a central breathing tube. The doctor inserts a lubricated tampon along the floor of the nose and, with the patient's head tilted backward, instills 5 to 10 mL of antibiotic or normal saline solution, *which causes the tampon to expand, stopping the bleeding.* The tampon should be moistened periodically, and the central breathing tube should be suctioned regularly.

In a child or a patient with blood dyscrasias, the doctor may fashion an absorbable pack by moistening a gauzelike, regenerated cellulose material with a vasoconstrictor. Applied to a visible bleeding point, this substance will swell to form a clot. The packing is absorbable and doesn't need removal.

container to the suction source. Test the suction equipment to make sure it works properly.

Perform hand hygiene. At the bedside, create a sterile field. (Use the sterile towels or the sterile tray.) Using sterile technique, label all medications and solutions and place all sterile equipment on the sterile field.[1]

If the doctor will inject a local anesthetic rather than spray it into the nose, place the 22G 1½″ needle attached to the 10-mL syringe on the sterile field. When the doctor readies the syringe, clean the stopper on the anesthetic vial with an alcohol pad, and hold the vial so he can withdraw the anesthetic. *This practice allows the doctor to avoid touching his sterile gloves to the nonsterile vial.*

Open the packages containing the sterile suction-connecting tubing and aspirating tip, and place them on the sterile field. Fill the sterile bowl with normal saline solution *so that the suction tubing can be flushed, as necessary.* Thoroughly lubricate the posterior packing with antibiotic ointment.

Implementation

- Verify the doctor's order.
- Confirm the patient's identity using at least two patient identifiers according to your facility's policy.[2]
- Explain the procedure to the patient, answer questions, and offer reassurance *to reduce his anxiety and promote cooperation.*
- Perform hand hygiene, put on sterile gloves and other personal protective equipment, and ensure that all people caring for the patient wear gowns, sterile gloves, and goggles during insertion of packing *to prevent possible contamination from splattered blood.*[3,4,5]
- Check the patient's vital signs, and observe for hypotension with postural changes. *Hypotension suggests significant blood loss.* Also monitor airway patency *because the patient will be at risk for aspirating or vomiting swallowed blood.*
- If ordered, administer a sedative using safe medication administration practices *to reduce the patient's anxiety and decrease sympathetic stimulation, which can exacerbate a nosebleed.*
- Help the patient sit with his head tilted forward *to minimize blood drainage into the throat and prevent aspiration.* Drape the patient.
- Make sure the suction regulator is on and attach the connecting tubing *so the doctor can aspirate the nasal cavity to remove clots before locating the bleeding source.*
- To inspect the nasal cavity, the doctor will use a nasal speculum and an external light source or a fiber-optic nasal endoscope. *To remove collected blood and help visualize the bleeding vessel,* he will use suction or cotton-tipped applicators. The nose may be treated before inspection with a topical vasoconstrictor such as phenylephrine *to slow bleeding and aid visualization.*
- Lubricate the soft catheters *to ease insertion in the posterior nasal cavity.*
- Instruct the patient to open his mouth and to breathe normally through his mouth during catheter insertion *to minimize gagging as the catheters pass through the nostril.*
- Help the doctor insert the packing, as directed. (See *Inserting anterior nasal packing* and *Inserting posterior nasal packing.*)
- Help the patient assume a comfortable position with his head elevated 45 to 90 degrees. Assess him for airway obstruction or any respiratory changes.
- Monitor the patient's vital signs regularly *to detect changes that may indicate hypovolemia or hypoxemia.*
- Check the posterior oropharynx frequently for bleeding into the back of the throat and for packing that has slipped out of position.
- *Because a patient with nasal packing must breathe through his mouth,* provide thorough oral care often. Artificial saliva, room humidification, and ample fluid intake also relieve dryness caused by mouth breathing.
- Assess the patient for pain.[6]

- As ordered, administer moderate doses of nonaspirin analgesics, decongestants, and sedatives using safe medication administration practices.
- Perform a follow-up pain assessment and notify the doctor if pain isn't adequately controlled.[6]
- Dispose of used and soiled equipment and supplies appropriately.
- Perform hand hygiene.[3,4,5]
- Document the procedure.[7]

Special considerations

- If mucosal oozing persists, apply a moustache dressing by securing a folded gauze pad over the nasal vestibules with tape or a commercial nasal dressing holder. Change the pad when soiled.
- Test the patient's call bell *to make sure he can summon help, if needed.* Also keep emergency equipment (flashlight, tongue depressor, syringe, and hemostats) at the patient's bedside *to speed packing removal if it becomes displaced and occludes the airway.*
- After the packing is in place, compile assessment data carefully *to help detect the underlying cause of nosebleeds.* Mechanical factors include a deviated septum, injury, and a foreign body. Environmental factors include drying and erosion of the nasal mucosa. Other possible causes are upper respiratory tract infection, anticoagulant or salicylate therapy, blood dyscrasias, cardiovascular or hepatic disorders, tumors of the nasal cavity or paranasal sinuses, chronic nephritis, and familial hemorrhagic telangiectasia.
- If significant blood loss occurs or if the underlying cause remains unknown, expect the doctor to order a complete blood count and coagulation profile as soon as possible. Blood transfusion may be necessary.
- After the procedure, the doctor may order arterial blood gas analysis *to detect any pulmonary complications* and arterial oxygen saturation monitoring *to assess for hypoxemia.* If necessary, prepare to administer supplemental humidified oxygen with a face mask.
- Until the pack is removed, the patient should be on modified bed rest.
- Nasal packing is usually removed in 2 to 5 days. After the packing is removed, instruct the patient to avoid blowing his nose forcefully for 48 hours, or as ordered.

Patient teaching

Tell the patient to expect reduced ability to detect smell and taste. Make sure he has a working smoke detector at home. Advise him to eat soft foods because his eating and swallowing abilities will be impaired. Instruct him to drink fluids often or to use artificial saliva to cope with dry mouth. Teach him measures to prevent nosebleeds, and instruct him to seek medical help if these measures fail to stop bleeding. (See *Preventing recurrent nosebleeds,* page 490.)

Complications

The pressure of a posterior pack on the soft palate may lead to hypoxemia. Patients with posterior packing are at special risk for aspiration of blood. Patients with underlying pulmonary conditions, such as chronic obstructive pulmonary disease and asthma,

---

Inserting posterior nasal packing

Posterior packing consists of a gauze roll shaped and secured by three sutures (one suture at each end and one in the middle) or a balloon-type catheter. To insert the packing, the doctor advances one or two soft catheters into the patient's nostrils (as shown). When the catheter tips appear in the nasopharynx, the doctor grasps them with a Kelly clamp or bayonet forceps and pulls them forward through the mouth. He secures the two end sutures to the catheter tip and draws the catheter back through the nostrils. This step brings the packing into place with the end sutures hanging from the patient's nostril. (The middle suture emerges from the patient's mouth to free the packing, when needed.)

The doctor may weight the nose sutures with a clamp. Then he will pull the packing securely into place behind the soft palate and against the posterior end of the septum (nasal choana).

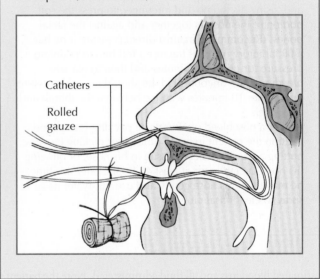

Catheters

Rolled gauze

---

are at special risk for exacerbation of the condition or for hypoxemia while nasal packing is in place. Hypoxemia can be detected with pulse oximetry. Signs and symptoms include tachycardia, confusion, cyanosis, and restlessness.

Airway obstruction may occur if a posterior pack slips backward. The patient may complain of difficulty swallowing, pain, or discomfort. In patients with posterior packs, otitis media may develop. Other possible complications include hematotympanum and pressure necrosis of nasal structures, especially the septum.

Sedation may cause hypotension in a patient with significant blood loss and may also increase the patient's risk of aspiration and hypoxemia.

Documentation

Record the type of pack used *to ensure its removal at the appropriate time.* On the intake-and-output record, document the

Preventing recurrent nosebleeds

Review these self-care guidelines with your patient to reduce his risk of developing recurrent nosebleeds.

■ *Because nosebleeds can result from dry mucous membranes,* suggest that the patient use a cool mist vaporizer or humidifier, as needed, especially in dry environments.

■ Teach the patient how to minimize pressure on nasal passages. Advise him, for instance, to avoid constipation and consequent straining during defecation. Recommend a fiber-rich diet and adequate fluid intake, and warn him to avoid extreme physical exertion for 24 hours after the nosebleed stops. Caution him to avoid aspirin (which has anticoagulant properties), alcoholic beverages, and tobacco for at least 5 days.

■ If the patient gets a nosebleed despite these precautions, tell him to keep his head higher than his heart and, using his thumb and forefinger, to press the soft portion of the nostrils together and against the facial bones. (Recommend against direct pressure if he has a facial injury or nasal fracture.) Tell him to maintain pressure for up to 10 minutes and then to reassess bleeding. If it's uncontrolled, he should reapply pressure for another 10 minutes with ice between the thumb and forefinger.

■ After a nosebleed or after nasal packing is removed, caution the patient to avoid rubbing or picking his nose, putting a handkerchief or tissue in his nose, or blowing his nose forcefully for at least 48 hours. After this time, he may blow his nose gently and use salt-water nasal spray to clear nasal clots.

estimated blood loss and all fluid administered. Note the patient's vital signs; his response to sedation, analgesics, or position changes; the results of any laboratory tests; and any drugs administered, including topical agents. Record any complications. Document patient teaching, discharge instructions, and clinical follow-up plans.

REFERENCES

1 The Joint Commission. (2012). Standard NPSG.03.04.01. *Comprehensive accreditation manual for hospitals: The official handbook.* Oakbrook Terrace, IL: The Joint Commission. (Level I)

2 The Joint Commission. (2012). Standard NPSG.01.01.01. *Comprehensive accreditation manual for hospitals: The official handbook.* Oakbrook Terrace, IL: The Joint Commission. (Level I)

3 The Joint Commission. (2012). Standard NPSG.07.01.01. *Comprehensive accreditation manual for hospitals: The official handbook.* Oakbrook Terrace, IL: The Joint Commission. (Level I)

4 Centers for Disease Control and Prevention. (October 2002). Guideline for hand hygiene in health-care settings. *Morbidity and Mortality Weekly Report, 51*(RR-16), 1–45. (Level I)

5 World Health Organization. (2009). *WHO guidelines on hand hygiene in health care: First global patient safety challenge. Clean care is safer care.* Geneva, Switzerland: World Health Organization. (Level I)

6 The Joint Commission. (2012). Standard PC.01.02.07. *Comprehensive accreditation manual for hospitals: The official handbook.* Oakbrook Terrace, IL: The Joint Commission. (Level I)

7 The Joint Commission. (2012). Standard RC.01.03.01. *Comprehensive accreditation manual for hospitals: The official handbook.* Oakbrook Terrace, IL: The Joint Commission. (Level I)

NASOENTERIC-DECOMPRESSION TUBE CARE

The nasoenteric-decompression tube is used to aspirate intestinal contents for analysis and to treat intestinal obstruction. The tube may also help to prevent nausea, vomiting, and abdominal distention after GI surgery.

After initial tube insertion, the patient lies on his right side for about 2 hours to promote the tube's passage. When the tube advances past the pylorus, it can be advanced 2″ (5 cm) per hour until it reaches the desired position. The tube is then secured to the patient's gown or bed linens, taped to his face, and connected to a suction machine.

The patient with a nasoenteric-decompression tube needs special care and continuous monitoring to ensure tube patency, maintain suction and bowel decompression, and detect such complications as fluid-electrolyte imbalances related to aspiration of intestinal contents. Offer the patient encouragement and support during insertion and removal of the tube and while the tube is in place. To promote comfort and to prevent skin breakdown, provide frequent mouth and nose care. Throughout treatment, keep precise intake and output records.

Equipment

Suction apparatus with intermittent suction capability ■ container of water ■ intake and output record sheets ■ mouthwash and water mixture ■ sponge swabs ■ petroleum jelly or water-soluble lubricant ■ cotton-tipped applicators ■ disposable irrigation set ■ irrigant ■ gloves and other personal protective equipment, as needed.

Preparation of equipment

Assemble the suction apparatus and set up the suction unit. If indicated, test the unit by turning it on and placing the end of the suction tubing in a container of water. If the tubing draws in water, the unit works.

Implementation

■ Verify the doctor's order.

■ Confirm the patient's identity using at least two patient identifiers according to your facility's policy.[1]

■ Perform hand hygiene, put on gloves as needed, and follow standard precautions as appropriate.[2,3,4]

TROUBLESHOOTING

Clearing a nasoenteric-decompression tube obstruction

If your patient's nasoenteric-decompression tube appears to be obstructed, notify the doctor right away. He may order measures such as those listed below *to restore patency quickly and efficiently.*

- Disconnect the tube from the suction source and irrigate with normal saline solution. Use gravity flow to help clear the obstruction unless ordered otherwise.
- If irrigation doesn't reestablish patency, the tube may be obstructed by its position against the gastric mucosa. To rectify this, tug slightly on the tube *to move it away from the mucosa.*
- If gentle tugging doesn't restore patency, the tube may be kinked and may need additional manipulation. Before proceeding, however, take these precautions:

– Never reposition or irrigate a nasoenteric-decompression tube (without a doctor's order) in a patient who has had GI surgery.
– Avoid manipulating a tube in a patient who had the tube inserted during surgery. *To do so may disturb new sutures.*
– Don't try to reposition a tube in a patient who was difficult to intubate (because of an esophageal stricture, for example).

- Explain to the patient and his family the purpose of the procedure. Answer questions clearly and thoroughly *to ease anxiety and enhance cooperation.*
- Check the suction machine at least every 2 hours *to confirm proper functioning and to ensure tube patency and bowel decompression. Excessive negative pressure may draw the mucosa into the tube openings, impair the suction's effectiveness, and injure the mucosa. By using intermittent suction, you may avoid these problems.* To check functioning in an intermittent suction unit, look for drainage in the connecting tube and dripping into the collecting container. Empty the container every 8 hours and measure the contents.
- Record intake and output accurately *to monitor fluid balance.*
- Watch for signs and symptoms of pneumonia related to the patient's inability to clear his pharynx or cough effectively with a tube in place. Be alert for fever, chest pain, tachypnea or labored breathing, and diminished breath sounds over the affected area.
- Observe drainage characteristics, including color, amount, consistency, odor, and any unusual changes.
- Provide oral care frequently (at least every 4 hours) *to increase patient comfort and promote a healthy oral cavity. If the tube remains in place for several days, mouth-breathing will leave the lips, tongue, and other tissues dry and cracked.* Encourage the patient to participate in oral care. (See "Oral care," page 524.)
- Lubricate the patient's lips with either sponge swabs or petroleum jelly applied with a cotton-tipped applicator.
- At least every 4 hours, gently clean and lubricate the patient's external nostrils with either petroleum jelly or water-soluble lubricant on a cotton-tipped applicator *to prevent skin breakdown.*
- Watch for peristalsis to resume, signaled by bowel sounds, passage of flatus, decreased abdominal distention and, possibly, a spontaneous bowel movement. *These signs may require tube removal.*
- After decompression and before extubation, as ordered, provide a clear- to full-liquid diet *to assess bowel function.*
- Discard gloves (if necessary) and perform hand hygiene.[2,3,4]
- Document the procedure.[5]

Special considerations

- If no drainage is accumulating in the collection container, suspect an obstruction in the tube. As ordered, irrigate the tube with the irrigation set to clear the obstruction. (See *Clearing a nasoenteric-decompression tube obstruction.*) Record the amount of instilled irrigant as "intake." Typically, normal saline solution supersedes water as the preferred irrigant *because water, which is hypotonic, may increase electrolyte loss, especially with frequent tube irrigation.*
- If your patient is ambulatory and his tube connects to a portable suction unit, he may move short distances while connected to the unit. Or, if feasible and ordered, the tube can be disconnected and clamped briefly while he moves about.
- If the tubing irritates the patient's throat or makes him hoarse, offer relief with mouthwash, gargles, viscous lidocaine, throat lozenges, an ice collar, sour hard candy, or gum, as appropriate.
- If the tip of the balloon falls below the ileocecal valve (confirmed by X-ray), the tube can't be removed nasally. It has to be advanced and removed through the anus.
- If the balloon at the end of the tube protrudes from the anus, notify the doctor. Most likely, the tube can be disconnected from suction, the proximal end severed, and the remaining tube removed gradually through the anus either manually or by peristalsis.

Complications

Besides fluid-volume deficit, electrolyte imbalance, and pneumonia, potential complications include intussusception of the bowel (from the weight of the balloon).

Documentation

Record the frequency and type of oral and nasal care given. Describe the therapeutic effect, if any. Document in your notes the amount, color, consistency, and odor of the drainage obtained each time you empty the collection container.

EQUIPMENT

Common types of nasoenteric-decompression tubes

The type of nasoenteric-decompression tube chosen for your patient will depend on the size of the patient and his nostrils, the estimated duration of intubation, and the reason for the procedure. For example, to remove viscous material from the patient's intestinal tract, the doctor may select a tube with a wide bore and a single lumen.

Whichever tube is used, you'll need to provide good mouth care and check the patient's nostrils often for signs of irritation. If you see any signs of irritation, retape the tube *so that it doesn't cause tension,* and then lubricate the nostril. Or check with the doctor to see if the tube can be inserted through the other nostril.

Most tubes are impregnated with a radiopaque mark *so that placement can easily be confirmed by X-ray or other imaging technique.*

Tubes, such as the pre-weighted Andersen Miller-Abbot type intestinal tube (shown below), have a tungsten-weighted inflatable latex balloon tip designed for temporary management of mechanical obstruction in the small or large intestines.

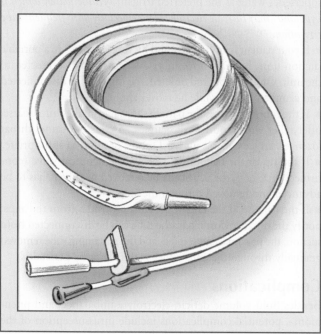

Record the amount of drainage on the intake and output sheet. Always record the amount of any irrigant or other fluid introduced through the tube or taken orally by the patient.

If the suction machine malfunctions, note the length of time it wasn't functioning and the nursing action taken. Document the amount and character of any vomitus. Also note the patient's tolerance of the tube's insertion and removal.

REFERENCES

1 The Joint Commission. (2012). Standard NPSG.01.01.01. *Comprehensive accreditation manual for hospitals: The official handbook.* Oakbrook Terrace, IL: The Joint Commission. (Level I)
2 The Joint Commission. (2012). Standard NPSG.07.01.01. *Comprehensive accreditation manual for hospitals: The official handbook.* Oakbrook Terrace, IL: The Joint Commission. (Level I)
3 Centers for Disease Control and Prevention. (October 2002). Guideline for hand hygiene in health-care settings. *Morbidity and Mortality Weekly Report, 51*(RR-16), 1–45. (Level I)
4 World Health Organization. (2009). *WHO guidelines on hand hygiene in health care: First global patient safety challenge. Clean care is safer care.* Geneva, Switzerland: World Health Organization. (Level I)
5 The Joint Commission. (2012). Standard RC.01.03.01. *Comprehensive accreditation manual for hospitals: The official handbook.* Oakbrook Terrace, IL: The Joint Commission. (Level I)

ADDITIONAL REFERENCE

Smeltzer, S.C., et al. (2010). *Brunner & Suddarth's textbook of medical-surgical nursing* (12th ed.). Philadelphia, PA: Lippincott Williams & Wilkins.

NASOENTERIC-DECOMPRESSION TUBE INSERTION AND REMOVAL

The nasoenteric-decompression tube is inserted nasally and advanced beyond the stomach into the intestinal tract. It's used to aspirate intestinal contents for analysis and to treat intestinal obstruction. The tube may also help to prevent nausea, vomiting, and abdominal distention after GI surgery. The doctor usually inserts or removes a nasoenteric-decompression tube; however, the nurse may remove it in an emergency.

The nasoenteric-decompression tube may have a pre-weighted tip and a balloon at one end of the tube that holds air or water to stimulate peristalsis and facilitate the tube's passage through the pylorus and into the intestinal tract. (See *Common types of nasoenteric-decompression tubes.*)

Equipment

For insertion

Nasoenteric-decompression tube ▪ suction-decompression equipment ▪ gloves ▪ towel or linen-saver pad ▪ water-soluble lubricant ▪ 4″ × 4″ gauze pad ▪ hypoallergenic tape ▪ bulb syringe or 60-mL catheter-tip syringe ▪ pH test paper ▪ penlight, as needed ▪ waterproof pen ▪ glass of water with straw ▪ Optional: labels for tube lumens, basin of ice or warm water, local anesthetic.

For removal

Sterile 10-mL syringe ▪ gloves ▪ towel or linen-saver pad ▪ clamp.

Preparation of equipment

Before insertion, stiffen a flaccid tube by chilling it in a basin of ice *to facilitate insertion.* To make a stiff tube flexible, dip it into warm water.

Air or water is added to the balloon either before or after insertion of the tube, depending on the type of tube used. Follow the manufacturer's recommendations.

Set up suction-decompression equipment, if ordered, and make sure it works properly.

Implementation

- Verify the doctor's order.
- Confirm the patient's identity using at least two patient identifiers according to your facility's policy.[1]
- Explain the procedure to the patient, forewarning him that he may experience some discomfort. Answer all questions *to decrease anxiety and increase cooperation.*
- Provide privacy and adequate lighting.
- Perform hand hygiene and put on gloves.[2,3,4]
- Position the patient as the doctor specifies, usually in semi-Fowler's or high Fowler's position. You may also need to help the patient hold his neck in a hyperextended position.
- Protect the patient's chest with a towel or linen-saver pad.

Inserting a nasoenteric-decompression tube

- Agree with the patient on a signal that can be used to stop the insertion briefly, if necessary.
- The doctor assesses the patency of the patient's nostrils. *To evaluate which nostril has better airflow in a conscious patient,* he holds one nostril closed and then the other as the patient breathes. In an unconscious patient, he examines each nostril with a penlight *to check for polyps, a deviated septum, or other obstruction.*
- *To decide how far the tube must be inserted to reach the stomach,* the doctor places the tube's distal end at the tip of the patient's nose and then extends the tube to the earlobe and down to the xiphoid process. He either marks the tube with a waterproof pen or holds it at this point.
- The doctor applies water-soluble lubricant to the first few inches of the tube *to reduce friction and tissue trauma and to facilitate insertion.*
- If the balloon already contains water, the doctor holds it so the fluid runs to the bottom. Then he pinches the balloon closed *to retain the fluid as the insertion begins.*
- Tell the patient to breathe through his mouth or to pant as the balloon enters his nostril. After the balloon begins its descent, the doctor releases his grip on it, allowing the weight of the fluid or the pre-weighted tip to pull the tube into the nasopharynx. When the tube reaches the nasopharynx, the doctor instructs the patient to lower his chin and to swallow. In some cases, the patient may sip water through a straw *to facilitate swallowing as the tube advances,* but not after the tube reaches the trachea *to prevents injury from aspiration.* The doctor continues to advance the tube slowly *to prevent it from curling or kinking in the stomach.*
- *To confirm the tube's passage into the stomach,* the doctor aspirates stomach contents with a bulb syringe or a catheter-tip syringe. Examine the aspirate and place several drops on a piece of pH paper to determine whether gastric contents are present. The desired gastric range is from 0 to 5, unless the patient is receiving acid-inhibiting agents; then the pH may increase to 6. The probability of gastric placement is increased if the aspirate has

a typical gastric fluid appearance (grassy green, clear and colorless with mucus, or brown) and the pH is less than 5.

- After the tube clears the pylorus, the doctor may direct you to advance it 2″ to 3″ (5 to 7.5 cm) every hour and to reposition the patient until the premeasured mark reaches the patient's nostril. Gravity and peristalsis will help advance the tube. (Notify the doctor if you can't advance the tube.)
- Keep the remaining premeasured length of tube well lubricated *to ease passage and prevent irritation.*
- After the tube progresses the necessary distance, the doctor will order an X-ray *to confirm tube positioning.*
- When the tube is in place, secure the external tubing with tape *to help prevent further progression.*

NURSING ALERT *Don't tape the tube while it advances to the premeasured mark unless the doctor asks you to do so.*

- Attach the tube to intermittent suction.
- Remove gloves and perform hand hygiene.[2,3,4]
- Document the procedure.[5]

Removing a nasoenteric-decompression tube

- Clamp the tube and disconnect it from the suction *to prevent the patient from aspirating any gastric contents that leak from the tube during withdrawal.*
- If your patient has a tube with an inflated balloon tip, attach a 10-mL syringe to the balloon port and withdraw the air or water. Don't deflate the balloon until you're ready to remove the tube.
- Slowly withdraw between 6″ and 8″ (15 and 20 cm) of the tube. Wait 10 minutes and withdraw another 6″ to 8″. Wait another 10 minutes. Continue this procedure until the tube reaches the patient's esophagus (with 18″ [45 cm] of the tube remaining inside the patient). At this point, you can gently withdraw the tube completely.
- Discard used equipment appropriately.
- Remove and discard gloves.
- Perform hand hygiene.[2,3,4]
- Document the procedure.[5]

Special considerations

- For a double- or triple-lumen tube, label which lumen accommodates balloon inflation and which accommodates drainage.
- Apply a local anesthetic, if ordered, to the nostril or the back of the throat *to dull sensations and the gag reflex for intubation.* Letting the patient gargle with a liquid anesthetic or holding ice chips in his mouth for a few minutes serves the same purpose.

Complications

Nasoenteric-decompression tubes may cause reflux esophagitis, nasal or oral inflammation, and nasal, laryngeal, or esophageal ulceration.

Documentation

Record the date and time the nasoenteric-decompression tube was inserted and by whom. Note the patient's tolerance of the procedure, the type of tube used, the suction type and amount, and the color, amount, and consistency of drainage.

Record the date and time of tube removal, the name of the person removing the tube, and the patient's tolerance of the removal procedure.

REFERENCES

1 The Joint Commission. (2012). Standard NPSG.01.01.01. *Comprehensive accreditation manual for hospitals: The official handbook.* Oakbrook Terrace, IL: The Joint Commission. (Level I)
2 The Joint Commission. (2012). Standard NPSG.07.01.01. *Comprehensive accreditation manual for hospitals: The official handbook.* Oakbrook Terrace, IL: The Joint Commission. (Level I)
3 Centers for Disease Control and Prevention. (October 2002). Guideline for hand hygiene in health-care settings. *Morbidity and Mortality Weekly Report, 51*(RR-16), 1–45. (Level I)
4 World Health Organization. (2009). *WHO guidelines on hand hygiene in health care: First global patient safety challenge. Clean care is safer care.* Geneva, Switzerland: World Health Organization. (Level I)
5 The Joint Commission. (2012). Standard RC.01.03.01. *Comprehensive accreditation manual for hospitals: The official handbook.* Oakbrook Terrace, IL: The Joint Commission. (Level I)

ADDITIONAL REFERENCE

Smeltzer, S.C., et al. (2010). *Brunner & Suddarth's textbook of medical-surgical nursing* (12th ed.). Philadelphia, PA: Lippincott Williams & Wilkins.

NASOGASTRIC TUBE CARE

Providing effective nasogastric (NG) tube care requires meticulous monitoring of the patient and the equipment. Monitoring the patient involves checking drainage from the NG tube and assessing GI function; monitoring the equipment involves verifying correct tube placement and function.

Equipment

Oral sponge swabs or toothbrush and toothpaste ▪ gloves ▪ petroleum jelly ▪ linen-saver pad, towel, or emesis basin ▪ ½″ or 1″ hypoallergenic tape ▪ water-soluble lubricant ▪ stethoscope ▪ graduated container ▪ Optional: screening test for occult blood.

Preparation of equipment

Make sure suction equipment works properly. (See *Common gastric suction devices.*) When using a Salem sump tube with suction, connect the larger, primary lumen (for drainage and suction) to the suction equipment and select the appropriate setting, as ordered (usually low constant suction). If the doctor doesn't specify the setting, follow the manufacturer's instructions. A Levin tube usually calls for intermittent low suction.

Implementation

▪ Confirm the patient's identity using at least two patient identifiers according to your facility's policy.[1]
▪ Explain the procedure to the patient and provide privacy.
▪ Perform hand hygiene and put on gloves.[2,3,4]

▪ Provide oral care once per shift, or as needed. Depending on the patient's condition, use oral sponge swabs to clean his teeth or assist him to brush his teeth with a toothbrush and toothpaste.
▪ Coat the patient's lips with petroleum jelly *to prevent dryness from mouth breathing.*
▪ Change the tape securing the tube, as needed or at least daily. Clean the skin, and apply fresh tape. Dab water-soluble lubricant on the nostrils, as needed.
▪ Regularly check the tape that secures the tube *because sweat and nasal secretions may loosen the tape.*
▪ Check the position of the NG tube periodically, according to facility policy and before instilling any type of solution into the tube.
▪ Irrigate the tube, as ordered or necessary.
▪ Assess bowel sounds regularly (every 4 to 8 hours) *to verify GI function.*
▪ Measure the drainage amount and update the intake and output record every 8 hours. Be alert for electrolyte imbalances with excessive gastric output.
▪ Inspect gastric drainage and note its color, consistency, odor, and amount. Normal gastric secretions have no color or appear yellow-green from bile and have a mucoid consistency. Immediately report any drainage with a coffee-bean color, *which may indicate bleeding.* If you suspect that the drainage contains blood, use a screening test (such as Hematest) for occult blood according to your facility's policy.
▪ Remove and discard gloves and perform hand hygiene.[2,3,4]
▪ Document the procedure.[5]

Special considerations

▪ NG tubes can become clogged or incorrectly positioned. Attempt to reposition the patient or rotate and reposition the tube. However, if the tube was inserted during surgery, avoid this maneuver *to ensure that the movement doesn't interfere with gastric or esophageal sutures.* Notify the doctor.
▪ If necessary, irrigate the NG tube and instill 30 mL of air into the vent tube *to maintain patency.* Don't attempt to stop reflux by clamping the vent tube. Unless contraindicated, elevate the patient's torso more than 30 degrees, and keep the vent tube above his midline *to prevent a siphoning effect.*
▪ If no drainage appears in the tube, check the suction equipment for proper function. Then, holding the NG tube over a linen-saver pad or an emesis basin, separate the tube and the suction source. Check the suction equipment by placing the suction tubing in an irrigant container. If the apparatus draws the water, check the NG tube for proper function. Be sure to note the amount of water drawn into the suction container on the intake-and-output record.
▪ If the patient is allowed to ambulate and you need to interrupt suction, disconnect the NG tube from the suction equipment. Clamp the tube *to prevent stomach contents from draining out of the tube.*

Complications

Epigastric or abdominal pain and vomiting may result from a clogged or improperly placed tube. Any NG tube—the Levin

EQUIPMENT

Common gastric suction devices

A variety of wall-mounted suction devices are available for applying negative pressure to nasogastric (NG) and other drainage tubes. Two common types are shown here.

Portable suction machine

In the portable suction machine, a vacuum created intermittently by an electric pump draws gastric contents up the NG tube and into the collecting bottle. This type of suction is becoming less commonly seen because of the prevalence of stationary, or wall-mounted, units.

Stationary suction machine

A stationary wall-unit apparatus can provide intermittent or continuous suction. On-off switches and variable power settings let you set and adjust the suction force on either machine.

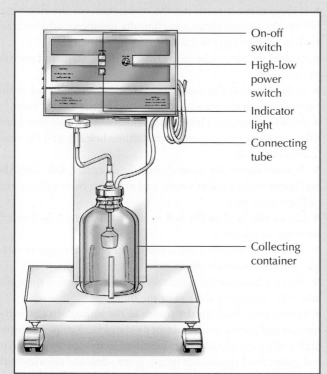

On-off switch
High-low power switch
Indicator light
Connecting tube
Collecting container

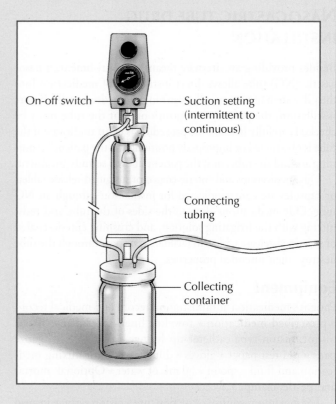

On-off switch
Suction setting (intermittent to continuous)
Connecting tubing
Collecting container

tube in particular—may move and aggravate esophagitis, ulcers, or esophageal varices, causing hemorrhage. Perforation may result from aggressive intubation. Dehydration and electrolyte imbalances may result from removing body fluids and electrolytes by suctioning. Pain, swelling, and salivary dysfunction may signal parotitis, which occurs in dehydrated, debilitated patients. Intubation can cause oral or nasal skin breakdown and discomfort and increased mucous secretions. Aspiration pneumonia may result from gastric reflux. Vigorous suction may damage the gastric mucosa and cause significant bleeding, possibly interfering with endoscopic assessment and diagnosis.

Documentation

Regularly confirm and record tube placement (usually every 4 to 8 hours). Keep a precise record of fluid intake and output. Describe drainage color, consistency, odor, and amount. Also note tape change times and the condition of the nares.

REFERENCES

1 The Joint Commission. (2012). Standard NPSG.01.01.01. *Comprehensive accreditation manual for hospitals: The official handbook*. Oakbrook Terrace, IL: The Joint Commission. (Level I)
2 The Joint Commission. (2012). Standard NPSG.07.01.01. *Comprehensive accreditation manual for hospitals: The official handbook*. Oakbrook Terrace, IL: The Joint Commission. (Level I)
3 Centers for Disease Control and Prevention. (October 2002). Guideline for hand hygiene in health-care settings. *Morbidity and Mortality Weekly Report, 51*(RR-16), 1–45. (Level I)
4 World Health Organization. (2009). *WHO guidelines on hand hygiene in health care: First global patient safety challenge. Clean care is safer care*. Geneva, Switzerland: World Health Organization. (Level I)

5 The Joint Commission. (2012). Standard RC.01.03.01. *Comprehensive accreditation manual for hospitals: The official handbook.* Oakbrook Terrace, IL: The Joint Commission. (Level I)

ADDITIONAL REFERENCES

Nettina, S.M. (2010). *Lippincott manual of nursing practice* (9th ed.). Philadelphia, PA: Lippincott Williams & Wilkins.

Taylor, C., et al. (2011). *Fundamentals of nursing: The art and science of nursing care* (7th ed.). Philadelphia, PA: Lippincott Williams & Wilkins.

NASOGASTRIC TUBE DRUG INSTILLATION

Besides providing an alternate means of nourishment, a nasogastric (NG) tube allows direct instillation of medication into the GI system of patients who can't ingest the drug orally. Before instillation, the patency and positioning of the tube must be checked carefully because the procedure is contraindicated if the tube is obstructed or improperly positioned, if the patient is vomiting around the tube, or if the patient's bowel sounds are absent.

Oily medications and enteric-coated or sustained-release tablets or capsules are contraindicated for instillation through an NG tube. Oily medications cling to the sides of the tube and resist mixing with the irrigating solution, and crushing enteric-coated or sustained-release tablets to facilitate transport through the tube destroys their intended properties.

Equipment

Patient's medication administration record and medical record ▪ prescribed medication ▪ towel or linen-saver pad ▪ 50- or 60-mL piston-type catheter-tip syringe ▪ two 4″ × 4″ gauze pads ▪ pH test paper ▪ gloves ▪ diluent ▪ cup for mixing medication and fluid ▪ spoon ▪ 50 mL of water ▪ Optional: mortar and pestle, clamp.

For maximum control of suction, use a piston syringe instead of a bulb syringe. The liquid for diluting the medication can be juice, water, or a nutritional supplement.

Preparation of equipment

Gather equipment for use at the bedside. Liquids should be at room temperature. *Administering cold liquids through an NG tube can cause abdominal cramping.* Although this isn't a sterile procedure, make sure the cup, syringe, spoon, and gauze are clean.

Implementation

▪ Verify the doctor's order.[1]
▪ Avoid distractions and interruptions when preparing and administering the medication to prevent medication errors.[2]
▪ Compare the medication label to the order and verify that the medication is correct.[3]
▪ Check the expiration date on the medication; don't give if the drug is expired.[3]

▪ Check the patient's medical record for an allergy to the prescribed medication. If an allergy is present, don't administer the medication and notify the doctor.[3]
▪ Discuss any unresolved concerns you may have with the patient's doctor.
▪ If the prescribed medication is in tablet form, crush the tablets with a mortar and pestle *to ready them for mixing in a cup with the diluting liquid.* Request liquid forms of medications, if available.
▪ Bring the medication and equipment to the patient's bedside.
▪ Perform hand hygiene and put on gloves.[4,5,6]
▪ Confirm the patient's identity using at least two patient identifiers according to your facility's policy.[7]
▪ If the patient is receiving the medication for the first time, inform the patient about any clinically significant adverse reactions or other concerns related to the new medication.[3]
▪ Explain the procedure to the patient, if necessary, and provide privacy.
▪ Make sure that the medication is being administered at the proper time, in the prescribed dose, and by the correct route.[3]
▪ If your facility uses a bar code scanning system, scan your identification badge, the patient's identification bracelet, and the medication's bar code.
▪ *To avoid soiling the sheets during the procedure,* fold back the bed linens to the patient's waist and drape his chest with a towel or linen-saver pad.
▪ Elevate the head of the bed so that the patient is in Fowler's position, as tolerated.
▪ Trace the tubing from the patient to its point of origin *to make sure you're accessing the proper tube.*[8]
▪ After unclamping the tube, take the 50- or 60-mL syringe and attach the syringe to the end of the tube.
▪ Gently draw back on the piston of the syringe. Examine the aspirate and place a small amount on the pH test strip. The probability of gastric placement is increased if the aspirate has a typical gastric fluid appearance (grassy green, clear and colorless with mucus shreds, or brown) and the pH is 5 or less. (However, only an X-ray can positively confirm the tube's position. A properly obtained and interpreted X-ray is recommended to confirm placement of any blindly inserted NG tube before its initial use for feedings or medication administration.[9]) If no gastric contents appear when you draw back on the syringe, the tube may have risen into the esophagus; you'll have to advance it before proceeding.[9]
▪ If you meet resistance when aspirating, stop the procedure. *Resistance may indicate a nonpatent tube or improper tube placement.* (Keep in mind that some smaller NG tubes may collapse when aspiration is attempted.) If the tube seems to be in the stomach, resistance probably means the tube is lying against the stomach wall. *To relieve resistance,* withdraw the tube slightly or turn the patient.
▪ After you have established that the tube is patent and in the correct position, clamp the tube, detach the syringe, and lay the end of the tube on a 4″ × 4″ gauze pad.
▪ Mix the crushed tablets or liquid medication with the diluent. If the medication is in capsule form, open the capsules and empty

their contents into the liquid. Pour liquid medications directly into the diluting liquid. Stir well with the spoon. (If the medication was in tablet form, make sure the particles are small enough to pass through the eyes at the distal end of the tube.)

■ Reattach the syringe, without the piston, to the end of the tube and open the clamp.

■ Deliver the medication slowly and steadily. (See *Giving medications through an NG tube.*)

■ If the medication flows smoothly, slowly add more until the entire dose has been given. If the medication doesn't flow properly, don't force it. Raise the syringe slightly. If it's too thick, dilute it with water. If you suspect that tube placement is inhibiting the flow, stop the procedure and reevaluate tube placement.

■ Watch the patient's reaction throughout the instillation. If he shows any sign of discomfort, stop the procedure immediately.

■ As the last of the medication flows out of the syringe, start to irrigate the tube by adding 30 to 50 mL of water. *Irrigation clears medication from the sides of the tube and from the distal end, reducing the risk of clogging.*

PEDIATRIC ALERT *For a child, irrigate the tube using only 15 to 30 mL of water.*

■ When the water stops flowing, quickly clamp the tube. Detach the syringe and dispose of it.

■ Remove the towel or linen-saver pad and replace the bed linens.

■ Leave the patient in Fowler's position, or have him lie on his right side with the head of the bed partially elevated. Have him maintain this position for at least 30 minutes after the procedure *to facilitate the downward flow of medication into the stomach and prevent esophageal reflux.*

■ Discard used supplies in the appropriate receptacle.

■ Remove and discard your gloves.

■ Perform hand hygiene.[4,5,6]

■ Document the procedure.[10]

Special considerations

■ *To prevent instillation of too much fluid* (more than 400 mL of liquid at one time for an adult), don't schedule the drug instillation with the patient's regular tube feeding, if possible.

■ If you must schedule a tube feeding and medication instillation simultaneously, give the medication first *to ensure that the patient receives the prescribed drug therapy even if he can't tolerate an entire feeding.* Remember to avoid giving foods that interact adversely with the drug. Tube feedings must be held 1 hour before and 1 hour after phenytoin administration.

■ If the patient receives continuous tube feedings, stop the feeding and check the gastric residual volume. If it's more than 500 mL, withhold the medication and feeding and notify the doctor. *An excessive amount of residual contents may indicate intestinal obstruction or paralytic ileus.*

■ If the NG tube is attached to suction, turn off the suction for 30 to 60 minutes after administering medication.

Patient teaching

If the patient will require an NG tube after discharge, give oral and written instructions for instilling medication through an NG tube to the patient and his family, as appropriate. Remain with

Giving medications through an NG tube

Holding the nasogastric (NG) tube at a level somewhat above the patient's nose, pour up to 30 mL of diluted medication into the syringe barrel. *To prevent air from entering the patient's stomach,* hold the tube at a slight angle and add more medication before the syringe empties. If necessary, raise the tube slightly higher *to increase the flow rate.*

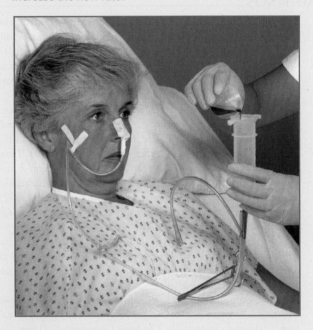

After you've delivered the entire dose, position the patient on her right side, head slightly elevated, *to minimize esophageal reflux.*

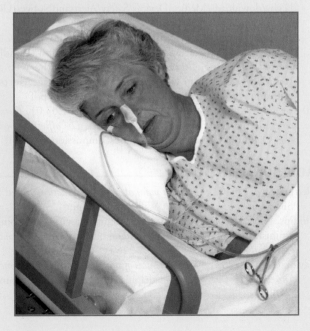

the patient when he performs the procedure for the first few times *so that you can provide assistance and answer any questions.* Encourage him and correct any errors in technique, as necessary.

Documentation

Record the instillation of medication, date and time of instillation, dose, and the patient's tolerance of the procedure. On his intake-and-output sheet, note the amount of fluid instilled. Document any patient teaching provided and whether the patient gave a return demonstration.

REFERENCES

1 The Joint Commission. (2012). Standard MM.04.01.01. *Comprehensive accreditation manual for hospitals: The official handbook.* Oakbrook Terrace, IL: The Joint Commission. (Level I)

2 Westbrook, J. et al. (2010). Association of interruptions with an increased risk and severity of medication administration errors. *Archives of Internal Medicine, 170*(8), 683–690.

3 The Joint Commission. (2012). Standard MM.06.01.01. *Comprehensive accreditation manual for hospitals: The official handbook.* Oakbrook Terrace, IL: The Joint Commission. (Level I)

4 The Joint Commission. (2012). Standard NPSG.07.01.01. *Comprehensive accreditation manual for hospitals: The official handbook.* Oakbrook Terrace, IL: The Joint Commission. (Level I)

5 Centers for Disease Control and Prevention. (October 2002). Guideline for hand hygiene in health-care settings. *Morbidity and Mortality Weekly Report, 51*(RR-16), 1–45. (Level I)

6 World Health Organization. (2009). *WHO guidelines on hand hygiene in health care: First global patient safety challenge. Clean care is safer care.* Geneva, Switzerland: World Health Organization. (Level I)

7 The Joint Commission. (2012). Standard NPSG.01.01.01. *Comprehensive accreditation manual for hospitals: The official handbook.* Oakbrook Terrace, IL: The Joint Commission. (Level I)

8 U.S. Food and Drug Administration. (2009). "Look. Check. Connect.: Safe Medical Device Connections Save Lives" [Online]. Accessed November 2011 via the Web at http://www.fda.gov/downloads/MedicalDevices/Safety/AlertsandNotices/UCM134873.pdf

9 American Association of Critical-Care Nurses (2009). "AACN Practice Alert: Verification of Feeding Tube Insertion (Blindly Inserted)" [Online]. Accessed October 2010 via the Web at http://www.aacn.org/WD/Practice/Docs/PracticeAlerts/Verification_of_Feeding_Tube_Placement_05-2005.pdf

10 The Joint Commission. (2012). Standard RC.01.03.01. *Comprehensive accreditation manual for hospitals: The official handbook.* Oakbrook Terrace, IL: The Joint Commission. (Level I)

ADDITIONAL REFERENCES

Nettina, S.M. (2010). *Lippincott manual of nursing practice* (9th ed.). Philadelphia, PA: Lippincott Williams & Wilkins.

Phillips, N.M., & Nay, R. (2008). A systematic review of nursing administration of medication via enteral tubes in adults. *Journal of Clinical Nursing, 17*(17), 2257–2265.

Taylor, C., et al. (2011). *Fundamentals of nursing: The art and science of nursing care* (7th ed.). Philadelphia, PA: Lippincott Williams & Wilkins.

Williams, N.T. (2008). Medication administration through enteral feeding tubes. *American Journal of Health-System Pharmacies, 65*(24), 2347–2357.

NASOGASTRIC TUBE INSERTION AND REMOVAL

Usually inserted to decompress the stomach, a nasogastric (NG) tube can prevent vomiting after major surgery. An NG tube is typically in place for 48 to 72 hours after surgery, by which time peristalsis usually resumes. It may remain in place for shorter or longer periods, however, depending on its use.

The NG tube has other diagnostic and therapeutic applications, especially in assessing and treating upper GI bleeding, collecting gastric contents for analysis, performing gastric lavage, aspirating gastric secretions, and administering medications and nutrients.

Inserting an NG tube requires close observation of the patient and verification of proper placement. The tube must be inserted with extra care in pregnant patients and in those with an increased risk of complications. For example, the doctor will order an NG tube for a patient with aortic aneurysm, myocardial infarction, gastric hemorrhage, or esophageal varices only if he believes that the benefits outweigh the risks of intubation.

Most NG tubes have a radiopaque marker or strip at the distal end so that the tube's position can be verified by X-ray. If the position can't be confirmed, the doctor may order fluoroscopy to verify placement.

The most common NG tubes are the Levin tube, which has one lumen, and the Salem sump tube, which has two lumens—one for suction and drainage and a smaller one for ventilation. Air flows through the vent lumen continuously, which protects the delicate gastric mucosa by preventing a vacuum from forming should the tube adhere to the stomach lining. (See *Types of NG tubes.*)

Equipment
For insertion

Tube (usually #12, #14, #16, or #18 French for a normal adult) ▪ towel or linen-saver pad ▪ facial tissues ▪ emesis basin ▪ penlight ▪ 1″ hypoallergenic tape ▪ alcohol pad ▪ gloves ▪ water-soluble lubricant ▪ cup or glass of water with straw (if appropriate) ▪ pH test strip or carbon dioxide detector ▪ tongue blade ▪ catheter-tip or bulb syringe or irrigation set ▪ safety pin ▪ ordered suction equipment ▪ Optional: rubber band and safety pin, basin of ice or warm water.

For removal

Stethoscope ▪ catheter-tip syringe ▪ normal saline solution ▪ towel or linen-saver pad ▪ adhesive remover ▪ gloves.

Preparation of equipment

Inspect the NG tube for defects, such as rough edges or partially closed lumens. Then check the tube's patency by flushing it with water. If you need to increase the tube's flexibility *to ease insertion,* coil it around your gloved fingers for a few seconds or dip it in

EQUIPMENT

Types of NG tubes

The doctor will choose the type and diameter of nasogastric (NG) tube that best suits the patient's needs, including lavage, aspiration, enteral therapy, and stomach decompression. Choices may include the Levin and Salem sump tubes.

Levin tube
The Levin tube is a rubber or plastic tube that has a single lumen, a length of 42″ to 50″ (106.5 to 127 cm), and holes at the tip and along the side.

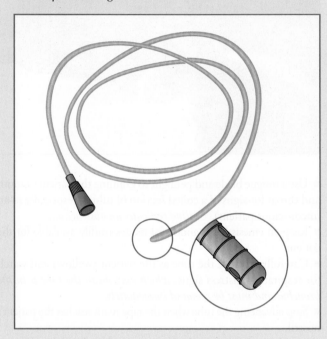

Salem sump tube
A Salem sump tube is a double-lumen tube that's made of clear plastic and has a blue sump port (pigtail) that allows atmospheric air to enter the patient's stomach. Thus, the tube floats freely and doesn't adhere to or damage gastric mucosa. The larger port of this 48″ (122-cm) tube serves as the main suction conduit. The tube has openings at 45, 55, 65, and 75 cm as well as a radiopaque line to verify placement.

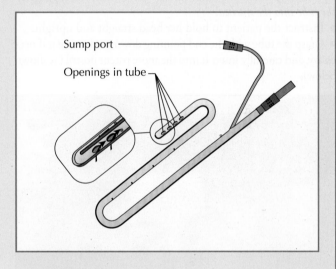

Sump port

Openings in tube

---

warm water. If the tube is too flaccid, stiffen it by filling the tube with water and then freezing it[1] or dipping the tube in ice water.

Implementation
- Verify the doctor's order.
- Perform hand hygiene and put on gloves.[2,3,4]
- Confirm the patient's identity using at least two patient identifiers according to your facility's policy.[5]
- Explain the procedure to the patient *to ease anxiety and promote cooperation*. Inform her that she may experience some nasal discomfort, that she may gag, and that her eyes may water.
- Agree on a signal that the patient can use if she wants you to stop briefly during the procedure.
- Provide privacy and help the patient into high Fowler's position unless contraindicated.
- Drape the towel or linen-saver pad over the patient's chest *to protect her gown and bed linens from spills.*

Inserting an NG tube
- Place the facial tissues and emesis basin well within the patient's reach.

- Help the patient face forward with her neck in a neutral position.
- Determine the length of the tube to be inserted to reach the stomach: hold the end of the tube at the tip of the patient's nose (as shown below) and extend the tube to the patient's earlobe and then down to the xiphoid process.

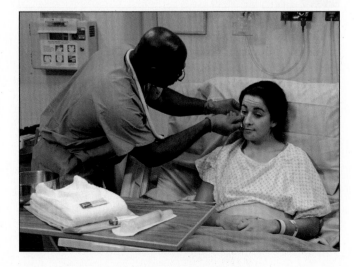

■ Mark this distance on the tubing with the tape. (Average measurements for an adult range from 22″ to 26″ [56 to 66 cm].) It may be necessary to add 2″ (5 cm) to this measurement in tall individuals *to ensure entry into the stomach.*

■ Determine which nostril will allow easier access; use a penlight and inspect for a deviated septum or other abnormalities. Ask the patient if she ever had nasal surgery or a nasal injury. Assess airflow in both nostrils by occluding one nostril at a time while the patient breathes through her nose. Choose the nostril with the better airflow. If the patient is able to respond, ask whether she has had an NG tube placed previously. If she has, then ask which nostril is better for insertion.

■ Lubricate the first 3″ (7.6 cm) of the tube with a water-soluble gel to minimize injury to the nasal passages. *Using a water-soluble lubricant prevents lipoid pneumonia, which may result from aspiration of an oil-based lubricant or from accidental slippage of the tube into the trachea.*

■ Instruct the patient to hold her head straight and upright.

■ Grasp the tube with the end pointing downward, curve it if necessary, and carefully insert it into the more patent nostril (as shown below).

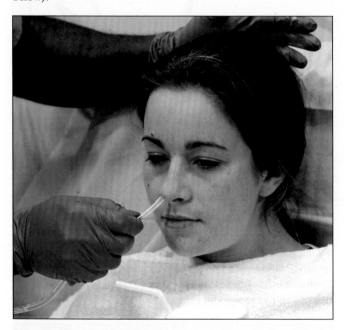

■ Aim the tube downward and toward the ear closer to the chosen nostril. Advance it slowly *to avoid pressure on the turbinates and resultant pain and bleeding.*

■ When the tube reaches the nasopharynx, you'll feel resistance. Instruct the patient to lower her head slightly *to close the trachea and open the esophagus.* Then rotate the tube 180 degrees toward the opposite nostril to redirect it *so that the tube won't enter the patient's mouth.*

■ Unless contraindicated, offer the patient a cup or glass of water with a straw. Direct her to sip and swallow as you slowly advance the tube *to help the tube pass to the esophagus* (as shown below). If you aren't using water, ask the patient to swallow.

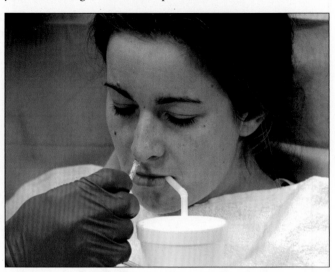

■ Use a tongue blade and penlight to examine the patient's mouth and throat for signs of a coiled section of tubing (especially in an unconscious patient). *Coiling indicates an obstruction.*

■ Keep an emesis basin and facial tissues readily available for the patient.

■ Carefully advance the tube as the patient swallows and watch for respiratory distress signs, *which may mean the tube is in the bronchus and must be removed immediately.*

■ Stop advancing the tube when the tape mark reaches the patient's nostril.

■ Attach a catheter-tip or bulb syringe to the tube and try to aspirate stomach contents (as shown below). If you don't obtain stomach contents, position the patient on her left side *to move the contents into the stomach's greater curvature,* and aspirate again. If you still can't aspirate stomach contents, advance the tube 1″ to 2″ (2.5 to 5 cm) and try to aspirate stomach contents again.

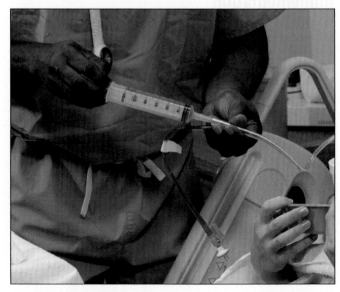

NURSING ALERT *When confirming tube placement, never place the tube's end in a container of water. If the tube should be malpositioned in the trachea, the patient may aspirate water. Water without bubbles doesn't confirm proper placement. Instead, the tube may be coiled in the trachea or the esophagus.*

■ Examine the aspirate and place several drops on a piece of pH paper *to determine whether gastric contents are present.* The desired gastric range is from 0 to 5, unless the patient is receiving acid-inhibiting agents; then the pH may increase to 6. The probability of gastric placement is increased if the aspirate has a typical gastric fluid appearance (grassy green, clear and colorless with mucus, or brown) and pH is less than 5.0. Alternately, use a carbon dioxide detector to confirm placement isn't in the lungs.

■ Anticipate an X-ray *to verify placement.*

■ Secure the NG tube to the patient's nose with hypoallergenic tape (or other designated tube holder or prepackaged product). If the patient's skin is oily, wipe the bridge of the nose with an alcohol pad and allow it to dry. You will need about 4″ (10 cm) of 1″ tape. Split one end of the tape up the center about 1¹⁄₂″ (3.8 cm). Make tabs on the split ends (by folding sticky sides together). Stick the uncut tape end on the patient's nose so that the split in the tape starts about ½″ (1.3 cm) to 1½″ from the tip of her nose. Crisscross the tabbed ends around the tube. Then apply another piece of tape over the bridge of the nose to secure the tube (as shown below).

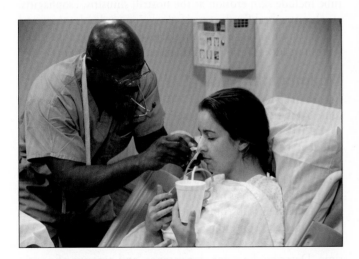

■ *To reduce discomfort from the weight of the tube,* tie a slipknot around the tube with a rubber band and then secure the rubber band to the patient's gown with a safety pin. Alternatively, wrap another piece of tape around the end of the tube and leave a tab. Then fasten the tape tab to the patient's gown.

■ Attach the tube to suction equipment, if ordered, and set the designated suction pressure.

■ Provide frequent nasal and oral care while the tube is in place.

■ Remove and discard gloves. Perform hand hygiene.[2,3,4]

■ Document the procedure.[6]

Removing an NG tube

■ Assess bowel function by auscultating for peristalsis or flatus.

■ Help the patient into semi-Fowler's position. Then drape a towel or linen-saver pad across her chest to protect her gown and bed linens from spills (as shown below).

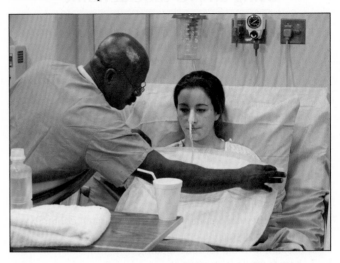

■ Using a catheter-tip syringe, flush the tube with 30 mL of air or normal saline solution (as shown below) *to ensure that the tube doesn't contain stomach contents that could irritate tissues during tube removal.*

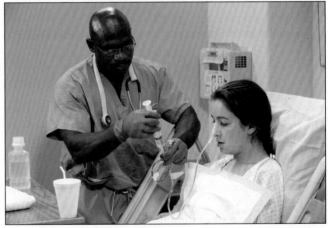

■ Untape the tube from the patient's nose, and then unpin it from her gown.

■ Clamp the tube by folding it in your hand (as shown below).

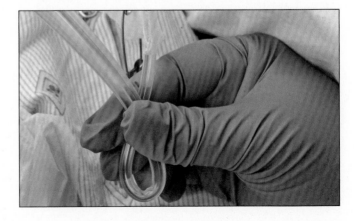

Using an NG tube at home

If your patient will need to have a nasogastric (NG) tube in place at home—for short-term feeding or gastric decompression, for example—find out who will insert the tube. If the patient will have a home care nurse, identify who it will be and, if possible, tell the patient when to expect the home care nurse.

If the patient or a family member will perform the procedure, you'll need to provide additional instruction and supervision. Using this checklist as a guide, teach the patient how to:

- obtain equipment needed for home intubation (including where to obtain equipment)
- insert the tube
- verify tube placement by aspirating stomach contents
- correct tube misplacement
- prepare formula for tube feeding
- store formula if appropriate
- administer formula through the tube
- remove and dispose of an NG tube
- clean and store a reusable NG tube
- use the NG tube for gastric decompression if appropriate
- set up and operate suctioning equipment
- troubleshoot suctioning equipment
- perform mouth care and other hygienic procedures.

- Ask the patient to hold her breath *to close the epiglottis.* Then withdraw the tube gently and steadily. (When the distal end of the tube reaches the nasopharynx, you can pull it quickly.)
- When possible, immediately cover and remove the tube *because its sight and odor may nauseate the patient.*
- Assist the patient with thorough oral care. (See "Oral care," page 524.)
- Clean the tape residue from the patient's nose with adhesive remover.
- Dispose of equipment in the appropriate receptacle.
- Remove and discard gloves. Perform hand hygiene.[2,3,4]
- Document the procedure.[6]

Special considerations

- If the patient has a deviated septum or other nasal condition that prevents nasal insertion, pass the tube orally after removing any dentures, if necessary. Sliding the tube over the tongue, proceed as you would for nasal insertion.
- When using the oral route, remember to coil the end of the tube around your hand *to help curve and direct the tube downward at the pharynx.*
- If your patient is unconscious, tilt the patient's chin toward the chest *to close the trachea.* Then advance the tube between respirations to ensure that it doesn't enter the trachea.

- While advancing the tube in an unconscious patient (or in a patient who can't swallow), stroke the patient's neck *to encourage the swallowing reflex and facilitate passage down esophagus.*
- While advancing the tube, observe for signs that it has entered the trachea, such as choking or breathing difficulties in a conscious patient and cyanosis in an unconscious patient or a patient without a cough reflex. If these signs occur, remove the tube immediately. Allow the patient time to rest; then try to reinsert the tube.
- If vomiting occurs after tube placement, suspect tubal obstruction or incorrect position. Assess immediately to determine the cause.
- For 48 hours after removal, monitor the patient for signs of GI dysfunction, including nausea, vomiting, abdominal distention, and food intolerance. GI dysfunction may necessitate reinsertion of the tube.

Patient teaching

An NG tube may be inserted at home. Indications for insertion include gastric decompression and short-term feeding. A home care nurse or the patient may insert the tube, deliver the feeding, and remove the tube. (See *Using an NG tube at home.*)

Complications

Potential complications of prolonged intubation with an NG tube include skin erosion at the nostril, sinusitis, esophagitis, esophagotracheal fistula, gastric ulceration, and pulmonary and oral infection. Additional complications that may result from suction include electrolyte imbalances and dehydration.

Documentation

Record the type and size of the NG tube and the date, time, and route of insertion. Include the method used to confirm placement of the tube. Also note the type and amount of suction, if used, and describe the drainage, including the amount, color, character, consistency, and odor. Note the patient's tolerance of the procedure. Include in your notes any signs and symptoms signaling complications, such as nausea, vomiting, and abdominal distention. Document subsequent placement assessments, irrigation procedures, and continuing problems after irrigation.

When you remove a nasogastric tube, record the date and time. Describe the color, consistency, and amount of gastric drainage. Note any unusual events following NG removal, such as nausea, vomiting, abdominal distention, and food intolerance. Note the patient's tolerance of the procedure.

References

1 Chun, D.H., et al. (2009). A randomized, clinical trial of frozen versus standard nasogastric tube placement. *World Journal of Surgery, 33*(9), 1789–1792. (Level II)

2 The Joint Commission. (2012). Standard NPSG.07.01.01. *Comprehensive accreditation manual for hospitals: The official handbook.* Oakbrook Terrace, IL: The Joint Commission. (Level I)

3 Centers for Disease Control and Prevention. (October 2002). Guideline for hand hygiene in health-care settings. *Morbidity and Mortality Weekly Report, 51*(RR-16), 1–45. (Level I)

4   World Health Organization. (2009). *WHO guidelines on hand hygiene in health care: First global patient safety challenge. Clean care is safer care.* Geneva, Switzerland: World Health Organization. (Level I)
5   The Joint Commission. (2012). Standard NPSG.01.01.01. *Comprehensive accreditation manual for hospitals: The official handbook.* Oakbrook Terrace, IL: The Joint Commission. (Level I)
6   The Joint Commission. (2012). Standard RC.01.03.01. *Comprehensive accreditation manual for hospitals: The official handbook.* Oakbrook Terrace, IL: The Joint Commission. (Level I)

ADDITIONAL REFERENCES

Craven, R.F., & Hirnle, C.J. (2012). *Fundamentals of nursing: Human health and function* (7th ed.). Philadelphia, PA: Lippincott Williams & Wilkins.
Durai, R., et al. (2009). Nasogastric tubes 1: Insertion technique and confirming the correct position. *Nursing Times, 105*(16), 12–13.
Meyer, P., et al. (2009). Colorimetric capnography to ensure correct nasogastric tube position. *Journal of Critical Care, 24*(2), 231–235.
Nettina, S.M. (2010). *Lippincott manual of nursing practice* (9th ed.). Philadelphia, PA: Lippincott Williams & Wilkins.
Taylor, C., et al. (2011). *Fundamentals of nursing: The art and science of nursing care* (7th ed.). Philadelphia, PA: Lippincott Williams & Wilkins.

NASOPHARYNGEAL AIRWAY INSERTION AND CARE

Insertion of a nasopharyngeal airway—a soft rubber or latex uncuffed catheter—establishes or maintains a patent airway. This airway is the typical choice for patients with airway obstruction or the risk for developing airway obstruction when conditions such as a clenched jaw or oral problems prevent placement of an oral airway.[1] It's also used to protect the nasal mucosa from injury when the patient needs frequent nasotracheal suctioning.

The airway follows the curvature of the nasopharynx, passing through the nose and extending from the nostril to the posterior pharynx. The bevel-shaped pharyngeal end of the airway facilitates insertion, and its funnel-shaped nasal end helps prevent slippage.

Insertion of a nasopharyngeal airway is preferred when an oropharyngeal airway is contraindicated or fails to maintain a patent airway. A nasopharyngeal airway is contraindicated if the patient has a pathologic nasopharyngeal deformity. An oropharyngeal airway is preferred when a basal skull fracture or severe coagulopathy is present or suspected.[1]

Equipment
For insertion

Nasopharyngeal airway of proper size ▪ tongue blade ▪ water-soluble lubricant ▪ gloves ▪ Optional: suction equipment; flashlight; mask for mouth-to-mask resuscitation, handheld resuscitation bag, or oxygen-powered breathing device.

For cleaning
Hydrogen peroxide ▪ water ▪ basin ▪ Optional: pipe cleaner.

Implementation

- Verify the doctor's order.
- Confirm the patient's identity using at least two patient identifiers according to your facility's policy.[2]
- Perform hand hygiene and put on gloves.[3,4,5]
- In nonemergency situations, explain the procedure to the patient *to decrease anxiety and increase cooperation.*
- Measure the diameter of the patient's nostril and the distance from the tip of his nose to his earlobe. Select an airway of slightly smaller diameter than the nostril and of slightly longer length (1″ [2.5 cm]) than measured. The sizes for this type of airway are labeled according to their internal diameter. The recommended airway size for a large adult is 8 to 9 mm; for a medium adult, 7 to 8 mm; for a small adult, 6 to 7 mm. Lubricate the distal half of the airway's surface with a water-soluble lubricant *to prevent traumatic injury during insertion.*
- Properly insert the airway. (See *Inserting a nasopharyngeal airway,* page 504.)
- Immediately after insertion, assess the patient's respirations. If absent or inadequate, initiate artificial positive-pressure ventilation with a mouth-to-mask technique, a handheld resuscitation bag, or an oxygen-powered breathing device.
- Check the airway regularly *to detect dislodgment or obstruction.*
- When the patient's natural airway is patent, remove the artificial airway in one smooth motion. If the airway sticks, apply lubricant around the nasal end of the tube and around the nostril; then gently rotate the airway until it's free.
- Remove your gloves and perform hand hygiene.[3,4,5]
- Document the procedure.[6]

Special considerations

- If the patient continues to cough or gag, the tube may be too long. If so, remove the airway and insert a shorter one.
- At least once every 8 hours, remove the airway *to check nasal mucous membranes for irritation or ulceration.*
- Clean the airway by placing it in a basin and rinsing it with hydrogen peroxide and then with water. If secretions remain, use a pipe cleaner to remove them. Reinsert the clean airway into the other nostril (if it's patent) *to avoid skin breakdown.*

Complications

Sinus infection may result from obstruction of sinus drainage. Insertion of the airway may injure the nasal mucosa and cause bleeding and, possibly, aspiration of blood into the trachea. Suction as necessary to remove secretions or blood. If the tube is too long, it may enter the esophagus and cause gastric distention and hypoventilation during artificial ventilation. Although semiconscious patients usually tolerate this type of airway better than conscious patients do, they may still experience laryngospasm and vomiting.

Inserting a nasopharyngeal airway

First, hold the airway beside the patient's face *to make sure it's the proper size* (as shown below). It should be slightly smaller than the patient's nostril diameter and slightly longer than the distance from the tip of his nose to his earlobe.

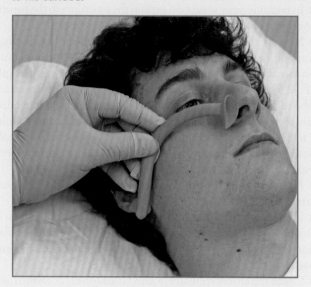

To insert the airway, hyperextend the patient's neck using a chin-lift or jaw-thrust technique *to anteriorly displace the patient's mandible* (unless contraindicated). Then push up the tip of his nose and pass the airway into his nostril (as shown below). Avoid pushing against any resistance *to prevent tissue trauma and airway kinking.*

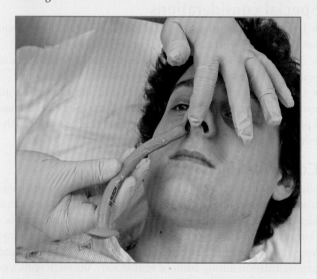

To check for correct airway placement, first close the patient's mouth. Then, place your finger over the tube's opening *to detect air exchange.* Also depress the patient's tongue with a tongue blade, and look for the airway tip behind the uvula.

Documentation

Record the date and time of the airway's insertion, size of the airway, removal and cleaning of the airway, shifts from one nostril to the other, condition of the mucous membranes, suctioning, complications and nursing action taken, and the patient's reaction to the procedure.

REFERENCES

1 American Heart Association. (2010). 2010 American Heart Association guidelines for cardiopulmonary resuscitation and emergency cardiovascular care. *Circulation, 122*(Suppl. 3), S729–767. (Level I)
2 The Joint Commission. (2012). Standard NPSG.01.01.01. *Comprehensive accreditation manual for hospitals: The official handbook.* Oakbrook Terrace, IL: The Joint Commission. (Level I)
3 The Joint Commission. (2012). Standard NPSG.07.01.01. *Comprehensive accreditation manual for hospitals: The official handbook.* Oakbrook Terrace, IL: The Joint Commission. (Level I)
4 Centers for Disease Control and Prevention. (October 2002). Guideline for hand hygiene in health-care settings. *Morbidity and Mortality Weekly Report, 51*(RR-16), 1–45. (Level I)
5 World Health Organization. (2009). *WHO guidelines on hand hygiene in health care: First global patient safety challenge. Clean care is safer care.* Geneva, Switzerland: World Health Organization. (Level I)
6 The Joint Commission. (2012). Standard RC.01.03.01. *Comprehensive accreditation manual for hospitals: The official handbook.* Oakbrook Terrace, IL: The Joint Commission. (Level I)

ADDITIONAL REFERENCES

Lynn-McHale Wiegand, D. (Ed.). (2011). *AACN procedure manual for critical care* (6th ed.). Philadelphia, PA: Saunders.
Taylor, C., et al. (2011). *Fundamentals of nursing: The art and science of nursing care* (7th ed.). Philadelphia, PA: Lippincott Williams & Wilkins.

NEBULIZER THERAPY

An established component of respiratory care, nebulizer therapy aids bronchial hygiene by restoring and maintaining mucous blanket continuity; hydrating dried, retained secretions; promoting expectoration of secretions; humidifying inspired oxygen; and delivering medications. Therapy may be administered through nebulizers that have a large or small volume, are connected to ventilator tubing, or are ultrasonic.

Large-volume nebulizers, such as the Venturi jet, are used to provide long-term 100% humidity for an artificial airway, such as with a tracheostomy or for certain pulmonary conditions such as cystic fibrosis. (See *Large-volume nebulizer.*) The aerosol mist can be delivered via mist tent, hood, mouthpiece, mask, T-piece, face tent, or tracheostomy collar.

In-line nebulizers are used to deliver medications to patients who are being mechanically ventilated. In this case, the nebulizer is placed in the inspiratory side of the ventilatory circuit as close to the endotracheal (ET) tube as possible.

Ultrasonic nebulizers are electrically driven and use high-frequency vibrations to break up surface water into particles. The resultant dense mist works to penetrate smaller airways and is useful for hydrating secretions, which induces a cough and sputum. The aerosol mist can be delivered to the patient via mist tent, hood, mouthpiece, mask, T-piece, face tent, or tracheostomy collar. Some ultrasonic nebulizers can also aerosolize medications, but this delivery system hasn't resulted in a demonstrably better clinical response to medication than a standard jet nebulizer.

Standard precautions for body fluid isolation should be used for all patients on nebulizer therapy. Special droplet precautions should be implemented for patients with known or suspected tuberculosis, including enclosing and containing aerosol administration and filtering aerosols that bypass or are exhaled by the patient.

Equipment

For large-volume nebulizer therapy

Pressurized gas source ▪ flowmeter ▪ patient interface device (such as a mask or collar) ▪ large-bore oxygen tubing ▪ nebulizer ▪ sterile distilled water ▪ heater, if ordered ▪ in-line thermometer, if using heater ▪ facial tissues and emesis basin or container for collecting or disposing of expectorated sputum ▪ suction source and supplies ▪ personal protective equipment ▪ Optional: oxygen blender (if a built-in adjustable oxygen controller isn't available).

For small-volume nebulizer therapy

Pressurized gas source ▪ flowmeter ▪ oxygen tubing ▪ nebulizer cup ▪ mouthpiece or mask ▪ normal saline solution ▪ prescribed medication ▪ facial tissues and emesis basin or container for collecting or disposing of expectorated sputum ▪ personal protective equipment ▪ Optional: suction source and supplies.

For in-line nebulizer therapy

Pressurized gas source ▪ flowmeter ▪ in-line nebulizer cup ▪ normal saline solution ▪ prescribed medication ▪ personal protective equipment.

For ultrasonic nebulizer therapy

Ultrasonic gas-delivery device ▪ large-bore oxygen tubing ▪ patient interface device (such as a mask or collar) ▪ nebulizer couplet compartment ▪ facial tissues and emesis basin or container for collecting or disposing of expectorated sputum ▪ inhaled bronchodilator ▪ Optional: suction source and supplies, personal protective equipment.

Preparation of equipment

Gather the appropriate equipment. Label all medications, medication containers, and other solutions and handle them using sterile technique.[1] Discard multidose containers after 24 hours.

For in-line nebulizer therapy, draw up the medication and diluent, open the nebulizer cup, inject the medication, and then replace the lid. Attach the cup to the gas source with attached tubing.

Large-volume nebulizer

The large-volume Venturi jet nebulizer works by passing air through a Venturi opening, drawing liquid up through feeding tubes, and nebulizing the solution.

Advantages
▪ Provides 100% humidity with cool or heated devices
▪ Provides oxygen and aerosol therapy
▪ Can be used for long-term therapy

Disadvantages
▪ Increases the risk of bacterial growth (in reusable units)
▪ Causes a collection of condensate in large-bore tubing
▪ May cause mucosal irritation from breathing hot, dry air (if water level isn't maintained correctly in reservoir)
▪ Increases the risk of overhydration from mist (in infants)

For ultrasonic nebulizer therapy, fill the couplet compartment on the nebulizer to the level indicated with the solution recommended by the manufacturer (typically tap water).

Implementation

▪ Verify the doctor's order.[2]
▪ Perform hand hygiene. Apply personal protective equipment, as appropriate.[3,4,5]
▪ Confirm the patient's identity using at least two patient identifiers according to facility policy.[6]
▪ Explain the procedure to the patient and answer all questions *to decrease anxiety and increase cooperation.*
▪ Take the patient's vital signs, and auscultate his lung fields *to establish a baseline.*[7]
▪ If possible, place the patient in a sitting or high Fowler's position *to encourage full lung expansion and promote aerosol dispersion.*

For large-volume nebulizer therapy

▪ Fill the water chamber to the indicated level with sterile distilled water. Avoid using saline solution *to prevent corrosion.* Add a heating device, if ordered, and place an in-line thermometer between the outlet port and the patient, as close to the patient as possible, *to monitor the actual temperature of the inhaled gas and to avoid burning the patient.*
▪ If the unit will supply oxygen, set the built-in adjustable oxygen regulator or adjust the external oxygen blender to the ordered oxygen concentration and analyze the flow at the patient's end of the tubing *to ensure delivery of the prescribed oxygen percentage.*
▪ Attach the delivery device to the patient.
▪ Encourage the patient to cough and expectorate, or suction as needed.

■ Check the water level in the nebulizer at frequent intervals and refill or replace, as indicated. When refilling a reusable container, discard the old water *to prevent infection from bacterial or fungal growth,* and refill the container to the indicator line with sterile distilled water.

■ If the nebulizer is heated, tell the patient to report warmth, discomfort, or hot tubing *because these may indicate a heater malfunction.* Use the in-line thermometer to monitor the temperature of the gas the patient is inhaling. If you turn off the flow for more than 5 minutes, unplug the heater *to avoid overheating the water and burning the patient when the aerosol is resumed.*

■ Auscultate the patient's lungs *to evaluate the effectiveness of therapy.*[7]

■ Remove and discard personal protective equipment and perform hand hygiene.[3,4,5]

■ Document the procedure.[8]

For small-volume nebulizer therapy

■ Draw up the prescribed medication, inject it into the nebulizer cup, and add the prescribed amount of saline solution or water.

■ After attaching the flowmeter to the gas source, attach the nebulizer to the flowmeter and then adjust the flow to at least 10 L/minute, but no more than 14 L/minute (as shown below), *to ensure adequate functioning while preventing excess venting.*

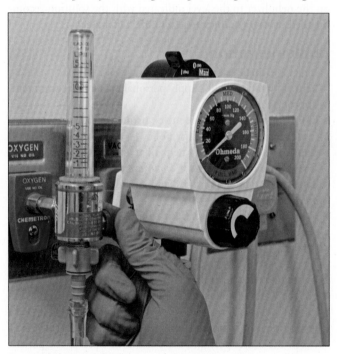

■ Check the outflow port *to ensure adequate misting.*

■ Assist the patient with mouthpiece or mask. Instruct the patient to grasp the mouthpiece securely with his teeth and lips

(as shown below). With either delivery system, the patient should inhale slowly through his mouth and hold each breath for 5 to 10 seconds before exhaling through his mouth.

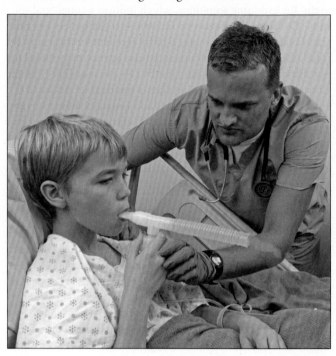

■ Remain with the patient during the treatment until all of the medication in the nebulizer cup has been aerosolized, about 15 to 20 minutes, and take his vital signs and assess lung sounds *to detect any adverse reaction to the medication.*

■ Encourage the patient to cough and expectorate, or suction as necessary.

■ Auscultate the patient's lungs *to evaluate the effectiveness of therapy.*[7]

■ Assist the patient with mouth care.

■ Clean and change the nebulizer cup and tubing according to your facility's policy *to prevent bacterial contamination.*

■ Dispose of waste appropriately. Remove and discard personal protective equipment and perform hand hygiene.[3,4,5]

■ Document the procedure.[8]

For in-line nebulizer therapy

■ Insert the nebulizer cup into the ventilatory circuit as close to the ET tube as possible.[9]

■ Remove the heat-moisture exchanger from the ventilator if it's attached.

■ Initiate gas flow to create a mist, or activate the ventilator's nebulizer adjunct.

■ If the patient is being ventilated using a spontaneous pressure mode, encourage him to take slow, even breaths during the treatment.

■ Remain with the patient during the treatment, which lasts 15 to 20 minutes, and monitor his vital signs, oximetry, and ventilator parameters *to detect any adverse reaction to the medication.*

■ Discontinue treatment when the medication is gone. Remove the nebulizer cup from the ventilatory circuit.

- Encourage the patient to cough, and suction excess secretions as necessary.
- Clean and store the nebulizer cup according to facility policy.
- Auscultate the patient's lungs *to evaluate the effectiveness of therapy.*[7]
- Remove and discard personal protective equipment and perform hand hygiene.[3,4,5]
- Document the procedure.[8]

For ultrasonic nebulizer therapy

- Before beginning, administer an inhaled bronchodilator (metered-dose inhaler or small-volume nebulizer) *to prevent bronchospasm, as ordered.*
- Encourage the patient to take slow, even breaths through his mouth.
- Turn on the nebulizer machine, and check the outflow port *to ensure proper misting.*
- Assist the patient with applying a mouthpiece or mask, as necessary, depending on the delivery system.
- Check the patient frequently during the procedure *to observe for adverse reactions.* Watch for labored respirations *because ultrasonic nebulizer therapy may hydrate retained secretions and obstruct airways.* Observe for wheezing resulting from irritation of the airways.
- Once again, take the patient's vital signs, and auscultate his lung fields.[7]
- Encourage the patient to cough and expectorate, or suction as needed.
- Dispose of sputum properly or send an ordered specimen to the laboratory immediately.
- Assist the patient with oral hygiene.
- Remove and discard personal protective equipment and perform hand hygiene.[3,4,5]
- Document the procedure.[8]

Special considerations

- Change the nebulizer unit and tubing according to your facility's policy *to prevent bacterial contamination.*
- When using a large-volume or high-output nebulizer (such as an ultrasonic nebulizer) on a pediatric patient or a patient with a delicate fluid balance, be alert for signs of overhydration (unexplained weight gain occurring over several days after the beginning of therapy), pulmonary edema, crackles, and electrolyte imbalance.
- Ventilator modes and settings can affect aerosol deposition. Lung-model studies suggest that low inspiratory flows, the use of decelerating flow instead of square wave, tidal volume greater than 500 mL, and increased duty cycle (inspiratory phase) are all associated with improved aerosol deposition. Spontaneous inspiration through the ventilator circuit increases lung deposition compared with controlled, assist/control, and pressure support ventilation.
- Placement of the aerosol device in the ventilator circuit affects the amount of drug delivered to the lungs. Placing the nebulizer 12″ (30 cm) from the ET tube is more efficient than placing it

between the patient and the ET tube *because the tubing acts as a reservoir for the accumulation of aerosol between inspirations.*[9]
- Adding gas from the nebulizer to the ventilator circuit may increase volumes, flows, and peak airway pressures, which in turn alters the intended pattern of ventilation. Ventilator setting adjustments made to accommodate the additional gas flow during nebulization must be reset at the end of treatment.[9]
- Adding gas from a nebulizer into the ventilator circuit may make the patient unable to trigger the ventilator during nebulization, leading to hypoventilation.
- If oxygen is being delivered concomitantly with nebulizer therapy, the fraction of inspired oxygen may be diluted if the flow isn't adequate; if the mist disappears when the patient inhales, increase the gas flow.
- After administering an in-line nebulizer treatment, remove the nebulizer cup from the ventilatory circuit between treatments *to prevent a pressure leak in the system.*
- With small-volume nebulizer treatments, a noseclip may be used if patient has difficulty remembering to breathe through his mouth.

Complications

Nebulized particulates can irritate the mucosa and cause bronchospasm and dyspnea.[9] Other complications include airway burns (when heating elements are used), infection from contaminated equipment (rare), overhydration, and adverse reactions to medications.

Documentation

Record the date, time, and duration of therapy; the type and amount of medication; FIO_2 or oxygen flow, if administered; baseline and subsequent vital signs and breath sounds; the patient's response to treatment; and any patient teaching provided.

REFERENCES

1 The Joint Commission. (2012). Standard NPSG.03.04.01. *Comprehensive accreditation manual for hospitals: The official handbook.* Oakbrook Terrace, IL: The Joint Commission. (Level I)
2 The Joint Commission. (2012). Standard MM.06.01.01. *Comprehensive accreditation manual for hospitals: The official handbook.* Oakbrook Terrace, IL: The Joint Commission. (Level I)
3 The Joint Commission. (2012). Standard NPSG.07.01.01. *Comprehensive accreditation manual for hospitals: The official handbook.* Oakbrook Terrace, IL: The Joint Commission. (Level I)
4 Centers for Disease Control and Prevention. (October 2002). Guideline for hand hygiene in health-care settings. *Morbidity and Mortality Weekly Report, 51*(RR-16), 1–45. (Level I)
5 World Health Organization. (2009). *WHO guidelines on hand hygiene in health care: First global patient safety challenge. Clean care is safer care.* Geneva, Switzerland: World Health Organization. (Level I)
6 The Joint Commission. (2012). Standard NPSG.01.01.01. *Comprehensive accreditation manual for hospitals: The official handbook.* Oakbrook Terrace, IL: The Joint Commission. (Level I)
7 American Association for Respiratory Care. (1995). AARC clinical practice guideline: Assessing response to bronchodilator therapy at point of care. *Respiratory Care, 40*(12), 1300–1307. (Level I)

8   The Joint Commission. (2012). Standard RC.01.03.01. *Comprehensive accreditation manual for hospitals: The official handbook.* Oakbrook Terrace, IL: The Joint Commission. (Level I)

9   American Association for Respiratory Care. (1999). AARC clinical practice guideline: Selection of device, administration of bronchodilator, and evaluation of response to therapy in mechanically ventilated patients. *Respiratory Care, 44*(1), 105–113. (Level I)

ADDITIONAL REFERENCES

American Association for Respiratory Care. (1996). AARC clinical practice guideline: Selection of a device for delivery of aerosol to the lung parenchyma. *Respiratory Care, 41*(7), 647–653.

Nettina, S.M. (2010). *Lippincott manual of nursing practice* (9th ed.). Philadelphia, PA: Lippincott Williams & Wilkins.

Taylor, C., et al. (2011). *Fundamentals of nursing: The art and science of nursing care* (7th ed.). Philadelphia, PA: Lippincott Williams & Wilkins.

NEGATIVE-PRESSURE WOUND THERAPY

Negative-pressure wound therapy enhances wound healing and helps with delayed or impaired wound healing. Treatment involves a special dressing placed in the wound or over a graft or flap and a pump that creates negative pressure within the wound bed. The negative-pressure device removes excess wound fluids that may cause maceration or delayed healing and stimulates the growth of healthy granulation tissue. Negative pressure also increases local blood flow, reduces edema, and draws the wound edges together. (See *Understanding negative-pressure wound therapy.*)

Negative-pressure wound therapy is indicated for acute and traumatic wounds, pressure ulcers, and chronic open wounds, such as diabetic ulcers, meshed grafts, and skin flaps.[1] It's contraindicated for fistulas that involve organs or body cavities, necrotic tissue with eschar, untreated osteomyelitis, malignant wounds, and wounds with exposed arteries and veins. This therapy should be used cautiously in patients with active bleeding, in those taking anticoagulants, and in those in whom achieving wound hemostasis has been difficult.

Equipment

Waterproof trash bag ■ goggles and gown, if indicated ■ emesis basin ■ sterile irrigating solution ■ gloves ■ sterile gloves ■ sterile scissors ■ linen-saver pad ■ irrigation kit with syringe ■ suction tubing ■ evacuation canister tubing ■ skin protectant wipe ■ evacuation canister ■ negative-pressure wound therapy unit ■ measuring tool and guide.

For foam packing

Foam packing ■ transparent dressing therapy drape.

For gauze packing

Nonadherent gauze ■ antimicrobial gauze packing moistened with sterile normal saline solution ■ drain ■ ostomy strip paste ■ transparent dressing(s).

Preparation of equipment

Assemble the negative-pressure wound therapy unit at the bedside according to the manufacturer's instructions. Set negative pressure according to the doctor's order (25 to 200 mm Hg) and the manufacturer's instructions. Prepare a place for the supplies within reach.

Warm the sterile irrigating solution to 90° to 95° F (32° to 35° C) *to reduce discomfort.* Pour irrigating solution into the container of the irrigation kit.

Implementation

■ Verify the doctor's order for frequency of dressing changes, type of negative-pressure unit, type of wound packing, and settings for the negative-pressure unit and assess the patient's condition.

■ Confirm the patient's identity using at least two patient identifiers according to your facility's policy.[2]

■ Explain the procedure to the patient. Answer all questions *to decrease anxiety and increase cooperation.*

■ Provide privacy.

■ Perform hand hygiene and put on gloves.[3,4,5] If necessary, put on a gown and goggles *to protect yourself from wound drainage and contamination.*

■ Assess the patient's condition. Medicate the patient for pain, if needed and as ordered, before beginning the procedure.

■ Place a linen-saver pad under the patient *to catch any spills and avoid linen changes.* Position the patient to allow maximum wound exposure. Place the emesis basin under the wound *to collect any drainage.*

■ Using sterile technique, prepare a sterile field and place all the supplies on the sterile field.

■ Remove the soiled dressing and discard it in the waterproof trash bag. Remove your gloves.

■ Perform hand hygiene[3,4,5] and put on a pair of sterile gloves.

■ Irrigate the wound thoroughly using the normal saline solution and the irrigation syringe. (See "Wound irrigation," page 795.)

■ Clean the area around the wound with normal saline solution; wipe intact skin with a skin protectant wipe and allow it to dry well. Remove and discard your gloves.

■ Put on a new pair of sterile gloves.

■ Assess the wound. Note the wound's precise location, tissue type and loss, size, color, odor, and drainage.

■ Measure the wound with your facility's measuring tool and guide. Measuring is usually done at baseline, with the first dressing change, weekly, and when negative-pressure wound therapy is discontinued.

■ If your gloves are contaminated, remove them and put on a new pair of gloves.

For foam packing

■ Using sterile scissors, cut the foam to the shape and measurement of the wound *to help maintain negative pressure to the entire wound.* More than one piece of foam may be necessary, depending on the size of the wound. Don't cut the foam directly over the wound *to prevent foam fragments from falling into the wound.* If a tunnel is present, cut the foam longer than the tunnel *to*

Understanding negative-pressure wound therapy

An option to consider when a wound fails to heal in a timely manner, negative-pressure wound therapy encourages healing by applying localized subatmospheric pressure at the site of the wound. The therapy reduces edema and bacterial colonization and stimulates the formation of granulation tissue.

Depending on the type of wound, the manufacturer's equipment, and the doctor's preference, gauze or foam packing will be ordered. Gauze is typically used in circumferential and tunneling wounds and explored fistulas because it fits most wounds and tends to be more comfortable for the patient during application and removal. Foam packing is typically used in wounds with a lot of exudate; it's available in various sizes to fit a wide range of wound types and can be cut to accommodate any wound size.

Wound with gauze packing

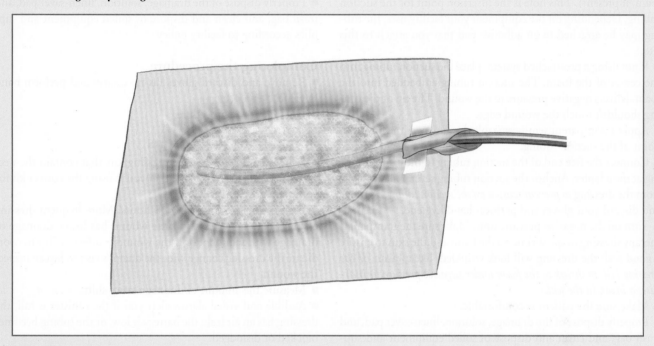

Wound with foam packing

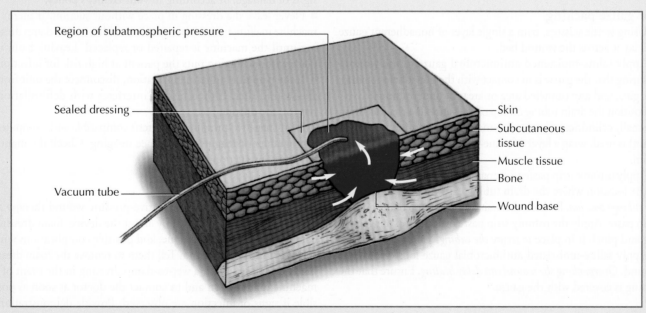

ensure the foam makes contact with the wound. Carefully place the foam in the wound, ensuring that the foam is in contact with the wound bed, margins, and any tunneled area or areas of undermining (if there's a groove in the foam, apply it with the groove side up). Don't pack the foam tightly into any areas of the wound *because doing so may delay healing.*

■ Apply the transparent therapy dressing drape over the foam leaving a 2″ (5-cm) margin of intact skin covered by the dressing around the wound *to ensure that the wound is covered completely and that the negative-pressure seal will be intact.*

■ Pierce a small hole, no bigger than ½″ (1.3 cm) in the center of the transparent therapy dressing drape (over the groove in the foam, if present). This hole is the insertion point for the suction tubing. Depending on the equipment your facility uses, the tubing may be attached to an adhesive pad that you attach to this site.

■ If not using a preattached system, place the suction tubing into the center of the foam. The suction tubing embedded into the foam delivers negative pressure to the wound. The tip of the tubing shouldn't touch the wound edge.

■ Apply a transparent semipermeable dressing over the insertion point of the suction tubing.

■ Connect the free end of the suction tubing to the canister tubing at the adapter. Anchor the suction tubing several inches away from the dressing *to prevent tension on the suction tubing.* Remove and discard your gloves and perform hand hygiene.

■ Turn on the negative-pressure unit. Make sure the transparent therapy dressing drape shrinks to the foam and the skin to ensure a good seal; the dressing will look wrinkled, like a raisin. *If the dressing fails to shrink to the foam under negative pressure, it indicates a break in the seal.*

■ Make sure the patient is comfortable.

■ Properly dispose of the drainage, solution, linen-saver pad, and trash bag, and clean and dispose of soiled equipment and supplies according to facility policy.

For gauze packing

■ Using sterile scissors, trim a single layer of nonadherent gauze and lay it across the wound bed.

■ Apply saline-moistened antimicrobial gauze to the wound, ensuring that the gauze is in contact with the nonadherent gauze, margins, and any tunneled area or areas of undermining.

■ Position the drain tubing on top of the gauze. If a channel drain (a small, cylindrical drain) or round drain (a round, perforated drain) is used, wrap a layer of saline-moistened gauze around the drain.

■ Apply ostomy strip paste to a small portion of the wound edge at the location where the drain tubing exits the wound *to secure the tubing's position.* Position the drain tubing on top of the ostomy strip paste. Apply the ostomy strip paste over the top of the tubing and pinch it in place *to secure the tubing's position.*

■ Apply saline-moistened antimicrobial gauze loosely into the wound. *Overpacking the wound can delay healing.* Ensure that the tubing is covered with the gauze.

■ Apply transparent semipermeable dressing(s) over the wound. Reinforce the seal by pinching the transparent occlusive film and ostomy strip paste together.

■ Connect the free end of the drain tubing to the canister tubing at the adapter. Anchor the drain tubing several inches away from the dressing *to prevent tension on the suction tubing.*

■ Turn on the negative-pressure unit. Make sure the transparent semipermeable dressing shrinks to the gauze and the skin to ensure a good seal; the dressing will look wrinkled, like a raisin. *If the dressing fails to shrink to the gauze under negative pressure, it indicates a break in the seal.*

■ Make sure the patient is comfortable.

■ Properly dispose of the drainage, solution, linen-saver pad, and trash bag, and clean and dispose of soiled equipment and supplies according to facility policy.

Completing the procedure

■ Remove and discard gloves (as necessary) and perform hand hygiene.[3,4,5]

■ Document the procedure.[6]

Special considerations

■ Many manufacturers have dressing kits that contain the necessary equipment. Make sure that you're using the correct kit for your patient's needs.

■ Change the dressing every 48 hours. More frequent dressing changes may be necessary if the wound has heavy drainage or drainage with sediment or if the wound is infected. Try to coordinate the dressing change with the doctor's visit so he can inspect the wound.

■ Measure the amount of drainage every shift.

■ Audible and visual alarms alert you if the canister is full, the dressing has an air leak, the battery is low, or the tubing becomes blocked or dislodged.

■ Change the canister once a week, when it's full, if it has any signs of damage, or according to your facility's policy.

■ Never leave the dressing in place without suction. If there's a machine malfunction, replace the foam with a wet-to-damp dressing until the machine is repaired or replaced. Leaving foam in place without suction puts the patient at high risk for infection.

■ If the patient requires defibrillation, disconnect the unit from the wound first. If the dressing interferes with defibrillation, remove the dressing.

■ Many negative-pressure units aren't compatible with computed tomography or magnetic resonance imaging. Check the manufacturer's instructions.

Patient teaching

If the patient will be using negative-pressure wound therapy at home, teach him and his family about the device, foam dressing changes using sterile technique, and possible complications with the machine or the wound. Tell them to remove the foam dressing and replace it with a wet-to-damp dressing in the event of a machine malfunction and to contact the doctor as soon as possible if signs of infection are observed. Provide demonstrations of dressing changes and observe return demonstrations. Answer their questions, and provide guidance and encouragement as needed.

Complications

Cleaning and care of wounds may temporarily increase the patient's pain and increases the risk of infection.

Documentation

Document the frequency and duration of therapy; the amount of negative pressure applied; the size and condition of the wound, including the location, tissue type and loss, odor, drainage, and measurement; and the patient's response to treatment. Document any patient teaching and the patient's response to the teaching.

REFERENCES

1 Andros, G., et al. (2006). Consensus statement on negative pressure wound therapy (V.A.C. Therapy) for the management of diabetic foot wounds. *Ostomy/Wound Management,* (Suppl.), 1–32. (Level I)
2 The Joint Commission. (2012). Standard NPSG.01.01.01. *Comprehensive accreditation manual for hospitals: The official handbook.* Oakbrook Terrace, IL: The Joint Commission. (Level I)
3 The Joint Commission. (2012). Standard NPSG.07.01.01. *Comprehensive accreditation manual for hospitals: The official handbook.* Oakbrook Terrace, IL: The Joint Commission. (Level I)
4 Centers for Disease Control and Prevention. (October 2002). Guideline for hand hygiene in health-care settings. *Morbidity and Mortality Weekly Report, 51*(RR-16), 1–45. (Level I)
5 World Health Organization. (2009). *WHO guidelines on hand hygiene in health care: First global patient safety challenge. Clean care is safer care.* Geneva, Switzerland: World Health Organization. (Level I)
6 The Joint Commission. (2012). Standard RC.01.03.01. *Comprehensive accreditation manual for hospitals: The official handbook.* Oakbrook Terrace, IL: The Joint Commission. (Level I)

ADDITIONAL REFERENCES

Ahn, C., & Salcido, R., (2008). Advances in wound photography and assessment methods. *Advances in Skin and Wound Care: The Journal of Prevention, 21*(2), 85–93.
Barker, D.E., et al. (2007). Experience with vacuum-pack temporary abdominal wound closure in 258 trauma and general and vascular surgical patients. *Journal of the American College of Surgeons, 204*(5), 784–792.
Bovill, E., et al. (2008). Topical negative pressure wound therapy: A review of its role and guidelines for its use in the management of acute wounds. *International Wound Journal, 5*(4), 511–529.
Chadwick, P. (2009). The use of negative pressure wound therapy in the diabetic foot. *British Journal of Nursing, 18*(20), S12, S14, S16.
Durai, R., et al. (2008). Indirect VAC: A novel technique of applying vacuum-assisted closure dressing. *Journal of Perioperative Practice, 18*(10), 437–439.
Ha, J., et al. (2008). A retrospective review of the outcomes of vacuum-assisted closure therapy in a vascular surgery unit. *Wounds, 20*(8), 221–229.
Langemo, D., et al. (2008). Measuring wound length, width, and area: Which technique? *Advances in Skin and Wound Care: The Journal of Prevention, 21*(1), 42–45.

Morris, G.S., et al. (2007). Negative pressure wound therapy activated by vacuum-assisted closure: Evaluating the assumptions. *Ostomy/Wound Management, 53*(1), 52–57.
Noble-Bell, G., & Forbes, A. (2008). A systematic review of the effectiveness of negative pressure wound therapy in the management of diabetes foot ulcers. *International Wound Journal, 5*(2), 233–242.
Preston, G. (2008). An overview of topical negative pressure therapy in wound care. *Nursing Standard, 23*(7), 62–64, 66, 68.
Scherer, S., et al. (2008). The mechanism of action of the vacuum-assisted closure device. *Plastic and Reconstructive Surgery, 122*(3), 786–797.
Sussman, C., & Bates-Jensen, B. (2007). *Wound care: A collaborative practice manual for health professionals.* Philadelphia, PA: Lippincott, Williams & Wilkins.
Thompson, G., (2008). An overview of negative pressure wound therapy (NPWT). *British Journal of Community Nursing, 13*(6), S23–S30.

NEPHROSTOMY AND CYSTOSTOMY TUBE DRESSING CHANGES

Two urinary diversion techniques—nephrostomy and cystostomy—ensure temporary or permanent drainage from the kidneys or bladder and help prevent urinary tract infection or kidney failure. (See *Urinary diversion techniques,* page 512.)

A nephrostomy tube drains urine directly from a kidney when a disorder inhibits the normal flow of urine. The tube is usually placed percutaneously, although sometimes it's surgically inserted through the renal cortex and medulla into the renal pelvis from a lateral flank incision. Tube placement is usually performed because of obstructive problems, such as ureteral or ureteropelvic junction calculi or tumors. Diverting urine with a nephrostomy tube also allows kidney tissue damaged from obstructive disease to heal.

A cystostomy tube drains urine from the bladder, diverting it from the urethra. This type of tube is used after certain gynecologic procedures, bladder surgery, prostatectomy, severe urethral strictures, or traumatic injury. The tube is inserted into the bladder approximately 2″ (5 cm) above the pubic symphysis and may be used alone or in addition to an indwelling urethral catheter.

Equipment

Antiseptic swabs ▪ linen-saver pad ▪ paper bag ▪ gloves ▪ sterile gloves ▪ precut 4″ × 4″ sterile drain dressings or transparent semipermeable dressings ▪ hypoallergenic adhesive tape.

Preparation of equipment

Gather the equipment at the patient's bedside. Open the skin cleaning swabs, the 4″ × 4″ sterile drain dressings, and sterile gloves. Open the paper bag and place it away from the other equipment *to avoid contaminating the sterile field.*

Urinary diversion techniques

A cystostomy or a nephrostomy can be used to create a permanent diversion, to relieve obstruction from an inoperable tumor, or to provide an outlet for urine after cystectomy. A temporary diversion can relieve obstruction from a calculus or ureteral edema.

In a *cystostomy*, a catheter is inserted percutaneously through the suprapubic area into the bladder. In a *nephrostomy*, a catheter is inserted percutaneously through the flank into the renal pelvis.

Cystostomy

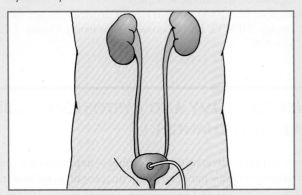

Nephrostomy

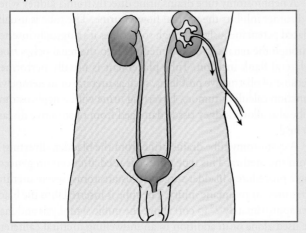

Implementation

- Verify the doctor's order.
- Confirm the patient's identity using at least two patient identifiers according to your facility's policy.[1]
- Provide privacy.
- Explain the procedure to the patient. Answer all questions *to decrease anxiety and increase cooperation.*
- Perform hand hygiene and put on gloves.[2,3,4]
- Position the patient *so you can clearly see the tube exit site.* If he has a nephrostomy tube, have him lie on his side opposite the tube. If the patient has a cystostomy tube, have him lie on his back.

- Place the linen-saver pad under the patient *to absorb excess drainage and keep him dry.*
- Carefully remove the tape around the tube, and remove the wet or soiled dressing.
- Discard the tape, dressings, and gloves in the paper bag.
- Note the markings on the tube at the insertion site *to check for accidental dislodgment.*
- Perform hand hygiene and put on sterile gloves. Use an antiseptic swab to clean the skin, wiping from the tube site outward.
- Discard the swab in the paper bag, being careful not to touch the bag and contaminate your gloves.
- Repeat the skin cleaning procedure, if needed.
- Pick up a sterile 4″ × 4″ drain dressing and place it around the tube. If necessary, overlap two drain dressings *for maximum absorption.* Or, depending on your facility's policy, apply a transparent semipermeable dressing over the tube and site *to allow for observation of the site without removing the dressing.*
- Secure the dressing with tape. Tape the tube to the patient's lateral abdomen *to prevent tension on the tube.*
- Dispose of all equipment appropriately.
- Remove your gloves and perform hand hygiene.[2,3,4]
- Help the patient to a comfortable position.
- Document the procedure.[5]

Special considerations

- Change the dressings once a day and as needed.
- Check a nephrostomy tube frequently for kinks or obstructions. Kinks are likely to occur if the patient lies on the insertion site. Suspect an obstruction when the amount of urine in the drainage bag decreases or the amount of urine around the insertion site increases. Pressure created by urine backing up in the tube can damage nephrons. Gently curve a cystostomy tube *to prevent kinks.*
- If you suspect that a blood clot or mucus plug obstructs a nephrostomy or cystostomy tube, try milking the tube *to restore its patency.* With your nondominant hand, hold the tube securely above the obstruction *to avoid pulling the tube out of the incision.* Then place the flat side of a closed hemostat under the tube just above the obstruction, pinch the tube against the hemostat, and slide both your finger and the hemostat toward you and away from the patient.
- Typically, cystostomy tubes for postoperative urologic patients should be checked hourly for 24 hours *to ensure adequate drainage and tube patency.* To check tube patency, note the amount of urine in the drainage bag and check the patient's bladder for distention.
- Keep the drainage bag below the level of the kidney at all times *to prevent urine reflux.*
- If the tube becomes dislodged, cover the site with a sterile dressing and notify the doctor immediately.
- The doctor may order the nephrostomy tube to be clamped *to determine the patient's readiness for removal.* While the tube is clamped, assess the patient for flank pain and fever, and monitor his urine output.

Patient teaching

Teach the home care patient and caregiver how to clean the tube insertion site with soap and water, check for skin breakdown, and change the dressing daily. Teach them how to change the drainage bag or leg bag. Explain that the patient can use a leg bag during the day and a larger drainage bag at night.

Stress the importance of reporting to the doctor any signs of infection (red skin or white, yellow, or green drainage at the insertion site), oral temperature greater than 100.4° F (38° C), or tube displacement (drainage that smells like urine).

Whether the patient uses a drainage bag or larger container, explain that he must wash it daily with a 1:3 vinegar-to-water solution and rinse and dry it thoroughly *to prevent crystalline buildup.* Encourage patients with unrestricted fluid intake to increase their daily intake to at least 3 qt (2.8 L) *to help flush the urinary system and reduce sediment formation.*

Complications

The patient has an increased risk of infection *because nephrostomy and cystostomy tubes provide a direct opening to the kidneys and bladder.*

Documentation

Describe the color and amount of drainage from the nephrostomy or cystostomy tube and record any color changes as they occur. Note the markings on the tube at the skin insertion site. If the patient has more than one tube, describe the drainage (color, amount, and character) from each separate tube. Note any complications and nursing actions taken. Document all patient teaching and the patient's response to the teaching.

REFERENCES

1 The Joint Commission. (2012). Standard NPSG.01.01.01. *Comprehensive accreditation manual for hospitals: The official handbook.* Oakbrook Terrace, IL: The Joint Commission. (Level I)
2 The Joint Commission. (2012). Standard NPSG.07.01.01. *Comprehensive accreditation manual for hospitals: The official handbook.* Oakbrook Terrace, IL: The Joint Commission. (Level I)
3 Centers for Disease Control and Prevention. (October 2002). Guideline for hand hygiene in health-care settings. *Morbidity and Mortality Weekly Report, 51*(RR-16), 1–45. (Level I)
4 World Health Organization. (2009). *WHO guidelines on hand hygiene in health care: First global patient safety challenge. Clean care is safer care.* Geneva, Switzerland: World Health Organization. (Level I)
5 The Joint Commission. (2012). Standard RC.01.03.01. *Comprehensive accreditation manual for hospitals: The official handbook.* Oakbrook Terrace, IL: The Joint Commission. (Level I)

ADDITIONAL REFERENCES

Hautmann, R. (2007). Urinary diversion. *Urology, 69*(1 Suppl.), 17–49.
Taylor, C., et al. (2011). *Fundamentals of nursing: The art and science of nursing care* (7th ed.). Philadelphia, PA: Lippincott Williams & Wilkins.

NEUROLOGIC ASSESSMENT

Neurologic vital signs supplement the routine measurement of temperature, pulse rate, blood pressure, and respirations by evaluating the patient's level of consciousness (LOC), pupillary activity, and orientation to time, place, and person. They provide a simple, indispensable tool for quickly checking the patient's neurologic status.

A measure of environmental awareness and self-awareness, LOC reflects cortical function and usually provides the first sign of central nervous system (CNS) deterioration. Changes in pupillary activity (pupil size, shape, equality, and response to light) may signal increased intracranial pressure (ICP) associated with a space-occupying lesion. Evaluating muscle strength and tone, reflexes, and posture also may help identify nervous system damage.

Changes in neurologic vital signs alone rarely indicate neurologic compromise; any changes should be evaluated in light of a complete neurologic assessment. But because these vital signs are controlled at the medullary level, changes in neurologic vital signs may signify ominous neurologic compromise.

Equipment

Penlight ▪ thermometer ▪ sterile cotton ball or cotton-tipped applicator ▪ stethoscope ▪ sphygmomanometer ▪ pupil size chart ▪ pencil or pen.

Implementation

▪ Confirm the patient's identity using at least two patient identifiers according to your facility's policy.[1]
▪ Explain the procedure to the patient, even if he's unresponsive. Answer all questions *to decrease anxiety and increase cooperation.*
▪ Perform hand hygiene and provide privacy.[2,3,4]

Assessing LOC and orientation

▪ Assess the patient's LOC by evaluating his responses. Use standard methods such as the Glasgow Coma Scale (see *Using the Glasgow Coma Scale,* page 514) and the Rancho Los Amigos Cognitive Scale (see *Using the Rancho Los Amigos Cognitive Scale,* page 515). Begin by measuring the patient's response to verbal, light tactile (touch), or painful (nail bed pressure) stimuli. First, ask the patient his full name. If he responds appropriately, assess his orientation to time, place, and person. Ask him where he is and then what day, season, and year it is. (Expect disorientation to affect the sense of date first, then time, place, caregivers and, finally, self.) When he responds verbally, assess the quality of replies. For example, garbled words indicate difficulty with the motor nerves that govern speech muscles. Rambling responses indicate difficulty with thought processing and organization.

Using the Glasgow Coma Scale

The Glasgow Coma Scale provides a standard reference for assessing or monitoring level of consciousness in a patient with a suspected or confirmed brain injury. This scale measures three responses to stimuli—eye opening, motor response, and verbal response—and assigns a number to each of the possible responses within these categories.

A score of 3 is the lowest and 15, the highest. A score of 7 or less indicates coma. This scale is commonly used in the emergency department, at the scene of an accident, and for evaluation of the hospitalized patient.

CHARACTERISTIC	RESPONSE/SCORE
Eye opening	■ Spontaneous—4 ■ To verbal command—3 ■ To pain—2 ■ No response—1

Best motor response	■ Obeys commands—6
	■ To painful stimuli:
	  – Localizes pain; pushes stimulus away—5
	  – Flexes and withdraws—4
	  – Abnormal flexion—3
	  – Abnormal extension response—2
	  – No response—1

Best verbal response (Arouse patient with painful stimuli, if necessary)	■ Oriented and converses—5 ■ Disoriented and converses—4 ■ Uses inappropriate words—3 ■ Makes incomprehensible sounds—2 ■ No response—1

Total: 3 to 15

■ Assess the patient's ability to understand and follow one-step commands that require a motor response. For example, ask him to open and close his eyes or stick out his tongue (as shown on next column top). Note whether the patient can maintain his LOC. If you must gently shake him to keep him focused on your verbal commands, he may be neurologically compromised.

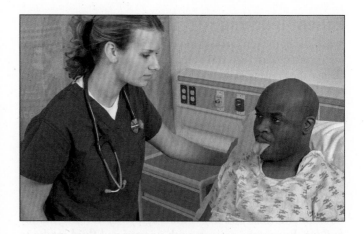

■ If the patient doesn't respond to commands or touch, apply a painful stimulus. Painful stimuli are classified as central (response via the brain) or peripheral (response via the spine). Apply a central stimulus first and note the patient's response. Acceptable central stimuli include squeezing the trapezius muscle, applying supraorbital or mandibular pressure, and rubbing the sternum. If the patient doesn't respond to central stimuli, apply a peripheral stimulus to all four extremities to establish a baseline. With moderate pressure, squeeze the nail beds on fingers and toes, and note his response. Check motor responses bilaterally *to rule out monoplegia (paralysis of a single area) and hemiplegia (paralysis of one side of the body).*

Examining pupils and eye movement

■ Ask the patient to open his eyes. If he doesn't respond, gently lift his upper eyelids. Inspect each pupil for size and shape, and compare the two for equality (as shown below). *To evaluate pupil size more precisely,* use a chart showing the various pupil sizes (in increments of 1 mm, with the normal diameter ranging from 2 to 6 mm). Remember, pupil size varies considerably, and some patients have normally unequal pupils (anisocoria). Also see if the pupils are positioned in, or deviated from, the midline. (See *Testing the pupils*, page 516.)

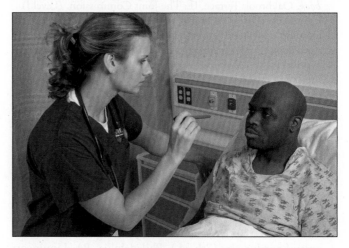

■ Test the patient's direct light response. First, darken the room. Then hold each eyelid open in turn, keeping the other eye covered. Swing the penlight from the patient's ear toward the midline of the

Using the Rancho Los Amigos Cognitive Scale

Widely used to classify brain-injured patients according to their behavior, the Rancho Los Amigos Cognitive Scale describes the phases of recovery—from coma to independent functioning—on a scale of I (unresponsive) to VIII (purposeful, appropriate, alert, and oriented). This chart is useful when assessing patients with posttraumatic amnesia.

LEVEL	RESPONSE	CHARACTERISTICS
I	None	The patient is unresponsive to any stimulus, including pain.
II	Generalized	The patient makes limited, inconsistent, nonpurposeful responses, often to pain only.
III	Localized	The patient can localize and withdraw from painful stimuli, can make purposeful responses and focus on presented objects, and may follow simple commands, but inconsistently and in a delayed manner.
IV	Confused and agitated	The patient is alert but agitated, confused, disoriented, and aggressive. He can't perform self-care and has no awareness of present events. Bizarre behavior is likely; agitation appears related to internal confusion.
V	Confused and inappropriate	The patient is alert and responds to commands but is easily distracted and can't concentrate on tasks or learn new information. He becomes agitated in response to external stimuli, and his behavior and speech are inappropriate. His memory is severely impaired and he can't carry over learning from one situation to another.
VI	Confused and appropriate	The patient has some awareness of himself and others but is inconsistently oriented. He can follow simple directions consistently with cueing and can relearn some old skills, such as activities of daily living, but continues to have serious memory problems (especially with short-term memory).
VII	Automatic and appropriate	The patient is consistently oriented with little or no confusion but frequently appears robotic when performing daily routines. His awareness of himself and his interaction with his environment increase, but he lacks insight, judgment, problem-solving skills, and the ability to plan realistically.
VIII	Purposeful and appropriate	The patient is alert and oriented, recalls and integrates past events, learns new activities, and performs activities of daily living independently; however, deficits in stress tolerance, judgment, and abstract reasoning persist. He may function in society at a reduced level.

face. Shine the light directly into the eye. Normally, the pupil constricts immediately. When you remove the penlight, the pupil should dilate immediately. Wait about 20 seconds before testing the other pupil *to allow it to recover from reflex stimulation.*

■ Now test consensual light response. Hold both eyelids open, but shine the light into one eye only. Watch for constriction in the other pupil, *which indicates proper nerve function of the optic chiasm.*

■ Brighten the room and have the conscious patient open his eyes. Observe the eyelids for ptosis or drooping. Then check extraocular movements. Hold up one finger, and ask the patient to follow it with his eyes alone. As you move the finger up, down, laterally, and obliquely, see if the patient's eyes track together to follow your finger (conjugate gaze). Watch for involuntary jerking or oscillating eye movements (nystagmus).

■ Check accommodation. Hold up one finger midline to the patient's face and several feet away. Have the patient focus on your finger. Gradually move your finger toward his nose while he focuses on your finger. This action should cause his eyes to converge and both pupils to constrict equally.

■ Test the corneal reflex by touching a wisp of cotton ball to the cornea. This test normally causes an immediate blink reflex. Repeat for the other eye.

NURSING ALERT *Excessive testing of the corneal reflex can cause corneal damage. Perform this assessment carefully.*

■ If the patient is unconscious, test the oculocephalic (doll's eye) reflex. Hold the patient's eyelids open. Then quickly but gently turn the patient's head to one side and then the other. If the

Testing the pupils

Slightly darken the room. Then test the pupils for direct response (reaction of the pupil you're testing) and consensual response (reaction of the opposite pupil) by holding a penlight about 20″ (51 cm) from the patient's eyes, directing the light at the eye from the side.

Next, test accommodation by placing your finger about 4″ (10 cm) from the bridge of the patient's nose. Ask him to look at a fixed object in the distance and then to look at your finger. His eyes should converge and his pupils should constrict.

Grading pupil size

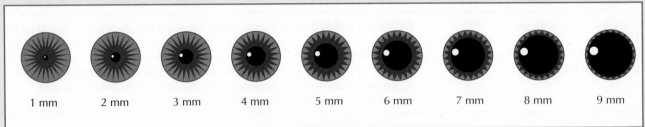

1 mm   2 mm   3 mm   4 mm   5 mm   6 mm   7 mm   8 mm   9 mm

---

patient's eyes move in the opposite direction from the side to which you turn the head, the reflex is intact.

NURSING ALERT *Never test the doll's eye reflex if you know or suspect that the patient has a cervical spine injury* because permanent spinal cord damage may result.

Evaluating motor function

■ If the patient is conscious, test his grip strength in both hands at the same time. Extend your hands, ask him to squeeze your fingers as hard as he can, and compare the strength of each hand. Grip strength is usually slightly stronger in the dominant hand.

■ Test arm strength by having the patient close his eyes and hold his arms straight out in front of him with the palms up (as shown below). See if either arm drifts downward or pronates, *indicating muscle weakness.*

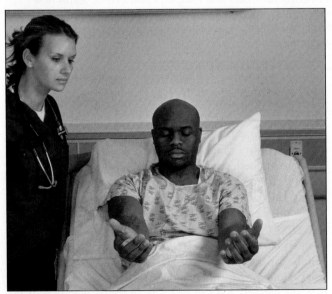

■ Test leg strength by having the patient raise his legs, one at a time, against gentle downward pressure from your hand. Gently push down on each leg at the midpoint of the thigh *to evaluate muscle strength* (as shown below).

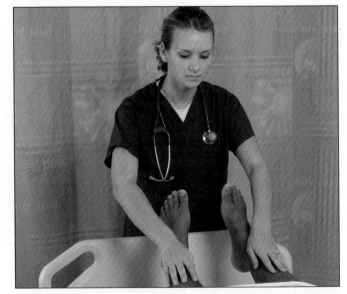

Identifying warning postures

Decorticate and decerebrate postures are ominous signs of central nervous system deterioration.

Decorticate (abnormal flexion)

In the decorticate posture, the patient's arms are adducted and flexed, with the wrists and fingers flexed on the chest. The legs may be stiffly extended and internally rotated, with plantar flexion of the feet.

The decorticate posture may indicate a lesion of the frontal lobe, internal capsule, or cerebral peduncles.

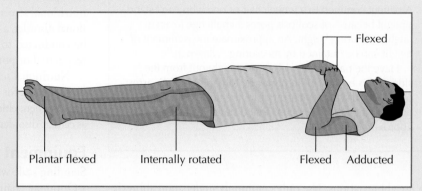

Flexed

Plantar flexed   Internally rotated   Flexed   Adducted

Decerebrate (extension)

In the decerebrate posture, the patient's arms are adducted and extended with the wrists pronated and the fingers flexed. One or both legs may be stiffly extended, with plantar flexion of the feet.

The decerebrate posture may indicate lesions of the upper brain stem.

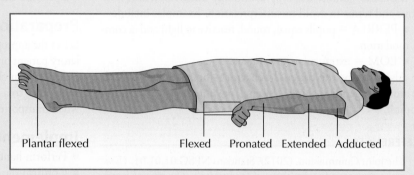

Plantar flexed   Flexed   Pronated   Extended   Adducted

NURSING ALERT *If decorticate or decerebrate posturing develops in response to stimuli, notify the doctor immediately. (See* Identifying warning postures.*)*

■ Flex and extend the extremities on both sides *to evaluate muscle tone.*

■ Test the plantar reflex in all patients. To do so, stroke the lateral aspect of the sole of the patient's foot with your thumbnail or another moderately sharp object (as shown below). Normally, this elicits flexion of all toes. Watch for a positive Babinski's sign—dorsiflexion of the great toe with fanning of the other toes—which indicates an upper motor neuron lesion.

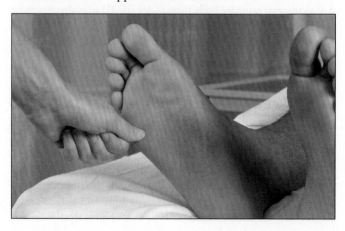

Completing the neurologic examination

■ Measure the patient's temperature, pulse rate, respiratory rate, and blood pressure. His pulse pressure—the difference between systolic pressure and diastolic pressure—is especially important *because widening pulse pressure can indicate increasing ICP.*

■ Document the procedure.[5]

Special considerations

NURSING ALERT *If a previously stable patient suddenly develops a change in neurologic or routine vital signs, further assess his condition, and notify the doctor immediately. One of the earliest changes that may occur with increased ICP is a change in the LOC. Changes in pulse and blood pressure do occur, but are generally seen late in the course of increasing ICP.*

■ If the patient is suspected of having a stroke, use the National Institutes of Health Stroke Scale to evaluate him according to your facility's policy.

Documentation

Baseline data require detailed documentation; subsequent notes can be brief unless the patient's condition changes. Record the patient's LOC and orientation, pupillary activity, motor function, and routine vital signs, as your facility's policy directs. To save time while keeping complete records, you may be allowed

---

Overcoming height measurement problems

A patient confined to a wheelchair or one who can't stand straight because of scoliosis poses a challenge to accurately measuring height. An approximate measurement of height can be obtained by measuring "wingspan."

Have the patient hold his arms straight out from the sides of his body. Children may be told to hold their arms out like bird wings. Measure from the tip of one middle finger to the tip of the other. That distance is the patient's approximate height.

---

to use abbreviations. Use only commonly understood abbreviations and terms to avoid misinterpretation. Examples include:

- PERRLA = pupils equal, round, reactive to light and accommodation
- EOM = extraocular movements.

Also describe the patient's behavior—for example, "difficult to arouse by gentle shaking," "sleepy," or "unresponsive to painful stimuli."

REFERENCES

1 The Joint Commission. (2012). Standard NPSG.01.01.01. *Comprehensive accreditation manual for hospitals: The official handbook.* Oakbrook Terrace, IL: The Joint Commission. (Level I)
2 The Joint Commission. (2012). Standard NPSG.07.01.01. *Comprehensive accreditation manual for hospitals: The official handbook.* Oakbrook Terrace, IL: The Joint Commission. (Level I)
3 Centers for Disease Control and Prevention. (October 2002). Guideline for hand hygiene in health-care settings. *Morbidity and Mortality Weekly Report, 51*(RR-16), 1–45. (Level I)
4 World Health Organization. (2009). *WHO guidelines on hand hygiene in health care: First global patient safety challenge. Clean care is safer care.* Geneva, Switzerland: World Health Organization. (Level I)
5 The Joint Commission. (2012). Standard RC.01.03.01. *Comprehensive accreditation manual for hospitals: The official handbook.* Oakbrook Terrace, IL: The Joint Commission. (Level I)

ADDITIONAL REFERENCES

American Association of Neuroscience Nurses (2007). "AANN Clinical Practice Guideline Series: Neurologic Assessment of the Older Adult. A Guide for Nurses" [Online]. Accessed January 2012 via the Web at http://www.aann.org/pdf/cpg/aannneuroassessmentolderadult.pdf
Caton-Richards, M. (2010). Assessing the neurological status of patients with head injuries. *Emergency Nursing, 17*(10), 28–31.
Hickey, J.V. (2009). *The clinical practice of neurological and neurosurgical nursing* (6th ed.). Philadelphia, PA: Lippincott Williams & Wilkins.
Lower, J. (2010). Using pain to assess neurologic response. *Nursing 2010 Critical Care, 5*(4), 11–12.
Taylor, C., et al. (2011). *Fundamentals of nursing: The art and science of nursing care* (7th ed.). Philadelphia, PA: Lippincott Williams & Wilkins.

NUTRITIONAL SCREENING

A patient's nutritional status is evaluated by examining information from several sources, such as the patient's medical history, physical assessment findings, and laboratory results. If the nutritional screening determines the patient is at risk for a nutritional disorder, a comprehensive nutritional assessment may then be conducted to set goals and determine interventions to correct actual or potential imbalances.

Nutritional screening also examines certain variables to determine the risk for problems in specific populations—such as pregnant women, elderly people, or those with certain disorders (such as cardiac disorders)—to detect deficiencies or potential imbalances.

Equipment

Standing scale with measuring bar ▪ nutritional screening form ▪ Optional: chair or bed scale, tape measure.

Preparation of equipment

Select the appropriate scale—usually, a standing scale for an ambulatory patient or a chair or bed scale for an acutely ill or debilitated patient. Then check to make sure the scale is balanced. Standing scales and, to a lesser extent, bed scales may become unbalanced when transported.

Implementation

- Perform hand hygiene.[1,2,3]
- Confirm the patient's identity using at least two patient identifiers according to your facility's policy.[4]
- Explain the purpose of and procedure for nutritional screening to the patient.
- Ask the patient to remove his shoes and obtain his weight using a scale. *Weight provides a rough estimate of body composition.*
- Ask about unplanned or unintentional weight loss. Determine how much weight the patient lost and over what period of time. *A weight loss of more than 5% in 30 days or 10% in 180 days places the patient at nutritional risk.*
- Measure the patient's height while he's standing erect without shoes, using the measuring bar on the scale. If the patient can't stand, approximate the height by measuring "wingspan." (See *Overcoming height measurement problems.*)
- Calculate or estimate body mass index (BMI) to evaluate weight in relation to height. (See *Calculating BMI.*)
- A BMI of 18.5 to 24.9 defines healthy weight; a BMI of 25 to 29.9 defines overweight; a BMI of 30 or more defines obesity.[5] (See *Determining BMI.*)
- Evaluate the patient's weight distribution by measuring his waist circumference around his abdomen at the level of the iliac crest. Before reading the tape measure, ensure that the tape is snug, but doesn't compress the skin and is parallel to the floor. If the measurement is greater than 35″ (89 cm) for a woman or 40″ (102 cm) for a man (with a normal BMI), the patient is at greater risk for health problems. People with a high distribution of fat around their waists as opposed to their hips and thighs are at greater risk for such diseases as type 2 diabetes, dyslipidemia, hypertension, and cardiovascular disease.[6]

Determining BMI

Body mass index (BMI) measures weight in relation to height. The BMI ranges shown here are for adults. They aren't exact ranges for healthy or unhealthy weights; however, they show that health risks increase at higher levels of overweight and obesity. To use the graph below, find your patient's weight along the bottom and then go straight up until you come to the line that matches his height. The shaded area indicates whether your patient is healthy, overweight, or obese.

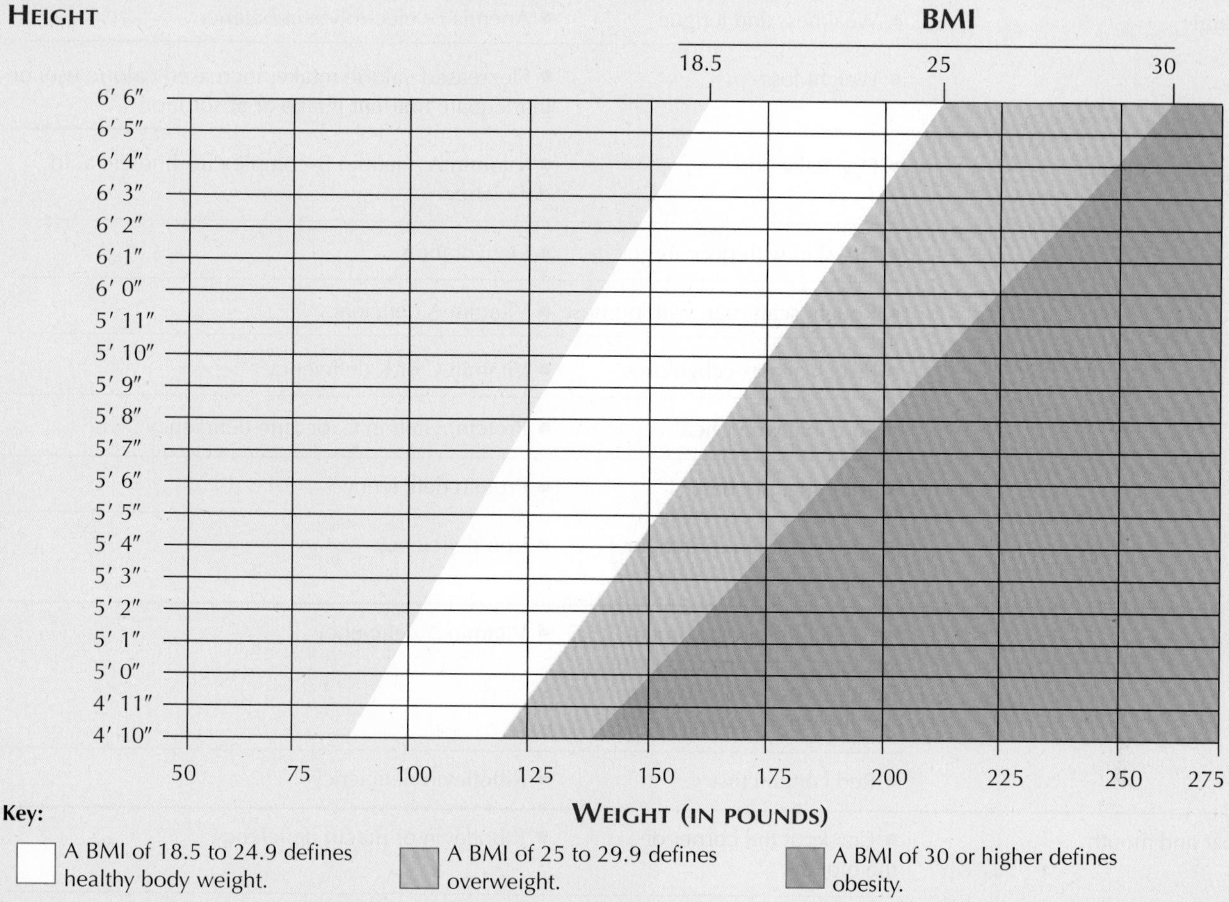

HEIGHT

BMI

Key:

- A BMI of 18.5 to 24.9 defines healthy body weight.
- A BMI of 25 to 29.9 defines overweight.
- A BMI of 30 or higher defines obesity.

Adapted from USDA. *Nutrition and Your Health: Dietary Guidelines for Americans* (5th ed.) Home and Garden Bulletin No. 232. (2000). Washington, D.C.: U.S. Department of Agriculture, U.S. Department of Health and Human Services.

■ Question the patient about his eating habits, living environment, and functional status *to determine whether he's at risk for nutritional problems.* A problem in any of these areas places the patient at risk and requires further nutritional assessment.

■ Examine the patient's laboratory values. A serum albumin level less than 3.5 mg/dL is a nonspecific indicator of poor nutrition. Prealbumin is the most accurate indicator because it reveals the most recent nutritional status (past 7 to 14 days). Serum transferrin reflects the patient's current protein status more accurately than albumin because of its shorter half-life. Elevated transferrin levels may indicate severe iron deficiency. Decreased hemoglobin levels and hematocrit suggest iron deficiency anemia. Decreased total lymphocyte count may indicate reduced protein stores.

■ Review the medical record and interview the patient *to determine whether his present illness or medical history places him at nutritional risk.*

Calculating BMI

Use one of the formulas below to calculate your patient's body mass index (BMI).

$$BMI = \left(\frac{\text{weight in pounds}}{\text{height in inches} \times \text{height in inches}} \right) \times 703$$

OR

$$BMI = \left(\frac{\text{weight in kilograms}}{\text{height in centimeters} \times \text{height in centimeters}} \right) \times 10,000$$

OR

$$BMI = \left(\frac{\text{weight in kilograms}}{\text{height in meters} \times \text{height in meters}} \right)$$

Evaluating nutritional disorders

This chart can help you interpret your nutritional assessment findings. Body systems are listed below, with signs or symptoms and the implications for each.

BODY SYSTEM OR REGION	SIGN OR SYMPTOM	IMPLICATIONS
General	■ Weakness and fatigue	■ Anemia or electrolyte imbalance
	■ Weight loss	■ Decreased calorie intake, increased calorie use, or inadequate nutrient intake or absorption
Skin, hair, and nails	■ Dry, flaky skin	■ Vitamin A, vitamin B-complex, or linoleic acid deficiency
	■ Dry skin with poor turgor	■ Dehydration
	■ Rough, scaly skin with bumps	■ Vitamin A deficiency
	■ Petechiae or ecchymoses	■ Vitamin C or K deficiency
	■ Sore that won't heal	■ Protein, vitamin C, or zinc deficiency
	■ Thinning, dry hair	■ Protein deficiency
	■ Spoon-shaped, brittle, or ridged nails	■ Iron deficiency
Eyes	■ Night blindness; corneal swelling, softening, or dryness; Bitot's spots (gray triangular patches on the conjunctiva)	■ Vitamin A deficiency
	■ Red conjunctiva	■ Riboflavin deficiency
Throat and mouth	■ Cracks at the corner of the mouth	■ Riboflavin or niacin deficiency
	■ Magenta tongue	■ Riboflavin deficiency
	■ Beefy, red tongue	■ Vitamin B_{12} deficiency
	■ Soft, spongy, bleeding gums	■ Vitamin C deficiency
	■ Swollen neck (goiter)	■ Iodine deficiency
Cardiovascular	■ Edema	■ Protein deficiency
	■ Tachycardia, hypotension	■ Fluid volume deficit
GI	■ Ascites	■ Protein deficiency
Musculoskeletal	■ Bone pain and bow legs	■ Vitamin D or calcium deficiency
	■ Muscle wasting	■ Protein, carbohydrate, and fat deficiency
Neurologic	■ Altered mental status	■ Dehydration and thiamine or vitamin B_{12} deficiency
	■ Paresthesia	■ Vitamin B_{12}, pyridoxine, or thiamine deficiency

■ Review physical assessment findings for signs of poor nutrition. (See *Evaluating nutritional disorders*.)

■ Make a referral to a registered dietitian if a nutritional screening suggests the patient is at risk for nutritional problems. A registered dietitian will then perform a comprehensive nutritional assessment.

■ Perform hand hygiene.[1,2,3]

■ Document the procedure.[7]

Special considerations

■ The nutritional screening is typically performed during the initial nursing history and physical assessment, but should be completed within 24 hours of admission.

■ When measuring height, note the growth of children as well as diminishing height of older adults. Growth of children may be noted on standardized charts to assess growth patterns for possible abnormalities. Diminishing height of older adults may be related to osteoporotic changes and should be investigated.

Documentation

Record the date and time of the nutritional screening. Place the patient's height and weight on the screening form as well as the graphic sheet or patient care flow sheet, according to your facility's policy. Note the type of scale used. Check off the appropriate patient responses on the screening tool for eating habits, living environment, and functional status. Calculate and record the patient's BMI. Use a progress note to record information that doesn't have a space on the screening tool. Record whether the patient has experienced any weight loss, the period of time over which the loss occurred, and how much weight was lost.

Make sure laboratory results are documented, including the name of anyone you notified of abnormal results, and whether orders were given. Note nutritional problems detected during the physical examination and review of the medical record. Include any patient teaching provided. For patients at nutritional risk, record the date and time, names of the people notified and whether they came to see the patient, orders given, nursing interventions taken, and the patient's response.

REFERENCES

1 The Joint Commission. (2012). Standard NPSG.07.01.01. *Comprehensive accreditation manual for hospitals: The official handbook*. Oakbrook Terrace, IL: The Joint Commission. (Level I)

2 Centers for Disease Control and Prevention. (October 2002). Guideline for hand hygiene in health-care settings. *Morbidity and Mortality Weekly Report, 51*(RR-16), 1–45. (Level I)

3 World Health Organization. (2009). *WHO guidelines on hand hygiene in health care: First global patient safety challenge. Clean care is safer care*. Geneva, Switzerland: World Health Organization. (Level I)

4 The Joint Commission. (2012). Standard NPSG.01.01.01. *Comprehensive accreditation manual for hospitals: The official handbook*. Oakbrook Terrace, IL: The Joint Commission. (Level I)

5 U.S. Department of Agriculture. (2010). "Dietary Guidelines for Americans: Report of the Dietary Guidelines Advisory Committee on the Dietary Guidelines for Americans, 2010" [Online]. Accessed October 2011 via the Web at http://www.cnpp.usda.gov/DGAs2010-DGACReport.htm

6 Kramer, C.K., et al. (2009). A prospective study of abdominal obesity and coronary artery calcium progression in older adults. *Journal of Clinical Endocrinology and Metabolism, 94*(12) 5039–5044.

7 The Joint Commission. (2012). Standard RC.01.03.01. *Comprehensive accreditation manual for hospitals: The official handbook*. Oakbrook Terrace, IL: The Joint Commission. (Level I)

ADDITIONAL REFERENCES

Bankhead, R., et al. (2009). Enteral nutrition practice recommendations. *Journal of Parenteral and Enteral Nutrition, 33*(2), 122–167.

Charney, P. (2008). Nutrition screening vs nutrition assessment: How do they differ? *Nutrition in Clinical Practice, 23*(4), 366–372.

Craven, R.F., & Hirnle, C.J. (2012). *Fundamentals of nursing: Human health and function* (7th ed.). Philadelphia, PA: Lippincott Williams & Wilkins.

Dunne, A. (2008). Malnutrition and the older adult: Care planning and management. *British Journal of Nursing, 17*(20), 1269–1273.

Nettina, S.M. (2010). *Lippincott manual of nursing practice* (9th ed.). Philadelphia, PA: Lippincott Williams & Wilkins.

Persenius, M.W., et al. (2008). Assessment and documentation of patients' nutritional status: Perceptions of registered nurses and their chief nurses. *Journal of Clinical Nursing, 17*(16), 2125–2136.

OMMAYA RESERVOIR DRUG INFUSION

Also known as a *subcutaneous cerebrospinal fluid (CSF) reservoir*, the Ommaya reservoir allows delivery of long-term drug therapy to the CSF by way of the brain's ventricles. The reservoir spares the patient repeated lumbar punctures to administer chemotherapeutic drugs, analgesics, antibiotics, and antifungals. It's most commonly used for chemotherapy and pain management, specifically for treating central nervous system (CNS) leukemia, malignant CNS disease, and meningeal carcinomatosis.

The reservoir is a mushroom-shaped silicone apparatus with an attached catheter. It's surgically implanted beneath the patient's scalp in the nondominant lobe, and the catheter is threaded into the ventricle through a burr hole in the skull. (See *How the Ommaya reservoir works*, page 522.) Besides providing convenient, comparatively painless access to CSF, the Ommaya reservoir permits consistent and predictable drug distribution throughout the subarachnoid space and CNS. It also allows for measurement of intracranial pressure (ICP).

Before reservoir insertion, the patient may receive a local or general anesthetic, depending on his condition and the doctor's preference. After an X-ray confirms placement of the reservoir, a pressure dressing is applied for 24 hours, followed by a gauze dressing for another day or two. The sutures may be removed in about 10 days. However, the reservoir can be used within 48 hours to deliver drugs, obtain CSF pressure measurements, drain CSF, and withdraw CSF specimens.

EQUIPMENT

How the Ommaya reservoir works

To insert an Ommaya reservoir, the doctor drills a burr hole and inserts the device's catheter through the patient's nondominant frontal lobe into the lateral ventricle. The reservoir, which has a self-sealing silicone injection dome, rests over the burr hole under a scalp flap. This creates a slight, soft bulge on the scalp about the size of a quarter. Usually, drugs are injected into the dome with a syringe.

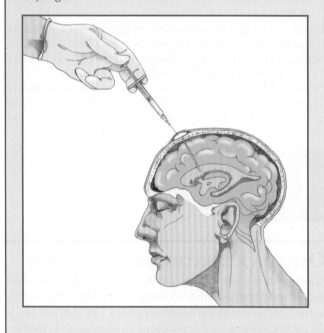

The doctor usually injects drugs into the Ommaya reservoir, but a specially trained nurse may perform this procedure if allowed by facility policy and the state's nurse practice act. This sterile procedure usually takes 15 to 30 minutes.

Equipment

Equipment varies but may include the following: Preservative-free prescribed drug ▪ personal protective equipment (sterile gloves, gown, mask, face shield, goggles) ▪ antiseptic solution (antiseptics containing alcohol or acetone should be avoided) ▪ sterile drape ▪ two 3-mL syringes ▪ 25G needle ▪ sterile gauze pad ▪ syringe containing preservative-free normal saline solution ▪ sterile label ▪ sterile marker ▪ CSF collection tubes.

For chemotherapy

Powder-free chemotherapy gloves ▪ nonlinting, nonabsorbent disposable gown ▪ face shield ▪ National Institute for Occupational Safety and Health–approved respirator mask (if aerosolization is likely) ▪ syringes with luer-lock connector ▪ chemotherapy sharps container ▪ hazardous waste container approved for cytotoxic waste ▪ chemotherapy spill kit.

Preparation of equipment

Make sure that a chemotherapy spill kit and emergency equipment are readily available if chemotherapy is being administered. Also ensure that the emergency equipment is functioning properly.

Implementation

▪ Verify the doctor's order in the patient's medical record and medication administration record.[1]
▪ Make sure that the doctor has obtained an informed consent and that the consent form is in the patient's medical record.[2,3]
▪ If administering a chemotherapeutic agent, become familiar with the information contained in the material safety data sheet specific to the prescribed drug.
▪ In collaboration with the patient's multidisciplinary team, review the patient's test results, specifically the complete blood count, blood urea nitrogen level, platelet count, and liver function studies.
▪ Check the patient's medication history for drugs that might interact with the prescribed medication.
▪ Determine whether the patient has received chemotherapy before and note the severity of any adverse effects.[2]
▪ Determine if the doctor has ordered any premedications *to combat adverse effects of the medication* and administer them as prescribed, following safe medication administration practices.
▪ Avoid distractions and interruptions when preparing and administering medication *to prevent medication administration errors.*[4]
▪ Verify that the drug is properly labeled when you receive it from the pharmacy and that this information includes the patient's full name and second identifier, full generic drug name, drug administration route, total dose to be given, total volume required to administer the dosage, date of administration, and the date and time of preparation and expiration. If the drug is a chemotherapeutic agent, make sure it also contains a label that clearly identifies the drug as hazardous. If you must prepare the drug yourself, make sure you label it properly.[2,5]
▪ Perform hand hygiene.[6,7,8]
▪ Confirm the patient's identity using at least two patient identifiers according to your facility's policy.[9]
▪ Confirm the treatment plan, drug route, and symptom management plan with the patient.[2]
▪ Assess the patient's physical condition, obtain vital signs *to use as a baseline for comparison*, and obtain his height and weight; double-check his body surface area.
▪ Recalculate the dose, as ordered, using the patient's body surface area; check your calculations against the written order.
▪ Position the patient so that he's either sitting or reclining.
▪ If your facility uses a bar code scanning system, scan your identification badge, the patient's identification bracelet, and the medication's bar code.
▪ Wash your hands using soap and water if the drug is a chemotherapeutic agent; perform hand hygiene if it isn't.

- Put on personal protective equipment. If you are administering a chemotherapeutic agent, wear two pairs of gloves, a gown, a mask, a face shield if splashing is likely, and a respirator, if necessary. Make sure your inner glove cuff is worn under the gown cuff and the outer glove cuff extends over the gown cuff *to fully protect your skin.* Inspect your gloves *to make sure they're physically intact.*
- Using a sterile drape, prepare a sterile field on a work surface close to the patient. Place the medication, CSF collection tubes, and preservative-free normal saline solution on the sterile field. Make sure that all medications on and off the sterile field are clearly labeled.[10]
- Remove and discard your gloves, wash your hands with soap and water (or perform hand hygiene), and put on sterile gloves.
- Prepare the patient's scalp with antiseptic solution, working in a circular motion from the center outward. Allow the solution to dry *to achieve its maximum affect.*

NURSING ALERT *Chemotherapeutic drugs are considered high-alert medications* because they can cause significant patient harm if used in error. *Never administer any chemotherapeutic drug without performing an independent double-check with another practitioner who is qualified to prepare or administer chemotherapy.*[11]

- Before administering the medication, have another practitioner who is qualified to prepare or administer chemotherapy perform an independent double-check according to your facility's policy *to verify the patient's identity and make sure that the correct drug is prepared in the prescribed concentration and volume; the drug hasn't expired; the drug's indication corresponds with the patient's diagnosis; the dosage calculations are correct and the dosing formula used to derive the final dose is correct; the route of administration is safe and proper for the patient; and the drug's integrity is intact.* Both of you should sign the patient's medical record indicating that the verification took place.
- After comparing results of the independent double-check with the other practitioner, begin administering the drug if there are no discrepancies. If discrepancies exist, rectify them before administering the drug.[12]
- Place the 25G needle at a 45-degree angle, insert it into the reservoir, and aspirate 3 mL of CSF into the attached syringe *to make sure it's clear and doesn't contain blood.*[13] If the aspirate isn't clear, notify the doctor before continuing. If laboratory studies are needed, clamp the tubing and discard the CSF, then withdraw the appropriate amount of CSF needed for any studies ordered.

NURSING ALERT *Don't use a Vacutainer to aspirate CSF; rapidly withdrawing CSF with this device could damage the ventricle's choroid plexus.*

- Continue to aspirate as many milliliters of CSF as the volume of drug to be instilled. Then detach the syringe from the needle hub, attach the drug syringe, and instill the medication slowly, monitoring the patient for headache, nausea, and dizziness. (Some facilities use the CSF instead of a preservative-free diluent to deliver the drug.)

- Pinch the tubing, detach the syringe, and attach the syringe containing preservative-free normal saline solution; slowly flush the reservoir according to your facility's policy.
- Withdraw the needle, cover the site with a sterile gauze pad, and apply gentle pressure for a moment or two until superficial bleeding stops.
- Discard the needle and syringe in an appropriate sharps container; make sure to use a chemotherapy sharps container if the medication was a chemotherapeutic agent.
- If laboratory testing is ordered, place the CSF reserved for laboratory testing in the collection tubes and label the tubes in the presence of the patient *to prevent mislabeling.* Discard the syringe in the appropriate sharps container.
- Instruct the patient to lie quietly for about 15 to 30 minutes after the procedure *to prevent meningeal irritation leading to nausea and vomiting.*
- Monitor the patient for adverse drug reactions and signs of increased ICP, such as nausea, vomiting, pain, and dizziness. Assess for adverse reactions every 30 minutes for 2 hours, every hour for 2 hours, and then every 4 hours or according to your facility policy.
- Remove and discard used supplies in the appropriate waste receptacles.
- Remove your personal protective equipment and discard in the appropriate receptacle.
- Wash your hands with soap and water if the drug was a chemotherapeutic agent;[2,5,8] perform hand hygiene if it wasn't.[6,7,8]
- Perform a comprehensive pain assessment using techniques appropriate for the patient's age, condition, and ability to understand.
- Administer pain medication as needed and prescribed, following safe medication administration practices.
- Perform hand hygiene.[6,7,8]
- Document the procedure.[14]

Special considerations

- If the prescribed medication is a chemotherapeutic agent, the order must be written and contain the patient's complete name and a second identifier; the date; the patient's diagnosis; any allergies; the regimen's name and number (if applicable), including the individual drug's generic name, treatment criteria, and dosage calculation method; the patient's height and weight; and any other variables used to calculate the dose. The order must also contain the dosage, route and rate of administration, schedule, duration of therapy, cumulative lifetime dose (if applicable), sequence of drug administration (if applicable), and any supportive care treatments appropriate for the regimen, such as premedications for hypersensitivity and nausea and hydration, if necessary. Have another practitioner qualified to prepare or administer chemotherapy do the same.[2,5]
- The doctor may prescribe an antiemetic to be administered 30 minutes before the procedure *to control nausea and vomiting.*
- If your patient is scheduled to receive an Ommaya reservoir, explain the procedure before reservoir insertion. Be sure that the patient and his family understand the potential complications, and answer any questions they may have. Reassure the patient

that any hair clipped for the implant will grow back and that only a coin-sized patch must remain clipped for injections. (Hair regrowth will be slower if the patient is receiving chemotherapy.)
■ After the reservoir is implanted, the site is commonly left open to air after the first 24 hours.[13] The patient may resume normal activities. Instruct him to protect the site from bumps and traumatic injury while the incision heals. Tell him that unless complications develop, the reservoir may function for years.

Patient teaching

Teach the patient and his family about measures to prevent health care facility–associated infections, including the importance of hand hygiene. Encourage them to remind health care workers who fail to perform hand hygiene before providing care.

Instruct the patient and his family to notify the doctor if any signs or symptoms of infection develop at the insertion site (for example, redness, swelling, tenderness, or drainage) or if the patient develops headache, neck stiffness, or fever, *which may indicate a systemic infection.*

Verify that the patient received written educational materials appropriate for his reading level and understanding that include information about his diagnosis, chemotherapy plan, possible long- and short-term adverse effects, risks associated with the regimen, reportable signs and symptoms, monitoring, sexual relations, contraception, special precautions, and follow-up care if the patient is receiving chemotherapy.

Complications

Infection may develop but can usually be treated successfully with antibiotics injected directly into the reservoir. Persistent infection may require removal of the reservoir.

Catheter migration or blockage may cause symptoms of increased ICP, such as headache and nausea. If the doctor suspects this problem, he may gently push and release the reservoir several times (a technique called *pumping*). With his finger on the patient's scalp, the doctor can feel the reservoir refill. Slow filling suggests catheter migration or blockage, which must be confirmed by a computed tomography scan. Surgical correction is required.

Documentation

Record the appearance of the reservoir insertion site before and after access, the patient's tolerance of the procedure, the amount of CSF withdrawn and its appearance, and the generic name and dose of the drug instilled. Note any adverse effects of the drug, the doctor who was notified, prescribed interventions, and the patient's response to the interventions. Document any patient and family teaching.

REFERENCES

1 The Joint Commission. (2012). Standard MM.06.01.01. *Comprehensive accreditation manual for hospitals: The official handbook.* Oakbrook Terrace, IL: The Joint Commission. (Level 1)
2 Polovich, M., et al. (Eds.). (2009). *Chemotherapy and biotherapy guidelines and recommendations for practice* (3rd ed.). Pittsburgh, PA: Oncology Nursing Society.
3 Centers for Medicare & Medicaid Services, Department of Health and Human Services. (2006). "Conditions of Participation: Patients' Rights" 42 CFR part 482.13 [Online]. Accessed November 2011 via the Web at https://www.cms.gov/CFCsAndCoPs/downloads/finalpatientrightsrule.pdf
4 Westbrook, J., et al. (2010). Association of interruptions with an increased risk and severity of medication administration errors. *Archives of Internal Medicine, 170*(8), 683–690.
5 Jacobson, J., et al. (2009). American Society of Clinical Oncology/Oncology Nursing Society chemotherapy administration safety standards. *Oncology Nursing Forum, 36*(6), 651–658.
6 Centers for Disease Control and Prevention. (October 2002). Guideline for hand hygiene in health-care settings. *Morbidity and Mortality Weekly Report, 51*(RR-16), 1–45. (Level I)
7 World Health Organization. (2009). *WHO guidelines on hand hygiene in health care: First global patient safety challenge. Clean care is safer care.* Geneva, Switzerland: World Health Organization. (Level I)
8 The Joint Commission. (2012). Standard NPSG.07.01.01. *Comprehensive accreditation manual for hospitals: The official handbook.* Oakbrook Terrace, IL: The Joint Commission. (Level 1)
9 The Joint Commission. (2012). Standard NPSG.01.01.01. *Comprehensive accreditation manual for hospitals: The official handbook.* Oakbrook Terrace, IL: The Joint Commission. (Level 1)
10 The Joint Commission. (2012). Standard NPSG.03.04.01. *Comprehensive accreditation manual for hospitals: The official handbook.* Oakbrook Terrace, IL: The Joint Commission. (Level 1)
11 Institute of Safe Medication Practices. "ISMP's List of High-Alert Medications." [Online]. Accessed August 2011 via the Web at http://www.ismp.org/tools/highalertmedications.pdf
12 Institute for Safe Medication Practices. (2008). "Conducting an Independent Double-check." *ISMP Medication Safety Alert! Nurse Advise-ERR, 6*(12), 1 [Online]. Accessed July 2011 via the Web at http://www.ismp.org/newsletters/nursing/Issues/NurseAdviseERR200812.pdf
13 Standard 58. Nonvascular infusion devices. Infusion nursing standards of practice. (2011). *Journal of Infusion Nursing, 34*(1S), S81–S82. (Level I)
14 The Joint Commission. (2012). Standard RC.01.03.01. *Comprehensive accreditation manual for hospitals: The official handbook.* Oakbrook Terrace, IL: The Joint Commission. (Level 1)

ORAL CARE

Oral care, which typically involves the nurse or patient brushing and flossing the patient's teeth and inspecting the mouth, is commonly performed in the morning, at bedtime, and after meals. Oral care removes soft plaque deposits and calculus from the teeth, cleans and massages the gums, reduces mouth odor, provides comfort, and reduces the risk of infection.

Patients who are intubated and receiving mechanical ventilation require oral care more frequently because mechanical ventilation dries the oral mucosa and affects salivary flow, increasing the risk for infection.[1] Oral care should be performed every 2 to 4 hours in these patients. In 2010, the Institute for Healthcare Improvement added daily oral care with chlorhexidine to its ventilator-associated pneumonia (VAP) prevention bundle because evidence shows that it helps prevent VAP when combined with the other bundle elements—elevating the head of the patient 30 to 45 degrees, interrupting sedation daily and assessing readiness to wean, and providing peptic ulcer disease and deep vein thrombosis prophylaxis, unless contraindicated.[2]

Equipment

Towel ■ facial tissues ■ emesis basin ■ trash bag ■ mouthwash (preferably alcohol-free) ■ toothbrush and toothpaste ■ cup ■ drinking straw ■ dental floss or interdental cleaner ■ gloves ■ dental floss holder, if available ■ small mirror, if necessary ■ Optional: oral irrigating device.

For a comatose or debilitated patient as needed

Linen-saver pad ■ bite block ■ petroleum jelly ■ oral suction equipment or gauze pads ■ sponge-tipped swab ■ Optional: mask, goggles, face shield.

For an intubated patient

Linen-saver pad ■ bite block or oropharyngeal airway ■ suction equipment ■ petroleum jelly ■ sponge-tipped swabs ■ 1.5% hydrogen peroxide solution ■ soft-bristle toothbrush ■ toothpaste ■ Optional: chlorhexidine mouth rinse.

Preparation of equipment

Bring a cup of water and other equipment to the patient's bedside. If you'll be using oral suction equipment, connect the tubing to the suction canister and suction catheter, turn on the suction apparatus, and check for correct operation.

Implementation

■ Perform hand hygiene and put on gloves as needed.[3,4,5]
■ Explain the procedure to the patient, and provide privacy.

Supervising oral care

■ For the bedridden patient capable of self-care, encourage her to perform her own mouth care.
■ If allowed, place the patient in Fowler's position. Place the overbed table in front of the patient, and arrange the equipment on it. Open the table and set up the built-in mirror, if available, or position a small mirror on the table (as shown below).

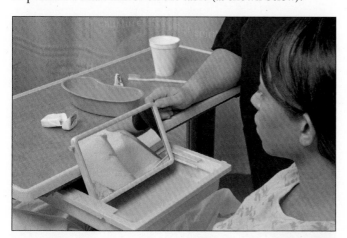

■ Drape a towel over the patient's chest *to protect her gown*. Instruct her to floss her teeth while looking into the mirror.
■ Observe the patient *to make sure she's flossing correctly*, and correct her if necessary. If the patient is using dental floss, tell her to wrap the floss around the second or third fingers of both hands. Starting with her front teeth and without injuring the gums, she should insert the floss as far as possible into the space between each pair of teeth (as shown below). Then she should clean the surfaces of adjacent teeth by pulling the floss up and down against the side of each tooth. After the patient flosses a pair of teeth, remind her to use a clean 1″ (2.5-cm) section of floss for the next pair.

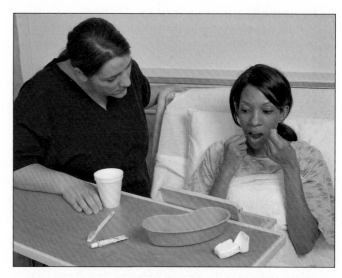

■ While the patient flosses, mix mouthwash and water in a glass, place a straw in the glass, and position the emesis basin nearby.
■ Instruct the patient to brush her teeth and gums while looking into the mirror. Encourage her to rinse frequently during brushing, and provide facial tissues for her to wipe her mouth.

Performing oral care

■ For a comatose patient or a conscious patient incapable of self-care, you'll perform oral care. If the patient wears dentures, clean them thoroughly. (See *Dealing with dentures*, page 526.) Some patients may benefit from an oral irrigating device. (See *Using an oral irrigating device*, page 527.)
■ Arrange the equipment on the overbed table or bedside stand, including the oral suction equipment, if necessary. Turn on the apparatus. If a suction apparatus isn't available, wipe the inside of the patient's mouth frequently with a moist, sponge-tipped swab.
■ Mix mouthwash and water in a glass and place a straw in it.

Dealing with dentures

Prostheses made of acrylic resins, vinyl composites, or both, dentures replace some or all of the patient's natural teeth. Dentures require proper care to remove soft plaque deposits and calculus and to reduce mouth odor. Such care involves removing and rinsing dentures after meals, daily brushing and removal of tenacious deposits, and soaking in a commercial denture cleaner. Dentures must be removed from the comatose or presurgical patient *to prevent possible airway obstruction*.

Equipment and preparation
Start by assembling the following equipment at the patient's bedside:
- Emesis basin
- Labeled denture cup
- Toothbrush or denture brush
- Gloves
- Toothpaste
- Commercial denture cleaner
- Paper towel
- Sponge-tipped swab
- Mouthwash (preferably alcohol-free)
- Gauze
- Optional: adhesive denture liner

Perform hand hygiene and put on gloves.[3,4,5]

Removing dentures
- To remove a full upper denture, grasp the front and palatal surfaces of the denture with your thumb and forefinger. Position the index finger of your opposite hand over the upper border of the denture and press *to break the seal between denture and palate*. Grasp the denture with gauze *because saliva can make it slippery*.
- To remove a full lower denture, grasp the front and lingual surfaces of the denture with your thumb and index finger and gently lift up.
- To remove partial dentures, first ask the patient or a caregiver how the prosthesis is retained and how to remove it. If the partial denture is held in place with clips or snaps,

then exert equal pressure on the border of each side of the denture. Avoid lifting the clasps, *which easily bend or break*.

Oral and denture care
- After removing dentures, place them in a properly labeled denture cup. Add warm water and a commercial denture cleaner *to remove stains and hardened deposits*. Follow package directions. Avoid soaking dentures in mouthwash containing alcohol *because it may damage a soft liner*.
- Instruct the patient to rinse with mouthwash *to remove food particles and reduce mouth odor*. Then stroke the palate, buccal surfaces, gums, and tongue with a soft toothbrush or sponge-tipped mouth swab *to clean the mucosa and stimulate circulation*. Inspect for irritated areas or sores *because they may indicate a poorly fitting denture*.
- Carry the denture cup, emesis basin, toothbrush, and toothpaste to the sink. Line the basin with a paper towel and fill it with water *to cushion the dentures in case you drop them*. Hold the dentures over the basin, wet them with warm water, and apply toothpaste to a denture brush or long-bristled toothbrush. Clean the dentures using only moderate pressure *to prevent scratches* and warm water *to prevent distortion*.
- Clean the denture cup, and place the dentures in it. Rinse the brush, and clean and dry the emesis basin. Return all equipment to the patient's bedside stand.

Inserting dentures
- If the patient desires, apply adhesive liner to the dentures and either insert them or have the patient insert them. You can moisten dentures with water, if necessary, *to reduce friction and ease insertion*.
- Encourage the patient to wear the dentures *to enhance appearance, facilitate eating and speaking, and prevent changes in the gum line that may affect denture fit*.

- Raise the bed to a comfortable working height *to prevent back strain*. Then lower the head of the bed, and position the patient on her side, with her face extended over the edge of the pillow (as shown on right column *to facilitate drainage and prevent fluid aspiration*.

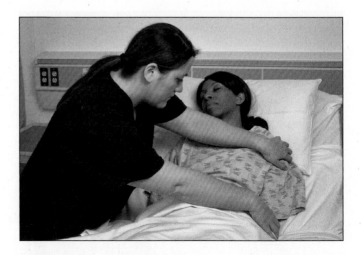

EQUIPMENT

Using an oral irrigating device

An oral irrigating device, such as the Water Pik, directs a pulsating jet of water around the teeth to massage gums and remove debris and food particles. It's especially useful for cleaning areas missed by brushing, such as around bridgework, crowns, and dental wires. Because this device enhances oral hygiene, it benefits patients undergoing head and neck irradiation, which can damage teeth and cause severe caries. The device also maintains oral hygiene in a patient with a fractured jaw or with mouth injuries that limit standard mouth care.

Equipment and preparation
To use the device, first assemble the following equipment:
- Oral irrigating device
- Towel
- Emesis basin
- Pharyngeal suction apparatus
- Salt solution or mouthwash (alcohol-free), if ordered
- Soap

Perform hand hygiene and put on gloves.[3,4,5]

Implementation
- Insert the oral irrigating device's plug into a nearby electrical outlet. Remove the device's cover, turn it upside down, and fill it with lukewarm water or with a mouthwash or salt solution, as ordered. When using a salt solution, dissolve the salt beforehand in a separate container. Then pour the solution into the cover. Salt solutions shouldn't be used in patients who have problems with dryness and dehydration *because salt solutions exacerbate these conditions.*
- Secure the cover to the base of the device. Remove the water hose handle from the base, and snap the jet tip into place. If necessary, wet the grooved end of the tip *to ease insertion.* Adjust the pressure dial to the setting most comfortable for the patient. If her gums are tender and prone to bleed, choose a low setting.
- Turn the patient to her side *to prevent aspiration of water.* Then place a towel under her chin and an emesis basin next to her cheek *to absorb or catch drainage.*
- Adjust the knurled knob on the handle *to direct the water jet,* place the jet tip in the patient's mouth, and turn on the device. Instruct the alert patient to keep her lips partially closed *to avoid spraying water.*

- Direct the water at a right angle to the gum line of each tooth and between teeth (as shown below). Avoid directing water under the patient's tongue *because this action may injure sensitive tissue.*

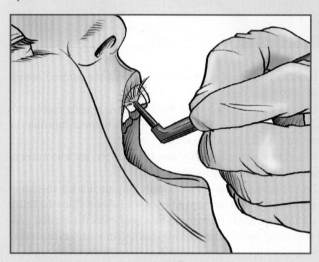

- After irrigating each tooth, pause briefly and instruct the patient to expectorate the water or solution into the emesis basin. If she's unable to do so, suction it from the sides of the mouth with the pharyngeal suction apparatus. After irrigating all teeth, turn off the device, and remove the jet tip from the patient's mouth.
- Empty the remaining water or solution from the cover, remove the jet tip from the handle, and return the handle to the base. Clean the jet tip with soap and water, rinse the cover, and dry them both and return them to storage.

- Place a linen-saver pad under the patient's chin and an emesis basin near her cheek (as shown on right column) *to absorb or catch drainage.*

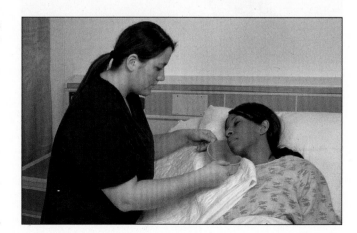

■ Lubricate the patient's lips with petroleum jelly (as shown below) *to prevent dryness and cracking.* Reapply lubricant, as needed, during oral care.

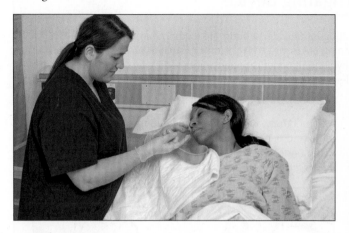

■ If necessary, insert the bite block *to hold the patient's mouth open during oral care.*

■ Using a dental floss holder, hold the floss against each tooth and direct it as close to the gum as possible without injuring the sensitive tissues around the tooth.

■ Wet the toothbrush with water. If necessary, use hot water *to soften the bristles.* Apply toothpaste.

■ Brush the patient's lower teeth from the gum line up; the upper teeth, from the gum line down (as shown below). Place the brush at a 45-degree angle to the gum line, and press the bristles gently into the gingival sulcus. Using short, gentle strokes *to prevent gum damage,* brush the facial surfaces (toward the cheek) and the lingual surfaces (toward the tongue) of the bottom teeth. Use just the tip of the brush for the lingual surfaces of the front teeth. Then, using the same technique, brush the facial and lingual surfaces of the top teeth. Next, brush the biting surfaces of the bottom and top teeth, using a back and forth motion. If possible, ask the patient to rinse frequently during brushing by taking the mouthwash solution through the straw. Hold the emesis basin steady under the patient's cheek, and wipe her mouth and cheeks with facial tissues, as needed.

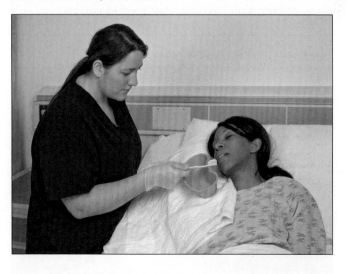

■ After brushing the patient's teeth, dip a sponge-tipped mouth swab into the mouthwash solution. Press the swab against the side of the glass to remove excess moisture. Gently stroke the gums, buccal surfaces, palate, and tongue (as shown below) *to clean the mucosa and stimulate circulation.* Replace the swab as necessary for thorough cleaning. Avoid inserting the swab too deeply *to prevent gagging and vomiting.*

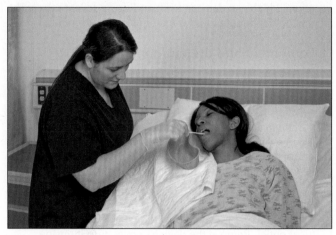

Performing oral care in an intubated patient

■ For an intubated patient, provide oral care according to your facility's policy. In addition to brushing twice daily, use sponge-tipped swabs with a 1.5% hydrogen peroxide solution to clean the patient's mouth every 2 to 4 hours. Use a chlorhexidine mouth rinse once daily, as prescribed, to prevent VAP.[1,2]

■ Assess the patient's level of consciousness and anxiety level to determine if sedation is necessary and whether the assistance of another staff member is needed.[2]

■ Administer sedation as ordered, if necessary, following safe medication administration practices.

■ Elicit the help of a coworker if needed.

■ Arrange the equipment on the overbed table or bedside stand, including the suction equipment.

■ Turn on the suction apparatus.

■ Raise the bed to a comfortable working position *to prevent back strain.*

■ Place the patient in high Fowler's position *to reduce the risk of aspiration.*

■ Place a linen-saver pad under the patient's chin *to absorb or catch drainage.*

■ If the patient is orally intubated, remove the bite block or oropharyngeal airway.[2]

■ Gently brush the patient's teeth using a soft-bristle toothbrush, toothpaste, and a small amount of water *to reduce oropharyngeal colonization and dental plaque, which increases the risk for VAP.*[2,5] Use short, gentle strokes *to prevent gum damage.*

■ Gently brush the surface of the tongue.

■ Perform deep suction *to remove oropharyngeal secretions and prevent aspiration of secretions.*[2]

■ In addition to brushing the patient's teeth, clean her mouth every 2 to 4 hours using a sponge-tipped swab with 1.5% hydrogen peroxide solution.[2]

■ Suction the patient's oropharynx *to remove secretions after cleaning.*[2]

■ If needed to prevent biting in the orally intubated patient, replace the bite block or oropharyngeal airway by inserting it along the endotracheal tube.[2]

■ Lubricate the patient's lips with petroleum jelly.

■ Reposition the patient for comfort, maintaining the head of the bed at 30 to 45 degrees, *to prevent aspiration and reduce the risk of VAP.*[2]

■ Return the patient's bed to the low position to maintain patient safety.

After oral care

■ Assess the patient's mouth for cleanliness and tooth and tissue condition.

■ Rinse the toothbrush, and clean the emesis basin and glass.

■ Remove your gloves and other personal protective equipment and perform hand hygiene.[3,4,5]

■ Place a clean suction catheter on the tubing. Return reusable equipment to the appropriate storage location, and properly discard disposable equipment in the trash bag.

■ Perform hand hygiene.[3,4,5]

■ Document the procedure.[6]

Special considerations

■ Use sponge-tipped mouth swabs to clean the teeth of a patient with sensitive gums. *These swabs produce less friction than a toothbrush but don't clean as well.*

■ Clean the mouth of a toothless comatose patient by wrapping a gauze pad around your index finger, moistening it with mouthwash, and gently swabbing the oral tissues.

■ Remember that mucous membranes dry quickly in the patient breathing through the mouth or receiving oxygen therapy. Moisten the patient's mouth and lips regularly with moistened sponge-tipped swabs or water.

Documentation

Record the date and time of oral care in your notes. Also document any unusual conditions, such as bleeding, edema, mouth odor, excessive secretions, or plaque on the tongue. Note the patient's tolerance of the procedure.

REFERENCES

1 Lynn-McHale Wiegand, D. (Ed.). (2011). *AACN procedure manual for critical care* (6th ed.). Philadelphia, PA: Saunders.

2 Institute for Healthcare Improvement. (2010). *5 million lives campaign getting started kit: Prevent ventilator-associated pneumonia.* Cambridge, MA: Institute for Healthcare Improvement. (Level I)

3 Centers for Disease Control and Prevention. (October 2002). Guideline for hand hygiene in health-care settings. *Morbidity and Mortality Weekly Report, 51*(RR-16), 1–45. (Level I)

4 World Health Organization. (2009). *WHO guidelines on hand hygiene in health care: First global patient safety challenge. Clean care is safer care.* Geneva, Switzerland: World Health Organization. (Level I)

5 The Joint Commission. (2012). Standard NPSG.07.01.01. *Comprehensive accreditation manual for hospitals: The official handbook.* Oakbrook Terrace, IL: The Joint Commission. (Level 1)

6 The Joint Commission. (2012). Standard RC.01.03.01. *Comprehensive accreditation manual for hospitals: The official handbook.* Oakbrook Terrace, IL: The Joint Commission. (Level 1)

ADDITIONAL REFERENCES

Craven, R.F., & Hirnle, C.J. (2012). *Fundamentals of nursing: Human health and function* (7th ed.). Philadelphia, PA: Lippincott Williams & Wilkins.

Feider, L.L., et al. (2010). Oral care practices for orally intubated critically ill adults. *American Journal of Critical Care, 19*(2), 175–183.

ORAL DRUG ADMINISTRATION

Because oral administration is usually the safest, most convenient, and least expensive method, most drugs are administered by this route. Drugs for oral administration are available in many forms: tablets, enteric-coated tablets, capsules, syrups, elixirs, oils, liquids, suspensions, powders, and granules. Some require special preparation before administration, such as mixing with juice to make them more palatable; oils, powders, and granules most often require such preparation.

Sometimes oral drugs are prescribed in higher dosages than their parenteral equivalents because after absorption through the GI system, they are immediately broken down by the liver before they reach the systemic circulation.

ELDER ALERT *Oral dosages normally prescribed for adults may be dangerous for elderly patients.*

Oral administration is contraindicated for unconscious patients; it may also be contraindicated in patients with nausea and vomiting and in those unable to swallow.

Equipment

Patient's medication record and chart ■ prescribed medication ■ medication cup ■ Optional: appropriate vehicle, such as jelly or applesauce, for crushed pills (commonly used with elderly patients), and juice, water, or milk for liquid medications; drinking straw; mortar and pestle for crushing pills; pill-cutting device for scored tablets.

Implementation

■ Avoid distractions and interruptions when preparing and administering medication to prevent medication administration errors.[1]

■ Compare the medication label to the order in the patient's medical record (as shown below).[1]

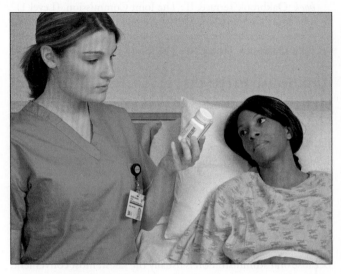

■ Verify that the medication hasn't expired and that no contraindications exist.
■ Visually inspect the medication for any loss of integrity.[2]
■ Verify that the medication is being administered at the proper time, in the prescribed dose, and by the correct route *to reduce the risk of medication errors.*[2]
■ Discuss any unresolved concerns about the medication with the patient's doctor.[2]
■ If the patient is receiving the medication for the first time, teach the patient about significant adverse reactions or other concerns related to the medication.[2]
■ Perform hand hygiene.[3,4,5]
■ Confirm the patient's identity using at least two patient identifiers according to your facility's policy.[6]
■ Assess the patient's condition to determine the need for the medication and the effectiveness of previous therapy.
■ Carefully observe the patient for a rash, pruritus, cough, or other signs of an adverse reaction to a previously administered drug.
■ Explain the procedure to the patient. Answer all questions to relieve anxiety and increase cooperation. Also provide information about why the medication is being administered.
■ Provide privacy.
■ If your facility uses a bar code scanning system, scan your identification badge, the patient's identification bracelet, and the medication's bar code according to your facility's policy.
■ Give the patient her medication (as shown on next column top) and an appropriate vehicle or liquid, as needed, *to aid swallowing, minimize adverse effects, or promote absorption.* For example, cyclophosphamide is given with fluids to minimize adverse effects; antitussive cough syrup is given without a fluid to avoid diluting its soothing effect on the throat. If appropriate, crush the medication *to facilitate swallowing.*

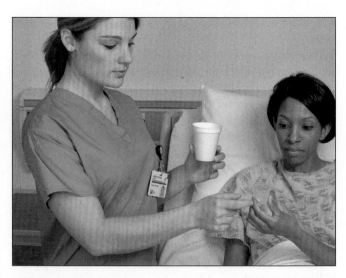

■ Stay with the patient until she has swallowed the drug. If she seems confused or disoriented, check her mouth *to make sure she has swallowed it.* Return and reassess the patient's response within 1 hour after giving the medication.[7]
■ Perform hand hygiene.[3,4,5]
■ Document the procedure.[8]

Special considerations

■ Notify the doctor about any medication withheld, unless parameters to hold are already written.
■ Use care in measuring out the prescribed dose of liquid oral medication. (See *Measuring liquid medications.*)
■ Don't give medication from a poorly labeled or unlabeled container. Don't attempt to label or reinforce drug labels yourself. *This must be done by a pharmacist.*[9]
■ Never give a medication prepared by someone else. Never allow your medication cart or tray out of your sight. *These precautions prevent anyone from rearranging the medications or taking one without your knowledge.* Never return unwrapped or prepared medications to stock containers. Instead, dispose of them and notify the pharmacy. Keep in mind that the disposal of any narcotic drug must be cosigned by another nurse, as mandated by law.
■ If the patient questions you about the medication or dosage, check the medication record again. If the medication is correct, reassure the patient. Make sure you explain any changes in the medication or dosage. As appropriate, teach about possible adverse effects. Ask the patient to report anything perceived as an adverse effect.
■ *To avoid damaging or staining the patient's teeth,* administer iron preparations through a straw. An unpleasant-tasting liquid can usually be made more palatable if taken through a straw *because the liquid contacts fewer taste buds.*
■ If the patient can't swallow a whole tablet or capsule, ask the pharmacist if the drug is available in liquid form or if it can be administered by another route. If not, ask him if you can crush the tablet or open the capsule and mix it with food. Keep in mind that many enteric-coated or time-release medications and gelatin

capsules shouldn't be crushed. Remember to contact the doctor for an order to change the route of administration when necessary.

Documentation

Note the drug administered, the dose, the date and time, and any adverse reactions. If adverse reactions occurred, document your interventions and the patient's response to those interventions. If the patient refuses a drug, document the refusal and notify the charge nurse and the patient's doctor, as needed. Also note if a drug was omitted or withheld for other reasons, such as radiology or laboratory tests, or if, in your judgment, the drug was contraindicated at the ordered time. Sign out all controlled substances given on the appropriate controlled substances central record. Document patient teaching.

REFERENCES

1 Westbrook, J., et al. (2010). Association of interruptions with an increased risk and severity of medication administration errors. *Archives of Internal Medicine, 170*(8), 683–690.

2 The Joint Commission. (2012). Standard MM.06.01.01. *Comprehensive accreditation manual for hospitals: The official handbook.* Oakbrook Terrace, IL: The Joint Commission. (Level 1)

3 The Joint Commission. (2012). Standard NPSG.07.01.01. *Comprehensive accreditation manual for hospitals: The official handbook.* Oakbrook Terrace, IL: The Joint Commission. (Level 1)

4 Centers for Disease Control and Prevention. (October 2002). Guideline for hand hygiene in health-care settings. *Morbidity and Mortality Weekly Report, 51*(RR-16), 1–45. (Level I)

5 World Health Organization. (2009). *WHO guidelines on hand hygiene in health care: First global patient safety challenge. Clean care is safer care.* Geneva, Switzerland: World Health Organization. (Level I)

6 The Joint Commission. (2012). Standard NPSG.01.01.01. *Comprehensive accreditation manual for hospitals: The official handbook.* Oakbrook Terrace, IL: The Joint Commission. (Level 1)

7 The Joint Commission. (2012). Standard MM.07.01.01. *Comprehensive accreditation manual for hospitals: The official handbook.* Oakbrook Terrace, IL: The Joint Commission. (Level 1)

8 The Joint Commission. (2012). Standard RC.01.03.01. *Comprehensive accreditation manual for hospitals: The official handbook.* Oakbrook Terrace, IL: The Joint Commission. (Level 1)

9 The Joint Commission. (2012). Standard MM.05.01.01. *Comprehensive accreditation manual for hospitals: The official handbook.* Oakbrook Terrace, IL: The Joint Commission. (Level 1)

ADDITIONAL REFERENCES

Craven, R.F., & Hirnle, C.J. (2012). *Fundamentals of nursing: Human health and function* (7th ed.). Philadelphia, PA: Lippincott Williams & Wilkins.

Nettina, S.M. (2010). *Lippincott manual of nursing practice* (9th ed.). Philadelphia, PA: Lippincott Williams & Wilkins.

Taylor, C., et al. (2011). *Fundamentals of nursing: The art and science of nursing care* (7th ed.). Philadelphia, PA: Lippincott Williams & Wilkins.

Measuring liquid medications

To pour liquids, hold the medication cup at eye level. Use your thumb to mark off the correct level on the cup (as shown below). Then set the cup down and read the bottom of the meniscus at eye level *to ensure accuracy.* If you've poured too much medication into the cup, discard the excess. Don't return it to the bottle.

Here are a couple of additional tips:

■ Hold the container so that the medication flows from the side opposite the label *so it won't run down the container and stain or obscure the label.* Remove drips from the lip of the bottle first and then from the sides, using a clean, damp paper towel.

■ For a liquid measured in drops, use only the dropper supplied with the medication.

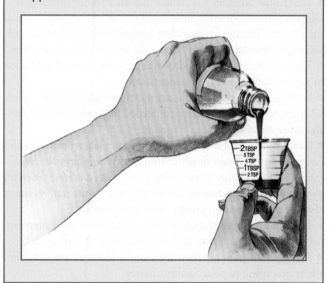

ORGAN DONOR, IDENTIFICATION

In 1984, the U.S. Congress passed the National Organ Transplant Act, which established the Organ Procurement and Transplant Network, a national registry for organ matching.[1] This act was created to address the critical shortage of organ donations and to improve the organ matching and placement process. With passage of this act, it's now a federal requirement to identify potential organ donors.

In addition to requirements of the National Organ Transplant Act, the U.S. Department of Health and Human Services requires U.S. hospitals to report every death or imminent death to the Organ Procurement Organization (OPO) as part of the hospital's condition of participation and eligibility to receive Medicare funds. The Joint Commission has also addressed organ donation in its accreditation requirements. As part of the process of identifying a potential organ donor, the doctor should make the family aware early on that organ donation should be considered to help elicit a more positive response from family members. The death pronouncement and the request to consider organ donation should never occur at the same time.[2] Ideally, referral to the OPO should occur when a patient scores less than 5 on the Glasgow Coma Scale or when two or more brain stem reflexes are absent.[2]

Equipment

Organ donation information materials ▪ brain death information (often dictated by state laws) ▪ blood sampling tubes and labels.

Preparation of equipment

Have information available regarding organ donation as well as the appropriate forms, including consent forms. Do your best to ensure the information is printed in a language the patient understands.

Implementation

▪ Determine whether the patient has an advance directive that addresses organ donation or is listed in a donor registry (such as on a driver's license) *because these legal documents, which are supported in most states, may influence the family's ultimate decision.*
▪ Keep the family informed of the patient's medical condition *to prepare them for realistic patient outcomes.*[2]
▪ Arrange for an interdisciplinary meeting with family in a quiet, nonthreatening environment, if needed, *to further help the family realize the diagnosis and prognosis.*
▪ Consult the OPO coordinator in your area when death is imminent and before brain death testing begins *to inform the coordinator that your facility is evaluating a potential candidate for organ donation so the coordinator can be present to guide staff members through the preparation process when appropriate.*
▪ Perform hand hygiene and put on personal protective equipment, including gloves, a gown, and eye protection, if indicated.[3,4,5]
▪ Confirm the patient's identity using at least two patient identifiers according to your facility's policy.[6]
▪ Collect laboratory samples as indicated *to provide data to assess organ function.* Tests may include complete blood count, liver and renal function tests, electrolyte levels, and human immunodeficiency virus testing.[2]
▪ Monitor vital signs and fluid status. *If there is decreased perfusion to organs, the patient may not be able to donate an organ.*[2]
▪ Assist with examining the patient for the determination of brain death.[7]
▪ As applicable, ensure that the patient's brain death has been declared appropriately. Many states have certain criteria that must be followed as well as guidelines on what type of doctor can make the declaration so that the OPO coordinator can then officially approach the family and determine willingness regarding organ donation.
▪ Contact the OPO coordinator if brain death is declared *so a coordinator can discuss possible organ donation with the family. An OPO coordinator is the best person to discuss organ donation with the family because it takes special knowledge, training, and experience to be able to deliver the appropriate message to families.*
▪ Encourage the family to be at the bedside as much as possible and keep them informed as procedures and preparations are taking place *to help promote family time and facilitate closure.*

▪ Make sure that the family knows what to expect when drugs are discontinued and the ventilator or other therapies are withdrawn *to help prevent additional grief or anxiety.*
▪ Discard used supplies in the appropriate manner.
▪ Perform hand hygiene after removing personal protective equipment and gloves.[3,4,5]
▪ Document the procedure.[8]

Special considerations

▪ Be aware of cultural and spiritual preferences that must also be considered when approaching the family about organ donation.
▪ If an ethical dilemma arises, consult your facility's ethics committee *to help clarify the decision-making process or offer viable alternatives for the family or staff.*

Complications

If communication with the OPO coordinator isn't established early enough, trust may be lost between the professional caregivers and the family, and successful organ donation may be denied. Other negative outcomes that may result include not honoring the patient's wishes, obtaining consent for organs that aren't viable, and identifying a donor who isn't medically suitable for organ donation.[2]

Documentation

Document any interactions you have with the family, such as multidisciplinary conferences and contact with the OPO coordinator. Document any family teaching provided and the family's understanding of the teaching. After brain death has been determined, document the date and time of the determination as well as the name of the doctor who made the declaration. Include all methods used to determine brain death. After the organ donation process is in place, any family contact, visitation, requests, or further teaching should be documented.

REFERENCES

1 U.S. Department of Health and Human Services. (2010). "U.S. Government Information on Organ and Tissue Donation and Transplantation" [Online]. Accessed October 2011 via the Web at http://www.organdonor.gov
2 Lynn-McHale Wiegand, D. (Ed.). (2011). *AACN procedure manual for critical care* (6th ed.). Philadelphia, PA: Saunders.
3 The Joint Commission. (2012). Standard NPSG.07.01.01. *Comprehensive accreditation manual for hospitals: The official handbook.* Oakbrook Terrace, IL: The Joint Commission. (Level 1)
4 Centers for Disease Control and Prevention. (October 2002). Guideline for hand hygiene in health-care settings. *Morbidity and Mortality Weekly Report, 51*(RR-16), 1–45. (Level I)
5 World Health Organization. (2009). *WHO guidelines on hand hygiene in health care: First global patient safety challenge. Clean care is safer care.* Geneva, Switzerland: World Health Organization. (Level I)
6 The Joint Commission. (2012). Standard NPSG.01.01.01. *Comprehensive accreditation manual for hospitals: The official handbook.* Oakbrook Terrace, IL: The Joint Commission. (Level 1)

7 Eelco, F.M., et al. (2010). "Evidence-based guideline update: Determining brain death in adults. Report of the Quality Standards Subcommittee of the American. Academy of Neurology" *Neurology*, *74*(23), 1911–18 [Online]. Accessed January 2012 via the Web at http://www.neurology.org/content/74/23/1911.full.html

8 The Joint Commission. (2012). Standard RC.01.03.01. *Comprehensive accreditation manual for hospitals: The official handbook*. Oakbrook Terrace, IL: The Joint Commission. (Level 1)

ADDITIONAL REFERENCES

Siegel, J.D., et al. "2007 Guideline for Isolation Precautions: Preventing Transmission of Infectious Agents in Healthcare Settings" [Online]. Accessed September 2011 via the Web at http://www.cdc.gov/hicpac/2007ip/2007isolationprecautions.html

U.S. Department of Health & Human Services Organ Procurement and Transplantation Network. "Policy Management: National Organ Transplant Act" [Online]. Accessed October 2011 via the Web at http://optn.transplant.hrsa.gov/policiesAndBylaws/nota.asp

ORONASOPHARYNGEAL SUCTION

Oronasopharyngeal suction removes secretions from the pharynx by a suction catheter inserted through the mouth or nostril. Used to maintain a patent airway, this procedure helps the patient who can't clear his airway effectively with coughing and expectoration, such as the unconscious or severely debilitated patient. The procedure should be done as often as necessary, depending on the patient's condition.

Because the catheter may inadvertently slip into the lower airway or esophagus, oronasopharyngeal suction is a sterile procedure that requires sterile equipment. However, clean technique may be used for a tonsil tip suction device. In fact, an alert patient can use a tonsil tip suction device himself to remove secretions.

Equipment

Wall suction or portable suction unit with connecting tubing ▪ water-soluble lubricant ▪ sterile normal saline solution ▪ disposable sterile container ▪ sterile suction catheter (a #10 to #16 French for an adult, #8 or #10 French for a child, or pediatric feeding tube for an infant) ▪ sterile gloves and personal protective equipment, as needed ▪ overbed table ▪ waterproof trash bag ▪ towel ▪ Optional: tongue blade, tonsil tip suction device, nasopharyngeal or oropharyngeal airway (optional for frequent suctioning).

A commercially prepared kit contains a sterile catheter, disposable container, and sterile gloves.

Preparation of equipment

Before beginning, check your facility's policy *to determine whether a doctor's order is required for oropharyngeal suctioning*. Also review the patient's blood gas or oxygen saturation values, and check vital signs. Evaluate the patient's ability to cough and deep breathe *to determine his ability to move secretions up the tracheobronchial tree*. Check his history for a deviated septum, nasal polyps, nasal obstruction, traumatic injury, epistaxis, or mucosal swelling.

If no contraindications exist, gather and place the suction equipment on the patient's overbed table or bedside stand. Position the table or stand on your preferred side of the bed *to facilitate suctioning*. Connect the tubing to the suctioning unit. Date and then open the bottle of normal saline solution. Open the waterproof trash bag.

Implementation

▪ Confirm the patient's identity using at least two patient identifiers according to your facility's policy.[1]

▪ Explain the procedure to the patient even if he's unresponsive. Inform him that suctioning may stimulate transient coughing or gagging, but tell him that coughing helps to mobilize secretions. If he has been suctioned before, just summarize the reasons for the procedure. Reassure him throughout the procedure *to minimize anxiety and fear, which can increase oxygen consumption*.

▪ Perform hand hygiene and put on your personal protective equipment, as appropriate.[2,3,4]

▪ Determine which nostril is more patent.

▪ Place the patient in semi-Fowler's or high Fowler's position, if tolerated, *to promote lung expansion and effective coughing*. If the patient is unconscious, position him on his side facing you *to help promote drainage of secretions*.

▪ Place a towel across the patient's chest.

▪ Turn on the suction from the wall or portable unit, and set the pressure according to your facility's policy. Usually, the pressure may be set between 100 and 120 mm Hg; *higher pressures cause excessive trauma without enhancing secretion removal*.[5]

▪ Occlude the end of the connecting tubing *to check suction pressure*.

▪ Using strict sterile technique, open the suction catheter kit or the packages containing the sterile catheter, container, and gloves. Put on the gloves; consider your dominant hand sterile and your nondominant hand nonsterile.

▪ Using your nondominant hand, pour the saline solution into the sterile container.

▪ With your nondominant hand, place a small amount of water-soluble lubricant on the sterile area of the catheter. *The lubricant is used to facilitate passage of the catheter during nasopharyngeal suctioning*.

▪ Pick up the catheter with your dominant (sterile) hand and attach it to the connecting tubing (as shown below). Use your nondominant hand to control the suction valve while your dominant hand manipulates the catheter.

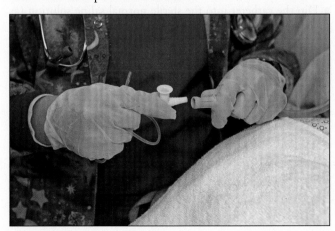

Tips on airway clearance

Deep breathing and coughing are vital for removing secretions from the lungs. Other techniques used to help clear the airways include diaphragmatic breathing and forced expiration. Here's how to teach these techniques to your patients.

Diaphragmatic breathing

First, tell the patient to lie supine, with his head elevated 15 to 20 degrees on a pillow. Tell him to place one hand on his abdomen and then inhale so that he can feel his abdomen rise. Explain that this is known as "breathing with the diaphragm."

Next, instruct the patient to exhale slowly through his nose—or, even better, through pursed lips—while letting his abdomen collapse. Explain that this action decreases his respiratory rate and increases his tidal volume.

Suggest that the patient perform this exercise for 30 minutes several times a day. After he becomes accustomed to the position and has learned to breathe using his diaphragm, he may apply abdominal weights of 8.8 to 11 lb (4 to 5 kg). The weights enhance the movement of the diaphragm toward the head during expiration.

To enhance the effectiveness of exercise, the patient may also manually compress the lower costal margins, perform straight-leg lifts, and coordinate the breathing technique with a physical activity such as walking.

Forced expiration

Explain to the patient that forced expiration (also known as *huff coughing*) helps clear secretions while causing less traumatic injury than does a cough. To perform the technique, tell the patient to forcefully expire without closing his glottis, starting with a middle to low lung volume. Tell him to follow this expiration with a period of diaphragmatic breathing and relaxation.

Inform the patient that if his secretions are in the central airways, he may have to use a more forceful expiration or a cough to clear them.

■ Dip the catheter into the sterile normal saline solution (as shown below) *to moisten the inside of the catheter.*

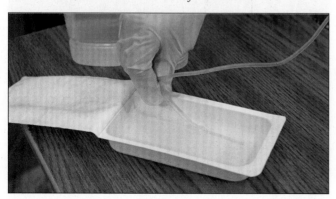

■ Instruct the patient to cough and breathe slowly and deeply several times before beginning suction. *Coughing helps loosen secretions and may decrease the amount of suction necessary, while deep breathing helps minimize or prevent hypoxia.* (See *Tips on airway clearance.*)

For nasal insertion

■ Raise the tip of the patient's nose with your nondominant hand *to straighten the passageway and facilitate insertion of the catheter.* Without applying suction, gently insert the suction catheter into the patient's nares (as shown below). Roll the catheter between your fingers *to help it advance through the turbinates.* Continue to advance the catheter approximately 5″ to 6″ (12.7 to 15.2 cm) until you reach the pool of secretions or the patient begins to cough.

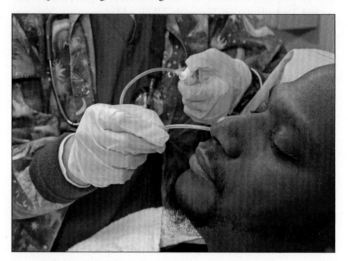

For oral insertion

■ Without applying suction, gently insert the catheter into the patient's mouth. Advance it 3″ to 4″ (7.5 to 10 cm) along the side of the patient's mouth until you reach the pool of secretions or the patient begins to cough. Suction both sides of the patient's mouth and pharyngeal area.

Completing the procedure

■ Using intermittent suction, withdraw the catheter from either the mouth or the nose with a continuous rotating motion *to minimize invagination of the mucosa into the catheter's tip and side ports.* Apply suction for no longer than 10 seconds at a time *to minimize tissue trauma.*

■ Between passes, wrap the catheter around your dominant hand *to prevent contamination.*

■ If secretions are thick, clear the lumen of the catheter by dipping it in normal saline solution and applying suction.

■ Repeat the procedure, up to three times, until gurgling or bubbling sounds stop and respirations are quiet. Allow 30 seconds to 1 minute *to allow reoxygenation and reventilation.*

■ After completing suctioning, pull your sterile glove off over the coiled catheter and discard them.

- Flush the connecting tubing with normal saline solution. Then discard the container of normal saline solution and remove your other glove.
- Take off other personal protective equipment and perform hand hygiene.
- Replace the used items *so they're ready for the next suctioning,* and perform hand hygiene.[2,3,4]
- Document the procedure.[6]

Special considerations

- If the patient has no history of nasal problems, alternate suctioning between nostrils *to minimize traumatic injury.*
- If repeated oronasopharyngeal suctioning is required, the use of a nasopharyngeal or oropharyngeal airway will help with catheter insertion, reduce traumatic injury, and promote a patent airway. *To facilitate catheter insertion for oropharyngeal suctioning,* depress the patient's tongue with a tongue blade, or ask another nurse to do so. *This technique helps you to visualize the back of the throat and also prevents the patient from biting the catheter.*
- If the patient has excessive oral secretions, consider using a tonsil tip catheter, *which allows the patient to remove oral secretions independently.*
- Let the patient rest after suctioning while you continue to observe him. The frequency and duration of suctioning depend on the patient's tolerance for the procedure and on any complications.

Patient teaching

Oronasopharyngeal suctioning may be performed in the home using a portable suction machine. Under these circumstances, suctioning is a clean rather than a sterile procedure.[7] Properly cleaned catheters can be reused, putting less financial strain on patients. Whether the patient requires disposable or reusable suction equipment, you should make sure that the patient and his caregivers have received proper teaching and support.[7]

Complications

Increased dyspnea caused by hypoxia and anxiety may result from this procedure. Hypoxia can result *because oxygen from the oronasopharynx is removed with the secretions.* The amount of oxygen removed varies, depending upon the duration of the suctioning, suction flow and pressure, the size of the catheter in relation to the size of the patient's airway, and the patient's physical condition.

In addition, bloody aspirate can result from prolonged or traumatic suctioning. Using water-soluble lubricant can help to minimize traumatic injury.

Documentation

Record the date, time, reason for suctioning, and technique used; amount, color, consistency, and odor (if any) of the secretions; the patient's respiratory status before and after the procedure; any complications and the nursing action taken; and the patient's tolerance for the procedure.

REFERENCES

1 The Joint Commission. (2012). Standard NPSG.01.01.01. *Comprehensive accreditation manual for hospitals: The official handbook.* Oakbrook Terrace, IL: The Joint Commission. (Level 1)
2 The Joint Commission. (2012). Standard NPSG.07.01.01. *Comprehensive accreditation manual for hospitals: The official handbook.* Oakbrook Terrace, IL: The Joint Commission. (Level 1)
3 Centers for Disease Control and Prevention. (October 2002). Guideline for hand hygiene in health-care settings. *Morbidity and Mortality Weekly Report, 51*(RR-16), 1–45. (Level I)
4 World Health Organization. (2009). *WHO guidelines on hand hygiene in health care: First global patient safety challenge. Clean care is safer care.* Geneva, Switzerland: World Health Organization. (Level I)
5 Lynn-McHale Wiegand, D. (Ed.). (2011). *AACN procedure manual for critical care* (6th ed.). Philadelphia, PA: Saunders.
6 The Joint Commission. (2012). Standard RC.01.03.01. *Comprehensive accreditation manual for hospitals: The official handbook.* Oakbrook Terrace, IL: The Joint Commission. (Level 1)
7 American Association for Respiratory Care. (1999). AARC clinical practice guideline: Suctioning of the patient in the home. *Respiratory Care, 44*(1), 99–104. (Level I)

ADDITIONAL REFERENCES

Centers for Disease Control and Prevention. (2004). Guidelines for preventing health-care- associated pneumonia, 2003. *Morbidity and Mortality Weekly Report, 53*(RR-03), 1–36.
Muscedere, J., et al. (2008). Comprehensive evidence-based clinical practice guidelines for ventilator-associated pneumonia: Prevention. *Journal of Critical Care, 23*(1), 126–137.
Taylor, C., et al. (2011). *Fundamentals of nursing: The art and science of nursing care* (7th ed.). Philadelphia, PA: Lippincott Williams & Wilkins.

OROPHARYNGEAL AIRWAY INSERTION AND CARE

An oropharyngeal airway, a curved plastic device, is inserted into the mouth to the posterior pharynx to establish or maintain a patent airway. In an unconscious patient, the tongue usually obstructs the posterior pharynx. The oropharyngeal airway conforms to the curvature of the palate, removing the obstruction and allowing air to pass around and through the tube. It also facilitates oropharyngeal suctioning. The oropharyngeal airway is intended for short-term use, as in the postanesthesia or postictal stage. It may be left in place longer as an airway adjunct to prevent the orally intubated patient from biting the endotracheal tube.

The oropharyngeal airway isn't the airway of choice for the patient with loose or avulsed teeth or who has undergone recent oral surgery.

NURSING ALERT *Inserting this airway in the conscious or semiconscious patient may stimulate vomiting and laryngospasm; use only in unresponsive patients who don't have a cough or gag reflex.*[1]

Inserting an oral airway

Unless this position is contraindicated, hyperextend the patient's head (as shown below) before using either the cross-finger or tongue blade insertion method.

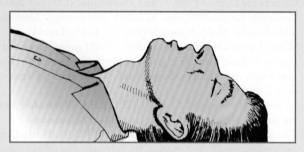

To insert an oral airway using the cross-finger method, place your thumb on the patient's lower teeth and your index finger on his upper teeth. Gently open his mouth by pushing his teeth apart (as shown below).

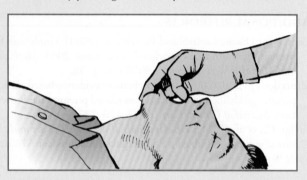

Insert the airway upside down *to avoid pushing the tongue toward the pharynx,* and slide it over the tongue toward the back of the mouth. Rotate the airway as it approaches the posterior wall of the pharynx so that it points downward (as shown below).

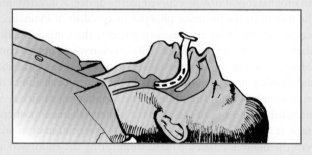

To use the tongue blade technique, open the patient's mouth and depress his tongue with the blade. Guide the airway over the back of the tongue as you did for the cross-finger technique.

Equipment

For insertion

Oral airway of appropriate size ▪ tongue blade ▪ padded tongue blade ▪ gloves ▪ tape ▪ Optional: suction equipment, handheld resuscitation bag or oxygen-powered breathing device.

For cleaning

Hydrogen peroxide ▪ water ▪ basin ▪ Optional: pipe cleaner.

For reflex testing

Cotton-tipped applicator.

Preparation of equipment

Select an airway of appropriate size for your patient; *an oversized airway can obstruct breathing by depressing the epiglottis into the laryngeal opening.* Usually, you'll select a medium size (size 4 or 5) for the average adult and a large size (size 6) for the large adult. Be sure to confirm the correct size of the airway by placing the airway flange beside the patient's cheek, parallel to his front teeth. If the airway is the right size, the airway curve should reach to the angle of the jaw.

Implementation

▪ Verify the doctor's order.
▪ Gather the appropriate equipment.
▪ Confirm the patient's identity using at least two patient identifiers according to your facility's policy.[2]
▪ Explain the procedure to the patient even though he may not appear to be alert.
▪ Provide privacy.
▪ Perform hand hygiene and put on gloves *to prevent contact with body fluids.*[3,4,5]
▪ If the patient is wearing dentures, remove them *so they don't cause further airway obstruction.*
▪ Suction the patient if necessary.
▪ Place the patient in the supine position with his neck hyperextended, if this isn't contraindicated.
▪ Insert the airway using the cross-finger or the tongue blade technique. (See *Inserting an oral airway.*)
▪ Auscultate the lungs *to ensure adequate ventilation.* Stridor, gasping respirations, or snoring may indicate inadequate airway placement.[6]
▪ After the airway is inserted and secured, position the patient on his side *to decrease the risk of aspiration of vomitus.*
▪ Perform mouth care every 2 to 4 hours, as needed. Begin by holding the patient's jaws open with a padded tongue blade and gently removing the airway. Place the airway in a basin and rinse it with hydrogen peroxide and then water. If secretions remain, use a pipe cleaner to remove them. Complete standard mouth care and reinsert the airway.
▪ While the airway is removed for mouth care, observe the mouth's mucous membranes *because tissue irritation or ulceration can result from prolonged airway use.*
▪ Frequently check the position of the airway *to ensure correct placement.*

- Remove and discard your gloves and perform hand hygiene.[4,5,6]
- Document the procedure.[7]

Special considerations

- Evaluate the patient's behavior *to provide the cue for airway removal*. The patient is likely to gag or cough as he becomes more alert, indicating that he no longer needs the airway.
- When the patient regains consciousness and can swallow, remove the airway by pulling it outward and downward, following the mouth's natural curvature.
- After the airway is removed, test the patient's cough and gag reflexes *to ensure that removal of the airway wasn't premature and that the patient can maintain his own airway*. To test for the gag reflex, use a cotton-tipped applicator to touch both sides of the posterior pharynx. To test for the cough reflex, gently touch the posterior oropharynx with the cotton-tipped applicator.

Complications

Tooth damage or loss, tissue damage, and bleeding may result from insertion. If the airway is too long, it may press the epiglottis against the entrance of the larynx, producing complete airway obstruction. If the airway isn't inserted properly, it may push the tongue posteriorly, aggravating the problem of upper airway obstruction. To prevent traumatic injury, make sure that the patient's lips and tongue aren't between his teeth and the airway.

If respirations are absent or inadequate immediately after inserting the airway, initiate artificial positive-pressure ventilation by using a mouth-to-mask technique, a handheld resuscitation bag, or an oxygen-powered breathing device. (See "Manual ventilation," page 465.)

Documentation

Record the date and time of the airway's insertion, size of the airway, removal and cleaning of the airway, condition of mucous membranes, any suctioning, any adverse reactions and the nursing action taken, and the patient's tolerance of the procedure.

REFERENCES

1 American Heart Association. (2010). 2010 American Heart Association guidelines for cardiopulmonary resuscitation and emergency cardiovascular care. *Circulation, 122*(Suppl. 3), S729–S767. (Level I)
2 The Joint Commission. (2012). Standard NPSG.01.01.01. *Comprehensive accreditation manual for hospitals: The official handbook.* Oakbrook Terrace, IL: The Joint Commission. (Level 1)
3 The Joint Commission. (2012). Standard NPSG.07.01.01. *Comprehensive accreditation manual for hospitals: The official handbook.* Oakbrook Terrace, IL: The Joint Commission. (Level 1)
4 Centers for Disease Control and Prevention. (October 2002). Guideline for hand hygiene in health-care settings. *Morbidity and Mortality Weekly Report, 51*(RR-16), 1–45. (Level I)
5 World Health Organization. (2009). *WHO guidelines on hand hygiene in health care: First global patient safety challenge. Clean care is safer care.* Geneva, Switzerland: World Health Organization. (Level I)
6 Lynn-McHale Wiegand, D. (Ed.). (2011). *AACN procedure manual for critical care* (6th ed.). Philadelphia, PA: Saunders.
7 The Joint Commission. (2012). Standard RC.01.03.01. *Comprehensive accreditation manual for hospitals: The official handbook.* Oakbrook Terrace, IL: The Joint Commission. (Level 1)

ADDITIONAL REFERENCE

Taylor, C., et al. (2011). *Fundamentals of nursing: The art and science of nursing care* (7th ed.). Philadelphia, PA: Lippincott Williams & Wilkins.

OXYGEN ADMINISTRATION

A patient will need oxygen therapy when hypoxemia results from a respiratory or cardiac emergency or an increase in metabolic function.

In a *respiratory emergency*, oxygen administration enables the patient to reduce his ventilatory effort. When conditions such as atelectasis or acute respiratory distress syndrome impair diffusion, or when lung volumes are decreased from alveolar hypoventilation, this procedure boosts alveolar oxygen levels.

In a *cardiac emergency*, oxygen therapy helps meet the increased myocardial workload as the heart tries to compensate for hypoxemia. Oxygen administration is particularly important for a patient whose myocardium is already compromised—for instance, from a myocardial infarction or cardiac arrhythmia.

When *metabolic demand* is high (in cases of massive trauma, burns, or high fever, for instance) oxygen administration supplies the body with enough oxygen to meet its cellular needs. This procedure also increases oxygenation in the patient with a reduced blood oxygen-carrying capacity, perhaps from carbon monoxide poisoning or sickle cell crisis.

The adequacy of oxygen therapy is determined by arterial blood gas (ABG) analysis, oximetry monitoring, and clinical examinations. The patient's disease, physical condition, and age help determine the most appropriate method of administration.

Equipment

The equipment needed depends on the type of delivery system ordered. (See *Guide to oxygen delivery systems*, pages 538 to 541.) Equipment includes selections from the following list: Oxygen source (wall unit, cylinder, liquid tank, or concentrator) ▪ flowmeter ▪ adapter, if using a wall unit, or a pressure-reduction gauge, if using a cylinder ▪ sterile humidity bottle and adapters ▪ sterile distilled water ▪ oxygen precaution sign ▪ appropriate oxygen delivery system (a nasal cannula, simple mask, or nonrebreather mask for low-flow and variable oxygen concentrations; a Venturi mask, aerosol mask, T tube, tracheostomy collar, tent, or oxygen hood for high-flow and specific oxygen concentrations) ▪ small-diameter or large-diameter connection tubing ▪ gauze pads and tape ▪ jet adapter for Venturi mask (if adding humidity) ▪ gloves ▪ stethoscope ▪ sphygmomanometer ▪ Optional: oxygen analyzer.

Preparation of equipment

Although a respiratory therapist typically is responsible for setting up, maintaining, and managing the equipment, you'll need a working knowledge of the oxygen system being used.

(Text continues on page 540.)

EQUIPMENT

Guide to oxygen delivery systems

Patients may receive oxygen through one of several administration systems. Each has its own benefits, drawbacks, and indications for use. The advantages and disadvantages of each system are compared below.

Nasal cannula
Oxygen is delivered through plastic cannulas in the patient's nostrils.

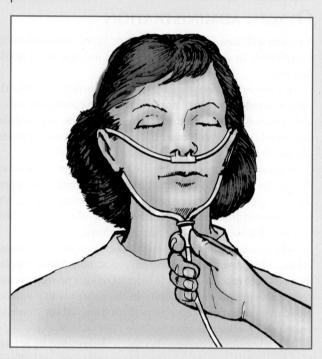

Advantages: Safe and simple; comfortable and easily tolerated; nasal prongs can be shaped to fit any face; effective for low oxygen concentrations; allows movement, eating, and talking; inexpensive and disposable.
Disadvantages: Can't deliver concentrations higher than 40%[7]; can't be used in complete nasal obstruction; may cause headaches or dry mucous membranes if flow rate exceeds 6 L/minute[7]; can dislodge easily.
Administration guidelines: Hook the cannula tubing behind the patient's ears and under the chin. Slide the adjuster upward under the chin to secure the tubing. If using an elastic strap to secure the cannula, position it over the ears and around the back of the head. Avoid applying it too tightly, which can result in excess pressure on facial structures and cannula occlusion as well. With a nasal cannula, oral breathers achieve the same oxygen delivery as nasal breathers.

Simple mask
Oxygen flows through an entry port at the bottom of the mask and exits through large holes on the sides of the mask.

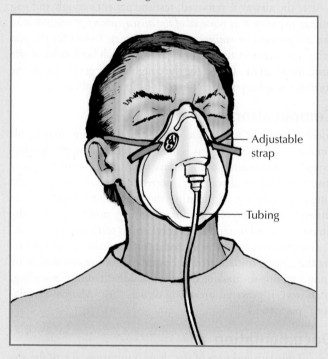

Adjustable strap

Tubing

Advantages: Can deliver concentrations of 35% to 50%.[7]
Disadvantages: Hot and confining; may irritate patient's skin; tight seal, which may cause discomfort, is required for higher oxygen concentration; interferes with talking and eating; impractical for long-term therapy because of imprecision.
Administration guidelines: Select the mask size that offers the best fit. Place the mask over the patient's nose, mouth, and chin, and mold the flexible metal edge to the bridge of the nose. Adjust the elastic band around the head to hold the mask firmly but comfortably over the cheeks, chin, and bridge of the nose. For elderly or cachectic patients with sunken cheeks, tape gauze pads to the mask over the cheek area to try to create an airtight seal. Without this seal, room air dilutes the oxygen, preventing delivery of the prescribed concentration. A minimum of 5 L/minute is required in all masks to flush expired carbon dioxide from the mask so that the patient doesn't rebreathe it.

Guide to oxygen delivery systems *(continued)*

Nonrebreather mask

On inhalation, the one-way valve opens, directing oxygen from a reservoir bag into the mask. On exhalation, gas exits the mask through the one-way expiratory valve and enters the atmosphere. The patient only breathes gas from the bag.

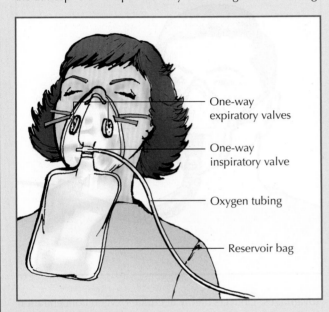

- One-way expiratory valves
- One-way inspiratory valve
- Oxygen tubing
- Reservoir bag

Advantages: Delivers the highest possible oxygen concentration (60% to 90%) short of intubation and mechanical ventilation; effective for short-term therapy; can be converted to a partial rebreather mask, if necessary, by removing the one-way valve.

Disadvantages: Requires a tight seal, which may be difficult to maintain and may cause discomfort; may irritate the patient's skin; interferes with talking and eating; impractical for long-term therapy.

Administration guidelines: Follow procedures listed for the simple mask. Make sure that the mask fits very snugly and that the one-way valves are secure and functioning. Because the mask excludes room air, valve malfunction can cause carbon dioxide buildup and suffocate an unconscious patient. If the reservoir bag collapses more than slightly during inspiration, raise the flow rate until you see only a slight deflation. Marked or complete deflation indicates an insufficient flow rate. Keep the reservoir bag from twisting or kinking. Ensure free expansion by making sure the bag lies outside the patient's gown and bedcovers.

CPAP mask

This system allows the spontaneously breathing patient to receive continuous positive airway pressure (CPAP) with or without an artificial airway.

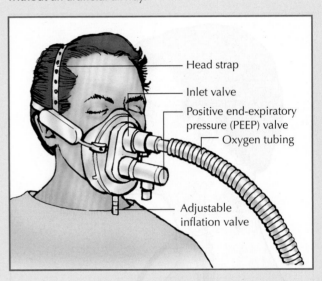

- Head strap
- Inlet valve
- Positive end-expiratory pressure (PEEP) valve
- Oxygen tubing
- Adjustable inflation valve

Advantages: Noninvasively improves arterial oxygenation by increasing functional residual capacity; allows the patient to avoid intubation; allows the patient to talk and cough without interrupting positive pressure.

Disadvantages: Requires a tight fit, which may cause discomfort; interferes with eating and talking; heightened risk of aspiration if the patient vomits; increased risk of pneumothorax, diminished cardiac output, and gastric distention; use cautiously in patients with chronic obstructive pulmonary disease, bullous lung disease, low cardiac output, or tension pneumothorax.

Administration guidelines: Place one strap behind the patient's head and the other strap over his head *to ensure a snug fit.* Attach one latex strap to the connector prong on one side of the mask. Then, use one hand to position the mask on the patient's face while using the other hand to connect the strap to the other side of the mask. After the mask is applied, assess the patient's respiratory, circulatory, and GI function every hour. Watch for signs of pneumothorax, decreased cardiac output, a drop in blood pressure, and gastric distention.

(continued)

EQUIPMENT

Guide to oxygen delivery systems *(continued)*

Transtracheal oxygen

The patient receives oxygen through a catheter inserted into the tracheal cartilage through a small permanent opening in the base of his neck in a simple outpatient procedure.

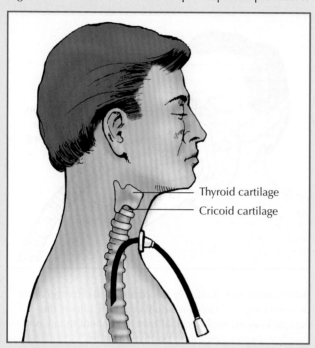

Thyroid cartilage
Cricoid cartilage

Advantages: Supplies oxygen to the lungs throughout the respiratory cycle; provides continuous oxygen without hindering mobility; doesn't interfere with eating or talking; doesn't dry mucous membranes; catheter can easily be concealed by a shirt or scarf.

Disadvantages: Not suitable for use in patients at risk for bleeding or those with severe bronchospasm, uncompensated respiratory acidosis, pleural herniation into the base of the neck, or high corticosteroid dosages.

Administration guidelines: After insertion, obtain a chest X-ray *to confirm placement.* Monitor the patient for bleeding, respiratory distress, pneumothorax, pain, coughing, or hoarseness. Don't use the catheter for about 1 week after insertion *to decrease the risk of subcutaneous emphysema.*

Venturi mask

The mask is connected to a Venturi device, which mixes a specific volume of air and oxygen.

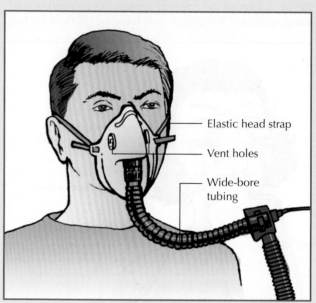

Elastic head strap
Vent holes
Wide-bore tubing

Advantages: Delivers highly accurate oxygen concentration despite patient's respiratory pattern because the same amount of air is always entrained; dilute jets can be changed or dial turned to change oxygen concentration; doesn't dry mucous membranes; humidity or aerosol can be added.

Disadvantages: Confining and may irritate skin; oxygen concentration may be altered if mask fits loosely, tubing kinks, oxygen intake ports become blocked, flow is insufficient, or patient is hyperpneic; interferes with eating and talking; condensate may collect and drip on the patient if humidification is used.

Administration guidelines: Make sure that the oxygen flow rate is set at the amount specified on each mask and that the Venturi valve is set for the desired fraction of inspired oxygen.

Check the oxygen outlet port *to verify flow.* Pinch the tubing near the prongs *to listen for a higher-pitched sound caused by the release of increased pressure.*

Implementation

- Verify the doctor's order for the oxygen therapy.[1]
- Perform hand hygiene and put on gloves.[2,3,4]
- Confirm the patient's identity using at least two patient identifiers according to your facility's policy.[5]

- Obtain a baseline physical assessment, including vital signs, lung sounds, oxygen saturation, and physical assessment. In an emergency, verify that the patient has a patent airway before administering oxygen.
- Explain the procedure to the patient, and let him know why he needs oxygen. He will need to be able to cooperate with the oxygen administration.

EQUIPMENT

Guide to oxygen delivery systems *(continued)*

Aerosols

A face mask, hood, tent, or tracheostomy tube or collar is connected to wide-bore tubing that receives aerosolized oxygen from a jet nebulizer. The jet nebulizer, which is attached near the oxygen source, adjusts air entrainment in a manner similar to the Venturi device.

Advantages: Administers high humidity; gas can be heated (when delivered through artificial airway) or cooled (when delivered through a tent).

Disadvantages: Condensate collected in the tracheostomy collar or T tube may drain into the tracheostomy; the weight of the T tube can put stress on the tracheostomy tube.

Administration guidelines: Guidelines vary with the type of nebulizer used—the ultrasonic, large-volume, small-volume, or in-line. When using a high-output nebulizer, watch for signs of overhydration, pulmonary edema, crackles, and electrolyte imbalance.

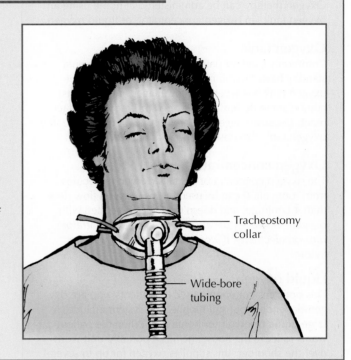

Tracheostomy collar

Wide-bore tubing

■ Check the patient's room *to make sure it's safe for oxygen administration.* Whenever possible, replace electrical devices with non-electrical ones.

PEDIATRIC ALERT *If the patient is a child and is in an oxygen tent, remove all toys that may produce a spark.* Oxygen supports combustion, and the smallest spark can cause a fire.

■ Place an oxygen precaution sign over the patient's bed and on the door to his room.

■ Help place the oxygen delivery device on the patient. Make sure it fits properly and is stable. Pad pressure areas, if needed.

■ Monitor the patient's response to oxygen therapy. Check his ABG values 20 to 30 minutes after initial adjustments of oxygen flow. When the patient is stabilized, you may use pulse oximetry instead. Check the patient frequently for signs of hypoxia, such as restlessness, decreased level of consciousness, increased heart rate, arrhythmias, perspiration, dyspnea, use of accessory muscles, yawning or flared nostrils, cyanosis, and cool, clammy skin. Obtain vital signs, as needed.

■ Observe the patient's skin integrity *to prevent skin breakdown on pressure points from the oxygen delivery device.* Wipe moisture or perspiration from the patient's face and from the mask as needed.

■ Remove and discard your gloves and perform hand hygiene.[2,3,4]

■ Document the procedure.[6]

Special considerations

NURSING ALERT *Never administer oxygen by nasal cannula at more than 2 L/minute to a patient with chronic lung disease*

unless you have a specific order to do so. Some patients with chronic lung disease are dependent on a state of hypercapnia and hypoxia to stimulate their respirations, and supplemental oxygen could cause them to stop breathing. *However, long-term oxygen therapy of 12 to 17 hours daily may help patients with chronic lung disease sleep better, survive longer, and experience a reduced incidence of pulmonary hypertension.*

■ If the patient will be receiving oxygen at a concentration above 60% for more than 24 hours, watch carefully for signs of oxygen toxicity. Prolonged high concentrations of oxygen can cause lung injury. Surfactant activity may be impaired, and increased capillary congestion, edema, interstitial space thickening, and fibrotic changes may occur. The patient may exhibit signs and symptoms of tracheobronchial irritation, such as coughing and substernal discomfort. Remind the patient to cough and deep-breathe frequently *to prevent atelectasis.* Also, *to prevent the development of serious lung damage,* measure ABG values repeatedly *to determine whether high oxygen concentrations are still necessary.*

Patient teaching

Before discharging a patient who will receive oxygen therapy at home, make sure you know the types of oxygen therapy, the kinds of services that are available, and the service schedules offered by local home suppliers. Together with the doctor and the patient, choose the device best suited to the patient. (See *Types of home oxygen therapy,* page 542.)

Types of home oxygen therapy

Oxygen therapy can be administered at home using an oxygen tank, an oxygen concentrator, or liquid oxygen.

Oxygen tank
Commonly used for patients who need oxygen on a standby basis or who need a ventilator at home, the oxygen tank has several disadvantages, including its cumbersome design and the need for frequent replacement. *Because oxygen is stored under high pressure,* the oxygen tank also poses a potential hazard.

Oxygen concentrator
The oxygen concentrator extracts oxygen molecules from room air. It can be used for low oxygen flow (less than 4 L/minute) and doesn't need to be refilled with oxygen. However, *because the oxygen concentrator runs on electricity,* it won't function during a power failure.

Liquid oxygen
This option is commonly used by patients who are oxygen-dependent but still mobile. The system includes a large liquid reservoir for home use. When the patient wants to leave the house, he fills a portable unit worn over the shoulder; this supplies oxygen for up to several hours, depending on the liter flow.

If the patient will be receiving transtracheal oxygen therapy, teach him how to properly clean and care for the catheter. Advise him to keep the skin surrounding the insertion site clean and dry *to prevent infection.*

No matter which device the patient uses, you'll need to evaluate his and his family members' ability and motivation to administer oxygen therapy at home. Make sure they understand the reason the patient is receiving oxygen and the safety issues involved in oxygen administration.

Teach them how to properly use and clean the equipment and supplies.

If the patient will be discharged with oxygen for the first time, make sure his health insurance covers home oxygen. If it doesn't, find out what criteria he must meet to obtain coverage. Without a third-party payer, the patient may not be able to afford home oxygen therapy.

Documentation
Record the date and time of oxygen administration; the type of delivery device; the oxygen flow rate; the patient's vital signs, skin color, respiratory effort, and lung sounds; subjective patient response before and after initiation of therapy; any complications and the nursing actions taken; and any patient or family teaching.

REFERENCES

1 The Joint Commission. (2012). Standard MM.04.01.01. *Comprehensive accreditation manual for hospitals: The official handbook.* Oakbrook Terrace, IL: The Joint Commission. (Level 1)
2 The Joint Commission. (2012). Standard NPSG.07.01.01. *Comprehensive accreditation manual for hospitals: The official handbook.* Oakbrook Terrace, IL: The Joint Commission. (Level 1)
3 Centers for Disease Control and Prevention. (October 2002). Guideline for hand hygiene in health-care settings. *Morbidity and Mortality Weekly Report, 51*(RR-16), 1–45. (Level I)
4 World Health Organization. (2009). *WHO guidelines on hand hygiene in health care: First global patient safety challenge. Clean care is safer care.* Geneva, Switzerland: World Health Organization. (Level I)
5 The Joint Commission. (2012). Standard NPSG.01.01.01. *Comprehensive accreditation manual for hospitals: The official handbook.* Oakbrook Terrace, IL: The Joint Commission. (Level 1)
6 The Joint Commission. (2012). Standard RC.01.03.01. *Comprehensive accreditation manual for hospitals: The official handbook.* Oakbrook Terrace, IL: The Joint Commission. (Level 1)
7 American Association for Respiratory Care. (1992). AARC clinical practice guideline: Pulse oximetry. *Respiratory Care, 37*(8), 891–897. (Level I)

ADDITIONAL REFERENCES

Nettina, S.M. (2010). *Lippincott manual of nursing practice* (9th ed.). Philadelphia, PA: Lippincott Williams & Wilkins.
Petterson, M.T., et al. (2007). The effect of motion of pulse oximetry and its clinical significance. *Anesthesia and Analgesia, 105* (6 Suppl.), 78–84.
Taenzer, A.H., et al. (2010). Impact of pulse oximetry surveillance on rescue events and intensive care unit transfers: A before-and-after concurrence study. *Anesthesiology, 112*(2), 282–287.
Taylor, C., et al. (2011). *Fundamentals of nursing: The art and science of nursing care* (7th ed.). Philadelphia, PA: Lippincott Williams & Wilkins.
Valdez-Lowe, C., et al. (2009). Pulse oximetry in adults. *AJN, 109*(6), 52–59; quiz 60.
Walters, T.P. (2007). Pulse oximetry knowledge and its effects on clinical practice. *British Journal of Nursing, 16*(21), 1332–1340.

PAIN MANAGEMENT

Considered the fifth vital sign, pain is defined as the sensory and emotional experience associated with actual or potential tissue damage. It includes not only the perception of an uncomfortable stimulus, but also the response to that perception.

The patient's self-report of pain is the most reliable indicator of the existence of pain. When a patient feels severe pain, he seeks medical help because he believes the pain signals a serious problem. This perception produces anxiety, which, in turn, increases the pain. To assess and manage pain properly, the nurse must depend on both the patient's subjective description and objective tools.

According to The Joint Commission, health care facilities are required to develop policies and procedures supporting the appropriate use of analgesics and other pain control therapies.[1]

Pain should be assessed at admission and reassessed at regular intervals. Pain assessment should include personal, cultural, spiritual, and ethnic beliefs. Patients and families should be educated about their role in pain management and informed about potential limitations and adverse effects of pain treatment.

Interventions used to manage pain include analgesics, emotional support, comfort measures, and complementary and alternative therapies such as cognitive techniques to distract the patient. Patients with severe pain typically require treatment with an opioid analgesic; such patients may also need invasive measures, such as epidural analgesia or patient-controlled analgesia (PCA).

Equipment

Pain assessment tool or scale ▪ oral hygiene supplies ▪ water ▪ nonopioid analgesic (such as aspirin or acetaminophen) ▪ Optional: PCA device; mild opioid (such as oxycodone or codeine); strong opioid (such as morphine or hydromorphone).

Implementation

▪ Perform hand hygiene.[2,3,4]
▪ Confirm the patient's identity using at least two patient identifiers according to your facility's policy.[5]
▪ Explain to the patient how pain medications work together with other pain management therapies to provide relief. Also explain that management aims to keep pain at a low level to permit optimal bodily function.[6]
▪ Assess the patient's pain by using a pain assessment tool or scale or by asking key questions and noting his response to the pain.[1] For instance, ask him to describe its duration, severity, and location. Look for physiologic or behavioral clues to the pain's severity.[7] (See *How to assess pain*.)
▪ Develop nursing diagnoses. Appropriate nursing diagnostic categories include acute or chronic pain, anxiety, activity intolerance, fear, risk for injury, deficient knowledge, and powerlessness.
▪ Work with the patient to develop a nursing care plan using interventions appropriate to the patient's lifestyle. These may include prescribed medications, emotional support, comfort measures, complementary and alternative therapies such as cognitive techniques, and education about pain and its management. Emphasize the importance of maintaining good bowel habits, respiratory functions, and mobility *because pain may exacerbate any problems in these areas*.
▪ Implement your care plan. *Because individuals respond to pain differently*, you'll find that what works for one person may not work for another.

Giving medications

▪ If the patient is allowed oral intake, begin with a nonopioid analgesic, such as acetaminophen or aspirin, every 4 to 6 hours as ordered.[8]

How to assess pain

To assess pain properly, you'll need to consider the patient's description and your observations of the patient's physical and behavioral responses. Start by asking this series of key questions (bearing in mind that the patient's responses will be shaped by his prior experiences, self-image, and beliefs about his condition):
▪ Where's the pain located? How long does it last? How often does it occur?
▪ Can you describe the pain?
▪ What brings the pain on?
▪ What relieves the pain or makes it worse?
Ask the patient to rank his pain on a scale of 0 to 10, with 0 denoting lack of pain and 10 denoting the worst pain level. *This rating helps the patient verbally evaluate pain therapies.*

Observe the patient's behavioral and physiologic responses to pain. Physiologic responses may be sympathetic or parasympathetic.

Behavioral responses
These include altered body position, moaning, sighing, grimacing, withdrawal, crying, restlessness, muscle twitching, and immobility.

Sympathetic responses
These are commonly associated with mild to moderate pain and include pallor, elevated blood pressure, dilated pupils, skeletal muscle tension, dyspnea, tachycardia, and diaphoresis.

Parasympathetic responses
These are commonly associated with severe, deep pain and include pallor, decreased blood pressure, bradycardia, nausea and vomiting, weakness, dizziness, and loss of consciousness.

Assess pain at least every 2 hours and during rest, activity, and through the night (when pain is usually heightened). Keep in mind that the ability to sleep doesn't indicate absence of pain.

▪ If the patient needs more relief than a nonopioid analgesic provides, you may give a mild opioid (such as oxycodone or codeine) as ordered.[8]
▪ If the patient needs still more pain relief, you may administer a strong opioid (such as morphine or hydromorphone) as prescribed. Administer oral medications if possible.[8] Check the appropriate drug information for each medication given.
▪ If ordered, teach the patient how to use a PCA device. *Such a device can help the patient manage his pain and decrease his anxiety.* (See "Patient-controlled analgesia," page 557.)
▪ Assess pain 30 minutes after parenteral medication administration; assess pain 60 minutes after oral medication administration. If the patient is still in pain, reassess him and alter your care plan as appropriate.[9]

Providing emotional support

■ Show your concern by spending time talking with the patient. Because of his pain and his inability to manage it, the patient may be anxious and frustrated. *Such feelings can worsen his pain.*

Performing comfort measures

■ Reposition the patient periodically *to reduce muscle spasms and tension and to relieve pressure on bony prominences.* Increasing the angle of the bed can reduce pull on an abdominal incision, diminishing pain. If appropriate, elevate a limb *to reduce swelling, inflammation, and pain.*
■ Splinting or supporting abdominal and chest incisions with a pillow when coughing or changing position helps decrease pain.
■ Apply cold compresses, as appropriate, *to decrease discomfort.*[7]
■ Give the patient a back massage *to help reduce tense muscles.*[7]
■ Perform passive range-of-motion exercises *to prevent stiffness and further loss of mobility, relax tense muscles, and provide comfort.*
■ Provide oral hygiene. Keep a fresh water glass or cup at the bedside *because many pain medications tend to dry the mouth.*
■ Wash the patient's face and hands *to soothe the patient, which may reduce his perception of pain.*

Using complementary and alternative therapies

■ Help the patient enhance the effect of analgesics by using such techniques as distraction, guided imagery, deep breathing, and relaxation.[7] You can easily use these "mind-over-pain" techniques at the bedside. Choose the method the patient prefers. If possible, start these techniques when the patient feels little or no pain. If he feels persistent pain, begin with short, simple exercises. Before beginning, dim the lights, loosen or remove the patient's restrictive clothing, and eliminate noise from the environment.
■ For *distraction,* have the patient recall a pleasant experience or focus his attention on an enjoyable activity. For instance, have him use music as a distraction by turning on the radio when the pain begins. Have him close his eyes and concentrate on listening, raising or lowering the volume as his pain increases or subsides. Note, however, that distraction is mainly helpful in relieving pain lasting for brief episodes or for painful procedures of short duration.
■ For *imagery,* help the patient concentrate on a peaceful, pleasant image, such as walking on the beach. Encourage him to concentrate on the details of the image he has selected by asking about its sight, sound, smell, taste, and touch. The positive emotions evoked by this exercise minimize pain.
■ For *deep breathing,* have the patient stare at an object, then slowly inhale and exhale as he counts aloud to maintain a comfortable rate and rhythm. Have him concentrate on the rise and fall of his abdomen. Encourage him to feel more and more weightless with each breath while he concentrates on the rhythm of his breathing or on any restful image.
■ For *muscle relaxation,* have the patient focus on a particular muscle group. Then ask him to tense the muscles and note the sensation. After 5 to 7 seconds, tell him to relax the muscles and concentrate on the relaxed state. Have him note the difference between the tense and relaxed states. After he tenses and relaxes one muscle group, have him proceed to another and then another until he's covered his entire body.

Completing the procedure

■ Perform hand hygiene.[2,3,4]
■ Document your findings and interventions.[10]

Special considerations

■ During periods of intense pain, the patient's ability to concentrate diminishes. If your patient is in severe pain, help him to select a cognitive technique that's easy to use. After he selects a technique, encourage him to use it consistently. Remind the patient that results of cognitive therapy techniques improve with practice. Help him through the initial sessions.
■ Pain shouldn't be considered a normal part of the aging process. Provide pain relief for the elderly patient using pharmacologic and nonpharmacologic approaches. Remember, safety is a special concern, especially the risk for falls due to impaired mobility from pain and from adverse effects of pain medications.
■ It's important to identify age-related factors that affect assessment and pain management in elderly patients. Because of adverse effects, certain medications such as meperidine and propoxyphene should be avoided.
■ Evaluate your patient's response to pain management. If he's still in pain, reassess him and alter your care plan as appropriate.[1,7,9]
■ Culture and beliefs affect behavioral responses to pain and treatment preferences; take into account the patient's expectations regarding pain relief when developing the care plan.[7]
■ Patients receiving opioid analgesics may be at risk for developing tolerance, dependence, or addiction. However, studies have demonstrated that addiction during acute pain treatment is less than one percent.[7]
■ Addiction is defined as psychological dependence characterized by a persistent pattern of dysfunctional drug use. The patient's behavior will be characterized by a craving for the drug to experience effects other than pain relief. A patient demonstrating such behavior usually has a preexisting problem that's exacerbated by the opioid use.[7] Discuss the addicted patient's problem with supportive personnel, and make appropriate referrals to experts.
■ Physical dependence is a physiologic state in which withdrawal signs and symptoms occur with abrupt cessation or reversal of the drug; it doesn't mean that addiction coexists. Signs and symptoms of physical dependence include anxiety, irritability, chills and hot flashes, excessive salivation and tearing, rhinorrhea, sweating, nausea, vomiting, and seizures. These signs and symptoms typically begin 6 to 12 hours after discontinuing the drug and peak in 24 to 72 hours. To reduce the risk of dependence, discontinue an opioid by decreasing the dose gradually each day. You may also switch to an oral opioid and decrease its dose gradually.
■ Tolerance is a neuroadaptive response that results in a decrease in one or more of the effects of the drug over time, such as decreased analgesia or sedation; it doesn't mean that addiction coexists.
■ If your patient has dementia or some other cognitive impairment, don't assume that he can't understand the pain scale or communicate about his pain. Experiment with several pain scales. A scale featuring faces, such as the Wong-Baker FACES scale, is

---

Visual pain rating scale

You can use nonverbal pain evaluate scales for pediatric patients age 3 and older and for adults with language difficulties. One such instrument is the Wong-Baker FACES pain rating scale; another, two simple faces such as the ones shown below. Ask the patient to choose the face that describes how he's feeling—either happy because he has no pain, or sad because he has some or a lot of pain. Alternatively, *to pinpoint varying levels of pain,* you can ask the patient to draw a face.

Wong-Baker FACES Scale

Hockenberry, M.J., et al. (2005). *Wong's essentials of pediatric nursing* (7th ed.). St. Louis, MO: Mosby, Inc. Reprinted with permission.

---

a good choice for many cognitively impaired patients and those with limited language skills. (See *Visual pain rating scale.*)

Complications

The most common adverse effects of analgesics include respiratory depression (the most serious), sedation, constipation, nausea, and vomiting.

Documentation

Document each step of the nursing process. Describe the subjective information you elicited from the patient, using his own words. Note the location, quality, and duration of the pain as well any precipitating factors.

Record your nursing diagnoses; include the pain-relief method selected and the patient's rating of the pain before and after pain management interventions. Use a flow sheet to document pain assessment findings. Summarize your actions, including the name and dosage of any medication given, and the patient's response. If the patient's pain wasn't relieved, note alternative treatments to consider the next time pain occurs. Also record any complications of drug therapy.

REFERENCES

1 The Joint Commission. (2012). Standard PC.01.02.07. *Comprehensive accreditation manual for hospitals: The official handbook.* Oakbrook Terrace, IL: The Joint Commission. (Level I)

2 The Joint Commission. (2012). Standard NPSG.07.01.01. *Comprehensive accreditation manual for hospitals: The official handbook.* Oakbrook Terrace, IL: The Joint Commission. (Level I)

3 Centers for Disease Control and Prevention. (October 2002). Guideline for hand hygiene in health-care settings. *Morbidity and Mortality Weekly Report, 51*(RR-16), 1–45. (Level I)

4 World Health Organization. (2009). *WHO guidelines on hand hygiene in health care: First global patient safety challenge. Clean care is safer care.* Geneva, Switzerland: World Health Organization. (Level I)

5 The Joint Commission. (2012). Standard NPSG.01.01.01. *Comprehensive accreditation manual for hospitals: The official handbook.* Oakbrook Terrace, IL: The Joint Commission. (Level I)

6 The Joint Commission. (2012). Standard PC.02.03.01. *Comprehensive accreditation manual for hospitals: The official handbook.* Oakbrook Terrace, IL: The Joint Commission. (Level I)

7 American Society of PeriAnesthesia Nurses. (2003). "ASPAN Pain and Comfort Clinical Guideline" [Online]. Accessed October 2011 via the Web at http://www.aspan.org/Portals/6/docs/ClinicalPractice/Guidelines/ASPAN_ClinicalGuideline_PainComfort.pdf

8 World Health Organization. (2010). "WHO's Pain Relief Ladder" [Online]. Accessed October 2011 via the Web at http://www.who.int/cancer/palliative/painladder/en

9 The Joint Commission. (2012). Standard PC.01.02.01. *Comprehensive accreditation manual for hospitals: The official handbook.* Oakbrook Terrace, IL: The Joint Commission. (Level I)

10 The Joint Commission. (2012). Standard RC.01.03.01. *Comprehensive accreditation manual for hospitals: The official handbook.* Oakbrook Terrace, IL: The Joint Commission. (Level I)

ADDITIONAL REFERENCES

American Society of Anesthesiologists Task Force on Chronic Pain Management and American Society of Regional Anesthesia and Pain Medicine. (2010). Practice guidelines for chronic pain management: An updated report. *Anesthesiology, 112*(4), 810–833.

Courtenay, M., & Carey, N. (2008). The impact and effectiveness of nurse-led care in the management of acute and chronic pain: A review of the literature. *Journal of Clinical Nursing, 17*(15), 2001–2013.

Fine, P.G., et al. (2009). Long-acting opioids and short-acting opioids: Appropriate use in chronic pain management. *Pain Medicine, 10*(Suppl. 2), S79–S88.

Helfand, M., & Freeman, M. (2009). Assessment and management of acute pain in adult medical inpatients: A systematic review. *Pain Medicine, 10*(7), 1183–1199.

Kelly, R.B. (2009). Acupuncture for pain. *American Family Physician, 80*(5), 481–484.

Martell, B.A., et al. (2007). Systematic review: Opioid treatment for chronic back pain: Prevalence, efficacy, and association with addiction. *Annals of Internal Medicine, 146*(2), 116–127.

Nwokeji, E.D., et al. (2007). Influences of attitudes on family physicians' willingness to prescribe long-acting opioid analgesics for patients with chronic nonmalignant pain. *Clinical Therapeutics, 29*(Suppl.), 2589–2602.

Samuels, J.G., & Fetzer, S.J. (2009). Evidence-based pain management: Analyzing the practice environment and clinical expertise. *Clinical Nurse Specialist, 23*(5), 245–251.

PARENTERAL NUTRITION ADMINISTRATION

When a patient can't meet his nutritional needs by oral or enteral feedings, he may require IV nutritional support, or parenteral nutrition. The patient's diagnosis, history, and prognosis determine the need for parenteral nutrition. Generally, this treatment is prescribed for any patient who can't absorb nutrients though the GI tract for more than 7 to 10 days.[1]

More specific indications include debilitating illness lasting longer than 2 weeks; loss of 10% or more of pre-illness weight; serum albumin level below 3.5 g/dL; excessive nitrogen loss from wound infection, fistulas, or abscesses; renal or hepatic failure; or a nonfunctioning GI tract for 5 to 7 days in a severely catabolic patient.

Common illnesses that can trigger the need for parenteral nutrition include inflammatory bowel disease, radiation enteritis, severe diarrhea, intractable vomiting, and moderate to severe pancreatitis. A massive small-bowel resection, bone marrow transplantation, high-dose chemotherapy or radiation therapy, and major surgery can also hinder a patient's ability to absorb nutrients, requiring parenteral nutrition.

Parenteral nutrition shouldn't be given to patients with a normally functioning GI tract, and it has limited value for well-nourished patients whose GI tract will resume normal function within 10 days. It also may be inappropriate for patients with a poor prognosis or if the risks of parenteral nutrition outweigh the benefits.

Parenteral nutrition may be given through a peripheral or central venous (CV) access device. Depending on the solution, it may be used to boost the patient's caloric intake, supply full caloric needs, or surpass the patient's caloric requirements.

The type of parenteral solution prescribed depends on the patient's condition and metabolic needs and on the administration route. The solution usually contains protein, carbohydrates, electrolytes, vitamins, and trace minerals. A lipid emulsion provides the necessary fat. (See *Types of parenteral nutrition.*)

Total parenteral nutrition (TPN) refers to any nutrient solution, including lipids, given through a CV access device. Peripheral parenteral nutrition (PPN), which is given through a peripheral catheter, supplies full caloric needs while avoiding the risks that accompany CV access. To keep from sclerosing the vein through which it's administered, the dextrose in PPN solution must be limited to 10% or less.[2] Therefore, the success of PPN depends on the patient's tolerance for the large volume of fluid necessary to supply his nutritional needs.

It's not uncommon for a patient to need an increase in the glucose content beyond the level a peripheral vein can handle. For example, most TPN solutions are six times more concentrated than blood; because of this, they must be delivered into a vein that has a high blood flow rate to dilute the solution.

The most common delivery route for TPN is through a CV access device into the superior vena cava.

Equipment

Bag or bottle of prescribed parenteral nutrition solution ▪ IV administration set ▪ sterile IV tubing ▪ 0.2-micron filter (or 1.2-micron filter if solution contains lipids or albumin)[2] ▪ time tape ▪ alcohol pads ▪ electronic infusion pump ▪ preservative-free normal saline solution ▪ intake-and-output record ▪ gloves ▪ Optional: mask.

Preparation of equipment

Remove the solution from the refrigerator 30 minutes to 1 hour before use.[2]

Implementation

▪ Verify the doctor's order[3] and make sure that the prescribed therapy is appropriate for the patient's age, condition, and access device and that the dose, rate, and route are appropriate for the patient.[2]

▪ Make sure that the solution container is labeled with the patient's identifiers and that the formula components have been added according to the doctor's order. Perform an independent double-check with another nurse if required by your facility.

▪ Inspect the integrity of the container and solution, and check the expiration date; return the solution to the pharmacy if the integrity of the container is compromised, the solution is cloudy or contains particles, or is expired.

▪ Perform hand hygiene and put on gloves and a mask, if required by your facility.[4,5,6]

▪ Confirm the patient's identity using at least two patient identifiers according to your facility's policy.[2,7]

▪ Explain the procedure to the patient and answer all questions *to allay his anxiety.*

▪ Compare the patient's name and second patient identifier on the solution container against the name on the patient's identification band.[7]

▪ If your facility uses a bar code scanning system, scan your identification badge, the patient's identification band, and the solution's bar code according to your facility's policy.

▪ Connect the IV infusion pump administration set and the micron filter (if the tubing doesn't contain an in-line filter); insert the filter as close to the catheter insertion site as possible.[8]

▪ Squeeze the IV drip chamber and, holding the drip chamber upright, insert the tubing spike into the IV bag or bottle. Then release the drip chamber.

▪ Prime the administration set tubing by inverting the filter at the distal end of the tubing and then opening the roller clamp. Let the solution fill the filter and the tubing; gently tap the tubing, filter, and Y-ports *to dislodge trapped air.*

Types of parenteral nutrition

TYPE	SOLUTION COMPONENTS/LITER	USES	SPECIAL CONSIDERATIONS
Total parenteral nutrition (TPN) by way of central venous (CV) access	■ Dextrose 15% in water (D$_{15}$W) to D$_{25}$W (1 L of dextrose 25% = 850 nonprotein calories) ■ Crystalline amino acids 2.5% to 8.5% ■ Electrolytes, vitamins, trace elements, and insulin, as ordered ■ Lipid emulsion 10% to 20% (usually infused as a separate solution)	■ For parenteral nutrition lasting 2 weeks or longer ■ For patients with large caloric and nutrient needs ■ Provides calories, restores nitrogen balance, and replaces essential vitamins, electrolytes, minerals, and trace elements ■ Promotes tissue synthesis, wound healing, and normal metabolic function ■ Allows the bowel to rest and heal; reduces activity in the gallbladder, pancreas, and small intestine ■ Improves tolerance of surgery	*Basic solution* ■ Nutritionally complete ■ Requires minor surgical procedure for CV access insertion and radiologic placement verification ■ Highly hypertonic solution ■ May cause metabolic complications (glucose intolerance, electrolyte imbalance, essential fatty acid deficiency) *IV lipid emulsion* ■ May not be used effectively in severely stressed patients (especially burn patients) ■ May interfere with immune mechanisms ■ Given through CV access device; irritates peripheral vein in long-term use
Total nutrient admixture	■ One day's nutrients contained in a single bag (also called *3:1 solution*) ■ Combines lipid emulsion with other parenteral solution components	■ For parenteral nutrition lasting 2 weeks or longer ■ For relatively stable patients ■ For other uses, see TPN (above)	■ See TPN (above) ■ Reduces need to handle bag, reducing the contamination risk ■ Decreases nursing time and reduces need for infusion sets and electronic devices, lowering facility costs, increasing patient mobility, and allowing easier adjustment to home care ■ Has limited use because not all types and amounts of components are compatible ■ Must use 1.2-micron filter
Peripheral parenteral nutrition	■ D$_5$W to D$_{10}$W ■ Crystalline amino acids 2.5% to 5% ■ Electrolytes, minerals, vitamins, and trace elements, as ordered ■ Lipid emulsion 10% or 20% (1 L of dextrose 10% and amino acids 3.5% infused at the same time as 1 L of lipid emulsion = 1,440 nonprotein calories)	■ For parenteral nutrition lasting 2 weeks or less ■ Provides up to 2,000 calories/day ■ Maintains adequate nutritional status in patients who can tolerate relatively high fluid volume, in those who usually resume bowel function and oral feedings after a few days, and in those susceptible to infections associated with CV access device	*Basic solution* ■ Nutritionally complete for a short time ■ Can't be used long term in nutritionally depleted patients ■ Used for weight maintenance, not weight gain ■ Avoids insertion and care of CV access device but requires adequate venous access ■ Delivers less hypertonic solutions than TPN ■ May cause phlebitis ■ Less chance of metabolic complications than with TPN *IV lipid emulsion* ■ As effective as dextrose for caloric source ■ Diminishes phlebitis if infused at the same time as basic nutrient solution

■ Attach the IV administration set tubing to the electronic infusion pump following the manufacturer's instructions, and set the infusion rate, concentration, and volume to be infused. Make sure that the infusion pump alarms are turned on and functioning. Label the container and IV tubing with the date, time, and your initials.

■ Thoroughly disinfect the access port with an alcohol pad using friction,[9] and then verify the patency of the access device by aspirating for a blood return *to reduce the risk for infiltration and extravasation.*[10]

■ Flush the catheter with preservative-free normal saline solution according to the catheter type and your facility's policy.[11,12]

■ Clamp the access device before disconnecting it *to prevent air from entering the catheter.* If the catheter is a CV access device and a clamp isn't available, ask the patient to perform Valsalva's maneuver just as you change the tubing, if possible. Or, if the patient is being mechanically ventilated, change the IV tubing immediately after the machine delivers a breath at peak inspiration. *Both of these measures increase intrathoracic pressure and prevent air embolism.*

■ Using sterile technique, attach the tubing to the designated luer-lock port.

■ Trace the tubing from the patient to its point of origin *to make sure that you've connected it to the proper port.*[13] After connecting the tubing, remove the clamp, if applicable. Secure all connections *to prevent harmful disconnections.*

NURSING ALERT *TPN solutions are considered "high-alert" medications* because they can cause significant harm when used in error.[14]

■ Before beginning the parenteral nutrition infusion, have another nurse perform an independent double-check according to your facility's policy to *verify the patient's identity and to make sure that the correct solution is hanging in the prescribed concentration; that the solution's indication corresponds with the patient's diagnosis; that the dosage calculations are correct and the dosing formula used to derive the final dose is correct; that the route of administration is safe and proper for the patient; that the pump settings are correct; and that the infusion line is attached to the correct port.*[15]

■ After comparing the results of the independent double-check with the other nurse, begin infusing the parenteral nutrition, as ordered, if there are no discrepancies. If discrepancies exist, rectify them before beginning the infusion.[15]

■ Remove and discard your gloves and mask, if worn, and perform hand hygiene.[4,5,6]

■ Document the procedure.[16]

Special considerations

■ Monitor the patient's glucose level every 6 hours, according to your facility's policy or the doctor's order. Insulin may be added to the parenteral nutrition solution; however, additional subcutaneous doses may also be needed.

■ Monitor intake and output and weigh the patient daily at the same time each morning after he voids, if possible. Suspect fluid imbalance if the patient gains more than 1 to 3 lb (0.5 kg to 1.4 kg) daily.

■ Don't perform routine site care and dressing changes if the patient has a short peripheral catheter; instead, change the dressing if it becomes damp or soiled or if it's no longer intact.[17,18]

■ If the patient has a short-term CV access device, routine dressing changes depend on the type of dressing. Change transparent semipermeable dressings at least every 7 days; change gauze dressings every 2 days. Change either type if it becomes damp or soiled or if it's no longer intact.[17,18] Dressing changes should also include cleaning the catheter-skin junction with an antiseptic solution and changing the stabilization device, if used.[17]

■ If lipids aren't being infused, change the administration tubing and filters that are used continuously no more frequently than every 96 hours; replace tubing every 24 hours if lipids are being administered continuously, or according to your facility's policy. If lipids are being administered intermittently, change the administration tubing with each new container. Change the administration tubing immediately if you suspect contamination or when the integrity of the product or system has been compromised. Hang time for a container of parenteral nutrition shouldn't exceed 24 hours; for lipids, it shouldn't exceed 12 hours.[19]

■ Monitor the patient's laboratory studies and report abnormalities to the doctor.

■ Closely monitor the catheter site for swelling, which may indicate infiltration. *Extravasation of parenteral nutrition solution can lead to tissue necrosis.* (See *Correcting common parenteral nutrition problems.*)

■ Take caution when using the parenteral nutrition line for other functions.[2] Don't use a single-lumen CV access device to infuse blood or blood products, to give a bolus injection, to administer simultaneous IV solutions, to measure CV pressure, or to draw blood for laboratory tests without a doctor's order.

■ Provide oral care regularly according to your facility's policy. Also provide emotional support. Keep in mind that patients commonly associate eating with positive feelings and can become disturbed when they can't eat.

Patient teaching

Teach the patient the potential adverse effects and complications of parenteral nutrition. Encourage him to inspect his mouth regularly for signs of parotitis, glossitis, and oral lesions. Tell him that he may have fewer bowel movements while receiving parenteral nutrition therapy. As appropriate, encourage him to remain physically active *to help his body use the nutrients more fully.*

Patients who require prolonged or indefinite parenteral nutrition may be able to receive the therapy at home. Home parenteral nutrition reduces the need for long hospitalizations and allows the patient to resume many of his normal activities. Make a home care referral and begin patient teaching before discharge *to make sure the patient knows how to perform the administration procedure and how to handle complications.*

Complications

Catheter-related sepsis is the most serious complication of parenteral nutrition. Although rare, a malpositioned subclavian or jugular vein catheter may lead to thrombosis or sepsis. An air embolism, a potentially fatal complication, can occur during IV

TROUBLESHOOTING

Correcting common parenteral nutrition problems

COMPLICATIONS	SIGNS AND SYMPTOMS	INTERVENTIONS
METABOLIC PROBLEMS		
Hepatic dysfunction	Elevated serum aspartate aminotransferase, alkaline phosphatase, and bilirubin levels	Reduce total caloric intake and dextrose intake, making up lost calories by administering lipid emulsion. Change to cyclical infusion. Use specific hepatic formulations only if the patient has encephalopathy.
Hypercapnia	Heightened oxygen consumption, increased carbon dioxide production, and measured respiratory quotient of 1 or greater	Reduce total caloric and dextrose intake, and balance dextrose and fat calories.
Hyperglycemia	Fatigue, restlessness, confusion, anxiety, weakness, polyuria, dehydration, elevated serum glucose levels and, in severe hyperglycemia, delirium or coma	Restrict dextrose intake by decreasing either the rate of infusion or the dextrose concentration. Compensate for calorie loss by administering lipid emulsion. Begin insulin therapy.
Hyperosmolarity	Confusion, lethargy, seizures, hyperosmolar hyperglycemic nonketotic syndrome, hyperglycemia, dehydration, and glycosuria	Discontinue dextrose infusion. Administer insulin and half-normal saline solution with 10 to 20 mEq/L of potassium to rehydrate the patient.
Hypocalcemia	Polyuria, dehydration, and elevated blood and urine glucose levels	Increase calcium supplements.
Hypoglycemia	Sweating, shaking, and irritability after the infusion has stopped	Increase dextrose intake or decrease exogenous insulin intake.
Hypokalemia	Muscle weakness, paralysis, paresthesia, and arrhythmias	Increase potassium supplements.
Hypomagnesemia	Tingling around the mouth, paresthesia in fingers, mental changes, and hyperreflexia	Increase magnesium supplements.
Hypophosphatemia "Refeeding syndrome"	Irritability, weakness, fluid retention, arrhythmias, cardiac failure, seizures, paresthesia, coma, and respiratory arrest; accompanied by drops in potassium and magnesium levels	Increase phosphate supplements.
Metabolic acidosis	Elevated serum chloride level and reduced serum bicarbonate level	Increase acetate and decrease chloride in parenteral nutrition solution.
Metabolic alkalosis	Reduced serum chloride level and elevated serum bicarbonate level	Decrease acetate and increase chloride in parenteral nutrition solution.
Zinc deficiency	Dermatitis, alopecia, apathy, depression, taste changes, confusion, poor wound healing, and diarrhea	Increase zinc supplements.
MECHANICAL PROBLEMS		
Clotted central venous (CV) access device	Interrupted flow rate and resistance to flushing and blood withdrawal	Attempt to aspirate the clot. If unsuccessful, instill a thrombolytic agent to clear the catheter lumen, as ordered.

(continued)

TROUBLESHOOTING

Correcting common parenteral nutrition problems *(continued)*

COMPLICATIONS	SIGNS AND SYMPTOMS	INTERVENTIONS
MECHANICAL PROBLEMS *(continued)*		
Cracked or broken tubing	Fluid leaking from the tubing	Apply a padded hemostat above the break to prevent air from entering the line. Change the tubing immediately.
Dislodged catheter	Catheter out of the vein	Apply pressure to the site with a sterile gauze pad.
Too-rapid infusion	Nausea, headache, and lethargy	Adjust the infusion rate and, if applicable, check the infusion pump.
OTHER PROBLEMS		
Air embolism	Apprehension, chest pain, tachycardia, hypotension, cyanosis, seizures, loss of consciousness, and cardiac arrest	Clamp the catheter. Place the patient in a steep, left lateral Trendelenburg position, if not contraindicated by another condition.[20] Administer oxygen, as ordered. If cardiac arrest occurs, begin cardiopulmonary resuscitation. When the catheter is removed, cover the insertion site with a dressing for 24 to 48 hours.
Extravasation	Swelling and pain around the insertion site	Stop the infusion. Estimate the volume of fluid that escaped into the tissues, based on the rate of infusion. Notify the doctor. Use a standardized scale to assess and document the extravasation.[21]
Infection	Erythema, edema, induration, or drainage from the insertion site, or chills, fever, and leukocytosis	Notify the doctor. Obtain peripheral blood cultures, as ordered. If a sample for blood culture is to be obtained from the catheter, change the needleless connector before obtaining the specimen. Make sure that blood cultures are obtained before initiating antibiotics. Immediate removal of a CV access device isn't recommended if temperature elevation is the only sign of infection. Send the catheter tip for culture if the device is suspected of being the cause of infection.[22]
Phlebitis	Pain, tenderness, redness, and warmth	Assess the vascular access site for signs and symptoms, and assess their severity using a standardized phlebitis scale. If the access device is a midline catheter or peripherally inserted central catheter, determine the possible cause (chemical, mechanical, bacterial, or postinfusion) and intervene accordingly. If the device used is a short peripheral catheter, remove it.[23] Notify the doctor. Apply gentle heat to the area, and elevate the insertion site, if possible.
Pneumothorax and hydrothorax	Dyspnea, chest pain, cyanosis, and decreased breath sounds	Assist with chest tube insertion and apply suction, as ordered.
Thrombosis	Erythema and edema at the insertion site; ipsilateral swelling of the arm, neck, face, and upper chest; pain at the insertion site and along the vein; malaise; fever; and tachycardia	Notify the doctor; a CV access device may or may not be removed. Systemic anticoagulation therapy may be prescribed.[24] Apply warm compresses to the insertion site, and elevate the affected extremity. Venous flow studies may be performed.

tubing changes if the tubing is inadvertently disconnected. It may also result from undetected hairline cracks in the tubing or hub. Extravasation of parenteral nutrition solution can cause necrosis and then sloughing of the epidermis and dermis.

Documentation

Document the type of the access device used; the parenteral nutrition formulation and additives; the volume of solution administered; the condition of the catheter insertion site; your assessment findings; the patient's response to therapy; and any complications and interventions and the patient's response to those interventions. (See *Documenting parenteral nutrition.*) Document any patient teaching provided and the patient's understanding of your teaching.

> ## Documenting parenteral nutrition[2]
>
> When documenting parenteral nutrition, make sure to include:
> ■ the type and location of the access device
> ■ the condition of the insertion site
> ■ the presence of blood return
> ■ the volume and rate of the solution infused
> ■ any additives added to the solution
> ■ your observations of any adverse reactions and your interventions
> ■ when you discontinue a central or peripheral IV catheter for parenteral nutrition
> ■ the date and time and the type of dressing applied after parenteral nutrition was discontinued
> ■ the appearance of the administration site.

REFERENCES

1 Mirtallo, J., et al. (2004). Safe practices for parenteral nutrition. *Journal of Parenteral and Enteral Nutrition, 28*(6), S65–S70. (Level I)

2 Standard 65. Parenteral nutrition. Infusion nursing standards of practice (2011). *Journal of Infusion Nursing, 34*(1S), S91–S93. (Level I)

3 The Joint Commission. (2012). Standard MM.06.01.01. *Comprehensive accreditation manual for hospitals: The official handbook.* Oakbrook Terrace, IL: The Joint Commission. (Level I)

4 Centers for Disease Control and Prevention. (October 2002). Guideline for hand hygiene in health-care settings. *Morbidity and Mortality Weekly Report, 51*(RR-16), 1–45. (Level I)

5 World Health Organization. (2009). *WHO guidelines on hand hygiene in health care: First global patient safety challenge. Clean care is safer care.* Geneva, Switzerland: World Health Organization. (Level I)

6 The Joint Commission. (2012). Standard NPSG.07.01.01. *Comprehensive accreditation manual for hospitals: The official handbook.* Oakbrook Terrace, IL: The Joint Commission. (Level I)

7 The Joint Commission. (2012). Standard NPSG.01.01.01. *Comprehensive accreditation manual for hospitals: The official handbook.* Oakbrook Terrace, IL: The Joint Commission. (Level I)

8 Standard 28. Filters. Infusion nursing standards of practice. (2011). *Journal of Infusion Nursing, 34*(1S), S33–S34. (Level I)

9 Standard 27. Needleless connectors. Infusion nursing standards of practice. (2011). *Journal of Infusion Nursing, 34*(1S), S32–S33. (Level I)

10 Standard 61. Parenteral medication and solution administration. Infusion nursing standards of practice. (2011). *Journal of Infusion Nursing, 34*(1S), S86–S87. (Level I)

11 Standard 45. Flushing and locking. Infusion nursing standards of practice. (2011). *Journal of Infusion Nursing, 34*(1S), S59–S63. (Level I)

12 Infusion Nurses Society. (2011). *Policies and procedures for infusion nursing* (4th ed.). Boston, MA: Infusion Nurses Society.

13 U.S. Food and Drug Administration. (2009). "Look. Check. Connect.: Safe Medical Device Connections Save Lives" [Online]. Accessed November 2011 via the Web at http://www.fda.gov/downloads/MedicalDevices/Safety/AlertsandNotices/UCM134873.pdf

14 Institute of Safe Medication Practices. "ISMP's List of High-Alert Medications." [Online]. Accessed October 2011 via the Web at http://www.ismp.org/tools/highalertmedications.pdf

15 Institute for Safe Medication Practices. (2008). "Conducting an Independent Double-check." *ISMP Medication Safety Alert! Nurse Advise-ERR, 6*(12), 1 [Online]. Accessed October 2011 via the Web at http://www.ismp.org/newsletters/nursing/Issues/NurseAdviseERR200812.pdf

16 The Joint Commission. (2012). Standard RC.01.03.01. *Comprehensive accreditation manual for hospitals: The official handbook.* Oakbrook Terrace, IL: The Joint Commission. (Level I)

17 Standard 46. Vascular access device site care and dressing changes. Infusion nursing standards of practice. (2011). *Journal of Infusion Nursing, 34*(1S), S63–S65. (Level I)

18 O'Grady, N.P., et al. (2011). "Guidelines for the Prevention of Intravascular Catheter-Related Infections" [Online]. Accessed November 2011 via the Web at http://www.cdc.gov/hicpac/pdf/guidelines/bsi-guidelines-2011.pdf (Level I)

19 Standard 43. Administration set change. Infusion nursing standards of practice. (2011). *Journal of Infusion Nursing, 34*(1S), S55–S57. (Level I)

20 Standard 50. Air embolism. Infusion nursing standards of practice. (2011). *Journal of Infusion Nursing, 34*(1S), S69–S70. (Level I)

21 Standard 48. Infiltration and extravasation. Infusion nursing standards of practice. (2011). *Journal of Infusion Nursing, 34*(1S), S66–S68. (Level I)

22 Standard 49. Infection. Infusion nursing standards of practice. (2011). *Journal of Infusion Nursing, 34*(1S), S68–S69. (Level I)

23 Standard 47. Phlebitis. Infusion nursing standards of practice. (2011). *Journal of Infusion Nursing, 34*(1S), S65–S66. (Level I)

24 Standard 52. Catheter-associated venous thrombosis. Infusion nursing standards of practice. (2011). *Journal of Infusion Nursing, 34*(1S), S71–S72. (Level I)

ADDITIONAL REFERENCE

Alexander, M., et al. (Eds.). (2010). *Infusion nursing: An evidence-based approach* (3rd ed.). Philadelphia, PA: Elsevier.

PARENTERAL NUTRITION MONITORING

Parenteral nutrition requires careful monitoring. Because the typical patient is in a protein-wasting state, parenteral nutrition therapy causes marked changes in fluid and electrolyte status and in glucose, amino acid, mineral, and vitamin levels. If the patient displays an adverse reaction or signs of complications, the parenteral nutrition regimen can be changed, as needed. (See "Parenteral nutrition administration," page 546.) Assessing a patient's nutritional status includes a physical examination as well as reviewing body weight, body composition, somatic and visceral protein stores, and laboratory values. Assessing the patient's condition to detect complications requires recognizing the signs and symptoms of such complications, understanding of laboratory test results, and keeping careful records.

Because the parenteral nutrition solution is high in glucose content, the infusion must start slowly to allow the patient's pancreatic beta cells to adapt to it by increasing insulin output. Within the first 3 to 5 days of parenteral nutrition, the typical adult patient can tolerate 3 L of solution daily without adverse reactions. Lipid emulsions also require monitoring.

Equipment

Gloves ▪ parenteral nutrition solution and administration equipment ▪ blood glucose meter ▪ stethoscope ▪ sphygmomanometer ▪ watch with second hand ▪ scale ▪ input and output chart ▪ additional equipment for nutritional assessment, as ordered ▪ Optional: face mask.

Preparation of equipment

For information on preparing the infusion pump and parenteral nutrition solution, see the appropriate procedures. Make sure each bag or bottle has a label listing the expiration date, glucose concentration, and total volume of solution. (If the bag or bottle is damaged and you don't have an immediate replacement, hang a bag of dextrose 10% in water until the new container is ready.)

Implementation

▪ Perform hand hygiene and put on gloves and mask, if required.[1,2,3]
▪ Confirm the patient's identity using at least two patient identifiers according to your facility's policy.[4,5]
▪ Explain the procedure to the patient *to diminish his anxiety and encourage cooperation.* Instruct him to inform you if he experiences any unusual sensations during the infusion.
▪ Record vital signs at least every 8 hours, or as ordered, *because temperature elevation may be a sign of intravascular catheter-related bloodstream infection.*
▪ Change the continuously used administration tubing and filters no more frequently than every 96 hours if lipids aren't being infused; replace tubing every 24 hours if lipids are being infused continuously, or according to your facility's policy. If lipids are administered intermittently, change the administration tubing with each new container. Change the administration tubing

immediately if contamination is suspected or if the integrity of the product or system has been compromised.[6,7]
▪ If the patient has a short peripheral catheter, don't perform routine site care; instead, change the dressing if it becomes damp or soiled or is no longer intact.[6,8] (See "IV catheter maintenance," page 431.)
▪ If the patient has a short-term central venous (CV) access device, routine dressing changes depend on the type of dressing. Change transparent semipermeable dressings at least every 7 days; change gauze dressings every 2 days. Change either dressing if it becomes damp or soiled or is no longer intact.[6,8] Dressing changes should also include cleaning the catheter-skin junction with an antiseptic solution and replacing the stabilizing device, if used.[6] (See "Central venous access catheter," page 133.)
▪ Physically assess the patient daily; monitor for signs of peripheral and pulmonary edema. Inspect the vascular catheter insertion site daily and palpate for tenderness through the intact dressing. Remove the dressing and thoroughly examine the site if fever, tenderness, or other findings that suggest a local or bloodstream infection exist.[6,8] If ordered, measure the patient's arm circumference and skin-fold thickness over the triceps.
▪ Weigh the patient at the same time each morning (after voiding), with the patient in similar-weight clothing, and on the same scale. Compare these data with his fluid intake and output record. *Weight gain, particularly early in treatment, may indicate fluid overload rather than increasing fat and protein stores.* A patient shouldn't gain more than 3 lb (1.4 kg) per week; a weight gain of 1 lb (0.5 kg) per week is a reasonable goal for most patients; suspect fluid imbalance if the patient gains more than 1 lb daily.
▪ Monitor the patient for signs and symptoms of glucose metabolism disturbance, fluid and electrolyte imbalances, and nutritional aberrations. Some patients may require supplemental insulin for the duration of parenteral nutrition; the pharmacy usually adds insulin directly to the parenteral nutrition solution. Monitor electrolyte levels frequently—daily at first. Monitor serum albumin weekly. (See *Laboratory monitoring of parenteral nutrition.*) Later, as the patient's condition stabilizes, you won't need to monitor these values quite as closely. (Be aware that in a severely dehydrated patient, albumin levels may actually drop initially as treatment restores hydration.)
▪ Monitor magnesium and calcium levels. If these electrolytes have been added to the parenteral nutrition solution, the dosage may need adjusting *to maintain normal serum levels.* Assess the patient for signs and symptoms of magnesium and calcium imbalances.
▪ Monitor serum glucose levels every 6 hours initially, then once per day, or according to your facility's policy. Watch for signs and symptoms of hyperglycemia, such as thirst, hunger, and polyuria. Periodically confirm blood glucose meter readings with laboratory tests.
▪ Assess renal function by monitoring blood urea nitrogen and creatinine levels; *increases can indicate excess amino acid intake.* Also assess nitrogen balance with 24-hour urine collection, as ordered.
▪ Assess liver function by periodically monitoring liver enzyme, bilirubin, triglyceride, and cholesterol levels. *Abnormal values may*

indicate an intolerance or excess of lipid emulsions or problems with metabolizing the protein or glucose in the parenteral nutrition formula.

■ Provide emotional support. *Patients tend to associate eating with positive feelings and can become disturbed when eating is prohibited.*[5]

■ Provide frequent oral care. (See "Oral care," page 524.)

■ Keep the patient active *to enable him to use nutrients more fully.*

■ When discontinuing parenteral nutrition, decrease the infusion rate slowly, depending on the patient's current glucose intake, *to minimize the risk of hyperinsulinemia and resulting hypoglycemia.* Weaning usually takes place over 24 to 48 hours but can be completed in 4 to 6 hours if the patient receives sufficient oral or IV carbohydrates.

■ While weaning the patient from parenteral nutrition, document his dietary intake and work with the nutritionist to determine the total calorie and protein intake. Also teach other health care staff members caring for the patient the importance of recording food intake. Use percentages of food consumed ("ate 50% of a baked potato") instead of subjective descriptions ("had a good appetite") *to provide a more accurate account of patient intake.*

■ Perform hand hygiene.[1,2,3]

■ Document the procedure.[9]

Special considerations

■ Always maintain strict sterile technique when handling the equipment used to administer therapy.[5] *Because the parenteral nutrition solution serves as a medium for bacterial growth and the CV access device provides systemic access,* the patient is at risk for infection and sepsis.

■ During daily multidisciplinary rounds, discuss the patient's readiness for enteral feeding; switch to enteral feedings as soon as the patient's condition warrants. Make sure the vascular access device is removed as soon as it's no longer needed *to reduce the risk of vascular catheter-related bloodstream infection.*[5,6]

■ Teach the patient about measures to prevent intravascular catheter-related infections, including the importance of hand hygiene.[10]

■ When using a filter, position it as close to the access site as possible.[11] Check the filter's porosity and psi capacity *to make sure it exceeds the psi exerted by the infusion pump.*

■ Don't allow parenteral nutrition solutions to hang for more than 24 hours; lipids should not exceed 12 hours.[5]

■ Be careful when using the parenteral nutrition access device for other functions.[5] If using a single-lumen CV access device, don't use the device to infuse blood or blood products, to give a bolus injection, to administer simultaneous IV solutions, to measure CV pressure, or to obtain blood samples for laboratory testing without a doctor's order. Never add medication to a parenteral nutrition solution container. Also, don't use a three-way stopcock, if possible, *because add-on devices increase the risk of infection.*

■ When a patient is severely malnourished, starting parenteral nutrition may spark refeeding syndrome, which includes a rapid drop in potassium, magnesium, and phosphorus levels. *To avoid compromising cardiac function,* initiate feeding slowly and

---

Laboratory monitoring of parenteral nutrition

These laboratory tests are usually ordered as part of monitoring for a patient receiving parenteral nutrition.

Baseline tests
Complete blood count (CBC), comprehensive metabolic panel (CMP)*, cholesterol, triglycerides, prothrombin time (PT), International Normalized Ratio (INR), lactate dehydrogenase (LD), magnesium phosphorus, transferrin

Daily tests
Weight, intake and output, glucose by fingerstick every 6 hours until stable, then as directed
Basic metabolic panel (BMP)** until stable, then three times a week

Weekly tests
CBC, CMP, cholesterol, triglycerides, PT, INR, LD, magnesium phosphorus, transferrin

*CMP includes blood urea nitrogen (BUN), creatinine, sodium, chloride, carbon dioxide (CO_2), glucose, potassium, calcium, albumin, total protein, alkaline phosphatase, alanine transaminase, aspartate transaminase, and bilirubin.
**BMP includes BUN, creatinine, sodium, chloride, CO_2, glucose, and potassium.

---

monitor the patient's blood values especially closely until they stabilize.

Complications

Catheter-related, metabolic, and mechanical complications can occur during parenteral nutrition administration.

Documentation

Document the type of access device used, the parenteral nutrition formulation, additives, the volume of solution, the rate of infusion, your assessment findings, and the patient's response to therapy. Record any adverse effects, date and time, name of the doctor notified, any prescribed interventions, and the patient's response to those interventions.[5] Document patient teaching provided.

REFERENCES

1 Centers for Disease Control and Prevention. (October 2002). Guideline for hand hygiene in health-care settings. *Morbidity and Mortality Weekly Report, 51*(RR-16), 1–45. (Level I)

2 World Health Organization. (2009). *WHO guidelines on hand hygiene in health care: First global patient safety challenge. Clean care is safer care.* Geneva, Switzerland: World Health Organization. (Level I)

3 The Joint Commission. (2012). Standard NPSG.07.01.01. *Comprehensive accreditation manual for hospitals: The official handbook.* Oakbrook Terrace, IL: The Joint Commission. (Level I)

4 The Joint Commission. (2012). Standard NPSG.01.01.01. *Comprehensive accreditation manual for hospitals: The official handbook.* Oakbrook Terrace, IL: The Joint Commission. (Level I)

5 Standard 65. Parenteral nutrition. Infusion nursing standards of practice (2011). *Journal of Infusion Nursing, 34*(1S), S91–S93. (Level I)

6 O'Grady, N.P., et al. (2011). "Guidelines for the Prevention of Intravascular Catheter-Related Infections" [Online]. Accessed November 2011 via the Web at http://www.cdc.gov/hicpac/pdf/guidelines/bsi-guidelines-2011.pdf (Level I)

7 Standard 43. Administration set change. Infusion nursing standards of practice. (2011). *Journal of Infusion Nursing, 34*(1S), S55–S57.

8 Standard 46. Vascular access device site care and dressing changes. Infusion nursing standards of practice. (2011). *Journal of Infusion Nursing, 34*(1S), S63–S65. (Level I)

9 The Joint Commission. (2012). Standard RC.01.03.01. *Comprehensive accreditation manual for hospitals: The official handbook.* Oakbrook Terrace, IL: The Joint Commission. (Level I)

10 The Joint Commission. (2012). Standard NPSG.07.04.01. *Comprehensive accreditation manual for hospitals: The official handbook.* Oakbrook Terrace, IL: The Joint Commission. (Level I)

11 Standard 28. Filters. Infusion nursing standards of practice. (2011). *Journal of Infusion Nursing, 34*(1S), S33–S34. (Level I)

ADDITIONAL REFERENCES

Alexander, M., et al. (Eds.). (2010). *Infusion nursing: An evidence-based approach* (3rd ed.). Philadelphia, PA: Elsevier.

Infusion Nurses Society. (2011). *Policies and procedures for infusion nursing* (4th ed.). Boston, MA: Infusion Nurses Society.

Mirtallo, J., et al. (2004). Safe practices for parenteral nutrition. *Journal of Parenteral and Enteral Nutrition, 28*(6), S39–S70.

Weinstein, S.M. (2007). *Plumer's principles and practices of intravenous therapy* (8th ed.). Philadelphia, PA: Lippincott Williams & Wilkins.

PASSIVE RANGE-OF-MOTION EXERCISES

Used to move the patient's joints through as full a range of motion (ROM) as possible, passive ROM exercises improve or maintain joint mobility and help prevent contractures. Performed by a nurse, a physical therapist, or a caregiver of the patient's choosing, these exercises are indicated for the patient with temporary or permanent loss of mobility, sensation, or consciousness. Properly performed passive ROM exercises require recognition of the patient's limits of motion and support of all joints during movement.

Exercises performed in the bed help with joint mobility, strength, and endurance and they prepare the patient for ambulating. During passive ROM exercises, another person moves the patient's extremities so that the joints move through a complete ROM, maximally stretching all muscle groups within each plane over each joint.

Passive ROM exercises are contraindicated in patients with septic joints, acute thrombophlebitis, severe arthritic joint inflammation, or recent trauma with possible hidden fractures or internal injuries.

ROM exercises require no special equipment other than gloves and personal protective equipment as indicated.

Implementation

■ Determine the joints that need ROM exercises, and consult the doctor or physical therapist about limitations or precautions for specific exercises.

■ The exercises below treat all joints, but they don't have to be performed in the order given or all at once. You can schedule them over the course of a day, whenever the patient is in the most convenient position. Remember to perform all exercises slowly and gently to the end of the normal ROM or to the point of pain, but no further. (See *Glossary of joint movements.*) Hold the position for 1 to 2 seconds.

■ Perform hand hygiene and put on gloves and other personal protective equipment as indicated.[1,2,3]

■ Confirm the patient's identity using at least two patient identifiers according to your facility's policy.[4]

■ Explain the procedure to the patient. Answer all questions *to decrease anxiety and increase cooperation.*

■ Raise the bed to a comfortable working height.

Exercising the neck

■ Support the patient's head with your hands and extend her neck, flex her chin to her chest, and tilt her head laterally toward each shoulder.

■ Rotate the patient's head from right to left (as shown below).

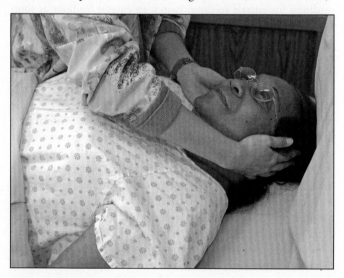

Exercising the shoulders

■ Support the patient's arm in an extended, neutral position; then extend her forearm and flex it back.

■ Abduct her arm outward from the side of her body, and adduct it back to the side.

■ Rotate the shoulder so that her arm crosses the midline, and bend the elbow so that her hand touches the opposite shoulder,

Glossary of joint movements

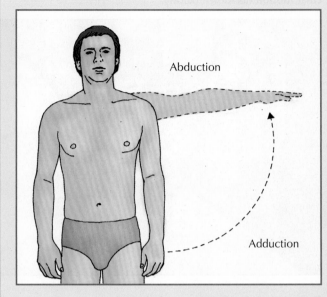

Abduction

Adduction

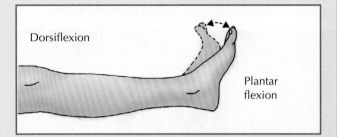

Dorsiflexion

Plantar flexion

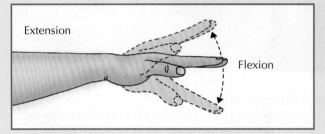

Extension

Flexion

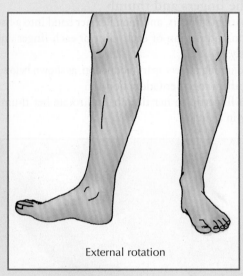

External rotation

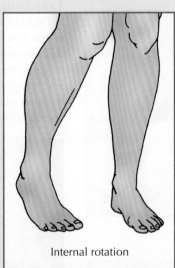

Internal rotation

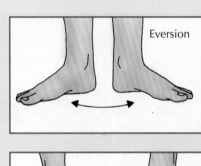

Eversion

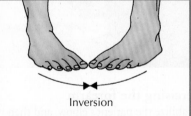

Inversion

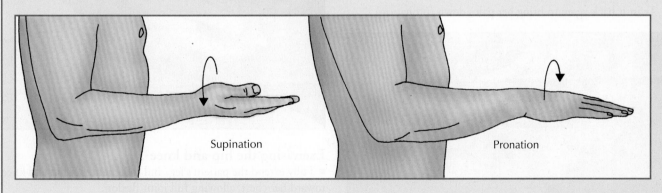

Supination

Pronation

then touches the mattress of the bed for complete internal rotation.

■ Return her shoulder to a neutral position and, with elbow bent, push her arm backward so that the back of her hand touches the mattress for complete external rotation (as shown below).

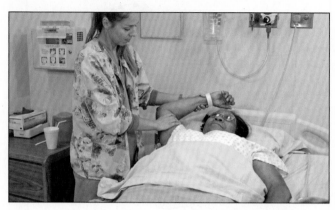

Exercising the elbow

■ Place the patient's arm at her side with her palm facing up.
■ Flex and extend her arm at the elbow (as shown below).

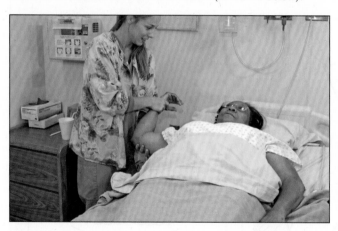

Exercising the forearm

■ Stabilize the patient's elbow, and then twist her hand to bring her palm up (supination, as shown below).
■ Twist it back again to bring her palm down (pronation).

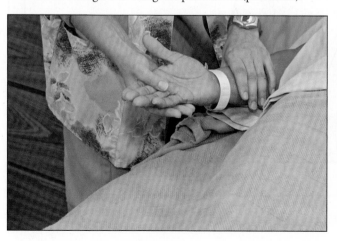

Exercising the wrist

■ Stabilize her forearm and flex and extend her wrist. Then rock her hand sideways for lateral flexion, and rotate her hand in a circular motion (as shown below).

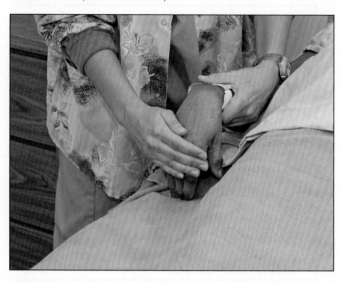

Exercising the fingers and thumb

■ Extend the patient's fingers, and then flex her hand into a fist; repeat extension and flexion of each joint of each finger and thumb separately.
■ Spread two adjoining fingers apart (abduction, as shown below), and then bring them together (adduction).
■ Oppose each fingertip to her thumb, and rotate her thumb and each finger in a circle.

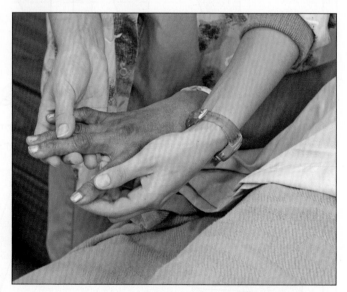

Exercising the hip and knee

■ Fully extend the patient's leg, and then bend her hip and knee toward her chest, allowing full joint flexion.
■ Next, move her straight leg sideways, out and away from her other leg (abduction), and then back, over, and across it (adduction).

■ Rotate her straight leg internally toward the midline (as shown below), then externally away from the midline.

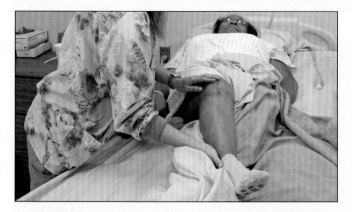

Exercising the ankle
■ Bend the patient's foot so that her toes push upward (dorsiflexion), and then bend her foot so that her toes push downward (plantar flexion).
■ Rotate her ankle in a circular motion (as shown below).
■ Invert her ankle so that the sole of her foot faces the midline, and evert her ankle so that the sole faces away from the midline.

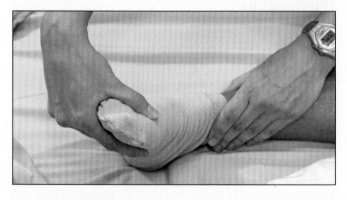

Exercising the toes
■ Flex the patient's toes toward the sole, and then extend them back toward the top of her foot.
■ Spread two adjoining toes apart (abduction, as shown below), and bring them together (adduction).
■ Remove your gloves and other personal protective equipment and discard. Perform hand hygiene.[1,2,3]
■ Document the procedure.[5]

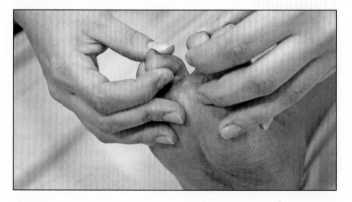

Special considerations
Because joints begin to stiffen within 24 hours of disuse, start passive ROM exercises as soon as possible, and perform them at least once each shift, usually while bathing or turning the patient. Use proper body mechanics, and repeat each exercise at least three times.
■ Patients who experience prolonged bed rest or limited activity without profound weakness can also be taught to perform ROM exercises on their own (called *active ROM exercises*), or they may benefit from isometric exercises. (See *Learning about isometric exercises,* page 558.)
■ If a disabled patient requires long-term rehabilitation after discharge, consult with a physical therapist and teach a family member or caregiver to perform passive ROM exercises.

Documentation
Record the joints exercised, the presence of edema or pressure areas, any pain resulting from the exercises, any limitation of ROM, and the patient's tolerance of the exercises.

REFERENCES

1 Centers for Disease Control and Prevention. (October 2002). Guideline for hand hygiene in health-care settings. *Morbidity and Mortality Weekly Report, 51*(RR-16), 1–45. (Level I)
2 World Health Organization. (2009). *WHO guidelines on hand hygiene in health care: First global patient safety challenge. Clean care is safer care.* Geneva, Switzerland: World Health Organization. (Level I)
3 The Joint Commission. (2012). Standard NPSG.07.01.01. *Comprehensive accreditation manual for hospitals: The official handbook.* Oakbrook Terrace, IL: The Joint Commission. (Level I)
4 The Joint Commission. (2012). Standard NPSG.01.01.01. *Comprehensive accreditation manual for hospitals: The official handbook.* Oakbrook Terrace, IL: The Joint Commission. (Level I)
5 The Joint Commission. (2012). Standard RC.01.03.01. *Comprehensive accreditation manual for hospitals: The official handbook.* Oakbrook Terrace, IL: The Joint Commission. (Level I)

ADDITIONAL REFERENCE

Craven, R.F., & Hirnle, C.J. (2012). *Fundamentals of nursing: Human health and function* (7th ed.). Philadelphia, PA: Lippincott Williams & Wilkins.

PATIENT-CONTROLLED ANALGESIA

Patient-controlled analgesia (PCA) is a drug delivery system providing IV analgesia, usually morphine, when the patient presses a call bell at the end of a cord. Analgesia is provided at the level and time needed by the patient. The device prevents the patient from accidentally overdosing by imposing a lockout time between doses, usually 6 to 10 minutes. During this interval, the patient won't receive any analgesic, even if he pushes the button.

PCA offers several advantages. It eliminates the need for IM analgesics, provides pain relief tailored to each patient's size and pain tolerance, gives the patient a sense of control over pain, and

Learning about isometric exercises

Patients can strengthen and increase muscle tone by contracting muscles against resistance (from other muscles or from a stationary object, such as a bed or a wall) without joint movement. These exercises require only a comfortable position—standing, sitting, or lying down—and proper body alignment. For each exercise, instruct the patient to hold each contraction for 2 to 5 seconds and to repeat it three to four times daily, below peak contraction level for the first week and at peak level thereafter.

Neck rotators
The patient places the heel of his hand above one ear. Then he pushes his head toward the hand as forcefully as possible, without moving the head, neck, or arm. He repeats the exercise on the other side.

Neck flexors
The patient places both palms on his forehead. Without moving his neck, he pushes his head forward while resisting with his palms.

Neck extensors
The patient clasps his fingers behind his head, then pushes his head against his clasped hands without moving his neck.

Shoulder elevators
Holding his right arm straight down at his side, the patient grasps his right wrist with his left hand. He then tries to shrug his right shoulder, but prevents it from moving by holding his arm in place. He repeats this exercise, alternating arms.

Shoulder, chest, and scapular musculature
The patient places his right fist in his left palm and raises both arms to shoulder height. He pushes his fist into his palm as forcefully as possible without moving either arm. Then, with his arms in the same position, he clasps his fingers and tries to pull his hands apart. He repeats the pattern, beginning with the left fist in the right palm.

Elbow flexors and extensors
With his right elbow bent 90 degrees and his right palm facing upward, the patient places his left fist against his right palm. He tries to bend his right elbow further while resisting with the left fist. He repeats the pattern, bending his left elbow.

Abdomen
The patient assumes a sitting position and bends slightly forward, with his hands in front of the middle of his thighs. He tries to bend forward further, resisting by pressing his palms against his thighs.

Alternatively, in the supine position, he clasps his hands behind his head. Then he raises his shoulders about 1" (2.5 cm), holding this position for a few seconds.

Back extensors
In a sitting position, the patient bends forward and places his hands under his buttocks. He tries to stand up, resisting with both hands.

Hip abductors
While standing, the patient squeezes his inner thighs together as tightly as possible. Placing a pillow between his knees supplies resistance and increases the effectiveness of this exercise.

Hip extensors
The patient squeezes his buttocks together as tightly as possible.

Knee extensors
The patient straightens his knee fully. Then he vigorously tightens the muscle above the knee so that it moves his kneecap upward. He repeats this exercise, alternating legs.

Ankle flexors and extensors
The patient pulls his toes upward, holding briefly. Then he pushes them down as far as possible, again holding briefly.

---

allows the patient to sleep at night with minimal daytime drowsiness. It also improves postoperative deep breathing, coughing, and ambulation and reduces opioid use compared with patients who don't receive PCA.

PCA is typically given to patients postoperatively as well as to terminal cancer patients and others with chronic diseases. To receive PCA therapy, a patient must be mentally alert, able to understand and comply with instructions and procedures, and have no history of allergy to the analgesic. PCA therapy is contraindicated in patients with limited respiratory reserve, a history of drug abuse or chronic sedative or tranquilizer use, or a psychiatric disorder.[1]

Equipment
PCA system and system-specific tubing ▪ syringe with prescribed medication ▪ alcohol pads ▪ compatible IV solution ▪ gloves ▪ tape ▪ naloxone ▪ oxygen administration setup and equipment.

Preparation of equipment
Several types of PCA systems are available, so follow the manufacturer's instructions for setting up the device. Obtain the medication and verify the medication order.[2] Gather equipment and bring it to the patient's bedside. Plug the PCA device into an electrical outlet; if the device is battery-operated, make sure that the battery is fully charged and working.

Implementation

- Perform hand hygiene and put on gloves.[3,4,5]
- Verify the doctor's order.[6]
- Connect the device tubing to the medication syringe and insert the syringe into the device. Make sure that the markings and labels on the syringe are readily visible. Prime the tubing to remove air from the system, *reducing the risk of an air embolism.*
- Program the device to deliver the prescribed parameters, such as loading dose, basal rate, bolus amount, and time lockout for boluses. Have a second nurse confirm the medication order and settings *to prevent possible errors.*[1,7]
- Confirm the patient's identity using at least two patient identifiers according to your facility's policy.[8]
- Provide privacy. Explain the procedure to the patient and answer all questions. Obtain baseline vital signs.
- Assess the patient's IV access site. If the patient doesn't have IV access, start an IV line, according to your facility's policy. Ensure the patency of the IV. (See "IV catheter insertion and removal," page 421.)
- Wipe the connection port on the patient's IV line with an alcohol pad, and then connect the PCA tubing to the patient's IV line or IV access device at the lowest possible port.[9]
- If your facility uses a bar code scanning system, log into the patient's electronic medication administration record and scan your identification badge, the patient's identification bracelet, and the medication's bar code.
- Label the PCA pump, PCA tubing, and IV infusion tubing with the date, the time, and your initials.
- Instruct the patient to push the button each time he has pain and needs relief.
- Monitor the patient's vital signs and oxygen saturation frequently during the initial loading dose and at least every 4 hours throughout therapy.[8] Be aware of the amount the patient will receive when he activates the device and the maximum amount the patient can receive within a specified time (if an adjustable device is used). Have naloxone and oxygen equipment readily available *in case the patient develops respiratory depression from the drug.*[7]
- Inspect the infusion site for changes; check the device function, including rate, periodically.
- Replace the medication syringe when empty.
- Remove gloves and discard used equipment appropriately. Perform hand hygiene.[3,4,5]
- Document the procedure.[10]

Special considerations

- Encourage the patient to cough and deep breath *to promote ventilation.*
- Monitor the IV insertion site for infiltration into subcutaneous tissues and for catheter occlusion, *which may cause the drug to back up into the primary IV tubing.*
- If the analgesic nauseates the patient, administer an antiemetic, as ordered.
- Assess the patient's pain using a pain-rating scale before therapy and then periodically during therapy. Notify the doctor if the patient's pain isn't being relieved.

- Perform an independent medication double-check with another nurse when handing over care of the patient.

Patient teaching

Before initiating PCA therapy, teach the patient how the device works.[7] Allow the patient to practice with a sample device, and reinforce that he should take enough analgesic to relieve acute pain but not enough to make him feel drowsy.

Be aware that PCA by proxy (someone other than the patient pressing the PCA dosing button) can have dangerous effects, including overdose. Provide education *to prevent unauthorized activation of the button.*[9]

Complications

Potential complications include respiratory depression (secondary to the drug) and IV infiltration.

Documentation

Record the date and time PCA therapy began, the IV access device used and its location, baseline vital signs and pain assessment, medication doses (loading dose, individual doses, and time interval), and your ongoing assessments of vital signs, pain, and the IV site. Document the patient's tolerance of the procedure. Note any patient teaching you provided and the patient's understanding of your teaching.

REFERENCES

1. Standard 64. Patient-controlled analgesia. Infusion nursing standards of practice. (2011). *Journal of Infusion Nursing, 34*(1S), S89–S91. (Level I)
2. The Joint Commission. (2012). Standard MM.06.01.01. *Comprehensive accreditation manual for hospitals: The official handbook.* Oakbrook Terrace, IL: The Joint Commission. (Level I)
3. Centers for Disease Control and Prevention. (October 2002). Guideline for hand hygiene in health-care settings. *Morbidity and Mortality Weekly Report, 51*(RR-16), 1–45. (Level I)
4. World Health Organization. (2009). *WHO guidelines on hand hygiene in health care: First global patient safety challenge. Clean care is safer care.* Geneva, Switzerland: World Health Organization. (Level I)
5. The Joint Commission. (2012). Standard NPSG.07.01.01. *Comprehensive accreditation manual for hospitals: The official handbook.* Oakbrook Terrace, IL: The Joint Commission. (Level I)
6. The Joint Commission. (2012). Standard MM.04.01.01. *Comprehensive accreditation manual for hospitals: The official handbook.* Oakbrook Terrace, IL: The Joint Commission. (Level I)
7. Institute for Safe Medication Practices. (2009). "Part II—How to Prevent Errors—Safety Issues with Patient-controlled Analgesia" [Online]. Accessed October 2011 via the Web at http://www.ismp.org/newsletters/acutecare/articles/20030724.asp (Level I)
8. The Joint Commission. (2012). Standard NPSG.01.01.01. *Comprehensive accreditation manual for hospitals: The official handbook.* Oakbrook Terrace, IL: The Joint Commission. (Level I)
9. D'Arcy, Y. (2008). Keep your patient safe during PCA. *Nursing, 38*(1), 50–55.

10 The Joint Commission. (2012). Standard RC.01.03.01. *Comprehensive accreditation manual for hospitals: The official handbook.* Oakbrook Terrace, IL: The Joint Commission. (Level I)

ADDITIONAL REFERENCES

Cranwell-Bruce, L.A. (2009). PCA delivery systems. *Med-Surg Nursing, 18*(2), 127–129, 133.

Nettina, S.M. (2010). *Lippincott manual of nursing practice* (9th ed.). Philadelphia, PA: Lippincott Williams & Wilkins.

Taylor, C., et al. (2011). *Fundamentals of nursing: The art and science of nursing care* (7th ed.). Philadelphia, PA: Lippincott Williams & Wilkins.

Voepel-Lewis, T., et al. (2008). The prevalence of and risk factors for adverse events in children receiving patient-controlled analgesia by proxy or patient-controlled analgesia after surgery. *Anesthesia and Analgesia, 107*(1), 70–75.

Wuhrman, E., et al. (2007). Authorized and unauthorized ('PCA by Proxy') dosing of analgesic infusion pumps: Position statement with clinical practice recommendations. *Pain Management Nursing, 8*(1), 4–11.

PERICARDIOCENTESIS, ASSISTING

Pericardiocentesis is a needle aspiration of pericardial fluid. This procedure is both therapeutic and diagnostic. It can be performed as an emergency measure to relieve cardiac tamponade and it can also provide a fluid sample to confirm and identify the cause of pericardial effusion (excess pericardial fluid) to help determine appropriate therapy.

Normally, small amounts of plasma-derived fluid within the pericardium lubricate the heart, reducing friction for the beating heart. Excess pericardial fluid may accumulate after inflammation, cardiac surgery, rupture, or trauma to the chest or pericardium. Rapidly forming effusions, such as those that develop after cardiac surgery or penetrating or blunt trauma, may induce cardiac tamponade, a potentially lethal syndrome marked by increased intrapericardial pressure, which prevents complete ventricular filling and thus reduces cardiac output. Slowly forming effusions, such as those that occur in pericarditis, typically pose less immediate danger because they allow the pericardium more time to adapt to the accumulating fluid.

The pericardium normally contains 10 to 50 mL of sterile fluid. Pericardial fluid is clear and straw colored, without evidence of pathogens, blood, or malignant cells. The white blood cell count in the fluid is usually less than $1,000/\mu l$. Its glucose concentration should approximate the glucose levels in blood. Pericardial effusions are typically classified as transudates or exudates. (See *Pericardial effusions: Transudates and exudates.*)

Equipment

Prepackaged pericardiocentesis tray ▪ pulse oximeter ▪ Kelly clamp ▪ alligator clips ▪ defibrillator and emergency drugs ▪ sterile gloves ▪ sterile marker ▪ sterile labels ▪ gloves ▪ protective eyewear ▪ surgical caps ▪ sterile gowns ▪ electrocardiograph or bedside monitor ▪ Optional: clippers, two-dimensional echocardiography equipment.

If a prepackaged equipment tray isn't available, you'll need the following: Antiseptic solution (chlorhexidine-based solution) ▪ 1% lidocaine for local anesthetic ▪ sterile needles (25G for anesthetic and 14G, 16G, and 18G 4″ or 5″ cardiac needles) ▪ 50-mL syringe with luer-lock tip ▪ sterile specimen container for culture ▪ specimen labels ▪ laboratory biohazard transport bags ▪ sterile drapes and towels ▪ 4″ × 4″ gauze pads ▪ sterile bandage ▪ vial of heparin 1:1,000 ▪ three-way stopcock.

Preparation of equipment

Needle insertion is generally guided by electrocardiogram (ECG) or echocardiogram. Connect the patient to the bedside monitor, and set to read lead V_1. Make sure a defibrillator and emergency drugs are nearby.

Implementation

▪ If able, conduct a preprocedure verification process *to make sure that all relevant documentation, related information, or equipment is available and correctly identified to the patient's identifiers.*[1]

▪ Verify that the laboratory and imaging studies have been completed as ordered and that the results are in the patient's medical record. Notify the doctor of any abnormal results.

▪ Make sure the patient has an informed consent form in his medical record, unless the procedure is being performed in an emergency situation.[2,3]

▪ Perform hand hygiene.[4,5,6]

▪ Confirm the patient's identity using at least two patient identifiers according to your facility's policy.[7]

▪ Explain the procedure to the patient and answer all questions *to ease his anxiety and ensure his cooperation.*

▪ Inform the patient that he may feel some pressure when the needle is inserted into the pericardial sac.

▪ Make sure the patient has had nothing by mouth for 6 to 8 hours before the procedure, except in an emergency situation.

▪ Verify patent IV access *in case fluids and medications are needed during the procedure.*

■ Administer sedation as ordered, following safe administration practices.

■ Immediately before the procedure, provide privacy.

■ Perform hand hygiene and put on sterile gloves.[4,5,6]

■ Open the equipment tray on an overbed table, being careful not to contaminate the sterile field when you open the wrapper. Label all medications, medication containers, and other solutions on and off the sterile field, maintaining sterility of the sterile field.[8]

■ Provide adequate lighting at the puncture site and adjust the height of the patient's bed *to allow the doctor to perform the procedure comfortably.*

■ Position the patient in the supine position with the head of the bed elevated 30 to 60 degrees to facilitate breathing and reduce the risk of aspiration of fluids.[9] Attach the cardiac monitoring leads, if not already done.

■ Remove and discard your gloves and perform hand hygiene again; assist the doctor, as necessary, with putting on protective eyewear, a mask, a cap, a sterile gown, and sterile gloves. Then put on the same equipment.

■ Conduct a time-out immediately before starting the procedure *to perform a final assessment that the correct patient, site, positioning, and procedure are identified and that, as applicable, all relevant information and necessary equipment are available.*[10]

■ The doctor cleans the skin with sterile gauze pads soaked in antiseptic solution from the left costal margin to the xiphoid process. Clipping the hair from the area may be necessary before applying the antiseptic solution.[11]

■ If no ampule of anesthetic is included on the equipment tray, clean the injection port of a multidose vial of anesthetic with an alcohol pad. Then invert the vial 45 degrees so that the doctor can insert a 25G needle and syringe and withdraw the anesthetic for injection.

■ Before the doctor injects the anesthetic, tell the patient he'll experience a transient burning sensation and local pain.

■ The doctor attaches a 50-mL syringe to one end of a three-way stopcock and the cardiac needle to the other.[9] The V_1 lead (precordial lead wire) of the ECG may be attached to the hub of the aspirating needle using the alligator clips *to help determine if the needle has come in contact with the epicardium during the procedure.*

■ Carefully observe the ECG tracing when the cardiac needle is being inserted; ST-segment elevation indicates that the needle has reached the epicardial surface and should be retracted slightly; an abnormally shaped QRS complex may indicate perforation of the myocardium. Premature ventricular contractions usually indicate that the needle has touched the ventricular wall.

■ The doctor will insert the needle through the chest wall into the pericardial sac, maintaining gentle aspiration until fluid appears in the syringe. The needle is angled 35 to 45 degrees toward the tip of the right scapula between the left costal margin and the xiphoid process. This subxiphoid approach minimizes the risk of lacerating the coronary vessels or the pleura.

■ If the procedure is guided by echocardiography, echocardiography contrast medium may be injected *to verify needle placement.*

■ When the needle is positioned properly, the doctor attaches a Kelly clamp to the skin surface *so it won't advance any further.*

■ Assist the doctor during aspiration of the pericardial fluid and labeling and numbering of the specimen tubes. (See *Aspirating pericardial fluid*, page 562.)

■ If bacterial culture and sensitivity tests are scheduled, record on the laboratory request any antimicrobial drugs the patient is receiving. If anaerobic organisms are suspected, consult the laboratory about proper collection technique *to avoid exposing the aspirate to air.*

■ Label all specimens clearly with the patient's name and the source of the specimen and send them to the laboratory immediately in a laboratory biohazard transport bag.

■ When the needle is withdrawn, immediately apply pressure to the site with sterile gauze pads for 3 to 5 minutes. Then apply a sterile bandage.

■ Remove and discard personal protective equipment and perform hand hygiene.[4,5,6]

■ Obtain a portable chest X-ray immediately after the procedure, as ordered.

■ Assess the patient for complications and monitor blood pressure, pulse, respirations, oxygen saturation, and heart sounds every 15 minutes until stable, then every half hour for 2 hours, every hour for 4 hours, and every 4 hours thereafter. Your facility may require more frequent monitoring. Reassure the patient that such monitoring is routine.

■ Monitor the puncture site for bleeding every 15 minutes until the patient's condition stabilizes and then every 4 hours for 24 hours, or according to your facility's policy.[9]

■ Monitor the patient continually for cardiac arrhythmias and document rhythm strips according to your facility's policy and procedure.

■ Return all equipment to the proper location and dispose of equipment according to your facility's policy.

■ Perform hand hygiene.[4,5,6]

■ Document the procedure.[12]

Special considerations

■ Watch for grossly bloody fluid aspirate, which may indicate inadvertent puncture of a cardiac chamber.

■ After the procedure, be alert for respiratory and cardiac distress. Watch especially for signs of cardiac tamponade, which include muffled and distant heart sounds, distended jugular veins, paradoxical pulse, and shock. Cardiac tamponade may result from rapid accumulation of pericardial fluid or puncture of a coronary vessel, causing bleeding into the pericardial sac.

Complications

Pericardiocentesis should be performed cautiously because of the risk of potentially fatal complications, such as laceration of a coronary artery or the myocardium. Other possible complications include ventricular fibrillation or vasovagal arrest, pleural infection, and accidental puncture of the lung, liver, or stomach.

To minimize the risk of complications, echocardiography should precede pericardiocentesis to determine the effusion site.

Aspirating pericardial fluid

In pericardiocentesis, a needle and syringe assembly is inserted through the chest wall into the pericardial sac (as illustrated below). Electrocardiographic (ECG) monitoring, with a leadwire attached to the needle and electrodes placed on the limbs (right arm [RA], right leg [RL], left arm [LA], and left leg [LL]), helps ensure proper needle placement and avoids damage to the heart.

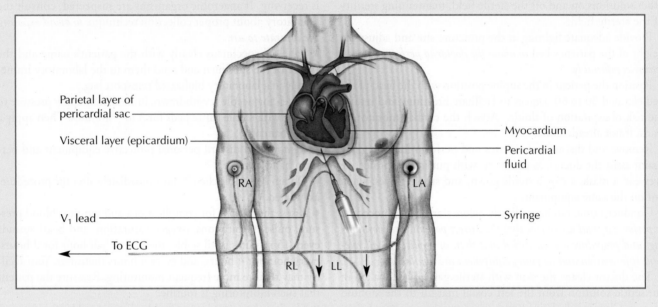

Documentation

Record the initiation and completion time of the procedure, the patient's response, vital signs, cardiac rhythm, and any medications administered. Also record and document ECG recording strips from before, during, and after the procedure. Document the amount, color, and consistency of the fluid; the number of specimen tubes collected; and the time of transport to the laboratory. Document any complications and interventions performed. Document patient and family teaching provided.

REFERENCES

1 The Joint Commission. (2012). Standard UP.01.01.01. *Comprehensive accreditation manual for hospitals: The official handbook.* Oakbrook Terrace, IL: The Joint Commission. (Level I)

2 The Joint Commission. (2012). Standard RI.01.03.01. *Comprehensive accreditation manual for hospitals: The official handbook.* Oakbrook Terrace, IL: The Joint Commission. (Level I)

3 Centers for Medicare & Medicaid Services, Department of Health and Human Services. (2006). "Conditions of Participation: Patients' Rights," 42 CFR part 482.13 [Online]. Accessed November 2011 via the Web at https://www.cms.gov/CFCsAndCoPs/downloads/finalpatientrightsrule.pdf

4 Centers for Disease Control and Prevention. (October 2002). Guideline for hand hygiene in health-care settings. *Morbidity and Mortality Weekly Report, 51*(RR-16), 1–45. (Level I)

5 World Health Organization. (2009). *WHO guidelines on hand hygiene in health care: First global patient safety challenge. Clean care is safer care.* Geneva, Switzerland: World Health Organization. (Level I)

6 The Joint Commission. (2012). Standard NPSG.07.01.01. *Comprehensive accreditation manual for hospitals: The official handbook.* Oakbrook Terrace, IL: The Joint Commission. (Level I)

7 The Joint Commission. (2012). Standard NPSG.01.01.01. *Comprehensive accreditation manual for hospitals: The official handbook.* Oakbrook Terrace, IL: The Joint Commission. (Level I)

8 The Joint Commission. (2012). Standard NPSG.03.04.01. *Comprehensive accreditation manual for hospitals: The official handbook.* Oakbrook Terrace, IL: The Joint Commission. (Level I)

9 Lynn-McHale Wiegand, D. (Ed.). (2011). *AACN procedure manual for critical care* (6th ed.). Philadelphia, PA: Saunders.

10 The Joint Commission. (2012). Standard UP.01.03.01. *Comprehensive accreditation manual for hospitals: The official handbook.* Oakbrook Terrace, IL: The Joint Commission. (Level I)

11 The Joint Commission. (2012). Standard NPSG.07.05.01. *Comprehensive accreditation manual for hospitals: The official handbook.* Oakbrook Terrace, IL: The Joint Commission. (Level I)

12 The Joint Commission. (2012). Standard RC.01.03.01. *Comprehensive accreditation manual for hospitals: The official handbook.* Oakbrook Terrace, IL: The Joint Commission. (Level I)

ADDITIONAL REFERENCES

Ben-Horin, S., et al. (2008). The composition of normal pericardial fluid and its implications for diagnosing pericardial effusions. *American Journal of Medicine, 118*(6), 636–640.

Woods, S., et al. (2010). *Cardiac nursing* (6th ed.). Philadelphia, PA: Lippincott Williams & Wilkins.

PERINEAL CARE

Perineal care, which includes care of the external genitalia and the anal area, should be performed during the daily bath and, if necessary, at bedtime and after urination and bowel movements. The procedure promotes cleanliness and prevents infection. It also removes irritating and odorous secretions, such as smegma, a cheeselike substance that collects under the foreskin of the penis. For the patient with perineal skin breakdown, frequent bathing followed by application of an ointment or cream aids healing.

Follow standard precautions when providing perineal care, and give great consideration to the patient's privacy.[1]

Equipment

Gloves ■ bath blanket ■ bathing supplies (disposable cleaning cloths, prepackaged bath product, or washcloths, a towel, and mild soap) ■ linen-saver pad ■ trash bag ■ Optional: facility-approved disinfectant, bath basin, toilet tissue, antiseptic soap, petroleum jelly, zinc oxide cream, vitamin A and D ointment, surgical pad.

After genital or rectal surgery, you may need to use sterile supplies, including sterile gloves, gauze, and cotton balls.

Preparation of equipment

Obtain ointment or cream as needed. If using a basin, fill it two-thirds full with warm water.

NURSING ALERT *Studies have shown that patients' bath basins are a reservoir for bacteria and may be a source of transmission of health care facility–acquired infections.[2] Follow your facility's policy regarding cleaning of bath basins. Many facilities require staff members to clean the basin with a facility-approved disinfectant before and after use.*

Implementation

■ Perform hand hygiene and put on gloves.[3,4,5]

■ Confirm the patient's identity using at least two patient identifiers according to facility policy.[6]

■ Gather the equipment at the patient's bedside and provide privacy.

■ Explain the procedure to the patient. Answer all questions *to decrease anxiety and increase cooperation.*

■ Adjust the bed to a comfortable working height *to prevent back strain,* and lower the head of the bed, if allowed.

■ Provide privacy and help the patient to a supine position. Place a linen-saver pad under the patient's buttocks *to protect the bed from stains and moisture.*

■ Drape the patient's legs, using a bath blanket, *to minimize exposure and embarrassment* and expose the genital area.

■ Wet the washcloth with warm water from a running spigot or the bath basin and apply mild soap. If using disposable cleaning cloths or a prepackaged bath product, open the packages and obtain the wet cloths.

For female patients

■ Ask the patient to bend her knees slightly and to spread her legs.

■ Separate her labia with one hand and wash with the other, using gentle downward strokes from the front to the back of the perineum *to prevent intestinal organisms from contaminating the urethra or vagina.* Avoid the area around the anus, and use a clean section of washcloth for each stroke by folding each used section inward. *This method prevents the spread of contaminated secretions or discharge.*

■ If using soap and water, wet a clean washcloth and rinse thoroughly from front to back *because soap residue can cause skin irritation.* Pat the area dry with a bath towel *because moisture can also cause skin irritation and discomfort.*

■ Turn the patient on her side to Sims' position, if possible, *to expose the anal area.*

■ Clean, rinse, and dry the anal area, starting at the posterior vaginal opening and wiping from front to back.

■ After cleaning the perineum, apply ointment or cream as needed (petroleum jelly, zinc oxide cream, or vitamin A and D ointment) *to prevent skin breakdown by providing a barrier between the skin and excretions.*

■ Reposition the patient comfortably. Remove the bath blanket and linen-saver pad, and then replace the bed linens.

■ If using a bath basin, clean it according to facility policy.

■ Dispose of soiled articles in the appropriate receptacle.[7]

■ Remove and discard your gloves and perform hand hygiene.[3,4,5]

■ Document the procedure.[8]

For male patients

■ Hold the shaft of the penis with one hand and wash with the other, beginning at the tip and working in a circular motion from the center to the periphery (as shown below) *to avoid introducing microorganisms into the urethra.* Use a clean section of washcloth for each stroke *to prevent the spread of contaminated secretions or discharge.*

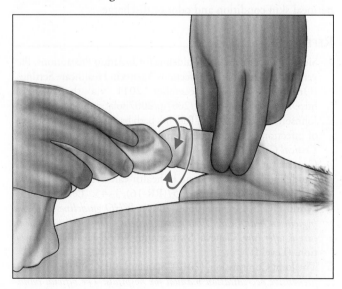

- If using soap and water, wet a clean washcloth and rinse thoroughly, using the same circular motion.
- For the uncircumcised patient, gently retract the foreskin and clean beneath it. If appropriate, rinse well but don't dry *because moisture provides lubrication and prevents friction when replacing the foreskin.* Replace the foreskin *to avoid constriction of the penis, which causes edema and tissue damage.*
- Wash the rest of the penis, using downward strokes toward the scrotum. If appropriate, rinse well and pat dry with a towel.
- Clean the top and sides of the scrotum; if appropriate, rinse thoroughly and pat dry. Handle the scrotum gently *to avoid causing discomfort.*
- Turn the patient on his side. Clean the bottom of the scrotum and the anal area. If appropriate, rinse well and pat dry.
- After cleaning the perineum, apply ointment or cream (petroleum jelly, zinc oxide cream, or vitamin A and D ointment), as needed, *to prevent skin breakdown by providing a barrier between the skin and excretions.*
- Reposition the patient comfortably. Remove the bath blanket and linen-saver pad, and then replace the bed linens.
- If using a bath basin, clean it according to facility policy.
- Dispose of soiled articles in the appropriate receptacle.[7]
- Remove your gloves and perform hand hygiene.[3,4,5]
- Document the procedure.[8]

Special considerations

- Give perineal care to a patient of the opposite gender in a matter-of-fact way *to minimize embarrassment.*
- If the patient is incontinent, first remove excess feces with toilet tissue. Then use a small amount of antiseptic soap and water *to clean the area.* Irrigate the perineal area with a peri bottle *to remove any remaining fecal matter.*

Documentation

Record perineal care and any special treatment in your notes. Document the need for continued treatment, if necessary. Describe perineal skin condition and odor or discharge.

REFERENCES

1 Siegel, J.D., et al. "2007 Guideline for Isolation Precautions: Preventing Transmission of Infectious Agents in Healthcare Settings" [Online]. Accessed December 2011 via the Web at http://www.cdc.gov/hicpac/2007ip/2007isolationprecautions.html
2 Johnson, D., et al. (2009). Patient's bath basins as potential sources of infection: A multicenter sampling study. *American Journal of Critical Care, 18*(1), 31–40. (Level III)
3 Centers for Disease Control and Prevention. (October 2002). Guideline for hand hygiene in health-care settings. *Morbidity and Mortality Weekly Report, 51*(RR-16), 1–45. (Level I)
4 World Health Organization. (2009). *WHO guidelines on hand hygiene in health care: First global patient safety challenge. Clean care is safer care.* Geneva, Switzerland: World Health Organization. (Level I)
5 The Joint Commission. (2012). Standard NPSG.07.01.01. *Comprehensive accreditation manual for hospitals: The official handbook.* Oakbrook Terrace, IL: The Joint Commission. (Level I)
6 The Joint Commission. (2012). Standard NPSG.01.01.01. *Comprehensive accreditation manual for hospitals: The official handbook.* Oakbrook Terrace, IL: The Joint Commission. (Level I)
7 Occupational Safety and Health Administration. "Bloodborne Pathogens, Standard Number 1910.1030" [Online]. Accessed October 2011 via the Web at http://www.osha.gov/pls/oshaweb/owadisp.show_document?p_table=STANDARDS&p_id=10051
8 The Joint Commission. (2012). Standard RC.01.03.01. *Comprehensive accreditation manual for hospitals: The official handbook.* Oakbrook Terrace, IL: The Joint Commission. (Level I)

ADDITIONAL REFERENCES

Craven, R.F., & Hirnle, C.J. (2012). *Fundamentals of nursing: Human health and function* (7th ed.). Philadelphia, PA: Lippincott Williams & Wilkins.

McGucklin, M., et al. (2008). Interventional patient hygiene model: Infection control and nursing share responsibility for patient safety, *American Journal of Infection Control 36*(1): 59–62.

PERIPHERALLY INSERTED CENTRAL CATHETER USE

A peripherally inserted central catheter (PICC) is a catheter that's inserted percutaneously into a peripheral vein. The catheter tip resides in the lower one-third of the superior vena cava, at the junction of the superior vena cava and right atrium. PICC placement is indicated for intermediate to long-term IV access for the administration of antibiotics, pain medications, chemotherapy or other vesicants, parenteral nutrition or other hyperosmolar solutions, or blood products. The early use of PICCS may also spare peripheral veins, limit the pain of repeated needle sticks, and help avoid complications that may occur with a central venous (CV) access device. PICCs are also used for patients receiving home care.

PICCs are made of silicone or polyurethane and vary in diameter and length. They're available in single, double, and triple-lumen versions, with and without valves. The type and size of PICC used depends on the patient's size and anatomic measurements as well as the therapy required; the patient receiving PICC therapy must also have a peripheral vein large enough to accept an introducer needle and catheter.

Most PICCs are manufactured with smooth, rounded tips to reduce trauma to the vein wall during insertion. Selecting a catheter length that's as close to the desired patient length measurement as possible avoids the need to trim the PICC (Groshong PICCs can't be trimmed). The catheter length should be subtracted from the total length of the PICC, with any extra length left outside the insertion site, safely secured.

Most PICCs have a preloaded stylet wire inside the catheter to add stiffness to the soft catheter, easing its advancement through the vein. The stylet terminates 1 to 2 cm away from the catheter tip. If the catheter length does require trimming, the stylet must be withdrawn and repositioned 1 to 2 cm from the cut end. The stylet should never be cut; it's removed after insertion.

PICC devices are easier to insert than other CV devices. A single catheter may be used for the entire course of therapy, resulting in greater convenience and reduced cost. A nurse trained in PICC insertion may perform the procedure if the state nurse practice act permits it, although the nurse may have to demonstrate competence every year.

Possible veins for PICC insertion include the basilic, median cubital, cephalic, and brachial. When selecting a site, avoid areas that are painful on palpation; veins compromised by bruising, infiltration, phlebitis, sclerosing, or cording; and, in patients with stage 4 or 5 chronic kidney disease, forearm and upper arm veins that could be used for vascular access. In a patient who has had breast surgery with axillary node dissection, don't use arm veins on the affected side; also avoid veins on the affected side in stroke patients, those undergoing radiation therapy, and those with lymphedema.[1] Use an ultrasound device to guide insertion *to increase your rate of success and reduce the risk for insertion-related complications.*[2] (See *Bedside ultrasound for PICC insertion.*) When inserted, the catheter is advanced until it reaches the superior vena cava near the junction of the right atrium.[2] To help prevent catheter-related bloodstream infections, use maximum sterile barriers during insertion.[3]

PICCs may be inserted with a through-the-introducer or modified Seldinger technique. The procedure below discusses the modified Seldinger technique.

PICC infusion and associated site care, including flushing of the catheter, may be performed by a nurse or appropriately trained parent or guardian. A PICC dressing should be changed at least every 7 days if a transparent semipermeable dressing is used.[2,4] If the patient is diaphoretic or the site is bleeding or oozing, a gauze dressing should be used instead of a semipermeable dressing; gauze dressings should be changed every 2 days. Replace either dressing if it becomes damp, loosened, or visibly soiled.[2,3]

PICCs are often used for administration of drugs, such as opioids, analgesics, antibiotics, parenteral nutrition, and chemotherapy. To prevent catheter-related bloodstream infections, wipe the injection surface with alcohol using friction and let it air-dry each time you access it.[3]

PICCs are removed when therapy is complete, if the catheter becomes damaged or broken and can't be repaired, if the patient has discomfort and pain, or, possibly, if the catheter becomes occluded. Measure the catheter after you remove it to ensure that the catheter has been removed intact.[5]

Equipment

For insertion
PICC insertion kit ▪ PICC catheter ▪ PICC insertion checklist ▪ chlorhexidine swabs ▪ sterile and clean measuring tape ▪ vial of normal saline solution ▪ syringes and needles of appropriate size ▪ sterile gauze pads ▪ linen-saver pad ▪ sterile drapes ▪ disposable skin marker ▪ tourniquet ▪ sterile marker ▪ sterile labels ▪ gloves ▪ sterile gloves ▪ sterile gown ▪ mask ▪ protective eyewear ▪ head cover ▪ 1% lidocaine without epinephrine ▪ catheter securement device, sterile tape, or sterile surgical strips ▪ sterile transparent semipermeable dressing ▪ Optional: bedside ultrasound

---

Bedside ultrasound for PICC insertion

Although special training is required, the use of bedside ultrasound helps provide safer, more efficient insertion of a peripherally inserted central catheter (PICC). Since the introduction of ultrasound, placing PICCs using visualization and palpation alone is rare.

Advantages of using ultrasound include:
▪ the ability to locate the exact position of veins that are neither visible nor palpable and detect possible anatomic variations or thrombosis in the vessel
▪ a successful cannulation rate of more than 90% on the first attempt
▪ the possibility of inserting a PICC in a location away from the antecubital fossa, which can limit or eliminate complications such as mechanical phlebitis
▪ a reduction in the complications related to traumatic placement.

---

equipment, sterile and clean disposable ultrasound probe cover, locator system, echogenic needle, heparin (10 units/mL).

Commercially prepared PICC insertion kits contain most of the equipment required to insert a PICC.

For flushing
Gloves ▪ syringe prefilled with appropriate flush solution[6] (heparinized saline or preservative-free normal saline solution as ordered) ▪ antiseptic pads (alcohol, tincture of iodine, or chlorhexidine-based).

For dressing change
Gloves ▪ sterile gloves ▪ masks ▪ sterile drape ▪ 2% chlorhexidine swabs ▪ transparent semipermeable dressing ▪ sterile disposable tape measure ▪ sterile tape, sterile surgical strips, or securement device ▪ label ▪ Optional: adhesive remover, chlorhexidine sponge disk, povidone-iodine swabs, 70% alcohol swabs, skin preparation adhesive, 2″ × 2″ gauze pads.

Many facilities stock a commercially prepared or facility-prepared sterile dressing change kit that contains the necessary supplies.

For drug administration
Patient's medication record ▪ gloves ▪ medication to be administered in an IV container with administration set (for infusion) or in a syringe (for IV bolus) ▪ two 10-mL syringes prefilled with normal saline solution ▪ heparin flush ▪ alcohol wipes.

For removal
Gloves ▪ linen-saver pad ▪ sterile occlusive dressing ▪ antiseptic ointment ▪ tape ▪ measuring tape ▪ warm, moist pack ▪ Optional: personal protective equipment.

Implementation
- Verify the doctor's order.
- Perform hand hygiene.[7,8,9]
- Confirm the patient's identity using at least two patient identifiers according to your facility's policy.[10]
- Explain the procedure to the patient and answer all questions *to decrease anxiety and increase cooperation.*

Inserting a PICC
- Make sure the doctor has obtained an informed consent and that it's documented in the medical record.[11,12]
- Conduct a preprocedure verification process *to make sure that all relevant documentation, related information, and equipment are available and correctly identified to the patient's identifiers.*[13]
- Check the patient's allergy status *to prevent anaphylaxis.*
- If you're using ultrasound, place a disposable cover on the bedside ultrasound probe. Then place a disposable tourniquet on the patient's selected upper arm and examine it for appropriate veins. Mark the expected insertion site with a disposable skin marker and remove the tourniquet.
- Using the clean measuring tape, determine catheter tip placement (the spot at which the catheter tip will rest after insertion).
- For placement in the superior vena cava, measure the distance from the insertion site to the shoulder and from the shoulder to the sternal notch (as shown below).

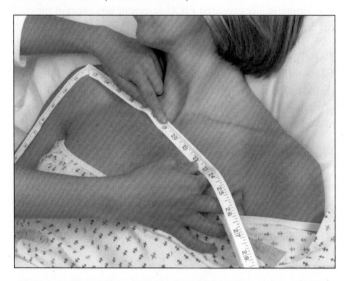

- Measure the midarm circumference of the selected extremity *to provide a baseline measurement.*
- Have the patient lie in a supine position with her arm at a 90-degree angle to her body. Place a linen-saver pad under her arm.
- Wash your hands for 60 seconds with antimicrobial soap and put on a surgical head cover, a gown, protective eyewear, and a mask.[14,15]
- Prepare a sterile field using a sterile drape and set up the PICC supplies on the sterile field.
- Put on sterile gloves.[14,15]

- Prepare the lidocaine and normal saline flush syringes. Label all medications, medication containers, and other solutions on and off the sterile field using sterile marker and labels.[16]
- If using ultrasound, ensure that a sterile probe cover is on the ultrasound probe *to prevent cross-contamination between patients.* If using a locator system, follow the manufacturer's directions regarding its use.
- Conduct a time-out immediately before starting the procedure *to determine that the correct patient, site, positioning, and procedure are identified, and confirm, as applicable, that relevant information and necessary equipment are available.*[17]
- Prepare the insertion site by scrubbing with chlorhexidine swabs using a back-and-forth motion for about 30 seconds. Allow the area to dry. Don't touch the intended insertion site.[2]
- Place a full body drape over the patient from head to toe. Cover everything except the insertion site.
- Place caps on the hub of each lumen of the catheter and prime each port. Always prepare the catheter according to the manufacturer's recommendations.
- If it's necessary to trim the PICC, pull the stylet wire back from the catheter tip. Using the sterile measuring tape, cut the distal end of the catheter to the appropriate premeasured length (as shown below).[18] Follow the manufacturer's recommendations and guidelines using the cutting equipment provided by the manufacturer. Then advance the stylet to 1 to 2 cm from the tip of the catheter and bend the stylet wire at the hub *to prevent movement of the wire, which could result in trauma upon insertion.* Place the catheter on the sterile field.

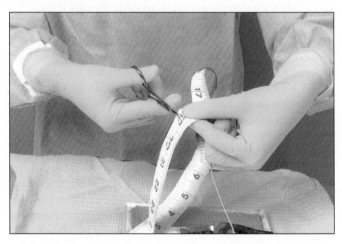

- Remove and discard your gloves. Then apply the tourniquet again about 4″ (10 cm) above the antecubital fossa.
- Put on a new pair of sterile gloves. Then place a sterile drape under the patient's arm, and drape the arm with a large sterile drape. Drop a sterile 4″ × 4″ gauze pad over the tourniquet.
- If using ultrasound, apply sterile ultrasound gel to the probe and use it to locate the appropriate vein.
- Anesthetize the area with lidocaine *to provide for patient comfort during insertion.*
- Perform a venipuncture using the appropriate needle. (An echogenic needle is used with ultrasound guidance.)

- Advance a guide wire 2″ to 4″ (5 to 10 cm) through the needle and secure it *to prevent embolization.*
- Remove the needle. If necessary, make a small skin nick at the insertion site *to facilitate the advancement of the introducer/dilator.*
- Thread the introducer/dilator over the guide wire until you're sure the tip is well within the vein. After successful vein entry, you should see a blood return.
- Carefully remove the guide wire and advance the introducer the rest of the way into the vein.
- Remove the dilator while holding the introducer still. *To minimize blood loss,* try applying finger pressure on the vein just beyond the distal end of the introducer sheath or place a finger over the opening of the introducer.
- Using sterile forceps, insert the catheter through the introducer into the vein and advance it 2″ to 4″.
- Remove the tourniquet using a sterile 4″ × 4″ gauze pad.
- If using a locator system, activate it now and follow the manufacturer's directions. Advance the catheter at a slow, steady pace until it's in position at the premeasured length.
- Grasp the tabs of the introducer sheath, and flex them toward its distal end *to split the sheath.* Peel the introducer while pulling away from the insertion site.
- Check for a blood return and flush the catheter with normal saline solution. If you're heparin locking the catheter, instill 5 mL of 10 units/mL heparin or follow your facility's policy.[19]
- Clean the site and secure the catheter with a catheter securement device, sterile tape, or sterile surgical strips.[20]
- If necessary, apply a sterile 2″ × 2″ gauze pad directly over the site and a sterile transparent semipermeable dressing over the gauze pad.[4] Leave this dressing in place for 24 hours.
- Label the dressing with the date, time, and your initials.[4]
- Dispose of used items properly.[3,21]
- Remove personal protective equipment and perform hand hygiene.[7,8,9]
- Obtain a chest X-ray *to verify proper placement.*[2]

Flushing a PICC
- Perform hand hygiene and put on gloves.[7,8,9]
- Thoroughly disinfect the needleless injection port with an antiseptic pad using friction and allow it to dry.[3,22]
- Attach the syringe of preservative-free normal saline solution, making sure that the clamp on the PICC is closed *to prevent accidental air embolism.*
- Open the clamp and slowly aspirate until a brisk blood return is obtained.[6,23]
- Slowly inject preservative-free normal saline solution into the catheter.
- Remove and discard the syringe and clamp the catheter *to prevent backflow of blood and potential clot formation.*[6,23]
- Administer IV fluid through the catheter as prescribed or proceed with locking the device.
- Thoroughly disinfect the needleless injection port with an antiseptic pad using friction and allow it to dry.[3,22]
- Attach the syringe of locking solution (heparin flush or preservative-free normal saline solution according to your facility's

policy) to the needleless injection port and slowly inject the solution into the catheter.[22,23]
- Clamp the device according to the needleless device used. For a positive-pressure needleless device, disconnect the syringe and then clamp the catheter. For a negative-pressure needleless device, clamp the catheter while maintaining pressure on the syringe plunger and then disconnect the syringe. For a neutral needleless device, clamp the catheter before or after removing the syringe.[23]
- Discard the syringe and other used supplies in the appropriate receptacles.[21]
- Remove and discard your gloves and perform hand hygiene.[8,9,10]
- Document the procedure.[7,24,25]

Performing a PICC dressing change
- Perform hand hygiene and put on a mask.[7,8,9]
- Position the patient with his arm extended away from his body at a 45- to 90-degree angle so that the insertion site is below heart level *to reduce the risk of air embolism.*
- Ask the patient to put on a mask or turn his head away from the site.
- Put on gloves, and remove the old dressing by holding your left thumb on the catheter and stretching the dressing parallel to the skin. Repeat the last step with your right thumb holding the catheter. Free the remaining section of the dressing from the catheter by peeling toward the insertion site from the distal end to the proximal end to prevent catheter dislodgment. If necessary, use adhesive remover or alcohol pads *to assist with loosening the old dressing.*
- Remove the tape and surgical strips or securement device that's anchoring the catheter.
- Temporarily secure the catheter with piece of tape *to prevent catheter migration.*
- Assess the site and skin for signs of inflammation or infection (redness, drainage, tenderness, ecchymosis, palpable cord, and streaking) and assess the arm for swelling, pain, or warmth. Check collateral circulation.
- Check the integrity of the catheter and hub *to detect any defects such as cracks or splits.*
- Remove your gloves and perform hand hygiene.[7,8,9]
- Using sterile technique open and prepare the necessary equipment (sterile dressing change kit, transparent semipermeable dressing, and securement tape or device).
- Put on sterile gloves.
- Clean the area thoroughly with chlorhexidine using a back-and-forth scrubbing motion for 30 seconds and allow it to fully dry *to be most effective against bacterial growth.* Alternatively, you may clean with povidone-iodine or 70% alcohol if indicated by your facility's policy.
- Apply a "window frame" of skin preparation solution around the catheter site, if needed, *to help the dressing stay in place.* If you plan on placing a chlorhexidine sponge at the insertion site, don't apply the skin protectant to the area the sponge will cover.
- Before redressing the site, use a sterile tape measure to measure the external length of the catheter from hub to skin entry *to ensure that the catheter hasn't migrated since originally inserted.* Compare

the measurement with the baseline external length documented at the time of insertion. Report a discrepancy of more than 2 cm to the doctor.

■ Apply the catheter securement device or use sterile tape or sterile surgical strips to secure the catheter. Make sure that any external catheter is looped away from the antecubital fossa and secured with tape before applying the dressing. *This precaution helps prevent kinking of the catheter during infusions.*

■ If applicable, place a chlorhexidine sponge disk at the catheter base.[3] To facilitate future removal, position the disk with the catheter resting on or near the radial slit of the disk. The edges of the slit must touch *to maximize antimicrobial action.* Always follow the manufacturer's directions.

NURSING ALERT *Don't use chlorhexidine sponge disks on patients younger than 2 months old or on patients sensitive to chlorhexidine* because the disk has constant contact with the skin.

■ Secure the chlorhexidine sponge disk with a transparent semipermeable dressing that has a high moisture vapor transmission rate. There should be continuous contact between the skin and the transparent semipermeable dressing or chlorhexidine sponge disk. You may instead use a sterile 4″ × 4″ gauze dressing in place of a transparent semipermeable dressing.[3,4]

■ Secure the tubing to the edge of the dressing *to prevent pulling and inadvertent removal of the tubing.*

■ Label dressing with the date, the time, and your initials.[4]

■ Discard supplies in the appropriate receptacle.

■ Remove your gloves and mask and perform hand hygiene.[7,8,9]

■ Document the procedure.[24,25]

Administering drugs using a PICC

■ Avoid distractions and interruptions when preparing and administering medications *to prevent medication errors.*[26]

■ Perform hand hygiene and put on gloves.[7,8,9]

■ If you'll be infusing medication, insert the administration set spike into the IV container, attach the needleless adapter, and prime the line. If you'll be giving an IV injection, fill a syringe with the prescribed drug or obtain the unit dose medication.

■ Verify the medication order, confirming that you have the right patient, medication, route, dose, and time of administration.[27]

■ If your facility uses a bar code scanning system, scan your identification badge, the patient's identification bracelet, and the medication's bar code, or follow the procedure for your facility's bar code system.

■ Discuss with the patient the medication to be administered, and answer his questions.

■ Clean the injection surface with alcohol using friction and allowing it to dry.[3,22]

■ Clamp the extension tubing, and connect the saline-filled syringe to the tubing.

■ Release the clamp and aspirate slowly *to verify blood return.*[6,23]

■ Then flush with 5 mL of normal saline solution *to clear the blood from the catheter.*

NURSING ALERT *Don't force the flush solution into the tubing* because the catheter may be occluded.

■ Remove the saline syringe.

■ Clean the injection surface with alcohol again using friction and allow it to dry; then administer the drug.[3,22]

Administering IV bolus injections

■ Insert the syringe with the medication for the IV bolus injection into the injection port of the PICC.

■ Inject the medication at the required rate. Then remove the syringe from the injection port.

■ Clean the injection port with alcohol using friction and allow it to dry.[3,22] Attach the second saline-filled syringe and flush with 5 mL of normal saline solution. (Remember to flush with normal saline solution between infusions of incompatible drugs or fluids.) Remove the syringe.

■ Clean the injection surface with alcohol using friction and allow it to dry.[3,22] Insert and inject the heparin flush solution (5 mL of 10 units/mL heparin) according to your facility's policy, *to prevent clotting in the device.*[22,23]

■ Close the clamp on the extension tubing.

■ Dispose of the equipment,[21] remove and discard your gloves, and perform hand hygiene.[7,8,9]

■ Document the procedure.[24,25]

Administering an infusion

■ Insert the administration set attached to the infusion bag.

■ Open the infusion line, and adjust the flow rate as necessary.

■ Infuse the medication for the prescribed length of time; then disconnect the tubing and clean the injection surface with alcohol using friction, and flush again with 5 mL of normal saline solution from the second 10-mL syringe. (Remember to flush with normal saline solution between infusions of incompatible drugs or fluids.) Remove the syringe.

■ Clean the injection surface with alcohol using friction and allow it to dry.[3,25] Insert and inject the heparin flush solution (5 mL of 10 units/mL heparin) according to your facility's policy, *to prevent clotting in the device.*[22,23]

■ Close the clamp on the tubing.

■ Dispose of the equipment,[21] remove and discard your gloves, and perform hand hygiene.[7,8,9]

■ Document the procedure.[24,25]

Removing a PICC

■ Perform hand hygiene and put on gloves and other personal protective equipment as indicated.[7,8,9]

■ Place a linen-saver pad under the patient's arm.

■ Remove the tape holding the extension tubing. Open two sterile gauze pads on a clean, flat surface.

■ Stabilize the catheter at the hub with one hand. Without dislodging the catheter, use your other hand to gently remove the dressing by pulling it toward the insertion site (as shown below).

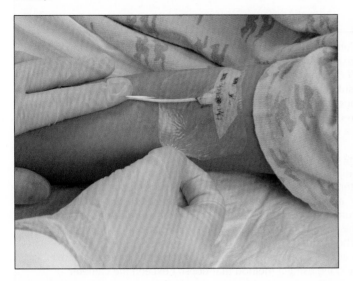

■ Next, withdraw the catheter with smooth, gentle pressure in small increments (as shown below). It should come out easily.

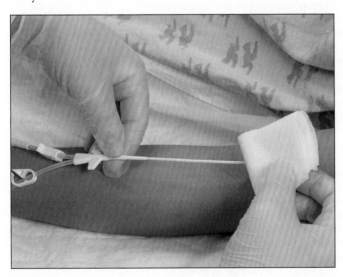

■ If you feel resistance, stop. Apply slight tension to the catheter by taping it down. Apply a warm, moist pack, and then try to remove the catheter again in a few minutes. If you still feel resistance after the second attempt, notify the doctor for further instructions.

■ When you successfully remove the catheter, apply manual pressure to the site with a sterile gauze pad until hemostasis is achieved.[28]

■ Measure and inspect the catheter (as shown below). If any part has broken off during removal, notify the doctor immediately, and monitor the patient for signs of distress.

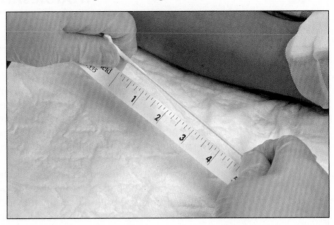

■ Cover the site with antiseptic ointment and a sterile occlusive dressing (as shown below).[28]

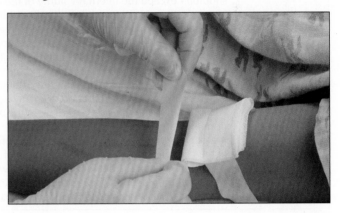

■ Dispose of used items properly. Remove and discard gloves and perform hand hygiene.[7,8,9]
■ Document the procedure.[24,25]

Special considerations

■ PICC therapy works best when introduced early in treatment; it shouldn't be considered a last resort for patients with sclerotic or repeatedly punctured veins.
■ Obtain a chest X-ray to confirm proper placement of the catheter tip before administering any IV solution.
■ Confirm a venous blood return and catheter patency before initiating any infusion.
■ For a patient receiving intermittent PICC therapy, flush the catheter with 5 mL of normal saline solution. If the catheter is to be heparin locked, instill 5 mL of heparin (10 units/mL) after each use according to your facility's policy. For catheters that aren't being used routinely, flush nonvalved catheters at least every 24 hours and valved catheters at least weekly.[19]
■ You can use a declotting agent to clear a clotted PICC, but make sure you read the manufacturer's recommendations first and follow facility policy. If you're still unable to flush the PICC, notify the doctor. (See *Troubleshooting a PICC*, page 570).

TROUBLESHOOTING

Troubleshooting a PICC

PROBLEM	INTERVENTION
Inability to flush or draw blood	■ Examine the peripherally inserted central catheter (PICC) *to ensure that clamps (if used or as part of extension tubing) are open and to confirm the catheter isn't kinked.* ■ If sutures are present, make sure they aren't causing obstruction. ■ Look for catheter occlusion, which may result from the patient's position; external or internal mechanical obstruction (such as a kink in the catheter under the dressing, catheter migration, precipitations, or thrombosis); nonthrombotic factors such as drug precipitates; thrombotic factors such as fibrin deposits or blood clots; catheter pinch-off resulting from an area of compression between the first rib and clavicle; or the medication itself and its compatibilities. ■ Note when the catheter was last functioning and when the last blood return was documented. ■ Extend or raise the patient's arm over his head. *This may help move the catheter away from the vessel wall.* If the catheter remains positional, notify the doctor. An X-ray may be needed to determine tip placement. ■ If you suspect occlusion from precipitation, attempt to aspirate to clear the catheter. If successful, flush the catheter with preservative-free 0.9% sodium chloride saline between all medications. If unsuccessful, obtain a doctor's order for an agent to treat the precipitate; consult with the pharmacy and check facility policy on who may perform this procedure. The instilled volume of the solution to clear precipitates shouldn't exceed the internal volume of the catheter to avoid pushing precipitate into the bloodstream. Installation, aspiration, and flushing should be done using a method that doesn't exceed the catheter manufacturer's maximum pressure limits *to avoid line rupture.* ■ If occlusion results from thrombosis, obtain a doctor's order for a thrombolytic declotting agent; follow the manufacturer's recommendations and check facility policy for who may administer the declotting agent.
Infiltration or extravasation (suspected or actual)	■ Always assess along the path of the catheter when performing IV site assessments. ■ Assess the extent of infiltration or extravasation using a standardized scale.[29] ■ Discontinue the infusion and remove the administration set but don't remove the PICC. Aspirate fluid from the catheter using a small syringe.[29] ■ Notify the doctor of the extravasation or infiltration; report the solution or medications infusing at the time of the complication, the estimated volume of fluid that escaped into the tissue,[29] and the site's appearance. ■ Obtain a doctor's order, in collaboration with the pharmacy, for an agent to treat the infiltration or extravasation if needed. Treatment depends on the properties of the infiltrated medication or solution, the manufacturer's guidelines for that agent, and the severity of the problem.
Phlebitis	■ Encourage limitation of movement at the PICC site. ■ Apply warm, moist soaks to the extremity *to ease discomfort.* ■ If signs and symptoms increase or if streak formation or a palpable cord is present, notify the doctor. ■ If pain at the access site and erythema or edema accompany the phlebitis, the PICC may need to be removed.
Catheter PICC migration (suspected or actual)	■ Catheter migration may result from excessive sneezing, coughing, or vomiting. Suspect migration of distally if the patient complains of chest pain or hears a noise during flushing of the PICC. ■ If migration is internal or external PICC migration is greater than 2 cm, notify the doctor. ■ Obtain an order for an X-ray to confirm tip placement. ■ External migration may require replacement of a PICC or a change in therapy. ■ Internal migration requires manipulation or removal.
Leaking or damaged catheter	■ Clamp and secure the catheter *to prevent migration and possible embolization of a catheter fragment.* Catheter embolization is an emergency and may require surgical intervention. ■ Determine the extent and location of damage. ■ A registered nurse competent in repairing the PICC line may perform this procedure by using the manufacturer's repair kit and guidelines. Note that not all PICC manufacturers provide repair kits; repair with other materials may lead to catheter separation and migration or embolization. ■ Inability to repair the PICC necessitates its removal. ■ Report a defective catheter according to your facility's policy.
Bleeding at Mild insertion site	■ Apply a gauze dressing after initial placement of the PICC, and change the first dressing in 24 hours. bleeding at the site may occur for the first 24 hours after PICC placement. ■ Limit movement of the extremity using an arm board as necessary. ■ If bleeding increases or persists past the first 24 hours, notify the doctor.

■ Assess the catheter insertion site through the transparent semipermeable dressing every shift. Look at the catheter and cannula pathway, and check for bleeding, redness, drainage, and swelling. Ask if the patient is having pain associated with therapy. Although oozing is common for the first 24 hours after insertion, excessive bleeding after that should be evaluated.

■ Patients who require repeated computerized axial tomography scans with contrast may have a PICC inserted that has been specially developed to withstand the high pressures of power injectors.

■ Chlorhexidine is the preferred skin disinfectant *because it has residual antibacterial activity that persists for hours after application*. Providone-iodine and 70% alcohol are also acceptable disinfectants.[4]

■ Application of catheter stabilization devices vary. Always follow the manufacturer's instructions.

■ If the dressing becomes damp, loose, or soiled, change it immediately. Maintaining a clean, dry, and occlusive dressing is important *to protect the catheter insertion site and reduce the risk for infection*.

■ If the catheter is inadvertently withdrawn by a significant amount during a dressing change, measure from the exit site to the hub, and reapply a sterile dressing. Notify the doctor, and prepare for a chest X-ray to determine the position of the PICC tip.

■ When administering flush solution or medication, always use a 10-mL syringe or larger *to prevent catheter rupture*.

■ If a portion of the catheter breaks during removal, immediately apply a tourniquet to the upper arm, close to the axilla, *to prevent advancement of the catheter piece into the right atrium*. Then check the patient's radial pulse. If you don't detect a pulse, the tourniquet is too tight; loosen it enough to detect a pulse. Keep the tourniquet in place until an X-ray can be obtained, the doctor is notified, and surgical retrieval is attempted.

■ After removal, change the PICC site dressing, and assess the site every 24 hours until the site has healed completely.[28]

Patient teaching

If the patient will be discharged with a PICC line, teach the patient or family members the proper technique for flushing the line. If possible, allow time for return demonstrations of the procedure.

Complications

PICC therapy causes fewer and less severe complications than conventional CV access devices, with catheter breakage on removal is among most common complication. Catheter tip migration may occur with vigorous flushing; patients receiving chemotherapy are most vulnerable to this complication *because of frequent nausea and vomiting and subsequent changes in intrathoracic pressure*. Catheter occlusion is also a relatively common complication.

Because infection is always a risk with a PICC, watch for such signs as swelling, redness or drainage at the site, or increased temperature.

Complications during removal include venospasm, thrombosis, and catheter breakage. If venospasm and thrombosis occur,

you'll feel resistance during removal; follow the appropriate interventions covered earlier in this entry if you encounter resistance or suspect catheter breakage during removal.

Air embolism is always a potential risk, but it poses less danger in PICC therapy than in traditional CV access devices *because the line is inserted below heart level*. To help prevent air embolism during removal, make sure to apply pressure to the site until bleeding stops.

Documentation

Document the entire procedure, including any problems that occur. For insertion, document the size, length, and type of catheter as well as the insertion location. Record the external length of the catheter at the time of placement. Note the lot number and manufacturer. Document any unexpected outcomes and your interventions.

For dressing change documentation, include the condition and length of the external catheter, the appearance of the site, and the patient's response, including any reports of pain or tenderness. Record the date and the time of the dressing change, any unexpected outcomes, and your interventions.

Document PICC removal interventions and the condition, length, and site of the catheter. Record all patient and family teaching and the patient's response.

REFERENCES

1 Standard 33. Site selection. Infusion nursing standards of practice. (2011). *Journal of Infusion Nursing, 34*(1S), S40–S43. (Level I)

2 Standard 35. Vascular access site preparation and device placement. Infusion nursing standards of practice. (2011). *Journal of Infusion Nursing, 34*(1S), S44–S45. (Level I)

3 O'Grady, N.P., et al. (2011). "Guidelines for the Prevention of Intravascular Catheter-Related Infections" [Online]. Accessed November 2011 via the Web at http://www.cdc.gov/hicpac/pdf/guidelines/bsi-guidelines-2011.pdf (Level I)

4 Standard 46. Vascular access device site care and dressing changes. Infusion nursing standards of practice. (2011). *Journal of Infusion Nursing, 34*(1S), S63–S65. (Level I)

5 Standard 44. Vascular access device removal. Infusion nursing standards of practice. (2011). *Journal of Infusion Nursing, 34*(1S), S57–S59. (Level I)

6 Standard 45. Flushing and locking. Infusion nursing standards of practice. (2011). *Journal of Infusion Nursing, 34*(1S), S59–S63. (Level I)

7 Centers for Disease Control and Prevention. (October 2002). Guideline for hand hygiene in health-care settings. *Morbidity and Mortality Weekly Report, 51*(RR-16), 1–45. (Level I)

8 World Health Organization. (2009). *WHO guidelines on hand hygiene in health care: First global patient safety challenge. Clean care is safer care.* Geneva, Switzerland: World Health Organization. (Level I)

9 The Joint Commission. (2012). Standard NPSG.07.01.01. *Comprehensive accreditation manual for hospitals: The official handbook.* Oakbrook Terrace, IL: The Joint Commission. (Level I))

10 The Joint Commission. (2012). Standard NPSG.01.01.01. *Comprehensive accreditation manual for hospitals: The official handbook.* Oakbrook Terrace, IL: The Joint Commission. (Level I)

11 Standard 12. Informed consent. Infusion nursing standards of practice. (2011). *Journal of Infusion Nursing, 34*(1S), S17. (Level I)

12 The Joint Commission. (2012). Standard RI.01.03.01. *Comprehensive accreditation manual for hospitals: The official handbook.* Oakbrook Terrace, IL: The Joint Commission. (Level I)

13 The Joint Commission. (2012). Standard UP.01.01.01. *Comprehensive accreditation manual for hospitals: The official handbook.* Oakbrook Terrace, IL: The Joint Commission. (Level I)

14 Standard 18. Infection prevention. Infusion nursing standards of practice. (2011). *Journal of Infusion Nursing, 34*(1S), S25. (Level I)

15 Standard 19. Hand hygiene. Infusion nursing standards of practice. (2011). *Journal of Infusion Nursing, 34*(1S), S26. (Level I)

16 The Joint Commission. (2012). Standard NPSG.03.04.01. *Comprehensive accreditation manual for hospitals: The official handbook.* Oakbrook Terrace, IL: The Joint Commission. (Level I)

17 The Joint Commission. (2012). Standard UP.01.03.01. *Comprehensive accreditation manual for hospitals: The official handbook.* Oakbrook Terrace, IL: The Joint Commission. (Level I)

18 Standard 32. Vascular access device selection: PICC. Infusion nursing standards of practice. (2011). *Journal of Infusion Nursing, 34*(1S), S38. (Level I)

19 Infusion Nurses Society. (2008). *Flushing protocols.* Boston, MA: Infusion Nurses Society. (Level I)

20 Standard 36. Vascular access device stabilization. Infusion nursing standards of practice. (2011). *Journal of Infusion Nursing, 34*(1S), S46. (Level I)

21 Standard 22. Safe handling and disposal of sharps, hazardous materials, and hazardous waste. Infusion nursing standards of practice. (2011). *Journal of Infusion Nursing, 34*(1S), S28. (Level I)

22 The Joint Commission. (2012). Standard RC.01.03.01. *Comprehensive accreditation manual for hospitals: The official handbook.* Oakbrook Terrace, IL: The Joint Commission. (Level I)

23 Standard 14. Documentation. Infusion nursing standards of practice. (2011). *Journal of Infusion Nursing, 34*(1S), S20. (Level I)

24 Standard 27. Needleless connectors. Infusion nursing standards of practice. (2011). *Journal of Infusion Nursing, 34*(1S), S32–S33. (Level I)

25 Nettina, S.M. (2010). *Lippincott manual of nursing practice* (9th ed.). Philadelphia, PA: Lippincott Williams & Wilkins.

26 Standard 61. Parenteral medication and solution administration. Infusion nursing standards of practice. (2011). *Journal of Infusion Nursing, 34*(1S), S86–S87. (Level I)

27 The Joint Commission. (2012). Standard MM.06.01.01. *Comprehensive accreditation manual for hospitals: The official handbook.* Oakbrook Terrace, IL: The Joint Commission. (Level I)

28 Lynn-McHale Wiegand, D. (Ed.). (2011). *AACN procedure manual for critical care* (6th ed.). Philadelphia, PA: Saunders.

29 Standard 48. Infiltration and extravasation. Infusion nursing standards of practice. (2011). *Journal of Infusion Nursing, 34*(1S), S66–S68. (Level I)

ADDITIONAL REFERENCES

Alexander, M., et al. (Eds.). (2010). *Infusion nursing: An evidence-based approach* (3rd ed.). Philadelphia, PA: Elsevier.

Association for Vascular Access. "Use of Modified Seldinger Technique for Peripherally Inserted Central Catheter Placement by Registered Nurses" [Online]. Accessed October 2011 via the Web at http:// www.avainfo.org/website/download.asp?id=193200

Association for Vascular Access. "Use of Real-time Imaging Modalities for Placement of Central Venous Access Devices" [Online]. Accessed October 2011 via the Web at http://www.avainfo.org/website/download.asp?id=193196

Camp-Sorrell, D. (Ed.). (2010). *Access device guidelines: Recommendations for nursing practice and education* (3rd ed.). Pittsburgh, PA: Oncology Nursing Society.

Hockley, S.J., et al. (2007). Efficacy of the CathRite system to guide bedside placement of peripherally inserted central venous catheters in critically ill patients: A pilot study. *Critical Care Resuscitation, 9*(3), 251–255.

Infusion Nurses Society. (2011). *Policies and procedures for infusion nursing* (4th ed.). Boston, MA: Infusion Nurses Society. (Level I)

Mimoz, O., et al. (2007). Chlorhexidine-based antiseptic solution vs. alcohol-based povidone-iodine for central venous catheter care. *Archives of Internal Medicine, 167*(19), 2066–2072.

Moureau, N.L. (2008). Using ultrasound to guide PICC and peripheral cannula insertion. *Nursing, 38*(10), 20–21.

Nichols, I., & Humphrey, J.P. (2008). The efficacy of upper arm placement of peripherally inserted central catheters using bedside ultrasound and microintroducer technique. *Journal of Infusion Nursing, 13*(3), 165–176.

Occupational Safety and Health Administration. "Bloodborne Pathogens, Standard Number 1910.1030" [Online]. Accessed October 2011 via the Web at http://www.osha.gov/pls/oshaweb/owadisp.show_document?p_table=STANDARDS&p_id=10051 (Level I)

Periard, D., et al. (2008). Randomized controlled trial of peripherally inserted central catheters vs. peripheral catheters for middle duration in-hospital intravenous therapy. *Journal of Thrombosis and Haemostasis, 6*(8), 1281–1288.

Westbrook, J. et al. (2010). Association of interruptions with an increased risk and severity of medication administration errors. *Archives of Internal Medicine, 170*(8), 683–690.

PERIPHERAL NERVE STIMULATION

Peripheral nerve stimulation assesses and monitors the depth of neuromuscular blockade in patients receiving neuromuscular-blocking drugs, which are administered to produce paralysis. Neuromuscular-blocking drugs may be given to help synchronize breathing and mechanical ventilation in patients with severe lung injury; assist with the treatment of severe muscle spasms in patients with seizures, tetanus, or drug overdose; and help in the management of increased intracranial pressure in patients with head injury.

A peripheral nerve stimulator (PNS) is used to evaluate the level of neuromuscular blockade and determine the lowest therapeutic dose of the neuromuscular-blocking drug needed to produce paralysis. The PNS works by stimulating a peripheral nerve with a series of brief electrical pulses to produce a muscle response or twitch.

The train of four (TOF) is the most commonly used method for monitoring neuromuscular blockade. Using this method, a series of four electrical impulses are delivered to a particular peripheral nerve. If four twitches occur, then 75% or less of the receptors are blocked. Three twitches occur when 80% of the receptors are blocked. One or two twitches correspond to 85% to 90% neuromuscular blockade. After the neuromuscular blockade drug is administered, it's titrated so that each set of four electrical impulses produces one or two muscle twitches.

Equipment

Peripheral nerve stimulator ∎ two electrode gel patches ∎ two lead-wires ∎ alcohol pads ∎ Optional: clippers.

Implementation

∎ Verify the doctor's order for peripheral nerve stimulation.
∎ Perform hand hygiene *to reduce the transmission of microorganisms.*[1,2,3]
∎ Confirm the patient's identity using at least two patient identifiers according to your facility's policy.[4]
∎ Explain the reasons for neuromuscular blockade and peripheral nerve stimulation to the patient and family *to increase their understanding and reduce anxiety.*
∎ Select a site for electrode placement that's accessible and is without edema, wounds, catheters, or dressings *to ensure optimum placement.* The preferred monitoring site is the ulnar nerve, but if it isn't accessible, other sites may be used.
∎ If the patient has excessive hair where an electrode is to be placed, remove the hair with clippers *to improve contact of the pad with the skin.*

Ulnar nerve stimulation

∎ Clean the site on the patient's arm where the electrodes are to be placed with an alcohol pad and allow it to dry *to reduce skin resistance.*
∎ Place the patient's arm in a relaxed position with the palm up so that the ulnar nerve is easily accessible.
∎ Place one electrode over the ulnar nerve at the crease of the wrist and the other electrode 1 to 2 cm away, parallel to the carpi ulnaris tendon (as shown below) *to ensure stimulation of the ulnar nerve.*

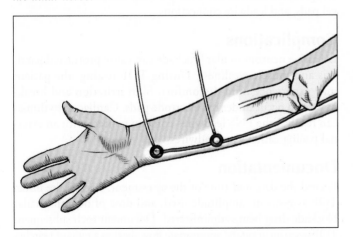

∎ Attach the leadwires to the PNS.
∎ Connect the black lead (negative) to the electrode nearest the wrist and the red lead (positive) to the electrode on the forearm.
∎ Switch the PNS on and choose a low milliampere (mA)—commonly 10 mA to 20 mA—*because higher current can cause overstimulation of the nerve and rhythmic nerve firing.*
∎ Press the TOF button to initiate the four impulses and count the number of twitches the stimulation produces. Visually count the number of thumb adductions or twitches while lightly feeling for twitches. Don't count finger movement that's caused by muscle stimulation.
∎ Turn off the PNS.

Facial nerve stimulation

∎ Clean the site on the patient's face where the electrodes are to be placed with an alcohol pad and allow it to dry *to reduce skin resistance.*
∎ Place one electrode near the outer canthus of the eye and a second electrode 2 cm below and at the level of the tragus of the ear (as shown below).

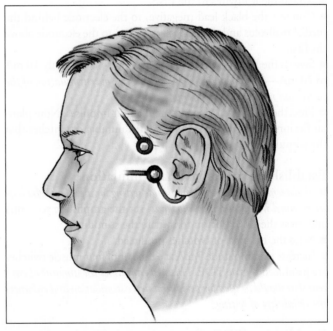

∎ Attach the leadwires to the PNS and connect the black lead (negative) to the electrode nearest the tragus and the red lead (positive) to the electrode near the outer canthus of the eye.
∎ Switch the PNS on and choose a low mA—commonly 10 mA to 20 mA—*because higher current can cause overstimulation of the nerve and rhythmic nerve firing.*
∎ Press the TOF button to initiate the four impulses and count the eyebrow twitches that the stimulation produces. Visually count the number of twitches while lightly feeling for twitches.
∎ Turn off the PNS.

Posterior tibial nerve stimulation

■ Clean the site on the patient's foot where the electrodes are to be placed with an alcohol pad and allow it to dry *to reduce skin resistance.*

■ Place one electrode 2 cm behind the medial malleolus and a second electrode 2 cm above the first electrode (as shown below).

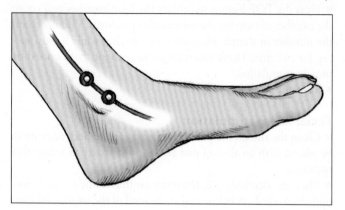

■ Attach the leadwires to the PNS.

■ Connect the black lead (negative) to the electrode behind the medial malleolus and the red lead (positive) to the electrode above the first.

■ Switch the PNS on and choose a low mA—commonly 10 mA to 20 mA—*because higher current can cause overstimulation of the nerve and rhythmic nerve firing.*

■ Press the TOF button to initiate the four impulses. Note plantar flexion of the great toe and count the number of twitches that the stimulation produces.

Establishing supramaximal stimulation

■ *To determine the baseline amplitude setting for a patient who hasn't received neuromuscular blockade,* set the amplitude to 5 mA and press the TOF button to initiate the stimulus.[5]

■ Note the number of twitches produced.

■ Increase the amplitude 5 mA at a time until four muscle twitches are produced by the TOF. *This step establishes the amount of current that should be used for peripheral nerve stimulation and enhances the reliability of testing.*[6]

Establishing TOF after neuromuscular blockade

■ Determine the TOF 10 to 15 minutes following a bolus dose or any change in neuromuscular drug administration to assess the level of neuromuscular blockade.

■ If you get zero twitches, troubleshoot the equipment. Next, increase the stimulating current and then retest another nerve. If there's still no response, check the neuromuscular blocker infusion rate, concentration, and dose, and then reduce the infusion rate, as ordered. Retest TOF in 10 to 15 minutes.

■ If you get one or two twitches, continue the current rate of the infusion.

■ If you get three or four twitches, increase the rate of the neuromuscular blockade. Retest TOF in 10 to 15 minutes.

Completing the procedure

■ Turn off the PNS.

■ Perform hand hygiene.[2,3,4]

■ Document the procedure.[6]

Ongoing care

■ Perform respiratory, cardiovascular, and neurologic assessments before any increase in the level of neuromuscular blockade.

■ Perform neurovascular checks hourly.

■ Change electrodes daily, or more frequently, if they become loose or the gel has dried out *to ensure optimum conduction.*

■ Assess the skin under the electrodes for signs of irritation or breakdown, which could impede conduction.

■ Reevaluate the level of neuromuscular blockade every 4 to 8 hours during therapy with neuromuscular blocking drugs, as ordered or according to facility policy, after the patient is stable and an adequate level of neuromuscular blockade is reached.

■ Document the procedure.[6]

Special considerations

■ *Because neuromuscular-blocking drugs don't produce amnesia, sedation, or analgesia,* sedative and analgesic drugs should always be administered before giving a neuromuscular blocking drug.[7]

■ When the neuromuscular blockade infusion is discontinued, check the TOF. Four of four muscle twitches should be present before discontinuing mechanical ventilation.

■ If the patient has hemiplegia, hemiparesis, or peripheral neuropathy (from diabetes), the motor response to PNS may not be as pronounced, which may cause the nurse to mistakenly believe that a higher dose of neuromuscular-blocking drugs is needed. With hemiplegia and hemiparesis, place the electrodes on the unaffected limb, if possible.

■ Check the site of electrode placement carefully *because incorrect placement can lead to muscle, rather than nerve, stimulation.*

■ If no twitches are elicited at a level that previously elicited a response, troubleshoot the PNS before decreasing the level of neuromuscular blockade. Check the polarity of the leads, battery charge, electrode contact with the skin, condition of electrode gel pads, and leadwire connections.

Complications

Excessive neuromuscular blockade can cause protracted paralysis and muscle weakness. During TOF testing, the patient may experience mild discomfort. Skin irritation and breakdown can occur under the electrode pads. Cardiac arrhythmias can result if the PNS leadwires come in contact with an external pacing catheter or leadwires.

Documentation

Record the date and time of the assessment. Record the initial TOF assessment, amplitude used, and dose of neuromuscular blockade drug being administered. Document each subsequent TOF assessment on the appropriate flow sheet as a ratio of twitches per four stimulations (for example, 0/4, 1/4, 2/4, 3/4, 4/4).

Note the current used as well as any bolus doses or changes in the rate of infusion of the neuromuscular-blocking drug. Record

How peritoneal dialysis works

Peritoneal dialysis works through a combination of diffusion and osmosis.

Diffusion

In diffusion, particles move through a semipermeable membrane from an area of high-solute concentration to an area of low-solute concentration.

In peritoneal dialysis, the water-based dialysate being infused contains glucose, sodium chloride, calcium, magnesium, acetate or lactate, and no waste products. Therefore, the waste products and excess electrolytes in the blood cross through the semipermeable peritoneal membrane into the dialysate. Removing the waste-filled dialysate and replacing it with fresh solution keeps the waste concentration low and encourages further diffusion.

Osmosis

In osmosis, fluids move through a semipermeable membrane from an area of low-solute concentration to an area of high-solute concentration. In peritoneal dialysis, dextrose is added to the dialysate to give it a higher solute concentration than the blood, creating a high osmotic gradient. Water migrates from the blood through the membrane at the beginning of each infusion, when the osmotic gradient is highest.

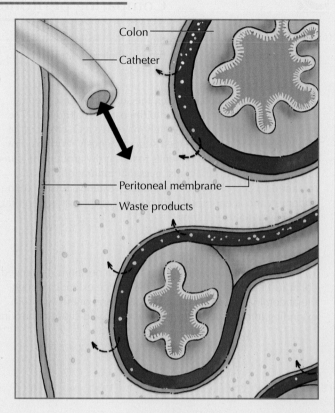

respiratory, cardiovascular, and neurologic assessments on a frequent assessment form. Note any adverse effects of neuromuscular blockade, the time and name of the doctor notified, orders given, nursing interventions performed, and the patient's response. Include any patient and family teaching.

REFERENCES

1 Centers for Disease Control and Prevention. (October 2002). Guideline for hand hygiene in health-care settings. *Morbidity and Mortality Weekly Report, 51*(RR-16), 1–45. (Level I)

2 World Health Organization. (2009). *WHO guidelines on hand hygiene in health care: First global patient safety challenge. Clean care is safer care.* Geneva, Switzerland: World Health Organization. (Level I)

3 The Joint Commission. (2012). Standard NPSG.07.01.01. *Comprehensive accreditation manual for hospitals: The official handbook.* Oakbrook Terrace, IL: The Joint Commission. (Level I)

4 The Joint Commission. (2012). Standard NPSG.01.01.01. *Comprehensive accreditation manual for hospitals: The official handbook.* Oakbrook Terrace, IL: The Joint Commission. (Level I)

5 Lynn-McHale Wiegand, D. (Ed.). (2011). *AACN procedure manual for critical care* (6th ed.). Philadelphia, PA: Saunders.

6 The Joint Commission. (2012). Standard RC.01.03.01. *Comprehensive accreditation manual for hospitals: The official handbook.* Oakbrook Terrace, IL: The Joint Commission. (Level I)

7 Murray, M.J., et al. (2002). Clinical practice guidelines for sustained neuromuscular blockade in the adult critically ill patient. *Critical Care Medicine, 30*(1), 142–156. (Level I)

PERITONEAL DIALYSIS

Peritoneal dialysis is indicated for patients with end-stage renal disease who are looking for an alternative to renal replacement therapy. Peritoneal dialysis can also be used in patients with vascular access issues, chronic heart failure, and ischemic heart disease.[1] In this procedure, dialysate—the solution instilled into the peritoneal cavity by a catheter—draws waste products, excess fluid, and electrolytes from the blood across the semipermeable peritoneal membrane. (See *How peritoneal dialysis works.*)

After a prescribed period, the dialysate is drained from the peritoneal cavity, removing impurities with it. The dialysis procedure is then repeated, using a new dialysate each time, until waste removal is complete and fluid, electrolyte, and acid-base balance has been restored. The procedure is also known as the dialysis cycle, consisting of the dialysate instillation phase, the dialysate dwell phase, and the dialysate drain phase.

Peritoneal dialysis is usually contraindicated in patients who have had extensive abdominal or bowel surgery or extensive

EQUIPMENT

Comparing peritoneal dialysis catheters

The first step in any type of peritoneal dialysis is insertion of a catheter *to allow instillation of dialyzing solution.* The surgeon may insert one of the three catheters described here.

Tenckhoff catheter

To implant a Tenckhoff catheter, the surgeon inserts the first 6¾" (17 cm) of the catheter into the patient's abdomen. The next 2¾" (7-cm) segment, which may have a Dacron cuff at one or both ends, is imbedded subcutaneously. Within a few days after insertion, the patient's tissues grow around the cuffs, forming a tight barrier against bacterial infiltration. The remaining 3⅞" (10 cm) of the catheter extends outside of the abdomen and is equipped with a metal adapter at the tip that connects to dialyzer tubing.

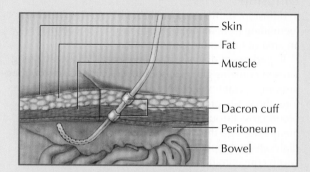

Skin
Fat
Muscle
Dacron cuff
Peritoneum
Bowel

Flanged-collar catheter

To insert this kind of catheter, the surgeon positions its flanged collar just below the skin so that the device extends through the abdominal wall. He keeps the distal end of the cuff from extending into the peritoneum, where it could cause adhesions.

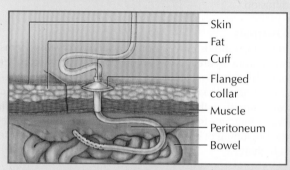

Skin
Fat
Cuff
Flanged collar
Muscle
Peritoneum
Bowel

Column-disk peritoneal catheter

To insert a column-disk peritoneal catheter (CDPC), the surgeon rolls up the flexible disk section of the implant, inserts it into the peritoneal cavity, and retracts it against the abdominal wall. The implant's first cuff rests just outside the peritoneal membrane, and its second cuff rests just underneath the skin.

Because the CDPC doesn't float freely in the peritoneal cavity, it keeps inflowing dialyzing solution from being directed at the sensitive organs, which increases patient comfort during dialysis.

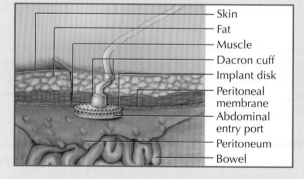

Skin
Fat
Muscle
Dacron cuff
Implant disk
Peritoneal membrane
Abdominal entry port
Peritoneum
Bowel

---

abdominal trauma, who are obese, or who have severe vascular disease or respiratory distress.

The catheter may be inserted in the operating room or under sterile conditions on the nursing unit. Dialysis can be performed either manually or using an automatic or semiautomatic cycle machine. (See *Comparing peritoneal dialysis catheters.*)

Equipment

Prescribed dialysate (1-L, 2-L, or 3-L bags with prescribed dextrose concentration) ▪ dialysate warmer ▪ medication vials, as ordered ▪ bowl of antiseptic solution, as needed ▪ two face masks ▪ goggles and gown ▪ dialysis administration set with drainage bag ▪ three pairs of sterile gloves ▪ IV pole ▪ antiseptic skin cleaning swabs ▪ hypoallergenic tape ▪ antiseptic pads ▪ precut sterile

drain dressings ▪ protective cap for catheter ▪ sterile 4" × 4" gauze pads ▪ small sterile plastic clamp ▪ 10-mL syringe with 22G 1½" needle, as needed ▪ specimen containers with labels, as needed ▪ laboratory request form, as needed ▪ straight catheterization kit, as needed.

Preparation of equipment

Place the dialysate bags in the commercial dialysate warmer set at 98.6° F (37° C) for about 1 hour *to ensure the dialysate is at body temperature. Warming the dialysate decreases the patient's discomfort during the procedure and reduces vasoconstriction of the peritoneal capillaries.* Dilated capillaries enhance blood flow to the peritoneal membrane surface, thus increasing waste clearance into the peritoneal cavity. Prescribed medications should be added to the dialysate bag immediately before the dialysate will be hung and used. Disinfect multidose vials by soaking them in a bowl of antiseptic solution for 5 minutes before use.

Implementation

- Verify the doctor's order for dialysis and dialysate to be used.[2]
- Perform hand hygiene, put on a gown, sterile gloves, and a face mask, and follow standard precautions.[3,4,5]
- Confirm the patient's identity using at least two patient identifiers according to your facility's policy.[6]
- Explain the procedure to the patient and answer all questions to *decrease anxiety and increase cooperation.*
- Obtain and record the patient's vital signs, weight, and abdominal girth *to establish baseline levels.*
- Review recent laboratory results (blood urea nitrogen, serum creatinine, sodium, potassium, complete blood count, hepatitis B virus, and human immunodeficiency virus status, if known.)
- Have the patient urinate, if possible, *to reduce the risk for bladder perforation during insertion of the peritoneal catheter.* If he can't urinate and assessment of the bladder suggests the presence of urine, obtain an order to perform a straight catheterization to empty his bladder.
- Place the patient in the supine position and have him put on one of the facemasks.
- Inspect the warmed dialysate, which should appear clear and colorless.
- Add any prescribed medication to the dialysate, using strict sterile technique *to avoid contaminating the solution.*
- Prepare the dialysis administration set as shown. (See *Setup for peritoneal dialysis.*)
- Close the clamps on all the lines. Place the drainage bag below the patient *to facilitate gravity drainage* and connect the drainage line to it. Connect the dialysate infusion lines to the first bag of dialysate using sterile technique. Hang the bag on the IV pole at the patient's bedside.
- Prime the tubing by opening the infusion lines and allowing the solution to flow until all the lines are primed. Close all of the clamps.
- Clean the catheter insertion site with antiseptic swabs according to your facility's policy.
- Connect the catheter to the administration set, using sterile technique *to prevent contamination of the catheter and the solution, which could cause peritonitis.*
- Open the drain dressing and the sterile 4″ × 4″ gauze pad packages.
- Remove and discard your gloves, perform hand hygiene,[3,4,5] and then put on the other pair of sterile gloves. Apply the precut drain dressings around the catheter. Cover them with the gauze pads and tape them securely.
- Unclamp the lines to the patient. Rapidly instill 500 mL of dialysate into the peritoneal cavity to test the catheter's patency.
- Clamp the lines to the patient. Immediately unclamp the lines to the drainage bag *to allow fluid to drain into the bag.* Outflow should be brisk.
- Having established the catheter's patency, clamp the lines to the drainage bag and unclamp the lines to the patient to infuse

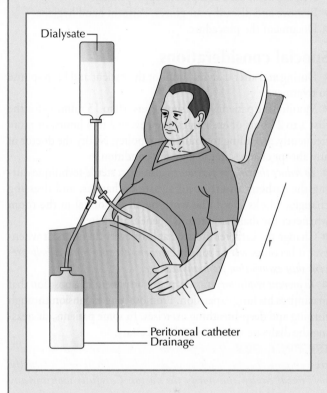

Setup for peritoneal dialysis

This illustration shows the proper setup for peritoneal dialysis.

Dialysate

Peritoneal catheter
Drainage

the prescribed volume of solution over a period of 5 to 10 minutes. As soon as the dialysate container empties, clamp the lines to the patient immediately *to prevent air from entering the tubing.*
- Allow the solution to dwell in the peritoneal cavity for the prescribed time (10 minutes to 4 hours). *This process lets excess fluid, electrolytes, and accumulated wastes move from the blood through the peritoneal membrane and into the dialysate.*
- Make sure the next dialysate bag is warming.
- At the end of the prescribed dwell time, unclamp the line to the drainage bag, and allow the solution to drain from the peritoneal cavity into the drainage bag (normally 20 to 30 minutes).
- Repeat the infusion-dwell-drain cycle immediately after the dialysate drains until the prescribed number of fluid exchanges has been completed.
- If the doctor (or your facility's policy) requires a dialysate specimen, you'll usually collect one after every 10 infusion-dwell-drain cycles (always during the drain phase) and after every 24-hour period, or as ordered. To do this, wipe the injection port with antiseptic (according to facility policy) and attach the 10-mL syringe to the 22G 1½″ needle and insert it into the injection port on the drainage line, using strict sterile technique, and aspirate the drainage sample. Transfer the sample to the specimen container, label it appropriately, and send it to the laboratory with a laboratory request form.

■ After completing the prescribed number of exchanges, clamp the catheter, remove and discard your gloves, perform hand hygiene, and put on another pair of sterile gloves. Disconnect the administration set from the peritoneal catheter. Place the sterile protective cap over the catheter's distal end.

■ Dispose of all used equipment appropriately.

■ Remove and discard your gloves. Perform hand hygiene.[3,4,5]

■ Document the procedure.[7]

Special considerations

■ During and after dialysis, monitor the patient and his response to treatment.

■ Monitor the patient's vital signs every 10 to 15 minutes for the first 1 to 2 hours of exchanges, then every 2 to 4 hours, or more frequently, according to your facility policy. Notify the doctor of any abrupt changes in the patient's condition.

■ *To reduce the risk for peritonitis,* use strict sterile technique during the catheter insertion, dialysate exchanges, and dressing changes. Masks should be worn by all personnel in the room whenever the dialysis system is opened or entered.

■ Change the catheter dressing at least every 24 hours or whenever it becomes wet or soiled. *Frequent dressing changes help prevent skin excoriation from any leakage.*

■ *To prevent respiratory distress,* place the patient in a position that maximizes his lung expansion. Promote lung expansion through turning and deep-breathing exercises. In some patients, decreasing the dialysate volume may be necessary.

NURSING ALERT *If the patient suffers severe respiratory distress during the dwell phase of dialysis, immediately drain the peritoneal cavity and notify the doctor. Carefully monitor any patient on peritoneal dialysis who's being weaned from a ventilator.*

■ *To prevent protein depletion,* the doctor may order a high-protein diet or a protein supplement. He will also monitor serum albumin levels.

■ Dialysate is available in three concentrations—4.25% dextrose, 2.5% dextrose, and 1.5% dextrose. The 4.25% solution usually removes the largest amount of fluid from the blood *because its glucose concentration is highest.* If your patient receives this concentrated solution, monitor him carefully *to prevent excess fluid loss.* Also, some of the glucose in the 4.25% solution may enter the patient's bloodstream, causing hyperglycemia severe enough to require an insulin injection or an insulin addition to the dialysate.

■ Patients with low serum potassium levels may require the addition of potassium to the dialysate solution *to prevent further losses.*

■ Heparin is typically added to the dialysate *to prevent accumulation of fibrin in the dialysis catheter.*

■ Monitor the patient's hemodynamic status. Note his fluid balance at the end of each infusion-dwell-drain cycle. (The patient's fluid balance is positive if he retains fluid at the end of an exchange and negative if you recover more fluid than was instilled with the exchange). Notify the doctor if the patient retains 500 mL or more of fluid for three consecutive cycles or if he loses 1 L of fluid for three consecutive cycles.

■ Weigh the patient daily *to help determine how much fluid is being removed during dialysis treatment.* Note the time and any variations in the weighing technique next to his weight on his chart.

■ If dialysate instillation or drainage is slow or absent, check all of the tubing for kinks. You can also try raising the IV pole or repositioning the patient *to increase the inflow rate.* Repositioning the patient or applying manual pressure to the lateral aspects of the patient's abdomen may also help increase drainage. If these maneuvers fail, notify the doctor. The catheter may be improperly positioned or an accumulation of fibrin may obstruct the catheter.

■ Always examine the drained fluid from each exchange (effluent) for color and clarity. Normally, the fluid is clear or pale yellow, but pink-tinged effluent may appear during the first three or four cycles. If the effluent remains pink-tinged or if it's grossly bloody, suspect bleeding into the peritoneal cavity and notify the doctor. Also notify the doctor if the effluent contains feces, which suggests bowel perforation, or if it's cloudy, which suggests peritonitis. Obtain a specimen for culture and Gram stain. Send the specimen in a labeled specimen container to the laboratory with a laboratory request form.

■ Patient discomfort at the start of the procedure is normal. If the patient experiences pain during the procedure, determine when it occurs, its quality and duration, and whether it radiates to other body parts, and notify the doctor. Pain during infusion usually results from a dialysate that's too cool or acidic. Pain may also result from rapid instillation; slowing the inflow rate may reduce the pain. Severe, diffuse pain with rebound tenderness and cloudy effluent may indicate peritoneal infection. Pain that radiates to the shoulder often results from air accumulation under the diaphragm. Severe, persistent perineal or rectal pain can result from improper catheter placement.

■ The patient undergoing peritoneal dialysis will require assistance in his daily care. *To minimize his discomfort,* perform daily care during a drain phase in the cycle, when the patient's abdomen is less distended.

Complications

Peritonitis, the most common complication, usually follows contamination of the dialysate, but it may develop if solution leaks from the catheter exit site and flows back into the catheter tract. Respiratory distress may result when dialysate in the peritoneal cavity increases pressure on the diaphragm, which decreases lung expansion.

Protein depletion may result from the diffusion of protein in the blood into the dialysate solution through the peritoneal membrane. As much as 14 g of protein may be lost daily—more in patients with peritonitis.

Constipation is a major cause of inflow-outflow problems and the patient may require laxatives or stool softeners.

Excessive fluid loss from the use of 4.25% solution may cause hypovolemia, hypotension, and shock. Excessive fluid retention may lead to blood volume expansion, hypertension, peripheral edema, and even pulmonary edema and heart failure.

Other possible complications include electrolyte imbalance and hyperglycemia, which can be identified by frequent blood tests.

Documentation

Record the amount of dialysate infused and drained, any medications added to the dialysate solution, and the color and character of the effluent. Record the patient's daily weight and fluid balance. Use a peritoneal dialysis flowchart to compute total fluid balance after each exchange. Note the patient's vital signs and tolerance of the treatment as well as other pertinent observations. Note any complications and nursing actions taken.

REFERENCES

1 National Kidney Foundation/KDOQI. (2006). "Clinical Practice Guidelines for Peritoneal Dialysis Adequacy, Update 2006" [Online]. Accessed August 2010 via the Web at http://www.kidney.org/professionals/KDOQI/guideline_eupHD_PD_VA/index.htm (Level I)
2 The Joint Commission. (2012). Standard MM.04.01.01. *Comprehensive accreditation manual for hospitals: The official handbook.* Oakbrook Terrace, IL: The Joint Commission. (Level I)
3 The Joint Commission. (2012). Standard NPSG.07.01.01. *Comprehensive accreditation manual for hospitals: The official handbook.* Oakbrook Terrace, IL: The Joint Commission. (Level I)
4 Centers for Disease Control and Prevention. (October 2002). Guideline for hand hygiene in health-care settings. *Morbidity and Mortality Weekly Report, 51*(RR-16), 1–45. (Level I)
5 World Health Organization. (2009). *WHO guidelines on hand hygiene in health care: First global patient safety challenge. Clean care is safer care.* Geneva, Switzerland: World Health Organization. (Level I)
6 The Joint Commission. (2012). Standard NPSG.01.01.01. *Comprehensive accreditation manual for hospitals: The official handbook.* Oakbrook Terrace, IL: The Joint Commission. (Level I)
7 The Joint Commission. (2012). Standard RC.01.03.01. *Comprehensive accreditation manual for hospitals: The official handbook.* Oakbrook Terrace, IL: The Joint Commission. (Level I)

ADDITIONAL REFERENCES

Nettina, S.M. (2010). *Lippincott manual of nursing practice* (9th ed.). Philadelphia, PA: Lippincott Williams & Wilkins.
Smeltzer, S.C., et al. (2010). *Brunner & Suddarth's textbook of medical-surgical nursing* (12th ed.). Philadelphia, PA: Lippincott Williams & Wilkins.

PERITONEAL LAVAGE, ASSISTING

Used mainly as a diagnostic procedure in a patient with blunt abdominal trauma, peritoneal lavage helps detect bleeding in the peritoneal cavity. When possible, abdominal ultrasound should be performed before peritoneal lavage to assess fluid in the abdominal cavity. Peritoneal lavage may also be used to warm the abdominal cavity in a patient with hypothermia, to obtain a cytology specimen in a patient with cancer, and for irrigation in a patient with peritonitis or an intraabdominal abscess.

The procedure may progress through several steps. Initially, the doctor inserts a catheter through the abdominal wall into the peritoneal cavity and aspirates the peritoneal fluid with a syringe. If he can't see blood in the aspirated fluid, he then infuses a balanced saline solution and siphons the fluid from the cavity. He inspects the siphoned fluid for blood and also sends fluid samples to the laboratory for microscopic examination.

The medical team maintains strict sterile technique throughout this procedure to avoid introducing microorganisms into the peritoneum and causing peritonitis. (See *Tapping the peritoneal cavity*, page 580.)

Peritoneal lavage is contraindicated in a patient who has had multiple abdominal operations (adhesions), who has an abdominal wall hematoma, who's unstable and needs immediate surgery, who has coagulopathies, or who can't be catheterized before the procedure. The procedure requires great caution and a different technique if the patient is pregnant.

Equipment

Indwelling urinary catheter insertion equipment ■ nasogastric (NG) tube insertion equipment ■ electric hair clippers ■ IV pole ■ macrodrip IV tubing ■ IV solutions (1 L of warmed, balanced saline solution, usually lactated Ringer's solution or normal saline solution) ■ peritoneal dialysis tray ■ two pairs of sterile gloves ■ gown ■ goggles ■ antiseptic solution ■ 3-mL syringe with 25G 1″ needle ■ 1% lidocaine with epinephrine, if needed ■ 8″ (20.3 cm) #14 intracatheter extension tubing and a small sterile hemostat (to clamp tubing) ■ 30-mL syringe ■ one 20G 1½″ needle ■ sterile towels ■ three containers for specimen collection, including one sterile tube for a culture and sensitivity specimen ■ labels ■ 4″ × 4″ sterile gauze pads ■ alcohol pads ■ 1″ hypoallergenic tape ■ 2-0 and 3-0 sutures.

Preparation of equipment

If using a commercially prepared peritoneal dialysis kit (containing a #15 peritoneal dialysis catheter, trocar, and extension tubing with roller clamp), make sure the macrodrip IV tubing doesn't have a reverse flow (or back-check) valve that prevents infused fluid from draining out of the peritoneal cavity. Label all medications, medication containers, and other solutions on and off the sterile field.[1]

Implementation

■ If able, conduct a preprocedure verification process *to make sure that all relevant documentation, related information, and equipment are available and correctly identified to the patient's identifiers.*[2]
■ Verify that the laboratory and imaging studies have been completed as ordered and that the results are in the patient's medical record. Notify the doctor of any abnormal results.
■ Make sure the patient has a signed informed consent form in his medical record, unless the procedure is being performed in an emergency.[3,4]
■ Perform hand hygiene.[5,6,7]
■ Confirm the patient's identity using at least two patient identifiers according to your facility's policy.[8]
■ Provide privacy and reinforce the doctor's explanation of the procedure. Answer all questions *to ease the patient's anxiety and ensure his cooperation.*
■ Put on a gown, sterile gloves, and goggles.

Tapping the peritoneal cavity

After preparing the patient's skin with an antiseptic solution and administering a local anesthetic to numb the area near the patient's navel, the surgeon will make a small incision (about ¾" [2 cm]) through the skin and subcutaneous tissues of the abdominal wall. He'll retract the tissue, ligate several blood vessels, and use 4" × 4" sterile gauze pads to absorb and keep incisional blood from entering the wound and producing a false-positive test result. Next, he'll direct the trocar through the incision into the pelvic midline until the instrument enters the peritoneum. Then he'll advance the peritoneal catheter (via the trocar) 6" to 8" (15 to 20 cm) into the pelvis. Using a syringe attached to the catheter, he'll aspirate fluid from the peritoneal cavity and look for blood or other abnormal findings.

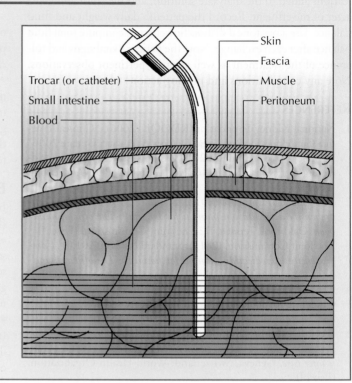

Trocar (or catheter)
Small intestine
Blood

Skin
Fascia
Muscle
Peritoneum

- Advise the patient to expect a sensation of abdominal fullness. Also inform him that he may experience a chill if the lavage solution isn't warmed or doesn't reach his body temperature.
- Catheterize the patient with the indwelling urinary catheter. *This step decreases the risk of the doctor accidentally perforating the bladder during the procedure.*
- Insert an NG tube. Attach this tube to the gastric suction machine (set for low intermittent suction) to drain the patient's stomach contents. Make sure placement is verified with an X-ray. *Decompressing the stomach prevents vomiting and subsequent aspiration and minimizes the possibility of bowel perforation during trocar or catheter insertion.*
- Clip the hair, as ordered, from the area between the patient's umbilicus and pubis.
- Set up the IV pole. Attach the macrodrip tubing to the lavage solution container, and clear air from the tubing *to avoid introducing air into the peritoneal cavity during the lavage.*
- Remove and discard your gloves and perform hand hygiene. Put on another pair of sterile gloves.
- Using sterile technique, open the peritoneal dialysis tray.
- Conduct a time-out immediately before starting the procedure *to determine that the correct patient, site, positioning, and procedure are identified and confirm, as applicable, that relevant information and necessary equipment are available.*[9]
- The doctor will wipe the patient's abdomen from the costal margin to the pubic area and from flank to flank with the antiseptic solution. He will drape the area with sterile towels from the dialysis tray *to create a sterile field.*

- Using sterile technique, hand the doctor the 3-mL syringe and the 25G 1" needle. If the peritoneal dialysis tray doesn't contain a sterile ampule of anesthetic, wipe the top of a multidose vial of 1% lidocaine with epinephrine with an alcohol pad, and invert the vial at a 45-degree angle *to allow the doctor to insert the needle and withdraw the anesthetic without touching the nonsterile vial.*
- The doctor injects the anesthetic directly below the umbilicus (or at an adjacent site if the patient has a surgical scar). After the area is numb, he makes an incision, inserts the catheter or trocar, withdraws fluid, and checks the findings. If findings are positive, the procedure will end and you'll prepare the patient for laparotomy and further measures. Even if retrieved fluid looks normal, lavage will continue. (See *Interpreting peritoneal lavage results.*)
- Trace the catheter extension tubing to its point of origin[10]; connect it to the IV tubing, if ordered; and instill 700 to 1,000 mL (10 mL/kg body weight) of the warmed IV solution into the peritoneal cavity over 10 to 15 minutes. Then clamp the tubing with the hemostat.[11]
- Unless contraindicated by the patient's injuries (such as a spinal cord injury, fractured ribs, or unstable pelvic fracture), gently tilt the patient from side to side *to distribute the fluid throughout the peritoneal cavity.* If the patient's condition contraindicates tilting, the doctor may gently palpate the sides of the abdomen *to distribute the fluid.*[11]
- After 5 to 10 minutes, place the IV container below the level of the patient's body, and open the clamp on the IV tubing. *Lowering the container helps excess fluid to drain.* Gently drain as much

of the fluid as possible from the peritoneal cavity to the container. Be careful not to disconnect the tubing from the catheter. The peritoneal cavity may take 20 to 30 minutes to drain completely.
- To obtain a fluid specimen, use a 30-mL syringe to withdraw between 25 and 30 mL of fluid from a port in the IV tubing. Clean the top of each specimen container with an alcohol pad. Deposit fluid specimens in the containers, and send the specimens to the laboratory for culture and sensitivity analysis, Gram stain, red and white blood cell counts, amylase and bile level determinations, and spun-down sediment evaluation. *Note:* If you didn't obtain the culture and sensitivity specimen first, change the needle before drawing this fluid sample *to avoid contaminating the specimen.*
- Label all the specimens in the presence of the patient, and send them to the laboratory immediately.[8] With positive test results, the doctor will usually perform a laparotomy. If test results are normal, the doctor will close the incision with sutures.
- Remove and discard your gloves and perform hand hygiene.[5,6,7]
- Put on sterile gloves, and dress the incision with a 4″ × 4″ sterile gauze pad secured with 1″ hypoallergenic tape.
- Discard disposable equipment, remove and discard your personal protective equipment, and perform hand hygiene.[5,6,7]
- Return reusable equipment to the appropriate department for cleaning and sterilization.[12]
- Document the procedure.[13]

Special considerations

- After lavage, monitor the patient's vital signs. Report signs and symptoms of shock (tachycardia, decreased blood pressure, diaphoresis, dyspnea or shortness of breath, and vertigo) at once. Assess the incisional site frequently for bleeding.
- If the doctor orders abdominal X-rays, they will probably precede peritoneal lavage. *X-ray films taken after lavage may be unreliable because of air introduced into the peritoneal cavity.*

Complications

Bleeding from lacerated blood vessels may occur at the incisional site or intra-abdominally. A visceral perforation causes peritonitis and requires laparotomy for repair. If the patient has respiratory distress, infusion of a balanced saline solution may cause additional stress and trigger respiratory arrest.

The bladder may be lacerated or punctured if it isn't emptied completely before peritoneal lavage. Infection may develop at the incision site without strict sterile technique.

Documentation

Record the type and size of the peritoneal dialysis catheter used, the type and amount of solution instilled and withdrawn from the peritoneal cavity, and the amount and color of fluid returned. Document whether the fluid flowed freely into and out of the abdomen. Note which specimens were obtained and sent to the laboratory. Also note any complications encountered and any interventions performed.

Interpreting peritoneal lavage results

If test findings in peritoneal lavage are abnormal, your patient may need laparotomy and further treatment. The most common abnormal findings include:
- unclotted blood, bile, or intestinal contents in aspirated peritoneal fluid (20 mL in an adult or 10 mL in a child)
- bloody or pinkish red fluid returned from lavage—dark enough to obscure reading newsprint through it (if you can read newsprint through the fluid, test results are considered negative, although the doctor may order more tests)
- green, cloudy, turbid, or milky peritoneal fluid return (normally appears clear to pale yellow)
- red blood cell count exceeding $100,000/mm^3$
- white blood cell count exceeding $500/mm^3$
- bacteria in fluid (identified by culture and sensitivity testing or Gram stain).

If the patient's condition is stable, borderline positive results may suggest the need for additional tests, such as echography and arteriography. If test results are questionable or inconclusive, the doctor may leave the catheter in place to repeat the procedure.

REFERENCES

1 The Joint Commission. (2012). Standard NPSG.03.04.01. *Comprehensive accreditation manual for hospitals: The official handbook.* Oakbrook Terrace, IL: The Joint Commission. (Level I)
2 The Joint Commission. (2012). Standard UP.01.01.01. *Comprehensive accreditation manual for hospitals: The official handbook.* Oakbrook Terrace, IL: The Joint Commission. (Level I)
3 The Joint Commission. (2012). Standard RI.01.03.01. *Comprehensive accreditation manual for hospitals: The official handbook.* Oakbrook Terrace, IL: The Joint Commission. (Level I)
4 Centers for Medicare & Medicaid Services, Department of Health and Human Services. (2006). "Conditions of Participation: Patients' Rights," 42 CFR part 482.13 [Online]. Accessed November 2011 via the Web at https://www.cms.gov/CFCsAndCoPs/downloads/finalpatientrightsrule.pdf
5 The Joint Commission. (2012). Standard NPSG.07.01.01. *Comprehensive accreditation manual for hospitals: The official handbook.* Oakbrook Terrace, IL: The Joint Commission. (Level I)
6 Centers for Disease Control and Prevention. (October 2002). Guideline for hand hygiene in health-care settings. *Morbidity and Mortality Weekly Report, 51*(RR-16), 1–45. (Level I)
7 World Health Organization. (2009). *WHO guidelines on hand hygiene in health care: First global patient safety challenge. Clean care is safer care.* Geneva, Switzerland: World Health Organization. (Level I)
8 The Joint Commission. (2012). Standard NPSG.01.01.01. *Comprehensive accreditation manual for hospitals: The official handbook.* Oakbrook Terrace, IL: The Joint Commission. (Level I)

Understanding pacemaker codes

A permanent pacemaker's three-letter (or sometimes five-letter) code simply refers to how it's programmed. The first letter represents the chamber that is paced; the second letter, the chamber that is sensed; and the third letter, how the pulse generator responds. The fourth letter describes rate modulation, and the fifth letter specifies the location or absence of multisite pacing. Typically, only the first three letters are shown.

FIRST LETTER	SECOND LETTER	THIRD LETTER
A = atrium	A = atrium	I = inhibited
V = ventricle	V = ventricle	T = triggered
D = dual (both chambers)	D = dual (both chambers)	D = dual (inhibited and triggered)
O = not applicable	O = not applicable	O = not applicable
S = single	S = single	

FOURTH LETTER	FIFTH LETTER
R = rate modulation—a sensor adjusts the programmed heart rate in response to patient activity. O = none	O = none A = atrium or atria V = ventricle or ventricles D = dual site

EXAMPLES OF TWO COMMON PROGRAMMING CODES:

DDD
Pace: atrium and ventricle
Sense: atrium and ventricle
Response: inhibited and triggered
This is a fully automatic, or universal, pacemaker.

VVI
Pace: ventricle
Sense: ventricle
Response: inhibited
This is a demand pacemaker, inhibited.

9 The Joint Commission. (2012). Standard UP.01.03.01. *Comprehensive accreditation manual for hospitals: The official handbook.* Oakbrook Terrace, IL: The Joint Commission. (Level I)

10 U.S. Food and Drug Administration. (2009). "Look. Check. Connect.: Safe Medical Device Connections Save Lives" [Online]. Accessed November 2011 via the Web at http://www.fda.gov/downloads/MedicalDevices/Safety/AlertsandNotices/UCM134873.pdf

11 Lynn-McHale Wiegand, D. (Ed.). (2011). *AACN procedure manual for critical care* (6th ed.). Philadelphia, PA: Saunders.

12 Rutala, W.A., et al. (2008). "Guideline for Disinfection and Sterilization in Healthcare Facilities, 2008" [Online]. Accessed October 2011 via the Web at http://www.cdc.gov/ncidod/dhqp/pdf/guidelines/Disinfection_Nov_2008.pdf

13 The Joint Commission. (2012). Standard RC.01.03.01. *Comprehensive accreditation manual for hospitals: The official handbook.* Oakbrook Terrace, IL: The Joint Commission. (Level I)

ADDITIONAL REFERENCE

Cha, J.Y., et al. (2009). Diagnostic peritoneal lavage remains a valuable adjunct to modern imaging techniques. *Journal of Trauma, 67*(2), 330–336.

PERMANENT PACEMAKER CARE

Designed to operate for 3 to 20 years, a permanent pacemaker is a self-contained device that the surgeon implants in a pocket beneath the patient's skin. This procedure is usually done in the operating room or cardiac catheterization laboratory. Nursing responsibilities involve monitoring the electrocardiogram (ECG) and maintaining sterile technique.

Permanent pacemakers function in the demand mode, allowing the patient's heart to beat on its own but preventing it from falling below a preset rate. Pacing electrodes can be placed in the atria, the ventricles, or both chambers (atrioventricular sequential, dual chamber). (See *Understanding pacemaker codes*.) The most common pacing codes are VVI for single-chamber pacing and DDD for dual-chamber pacing.

Candidates for permanent pacemakers include patients with myocardial infarction and persistent bradyarrhythmia and patients with complete heart block or slow ventricular rates stemming from congenital or degenerative heart disease or cardiac surgery.[1] Patients who suffer from Stokes-Adams, Wolff-Parkinson-White, or sick sinus syndrome may also benefit from permanent pacemaker implantation.

Permanent pacemakers are also used in patients other than those with symptomatic bradycardia. These include patients with hypertrophic obstructive cardiomyopathy, dilated cardiomyopathy, atrial fibrillation, neurocardiogenic syndrome, and long-QT syndrome.

A biventricular pacemaker is effective in patients with heart failure who have intraventricular conductor defects. This device differs from a standard pacemaker in that it has three leads instead of one or two. One lead is placed in the right atrium and the others are placed in each of the ventricles, where they simultaneously stimulate the right and left ventricle. This allows the ventricles to coordinate their pumping action, making the heart more efficient.

Equipment

Sphygmomanometer ▪ stethoscope ▪ ECG monitor and strip-chart recorder ▪ antiseptic ointment ▪ gloves ▪ sterile gauze dressing ▪ hypoallergenic tape ▪ IV catheter insertion equipment ▪ prescribed medications.

Implementation

▪ Conduct a preprocedure verification process *to make sure that all relevant documentation, related information, and equipment are available and correctly identified to the patient's identifiers.*[2]
▪ Verify that the laboratory and imaging studies have been completed as ordered and that the results are in the patient's medical record. Notify the doctor of any abnormal results.
▪ Make sure the patient has a signed informed consent form in his medical record, unless the procedure is being performed in an emergency.[3,4]
▪ Perform hand hygiene.[5,6,7]
▪ Confirm the patient's identity using at least two patient identifiers according to your facility's policy.[8]
▪ Provide privacy and reinforce the doctor's explanation of the procedure. Answer all questions *to ease his anxiety and ensure his cooperation.* Provide and review literature from the manufacturer or the American Heart Association so the patient can learn about the pacemaker and how it works. Emphasize that the pacemaker merely augments his natural heart rate.
▪ Ask the patient if he's allergic to anesthetics or iodine.

Preoperative care

▪ Perform hand hygiene and put on gloves.[5,6,7]
▪ Establish an IV line at a keep-vein-open rate. (See "IV catheter insertion and removal," page 421.)
▪ Obtain baseline vital signs and a baseline ECG.
▪ Administer antibiotics, as ordered.[9]
▪ Provide sedation, as ordered.
▪ Discard used supplies and perform hand hygiene.[5,6,7]
▪ Document the procedure.[10]

Postoperative care

▪ Monitor the patient's ECG *to check for arrhythmias and to ensure correct pacemaker functioning*
▪ Monitor the IV flow rate; the IV line is usually kept in place for 24 to 48 hours postoperatively *to allow for possible emergency treatment of arrhythmias.*

▪ Perform hand hygiene and put on gloves.[5,6,7]
▪ Check the dressing for signs of bleeding and infection (swelling, redness, or exudate).
▪ Change the dressing and apply antiseptic ointment at least once every 24 to 48 hours, or according to doctor's orders and facility policy. If the dressing becomes soiled or the site is exposed to air, change the dressing immediately, regardless of when you last changed it.
▪ Check vital signs and level of consciousness (LOC) every 15 minutes for the first hour, every hour for the next 4 hours, every 4 hours for the next 48 hours, and then once every shift or according to your facility policy.
▪ Discard used supplies and perform hand hygiene.[5,6,7]
▪ Document the procedure.[10]

ELDER ALERT *Confused, elderly patients with second-degree heart block won't show immediate improvement in LOC.*

Special considerations

▪ Provide the patient with an identification card that lists the pacemaker type and manufacturer, serial number, pacemaker rate setting, date implanted, and the doctor's name. (See *Teaching the patient who has a permanent pacemaker,* page 584.)
▪ Watch for signs of pacemaker malfunction.

Complications

NURSING ALERT *Watch for signs and symptoms of a perforated ventricle, with resultant cardiac tamponade: persistent hiccups, distant heart sounds, pulsus paradoxus, hypotension with narrow pulse pressure, increased venous pressure, cyanosis, distended jugular veins, decreased urine output, restlessness, or complaints of fullness in the chest. If the patient develops any of these, notify the doctor immediately.*

Insertion of a permanent pacemaker also places the patient at risk for infection, lead displacement, or a lead fracture and disconnection.

Documentation

Document the type of pacemaker used, the serial number and the manufacturer's name, the pacing rate, the date of implantation, and the doctor's name. Note whether the pacemaker successfully treated the patient's arrhythmias and the condition of the incision site. Document any patient teaching provided.

REFERENCES

1 Gregoratos, G., et al. (2002). ACC/AHA/NASPE 2002 guideline update for implantation of cardiac pacemakers and antiarrhythmia devices: Summary article. *Circulation, 106*(16), 2145–2161. (Level I)
2 The Joint Commission. (2012). Standard UP.01.01.01. *Comprehensive accreditation manual for hospitals: The official handbook.* Oakbrook Terrace, IL: The Joint Commission. (Level I)
3 The Joint Commission. (2012). Standard RI.01.03.01. *Comprehensive accreditation manual for hospitals: The official handbook.* Oakbrook Terrace, IL: The Joint Commission. (Level I)

PATIENT TEACHING

Teaching the patient who has a permanent pacemaker

If your patient is going home with a permanent pacemaker, teach him about daily care, safety and activity guidelines, and other precautions.

Daily care

■ Clean your pacemaker site gently with soap and water when you take a shower or a bath. Leave the incision exposed to the air.

■ Inspect your skin around the incision. A slight bulge is normal, but call your doctor if you feel discomfort or notice swelling, redness, a discharge, or other problems.[1]

■ Check your pulse for 1 minute as your nurse or doctor showed you—on the side of your neck, inside your elbow, or on the thumb side of your wrist. Your pulse rate should be the same as your pacemaker rate or slightly faster. Contact your doctor if you think your heart is beating too fast or too slow.

■ Take your medications, including those for pain, as prescribed. Even with a pacemaker, you still need the medication your doctor ordered.

Safety and activity

■ Keep your pacemaker instruction booklet handy, and carry your pacemaker identification card at all times. This card has your pacemaker model number and other information needed by health care personnel who treat you.

■ You can resume most of your usual activities when you feel comfortable doing so, but don't drive until the doctor gives you permission. Also avoid heavy lifting and stretching exercises for at least 6 to 8 weeks or as directed by your doctor.

■ Try to use both arms equally to prevent stiffness. Check with your doctor before you golf, swim, play tennis, or perform other strenuous activities.

Electromagnetic interference

■ Today's pacemakers are designed and insulated to eliminate most electrical interference. You can safely operate common household electrical devices, including microwave ovens, razors, and sewing machines. And you can ride in or operate a motor vehicle without it affecting your pacemaker.

■ Take care to avoid direct contact with large running motors, high-powered CB radios and other similar equipment, welding machinery, and radar devices.

■ If your pacemaker activates the metal detector in an airport, show your pacemaker identification card to the security official.

■ Because the metal in your pacemaker makes you ineligible for certain diagnostic studies, such as magnetic resonance imaging, be sure to inform your doctors, dentist, and other health care personnel that you have a pacemaker.

Special precautions

■ If you feel light-headed or dizzy when you're near any electrical equipment, moving away from the device should restore normal pacemaker function. Ask your doctor about particular electrical devices.

■ Notify your doctor if you experience any signs of pacemaker failure, such as palpitations, a fast heart rate, a slow heart rate (5 to 10 beats less than the pacemaker's setting), dizziness, fainting, shortness of breath, swollen ankles or feet, anxiety, forgetfulness, or confusion.

■ If you feel like you're going to faint, immediately call 911 and lie down to prevent falling.

Checkups

■ Be sure to schedule a follow-up visit, and keep regular checkup appointments with your doctor.

■ If your doctor checks your pacemaker status by telephone, keep your transmission schedule and instructions in a handy place.

4   Centers for Medicare & Medicaid Services, Department of Health and Human Services. (2006). "Conditions of Participation: Patients' Rights," 42 CFR part 482.13 [Online]. Accessed November 2011 via the Web at https://www.cms.gov/CFCsAndCoPs/downloads/finalpatientrightsrule.pdf

5   The Joint Commission. (2012). Standard NPSG.07.01.01. *Comprehensive accreditation manual for hospitals: The official handbook.* Oakbrook Terrace, IL: The Joint Commission. (Level I)

6   Centers for Disease Control and Prevention. (October 2002). Guideline for hand hygiene in health-care settings. *Morbidity and Mortality Weekly Report, 51*(RR-16), 1–45. (Level I)

7   World Health Organization. (2009). *WHO guidelines on hand hygiene in health care: First global patient safety challenge. Clean care is safer care.* Geneva, Switzerland: World Health Organization. (Level I)

8   The Joint Commission. (2012). Standard NPSG.01.01.01. *Comprehensive accreditation manual for hospitals: The official handbook.* Oakbrook Terrace, IL: The Joint Commission. (Level I)

9 Baddour, L.M., et al. (2010). Update on cardiovascular implantable electronic device infections and their management: A scientific statement from the American Heart Association. *Circulation, 121*(3), 458–477. (Level I)
10 The Joint Commission. (2012). Standard RC.01.03.01. *Comprehensive accreditation manual for hospitals: The official handbook.* Oakbrook Terrace, IL: The Joint Commission. (Level I)

ADDITIONAL REFERENCE

Lynn-McHale Wiegand, D. (Ed.). (2011). *AACN procedure manual for critical care* (6th ed.). Philadelphia, PA: Saunders.

PERSONAL PROTECTIVE EQUIPMENT

Isolation procedures may be implemented to prevent the spread of infection from patient to patient, from patients to health care workers, or from health care workers to patients. Central to the success of these procedures is the selection of the proper personal protective equipment and adequate training of those who use it.

Equipment
Materials for isolation
Personal protective equipment ▪ isolation cart or anteroom for storing equipment ▪ door card or sign alerting staff members and others entering the room that isolation precautions are in effect.

Personal protective equipment
Fluid-resistant gowns ▪ gloves ▪ goggles or face shield ▪ masks or respirators.

Each staff member must be trained in the proper use of personal protective equipment.

Preparation of equipment
Remove the cover from the isolation cart if necessary, and set up the work area. Check the cart or anteroom *to make sure an adequate amount of the proper isolation supplies are available for the designated isolation category.*

Implementation
▪ Remove your watch (or push it well up on your arm) and your rings, according to facility policy. *These actions help to prevent the spread of microorganisms hidden under your watch or rings.*
▪ Perform hand hygiene.[1,2,3]
▪ Take the gown and allow it to unfold in front of you. Put on the gown and wrap it around the back of your uniform, making sure it overlaps and completely covers your uniform *to prevent contact with the patient or his environment.*[4] Tie the strings or fasten the snaps or pressure-sensitive tabs at the neck. Then tie the waist strings.
▪ Place the mask snugly over your nose and mouth. Secure the ear loops around your ears or tie the strings at the middle of the back of your head and neck *so the mask won't slip off.* If the mask has a metal strip, squeeze it to fit your nose firmly but comfort-

Putting on a face mask

To avoid spreading airborne particles, wear a face mask. Position the mask to cover your nose and mouth, and secure it high enough to ensure stability. Tie the top strings at the back of your head above the ears. Then tie the bottom strings at the base of your neck.[3]

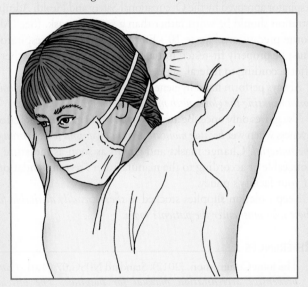

Adjust the metal nose strip if the mask has one.[3]

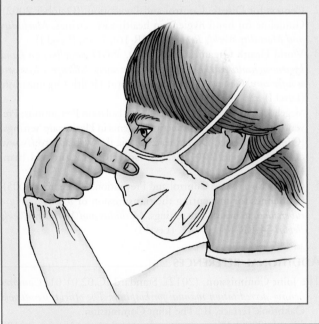

ably.[4] (See *Putting on a face mask.*) If you wear eyeglasses, tuck the upper edge of the mask under the lower edge of the glasses.
▪ Choose eye protection according to your risk of exposure. Although goggles provide eye protection, they don't protect the rest of the face from splashing of potentially infectious substances.

Wear a face shield for any procedures that may involve spraying or splashing of respiratory secretions or other body fluids.[4]

- Select gloves according to your hand size *to make sure they fit securely.* Put on the gloves and pull them over the cuffs of your gown *to cover the edges of the gown's sleeves.*[4]

Special considerations

- If airborne precautions are required, an N95 particulate respirator approved by the Occupational Safety and Health Administration should be worn rather than a surgical mask. (See "Airborne precautions," page 10.) Employees who wear respirators must be properly fit-tested initially, and then periodically thereafter according to federal, state, and local regulations.[5]
- Always perform hand hygiene before putting on gloves *to avoid contaminating the gloves with microorganisms from your hands.*[1,2,3]
- Use gloves only once. Be aware that isolation garb loses its effectiveness when wet *because moisture permits organisms to seep through the material.* Change masks and gowns as soon as moisture is noticeable or according to the manufacturer's recommendations or your facility's policy.
- Keep isolation supplies stocked *so they're readily available for those who must enter the patient's room.*

REFERENCES

1 The Joint Commission. (2012). Standard NPSG.07.01.01. *Comprehensive accreditation manual for hospitals: The official handbook.* Oakbrook Terrace, IL: The Joint Commission. (Level I)

2 Centers for Disease Control and Prevention. (October 2002). Guideline for hand hygiene in health-care settings. *Morbidity and Mortality Weekly Report, 51*(RR-16), 1–45. (Level I)

3 World Health Organization. (2009). *WHO guidelines on hand hygiene in health care: First global patient safety challenge. Clean care is safer care.* Geneva, Switzerland: World Health Organization. (Level I)

4 Siegel, J.D., et al. "2007 Guideline for Isolation Precautions: Preventing Transmission of Infectious Agents in Healthcare Settings" [Online]. Accessed December 2011 via the Web at http://www.cdc.gov/hicpac/2007ip/2007isolationprecautions.html (Level I)

5 Centers for Disease Control and Prevention. (December 2005). Guidelines for preventing the transmission of *Mycobacterium tuberculosis* in health care settings. *Morbidity and Mortality Weekly Report 54*(RR-17), 1–141. (Level I)

ADDITIONAL REFERENCES

The Joint Commission. (2012). Standard IC.02.01.01. *Comprehensive accreditation manual for hospitals: The official handbook.* Oakbrook Terrace, IL: The Joint Commission.

Rushing, J. (2006). Wearing personal protective gear. *Nursing, 36*(10), 56–57.

Snyder, G.M., et al. (2008). Detection of methicillin-resistant *Staphylococcus aureus* and vancomycin-resistant enterococci on the gowns and gloves of healthcare workers. *Infection Control and Hospital Epidemiology, 29*(7), 583–589.

PNEUMATIC ANTISHOCK GARMENT APPLICATION

A pneumatic antishock garment (PASG), also known as *medical antishock trousers* or a *MAST suit,* consists of inflatable bladders sandwiched between double layers of fabric. When inflated, a PASG places external pressure on the lower extremities and abdomen, creating an autotransfusion effect that squeezes blood superiorly and increases blood volume to the heart, lungs, and brain by up to 30%.

A PASG is used to treat shock when systolic blood pressure falls below 80 mm Hg or below 100 mm Hg when accompanied by signs of shock. It can control abdominal and lower extremity hemorrhage as well as help stabilize and splint pelvic and femoral fractures.

Use of a PASG is contraindicated in patients with cardiogenic shock, heart failure, pulmonary edema, tension pneumothorax, or increased intracranial pressure. The device should be used cautiously during pregnancy.

Equipment
For application
Gloves ▪ PASG ▪ foot pump ▪ Optional: resuscitation equipment, personal protective equipment.

For removal
Gloves ▪ PASG ▪ resuscitation equipment ▪ hospital-grade disinfectant.

PASGs come in a pediatric size for patients 3½′ to 5′ (1 to 1.5 m) tall and an adult size for patients taller than 5′.

Preparation of equipment
Before applying, spread open the PASG on a smooth surface or blanket *to avoid puncturing it.* Make sure all the stopcock valves are open. Attach the foot pump.

Implementation
- Verify the doctor's order.
- Perform hand hygiene and put on gloves.[1,2,3]
- Confirm the patient's identity using at least two patient identifiers according to your facility's policy.[4]
- Explain the procedure to the patient and answer all questions *to allay his fears and ensure his cooperation.*

Applying a PASG
- Take the patient's vital signs *to establish baseline measurements.* Assess his physical condition *to ensure that there are no contraindications to the use of the PASG.*
- Assess the patient's injuries *to see whether he can be turned from side to side.* If he can't be turned, slide the PASG under him. If he can be turned, place the PASG next to him and logroll him onto it. You can also set up the PASG on a stretcher and place the patient on it in a supine position. (See *Applying a pneumatic antishock garment.*)
- Examine the patient for sharp objects *that could injure him or the garment* such as pieces of glass.

Applying a pneumatic antishock garment

After taking the patient's baseline vital signs and explaining the treatment, prepare to apply the antishock garment. On a smooth surface, open the garment with Velcro fasteners down.

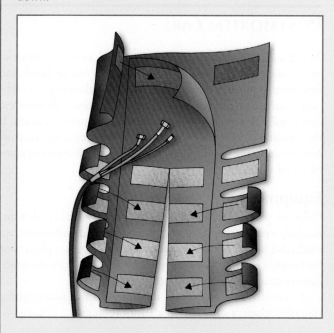

Open all stopcock valves; then attach the foot pump tubing to the valve on the pressure control unit. Determine if the patient be turned from side to side. If not, slide the garment under him. If he can be turned, place the garment next to him and, with assistance, move him onto it.

Before closing the garment, remove any sharp objects, such as pieces of glass, stones, keys, or a buckle, *that could injure the patient or tear the garment.* As appropriate, pad pressure points and apply lanolin *to protect the patient's skin from irritation.*

Place the upper edge of the garment just below the patient's lowest rib. Wrap the right leg compartment around the patient's right leg. Secure the compartment by fastening all the Velcro straps from ankle to thigh. Repeat this procedure for the left leg; then wrap the abdomen. Double-check that all valves are properly positioned.

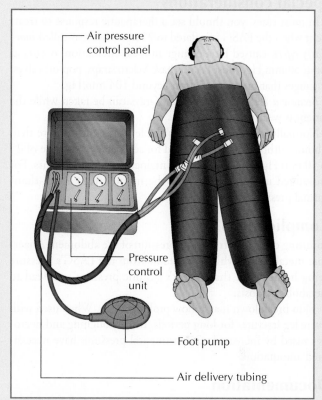

Air pressure control panel

Pressure control unit

Foot pump

Air delivery tubing

■ Double-check the stopcocks to ensure they're all open *so the PASG will inflate uniformly.*
■ Inflate the legs of the garment first, then the abdominal segment, to about 20 to 30 mm Hg initially.
■ Monitor the patient's blood pressure and pulse rate. Continue to inflate the garment slowly while monitoring vital signs. Stop inflating when the patient's systolic blood pressure reaches the desired level, usually 100 mm Hg.
■ Close all stopcocks *to prevent accidental air loss.*
■ Monitor the patient's blood pressure, pulse rate, and respirations every 5 minutes *to determine his response to application of the PASG.* Check his pedal pulses and temperature periodically. Notify the doctor if the circulation in the feet seems impaired.
■ Remove and discard your gloves and perform hand hygiene.[1,2,3]
■ Document the procedure.[5]

Removing a PASG
■ Before deflation, make sure IV lines are patent, a doctor is in attendance, and emergency resuscitation equipment is immediately available. *Removing a PASG may cause the patient's blood pressure to drop rapidly.*
■ Open the abdominal stopcock and start releasing small amounts of air. Closely monitor the patient's systolic blood pressure as you do this. If it drops 5 mm Hg, close the stopcock.
NURSING ALERT *Deflating the garment too quickly can allow circulating blood to rush to the abdomen or extremities, causing potentially irreversible shock.*
■ If a drop in blood pressure requires you to stop deflating the PASG, increase the flow rate of IV solutions *to help stabilize blood pressure.*

- If blood pressure is stable, continue to deflate the PASG slowly. After deflating the abdominal section, deflate the legs simultaneously.
- When the PASG is loose enough, gently pull it off.
- Disinfect the PASG, as required, but don't autoclave it or use solvents.
- Remove and discard your gloves and perform hand hygiene.[1,2,3]
- Document the procedure.[5]

Special considerations

- In most cases, you should see a therapeutic response to treatment when the PASG is inflated to 25 mm Hg. A so-called *morbidity effect,* caused by a change in local circulation, occurs at about 50 mm Hg. Most PASGs have Velcro straps, pop-off valves, or gauges that prevent inflation beyond 104 mm Hg.
- *Because a PASG is radiolucent,* X-rays can be taken while the patient is wearing it.
- Normally, the PASG shouldn't be left inflated for more than 2 hours, although it may be used for several days. A range of 25 to 50 mm Hg can usually be maintained for up to 48 hours. For prolonged use, the PASG may be inflated to a lower-than-normal pressure.

Complications

Vomiting can result from compression of the abdomen. Anaerobic metabolism, which can result from the PASG's pressure being higher than the patient's systolic pressure, can lead to metabolic acidosis.

Skin breakdown may follow prolonged use. When used with severe leg fractures for long periods, tissue sloughing and necrosis caused by increased compartmental pressures have necessitated amputation.

Documentation

Record the time of application and the patient's vital signs before application and during treatment. Record the time of removal and the patient's vital signs.

REFERENCES

1 Centers for Disease Control and Prevention. (October 2002). Guideline for hand hygiene in health-care settings. *Morbidity and Mortality Weekly Report, 51*(RR-16), 1–45. (Level I)
2 World Health Organization. (2009). *WHO guidelines on hand hygiene in health care: First global patient safety challenge. Clean care is safer care.* Geneva, Switzerland: World Health Organization. (Level I)
3 The Joint Commission. (2012). Standard NPSG.07.01.01. *Comprehensive accreditation manual for hospitals: The official handbook.* Oakbrook Terrace, IL: The Joint Commission. (Level I)
4 The Joint Commission. (2012). Standard NPSG.01.01.01. *Comprehensive accreditation manual for hospitals: The official handbook.* Oakbrook Terrace, IL: The Joint Commission. (Level I)
5 The Joint Commission. (2012). Standard RC.01.03.01. *Comprehensive accreditation manual for hospitals: The official handbook.* Oakbrook Terrace, IL: The Joint Commission. (Level I)

ADDITIONAL REFERENCE

Dickinson, K., & Roberts, I. (2000). Medical anti-shock trousers (pneumatic anti-shock garments) for circulatory support in patients with trauma. *Cochrane Database of Systemic Reviews* (2), CD001856.

POSTMORTEM CARE

After a patient dies, care includes preparing him for family viewing, arranging transportation to the morgue or funeral home, and determining the disposition of the patient's belongings. In addition, postmortem care entails comfortin their privacy. Postmortem care usually begins after a doctor certifies the patient's death. If the patient died violently or under suspicious circumstances, postmortem care may be postponed until the medical examiner completes an autopsy.

Equipment

Gauze or soft string ties ▪ gloves ▪ chin straps ▪ ABD pads ▪ cotton balls ▪ plastic shroud or body wrap ▪ three identification tags ▪ adhesive bandages to cover wounds or punctures ▪ plastic bag for patient's belongings ▪ water-filled basin ▪ soap ▪ towels ▪ washcloths ▪ stretcher ▪ personal protective equipment.

A commercial morgue pack usually contains gauze or string ties, chin straps, a shroud, and identification tags.

Implementation

- Notify the appropriate facility personnel, such as the nursing supervisor, that the patient has been pronounced dead.
- Notify the clergyperson or social worker according to your facility's policy if he hasn't already been notified.
- Notify your local organ procurement agency of the patient's death, according to federal regulations and your facility's policy.[1]
- Provide privacy. Offer support to family members if they're present.
- Perform hand hygiene and put on gloves and other personal protective equipment according to standard precautions, or maintain isolation precautions if they were being used.[2,3,4]
- Place the body in the supine position, with the arms at the sides and the head on a pillow. Then elevate the head of the bed 30 degrees *to prevent discoloration from blood settling in the face.*
- If the patient wore dentures and your facility's policy permits, gently insert them; then close the mouth. Close the eyes by gently pressing on the lids with your fingertips. If they don't stay closed, place moist cotton balls on the eyelids for a few minutes, and then try again to close them. Place a folded towel under the chin *to keep the jaw closed.*
- Remove all indwelling urinary catheters, tubes, and tape, and apply adhesive bandages to puncture sites, if the patient is not to have an autopsy performed. Replace soiled dressings.
- Collect all the patient's valuables *to prevent loss.* If you're unable to remove a ring, cover it with gauze, tape it in place, and tie the gauze to the wrist *to prevent slippage and subsequent loss.*

- Clean the body thoroughly, using soap, a basin, and washcloths. Place one or more ABD pads between the buttocks *to absorb rectal discharge or drainage.*
- Cover the body up to the chin with a clean sheet.
- Offer comfort and emotional support to the family and intimate friends. Ask if they wish to see the patient. If they do, allow them to do so in privacy. Ask if they would prefer to leave the patient's jewelry on the body. Give belongings to the family, if possible.
- Have the family sign body release forms, as appropriate, according to your facility's policy.
- After the family leaves, remove the towel from under the chin of the deceased patient. Pad the chin, and wrap chin straps under the chin and tie them loosely on top of the head. Then, pad the wrists and ankles *to prevent bruises,* and tie them together with gauze or soft string ties.
- Fill out the three identification tags. Each tag should include the deceased patient's name, room and bed numbers, date and time of death, and doctor's name. Tie one tag to the deceased patient's hand or foot, but don't remove his identification bracelet *to ensure correct identification.*
- Place the shroud or body wrap on the morgue stretcher and, after obtaining assistance, transfer the body to the stretcher. Wrap the body, and tie the shroud or wrap with the string provided. Then, attach another identification tag to the front of the shroud or wrap; then cover the shroud or wrap with a clean sheet. If a shroud or wrap isn't available, dress the deceased patient in a clean gown and cover the body with a sheet.
- Place the deceased patient's personal belongings, including valuables, in a bag and attach the third identification tag to it.
- If the patient was in isolation, follow facility policy for isolation precautions.
- Remove and discard your gloves and perform hand hygiene.[2,3,4]
- Close the doors of adjoining rooms if possible. Then take the body to the morgue, if your facility follows this process. Use corridors that aren't crowded and, if possible, use a service elevator. Otherwise, leave the body in the room until picked up by the funeral home personnel.
- Perform hand hygiene.[2,3,4]
- Document the procedure.[5]

Special considerations

- Give the deceased patient's personal belongings to his family or bring them to the morgue. If you give the family jewelry or money, make sure a coworker is present as a witness. Obtain the signature of an adult family member *to verify receipt of valuables or to state their preference that jewelry remain on the patient.*
- Offer to call clergy or a social worker *to assist the family, as necessary.*

Documentation

Document that postmortem care was provided. Although the extent of documentation varies among facilities, always record the disposition of the patient's possessions, especially jewelry and money. Also note the date and time the deceased patient was transported to the morgue.

REFERENCES

1 Centers for Medicare & Medicaid Services, Department of Health and Human Services. (1998, revised 2004). Title 42 CFR Public Health, Volume 3, Chapter IV, Part 482—Conditions of Participation for Hospitals. Subpart C—Basic Hospital Functions, Section 482.45—Condition of Participation: Organ, Tissue, and Eye Procurement. Washington, D.C.: U.S. Government Printing Office.
2 Centers for Disease Control and Prevention. (October 2002). Guideline for hand hygiene in health-care settings. *Morbidity and Mortality Weekly Report, 51*(RR-16), 1–45. (Level I)
3 World Health Organization. (2009). *WHO guidelines on hand hygiene in health care: First global patient safety challenge. Clean care is safer care.* Geneva, Switzerland: World Health Organization. (Level I)
4 The Joint Commission. (2012). Standard NPSG.07.01.01. *Comprehensive accreditation manual for hospitals: The official handbook.* Oakbrook Terrace, IL: The Joint Commission. (Level I)
5 The Joint Commission. (2012). Standard RC.01.03.01. *Comprehensive accreditation manual for hospitals: The official handbook.* Oakbrook Terrace, IL: The Joint Commission. (Level I)

ADDITIONAL REFERENCES

Craven, R.F., & Hirnle, C.J. (2012). *Fundamentals of nursing: Human health and function* (7th ed.). Philadelphia, PA: Lippincott Williams & Wilkins.
Kuebler, K.K. (2007). *Palliative and end of life care: Clinical practice guidelines* (2nd ed.). Philadelphia, PA: Mosby.
Taylor, C., et al. (2011). *Fundamentals of nursing: The art and science of nursing care* (7th ed.). Philadelphia, PA: Lippincott Williams & Wilkins.

POSTOPERATIVE CARE

Postoperative care begins when the patient arrives on the postanesthesia care unit (PACU) and continues as he moves to the short procedure unit, medical-surgical unit, or critical care area. The purpose of postoperative care is to minimize postoperative complications, such as pain, inadequate oxygenation, or adverse physiologic effects of sudden movement, through early detection and prompt treatment.

Recovery from general anesthesia takes longer than its induction because the anesthetic is retained in fat and muscle. Because fat has a meager blood supply, it releases the anesthetic slowly, providing enough anesthesia to maintain adequate blood and brain levels during surgery. The patient's recovery time varies with his amount of body fat, his overall condition, his premedication regimen, and the type, dosage, and duration of anesthesia.

Equipment

Thermometer ■ watch with second hand ■ stethoscope ■ sphygmomanometer ■ postoperative flowchart or other documentation tool ■ medications, as ordered.

Implementation

- Gather the necessary equipment at the patient's bedside.
- Perform hand hygiene and put on gloves.[1,2,3]
- Receive hand-off communication about the procedure and the patient's condition from the perioperative nurse.[4] This record should include a summary of operative procedures and pertinent findings; type of anesthesia; vital signs (preoperative, intraoperative, and postoperative); medical history; medication history, including preoperative, intraoperative, and postoperative medications; fluid therapy, including estimated blood loss, type and number of drains, catheters, and amount and characteristics of drainage; and notes on the condition of the surgical wound. For example, if the patient had vascular surgery, knowing the location and duration of blood vessel clamping can prevent postoperative complications.[4,5]
- Confirm the patient's identity using at least two patient identifiers according to your facility's policy.[6]
- Explain all actions to the patient *to decrease anxiety and increase cooperation.*
- Transfer the patient from the PACU stretcher to the bed, and position him properly. Get a coworker to help, if necessary. When moving the patient, keep transfer movements smooth *to minimize pain and postoperative complications and avoid back strain among team members.* Use a transfer board as needed.
- Raise the bed's side rails *to ensure the patient's safety.*
- **NURSING ALERT** *If the patient has had orthopedic surgery, always get a coworker to help transfer him. Ask the coworker to move only the affected extremity. If the patient is in skeletal traction, you may receive special orders for moving him. If you must move him, have a coworker move the weights as you and another coworker move the patient.*
- Monitor the patient's respiratory status by assessing his airway. Note breathing rate and depth, and auscultate for breath sounds. Provide oxygen *to maintain an oxygen saturation of greater than 94%.* Simple face masks are generally used until the patient is more awake.[7]
- Monitor the patient's pulse rate. It should be strong and easily palpable. The heart rate should be within 20% of the preoperative heart rate.
- Compare postoperative blood pressure to preoperative blood pressure. It should be within 20% of the preoperative level unless the patient suffered a hypotensive episode during surgery.
- Elevate the head of the bed, if acceptable from a surgical standpoint, *to improve ventilation and to prevent aspiration of secretions.*[5]
- Assess the patient's level of consciousness, skin color, and mucous membranes.
- Obtain the patient's core body temperature *because anesthesia lowers body temperature.* A patient with a temperature lower than 96.8° F (36° C), shivering, or other symptoms of hypothermia should be treated with active rewarming. (See "Hyperthermia-hypothermia blanket use," page 348.) *Hypothermia has deleterious effects on many systems and inhibits the metabolism of inhaled, IV, and regional anesthetics.*[5,8]
- Perform a neurologic assessment, particularly in a patient who has undergone a surgical procedure involving components of the neurologic system.

- Complete a GI assessment and verify the patency of any nasogastric or orogastric drainage tubes that are present. Also verify whether they should be connected to suction. Assess the patient's bowel sounds, especially if surgery involving the abdomen has occurred. Perform a nausea assessment as soon as the patient awakens and regularly thereafter; nausea and vomiting should be treated early and aggressively.[8]
- Perform a genitourinary assessment, including whether an indwelling urinary catheter is present and the color, quantity, and quality of urine. Some patients who undergo urinary tract surgery may have continuous bladder irrigation to control bleeding and reduce the chance of blockage or clots forming in the bladder. Maintain continuous bladder irrigation as ordered by the doctor.[9]
- Assess the patient's pain intensity using a self-reporting 0-to-10 scale whenever possible. Assess pain type, location, frequency, and duration. Also assess other sources of discomfort, such as nausea, vomiting, positioning, and anxiety.
- Provide pain medication as ordered. Assess the patient's pain level before and after administration according to facility policy.
- Assess the patient's infusion sites for redness, pain, swelling, or drainage. *These findings indicate infiltration and require discontinuing the IV and restarting it at another site.*
- Assess surgical wound dressings; they should be clean and dry. If they're soiled, assess the characteristics of the drainage and outline the soiled area. Note the date and time of assessment on the dressing. Assess the soiled area frequently; if it enlarges, reinforce the dressing and alert the doctor.
- Note the presence and condition of any drains and tubes. Note the color, type, odor, and amount of drainage. Make sure all drains are properly connected and free from kinks and obstructions.
- If the patient has had vascular or orthopedic surgery, assess the appropriate extremity—or all extremities—depending on the surgical procedure. Perform neurovascular assessments; assess color, temperature, sensation, movement, and presence and quality of pulses; and notify the doctor of any abnormalities.
- Continue deep vein thrombosis prophylaxis, such as using sequential compression sleeves or boots, according to the doctor's order or facility protocol.[5]
- As the patient recovers from anesthesia, monitor his respiratory and cardiovascular status closely. Be alert for signs of airway obstruction and hypoventilation caused by laryngospasm, or for sedation, which can lead to hypoxemia. *Cardiovascular complications—such as arrhythmias and hypotension—may result from the anesthetic agent or the operative procedure.*
- Encourage coughing and deep-breathing exercises (unless the patient has just had nasal, ophthalmic, or neurologic surgery) *to avoid increasing intracranial pressure.*
- Assess for nausea and vomiting.
- Administer postoperative medications, such as antibiotics, analgesics, antiemetics, or reversal agents, as ordered and appropriate.
- Remove all fluids from the patient's bedside until he is alert enough to eat and drink. Before giving him liquids, assess his gag reflex *to prevent aspiration.* To do this, lightly touch the back of

his throat with a cotton swab; the patient will gag if the reflex has returned. Do this test quickly *to prevent a vagal reaction*.

■ Monitor the patient's intake and output.

■ Assess for the presence of bowel sounds and passage of flatus before allowing the patient to have food.

■ Remove and discard your gloves. Perform hand hygiene.[1,2,3]

■ Document the procedure.[10]

Special considerations

■ Fear, pain, anxiety, hypothermia, confusion, and immobility can upset the patient and jeopardize his safety and postoperative status. Offer emotional support to the patient and his family. Keep in mind that the patient who has lost a body part or who has been diagnosed with an incurable disease will need ongoing emotional support. Refer him and his family for counseling as needed.

■ As the patient recovers from general anesthesia, reflexes appear in reverse order to that in which they disappeared. Hearing recovers first, so avoid holding inappropriate conversations.

■ The patient under general anesthesia can't protect his own airway *because of muscle relaxation*. As he recovers, his cough and gag reflexes reappear. If he can lift his head without assistance, he's usually able to breathe on his own.

■ If the patient received spinal anesthesia, he may need to remain supine with the bed adjusted to between 0 and 20 degrees for at least 6 hours *to reduce the risk of spinal headache from leakage of cerebrospinal fluid*. Check your facility's policy and procedure for activity restriction after spinal anesthesia. The patient won't be able to move his legs, so be sure to reassure him that sensation and mobility will return. (See *Assessing level of blockade from spinal anesthesia*, page 592.)

■ If the patient has epidural analgesia infusion for postoperative pain control, monitor his respiratory status closely. *Respiratory arrest may result from the respiratory depressant effects of the opioid.* Also monitor the patient's blood pressure, heart rate, and arterial oxygen saturation according to your facility's policy. He may also suffer nausea, vomiting, or itching. Epidural analgesia may also include administering a local anesthetic with the opioid. (See "Epidural analgesic administration," page 280.) Assess the patient's lower-extremity motor strength every 2 to 4 hours. If sensori-motor loss occurs (numbness or weakness of the legs), notify the doctor *because the dosage may need to be decreased*.

■ If the patient will be using a patient-controlled anesthesia (PCA) unit, make sure he understands how to use it. Caution him to activate it only when he has pain, not when he feels sleepy or is pain-free. Review your facility's criteria for PCA use.

ELDER ALERT *If the patient is older, be aware of age-related changes that will alter your assessment. Monitor cardiovascular status carefully* because blood loss, pain, bed rest, and fluid and electrolyte imbalances can alter it. *Respiratory status also should be monitored carefully* because ventilation and oxygenation can be altered by age-related changes or years of smoking or chronic diseases. *Monitor level of consciousness and pain carefully* because mental status changes can affect these and make pain control more difficult. Drug metabolism slows with age, *so monitor the older adult's risk for drug reactions, toxicity, and interactions.*

Monitor intake and output carefully and watch for urinary tract infections because of decreased renal functioning and decreased bladder capacity. *Be careful when positioning the older patient and prevent postoperative falls* because the patient may have osteoporosis and may be prone to fractures. *Also monitor for signs and symptoms of infection* because the risk of infection increases with age.

Complications

Postoperative complications may include cardiac arrhythmias, hypotension, hypovolemia, septicemia, septic shock, atelectasis, pneumonia, thrombophlebitis, pulmonary embolism, urine retention, wound infection, wound dehiscence, evisceration, abdominal distention, paralytic ileus, constipation, altered body image, and postoperative psychosis.

Recovery from anesthesia isn't a linear progression. Patients can, and often do, regress to a less awake status, occlude their airways, become unstable because of slow bleeding or sepsis, have spikes or dips in blood pressure and heart rate due to peaking or wearing off of medication, or become suddenly nauseated with severe emesis that puts them at risk for aspiration. Hypothermia, hypoxemia, hypoventilation, and airway obstruction are the primary complications monitored for in the PACU.[11]

Documentation

Document vital signs on the appropriate flowchart. Record the condition of dressings and drains and characteristics of drainage. Document all assessment findings, any conditions reported to the doctor, and interventions required to address abnormal findings. Document all interventions taken to alleviate pain and anxiety and the patient's responses to them. Document any complications and interventions taken.

REFERENCES

1 The Joint Commission. (2012). Standard NPSG.07.01.01. *Comprehensive accreditation manual for hospitals: The official handbook.* Oakbrook Terrace, IL: The Joint Commission. (Level I)

2 Centers for Disease Control and Prevention. (October 2002). Guideline for hand hygiene in health-care settings. *Morbidity and Mortality Weekly Report, 51*(RR-16), 1–45. (Level I)

3 World Health Organization. (2009). *WHO guidelines on hand hygiene in health care: First global patient safety challenge. Clean care is safer care.* Geneva, Switzerland: World Health Organization. (Level I)

4 Recommended practices for transfer of patient care information. (2011). In R. Conner, et al. (Eds). *Perioperative standards and recommended practices.* Denver, CO: AORN.

5 AORN guidance statement: Safe patient handling and movement in the perioperative setting. (2011). In R. Conner, et al. (Eds.). *Perioperative standards and recommended practices.* Denver, CO: AORN.

6 The Joint Commission. (2012). Standard NPSG.01.01.01. *Comprehensive accreditation manual for hospitals: The official handbook.* Oakbrook Terrace, IL: The Joint Commission. (Level I)

7 Gali, B., et al. (2009). Identification of patients at risk for postoperative respiratory complications using a preoperative obstructive sleep apnea screening tool and postanesthesia care assessment. *Anesthesiology, 110*(4), 1869–1877.

Assessing level of blockade from spinal anesthesia

Spinal anesthesia produces a sympathetic, sensory, and motor block. If your patient received spinal anesthesia, be ready to assess the downward progression of the level of blockade. Using a dermatome chart aids this assessment. Each dermatome represents a specific body area supplied with nerve fibers from an individual spinal root (cervical, thoracic, lumbar, or sacral). To document the patient's sensory and motor function, mentally divide his body into dermatomes. Anatomic reference points include the nipple line at T4, xiphoid at T6, umbilicus at T10, and groin at L1.

Anterior view

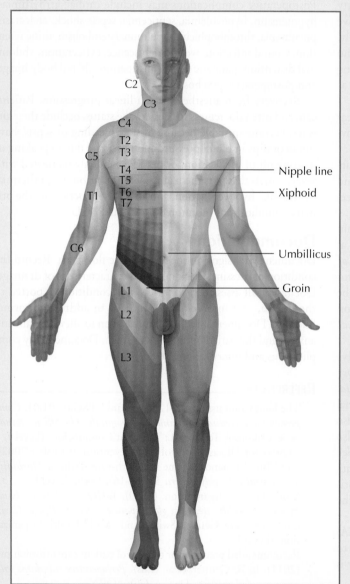

Posterior view

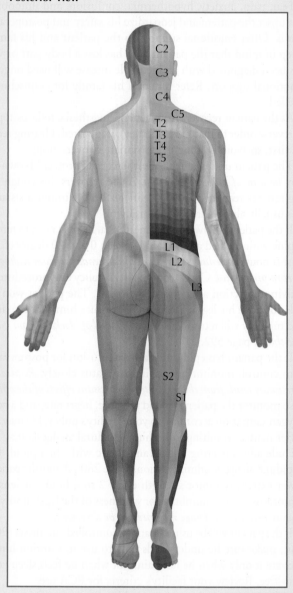

8 American Society of Peri Anesthesia Nurses. (2010). Clinical guideline for the promotion of perioperative normothermia. In *Perianesthesia nursing standards and practice recommendations: 2010–2012*. Cherry Hill, NJ: American Society of PeriAnesthesia Nurses.

9 Feliciano, T., et al. (2008). A retrospective, descriptive, exploratory study evaluating incidence of postoperative urinary retention after spinal anesthesia and its effect on PACU discharge. *Journal of Perianesthesia Nursing, 23*(6), 394–400.

10 The Joint Commission. (2012). Standard RC.01.03.01. *Comprehensive accreditation manual for hospitals: The official handbook*. Oakbrook Terrace, IL: The Joint Commission. (Level I)

11 Flockton, E., et al. (2008). Reversal of rocuronium-induced neuromuscular block with sugammadex is faster than reversal of cisatracurium-induced block with neostigmine. *British Journal of Anaesthesia, 100*(5), 622–630.

ADDITIONAL REFERENCE

Pedoto, A., & Heerdt, P.M. (2009). Postoperative care after pulmonary resection: Postanesthesia care unit versus intensive care unit. *Current Opinion in Anaesthesiology, 22*(1), 50–55.

PREOPERATIVE CARE

Preoperative care begins when surgery is planned and ends with the administration of anesthesia. This phase of care includes a preoperative interview and assessment to collect baseline subjective and objective data from the patient and his family; diagnostic tests such as urinalysis, electrocardiogram, and chest radiography; preoperative teaching; securing informed consent from the patient; and physical preparation.

Equipment

Thermometer ▪ sphygmomanometer ▪ stethoscope ▪ watch with second hand ▪ weight scale ▪ tape measure.

Preparation of equipment

Gather all equipment needed at the patient's bedside or in the admission area.

Implementation

▪ Review the patient's preadmission findings.[1]
▪ Make sure the patient has a signed informed consent form in his medical record (See *Obtaining informed consent.*)[2,3]
▪ Perform hand hygiene.[4,5,6]
▪ Confirm the patient's identity using at least two patient identifiers according to your facility's policy.[7]
▪ If the patient is having same-day surgery, make sure he knows ahead of time not to eat or drink anything for 8 hours before surgery. Confirm with him what time he's scheduled to arrive at the facility, and tell him to leave all jewelry and valuables at home. Also make sure the patient has arranged for someone to accompany him home after surgery.
▪ Obtain a health history and assess the patient's knowledge, perceptions, and expectations about his surgery. Ask about previous medical and surgical interventions. Also determine the patient's psychosocial needs; ask about occupational well-being, financial matters, support systems, mental status, and cultural beliefs. Use your facility's preoperative surgical assessment database, if available, to gather this information.[1]
▪ Obtain a drug history and anesthetic history. Ask about current prescriptions, over-the-counter medications (including any supplements and herbal preparations), and known allergies to foods, drugs, and latex.[1]
▪ Obtain results of X-ray examinations or other preoperative tests.[1,8]

Obtaining informed consent

Informed consent means that the patient is entitled to a full explanation of the procedure, its risks and complications, and the risk if the procedure isn't performed at this time. Although obtaining informed consent is the doctor's responsibility, the nurse is responsible for verifying that this step has been taken.

You may be asked to witness the patient's signature. However, if you didn't hear the doctor's explanation to the patient, you must sign that you are witnessing the patient's signature only.

Consent forms must be signed before the patient receives his preoperative medication because forms signed after sedatives are given are legally invalid. Adults and emancipated minors can sign their own consent forms. Children's consent forms, or those of adults with impaired mental status, must be signed by a parent or guardian.

▪ Ask if the patient has an advance directive. Provide information about advance directives as appropriate. (See "Advance directives," page 6.)
▪ Measure the patient's height, weight, and vital signs.
▪ Identify risk factors that may interfere with a positive expected outcome. Be sure to consider age, general health, medications, mobility, nutritional status, fluid and electrolyte disturbances, and lifestyle. Also consider the location, nature, and the extent of the surgical procedure.
▪ Explain preoperative procedures to the patient. Include typical events that the patient can expect. Discuss equipment that may be used postoperatively, such as nasogastric tubes and IV equipment. Explain the typical incision, dressings, and staples or sutures that will be used. *Preoperative teaching can help reduce postoperative anxiety and pain, increase patient compliance, hasten recovery, and decrease length of stay.*
▪ Discuss postoperative pain management. Teach the patient how to use a pain scale of 0 to 10 to rate his pain. Find out what his goals and expectations for pain relief are. Explore his previous pain experiences and those pain interventions that were most effective. Ask about his analgesic history.[9]
▪ Talk the patient through the sequence of events from operating room to recovery room (postanesthesia care unit [PACU]) back to the patient's room. Some patients may be transferred from the PACU to an intensive care unit or surgical care unit. Your patient may also benefit from a tour of the areas he'll see during the perioperative events.
▪ When discussing transfer procedures and techniques, describe sensations the patient will experience. Tell him that he'll be taken to the operating room on a stretcher and transferred from the stretcher to the operating room table. *For his own safety,* he'll be held securely to the table with soft restraints. The operating room nurses will check his vital signs frequently.

■ Tell the patient that the operating room may feel cool. Electrodes may be put on his chest to monitor his heart rate during surgery. Describe the drowsy floating sensation he'll feel as the anesthetic takes effect. Tell him it's important that he relax at this time.

■ Tell the patient about exercises that he may be expected to perform after surgery, such as deep breathing, coughing (while splinting the incision if necessary), extremity exercises and movement, and ambulation *to minimize respiratory and circulatory complications.* If the patient will undergo ophthalmic or neurologic surgery, he won't be asked to cough *because coughing increases intracranial pressure.*

■ On the day of surgery, important interventions include providing for morning care, administering ordered preoperative medications, completing the preoperative checklist and chart, and providing support to the patient and his family.

■ Other immediate preoperative interventions may include preparing the GI tract (restricting food and fluids for about 8 hours before surgery) *to reduce vomiting and the risk of aspiration,* using enemas before abdominal or GI surgery *to clean the lower GI tract of fecal material,* and giving antibiotics for 2 or 3 days preoperatively *to prevent contamination of the peritoneal cavity by GI bacteria.*

■ Just before the patient is moved to the surgical area, make sure he is wearing a hospital gown, has his identification band in place, and has his vital signs recorded. Check to see that hairpins, nail polish, and jewelry have been removed. Note whether dentures, contact lenses, or prosthetic devices have been removed or left in place.

■ Verify with the patient that the correct surgical site has been marked.

■ Provide face-to-face hand-off communication about the patient's status and care to the person who will assume responsibility for the patient's care in the operating room. Allow time for questions and clarification of any information.[10]

■ Perform hand hygiene.[4,5,6]

■ Document the procedure.[11]

Special considerations

■ Preoperative medications must be given on time *to enhance the effect of ordered anesthesia.* The patient should take nothing by mouth preoperatively. Don't give oral medications unless ordered. Be sure to raise the bed's side rails immediately after giving preoperative medications.[1]

■ If family or others are present, direct them to the appropriate waiting area and offer support as needed.

Documentation

Complete the preoperative checklist used by your facility. Record all nursing care measures and preoperative medications, results of diagnostic tests, and the time the patient is transferred to the surgical area. The chart and the surgical checklist must accompany the patient to surgery.

REFERENCES

1 AORN guidance statement: Preoperative patient care in the ambulatory surgery setting. (2011). In R. Conner, et al. (Eds.). *Perioperative standards and recommended practices.* Denver, CO: AORN.

2 The Joint Commission. (2012). Standard RI.01.03.01. *Comprehensive accreditation manual for hospitals: The official handbook.* Oakbrook Terrace, IL: The Joint Commission. (Level I)

3 Centers for Medicare & Medicaid Services, Department of Health and Human Services. (2006). "Conditions of Participation: Patients' Rights," 42 CFR part 482.13 [Online]. Accessed November 2011 via the Web at https://www.cms.gov/CFCsAndCoPs/downloads/finalpatientrightsrule.pdf

4 The Joint Commission. (2012). Standard NPSG.07.01.01. *Comprehensive accreditation manual for hospitals: The official handbook.* Oakbrook Terrace, IL: The Joint Commission. (Level I)

5 Centers for Disease Control and Prevention. (October 2002). Guideline for hand hygiene in health-care settings. *Morbidity and Mortality Weekly Report, 51*(RR-16), 1–45. (Level I)

6 World Health Organization. (2009). *WHO guidelines on hand hygiene in health care: First global patient safety challenge. Clean care is safer care.* Geneva, Switzerland: World Health Organization. (Level I)

7 The Joint Commission. (2012). Standard NPSG.01.01.01. *Comprehensive accreditation manual for hospitals: The official handbook.* Oakbrook Terrace, IL: The Joint Commission. (Level I)

8 The Joint Commission. (2012). Standard UP.01.01.01. *Comprehensive accreditation manual for hospitals: The official handbook.* Oakbrook Terrace, IL: The Joint Commission. (Level I)

9 American Society of PeriAnesthesia Nurses. (2010) Pain and comfort clinical guideline. In *Perianesthesia nursing standards and practice recommendations: 2010–2012.* Cherry Hill, NJ: American Society of Perianesthesia Nurses.

10 Recommended practices for transfer of patient care information. (2011). In R. Conner, et al. (Eds.). *Perioperative standards and recommended practices.* Denver, CO: AORN.

11 The Joint Commission. (2012). Standard RC.01.03.01. *Comprehensive accreditation manual for hospitals: The official handbook.* Oakbrook Terrace, IL: The Joint Commission. (Level I)

ADDITIONAL REFERENCE

Williams, J., et al. (2007). The chemical control of preoperative anxiety. *Psychophysiology, 12*(1), 46–49.

PREOPERATIVE SKIN PREPARATION

Proper preparation of the patient's skin for surgery renders it as free as possible from microorganisms, which reduces the risk of infection at the incision site.[1] This procedure doesn't duplicate or replace the full sterile preparation that immediately precedes surgery. Before any surgical procedure, the patient should have two preoperative showers with chlorhexidine gluconate to reduce the number of microorganisms on the skin and decrease the risk of contaminating the surgical incision.[1]

Hair should not be removed from the area surrounding the operative site unless it's thick enough to interfere with surgery because hair removal may increase the risk of infection. If hair is removed, use electric clippers. Clipping hair should occur immediately before an operation to decrease the risk of surgical

Where to remove hair for surgery

Shoulder and upper arm
On operative side, remove hair from fingertips to hairline and center chest to center spine, extending to iliac crest and including the axilla.

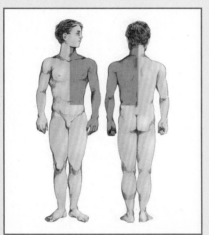

Forearm, elbow, and hand
On operative side, remove hair from fingertips to shoulder. Include axilla unless surgery is for hand.

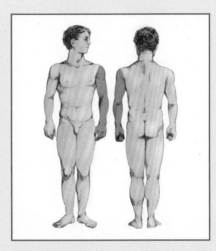

Thigh
On operative side, remove hair from toes to 3″ (7.6 cm) above umbilicus and from midline front to midline back, including pubis.

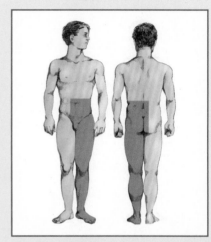

Chest
Remove hair from chin to iliac crests and to midline of back on operative side (2″ [5 cm] beyond midline of back for thoracotomy). Include axilla and entire arm to elbow on operative side.

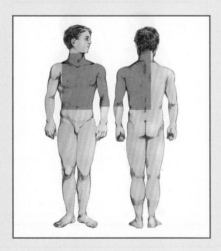

Abdomen
Remove hair from 3″ above nipples to upper thighs, including pubic area.

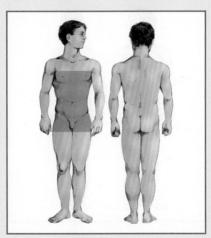

Lower abdomen
Remove hair from 2″ above umbilicus to midthigh, including pubic area; for femoral ligation, to midline of thigh in back; for hernioplasty and embolectomy, to costal margin and down to knee.

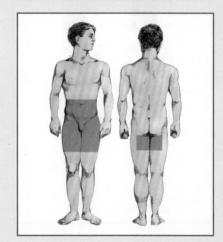

(continued)

site infection.[1,2,3,4] Each facility has a hair removal policy. (See *Where to remove hair for surgery.*)

The area of preparation always exceeds that of the expected incision to minimize the number of microorganisms in the areas adjacent to the proposed incision and to allow surgical draping of the patient without contamination.[1]

Equipment
Chlorhexidine gluconate antiseptic skin cleaner ▪ gloves ▪ tap water ▪ bath blanket ▪ basins ▪ linen-saver pad ▪ electric or battery-operated clippers, single use or with a reusable head that can be disinfected ▪ adjustable light ▪ Optional: 4″ × 4″ gauze

Where to remove hair for surgery *(continued)*

Hip
On operative side, remove hair from toes to nipples and at least 3″ beyond midline back and front, including pubis.

Knee and lower leg
On operative side, remove hair from toes to groin.

Ankle and foot
On operative side, remove hair from toes to 3″ above knee.

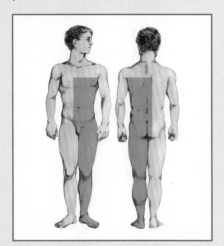

Flank
On operative side, remove hair from nipples to pubis, 3″ beyond midline in back, 2″ past abdominal midline. Include pubic area and, on affected side, upper thigh and axilla.

Perineum
Remove hair from pubis, perineum, and perianal area, and from waist to at least 3″ below groin in front and at least 3″ below buttocks in back.

Spine
Remove hair from axillae and back, including shoulders and neck to hairline, down to both knees.

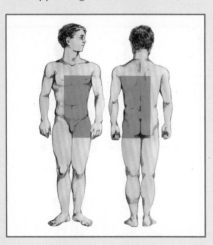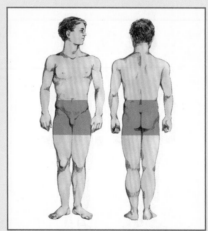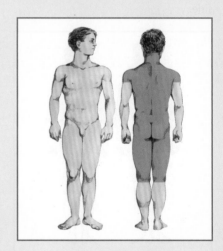

pads, cotton-tipped applicators, nail polish remover, depilatory cream, orangewood stick, trash bag, towel.

Preparation of equipment

Use warm tap water *because heat reduces the skin's surface tension and facilitates removal of soil and hair.* Pour plain warm water into the basin *for rinsing.*

Implementation

- Perform hand hygiene and put on gloves.[5,6,7]
- Confirm the patient's identity using at least two patient identifiers according to your facility's policy.[8]
- Verify the doctor's order, provide privacy, and explain the procedure to the patient, including the reason for the extensive preparations *to avoid causing undue anxiety.*

- Place the patient in a comfortable position, drape him with the bath blanket, and expose the preparation area. For most surgeries, this area extends 12″ (30.5 cm) in each direction from the expected incision site. However, *to ensure privacy and avoid chilling the patient,* expose only one small area at a time while performing skin preparation.
- Position a linen-saver pad beneath the patient *to catch spills and avoid linen changes.* Adjust the light to illuminate the preparation area.
- Assess skin condition in the preparation area, and report any rash, abrasion, or laceration to the doctor before beginning the procedure. *Any break in the skin increases the risk of infection and could cause cancellation of planned surgery.*[1]
- Have the patient remove all jewelry in or near the operative site.
- Begin removing hair from the preparation area, if necessary, by clipping any long hairs with clippers to remove microorganisms. Perform the procedure as near to the time of surgery as possible *so that microorganisms will have minimal time to proliferate.*[1,3]
- Proceed with a 10-minute scrub *to ensure a clean preparation area.* Wash the area with a chlorhexidine gluconate antiseptic skin cleaner. Using a circular motion, start at the expected incision site and work outward toward the periphery of the area *to avoid recontaminating the clean area.* Apply light friction while washing *to improve the antiseptic effect of the solution.*[1,3]
- Carefully clean skin folds and crevices *because they harbor greater numbers of microorganisms.* Scrub the perineal area last, if it's part of the preparation area, for the same reason. Pull loose skin taut.
- If necessary, use cotton-tipped applicators to clean the umbilicus and an orangewood stick to clean under nails. Remove any nail polish *because the anesthetist uses nail bed color to determine adequate oxygenation and may place a probe on the nail to measure oxygen saturation.*
- Dry the area with a clean towel, and remove the linen-saver pad.
- Give the patient any special instructions for care of the prepared area, and remind him to keep the area clean for surgery. Make sure the patient is comfortable.
- Properly dispose of solutions and the trash bag, and clean or dispose of soiled equipment and supplies according to your facility's policy.
- Remove and discard your gloves an perform hand hygiene.[5,6,7]
- Document the procedure.[9]

Special considerations

- Avoid removing facial or neck hair on women and children unless ordered. Scalp hair removal is usually performed in the operating room, but if you're required to prepare the patient's scalp, put all hair in a plastic or paper bag and store it with the patient's possessions.
- Depilatory cream can also be used to remove hair. Although this method produces clean, intact skin without risking lacerations or abrasions, it can cause skin irritation or rash, especially in the groin area.[1,3] A skin test must first be performed *to determine the risk for skin irritation.*[1] If possible, cut long hairs with scissors before applying the cream *because removal of remaining*

hair then requires less cream. Then use a glove to apply the cream in a layer ½″ (1.3 cm) thick. After about 10 minutes, remove the cream with moist gauze pads. Next, wash the area with antiseptic soap solution, rinse, and pat dry.

Complications

Rashes, nicks, lacerations, and abrasions are the most common complications of skin preparation. They also increase the risk of postoperative infection.

Documentation

Documentation should include the date, time, and area prepared as well as the condition of the skin before and after preparation. Include documentation about hair removal, if performed, including the time, method, and area of removal.[1]

REFERENCES

1 Recommended practices for preoperative patient skin antisepsis. (2011). In R. Conner, et al. (Eds.). *Perioperative standards and recommended practices.* Denver, CO: AORN. (Level VII)
2 Anderson, D.J. (2008). Strategies to prevent surgical site infections in acute care hospitals. *Infection Control and Hospital Epidemiology, 29*(S1), S51–S61. (Level I)
3 Mangram, A.J., et al. "Guideline for Prevention of Surgical Site Infection, 1999" [Online]. Accessed March 2012 via the Web at http://www.cdc.gov/hicpac/pdf/guidelines/SSI_1999.pdf
4 Olson, M.M., et al. (1986). Preoperative hair removal with clippers does not increase infection rate in clean surgery wounds. *Surgery, Gynecology, and Obstetrics, 162*(2), 181–182.
5 Centers for Disease Control and Prevention. (October 2002). Guideline for hand hygiene in health-care settings. *Morbidity and Mortality Weekly Report, 51*(RR-16), 1–45. (Level I)
6 The Joint Commission. (2012). Standard NPSG.07.01.01. *Comprehensive accreditation manual for hospitals: The official handbook.* Oakbrook Terrace, IL: The Joint Commission. (Level I)
7 World Health Organization. (2009). *WHO guidelines on hand hygiene in health care: First global patient safety challenge. Clean care is safer care.* Geneva, Switzerland: World Health Organization. (Level I)
8 The Joint Commission. (2012). Standard NPSG.01.01.01. *Comprehensive accreditation manual for hospitals: The official handbook.* Oakbrook Terrace, IL: The Joint Commission. (Level I)
9 The Joint Commission. (2012). Standard RC.01.03.01. *Comprehensive accreditation manual for hospitals: The official handbook.* Oakbrook Terrace, IL: The Joint Commission. (Level I)

PRESSURE DRESSING APPLICATION

For effective control of capillary or small-vein bleeding, temporary application of pressure directly over a wound may be achieved with a bulk dressing held by a glove-protected hand, bound into place with a pressure bandage, or held under pressure by an inflated air splint. A pressure dressing requires frequent checks for wound drainage to determine its effectiveness in controlling bleeding. The wound shouldn't be cleaned until the bleeding stops.

Equipment

Two or more sterile gauze pads ▪ roller gauze ▪ adhesive tape ▪ gloves ▪ metric ruler ▪ Optional: clean cloth.

Preparation of equipment

Obtain the pressure dressing quickly *to avoid excessive blood loss.* Use clean cloth for the dressing if sterile gauze pads are unavailable.

Implementation

▪ Perform hand hygiene and put on gloves.[1,2,3]
▪ Quickly explain the procedure to the patient *to help decrease his anxiety.*
▪ Elevate the injured body part, if possible, *to help reduce bleeding.*
▪ Place enough gauze pads over the wound to cover it.
▪ For an extremity or a trunk wound, hold the dressing firmly over the wound and wrap the roller gauze tightly across it and around the body part *to provide pressure on the wound.* Secure the bandage with adhesive tape.
▪ To apply a dressing to the neck, the shoulder, or another location that can't be tightly wrapped, don't use roller gauze. Instead, apply tape directly over the dressings *to provide the necessary pressure at the wound site.*
▪ Check pulse, temperature, and skin condition distal to the wound site *because excessive pressure can obstruct normal circulation.*
▪ Check the dressing frequently *to monitor wound drainage.* Use the metric standard of measurement to determine the amount of drainage, and document these serial measurements for later reference. Don't circle a potentially wet dressing with ink *because such markings don't provide permanent documentation in the medical record and also risk contaminating the dressing.*
▪ If the dressing becomes saturated, don't remove it; *removal would interfere with the pressure.* Instead, apply an additional dressing over the saturated one and continue to monitor and record drainage.
▪ Obtain additional medical care as soon as possible.
▪ Remove and discard gloves and perform hand hygiene.[1,2,3]
▪ Document the procedure.[4]

Special considerations

▪ Apply pressure directly to the wound with your gloved hand if sterile gauze pads and clean cloth are unavailable.
▪ Avoid using an elastic bandage to bind the dressing *because it can't be wrapped tightly enough to create pressure on the wound site.*

Complications

A pressure dressing that's applied too tightly can impair circulation.

Documentation

When the bleeding is controlled, record the date and time of dressing application, presence or absence of distal pulses, integrity of distal skin, and amount of wound drainage as well as any complications.

REFERENCES

1 Centers for Disease Control and Prevention. (October 2002). Guideline for hand hygiene in health-care settings. *Morbidity and Mortality Weekly Report, 51*(RR-16), 1–45. (Level I)
2 The Joint Commission. (2012). Standard NPSG.07.01.01. *Comprehensive accreditation manual for hospitals: The official handbook.* Oakbrook Terrace, IL: The Joint Commission. (Level I)
3 World Health Organization. (2009). *WHO guidelines on hand hygiene in health care: First global patient safety challenge. Clean care is safer care.* Geneva, Switzerland: World Health Organization. (Level I)
4 The Joint Commission. (2012). Standard RC.01.03.01. *Comprehensive accreditation manual for hospitals: The official handbook.* Oakbrook Terrace, IL: The Joint Commission. (Level I)

PRESSURE ULCER CARE

As the name implies, pressure ulcers result when pressure—applied with great force for a short period or with less force over a long period—impairs circulation, depriving tissues of oxygen and other life-sustaining nutrients. This process damages skin and underlying structures. Untreated, resulting ischemic lesions can lead to serious infection.

Most pressure ulcers develop over bony prominences, where friction and shearing force combine with pressure to break down skin and underlying tissues. Persistent pressure on bony prominences obstructs capillary blood flow, leading to tissue necrosis. Common sites include the sacrum, coccyx, ischial tuberosities, and greater trochanters. Other common sites include the skin over the vertebrae, scapulae, elbows, knees, and heels in bedridden and relatively immobile patients.

Successful pressure ulcer treatment involves relieving pressure, restoring circulation, promoting adequate nutrition and, if possible, resolving or managing related disorders. Typically, the effectiveness and duration of treatment depend on the pressure ulcer's characteristics.[1] (See *Staging pressure ulcers.*)

Ideally, prevention is the key to avoiding extensive therapy. Preventive measures include off-loading pressure, maintaining adequate nourishment, and ensuring mobility to relieve pressure and promote circulation.[2] Performing a risk assessment is necessary to implement effective prevention strategies.[2] (See *Braden scale: Predicting pressure ulcer risk*, pages 602 and 603.)

When a pressure ulcer develops despite preventive efforts, treatment includes methods to decrease pressure, such as frequent repositioning to shorten pressure duration and the use of special equipment to reduce pressure intensity. Treatment also may involve pressure-reducing devices, such as special beds, mattresses, mattress overlays, and chair cushions.

Equipment

Pressure-redistribution device ▪ pillows ▪ lotion ▪ protective moisture barrier ▪ gloves.

(Text continues on page 601.)

Staging pressure ulcers[1]

Pressure ulcer staging reflects the depth and extent of tissue involvement. The classification system developed by the National Pressure Ulcer Advisory Panel is the most widely used system and categorizes pressure ulcers into four stages and two additional categories—suspected deep tissue injury and unstageable pressure ulcers.

Suspected deep tissue injury

Deep tissue injury is characterized by a purple or maroon localized area of intact skin or blood-filled blister caused by damage of underlying soft tissue from pressure or shear. It may be preceded by tissue that's painful, firm, mushy, boggy, or warm or cool compared with adjacent tissue. The depth of the suspected deep tissue injury is unknown. It may be difficult to detect in individuals with dark skin tones. It may initially appear as a thin blister over a dark wound bed.

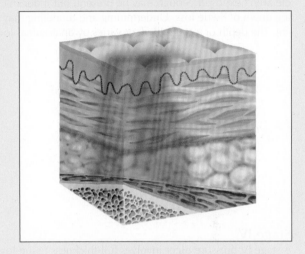

Stage I

Stage I ulcers are characterized by intact skin with nonblanchable redness of a localized area, usually over a bony prominence. The area may be warmer or cooler than adjacent tissue or painful and firm or soft. Darkly pigmented skin may not have visible blanching, but its color and temperature may differ from the surrounding area.

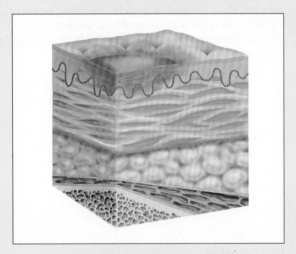

Stage II

A stage II pressure ulcer is characterized by partial-thickness loss of the dermis, presenting as a shallow, open ulcer with a red-pink wound bed without slough. It may also present as an intact or open serum-filled blister. This stage shouldn't be used to describe skin tears, tape burns, excoriation, perineal dermatitis, or maceration.

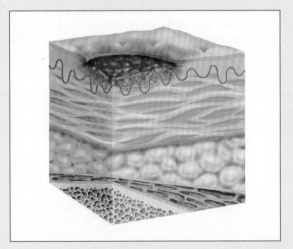

(continued)

Staging pressure ulcers *(continued)*

Stage III

A stage III pressure ulcer is characterized by full-thickness tissue loss. Subcutaneous fat may be visible, but bone, tendon, and muscle aren't exposed. Slough may be present, but it doesn't obscure the depth of tissue loss. Undermining and tunneling may be present. The depth of a stage III ulcer varies by anatomical location.

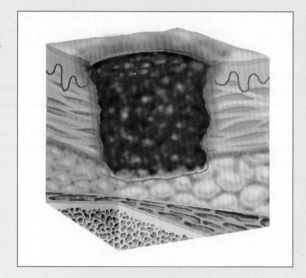

Stage IV

A stage IV pressure ulcer involves full-thickness tissue loss with exposed bone, tendon, or muscle. Slough or eschar may be present on some parts of the wound bed. Undermining and tunneling are also common. The depth of a stage IV ulcer varies by anatomic location.

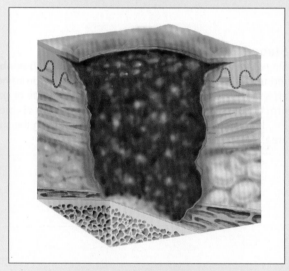

Unstageable

An unstageable ulcer is characterized by full-thickness tissue loss, in which the base of the ulcer in the wound bed is covered by slough, eschar, or both. Until enough slough or eschar is removed to expose the base of the wound, the true depth, and therefore stage, can't be determined.

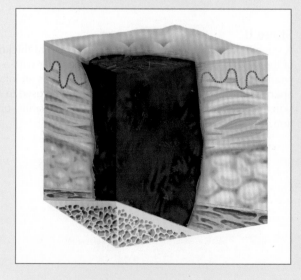

Implementation

■ Perform hand hygiene and put on gloves.[3,4,5]

■ Confirm the patient's identity using at least two patient identifiers according to your facility's policy.[6]

■ Explain the procedure to the patient. Answer any questions *to decrease anxiety and increase cooperation.*

■ Turn and reposition the patient every 1 to 2 hours, unless contraindicated. For patients with limited mobility, use a pressure-redistribution device, such as air, gel, or a 4″ (10.2 cm) foam mattress overlay.[7] Low- or high-air-loss bed therapy may be indicated *to redistribute excessive pressure and promote evaporation of excess moisture.*

■ When turning the patient, lift him rather than slide him *because sliding increases friction and shear.*[2,8] Use a turning sheet and get help from coworkers, if necessary.

NURSING ALERT *Avoid placing the patient directly on his trochanter.*[2] *Instead, place him on his side, at about a 30-degree angle.*[8]

■ Use pillows *to position the patient and increase his comfort.* Be sure to eliminate sheet wrinkles that could increase pressure and cause discomfort. Make sure the patient's heels don't rest on the bed.[2,8]

■ Post a turning schedule at the patient's bedside. Adapt position changes to his situation. Emphasize the importance of regular position changes to the patient and his family, and encourage their participation in the treatment and prevention of pressure ulcers by having them perform a position change correctly, after you have demonstrated how.

■ As appropriate, implement active or passive range-of-motion exercises *to redistribute pressure and promote circulation. To save time,* combine these exercises with bathing, if applicable.

■ Direct the patient confined to a chair or wheelchair to shift his weight every 15 minutes *to promote blood flow to compressed tissues.*[2,8] Show a paraplegic patient how to shift his weight by doing push-ups in the wheelchair. If the patient needs your help, sit next to him and help him shift his weight to one buttock for 60 seconds; then repeat the procedure on the other side. Provide him with pressure-redistribution cushions, as appropriate. However, avoid seating the patient on a rubber or plastic doughnut, *which can increase localized pressure at vulnerable points.*

■ If a patient confined to a chair or wheelchair can stand, assist the patient into a standing position every hour, if possible.

■ Adjust or pad appliances, casts, or splints, as needed, *to ensure proper fit and avoid increased pressure and impaired circulation.*

■ Tell the patient to avoid heat lamps and harsh soaps *because they dry the skin.* Applying lotion after bathing will help keep his skin hydrated.[2] Also tell him to avoid vigorous massage *because it can damage capillaries.*

■ If the patient's condition permits, recommend a diet that includes adequate calories, protein, and vitamins.[2] Dietary therapy may involve nutritional consultation, food supplements, enteral feeding, or total parenteral nutrition.

■ If diarrhea develops or if the patient is incontinent, clean and dry soiled skin. Then apply a protective moisture barrier *to prevent incontinence-associated dermatitis.*[2]

■ Document the procedure.[9]

Special considerations

■ Except for brief periods, avoid raising the head of the bed more than 30 degrees *to prevent shearing forces.*[2]

■ Avoid using elbow and heel protectors that fasten with a single narrow strap. *The strap may impair neurovascular function in the involved hand or foot.*

■ Avoid using artificial sheepskin. *It doesn't reduce pressure, and it may create a false sense of security.*

■ Repair of stage III and stage IV ulcers may require surgical intervention—such as direct closure, skin grafting, and flaps—depending on the patient's needs.

Patient teaching

Make sure the patient, family members, and caregivers learn pressure ulcer prevention and treatment strategies so that they understand the importance of care, the available choices, the rationales for treatments, and their own role in selecting goals and shaping the care plan.[2]

Complications

Infection may cause foul-smelling drainage, persistent pain, severe erythema, induration, and elevated skin and body temperatures. Advancing infection or cellulitis can lead to septicemia. Severe erythema may signal worsening cellulitis, which indicates that the offending organisms have invaded the tissue and are no longer localized.

Documentation

Update the care plan, as required. On the clinical record, document interventions used to prevent pressure ulcers and the patient's response. If a pressure ulcer develops, note changes in the condition or size of the pressure ulcer and elevations of skin temperature. Document when the doctor was notified of pertinent abnormal observations. Record the patient's temperature daily on the graphic sheet to allow easy assessment of body temperature patterns.

REFERENCES

1 National Pressure Ulcer Advisory Panel. (2007). "Pressure Ulcer Stages Revised by NPUAP" [Online]. Accessed August 2010 via the Web at www.npuap.org/pr2.htm (Level V)

2 Institute for Clinical Systems Improvement. (2010). "Health Care Protocol: Pressure Ulcer Prevention and Treatment Protocol" (2nd ed.) [Online]. Accessed August 2010 via the Web at http://www.icsi.org/pressure_ulcer_treatment_protocol review_and_comment_/pressure_ulcer_treatment_protocol_.html (Level V)

3 Centers for Disease Control and Prevention. (October 2002). Guideline for hand hygiene in health-care settings. *Morbidity and Mortality Weekly Report, 51*(RR-16), 1–45. (Level I)

4 The Joint Commission. (2012). Standard NPSG.07.01.01. *Comprehensive accreditation manual for hospitals: The official handbook.* Oakbrook Terrace, IL: The Joint Commission. (Level I)

5 World Health Organization. (2009). *WHO guidelines on hand hygiene in health care: First global patient safety challenge. Clean care is safer care.* Geneva, Switzerland: World Health Organization. (Level I)

Braden scale: Predicting pressure ulcer risk

The Braden scale is the most reliable of several instruments used to assess the risk of developing pressure ulcers. The numbers to the left of each description are the points to be tallied; the lower the score, the greater the risk.

Patient's name: _____

Evaluator's name: _____

Sensory perception Ability to respond meaningfully to pressure-related discomfort	**1. Completely limited** Patient is unresponsive (doesn't moan, flinch, or grasp in response) to painful stimuli because of diminished level of consciousness or sedation. OR Patient has a limited ability to feel pain over most of body's surface.	**2. Very limited** Patient responds only to painful stimuli; can't communicate discomfort except through moaning or restlessness. OR Patient has a sensory impairment that limits ability to feel pain or discomfort over half of body.
Moisture Degree to which skin is exposed to moisture	**1. Constantly moist** Patient's skin is kept moist almost constantly by perspiration or urine; dampness is detected every time he's moved or turned.	**2. Very moist** Patient's skin is usually but not always moist; linen must be changed at least once per shift.
Activity Degree of physical activity	**1. Bedfast** Patient is confined to bed.	**2. Chairfast** Patient's ability to walk is severely limited or nonexistent; can't bear own weight and must be assisted into a chair or wheelchair.
Mobility Ability to change and control body position	**1. Completely immobile** Patient doesn't make even slight changes in body or extremity position without assistance.	**2. Very limited** Patient makes occasional slight changes in body or extremity position but can't make frequent or significant changes independently.
Nutrition Usual food intake pattern	**1. Very poor** Patient never eats a complete meal; rarely eats more than one-third of any food offered; eats two servings or less of protein (meat or dairy products) per day; takes fluids poorly; doesn't take a liquid dietary supplement. OR Patient is NPO or maintained on clear liquids or IV fluids for more than 5 days.	**2. Probably inadequate** Patient rarely eats a complete meal and generally eats only about one-half of any food offered; protein intake includes only three servings of meat or dairy products per day; occasionally will take a dietary supplement. OR Patient receives less than optimum amount of liquid diet or tube feeding.
Friction and shear	**1. Problem** Patient requires moderate to maximum assistance in moving; complete lifting without sliding against sheets is impossible; frequently slides down in bed or chair, requiring frequent repositioning with maximum assistance; spasticity, contractures, or agitation leads to almost constant friction.	**2. Potential problem** Patient moves feebly or requires minimum assistance during a move; skin probably slides to some extent against sheets, chair restraints, or other devices; maintains relatively good position in chair or bed most of the time but occasionally slides down.

© Barbara Braden and Nancy Bergstrom, 1988.

Date of Assessment: _____

| | | Score |

3. Slightly limited
Patient responds to verbal commands but can't always communicate discomfort or the need to be turned.
OR
Patient has some sensory impairment that limits ability to feel pain or discomfort in one or two extremities.

4. No impairment
Patient responds to verbal commands; has no sensory deficit that would limit ability to feel or voice pain or discomfort.

Score

3. Occasionally moist
Patient's skin is occasionally moist; linen requires an extra change approximately once per day.

4. Rarely moist
Patient's skin is usually dry; linen requires changing only at routine intervals.

Score

3. Walks occasionally
Patient walks occasionally during the day, but for very short distances, with or without assistance; spends majority of each shift in a bed or chair.

4. Walks frequently
Patient walks outside room at least twice per day and inside room at least once every 2 hours during waking hours.

Score

3. Slightly limited
Patient makes frequent (although slight) changes in body or extremity position independently.

4. No limitations
Patient makes major and frequent changes in body or extremity position without assistance.

Score

3. Adequate
Patient eats more than one-half of most meals; eats four servings of protein (meat and dairy products) per day; occasionally refuses a meal but will usually take a supplement if offered.
OR
Patient is on a tube feeding or total parenteral nutrition regimen that probably meets most nutritional needs.

4. Excellent
Patient eats most of every meal and never refuses a meal; usually eats four or more servings of meat and dairy products per day; occasionally eats between meals; doesn't require supplementation.

Score

3. No apparent problem
Patient moves in bed and in chair independently and has sufficient muscle strength to lift up completely during move; maintains good position in bed or chair at all times.

Score

Total Score

6   The Joint Commission. (2012). Standard NPSG.01.01.01. *Comprehensive accreditation manual for hospitals: The official handbook*. Oakbrook Terrace, IL: The Joint Commission. (Level I)

7   Cullum, N., et al. (2004). Support surfaces for pressure ulcer prevention. *Cochrane Database of Systematic Reviews* (3), CD001735. (Level I)

8   European Pressure Ulcer Advisory Panel and National Pressure Ulcer Advisory Panel. (2009). "Pressure Ulcer Prevention: Quick Reference Guide" [Online]. Accessed October 2011 via the Web at http://www.npuap.org/Final_Quick_Prevention_for_web_2010.pdf (Level VII)

9   The Joint Commission. (2012). Standard RC.01.03.01. *Comprehensive accreditation manual for hospitals: The official handbook*. Oakbrook Terrace, IL: The Joint Commission. (Level I)

ADDITIONAL REFERENCES

Baranoski, S., & Ayello, E.A. (2008). *Wound care essentials: Practice principles* (2nd ed.). Philadelphia, PA: Lippincott Williams & Williams.

Keast, D.H., et al. (2007). Best practice recommendations for the prevention and treatment of pressure ulcers: Update 2006. *Advances in Skin and Wound Care, 20*(8), 447–460.

PROGRESSIVE AMBULATION

After surgery or a period of bed rest, patients must begin the gradual return to full ambulation. When it's begun promptly and properly, progressive ambulation thwarts many of the complications of prolonged inactivity.

Complications prevented by early progressive ambulation include respiratory stasis and hypostatic pneumonia; circulatory stasis, thrombophlebitis, and emboli; urine retention, urinary tract infection, urinary stasis, and calculus formation; abdominal distention, constipation, and decreased appetite; and sensory deprivation.[1] Progressive ambulation also helps restore the patient's sense of equilibrium and enhances his self-confidence and self-image.

Progressive ambulation begins with dangling the patient's feet over the edge of the bed and progresses to seating him in an armchair or wheelchair, walking around the room with him, and then walking with him in the halls until he can walk by himself. The patient's progress depends on his physical condition and his tolerance. Successful return to full ambulation requires correct body mechanics, careful patient observation, and open communication between patient, doctor, and nurse.

Equipment

Robe ■ chair or wheelchair ■ nonskid slippers or hard-soled shoes ■ assistive device (cane, crutches, walker), if necessary.

If the patient requires an assistive device, the physical therapist usually selects the appropriate one and teaches its use.

Implementation

■ Check the patient's history, diagnosis, and therapeutic regimen.
■ Perform hand hygiene.[2,3,4]

■ Confirm the patient's identity using at least two patient identifiers according to your facility's policy.[5]
■ Ask the patient whether he's in pain or feels weak; if necessary, give an analgesic, as ordered, and wait 30 to 60 minutes for it to take effect before trying ambulation. Remember that a medicated patient may develop hypotension, dizziness, or drowsiness.
■ Explain the goal of ambulation. (See *Helping the patient regain mobility*.) Provide encouragement *because he may be hesitant or fearful*; reassure him that he need not attempt more than he can reasonably do. If he fears pain in an incision, show him how to support it by placing a hand alongside or gently over the dressing site, or splint the incision for him.
■ Remove equipment or other objects *to provide a clear path and prevent falls*.
■ Lock the wheels on the bed or chair, if appropriate.

Dangle the patient's legs
■ Position the bed horizontally and the patient laterally, facing you. Move his legs over the side of the bed and grasp his shoulders, standing with your feet apart so you have a wide base of support. Ask him to help by pushing up from the bed with his arms. Then shift your weight from the foot closest to his head to the other foot as you steadily raise him to the sitting position. Pull with your whole body, not just your arms, *to avoid straining your back and jostling the patient*. Alternatively, you can raise the head of the bed to a 45-degree angle *to allow easier elevation of the patient*. Don't use this method if the patient has trouble balancing himself while sitting. Ask a coworker for assistance whenever necessary.
■ While the patient adjusts to an upright position, continue to stand facing him *to keep him from falling*, and observe him closely. Be alert for signs and symptoms of orthostatic hypotension, such as fainting, dizziness, and complaints of blurred vision. If desired, check the patient's pulse rate and blood pressure. If the pulse rate increases more than 20 beats/minute, allow the patient to rest before slowly progressing.

Help the patient stand
■ After the patient can dangle his legs and support his weight on them, have him attempt the standing position. Help the patient put on a robe and nonskid slippers or shoes.
■ Don't allow a robe, a drainage tube, or anything else to dangle around the patient's feet.
■ If the patient is alert and fairly strong, place his feet flat on the floor and allow him to stand by himself. As he stands, place one hand under his axilla and the other hand around his waist *to prevent falls*. Help him stand fully erect. Encourage him to look forward and not at the floor *to help maintain his balance*.
■ If the patient needs help standing up, face him and position your knees at either side of his. Bend your knees, put your arms around his waist, and instruct him to push up from the bed with his arms. Then straighten your knees and pull the patient with you while rising to an erect position. *This technique helps you avoid back strain*.

Help the patient sit or walk

■ Once the patient stands, you can pivot and lower him into an armchair or wheelchair, or you can begin to walk with him.

■ If you've decided to seat him, make sure the chair is secure and won't slip as you lower the patient into it. Place his lower back against the rear of the chair and his feet flat on the floor. Position his hips and knees at right angles, and keep his upper body straight. Then flex his elbows and place his forearms on the arms of the chair.

■ If the patient can walk safely only with your assistance, stand to the side and slightly behind him, placing one hand under his axilla and the other hand around his waist. If the patient has weakness or paralysis on one side, stand on the affected side and stabilize him by putting one arm around his waist.

■ If necessary, ask a coworker to help you. Stand on opposite sides of the patient and place one hand under his arm or on his elbow.

■ Give the patient verbal and tactile cues *to encourage him.* Stay close to a railed wall or another supportive structure and, if necessary, allow the patient to rest in a chair before attempting to walk back to his room. If he can't walk back, tell him to remain seated while you summon assistance or obtain a wheelchair. Don't leave the patient unattended if you have any reason to think he may fall. If you can't find a chair nearby, have the patient lean against the wall and call for assistance as you help support him. If necessary, steady him as he slides down the wall to sit on the floor.

■ Perform hand hygiene.[2,3,4]

■ Document the procedure.[6]

Special considerations

■ Patients on medications such as beta-adrenergic blockers and vasodilators may be subject to episodes of bradycardia and hypotension.

■ If early ambulation is impossible, encourage bed exercises. Don't let the use of catheters and IV tubing discourage ambulation; secure these devices so they are easily portable, and check dressings and tubes carefully afterward for proper position and changes in drainage. If appropriate, measure pulse, respiratory rate, and blood pressure. When leaving the patient sitting up in a chair, make sure he has a call bell or signal device.

■ If the patient begins to fall, try to break his fall by easing him to the bed, chair, or floor, making sure he doesn't strike his head. Then summon help. Don't leave the patient alone—he needs your comfort and reassurance.

■ If the patient experiences dyspnea, diaphoresis, or orthostatic hypotension, stabilize his position and take vital signs. Place him in semi-Fowler's position *to facilitate breathing.* If his condition doesn't improve rapidly, notify the doctor.

Documentation

Record the type of transfer and assistance needed; the duration of sitting, standing, or walking; the distance walked, if appropriate; the patient's response to ambulation; and any significant changes in blood pressure, pulse, and respiration.

Helping the patient regain mobility

Dangling legs

To help the patient support himself in a dangling position, move an overbed table in front of him and place a pillow on it.

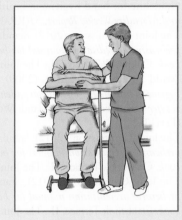

Sitting

Seat the patient in a chair with armrests and a straight back, with his lower back against the rear of the chair, feet flat on the floor, hips and knees at right angles, and upper body straight. Rest his forearms on the armrests.

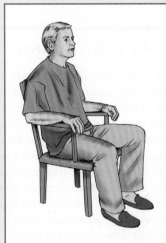

Walking

Provide a path unimpeded by equipment and other objects, and avoid overexertion. If necessary, hold the patient *so you can control his upper and lower body and any lateral movements.*

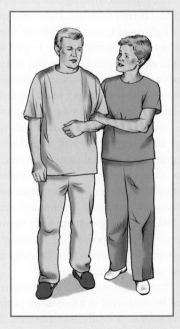

References

1 Hirsh, J., et al. (2008). Prevention of venous thromboembolism: The Eighth ACCP Conference on Antithrombotic and Thrombolytic Therapy. *Chest, 133*(6), 1105–1125.

2 Centers for Disease Control and Prevention. (October 2002). Guideline for hand hygiene in health-care settings. *Morbidity and Mortality Weekly Report, 51*(RR-16), 1–45. (Level I)

3 The Joint Commission. (2012). Standard NPSG.07.01.01. *Comprehensive accreditation manual for hospitals: The official handbook.* Oakbrook Terrace, IL: The Joint Commission. (Level I)

4 World Health Organization. (2009). *WHO guidelines on hand hygiene in health care: First global patient safety challenge. Clean care is safer care.* Geneva, Switzerland: World Health Organization. (Level I)

5 The Joint Commission. (2012). Standard NPSG.01.01.01. *Comprehensive accreditation manual for hospitals: The official handbook.* Oakbrook Terrace, IL: The Joint Commission. (Level I)

6 The Joint Commission. (2012). Standard RC.01.03.01. *Comprehensive accreditation manual for hospitals: The official handbook.* Oakbrook Terrace, IL: The Joint Commission. (Level I)

Prone positioning

Prone positioning is a therapeutic maneuver to improve oxygenation and pulmonary mechanics in patients with acute lung injury or mechanically ventilated patients with acute respiratory distress syndrome (ARDS) who require high concentrations of inspired oxygen. Also known as *proning*, the procedure involves physically turning a patient from a supine position (on the back) to a facedown position (prone position).

The recommended criteria for using prone positioning include patients with ARDS who require high plateau pressure or a high fraction of inspired oxygen, which make mechanical ventilation potentially damaging to the lungs.[1]

The physical challenges of prone positioning have been a traditional barrier to its use. However, equipment innovations (such as a lightweight, cushioned frame that straps to the front of the patient before turning) have helped to minimize the risks associated with moving patients and maintaining them in the prone position for several hours at a time. With the appropriate equipment, prone positioning may also facilitate better movement of the diaphragm by allowing the abdomen to expand more fully.

Prone positioning is usually performed for 6 or more hours a day, for as long as 10 days, until the requirement for a high concentration of inspired oxygen resolves. Aside from early intervention, factors predictive of patients' responses aren't consistent among studies, and patients' initial responses aren't always predictive of their subsequent responses. Patients with extrapulmonary ARDS (such as ARDS resulting from multiple trauma) appear to respond consistently to prone positioning.[2] Although research has demonstrated improved oxygenation with proning, it's unclear whether the survival rate is increased.[3]

Prone positioning is contraindicated in patients whose heads can't be supported in a face-down position as well as in those who can't tolerate a head-down position. Relative contraindications include increased intracranial pressure; unstable spine, chest, or pelvis; unstable bone fractures; left-sided heart failure (nonpulmonary respiratory failure); shock; abdominal compartment syndrome; abdominal surgery; extreme obesity (greater than 300 lb [136 kg]); and pregnancy. Hemodynamically unstable patients (systolic blood pressure less than 90 mm Hg), despite aggressive fluid resuscitation and vasopressors, should be evaluated thoroughly before prone positioning is initiated.

Equipment

Vollman prone positioner (Hill-Rom) or other prone-positioning device ▪ gloves ▪ minimum of three trained staff members ▪ drawsheet ▪ small towel for under the patient's head to catch secretions ▪ small pillows or rolled towels for positioning ▪ suction, as needed ▪ oral care supplies (see "Oral care," page 524) ▪ eye lubricant ▪ tape ▪ Optional: personal protective equipment.

Preparation of equipment

Clean the positioner, according to facility policy, between positioning turns and when discontinuing prone positioning.

Implementation

▪ Verify the doctor's order.
▪ Perform hand hygiene.[4,5,6]
▪ Confirm the patient's identity using at least two patient identifiers according to your facility's policy.[7]

Assessing the patient

▪ Assess the patient's hemodynamic status *to determine whether the patient can tolerate the prone position.*
▪ Assess the patient's neurologic status before prone positioning. Generally, the patient will be sedated heavily. Although agitation isn't a contraindication for the procedure, it must be managed effectively.
▪ Determine whether the patient's size and weight will allow a 180-degree turn on a narrow critical care bed. Consider obtaining a wider specialty bed if needed.
▪ Explain the procedure to the patient and family members and answer all questions to allay their anxiety and promote cooperation.

Before turning the patient

▪ Gather the equipment.
▪ Obtain the help of two coworkers. *A minimum of three trained staff members is required.*
▪ Perform hand hygiene[4,5,6] and put on gloves or other protective equipment, as appropriate.[9]
▪ Provide eye care, including lubrication and horizontal taping of eyelids, if indicated.[1]
▪ Ensure that the patient's tongue is inside the mouth; if it's edematous or protruding, insert a bite block.[1]
▪ Secure the patient's endotracheal (ET) tube or tracheotomy tube *to prevent accidental dislodgment.*[1]
▪ Perform anterior body wound care and dressing changes.[1]
▪ Empty ileostomy or colostomy drainage bags.[1]
▪ Remove anterior chest wall electrocardiogram (ECG) monitoring leads, making sure the patient's cardiac rate and rhythm

can still be monitored; these leads will be repositioned on the patient's back after she's prone.[1]

■ Ensure that the brake of the bed is engaged.

■ Attach the surface of the prone positioner to the bed frame, as recommended by the manufacturer.

■ Position the three staff members appropriately: one on either side of the bed and one at the head of the bed.[1]

NURSING ALERT *The staff member at the head of the bed is responsible for monitoring the ET tube and mechanical ventilator tubing.*

■ Adjust all patient tubing and invasive monitoring lines *to prevent dislodging, kinking, disconnection, or contact with the patient's body during the turning procedure and while the patient remains in the prone position.*

NURSING ALERT *Place all lines inserted in the upper torso over the right or left shoulder (as shown below), with the exception of chest tubes, which are placed at the foot of the bed. All lines inserted in the lower torso are positioned at the foot of the bed.[1]*

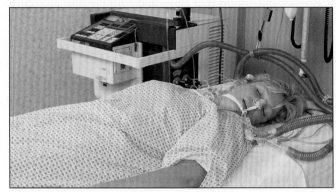

■ Turn the patient's face away from the ventilator, placing the ET tubing on the side of the patient's face that's turned away from the ventilator.[1] Loop the remaining tubing above the patient's head to *prevent disconnection of the ventilator tubing or kinking of the ET tube.*

■ Place the straps of the prone positioner under the patient's head, chest, and pelvic area.[1]

■ Attach the prone-positioning device to the patient by placing the frame on top of the patient.[1]

■ Position the nonmovable chest piece, which acts as a marker for proper device placement, so that it's resting between the patient's clavicles and sixth ribs.[1]

NURSING ALERT *If the patient has a short neck or limited neck range of motion, align the chest piece lower—at the third intercostal space; move both head pieces up to the top of the frame so that only the forehead is supported by the head cushion and the chin is suspended to reduce the risk of skin breakdown.*

■ Adjust the pelvic piece of the device so that it rests ½" above the iliac crest.[1]

■ Evaluate the distance between the chest and pelvic pieces to ensure suspension of the abdomen, while preventing bowing of the patient's back.

■ Adjust the chin and forehead pieces of the device so that facial support is provided in either a facedown or side-lying position without interfering with the ET tube.[1]

■ Secure the positioning device to the patient by fastening all the soft adjustable straps on one side before tightening them on the opposite side (as shown below).[1]

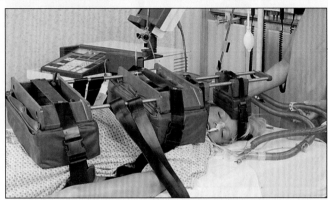

■ Once secured, lift the positioner *to ensure a secure fit.* Look for cushion compression. If the frame isn't tightly secured, shear and friction injuries to the chest and pelvic area may occur.[1]

Turning the patient

■ Lower the side rails of the bed and move the patient to the edge of the bed farthest away from the ventilator by using a drawsheet. The person closest to the patient maintains body contact with the bed at all times, serving as a side rail.[1]

■ Tuck the straps attached to the steel bar closest to the center of the bed underneath the patient. Then tuck the patient's arm and hand that are resting in the center of the bed under her buttocks. Cross the leg closest to the edge of the bed over the opposite leg at the ankle, *which will help with forward motion when the turning process begins.*[1]

NURSING ALERT *If the patient's arm can't be straightened and tucked under her buttocks, tuck the arm into the open space between the chest and pelvic pads.*

■ Turn the patient toward the ventilator at a 45-degree angle.[1]

NURSING ALERT *Always turn the patient in the direction of the mechanical ventilator.*

■ The person on the side of the bed with the ventilator grasps the upper steel bar. The person on the other side of the bed grasps the lower steel bar or turning straps of the device.[1]

■ Lift the patient by the frame into the prone position on the count of three.[1]

■ Gently move the patient's tucked arm and hand *so they are parallel to her body and comfortable* (as shown below).

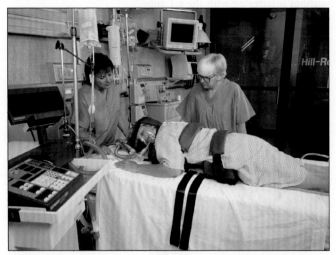

NURSING ALERT To prevent placing stress on the shoulder capsule, *don't extend the arm to a 90-degree angle.*

■ Loosen the straps if the patient is clinically stable.[1]

NURSING ALERT *Keeping the straps securely fastened in an unstable patient allows for rapid supine repositioning in an emergency.*[1]

■ Support the patient's feet with a pillow or towel roll *to provide correct flexion while she's prone.*[1]

■ Pad the patient's elbows *to prevent ulnar nerve compression.*

■ Monitor the patient's response to the prone position by assessing vital signs, pulse oximetry, and mixed venous oxygen saturation. The patient's vital signs should return to normal within 10 minutes of initiating the prone position. Arterial blood gas levels should be obtained within ½ hour of proning and within ½ hour before returning the patient to the supine position.[1]

■ Reposition the patient's head hourly while in the prone position *to prevent facial breakdown.* As one person lifts the patient's head, the second person moves the headpieces to provide head support in a different position.[1]

■ Perform range-of-motion exercises to the shoulders, arms, and legs every 2 hours.

■ Give oral care and suction the patient's airway, as needed. *The prone position promotes postural drainage.*

■ After the patient is prone, restart the patient's tube feeding as ordered and tolerated; *there is a minimal risk for aspiration because the patient is in a head-down position.*[1]

■ Remove and discard your gloves and other personal protective equipment, if worn, and perform hand hygiene.[4,5,6]

Returning the patient to the supine position

■ Perform hand hygiene[4,5,6] and put on gloves and other personal protective equipment as needed.[8]

■ Remove the posterior chest ECG leads while ensuring the ability to monitor the patient's cardiac rate and rhythm. The leads will be repositioned on to the patient's chest once he's supine.

■ Position the patient on the edge of the bed closest to the ventilator.[1]

■ Adjust all patient tubing and monitoring lines *to prevent dislodging.*[1]

■ Place one staff member on either side of the patient and one at his head.

■ Straighten the patient's arms and rest them on either side. Cross the leg closest to the edge of the bed over the opposite leg.[1]

■ Fasten the straps tightly.[1]

■ Using the steel bars of the device, turn the patient to a 45-degree angle away from the ventilator and then roll him to the supine position.[1]

■ Position the patient's arms parallel to his body.

■ Unfasten the positioning device and remove it from the patient; the straps may be left in place under the patients for future turning.[1]

■ Assess the patient's response.

■ Remove and discard your gloves and other personal protective equipment, if worn, and perform hand hygiene.[4,5,6]

■ Document the procedure.[9]

Special considerations

■ A doctor's order is usually required before prone positioning of a critically ill patient.

■ The procedure requires special training and established guidelines *to ensure patient safety.*

■ Not all patients with ARDS respond favorably to prone positioning, and the benefit sometimes decreases over time.

■ The patient may not have an immediate positive response to the prone position. Maximum response to the position may take up to 6 hours in some patients.

■ Some patients may require increased sedation during the procedure.

■ *To reduce the risk of aspirating gastric contents during the turning procedure,* it's recommended that the tube feedings be turned off 1 hour before initiating the position. The tube feedings can safely be restarted after the patient is positioned.

■ The prone-positioning schedule is generally determined by the patient's ability to maintain improvements in partial pressure of arterial oxygen while in the prone position; however, a schedule of every 6 hours in the prone position is recommended. Recent studies show that 12 to 20 hours within a 24-hour period is the typical amount of time patients are placed prone.[1]

■ Other methods for prone positioning include the KCI Roto-Prone Therapy System and, for smaller patients, using pillows and blankets.

■ Use continuous waveform capnography, if possible, *to detect dislodgement of the ET tube.*

■ Discontinue the procedure when the patient no longer demonstrates improved oxygenation with the position change.

NURSING ALERT *Lateral rotation therapy is strongly recommended with prone positioning.*

Complications

Potential complications of prone positioning include inadvertent ET extubation; airway obstruction; decreased oxygen saturation;

apical atelectasis; obstructed chest tube; pressure injuries on the weight-bearing parts of the body, including the knees and chest; hemodynamic instability; dislodgment of central venous access; transient arrhythmias; reversible dependent edema of the face (forehead, eyelids, conjunctiva, lips, and tongue) and anterior chest wall; contractures; enteral feeding intolerance; aspiration of enteral feeding when repositioned; and corneal ulceration.

NURSING ALERT *Critically ill patients with active intra-abdominal processes, regardless of position, are at risk for sepsis and septic shock.*

Documentation

Document the patient's response to therapy, ability to tolerate the turning procedure, length of time in the position, and positioning schedule. Also document monitoring, any complications, and any nursing interventions.

REFERENCES

1 Lynn-McHale Wiegand, D. (Ed.). (2011). *AACN procedure manual for critical care* (6th ed.). Philadelphia, PA: Saunders.

2 Alsaghir, A.H., & Martin, C.M. (2008). Effect of prone positioning in patients with acute respiratory distress syndrome: A meta-analysis. *Critical Care Medicine, 36*(2), 603–609. (Level I)

3 Sud, S., et al. (2008). Effect of mechanical ventilation in the prone position on clinical outcomes in patients with acute hypoxemic respiratory failure: A systematic review and meta-analysis. *Canadian Medical Association Journal, 178*(9), 1153–1161. (Level I)

4 Centers for Disease Control and Prevention. (October 2002). Guideline for hand hygiene in health-care settings. *Morbidity and Mortality Weekly Report, 51*(RR-16), 1–45. (Level I)

5 The Joint Commission. (2012). Standard NPSG.07.01.01. *Comprehensive accreditation manual for hospitals: The official handbook.* Oakbrook Terrace, IL: The Joint Commission. (Level I)

6 World Health Organization. (2009). *WHO guidelines on hand hygiene in health care: First global patient safety challenge. Clean care is safer care.* Geneva, Switzerland: World Health Organization. (Level I)

7 The Joint Commission. (2012). Standard NPSG.01.01.01. *Comprehensive accreditation manual for hospitals: The official handbook.* Oakbrook Terrace, IL: The Joint Commission. (Level I)

8 Siegel, J.D., et al. "2007 Guideline for Isolation Precautions: Preventing Transmission of Infectious Agents in Healthcare Settings" [Online]. Accessed September 2011 via the Web at http://www.cdc.gov/hicpac/2007ip/2007isolationprecautions.html

9 The Joint Commission. (2012). Standard RC.01.03.01. *Comprehensive accreditation manual for hospitals: The official handbook.* Oakbrook Terrace, IL: The Joint Commission. (Level I)

ADDITIONAL REFERENCES

Fernandez, R., et al. (2008). Prone positioning in acute respiratory distress syndrome: A multicenter randomized clinical trial. *Intensive Care Medicine, 34*(8), 1487–1491.

Fessler, H.E. & Talmor, D.S. (2010). Should prone positioning be routinely used for lung protection during mechanical ventilation? *Respiratory Care, 55*(1), 88–99.

Kopterides, P., et al. (2009). Prone positioning in hypoxemic respiratory failure: Meta-analysis of randomized controlled trials. *Journal of Critical Care, 24*(1), 89–100.

Morrell, N. (2010). Prone positioning in patients with acute respiratory distress syndrome. *Nursing Standard, 24*(21), 42–45.

Taccone, P., et al. (2009). Prone positioning in patients with moderate and severe acute respiratory distress syndrome: A randomized controlled trial. *JAMA, 302*(18), 1977–1984.

PROTECTIVE ENVIRONMENT GUIDELINES

The Centers for Disease Control and Prevention recommends that patients undergoing allogenic hematopoietic stem cell transplant (in which bone marrow is taken from a person other than the recipient) be placed in a protective environment room for the prevention of fungal infections.[1,2,3]

An effective protective environment requires a positive-pressure room with the door kept closed to maintain the proper air pressure balance between the isolation room and the adjoining hallway (12 air exchanges per hour). Positive air pressure must be monitored daily with smoke tubes or flutter strips. The incoming air is filtered through high-efficiency particulate air (HEPA) filtration before circulation.[1,4,5]

Equipment

Gloves ■ gowns ■ masks ■ N-95 respirator masks ■ positive-pressure room with HEPA filter ■ new thermometer ■ new blood pressure cuff ■ new stethoscope.

Equipment should be restricted to the patient's room.

Preparation of equipment

Ensure that all equipment taken into the room is properly cleaned with facility- and Environmental Protection Agency—approved disinfectant before entering the room.[5]

Implementation

■ Place the patient in the protective environment room and explain the protective environment requirements to the patient and his family *to reduce patient anxiety and promote cooperation.*

■ Screen visitors *to prevent anyone with a known or suspected infection from entering the room.*

■ Perform hand hygiene before putting on gloves, after removing gloves, and as indicated during patient care.[2,5,6,7,8]

■ Wear gloves, a gown, and a mask according to standard precautions and other precautions (droplet, contact, and airborne) as indicated.[3]

■ Ensure daily room cleaning with techniques that minimize dust, such as wet-dusting horizontal surfaces.[5]

■ Avoid transporting the patient out of the room; if the patient must be moved, make sure he wears an N-95 mask *to protect the patient from breathing in small particles that may cause infection.*[3]

■ Notify the receiving department that the patient is on protective environment requirements and that the patient must be returned to his room promptly.

■ Prohibit fresh or dried flowers or potted plants in protective environment rooms or areas. *Cut flowers in water, dry flowers, and potted plants are sources for bacterial and fungal growth.*[5]

■ Document the procedure.[9]

Special considerations

- If the patient requires airborne precautions, implement them in the protective environment room if an anteroom is present. Air in the anteroom is filtered by a portable HEPA filtration unit. If there is no anteroom, the patient may be placed in an airborne infection isolation room with portable ventilation units and HEPA filters *to increase the filtration of fungal spores.*

Documentation

Record the need for a protective environment in the nursing care plan and as otherwise indicated by your facility's policy. Document initiation and maintenance, the patient's tolerance of the procedure, and any patient or family teaching done. Also document the date the protective environment was discontinued.

REFERENCES

1 Barclay, L. (2007). "CDC Revises Guidelines for Infection Prevention in Hospitals and Healthcare Settings" [Online]. Accessed January 2012 via the Web at http://www.medscape.org/viewarticle/ 559217 (Level I)
2 Duffy, L. (2009). Care of immunocompromised patients in the hospital. *Nursing Standard, 23*(6), 35–41.
3 Siegel, J.D., et al. "2007 Guideline for Isolation Precautions: Preventing Transmission of Infectious Agents in Healthcare Settings" [Online]. Accessed December 2011 via the Web at http://www.cdc.gov/hicpac/2007ip/2007isolationprecautions.html
4 Carico, R., et al. (2009). *APIC text of infection control and epidemiology* (Vol. 1). Washington, D.C.: Association for Professionals in Infection Control and Epidemiology.
5 Riley, M., et al. (2009). Are your isolation precautions up to date? *Nursing Critical Care, 4*(3), 8–10.
6 Centers for Disease Control and Prevention. (October 2002). Guideline for hand hygiene in health-care settings. *Morbidity and Mortality Weekly Report, 51*(RR-16), 1–45. (Level I)
7 The Joint Commission. (2012). Standard NPSG.07.01.01. *Comprehensive accreditation manual for hospitals: The official handbook.* Oakbrook Terrace, IL: The Joint Commission. (Level I)
8 World Health Organization. (2009). *WHO guidelines on hand hygiene in health care: First global patient safety challenge. Clean care is safer care.* Geneva, Switzerland: World Health Organization. (Level I)
9 The Joint Commission. (2012). Standard RC.01.03.01. *Comprehensive accreditation manual for hospitals: The official handbook.* Oakbrook Terrace, IL: The Joint Commission. (Level I)

PULMONARY ARTERY PRESSURE AND PULMONARY ARTERY WEDGE PRESSURE MONITORING

Continuous pulmonary artery pressure (PAP) and intermittent pulmonary artery wedge pressure (PAWP) measurements provide important information about left ventricular function and preload. You can use this information not only for monitoring but also for aiding diagnosis, refining your assessment, guiding interventions, and projecting patient outcomes.

Nearly all acutely ill patients are candidates for PAP monitoring—especially those who are hemodynamically unstable, need fluid management or continuous cardiopulmonary assessment, or are receiving multiple or frequently administered cardioactive drugs. Use of a pulmonary artery (PA) catheter is generally recommended for assessing intravascular volume, particularly in patients with severe pulmonary edema, heart failure, or oliguric renal failure; guiding therapy in severe refractory shock or multiple-organ-dysfunction syndrome; and guiding therapy to maximize oxygen delivery to tissues in some selected patients.

A PA catheter can have up to six lumens, allowing more hemodynamic information to be gathered. In addition to distal and proximal lumens used to measure pressures, a PA catheter has a balloon inflation lumen that inflates the balloon for PAWP measurement and a thermistor connector lumen that allows cardiac output measurement. Some catheters also have a pacemaker wire lumen that provides a port for pacemaker electrodes and measures continuous mixed venous oxygen saturation. (See *PA catheters: From basic to complex.*)

The PA catheter is inserted into the heart's right side with the distal tip lying in the pulmonary artery. Left-sided pressures can be assessed indirectly.

No specific contraindications for PAP monitoring exist. However, some patients undergoing it require special precautions. These include elderly patients with pulmonary hypertension, those with left bundle-branch heart block, and those for whom a systemic infection would be life-threatening.

Equipment

1.5-mL syringe that's attached to balloon port or catheter.

Implementation

- Perform hand hygiene.[1,2,3]
- Confirm the patient's identity using at least two patient identifiers according to your facility's policy.[4]
- Explain the procedure to the patient and answer all questions *to decrease anxiety and increase cooperation.*

Taking a PAP reading

- After assisting with catheter insertion and recording initial pressure readings, record subsequent PAP values and monitor waveforms. These values will be used to calculate other important hemodynamic indices. *To ensure accurate values,* make sure the transducer is properly leveled and zeroed at the phlebostatic axis.[5]
- Perform a dynamic response measurement or square wave test and document it every 8 to 12 hours *to assess and validate optimal waveforms.*[5,6] (See *Square wave test,* page 612.)
- If possible, obtain PAP values at end expiration (when the patient completely exhales).[5] *At this time, intrathoracic pressure approaches atmospheric pressure and has the least effect on PAP.* If you obtain a reading during other phases of the respiratory cycle, respiratory interference may occur. For instance, during inspiration, when intrathoracic pressure drops, PAP may be falsely low because the negative pressure is transmitted to the catheter. During expiration, when intrathoracic pressure rises, PAP may be falsely high.

EQUIPMENT

PA catheters: From basic to complex

Depending on the intended use, a pulmonary artery (PA) catheter may be basic or complex. The basic PA catheter has a distal and proximal lumen, a thermistor, and a balloon inflation gate valve. The distal lumen, which exits in the pulmonary artery, monitors PA pressure. Its hub usually is marked "P distal" or is color-coded yellow. The proximal lumen exits in the right atrium or vena cava, depending on the size of the patient's heart. It monitors right atrial pressure and can be used as the injected solution lumen for cardiac output determination and for infusing solutions. The proximal lumen hub usually is marked "Proximal" or is color-coded blue.

The thermistor, located about 1½" (4 cm) from the distal tip, measures temperature (aiding core temperature evaluation) and allows cardiac output measurement. The thermistor connector attaches to a cardiac output connector cable and then to a cardiac output monitor. Typically, it's red.

The balloon inflation gate valve is used for inflating the balloon tip with air. A stopcock connection, typically color-coded red, may be used.

Additional lumens

Some PA catheters have additional lumens used to obtain other hemodynamic data or permit certain interventions. For instance, a proximal infusion port, which exits in the right atrium or vena cava, allows additional fluid administration. A right ventricular lumen, exiting in the right ventricle, allows fluid administration, right ventricular pressure measurement, or use of a temporary ventricular pacing lead.

Some catheters have additional right atrial and right ventricular lumens for atrioventricular pacing. A right

ventricular ejection fraction test-response thermistor, with PA and right ventricular sensing electrodes, allows volumetric and ejection fraction measurements. Fiber-optic filaments, such as those used in pulse oximetry, exit into the pulmonary artery and permit measurement of continuous mixed venous oxygen saturation.

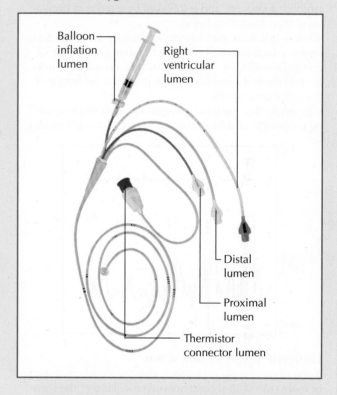

- For patients with a rapid respiratory rate and subsequent variations, you may have trouble identifying end expiration. The monitor displays an average of the digital readings obtained over time, as well as those readings obtained during a full respiratory cycle. If possible, obtain a printout. Use the averaged values obtained through the full respiratory cycle.

- *To analyze trends accurately,* be sure to record values at consistent times during the respiratory cycle.

Taking a PAWP reading

- PAWP is recorded by inflating the balloon and letting it float in a distal artery. Some facilities allow only doctors or specially trained nurses to take a PAWP reading *because of the risk of pulmonary artery rupture*—a rare but life-threatening complication. If your facility permits you to perform this procedure, do so with extreme caution and make sure you're thoroughly familiar with intracardiac waveform interpretation.

- To begin, verify that the transducer is properly leveled and zeroed. Detach the syringe from the balloon inflation hub. Draw

1.5-mL of air into the syringe, and then reattach the syringe to the hub. Watching the monitor, inject the air through the hub slowly and smoothly. When you see a wedge tracing on the monitor, immediately stop inflating the balloon. *Never inflate the balloon beyond the volume needed to obtain a wedge tracing.* (See *Observing the PAWP waveform,* page 613.)

NURSING ALERT *Never leave the balloon inflated* because this may cause a pulmonary infarction.

- Take the pressure reading at end expiration. Note the amount of air needed to change the PA tracing to a wedge tracing (normally, 1.25 to 1.5 mL). If the wedge tracing appeared with the injection of less than 1.25 mL, suspect that the catheter has migrated into a more distal branch and requires repositioning. If the balloon is in a more distal branch, the tracings may move up the oscilloscope, indicating that the catheter tip is recording balloon pressure rather than PAWP, which may lead to pulmonary artery rupture.

- Detach the syringe from the balloon inflation port and allow the balloon to deflate on its own. Observe the waveform tracing

Square wave test[6]

When using a pressure monitoring system, you must ensure and document the system's accuracy. Along with leveling and zeroing the system to atmospheric pressure at the phlebostatic axis and interpreting waveforms, you can ensure accuracy by performing the square wave test (or dynamic response test).

To perform the test, take the following steps:

■ Activate the fast-flush device for 1 second, and then release. Obtain a graphic printout.
■ Observe for the desired response: The pressure wave rises rapidly, squares off, and is followed by a series of oscillations. (See illustration below.)
■ Know that these oscillations should have an initial downstroke, which extends below the baseline and just 1 to 2 oscillations after the initial downstroke. Usually, but not always, the first upstroke is about one-third the height of the initial downstroke.
■ Be aware that the intervals between oscillations should be no more than 0.04 to 0.08 second (1 to 2 small boxes).

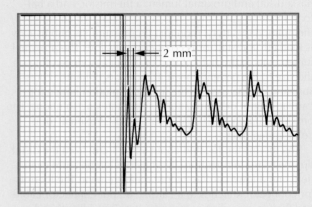

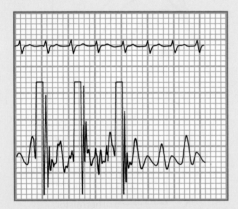

Underdamped square wave

If you observe extra oscillations after the initial downstroke or more than 0.08 second between oscillations, the waveform is underdamped. (See illustration at right column top.) This can cause falsely high pressure readings and artifact in the waveforms. It can be corrected by:

■ removing excess tubing or extra stopcocks from the system
■ inserting a damping device (available from pressure tubing companies).

Repeat the square wave test and read the pressure waveform.

Overdamped square wave

If you observe a slurred upstroke at the beginning of the square wave and a loss of oscillations after the initial downstroke, the waveform is overdamped. (See illustration below.) This can cause falsely low pressure readings, and you can lose the sharpness of waveform peaks and the dicrotic notch. It can be corrected by:

■ clearing the line of any blood or air
■ checking to make sure there are no kinks or obstructions in the line
■ ensuring that you're using short, low-compliance tubing.

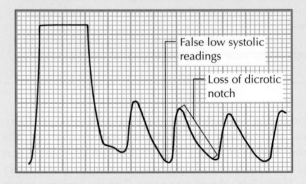

False low systolic readings

Loss of dicrotic notch

Adapted with permission from Quaal, S.J. (2001). Improving the accuracy of pulmonary artery catheter measurements. *Journal of Cardiovascular Nursing, 15*(2), 71–82.

and make sure the tracing returns from the wedge tracing to the normal PA tracing.

Completing the procedure
■ Perform hand hygiene.[1,2,3]
■ Document the procedure.[7]

Special considerations

■ Advise the patient to use caution when moving about in bed *to avoid dislodging the catheter.*
■ Never inflate the balloon with more than the recommended air volume (specified on the catheter shaft) *because this action may cause loss of elasticity or balloon rupture.* With appropriate inflation volume, the balloon floats easily through the heart

Observing the PAWP waveform

Upon balloon inflation, you should see the normal pulmonary artery pressure (PAP) waveform flatten to the characteristic pulmonary artery wedge pressure (PAWP) waveform. Balloon inflation should be halted upon observation of this waveform. Upon balloon deflation, the PAP waveform should immediately reappear.

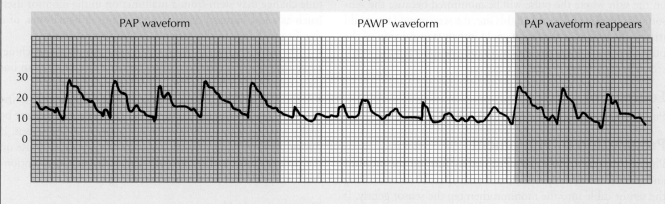

chambers and rests in the main branch of the pulmonary artery, producing accurate waveforms. Never inflate the balloon with fluids *because they may not be able to be retrieved from inside the balloon, preventing deflation.*

■ Be aware that the catheter may slip back into the right ventricle. *Because the tip may irritate the ventricle and cause arrhythmias,* check the monitor for a right ventricular waveform to detect this problem promptly.

■ *To minimize valvular trauma,* make sure the balloon is deflated whenever the catheter is withdrawn from the pulmonary artery to the right ventricle or from the right ventricle to the right atrium.

■ Change the dressing whenever it's moist or every 48 hours for a gauze dressing and at least every 7 days for a transparent dressing. Redress the site according to your facility's policy. Change the pressure tubing and flush solution every 96 hours, or as needed.[5,8]

Complications

Complications of PA catheter insertion include pulmonary artery perforation, pulmonary infarction, catheter knotting, local or systemic infection, cardiac arrhythmias, and heparin-induced thrombocytopenia.

Documentation

Document the date and time the measurements were taken, the results of the dynamic response or square wave test, the measurement results, and the patient's response.

REFERENCES

1 The Joint Commission. (2012). Standard NPSG.07.01.01. *Comprehensive accreditation manual for hospitals: The official handbook.* Oakbrook Terrace, IL: The Joint Commission. (Level I)

2 Centers for Disease Control and Prevention. (October 2002). Guideline for hand hygiene in health-care settings. *Morbidity and Mortality Weekly Report, 51*(RR-16), 1–45. (Level I)

3 World Health Organization. (2009). *WHO guidelines on hand hygiene in health care: First global patient safety challenge. Clean care is safer care.* Geneva, Switzerland: World Health Organization. (Level I)

4 The Joint Commission. (2012). Standard NPSG.01.01.01. *Comprehensive accreditation manual for hospitals: The official handbook.* Oakbrook Terrace, IL: The Joint Commission. (Level I)

5 American Association of Critical-Care Nurses. (2009). "AACN Practice Alert: Pulmonary Artery/Central Venous Pressure Monitoring" [Online]. Accessed October 2011 via the Web at http://www.aacn.org/WD/Practice/Docs/PracticeAlerts/PAP_Measurement_05-2004.pdf (Level I)

6 Quaal, S.J. (2001). Improving the accuracy of pulmonary artery catheter measurements. *Journal of Cardiovascular Nursing, 15*(2), 71–82. (Level VI)

7 The Joint Commission. (2012). Standard RC.01.03.01. *Comprehensive accreditation manual for hospitals: The official handbook.* Oakbrook Terrace, IL: The Joint Commission. (Level I)

8 O'Grady, N.P., et al. (2011). "Guidelines for the Prevention of Intravascular Catheter-Related Infections" [Online]. Accessed November 2011 via the Web at http://www.cdc.gov/hicpac/pdf/guidelines/bsi-guidelines-2011.pdf (Level I)

PULSE AMPLITUDE MONITORING

Determining the presence and strength of peripheral pulses, an essential part of cardiovascular assessment, helps you to evaluate the adequacy of peripheral perfusion. A pulse amplitude monitor simplifies this procedure. A sensor taped to the patient's skin over a pulse point sends signals to a monitor, which measures the amplitude of the pulse and displays it as a waveform on a screen. The system continuously monitors the patient's peripheral pulse so you can perform other patient care duties.

The pulse amplitude monitor can be used after peripheral vascular reconstruction on the upper or lower extremities or after percutaneous transluminal peripheral or coronary angioplasty (either with the sheaths in place or after they've been removed).

Because the sensor monitors only relatively flat pulse points, it can't be used for the posterior tibial pulse point. Also, movement distorts the waveform, so the patient must stay as still as possible during monitoring. The patient shouldn't have lesions on the skin where the pulse will be monitored because the sensor must be placed directly on this site; the sensor and tape could irritate the lesion, or the lesion could impair transmission of the pulse amplitude. If the patient has a strong peripheral pulse, you'll see an adequate waveform.

Equipment

Pulse amplitude display monitor with sensor.

Preparation of equipment

Plug the monitor into a grounded outlet. Turn on the monitor and allow it to warm up, which may take up to 10 seconds. Plug the sensor cable into the monitor; then tap the sensor gently. If tapping causes interference on the display screen, you can assume the sensor-monitor connection is functioning properly.

Implementation

- Perform hand hygiene.[1,2,3]
- Confirm the patient's identity using at least two patient identifiers according to your facility's policy.[4]
- Explain to the patient how the pulse amplitude monitor works. Answer all *questions to decrease anxiety and increase cooperation.*
- Locate the pulse you want to monitor. Mention that you'll tape the sensor to a selected site, usually the foot.
- Place the sensor over the strongest point of the pulse you're going to monitor. While observing the display screen, move the sensor until you see a strong upright waveform.
- Without moving the sensor from this site, peel off the adhesive strips and affix the sensor securely to the patient's foot. The sensor must maintain proper skin contact, so be sure to tape it firmly.
- Adjust the height of the pulse wave signal to half the height of the display screen. *This will give the waveform room to fluctuate as the pulse amplitude increases and decreases.*
- Set the low and high waveform amplitude alarms *so you'll be alerted to any waveform changes.*

Discontinuing monitor use

- Peel the sensor tapes from the patient's skin.
- Turn the machine off but keep it plugged in.
- Discard the sensor and, if necessary, wipe the monitor with a mild soap solution.
- Perform hand hygiene.[1,2,3]
- Document the procedure.[5]

Special considerations

- Be aware that although the waveform displayed by a pulse amplitude monitor may resemble an electrocardiogram or blood pressure waveform, it's not the same.

- Don't apply much pressure on the pulse sensor film or press on it with a sharp object *because such stress may warp or destroy the sensor.*
- Never place the sensor over an open wound or ulcerated skin.
- If waveform amplitude decreases, assess the patient's leg for capillary refill time, temperature, color, and sensation. The amplitude change may stem from a malfunction in the monitor itself (such as a low battery) or from a thrombus, a hematoma, or a significant change in the patient's hemodynamic status.
- If the display screen is blank when you turn on the machine, make sure that the monitor is plugged in. If it's plugged in but the screen remains blank, the screen may need repair.
- If the screen is functioning but no waveform appears on it, first check the sensor-monitor connection. Then check the sensor by gently tapping it to see if interference appears on the screen. If the sensor is working properly, relocate the peripheral pulse on the patient's foot, and reapply the sensor. If your interventions don't work, the screen may need servicing.

Documentation

Print out a strip of the patient's waveform, and place the strip in the patient's medical record during every shift and whenever you note a change in the waveform or the patient's condition. Along the left side of the strip, you'll see a reference scale used to measure pulse amplitude height. Include this scale in your documentation. Indicate the site where the sensor was placed.

REFERENCES

1 Centers for Disease Control and Prevention. (October 2002). Guideline for hand hygiene in health-care settings. *Morbidity and Mortality Weekly Report, 51*(RR-16), 1–45. (Level I)
2 The Joint Commission. (2012). Standard NPSG.07.01.01. *Comprehensive accreditation manual for hospitals: The official handbook.* Oakbrook Terrace, IL: The Joint Commission. (Level I)
3 World Health Organization. (2009). *WHO guidelines on hand hygiene in health care: First global patient safety challenge. Clean care is safer care.* Geneva, Switzerland: World Health Organization. (Level I)
4 The Joint Commission. (2012). Standard NPSG.01.01.01. *Comprehensive accreditation manual for hospitals: The official handbook.* Oakbrook Terrace, IL: The Joint Commission. (Level I)
5 The Joint Commission. (2012). Standard RC.01.03.01. *Comprehensive accreditation manual for hospitals: The official handbook.* Oakbrook Terrace, IL: The Joint Commission. (Level I)

PULSE ASSESSMENT

Blood pumped into an already-full aorta during ventricular contraction creates a fluid wave that travels from the heart to the peripheral arteries. This recurring wave—called a *pulse*—can be palpated at locations on the body where an artery crosses over bone on firm tissue. In adults and children older than age 3 and in adults with a suspected cardiac disorder that affects the patient's heart rate and rhythm, the radial artery in the wrist is the most common palpation site. (See *Pulse points.*) In infants and children younger than age 3, a stethoscope is used to listen to the heart itself rather than palpating a pulse. Because auscultation is done at the heart's apex, this is called the apical pulse.

An apical-radial pulse is taken by simultaneously counting apical and radial beats—the first by auscultation at the apex of the heart, the second by palpation at the radial artery. Some heart-beats detected at the apex can't be detected at peripheral sites. When this occurs, the apical pulse rate is higher than the radial; the difference is the pulse deficit.

Pulse taking involves determining the rate (number of beats per minute), rhythm (pattern or regularity of the beats), and volume (amount of blood pumped with each beat). If the pulse is faint or weak, use a Doppler ultrasound blood flow detector if available.

Equipment

Watch with second hand ▪ stethoscope (for auscultating apical pulse) ▪ alcohol pad.

Preparation of equipment

If you aren't using your own stethoscope, disinfect the earpieces with an alcohol pad before and after use *to prevent cross-contamination.*[1]

Implementation

▪ Perform hand hygiene.[2,3,4]
▪ Confirm the patient's identity using at least two patient identifiers according to your facility's policy.[5]
▪ Tell the patient that you intend to take his pulse.
▪ Make sure the patient is comfortable and relaxed *because an awkward, uncomfortable position may affect the heart rate.*

Taking a radial pulse

▪ Place the patient in a sitting or supine position, with his arm at his side or across his chest.
▪ Gently press your index, middle, and ring fingers on the radial artery, inside the patient's wrist (as shown below). You should feel a pulse with only moderate pressure; *excessive pressure may obstruct blood flow distal to the pulse site.* Don't use your thumb to take the patient's pulse *because your thumb's own strong pulse may be confused with the patient's pulse.*

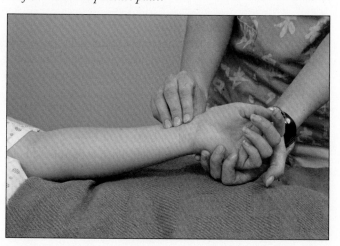

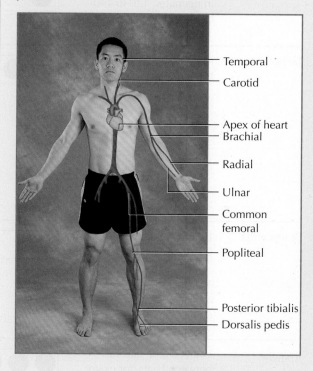

Pulse points

Shown below are anatomic locations where an artery crosses bone or firm tissue and can be palpated for a pulse.

Temporal
Carotid
Apex of heart
Brachial
Radial
Ulnar
Common femoral
Popliteal
Posterior tibialis
Dorsalis pedis

▪ After locating the pulse, count the beats for 60 seconds, or count for 30 seconds and multiply by 2. *Counting for a full minute provides a more accurate picture of irregularities.* While counting the rate, assess pulse rhythm and volume by noting the pattern and strength of the beats. If you detect an irregularity, repeat the count, and note whether it occurs in a pattern or randomly. If you're still in doubt, take an apical pulse. (See *Identifying pulse patterns,* page 616.)

Taking an apical pulse

▪ Help the patient to a supine position and drape him if necessary.
▪ Warm the diaphragm or bell of the stethoscope in your hand. *Placing a cold stethoscope against the skin may startle the patient and momentarily increase the heart rate.* Keep in mind that the bell transmits low-pitched sounds more effectively than the diaphragm.

Identifying pulse patterns

TYPE	RATE	RHYTHM (PER 3 SECONDS)	CAUSES AND INCIDENCE
Normal	60 to 100 beats/minute; in neonates, 120 to 140 beats/minute	● ● ● ●	▪ Varies with such factors as age, physical activity, and gender (men usually have lower pulse rates than women)
Tachycardia	More than 100 beats/minute	●●●●●●	▪ Accompanies stimulation of the sympathetic nervous system by emotional stress, such as anger, fear, or anxiety, or by the use of certain drugs such as caffeine ▪ May result from exercise and from certain health conditions, such as heart failure, anemia, and fever (which increases oxygen requirements and therefore pulse rate)
Bradycardia	Less than 60 beats/minute	● ● ●	▪ Accompanies stimulation of the parasympathetic nervous system by drug use, especially digoxin, and such conditions as cerebral hemorrhage and heart block ▪ May also be present in fit athletes
Irregular	Uneven time intervals between beats (for example, periods of regular rhythm interrupted by pauses or premature beats)	●●●● ●●●	▪ May indicate cardiac irritability, hypoxia, digoxin toxicity, potassium imbalance, or sometimes more serious arrhythmias if premature beats occur frequently ▪ Occasional premature beats are normal

▪ Place the diaphragm or bell of the stethoscope over the apex of the heart (normally located at the fifth intercostal space left of the midclavicular line). Then insert the earpieces into your ears. Count the beats for 60 seconds (as shown below), and note their rhythm, volume, and intensity (loudness).

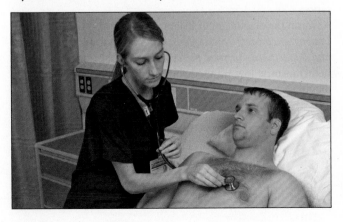

▪ Remove the stethoscope and make the patient comfortable.
▪ Clean the stethoscope with an alcohol pad *to prevent cross-contamination.*

Taking an apical-radial pulse

▪ Two nurses work together to obtain the apical-radial pulse; one palpates the radial pulse while the other auscultates the apical pulse with a stethoscope. Both must use the same watch when counting beats.
▪ Help the patient to a supine position and drape him if necessary.
▪ Locate the apical and radial pulses.
▪ Determine a time to begin counting. Then each nurse should count beats for 60 seconds.
▪ Clean and disinfect the stethoscope using a hospital-grade disinfectant, according to your facility's policy.[1]

Completing the procedure
- Perform hand hygiene.[2,3,4]
- Document the procedure.[6]

Special considerations
- When the peripheral pulse is irregular, take an apical pulse to measure the heartbeat more directly. If the pulse is faint or weak, use a Doppler ultrasound blood flow detector if available. (See "Doppler use," page 232.)
- If another nurse isn't available for an apical-radial pulse, hold the stethoscope in place with the hand that holds the watch while palpating the radial pulse with the other hand. You can then feel any discrepancies between the apical and radial pulses.

Documentation
Record pulse rate, rhythm, and volume as well as the time of measurement. "Full" or "bounding" describes a pulse of increased volume; "weak" or "thready," decreased volume. When recording the apical pulse, include intensity of heart sounds. When recording the apical-radial pulse, chart the rate according to the pulse site—for example, A/R pulse of 80/76.

REFERENCES
1 Rutala, W.A., et al. (2008). "Guideline for Disinfection and Sterilization in Healthcare Facilities, 2008" [Online]. Accessed October 2011 via the Web at http://www.cdc.gov/ncidod/dhqp/pdf/guidelines/Disinfection_Nov_2008.pdf
2 Centers for Disease Control and Prevention. (October 2002). Guideline for hand hygiene in health-care settings. *Morbidity and Mortality Weekly Report, 51*(RR-16), 1–45. (Level I)
3 The Joint Commission. (2012). Standard NPSG.07.01.01. *Comprehensive accreditation manual for hospitals: The official handbook.* Oakbrook Terrace, IL: The Joint Commission. (Level I)
4 World Health Organization. (2009). *WHO guidelines on hand hygiene in health care: First global patient safety challenge. Clean care is safer care.* Geneva, Switzerland: World Health Organization. (Level I)
5 The Joint Commission. (2012). Standard NPSG.01.01.01. *Comprehensive accreditation manual for hospitals: The official handbook.* Oakbrook Terrace, IL: The Joint Commission. (Level I)
6 The Joint Commission. (2012). Standard RC.01.03.01. *Comprehensive accreditation manual for hospitals: The official handbook.* Oakbrook Terrace, IL: The Joint Commission. (Level I)

ADDITIONAL REFERENCE
Craven, R.F., & Hirnle, C.J. (2012). *Fundamentals of nursing: Human health and function* (7th ed.). Philadelphia, PA: Lippincott Williams & Wilkins.

PULSE OXIMETRY
Performed intermittently or continuously, pulse oximetry is a relatively simple procedure used to monitor arterial oxygen saturation noninvasively. Pulse oximeters usually denote arterial oxygen saturation values with the symbol SpO_2, whereas invasively measured arterial oxygen saturation values are denoted by the symbol SaO_2.

In this procedure, two diodes send red and infrared light through a pulsating arterial vascular bed, like the one in the fingertip. A photodetector slipped over the finger measures the transmitted light as it passes through the vascular bed, detects the relative amount of color absorbed by arterial blood, and calculates the arterial oxygen saturation without interference from surrounding venous blood, skin, connective tissue, or bone. Using the ear probe, oximetry works by monitoring the transmission of light waves through the vascular bed of a patient's earlobe. Results will be inaccurate if the patient's earlobe is poorly perfused, as from a low cardiac output. (See *How oximetry works*, page 618.)

Equipment
Oximeter ▪ finger or ear probe ▪ alcohol pads ▪ nail polish remover, if necessary.

Implementation
- Perform hand hygiene.[1,2,3]
- Confirm the patient's identity using at least two patient identifiers according to your facility's policy.[4]
- Explain the procedure to the patient. Answer all questions *to decrease anxiety and increase cooperation.*

For pulse oximetry using a finger probe
- Select a finger for the test. Although the index finger is commonly used, a smaller finger may be selected if the patient's fingers are too large for the equipment. Make sure the patient isn't wearing false fingernails, and remove any nail polish from the test finger. Place the transducer (photodetector) probe over the patient's finger so that light beams and sensors oppose each other (as shown below). If the patient has long fingernails, position the probe perpendicular to the finger, if possible, or clip the fingernail. Always position the patient's hand at heart level *to eliminate venous pulsations and to promote accurate readings.*

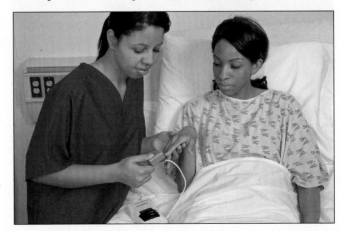

EQUIPMENT

How oximetry works

The pulse oximeter (shown below) allows noninvasive monitoring of the percentage of hemoglobin saturated by oxygen, or SpO₂ levels, by measuring the absorption (amplitude) of light waves as they pass through areas of the body that are highly perfused by arterial blood. Oximetry also monitors pulse rate and amplitude.

Light-emitting diodes in a transducer (photodetector) attached to the patient's body (shown below on the index finger) send red and infrared light beams through tissue. The photodetector records the relative amount of each color absorbed by arterial blood and transmits the data to a monitor, which displays the information with each heartbeat. If the SpO₂ level or pulse rate varies from preset limits, the monitor triggers visual and audible alarms.

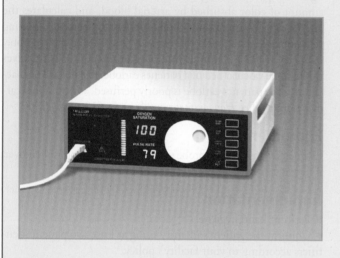

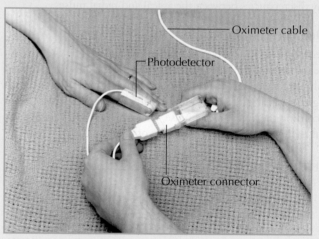

PEDIATRIC ALERT *If you're testing a neonate or small infant, wrap the probe around the foot so that light beams and detectors oppose each other. For a large infant, use a probe that fits on the great toe and secure it to the foot.*

■ Turn on the power switch (as shown below). If the device is working properly, a beep will sound, a display will light momentarily, and the pulse searchlight will flash. The SpO₂ and pulse rate displays will show stationary zeros. After four to six heartbeats, the SpO₂ and pulse rate displays will supply information with each beat, and the pulse amplitude indicator will begin tracking the pulse.

For pulse oximetry using an ear probe

■ Using an alcohol pad, massage the patient's earlobe for 10 to 20 seconds and allow it to dry. Mild erythema indicates adequate vascularization.

■ Following the manufacturer's instructions, attach the ear probe to the patient's earlobe or pinna (as shown below). Use the ear probe stabilizer for prolonged or exercise testing. Be sure to establish good contact on the ear; *an unstable probe may set off the low-perfusion alarm.*

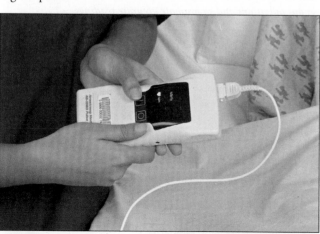

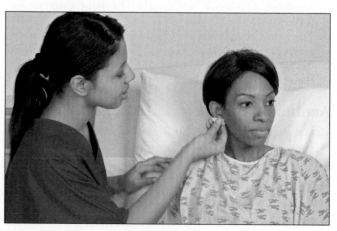

■ After the probe has been attached for a few seconds, a saturation reading and pulse waveform will appear on the oximeter's screen.

■ Leave the ear probe in place for 3 or more minutes until readings stabilize at the highest point, or take three separate readings and average them. Make sure you revascularize the patient's earlobe each time.

Completing the procedure

■ Remove the probe, turn off and unplug the unit, and clean the probe by gently rubbing it with an alcohol pad.

■ Document the procedure.[5]

Special considerations

■ Remember: The pulse rate on the pulse oximeter should correspond to the patient's actual pulse. If the rates don't correspond, the saturation reading can't be considered accurate. You should assess the patient, check the oximeter, and reposition the probe, if necessary.

■ If oximetry has been performed properly, readings are typically accurate. However, certain factors may interfere with accuracy. For example, elevated carboxyhemoglobin or methemoglobin levels (such as occur in heavy smokers and urban dwellers) can cause a falsely elevated SpO_2 reading. Certain intravascular substances, such as lipid emulsions and dyes, can also prevent accurate readings. Other factors that may interfere with accurate results include excessive light (for example, from phototherapy, surgical lamps, direct sunlight, and excessive ambient lighting), excessive patient movement, excessive ear pigment, hypothermia, hypotension, and vasoconstriction.

■ If the patient has compromised circulation in the extremities, you can place a photodetector across the bridge of the nose.

■ If SpO_2 is used to guide weaning the patient from forced inspiratory oxygen, obtain samples for arterial blood gas analysis occasionally to correlate SpO_2 readings with SaO_2 levels.

■ If an automatic blood pressure cuff is used on the same extremity that's used for measuring SpO_2, the cuff will interfere with SpO_2 readings during inflation.

■ If light is a problem, cover the probes; if patient movement is a problem, move the probe or select a different probe; and if ear pigment is a problem, reposition the probe, revascularize the site, or use a finger probe. (See *Diagnosing pulse oximeter problems*.)

■ Normal SpO_2 levels for pulse oximetry are 95% to 100% for adults and 93.8% to 100% by 1 hour after birth for healthy, full-term neonates. Lower levels may indicate hypoxemia that warrants intervention. For such patients, follow your facility's policy or the doctor's orders, which may include increasing oxygen therapy. If SpO_2 levels decrease suddenly, you may need to resuscitate the patient immediately. Notify the doctor of any significant change in the patient's condition.

Documentation

Document the date, time, procedure type, patient's activity level and position, probe site, amount of supplemental oxygen, oxygen saturation, and any action taken. Record readings on appropriate flowcharts if indicated.

TROUBLESHOOTING

Diagnosing pulse oximeter problems

To maintain a continuous display of arterial oxygen saturation (SpO2) levels, you'll need to keep the monitoring site clean and dry. Make sure the skin doesn't become irritated from adhesives used to keep disposable probes in place. You may need to change the site if this happens. Disposable probes that irritate the skin also can be replaced by nondisposable models.

Another common problem with pulse oximeters is the failure of the devices to obtain a signal. Your first reaction if this happens should be to check the patient's vital signs. If they're sufficient to produce a signal, check for the following problems.

Poor connection
See if the sensors are properly aligned. Make sure that wires are intact and securely fastened and that the pulse oximeter is plugged into a power source.

Inadequate or intermittent blood flow to the site
Check the patient's pulse rate and capillary refill time and take corrective action if blood flow to the site is decreased by loosening restraints, removing tight-fitting clothes, taking off a blood pressure cuff, or checking arterial and IV lines. If none of these interventions works, you may need to find an alternate site. Finding a site with proper circulation may also prove challenging when a patient is receiving vasoconstrictive drugs.

Equipment malfunctions
Remove the pulse oximeter from the patient, set the alarm limits according to your facility's policy, and try the instrument on yourself or another healthy person. This test will tell you if the equipment is working correctly.

REFERENCES

1 Centers for Disease Control and Prevention. (October 2002). Guideline for hand hygiene in health-care settings. *Morbidity and Mortality Weekly Report, 51*(RR-16), 1–45. (Level I)

2 The Joint Commission. (2012). Standard NPSG.07.01.01. *Comprehensive accreditation manual for hospitals: The official handbook.* Oakbrook Terrace, IL: The Joint Commission. (Level I)

3 World Health Organization. (2009). *WHO guidelines on hand hygiene in health care: First global patient safety challenge. Clean care is safer care.* Geneva, Switzerland: World Health Organization. (Level I)

4 The Joint Commission. (2012). Standard NPSG.01.01.01. *Comprehensive accreditation manual for hospitals: The official handbook.* Oakbrook Terrace, IL: The Joint Commission. (Level I)

5 The Joint Commission. (2012). Standard RC.01.03.01. *Comprehensive accreditation manual for hospitals: The official handbook.* Oakbrook Terrace, IL: The Joint Commission. (Level I)

ADDITIONAL REFERENCES

Lynn-McHale Wiegand, D. (Ed.). (2011). *AACN procedure manual for critical care* (6th ed.). Philadelphia, PA: Saunders.

Pullen, R.L., Jr. (2010). Using pulse oximetry accurately. *Nursing, 40*(4), 63.

Taenzer, A.H., et al. (2010). Impact of pulse oximetry surveillance on rescue events and intensive care unit transfers: A before-and-after concurrence study. *Anesthesiology, 112*(2), 282–287.

Valdez-Lowe, C., et al. (2009). Pulse oximetry in adults. *AJN, 109*(6), 52–59; quiz 60.

RADIATION IMPLANT THERAPY

For this treatment, also called *brachytherapy,* the doctor uses implants of radioactive isotopes (encapsulated in seeds, needles, or sutures) to deliver ionizing radiation within a body cavity or interstitially to a tumor site. Implants can deliver a continuous radiation dose over several hours or days to a specific site while minimizing exposure to adjacent tissues. The implants may be permanent or temporary. Isotopes such as cesium 137 and 131, gold 198, iodine 125, iridium 192, palladium 103, and phosphorus 32 (^{32}P) are used to treat cancers. (See *Radioisotopes and their uses.*)

Common implant sites include the brain, breast, cervix, endometrium, lung, neck, oral cavity, prostate, and vagina. Radiation implant therapy is commonly combined with external radiation therapy (teletherapy) for increased effectiveness.

For treatment, the patient is usually placed in a private room (with its own bathroom) located as far away from high-traffic areas as practical. If monitoring shows an increased radiation hazard, adjacent rooms and hallways may also need to be restricted. Consult your facility's radiation safety policy for specific guidelines.

Equipment

Film badge or pocket dosimeter ▪ radiation precaution sign for door ▪ radiation precaution warning labels ▪ masking tape ▪ lead-lined container ▪ long-handled forceps ▪ Optional: lead shield and lead strip.

For implants inserted in the oral cavity or neck

Emergency tracheotomy tray.

For implants inserted in the anal cavity or vagina

Male T-binder ▪ sanitary napkins.

Preparation of equipment

Place the lead-lined container and long-handled forceps in a corner of the patient's room. Mark a "safe line" on the floor with masking tape 6′ (1.8 m) from the patient's bed *to warn visitors to keep clear of the patient to minimize their radiation exposure.* If desired, place a portable lead shield in the back of the room *to use when providing care.*

Place an emergency tracheotomy tray in the room if an implant will be inserted in the oral cavity or neck.

Implementation

▪ Make sure that an informed consent has been obtained and is documented in the patient's medical record.[1]

▪ Perform hand hygiene.[2,3,4]

▪ Confirm the patient's identity using at least two patient identifiers according to your facility's policy.[5]

▪ Explain the treatment and its goals to the patient. Before treatment begins, review radiation safety procedures, visitation policies, potential adverse effects, and interventions for those effects. Also review long-term concerns and home care issues.

▪ Place the radiation precaution sign on the door.

▪ Make sure that all laboratory tests are performed before beginning treatment. If laboratory work is required during treatment, a technician (equipped with a film badge) should obtain the specimen, label the collection tube with a radiation precaution label, and alert the laboratory personnel before taking the samples to the laboratory. If urine tests are needed for ^{32}P therapy, ask the radiation oncology department or laboratory technician how to transport these specimens safely.

▪ Affix a radiation precaution warning label to the patient's identification wristband.

▪ Affix warning labels to the patient's chart and Kardex *to ensure staff awareness of the patient's radioactive status.*

▪ Alert staff members that the patient is receiving radiation implant therapy by placing a radiation precaution warning in the patient's medical record *to prevent accidental exposure to radiation.*

▪ Wear a film badge or dosimeter at or above waist level during the entire shift. Turn in the radiation badge monthly or according to your facility's protocol. *Pocket dosimeters measure immediate exposures.* In many facilities, these measurements aren't part of the permanent exposure record but are used to ensure that nurses receive the lowest possible exposure.

▪ Each nurse must have a personal, nontransferable film badge or ring badge that's worn only within the work environment.[6] *Badges document each person's cumulative lifetime radiation exposure.* Only primary caregivers are badged and allowed into the patient's room.

▪ *To minimize exposure to radiation,* use the three principles of time, distance, and shielding: Time—plan to give care in the shortest time possible. *Less time equals less exposure.* Distance—work as far away from the radiation source as possible. Give care from the side opposite the implant or from a position allowing the greatest working distance possible. *The intensity of radiation exposure varies inversely as the square of the distance from the source.* Shielding—use a portable shield, if needed and desired.[6]

Radioisotopes and their uses

Unstable elements, radioisotopes emit three kinds of energy particles as they decay to a stable state. These particles are ranked by their penetrating power. *Alpha particles* possess the lowest energy level and are easily stopped by a sheet of paper. More powerful *beta particles* can be stopped by the skin's surface. *Gamma rays,* the most powerful, can be stopped only by dense shielding, such as lead. Some isotopes commonly used in cancer treatments are listed below.

RADIOISOTOPE	KEY FACTS	NURSING INTERVENTIONS
Cesium 137 (^{137}Cs) Gynecologic cancers, head and neck cancers, rectal cancers, and esophageal cancers	■ 30-year half-life ■ Emits gamma particles ■ Encased in steel capsules that are placed temporarily in the patient in the operating room	■ Elevate the head of the bed no more than 45 degrees. ■ Encourage fluids and implement a low-residue diet. ■ Encourage quiet activities; enforce strict bed rest, as ordered.
Iodine 125 (^{125}I) Localized or unresectable tumors, slow-growing tumors, and recurrent disease	■ 60-day half-life ■ Emits gamma particles ■ Permanently implanted as tiny seeds or sutures directly into the tumor or tumor bed	■ Because seeds may become dislodged, no linens, body fluids, instruments, or utensils may leave the patient's room until they're monitored. ■ If a seed is dislodged and found, call the radiation oncology department; use long-handled forceps to put it in a lead-lined container in the room. ■ Monitor body fluids to detect displaced seeds. Give the patient a 24-hour urine container that can be closed.
Iridium 192 (^{192}Ir) Gynecologic cancers and tumors of the prostate, brain, head, neck, rectum, and breast	■ 74-day half-life ■ Emits gamma particles ■ Temporarily implanted as seeds strung inside special catheters that are implanted around the tumor	■ If a catheter is dislodged, call the radiation oncology department; use long-handled forceps to put the implant in a lead-lined container in the room.
Palladium 103 (^{103}Pd) Prostate cancer	■ 17-day half-life ■ Emits gamma particles ■ Permanently implanted as seeds in the tumor or tumor bed	■ See interventions for ^{125}I.
Phosphorus 32 (^{32}P) Polycythemia, leukemia, bone metastasis, and malignant ascites	■ 14-day half-life ■ Emits beta particles ■ Used as an IV solution rather than an implant because of its low energy level	■ No shielding is required other than a Lucite syringe shield. ■ Patients receiving ^{32}P are placed in a private room with a separate bathroom.
Gold 198 (^{198}Au) Localized male genitourinary tumors	■ 3-day half-life ■ Emits gamma particles ■ Permanently implanted as tiny seeds directly into the tumor or tumor bed	■ If you find a dislodged seed, call the radiation oncology department for disposal.
Cesium 131 (^{131}Cs) Prostate, liver, head, and neck tumors	■ 10-day half-life ■ Permanently implanted as tiny seeds directly into the tumor bed ■ Emits gamma particles	■ See ^{198}Au.

■ Provide essential nursing care only, limiting time in the patient's room. Make sure that perineal wipes, sanitary pads, and similar items are bagged correctly and monitored (refer to your facility's radiation policy).

■ Keep soiled linens in the patient's room until scanned and cleared by the radiation officer.[6]

■ Dressing changes over an implanted area must be supervised by the radiation technician or another designated caregiver.

■ Perform hand hygiene.[2,3,4]

■ Document the procedure.[7]

Special considerations

■ Before discharge, a patient's temporary implant must be removed and properly stored by the radiation oncology department. A patient with a permanent implant may not be released until his radioactivity level drops below 5 millirems/hour at 1 m.

■ Nurses and visitors who are pregnant or trying to conceive or father a child must not attend patients receiving radiation implant therapy *because the gonads and developing embryo and fetus are highly susceptible to the damaging effects of ionizing radiation.*

■ If the patient must be moved out of his room, notify the appropriate department of the patient's status *to give receiving personnel time to make appropriate preparations to receive the patient.* When moving the patient, make sure that the route is clear of equipment and other people and that the elevator, if there is one, is keyed and ready to receive the patient. Move the patient in a bed or wheelchair, accompanied by two badged caregivers. If the patient is delayed along the way, stand as far away from the bed as possible until you can continue.

■ The patient's room must be monitored daily by the radiation oncology department, and disposables must be monitored and removed according to facility guidelines.

■ If a code is called on a patient with an implant, follow your facility's code procedures as well as these steps: Notify the code team of the patient's radioactive status *to exclude any team member who is pregnant or trying to conceive or father a child.* Also notify the radiation oncology department. Cover the implant site with a strip of lead shielding if possible. Don't allow anything to leave the patient's room until it's monitored for radiation. Limit those entering the room to those essential personnel to perform code procedures. The primary care nurse must remain in the room (as far away from the patient as possible) *to act as a resource person for the patient and to provide film badges or dosimeters to code team members.*

■ If an implant becomes dislodged, notify the radiation oncology department staff members and follow their instructions. Typically, the dislodged implant is collected with long-handled forceps and placed in a lead-shielded canister.

■ Tell the patient who has had a cervical implant to expect slight to moderate vaginal bleeding after being discharged. This flow normally changes color from pink to brown to white. Instruct her to notify the doctor if bleeding increases, persists for more than 48 hours, or has a foul odor. Explain to the patient that she may resume most normal activities but should avoid sexual intercourse and the use of tampons until after her follow-up visit to the doctor (about 6 weeks after discharge). Instruct her to take showers rather than baths for 2 weeks, to avoid douching unless allowed by the doctor, and to avoid activities that cause abdominal strain for 6 weeks.

■ Refer the patient for sexual or psychological counseling if needed.

■ If a patient with an implant dies on the unit, notify the radiation oncology department *so they can remove a temporary implant and store it properly.* If the implant was permanent, radiation oncology staff members will determine which precautions to follow before postmortem care can be provided and before the body can be moved to the morgue.

Complications

Depending on the implant site and total radiation dose, complications of implant therapy may include dislodgment of the radiation source or applicator, tissue fibrosis, xerostomia, radiation pneumonitis, muscle atrophy, sterility, vaginal dryness or stenosis, fistulas, hypothyroidism, altered bowel habits, infection, airway obstruction, diarrhea, cystitis, myelosuppression, neurotoxicity, and secondary cancers. Encourage the patient and family members to keep in contact with the radiation oncology department and to call them if concerns or physical changes occur.

Documentation

Record radiation precautions taken during treatment, adverse effects of therapy, teaching given to the patient and family and their responses to it, the patient's tolerance of isolation procedures and the family's compliance with procedures, and referrals to local cancer services.

REFERENCES

1 The Joint Commission. (2012). Standard RI.01.03.01. *Comprehensive accreditation manual for hospitals: The official handbook.* Oakbrook Terrace, IL: The Joint Commission. (Level I)

2 The Joint Commission. (2012). Standard NPSG.07.01.01. *Comprehensive accreditation manual for hospitals: The official handbook.* Oakbrook Terrace, IL: The Joint Commission. (Level I)

3 Centers for Disease Control and Prevention. (October 2002). Guideline for hand hygiene in health-care settings. *Morbidity and Mortality Weekly Report, 51*(RR-16), 1–45. (Level I)

4 World Health Organization. (2009). *WHO guidelines on hand hygiene in health care: First global patient safety challenge. Clean care is safer care.* Geneva, Switzerland: World Health Organization. (Level I)

5 The Joint Commission. (2012). Standard NPSG.01.01.01. *Comprehensive accreditation manual for hospitals: The official handbook.* Oakbrook Terrace, IL: The Joint Commission. (Level I)

6 Polovich, M., et al. (Eds.). (2009). *Chemotherapy and biotherapy guidelines and recommendations for practice* (3rd ed.). Pittsburgh, PA: Oncology Nursing Society.

7 The Joint Commission. (2012). Standard RC.01.03.01. *Comprehensive accreditation manual for hospitals: The official handbook.* Oakbrook Terrace, IL: The Joint Commission. (Level I)

ADDITIONAL REFERENCES

Bruner, D., et al. (Eds.). (2011). *Manual for radiation oncology nursing practice and education* (4th ed.). Pittsburgh, PA: Oncology Nursing Society.

Cash J., et al. (2009). Combined modality treatment for prostate cancer with dynamic adaptive radiation therapy using four-dimensional image-guided intensity-modulated radiation therapy and brachytherapy. *Journal of Radiology Nursing, 28*(3), 87–95.

I-Chow, H, et al. (2008). "American Brachytherapy Society: Prostate High-Dose Rate Task Group" [Online]. Accessed November 2011 via the Web at http://www.americanbrachytherapy.org/guidelines/HDRTaskGroup.pdf

Keisch, M., et al. (2007). "American Brachytherapy Society: Breast Brachytherapy Task Group" [Online]. Accessed November 2011 via the Web at http://www.americanbrachytherapy.org/guidelines/ abs_breast_brachytherapy_taskgroup.pdf

Kwekkeboom, K.L., et al. (2009). Patterns of pain and distress during high-dose-rate intracavity brachytherapy for cervical cancer. *Journal of Supportive Oncology, 7*(3), 108–114.

Merrick, G.S., et al. "American Brachytherapy Society: Prostate Low-Dose Rate Task Group" [Online]. Accessed November 2011 via the Web at http://www.americanbrachytherapy.org/guidelines/prostate_ low-doseratetaskgroup.pdf

Phan, T.P., et al. (2007). High dose rate brachytherapy as a boost for the treatment of localized prostate cancer. *The Journal of Urology, 177*(1), 123–127.

So, W.K., & Chui, Y.Y. (2007). Women's experience of internal radiation treatment for uterine cervical cancer. *Journal of Advanced Nursing, 60*(2), 154–161.

Viswanathan, A.N., et al. "American Brachytherapy Society: Cervical Cancer Brachytherapy Task Group" [Online]. Accessed November 2011 via the Web at http://www.americanbrachytherapy.org/guidelines/cervical_cancer_taskgroup.pdf

RADIATION THERAPY, EXTERNAL

About 60% of all cancer patients are treated with some form of external radiation therapy. Also called radiotherapy, this treatment delivers radiation—X-rays or gamma rays—directly to the cancer site.

Radiation doses are based on the type, stage, and location of the tumor as well as on the patient's size, condition, and overall treatment goals. Doses are given in increments, usually 3 to 5 times a week, until the total dose is reached.

The goals of radiation therapy include *cure,* in which the cancer is completely destroyed and not expected to recur; *control,* in which the cancer doesn't progress or regress but is expected to progress at some later time; or *palliation,* in which radiation is given to relieve signs and symptoms (such as bone pain, seizures, bleeding, and headache) caused by the cancer.

External beam radiation therapy is delivered by machines that aim a concentrated beam of high-energy particles (photons and gamma rays) at the target site. Two types of machines are commonly used: units containing cobalt or cesium as radioactive sources for gamma rays, and linear accelerators that use electricity to produce X-rays. Linear accelerators produce high energy with great penetrating ability.

Radiation therapy may be augmented by chemotherapy, radiation implant therapy (brachytherapy), or surgery, as needed.

Equipment

Radiation therapy machine.

Implementation

- Verify the doctor's order.
- Verify that the radiation oncology department has obtained informed consent and that the form is documented in the patient's medical record.[1]
- Perform hand hygiene.[2,3,4]
- Confirm the patient's identity using at least two patient identifiers according to your facility's policy.[5]
- Explain the treatment to the patient and his family. Review the treatment goals, and discuss the range of potential adverse effects as well as interventions to minimize them. Also discuss possible long-term complications and treatment issues. Educate the patient and his family about local cancer services. Answer all questions *to decrease anxiety and increase cooperation.*
- Review the patient's clinical record for recent laboratory and imaging results, and alert the radiation oncology staff to any abnormalities or pertinent results (such as myelosuppression, paraneoplastic syndromes, oncologic emergencies, and tumor progression).
- Transport the patient to the radiology oncology department.
- The patient begins by undergoing simulation (treatment planning), in which the target area is mapped out on his body using a machine similar to the radiation therapy machine. Then the target area is tattooed or marked in ink on his body *to ensure accurate treatments.*
- The doctor and radiation oncologist determine the duration and frequency of treatments, depending on the patient's body size, size of portal, extent and location of cancer, and treatment goals.
- The patient is positioned on the treatment table beneath the machine. Treatments last from a few seconds to a few minutes. Reassure the patient that he won't feel anything and that he will not be radioactive. After treatment is complete, the patient may return home or to his room.
- Perform hand hygiene.[2,3,4]
- Document the procedure.[6]

Special considerations

- Emphasize the importance of keeping follow-up appointments with the doctor.
- Refer the patient to a support group, such as a local chapter of the American Cancer Society.

Patient teaching

Teach the patient and his family proper skin care and management of the possible adverse effects of treatment. Explain to the patient that the full benefit of radiation treatments may not occur until several weeks or months after treatments begin. Instruct him to report any long-term adverse effects.

Instruct the patient about the importance of leaving the target area markings intact *to ensure treatment accuracy.*

Complications

Adverse effects arise gradually and diminish gradually after treatments. They may be acute, subacute (accumulating as treatment progresses), chronic (following treatment), or long-term (arising months to years after treatment). Adverse effects are localized to the area of treatment, and their severity depends on the total radiation dosage, underlying organ sensitivity, and the patient's overall condition.

Common acute and subacute adverse effects can include altered skin integrity, altered GI and genitourinary function, altered fertility and sexual function, altered bone marrow production, fatigue, and alopecia.

Long-term complications or adverse effects may include radiation pneumonitis, neuropathy, skin and muscle atrophy, telangiectasia, fistulas, altered endocrine function, and secondary cancers. Other complications of treatment include headache, alopecia, xerostomia, dysphagia, stomatitis, altered skin integrity (wet or dry desquamation), nausea, vomiting, heartburn, diarrhea, cystitis, and fatigue.

Documentation

Record radiation precautions taken during treatment, interventions used and evaluation of the interventions, grading of adverse effects, teaching given to the patient and family and their responses to it, the patient's tolerance of isolation procedures and the family's compliance with procedures, discharge plans and teaching, and referrals to local cancer services, if any.

REFERENCES

1 The Joint Commission. (2012). Standard RI.01.03.01. *Comprehensive accreditation manual for hospitals: The official handbook.* Oakbrook Terrace, IL: The Joint Commission. (Level I)
2 The Joint Commission. (2012). Standard NPSG.07.01.01. *Comprehensive accreditation manual for hospitals: The official handbook.* Oakbrook Terrace, IL: The Joint Commission. (Level I)
3 Centers for Disease Control and Prevention. (October 2002). Guideline for hand hygiene in health-care settings. *Morbidity and Mortality Weekly Report, 51*(RR-16), 1–45. (Level I)
4 World Health Organization. (2009). *WHO guidelines on hand hygiene in health care: First global patient safety challenge. Clean care is safer care.* Geneva, Switzerland: World Health Organization. (Level I)
5 The Joint Commission. (2012). Standard NPSG.01.01.01. *Comprehensive accreditation manual for hospitals: The official handbook.* Oakbrook Terrace, IL: The Joint Commission. (Level I)
6 The Joint Commission. (2012). Standard RC.01.03.01. *Comprehensive accreditation manual for hospitals: The official handbook.* Oakbrook Terrace, IL: The Joint Commission. (Level I)

ADDITIONAL REFERENCES

Bruner, D., et al. (Eds.). (2011). *Manual for radiation oncology nursing practice and education* (4th ed.). Pittsburgh, PA: Oncology Nursing Society.

Cash J., et al. (2009). Combined modality treatment for prostate cancer with dynamic adaptive radiation therapy using four-dimensional image-guided intensity-modulated radiation therapy and brachytherapy. *Journal of Radiology Nursing, 28*(3), 87–95.

RADIOACTIVE IODINE THERAPY

Because the thyroid gland concentrates iodine, radioactive iodine 131 (^{131}I) can be used to treat thyroid cancer. Usually administered orally, this isotope is used to treat postoperative residual cancer, recurrent disease, inoperable primary thyroid tumors, invasion of the thyroid capsule, or thyroid ablation as well as cancers that have metastasized to cervical or mediastinal lymph nodes or other distant sites.

Because ^{131}I is absorbed systemically, all body secretions, especially urine, must be considered radioactive. For ^{131}I treatments, the patient usually is placed in a private room (with its own bathroom) located as far away from high-traffic areas as practical. Adjacent rooms and hallways may also need to be restricted. Consult your facility's radiation safety policy for specific guidelines.

In lower doses, ^{131}I also may be used to treat hyperthyroidism. Most patients receive this treatment on an outpatient basis and are sent home with appropriate home care instructions.

Equipment

Film badges, pocket dosimeters, or ring badges ■ radiation precaution sign for door ■ radiation precaution warning labels ■ waterproof gowns ■ gloves ■ clear and red plastic bags for contaminated articles ■ plastic wrap ■ absorbent plastic-lined pads ■ masking tape ■ radioresistant gloves ■ trash cans ■ emergency tracheotomy tray ■ Optional: portable lead shield.

Preparation of equipment

Assemble all necessary equipment in the patient's room. Keep an emergency tracheotomy tray just outside the room or in a handy place at the nurses' station. Place the radiation precaution sign on the door. Affix warning labels to the patient's chart and Kardex *to ensure staff awareness of the patient's radioactive status.*

Place an absorbent plastic-lined pad on the bathroom floor and under the sink; if the patient's room is carpeted, cover it with such a pad as well. Place an additional pad over the bedside table. Secure plastic wrap over the telephone, television controls, bed controls, mattress, call bell, toilet seat, and flush handle. *These measures prevent radioactive contamination of working surfaces.* Keep a hazardous waste container lined with a clear and then a red leak-proof bag in the patient's room. Keep objects in the patient's room until they've been scanned and cleared by the radiation safety officer.[1]

Notify the dietitian to supply foods and beverages in disposable containers only and to provide disposable utensils.

Implementation

■ Review the patient's health history for vomiting, diarrhea, productive cough, and sinus drainage, *which could increase the risk of radioactive secretions.*

■ Verify that the doctor has obtained informed consent and that the form is documented in the patient's medical record.[2]

■ Perform hand hygiene.[3,4,5]

■ Confirm the patient's identity using at least two patient identifiers according to your facility's policy.[6]

■ Explain the procedure and review treatment goals with the patient and his family. Before treatment begins, review your facility's radiation safety procedures and visitation policies, potential adverse effects, interventions, and home care procedures.

■ Check for allergies to iodine-containing substances, such as contrast media and shellfish. Review the patient's medication history for thyroid-containing or thyroid-altering drugs and for lithium carbonate, *which may increase ^{131}I uptake.*

■ Review the patient's health history for vomiting, diarrhea, productive cough, and sinus drainage, *which could increase the risk of radioactive secretions.*

■ If necessary, remove the patient's dentures *to avoid contaminating them and to reduce radioactive secretions.* Tell him they'll be returned 48 hours after treatment.

■ Affix a radiation precaution label to the patient's identification wristband.

■ Encourage the patient to use the toilet rather than a bedpan or urinal and to flush it three times after each use *to reduce radiation levels. To help avoid splash and aerosol contamination,* close the lid or cover the toilet before flushing.

■ Tell the patient to remain in his room except for tests or procedures. Allow him to ambulate.

■ Unless contraindicated, instruct the patient to increase his fluid intake to 3 qt (3 L) daily.

■ Encourage the patient to chew or suck on hard candy *to keep salivary glands stimulated and prevent them from becoming inflamed (which may develop in the first 24 hours).*

■ Ensure that all laboratory tests are performed before beginning treatment. If laboratory work is required, the laboratory technician equipped with a radiation badge obtains the specimen, labels the collection tube with a radiation precaution warning label, and alerts the laboratory personnel before transporting it. If urine tests are needed, ask the radiation oncology department or laboratory technician how to transport the specimens safely.

■ Wear a film badge or dosimeter at or above waist level during the entire shift. Turn in the radiation badge monthly or according to your facility's protocol, and be sure to record your exposures accurately. *Pocket dosimeters measure immediate exposures.* These measurements may not be part of the permanent exposure record, but they help ensure that nurses receive the lowest possible exposure.

■ Each nurse must have a personal, nontransferable film badge or ring badge. *Badges document each person's cumulative lifetime radiation exposure.* Only primary caregivers are badged and allowed into the patient's room.[1]

■ Wear gloves to touch the patient or objects in his room.

■ Wear a waterproof gown and gloves when handling the patient's body secretions (for example, when moving his emesis basin).

■ Allow visitors to stay no more than 30 minutes every 24 hours with the patient or according to your facility policy. Stress that no visitors who are pregnant or trying to conceive or father a child will be allowed.

PEDIATRIC ALERT *Visitors younger than age 18 aren't allowed for their protection.*

■ Restrict direct contact to no more than 30 minutes or 20 millirems per day. If the patient is receiving 200 millicuries of ^{131}I, remain with him only 2 to 4 minutes and stand no closer than 1′ (30 cm) away. If standing 3′ (1 m) away, the time limit is 20 minutes; if standing 5′ (1.5 m) away, the limit is 30 minutes.

■ Give essential nursing care only; omit bed baths. If ordered, provide perineal care, making sure that wipes, sanitary pads, and similar items are bagged correctly.

■ If the patient vomits or urinates on the floor, notify the nuclear medicine department and use nondisposable radioresistant gloves when cleaning the floor. After cleanup, wash your gloved hands, remove the gloves and leave them in the room, and then rewash your hands.

■ If the patient must be moved from his room, notify the appropriate department of his status *so that receiving personnel can make appropriate arrangements to receive him.* When moving the patient, ensure that the route is clear of equipment and other people and that the elevator, if there is one, is keyed and ready to receive the patient. Move the patient in a bed or wheelchair, accompanied by two badged caregivers. If delayed, stand as far away from him as possible until you can continue.

■ The patient's room must be cleaned by the radiation oncology department, not by housekeeping. The room must be monitored daily, and disposables must be monitored and removed according to facility guidelines.

■ Perform hand hygiene.[3,4,5]

■ Document the procedure.[7]

Special considerations

■ Nurses and visitors who are pregnant or trying to conceive or father a child must not attend or visit patients receiving ^{131}I therapy *because the gonads and developing embryo and fetus are highly susceptible to the damaging effects of ionizing radiation.*

■ If a code is called on a patient undergoing ^{131}I therapy, follow your facility's code procedures as well as these steps. Notify the code team of the patient's radioactive status *to exclude any team member who is pregnant or trying to conceive or father a child.* Also notify the radiation oncology department. Don't allow anything out of the patient's room until it's monitored. The primary care nurse must remain in the room (as far as possible from the patient) *to act as a resource person and to provide film badges or dosimeters to code team members.*

■ If the patient dies on the unit, notify the radiology safety officer, who will determine which precautions to follow before postmortem care is provided and before the body can be removed to the morgue.

Patient teaching

At discharge, schedule the patient for a follow-up examination. Also arrange for a whole-body scan approximately 7 to 10 days after ^{131}I treatment.

What to do after
¹³¹I treatment

Instruct the patient to report any long-term adverse reactions. In particular, review signs and symptoms of hypothyroidism and hyperthyroidism. Also ask him to report any signs and symptoms of thyroid cancer, such as enlarged lymph nodes, dyspnea, bone pain, nausea, vomiting, and abdominal discomfort.

Although the patient's radiation level at discharge will be safe, suggest that he take extra precautions during the first week, such as using separate eating utensils, sleeping in a separate bedroom, and avoiding body contact.

Sexual intercourse may be resumed 1 week after ¹³¹I treatment. However, urge a female patient to avoid pregnancy for 6 months after treatment, and tell a male patient to avoid impregnating his partner for 3 months after treatment.

Teach the patient precautions he should follow at home as well as signs and symptoms to report. (See *What to do after ¹³¹I treatment*.) Inform the patient and his family of community support services for cancer patients.

Complications

Myelosuppression is common in patients who undergo repeated ¹³¹I treatments. Radiation pulmonary fibrosis may develop if extensive lung metastasis was present when ¹³¹I was administered.

Other complications may include nausea, vomiting, headache, radiation thyroiditis, fever, sialadenitis, and pain and swelling at metastatic sites.

Documentation

Record radiation precautions taken during treatment, teaching given to the patient and family, the patient's tolerance of (and the family's compliance with) isolation procedures, and referrals to local cancer counseling services.

REFERENCES

1 Polovich, M., et al. (Eds.). (2009). *Chemotherapy and biotherapy guidelines and recommendations for practice* (3rd ed.). Pittsburgh, PA: Oncology Nursing Society.
2 The Joint Commission. (2012). Standard RI.01.03.01. *Comprehensive accreditation manual for hospitals: The official handbook.* Oakbrook Terrace, IL: The Joint Commission. (Level I)
3 The Joint Commission. (2012). Standard NPSG.07.01.01. *Comprehensive accreditation manual for hospitals: The official handbook.* Oakbrook Terrace, IL: The Joint Commission. (Level I)
4 Centers for Disease Control and Prevention. (October 2002). Guideline for hand hygiene in health-care settings. *Morbidity and Mortality Weekly Report, 51*(RR-16), 1–45. (Level I)
5 World Health Organization. (2009). *WHO guidelines on hand hygiene in health care: First global patient safety challenge. Clean care is safer care.* Geneva, Switzerland: World Health Organization. (Level I)
6 The Joint Commission. (2012). Standard NPSG.01.01.01. *Comprehensive accreditation manual for hospitals: The official handbook.* Oakbrook Terrace, IL: The Joint Commission. (Level I)
7 The Joint Commission. (2012). Standard RC.01.03.01. *Comprehensive accreditation manual for hospitals: The official handbook.* Oakbrook Terrace, IL: The Joint Commission. (Level I)

ADDITIONAL REFERENCE

Bruner, D., et al. (Eds.). (2011). *Manual for radiation oncology nursing practice and education* (4th ed.). Pittsburgh, PA: Oncology Nursing Society.

RECTAL SUPPOSITORIES AND OINTMENTS

A rectal suppository is a small, solid, medicated mass, usually cone-shaped, with a cocoa butter or glycerin base. It may be inserted to stimulate peristalsis and defecation or to relieve pain, vomiting, and local irritation. Rectal suppositories commonly contain drugs that reduce fever, relieve constipation, induce relaxation, interact poorly with digestive enzymes, or have a taste too offensive for oral use. Rectal suppositories melt at body temperature and are absorbed slowly.

Because insertion of a rectal suppository may stimulate the vagus nerve, this procedure is contraindicated in patients with potential cardiac arrhythmias. It may also have to be avoided in patients with active rectal bleeding or who have undergone recent rectal or prostate surgery because of the risk of local trauma or discomfort during insertion.

An ointment is a semisolid medication used to produce local effects. It may be applied externally to the anus or internally to the rectum. Rectal ointments commonly contain drugs that reduce inflammation or relieve pain and itching.

Equipment

Rectal suppository or ointment ■ applicator ■ patient's medication record and chart ■ gloves ■ water-soluble lubricant ■ 4″ × 4″ gauze pads ■ Optional: bedpan.

Preparation of equipment

Store rectal suppositories in the refrigerator until needed *to prevent softening and, possibly, decreased effectiveness of the medication. A softened suppository is also difficult to handle and insert.* To harden a softened suppository, hold the suppository (in its wrapper) under cold running water.

Implementation

■ Avoid distractions and interruptions when preparing and administering the medications to prevent medication administration errors.

■ Verify the order on the patient's medication record by checking it against the doctor's order.[2]

■ Compare the medication label to the doctor's order to verify the correct medication, indication, dose, route, and time of administration.[2]

■ Check the expiration date on the medication; don't give the drug is it's expired.[2]

■ Perform hand hygiene and put on gloves.[3,4,5]

■ Confirm the patient's identity using at least two patient identifiers according to your facility's policy.[6]

■ Provide privacy.

■ Explain the procedure and the purpose of the medication to the patient. If the patient is receiving the medication for the first time, inform the patient or his family about the significance of adverse reactions or other concerns related to administering the medication.[2]

■ Visually inspect the medication for discoloration or any other loss of integrity. Don't give the medication if its integrity is compromised.[2]

■ If your facility uses a bar code scanning system, be sure to scan your identification badge, the patient's identification bracelet, and the medication's bar code.

■ Place the patient on his left side in Sims' position. Drape him with the bedcovers to expose only the buttocks.

Rectal suppository administration

■ Remove the suppository from its wrapper and lubricate it with water-soluble lubricant.

■ Lift the patient's upper buttock with your nondominant hand *to expose the anus.*

■ Instruct the patient to take several deep breaths through his mouth *to help relax the anal sphincters and reduce anxiety or discomfort during insertion.*

■ Using the index finger of your dominant hand, insert the suppository—tapered end first—about 3″ (7.6 cm), until you feel it pass the internal anal sphincter. Try to direct the tapered end toward the side of the rectum *so that it contacts the membranes.* (See *How to administer a rectal suppository.*)

■ Ensure the patient's comfort. Encourage him to lie quietly and, if applicable, to retain the suppository for the appropriate length of time. If the suppository is administered to relieve constipation, tell the patient to retain it as long as possible (at least 20 minutes) to be effective. Press on the anus with a gauze pad if necessary until the urge to defecate passes.

Rectal ointment administration

■ To apply externally, use gloves or a gauze pad to spread medication over the anal area.

■ To apply internally, attach the applicator to the tube of ointment and coat the applicator with water-soluble lubricant.

■ Expect to use about 1″ (2.5 cm) of ointment. *To gauge how much pressure to use during application,* squeeze a small amount from the tube before you attach the applicator.

■ Lift the patient's upper buttock with your nondominant hand *to expose the anus.*

How to administer a rectal suppository

When inserting a suppository, direct its tapered end toward the side of the rectum so that it contacts the membranes, encouraging absorption of the medication.

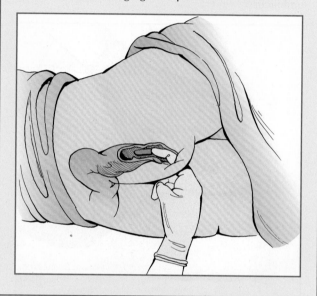

■ Instruct the patient to take several deep breaths through his mouth *to relax the anal sphincters and reduce anxiety or discomfort during insertion.*

■ Gently insert the applicator, directing it toward the umbilicus. (See *How to administer rectal ointment,* page 628.)

■ Slowly squeeze the tube to eject the medication.

■ Remove the applicator and place a folded 4″ × 4″ gauze pad between the patient's buttocks to absorb *excess ointment.*

■ Detach the applicator from the tube and recap the tube. Then clean the applicator thoroughly with soap and warm water.

Completing the procedure

■ Remove and discard your gloves. Perform hand hygiene.[3,4,5]

■ Document the procedure.[7]

Special considerations

■ Because the intake of food and fluid stimulates peristalsis, a suppository for relieving constipation should be inserted about 30 minutes before mealtime *to help soften the feces in the rectum and facilitate defecation.* A medicated retention suppository should be inserted between meals.

■ Instruct the patient to avoid expelling the suppository. If he has difficulty retaining it, place him on a bedpan.

■ Make sure the patient's call bell is handy, and watch for his signal *because he may be unable to suppress the urge to defecate.* For example, a patient with proctitis has a highly sensitive rectum and may not be able to retain a suppository for long.

How to administer rectal ointment

When applying a rectal ointment internally, be sure to lubricate the applicator *to minimize pain on insertion*. Direct the applicator tip toward the patient's umbilicus.

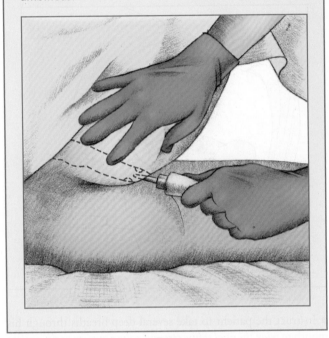

■ Be sure to inform the patient that the suppository may discolor his next bowel movement. For example, hydrocortisone (Anusol) suppositories can give feces a silver-gray pasty appearance.
■ Advise the patient to report any increase in itching or burning at the rectal area. *This may indicate increased irritation.*
■ Some nonprescription rectal ointments are available. Instruct the patient how to self-administer the ointment, if appropriate.

Complications

Complications may be related to the action of the medication. Occasionally, vagal nerve stimulation may occur, causing a vagal reaction. Irritation of the tissue may occur.

Documentation

Record the time and date, dosage, route, and site of administration. Document the effect of the medication, the patient's tolerance of the procedure, complications, and nursing actions taken. Note patient teaching and the patient's understanding of your teaching.

REFERENCES

1 Westbrook, J. et al. (2010). Association of interruptions with an increased risk and severity of medication administration errors. *Archives of Internal Medicine, 170*(8), 683–690.

2 The Joint Commission. (2012). Standard MM.06.01.01. *Comprehensive accreditation manual for hospitals: The official handbook.* Oakbrook Terrace, IL: The Joint Commission. (Level I)
3 The Joint Commission. (2012). Standard NPSG.07.01.01. *Comprehensive accreditation manual for hospitals: The official handbook.* Oakbrook Terrace, IL: The Joint Commission. (Level I)
4 Centers for Disease Control and Prevention. (October 2002). Guideline for hand hygiene in health-care settings. *Morbidity and Mortality Weekly Report, 51*(RR-16), 1–45. (Level I)
5 World Health Organization. (2009). *WHO guidelines on hand hygiene in health care: First global patient safety challenge. Clean care is safer care.* Geneva, Switzerland: World Health Organization. (Level I)
6 The Joint Commission. (2012). Standard NPSG.01.01.01. *Comprehensive accreditation manual for hospitals: The official handbook.* Oakbrook Terrace, IL: The Joint Commission. (Level I)
7 The Joint Commission. (2012). Standard RC.01.03.01. *Comprehensive accreditation manual for hospitals: The official handbook.* Oakbrook Terrace, IL: The Joint Commission. (Level I)

ADDITIONAL REFERENCES

Bradshaw, A., & Price, L. (2007). Rectal suppository insertion: The reliability of the evidence as a basis for nursing practice. *Journal of Clinical Nursing, 16*(1), 98–103.
Nettina, S.M. (2010). *Lippincott manual of nursing practice* (9th ed.). Philadelphia, PA: Lippincott Williams & Wilkins.
Taylor, C., et al. (2011). *Fundamentals of nursing: The art and science of nursing care* (7th ed.). Philadelphia, PA: Lippincott Williams & Wilkins.

RECTAL TUBE INSERTION AND REMOVAL

Whether GI hypomotility simply slows the normal release of gas and feces or results in paralytic ileus, inserting a rectal tube may relieve the discomfort of distention and flatus. Decreased motility may result from various medical or surgical conditions, certain medications (such as atropine), or even swallowed air. Conditions that contraindicate using a rectal tube include recent rectal or prostatic surgery, recent myocardial infarction, and diseases of the rectal mucosa.

Equipment

Stethoscope ■ linen-saver pads ■ drape ■ water-soluble lubricant ■ commercial kit or #22 to #34 French rectal tube of soft rubber or plastic ■ container (emesis basin, plastic bag, or water bottle with vent) ■ tape ■ gloves ■ equipment for performing perineal care.

Implementation

■ Gather all the equipment at the patient's bedside.
■ Perform hand hygiene and put on gloves.[1,2,3] Put on other personal protective equipment if needed.
■ Confirm the patient's identity using at least two patient identifiers according to your facility's policy.[4]
■ Provide privacy and explain the procedure. Answer all questions *to decrease anxiety and increase cooperation.*

■ Check for abdominal distention. Using the stethoscope, auscultate for bowel sounds.

■ Place the linen-saver pads under the patient's buttocks *to absorb any drainage that may leak from the tube.*

■ Position the patient in left-lateral Sims' position *to facilitate rectal tube insertion.*

■ Drape the patient's exposed buttocks.

■ Lubricate the rectal tube tip with water-soluble lubricant *to ease insertion and prevent rectal irritation.*

■ Lift the patient's right buttock *to expose the anus.*

■ Insert the rectal tube tip into the anus, advancing the tube 2″ to 4″ (5 to 10 cm) into the rectum (as shown below). Direct the tube toward the umbilicus along the anatomic course of the large intestine.

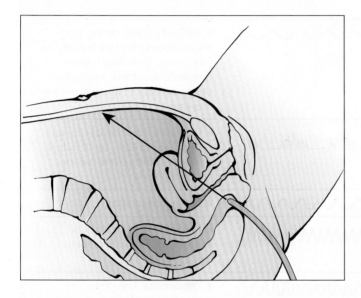

■ As you insert the tube, tell the patient to breathe slowly and deeply, or suggest that he bear down as he would for a bowel movement *to relax the anal sphincter and ease insertion.*

■ Using tape, secure the rectal tube to the buttocks. Then attach the tube to the container *to collect possible leakage.*

■ Remove the tube after 15 to 20 minutes. If the patient reports continued discomfort or if gas wasn't expelled, you can repeat the procedure in 2 or 3 hours if ordered.

■ Clean the patient, and replace soiled linens and the linen-saver pad. Make sure the patient feels as comfortable as possible.

■ Check for abdominal distention and listen for bowel sounds.

■ If you will reuse the equipment, clean it and store it in the bedside cabinet; otherwise discard the tube.

■ Remove and discard your gloves and other personal protective equipment if worn; perform hand hygiene.[1,2,3]

■ Document the procedure.[5]

Special considerations

■ Fastening a plastic bag to the external end of the tube lets you observe gas expulsion (like a balloon).

■ Leaving a rectal tube in place indefinitely does little to promote peristalsis, can reduce sphincter responsiveness, and may lead to permanent sphincter damage or pressure necrosis of the mucosa.

■ Repeat insertion periodically *to stimulate GI activity.* If the tube fails to relieve distention, notify the doctor.

Documentation

Record the date and time that you inserted the tube. Write down the amount, color, and consistency of any evacuated matter. Describe the patient's abdomen—hard, distended, soft, or drumlike on percussion. Note bowel sounds before and after insertion and the patient's tolerance of the procedure.

REFERENCES

1 The Joint Commission. (2012). Standard NPSG.07.01.01. *Comprehensive accreditation manual for hospitals: The official handbook.* Oakbrook Terrace, IL: The Joint Commission. (Level I)

2 Centers for Disease Control and Prevention. (October 2002). Guideline for hand hygiene in health-care settings. *Morbidity and Mortality Weekly Report, 51*(RR-16), 1–45. (Level I)

3 World Health Organization. (2009). *WHO guidelines on hand hygiene in health care: First global patient safety challenge. Clean care is safer care.* Geneva, Switzerland: World Health Organization. (Level I)

4 The Joint Commission. (2012). Standard NPSG.01.01.01. *Comprehensive accreditation manual for hospitals: The official handbook.* Oakbrook Terrace, IL: The Joint Commission. (Level I)

5 The Joint Commission. (2012). Standard RC.01.03.01. *Comprehensive accreditation manual for hospitals: The official handbook.* Oakbrook Terrace, IL: The Joint Commission. (Level I)

ADDITIONAL REFERENCES

Nettina, S.M. (2010). *Lippincott manual of nursing practice* (9th ed.). Philadelphia, PA: Lippincott Williams & Wilkins.

Taylor, C., et al. (2011). *Fundamentals of nursing: The art and science of nursing care* (7th ed.). Philadelphia, PA: Lippincott Williams & Wilkins.

RESPIRATION ASSESSMENT

Controlled by the respiratory center in the lateral medulla oblongata, respiration is the exchange of oxygen and carbon dioxide between the atmosphere and body cells. External respiration, or breathing, is accomplished by the diaphragm and chest muscles and delivers oxygen to the lower respiratory tract and alveoli.

Four measures of respiration—rate, rhythm, depth, and sound—reflect the body's metabolic state, diaphragm and chest-muscle condition, and airway patency. Respiratory rate is recorded as the number of cycles (with cone cycle consisting of inspiration and expiration) per minute; rhythm, as the regularity of these cycles; depth, as the volume of air inhaled and exhaled with each respiration; and sound, as the audible digression from normal, effortless breathing.

The best time to assess your patient's respirations is immediately after taking the pulse rate.

Equipment

Watch with second hand ■ stethoscope, as needed ■ alcohol pad.

Identifying respiratory patterns

The table below shows several common types of respiratory patterns and their possible causes. Assess the patient both for the underlying cause and for the effect on the patient.

TYPE	CHARACTERISTICS	PATTERN	POSSIBLE CAUSES
Apnea	Periodic absence of breathing		■ Mechanical airway obstruction ■ Conditions affecting the brain's respiratory center in the lateral medulla oblongata
Apneustic	Prolonged, gasping inspiration followed by extremely short, inefficient expiration		■ Lesions of the respiratory center
Bradypnea	Slow, regular respirations of equal depth		■ Normal pattern during sleep ■ Conditions affecting the respiratory center, including tumors, metabolic disorders, respiratory decompensation, and use of opiates and alcohol
Cheyne-Stokes	Fast, deep respirations punctuated by periods of apnea lasting 20 to 60 seconds		■ Increased intracranial pressure, severe heart failure, renal failure, meningitis, drug overdose, or cerebral anoxia
Eupnea	Normal rate and rhythm		■ Normal respiration
Kussmaul's	Fast (over 20 breaths/minute), deep (resembling sighs), labored respirations without pause		■ Renal failure or metabolic acidosis, particularly diabetic ketoacidosis
Tachypnea	Rapid respirations; rate rises with body temperature at a rate of about four breaths/minute for every degree Fahrenheit above normal		■ Pneumonia, compensatory respiratory alkalosis, respiratory insufficiency, lesions of the respiratory center, or salicylate poisoning

Implementation

■ Perform hand hygiene.[1,2,3]
■ Confirm the patient's identity using at least two patient identifiers according to your facility's policy.[4]
■ Provide privacy and explain the procedure. Answer all questions *to decrease anxiety and increase cooperation.*
■ Keep your fingertips over the radial artery, and don't tell the patient you're counting respirations. *If you tell him, he'll become conscious of his respirations and the rate may change.*
■ Count respirations by observing the rise and fall of the patient's chest as he breathes. Alternatively, position the patient's opposite arm across his chest and count respirations by feeling its rise and fall. Consider one rise and one fall as one respiration.
■ Count respirations for 30 seconds and multiply by 2 or count for 60 seconds if respirations are irregular *to account for variations in respiratory rate and pattern.*

■ As you count respirations, be alert for and record such breath sounds as stertor, stridor, wheezing, and an expiratory grunt. *Stertor* is a snoring sound resulting from secretions in the trachea and large bronchi. Listen for it in patients with neurologic disorders and in those who are comatose. *Stridor* is an inspiratory crowing sound that occurs with upper airway obstruction in laryngitis, croup, or the presence of a foreign body. *Wheezing* is caused by partial obstruction in the smaller bronchi and bronchioles. This high-pitched, musical sound is common in patients with emphysema or asthma.
ELDER ALERT *In older patients, an* expiratory grunt *may result from partial airway obstruction or neuromuscular reflex.*
■ Observe chest movements for depth of respirations. If the patient inhales a small volume of air, record this as shallow; if he inhales a large volume, record this as deep.
■ Listen to breathing *to determine the rhythm and sound of respirations.* (See *Identifying respiratory patterns.*)

- To detect breath sounds—such as crackles and rhonchi—or the lack of sound in the lungs, use a cleaned and disinfected stethoscope.[5]
- Observe the patient for use of accessory muscles, such as the scalene, sternocleidomastoid, trapezius, and latissimus dorsi. Using these muscles reflects a weakness of the diaphragm and the external intercostal muscles, the major muscles of respiration.
- Clean and disinfect your stethoscope using an alcohol pad.[5]
- Perform hand hygiene.[1,2,3]
- Document your findings.[6]

Special considerations

- Respiratory rates of less than 8 or more than 40 breaths/minute usually are considered abnormal; report the sudden onset of such rates promptly. Observe the patient for signs of dyspnea, such as an anxious facial expression, flaring nostrils, a heaving chest wall, and cyanosis. To detect cyanosis, look for characteristic bluish discoloration in the nail beds or the lips, under the tongue, in the buccal mucosa, or in the conjunctiva.
- In assessing the patient's respiratory status, consider his personal and family history. Ask if he smokes; if he does, ask how many years he's smoked and how many packs a day.

Documentation

Record the rate, depth, rhythm, and sound of the patient's respirations.

REFERENCES

1 The Joint Commission. (2012). Standard NPSG.07.01.01. *Comprehensive accreditation manual for hospitals: The official handbook.* Oakbrook Terrace, IL: The Joint Commission. (Level I)
2 Centers for Disease Control and Prevention. (October 2002). Guideline for hand hygiene in health-care settings. *Morbidity and Mortality Weekly Report, 51*(RR-16), 1–45. (Level I)
3 World Health Organization. (2009). *WHO guidelines on hand hygiene in health care: First global patient safety challenge. Clean care is safer care.* Geneva, Switzerland: World Health Organization. (Level I)
4 The Joint Commission. (2012). Standard NPSG.01.01.01. *Comprehensive accreditation manual for hospitals: The official handbook.* Oakbrook Terrace, IL: The Joint Commission. (Level I)
5 Rutala, W.A., et al. (2008). "Guideline for Disinfection and Sterilization in Healthcare Facilities, 2008" [Online]. Accessed November 2011 via the Web at http://www.cdc.gov/ncidod/dhqp/pdf/guidelines/Disinfection_Nov_2008.pdf (Level I)
6 The Joint Commission. (2012). Standard RC.01.03.01. *Comprehensive accreditation manual for hospitals: The official handbook.* Oakbrook Terrace, IL: The Joint Commission. (Level I)

RESTRAINT APPLICATION

The Centers for Medicare and Medicaid Services (CMS) and The Joint Commission define restraints as devices that immobilize or reduce the ability of a patient to move the arms, legs, body, or head freely, except in situations involving orthopedic devices, surgical bandages, and similar devices required for the patient's care.

A vest restraint can be used to prevent self–injury from falls or to immobilize a patient to assist medical treatment. It's applied to a patient's torso over his hospital gown or clothing. The straps are then secured to the patient's bed frame or chair.

A limb restraint is a device consisting of a cuff, typically made of padded fabric or foam, that's applied to a patient's wrists or ankles, and straps that are secured to the patient's bed frame or chair. Limb restraints may be used to prevent self-injury or to prevent the removal of therapeutic equipment, such as IV lines, indwelling catheters, and nasogastric tubes.

A mitt restraint is a pocket enclosure that's applied over a patient's hand to prevent self-injury or removal of therapeutic equipment, such as IV lines, indwelling catheters, and nasogastric tubes. Mitt restraints may be padded or rigid and may include finger separators or leave the fingers exposed. Optional straps that can be secured to the patient's bed frame or chair may be included with the device or may need to be ordered separately if indicated. Most mitt restraints can be applied to either hand.

A belt restraint consists of a strip of material—usually cotton fabric or mesh—that's applied over a patient's gown or clothing, around the waist or lap, and then secured to the bed frame or chair. The straps are then secured to the patient's bed frame or chair. Belt restraints can be used to prevent self-injury from falls or to immobilize a patient to assist with medical treatment.

A leather or leather-like restraint is made of leather or a synthetic substitute for leather, such as polyurethane or vinyl, and is applied to a patient's wrists or ankles and then secured to the bed frame or chair. It can be used to prevent self-injury or injury to others or to immobilize a patient for medical treatment. Although some facilities prefer to use traditional leather restraints because of the perceived strength of the material, synthetic materials offer the advantage of being easier to clean and sanitize.

The CMS and The Joint Commission recognize the rights of patients to be free from restraint or seclusion, of any form, imposed as a means of coercion, discipline, convenience, or retaliation by staff members. Therefore, restraint or seclusion may only be used to ensure the immediate physical safety of the patient, a staff member, or others and should only be used when all other methods have failed to keep the patient from harming himself or others. This standard has been established with the intent of reducing the overall use of restraints. If restraints must be used, the health care provider must choose a restraint that's the least restrictive to the patient and discontinue restraint use at the earliest possible time.[1,2]

Only staff members trained in the use of restraints and the use of less restrictive techniques aimed at avoiding restraint are permitted to evaluate the need for restraints, apply restraints, and monitor patients who are restrained. Always check your facility's policy on restraints before applying them to a patient.[1,3]

Equipment

Restraint device (vest, limb, mitt, belt, or leather) ▪ key ▪ cuff liners (if recommended by the manufacturer).

Preparation of equipment

Because there are various types of body restraints, always refer to the manufacturer's preparation and application instructions. For example, some vest restraints wrap around the patient with the straps crossing in the front, whereas other types close with a zipper at the patient's back. Check to see that you have obtained the correct size for the patient's build and weight. Some devices require that the straps be fed through the cuff before application. Because there are various types of belt restraints, make sure you've chosen a restraint that's appropriate for your patient. For example, a restraint may hold a patient in a stationary position or allow the patient to roll from side to side, may wrap around the pelvis in addition to the waist for additional security when sitting up, or be padded or unpadded. Some belt restraints wrap around the patient with the straps crossing in the back; others have straps that cross in the front.

If using leather restraints, make sure the straps are unlocked and the key fits the lock.

Check the device for damage before use; obtain a new device if necessary.

Implementation

■ Obtain a doctor's order for the restraint. In an emergency situation, obtain an order as soon as possible after applying the restraints according to your facility's policy.[1,4]
■ Perform hand hygiene.[5,6,7]

NURSING ALERT *If the patient is being restrained because of violent or self-destructive behavior that jeopardizes the physical safety of the patient, staff members, or others, the doctor or other licensed independent practitioner responsible for the patient's care must conduct an in-person evaluation within 1 hour of initiating the restraint. No as-needed or standing orders for restraints can be used.*[1]

■ Tell the patient that you're applying a restraint. Assure him that the restraint is being used to protect him from injury rather than to punish him. Emphasize that the restraint will be removed as soon as it is safe to do so, and tell him the criteria you'll use for discontinuing restraints.
■ If necessary, obtain the assistance of additional staff members to apply the restraints.

Applying a vest restraint
■ If the patient's condition permits, assist the patient to a sitting position. If the patient is unable to sit, apply the vest restraint by rolling the patient side to side.
■ Smooth out the patient's gown or clothing *to remove as many wrinkles as possible.*
■ Slip the vest over the patient's gown or clothing.
■ Assist the patient in putting his arms through the armholes.
■ For a criss-cross vest restraint, check that the V-shape neck is in front. Criss-cross the straps in the front of the vest. Never criss-cross the flaps in the back *because doing so may cause the patient to choke if he tries to squirm out of the vest.* Feed the straps through the holes in the front of the vest as indicated by manufacturer's instructions.
■ For a zipper vest restraint, make sure that the zipper is in the back. Zip up the back of the restraint.
■ Adjust the vest for a comfortable fit. Make sure the restraint doesn't compromise breathing or circulation. You should be able to slip an open, flat hand between the vest and the patient.

Applying a limb restraint
■ Position the patient's wrist or ankle in the soft padded cuff portion of the restraint by slipping the cuff over the patient's hand or foot. If using a wrap type device, wrap the wrist or ankle so that the fasteners are on the outside of the device.
■ If indicated, fasten the buckle or Velcro fastener.
■ Adjust the straps for a snug fit that doesn't compromise the patient's circulation. You should be able to slip one or two fingers between the restraint and the patient's skin. *Applying the restraint too tightly may impair circulation distal to the restraint.*

Applying a mitt restraint
■ Assess for baseline hand and finger circulation *to determine the appropriateness of the device and to determine whether circulatory changes may occur after application.*
■ Insert the patient's hand into the mitt with his palm facing down according to the manufacturer's instructions. If finger separators are available in the device, separate each finger into its own slot.
■ Wrap the strap over the mitt and around the patient's wrist *to secure the mitt to the patient.*
■ Secure the strap with the device's fastener, which may be Velcro or some other type of fastener.
■ Adjust the straps for a snug fit that doesn't compromise the patient's circulation. You should be able to slip one or two fingers between the restraint and the patient's skin. *Applying the restraint too tightly may impair circulation distal to the restraint.*

Applying a belt restraint
Restraining a patient in a chair
■ Position the patient as far back in the seat as possible.
■ Wrap the device around the patient's hips and over his smoothed-out gown or clothing so that the straps end up at the back of the chair.
■ If the belt is padded, place the padded side toward the patient.
■ If the device includes a pelvic holder, place the narrow side to the back of the chair and bring the wide part of the holder up between the patient's legs and connect the straps.
■ Criss-cross the straps at the back of the chair *for added security.*
■ Adjust the belt for a snug but comfortable fit that doesn't compromise the patient's breathing or circulation. You should be able to slip an open, flat hand between the device and the patient. *If the belt is too loose, it may pose a choking hazard to the patient if he tries to squirm out of it.*

Restraining a patient in a bed
■ Position the belt under the patient at waist level.
■ Thread the straps through the slots at either the front or back of the patient according to the manufacturer's directions and the desired movement limitation.
■ Adjust the belt for a snug but comfortable fit that doesn't compromise the patient's breathing or circulation. You should be able to slip an open, flat hand between the device and the patient. *If the belt is too loose, it may pose a choking hazard to patient if he tries to squirm out of it.*

Tying a quick-release knot

A quick-release knot allows you to quickly release the knot, using one hand, if the patient is in distress or has an emergency. Follow the steps below to tie a quick-release knot.

1. Wrap the attachment strap once around the bed frame leaving at least an 8″ (20 cm) tail. Fold the loose end in half to create a loop (as shown).

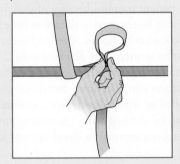

2. Cross the loop over the other end of the tie (as shown)

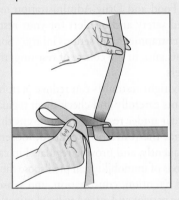

3. Insert the folded strap where the straps cross over each other. This step will feel like when you are tying your shoes.

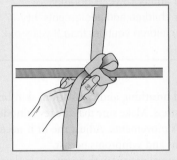

4. Pull on the loop to tighten.

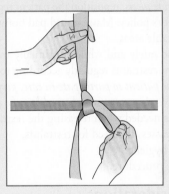

Applying a leather restraint

NURSING ALERT *Never attempt to apply leather restraints to a patient alone. Give each staff member a specific task to immobilize the patient before applying the restraints.*

■ Position the patient supine on the bed, with each arm and leg securely held down *to minimize combative behavior and to prevent injury to the patient and others.* Immobilize the patient's arms and legs above and below the joints—knee, ankle, shoulder, and wrist—*to minimize his movement without exerting excessive force.*

■ If indicated by the manufacturer, apply cuff liners to the restraint cuffs *to reduce friction between the skin and the restraint, preventing skin irritation and breakdown.*

■ Wrap the restraint around the extremity and adjust it to fit. Apply the restraints securely but not too tightly. You should be able to slip one finger between the restraint and the patient's skin. *A tight restraint can compromise circulation; a loose one can slip off or move up the patient's arm or leg, causing skin irritation and breakdown.*

■ Secure the locking mechanism and make sure that it clicks. Tug it gently *to be sure it's secure.* Attach the connecting strap and secure the strap to the bed frame, out of the patient's reach. Once the restraint is secure, a coworker can release the arm or leg. Check the restraint for proper fit. Flex the patient's arm or leg slightly before locking the strap *to allow room for movement and to prevent frozen joints and dislocations.*

■ Place the key in an accessible location at the nurse's station.

Completing the procedure

■ Tie or secure the straps of the restraints to the frame of the bed, chair, or wheelchair and out of the patient's reach. Some restraints are equipped with quick-release buckles that must be attached to the bed frame or chair according to manufacturer's instructions. Never secure the restraint to a bed rail or other movable part of the equipment. Use a bow or a knot that can be released quickly and easily in an emergency. (See *Tying a quick-release knot.*) Never tie a regular knot to secure the straps. Leave 1″ to 2″ (2.5 to 5 cm) of slack in the straps *to allow room for movement.*

■ Continuously assess the patient according to the parameters and frequency dictated by your facility's policy, the patient's condition, and the type of device used. Be alert for complications,

---

Restraint orders

If the patient is being restrained because of violent or self-destructive behavior, follow The Joint Commission and Centers for Medicare and Medicaid Services guidelines for order limits (or your facility's policy if it's more restrictive). Restraints should be limited to:

- 4 hours for adults 18 years or older
- 2 hours for children and adolescents 9 to 17 years old
- 1 hour for children younger than 9 years old.[1]

---

such as impaired breathing and circulation, skin breakdown, or psychological distress. Make sure that the restraint doesn't tighten with the patient's movements. Adjust the fit if necessary. Notify the doctor if signs and symptoms persist.[8,9]

- Assist the restrained patient with nutrition, hydration, hygiene, elimination, pain control, and comfort measures.[9]
- *To prevent pressure ulcers,* reposition the patient regularly according to your facility's policy. Massage and pad bony prominences and other vulnerable areas.
- If able to do so safely and while continually monitoring the patient, release the restraints regularly according to your facility's policy *to allow the patient to participate in care, perform range-of-motion (ROM) exercises, turn, stretch, and breathe deeply.* Have a coworker assist as needed when releasing the restraint.[9]
- Continue to reassess the need for restraints.
- Perform hand hygiene.[5,6,7]
- Document the procedure.[10]

Special considerations

- Know the latest Joint Commission and CMS standards for applying restraints as well as your facility's policy for restraint use. Make sure that less restrictive measures have been attempted before implementation. Aim to discontinue restraints at the earliest safe opportunity.[2,11]
- A vest restraint should be used with caution in patients with heart failure or respiratory disorders.
- When the patient is at high risk for aspiration, restrain him on his side. Never secure all four restraints to one side of the bed *because the patient may fall out of bed.*
- Don't apply a limb or mitt restraint above an IV site *because the constriction may occlude the infusion or cause infiltration into surrounding tissue.*
- Never secure restraints to the side rails *because someone might inadvertently lower the rail before noticing the attached restraint. This movement may jerk the patient's limb or body, causing him discomfort and trauma.* Never secure restraints to the fixed frame of the bed if the patient's position is to be changed.
- Don't restrain a patient in the prone position. *This position limits his field of vision, intensifies feelings of helplessness and vulnera-*

bility, and impairs respiration, especially if the patient has been sedated.*

- If the patient continues to require restraint, obtain a new order from the doctor in accordance with your facility's policy and at least within 24 hours of the previous order. The doctor will need to evaluate the patient before writing a new restraint order.
- If the patient consented to have his family informed of his care, notify them of the use of restraints, how the patient will be monitored while restrained, and the criteria for discontinuing restraints.
- Orders for patient restraint because of violent or self-destructive behavior may be renewed to the above time limits for a maximum of 24 consecutive hours. After 24 hours, a new order for restraint must be written. (See *Restraint orders.*)[4]
- When restraints are discontinued, sanitize them according to the manufacturer's instructions. Synthetic restraints may be machine washed or wiped down with a sanitizer. Soiled leather restraints may be cleaned with a sanitizer; however if leather restraints have been exposed to blood or body fluids, they must be discarded.

Complications

Follow U.S. Food and Drug Administration recommendations regarding bed safety and be alert for your restrained patient's potential for entrapment and serious injury.[12] Some patients may resist restraints and, in the course of resisting, may injure themselves or others.

Excessively tight restraints can reduce peripheral circulation. Apply restraints carefully and check them regularly. Skin breakdown can occur under restraints. To prevent this complication, make sure that the restraint is padded, loosen or remove the restraints frequently, and provide regular skin care.

Long periods of immobility can predispose the patient to pneumonia, urine retention, constipation, and sensory deprivation. Reposition the patient and attend to his elimination requirements as needed.

Documentation

Document each episode of the use of restraint, including the date and time the restraint was initiated. Document the patient's signs and symptoms, the less restrictive interventions you tried first, your assessment of the need for restraint, and the doctor or other licensed independent practitioner who evaluated the patient and ordered the restraints, according to your facility's policy. Document the patient's response to the restraints. Include the conditions or behaviors necessary for discontinuing the restraint and whether these conditions were communicated to the patient.[9,13]

Document each in-person evaluation by the doctor or other licensed independent practitioner.[13]

According to your facility's policy, record regular assessments of the patient, including signs of injury, nutrition, hydration, circulation, ROM, vital signs, hygiene, elimination, comfort, physical and psychological status, and readiness for removing restraints. Record your interventions to help the patient meet the conditions for removing the restraint; you may use a flow sheet to record frequent assessments. Document any injuries or complications and the time and name of the practitioner notified of your interventions.[9,13]

REFERENCES

1 Centers for Medicare & Medicaid Services, Department of Health and Human Services. (2006). "Conditions of Participation: Patients' Rights," 42 CFR part 482.13 [Online]. Accessed November 2011 via the Web at https://www.cms.gov/CFCsAndCoPs/downloads/finalpatientrightsrule.pdf

2 The Joint Commission. (2012). Standard PC.03.05.01. *Comprehensive accreditation manual for hospitals: The official handbook*. Oakbrook Terrace, IL: The Joint Commission. (Level I)

3 The Joint Commission. (2012). Standard PC.03.05.17. *Comprehensive accreditation manual for hospitals: The official handbook*. Oakbrook Terrace, IL: The Joint Commission. (Level I)

4 The Joint Commission. (2012). Standard PC.03.05.05. *Comprehensive accreditation manual for hospitals: The official handbook*. Oakbrook Terrace, IL: The Joint Commission. (Level I)

5 Centers for Disease Control and Prevention. (October 2002). Guideline for hand hygiene in health-care settings. *Morbidity and Mortality Weekly Report, 51*(RR-16), 1–45. (Level I)

6 World Health Organization. (2009). *WHO guidelines on hand hygiene in health care: First global patient safety challenge. Clean care is safer care*. Geneva, Switzerland: World Health Organization. (Level I)

7 The Joint Commission. (2012). Standard NPSG.07.01.01. *Comprehensive accreditation manual for hospitals: The official handbook*. Oakbrook Terrace, IL: The Joint Commission. (Level I)

8 The Joint Commission. (2012). Standard PC.03.05.07. *Comprehensive accreditation manual for hospitals: The official handbook*. Oakbrook Terrace, IL: The Joint Commission. (Level I)

9 The Joint Commission. (2012). Standard PC.03.05.09. *Comprehensive accreditation manual for hospitals: The official handbook*. Oakbrook Terrace, IL: The Joint Commission. (Level I)

10 The Joint Commission. (2012). Standard RC.01.03.01. *Comprehensive accreditation manual for hospitals: The official handbook*. Oakbrook Terrace, IL: The Joint Commission. (Level I)

11 The Joint Commission. (2012). Standard PC.03.05.11. *Comprehensive accreditation manual for hospitals: The official handbook*. Oakbrook Terrace, IL: The Joint Commission. (Level I)

12 U.S. Food and Drug Administration. (2011). "Hospital Beds" [Online]. Accessed November 2011 via the Web at http://www.fda.gov/MedicalDevices/ProductsandMedicalProcedures/GeneralHospitalDevicesandSupplies/HospitalBeds/default.htm

13 The Joint Commission. (2012). Standard PC.03.05.15. *Comprehensive accreditation manual for hospitals: The official handbook*. Oakbrook Terrace, IL: The Joint Commission. (Level I)

RING REMOVAL

A ring can become excessively tight on a patient's finger after an injury such as a sprain or from some other cause of swelling such as the swelling that can occur in a localized allergic reaction. Very tight-fitting rings can obstruct lymphatic drainage, causing swelling and further constriction. Removal may be necessary to relieve chronic or acute edema and to prevent vascular compromise in a finger or toe constricted by a ring or metal or plastic band.

Equipment

Ice ■ soap and water ■ towel ■ lubricant (petroleum jelly, lotion) ■ rubber tourniquet or Penrose drain ■ Optional: local anesthetic without epinephrine, syringe, needles, alcohol pads.

Coiled-string method

String, umbilical tape, ribbon gauze, or thick suture material.

Ring-cutter method

Lubricant (some cutters require a water-soluble lubricant) ■ ring cutter (manual, battery, or electric-powered) ■ pliers, hemostat, or ring spreader ■ protective eyewear ■ 20-mL syringe filled with water.

Implementation

■ Perform hand hygiene and put on gloves.[1,2,3]

■ Confirm the patient's identity using at least two patient identifiers according to your facility's policy.[4]

■ Explain the procedure to the patient. Answer all questions *to decrease anxiety and increase cooperation.*

■ Inspect the digit for wounds, lacerations, fractures, or dislocations. Assess the digit's capillary refill, sensation, and movement.

NURSING ALERT *If vascular compromise is present, the ring should be removed with a ring cutter as quickly as possible.*

■ Assess the patient's pain level.

■ Obtain an X-ray of the digit, if ordered, and report abnormal findings to the doctor.

■ *To limit further swelling,* apply ice and elevate the affected extremity above heart level. You can also wrap a rubber tourniquet or Penrose drain circumferentially in a distal-to-proximal direction *to reduce swelling.* Leave the wrap in place for 5 minutes, and then remove it.

■ Lubricate the skin beneath the ring with soap and water or a lubricant *to allow the ring to be slipped off of the finger or toe.* Hold the ring with a towel, and pull with a rocking motion in an attempt to remove the ring.

NURSING ALERT *Even if the patient tells you he has tried to remove the object from the finger at home, it's generally worthwhile to attempt removal with soap and water or a lubricant before trying other techniques. The pain from constriction often prevents the patient from applying adequate circular traction to remove the ring.*

■ If the ring can't be removed, use one of the methods below.

Coiled-string method

NURSING ALERT *Don't use the coiled-string method if the patient has any lacerations, fractures, or dislocations involving the affected digit; use a ring cutter instead.*

■ While the affected digit is elevated, slip the end of a long strip of string under the ring. Use a hemostat, if necessary, to thread the string under the ring.

■ Anchor the string with your nondominant hand, or ask the patient to anchor it.

■ Wrap the string around the digit, beginning adjacent to the ring margin. Wrap the string in a snug, smooth, single layer in a clockwise fashion, slightly overlapping the previous layer, progressing from proximal to distal until it covers the area of greatest swelling. *Because the area of the proximal interphalangeal joint is the most difficult area to slip the ring over,* make sure that you wrap this area firmly (as shown below).

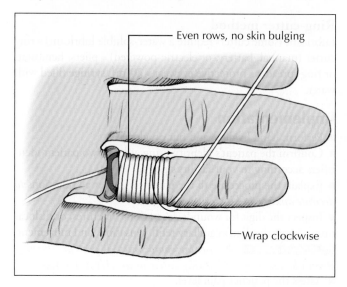

Even rows, no skin bulging

Wrap clockwise

■ When the wrapping is complete, pull the proximal end of the string against the ring and then start to unwrap the string in a clockwise direction, moving the ring toward the tip of the finger (as shown below). If needed, place a small amount of lubricant over the string *to facilitate sliding the ring.*

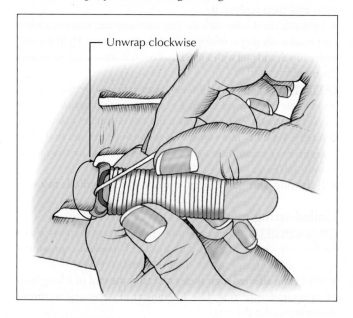

Unwrap clockwise

NURSING ALERT *Moving the ring over the proximal interphalangeal joint will be the most difficult and may cause the most pain to the patient. It's not uncommon to cause abrasions to the skin during this procedure.*

Ring-cutter method
Manual ring cutter
■ Obtain written consent for cutting and removing the ring.
■ Put on protective eyewear *to avoid possible injury caused by metal fragments.*
■ Slip the curved finger guard of the ring cutter under the ring. Use lubricant if necessary. Rotate the ring, if possible, so that the thinnest part of the band is located under the saw blade (as shown below).

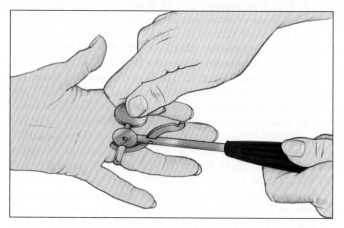

■ Clamp the cutting disk down firmly on the ring, and use the turnkey to manually turn the cutting disk until the ring is severed.
■ After the ring has been cut through, bend the ring apart with pliers, a hemostat, or a ring spreader (as shown below) *to allow removal.*

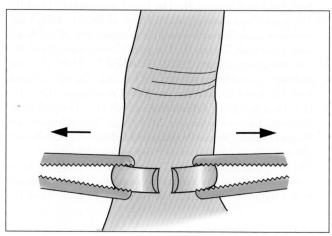

■ If the ring is a wide band, it may be necessary to make a second cut *to remove a wedge from the ring.*
■ Irrigate the skin with water *to remove any metal particles.*
■ Remove protective eyewear.

Battery or electric-powered ring-cutter method
■ Obtain written consent for cutting and removing the ring.
■ Put on protective eyewear *to avoid possible injury caused by metal fragments.*

■ Ensure that the correct cutting blade is in place. Some manufacturers supply different blades for different types of metals. Always follow the manufacturer's instructions.

■ Place the finger guard of the ring cutter under the ring. Use lubricant if necessary. Rotate the ring, if possible, so that the thinnest part of the band is located under the saw blade.

■ Turn on the power to the cutting blade so that it's rotating before it makes contact with the ring.

■ Apply gentle pressure to make contact between the rotating blade and the ring.

NURSING ALERT *The friction caused by cutting may produce an uncomfortable amount of heat in the ring and the patient's hand. Ask the patient if he's comfortable, and regularly check the temperature of the ring and cutter blade with your fingers. Stop briefly to allow the ring and cutter to cool down if necessary.*

■ After the ring has been cut through, bend the ring apart with pliers, a hemostat, or a ring spreader *to allow removal* or make a second cut on the opposite side of the ring and remove the wedge.

■ Irrigate the skin with water *to remove any metal particles.*

Completing the procedure

■ Remove protective eyewear.
■ Reassess the neurovascular status of the digit.
■ Elevate the digit and apply cold packs, as ordered.
■ Discard the supplies, remove your gloves, and perform hand hygiene.[1,2,3]
■ Document the procedure.[5]

Special considerations

■ Some rings are made of tungsten carbide, ceramic, or natural stone; these rings can be removed with locking pliers (vise-grip pliers). (See *Using locking pliers.*)

■ Return all pieces of the removed ring to the patient.

■ If required, assist the doctor with administering digital anesthesia using a local anesthetic without epinephrine.

NURSING ALERT *Never use products containing epinephrine on a finger or toe because epinephrine exerts a vasoconstrictive effect.*

■ Reassess the neurovascular status frequently after ring removal. Notify the doctor immediately of any abnormalities.

■ Assess the patient's pain level, and administer analgesics as ordered following safe medication administration practices.

■ Clean any open wounds, and cover them with a sterile dressing *to prevent infection.*

■ Administer tetanus immunization, as indicated and ordered, following safe medication administration practices.

■ When removing rings or other objects from children, use age-appropriate terms. Allow the parent to stay and hold the child during the procedure. Allow the child to examine the equipment, if appropriate.

Using locking pliers

Tungsten carbide, ceramic, and natural stone rings made of onyx or jade are removed by cracking them into pieces with standard locking pliers. Follow these steps:

■ Place the locking pliers over the band, and adjust the jaws to clamp lightly.

■ Release the clamp and then readjust the jaws, tightening the screw $1/4$ turn to clamp it again.

■ Repeat this process until a crack is heard. The ring will break into two or more pieces.

■ Take care when removing the pieces. *Because the cracked edges are sharp,* don't rotate the cracked ring on the finger.

Complications

If a ring remains in place on an injured finger, the constricting effects of the circumferential object can lead to obstruction of lymphatic drainage, which in turn leads to more swelling and further constriction. Venous and, eventually, arterial circulation can be compromised by this constriction. Skin on the affected digit can be cut by string removal technique or by a ring cutter.

Patient teaching

Inform the patient that pain should dissipate in 1 to 2 hours and that edema should resolve within 24 hours (or as indicated by initial trauma to the digit). Usually, all signs and symptoms should resolve within 48 hours. Tell the patient that no follow-up is needed unless complications arise. Instruct him to apply an ice pack to the digit for 20 minutes four times daily for 36 to 48 hours *to relieve edema and pain.* Caution the patient to avoid wearing constricting objects on fingers and toes and to remove rings from digits whenever edema is possible. Instruct the patient to contact the doctor promptly if he experiences signs and symptoms of infection (warmth, increased edema, and pain).

Documentation

Document your assessment findings, including the skin condition and neurovascular status of the digit before and after ring removal. Document the methods used to facilitate removal of the ring, the success achieved, and the disposition of the ring. Record the patient's pain status and interventions provided. Record any patient teaching and discharge instructions provided, questions asked by the patient and your responses, and the patient's understanding of digit care.

EQUIPMENT

Understanding the Roto Rest bed

Driven by a silent motor, this bed turns the immobilized patient slowly and continuously. The motion provides constant passive exercise and peristaltic stimulation without depriving the patient of sleep or risking further injury. The bed is radiolucent, permitting X-rays to be taken through it without moving the patient. It also has a built-in cooling fan, and allows access for surgery on patients with multiple trauma without disrupting spinal alignment or traction.

The bed's hatches give access to various parts of the patient's body. Arm hatches permit full range of motion and have holes for chest tubes. Leg hatches allow full hip extension. The perineal hatch provides access for bowel and bladder care, the thoracic hatch for chest auscultation and lumbar puncture, and the cervical hatch for wound care, bathing, and shampooing.

Top view

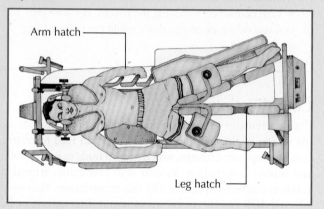

Arm hatch

Leg hatch

Back view

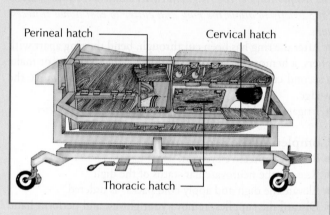

Perineal hatch

Cervical hatch

Thoracic hatch

REFERENCES

1   The Joint Commission. (2012). Standard NPSG.07.01.01. *Comprehensive accreditation manual for hospitals: The official handbook.* Oakbrook Terrace, IL: The Joint Commission. (Level I)
2   Centers for Disease Control and Prevention. (October 2002). Guideline for hand hygiene in health-care settings. *Morbidity and Mortality Weekly Report, 51*(RR-16), 1–45. (Level I)
3   World Health Organization. (2009). *WHO guidelines on hand hygiene in health care: First global patient safety challenge. Clean care is safer care.* Geneva, Switzerland: World Health Organization. (Level I)
4   The Joint Commission. (2012). Standard NPSG.01.01.01. *Comprehensive accreditation manual for hospitals: The official handbook.* Oakbrook Terrace, IL: The Joint Commission. (Level I)
5   The Joint Commission. (2012). Standard RC.01.03.01. *Comprehensive accreditation manual for hospitals: The official handbook.* Oakbrook Terrace, IL: The Joint Commission. (Level I)

ADDITIONAL REFERENCES

Bothner, J. (2011). Ring removal techniques [Online]. Accessed January 2012 via the Web at http://www.uptodate.com/contents/ring-removal-techniques
Proehl, J.A. (2009). *Emergency nursing procedures* (4th ed.). St. Louis, MO: Mosby Elsevier.

ROTATION BEDS

Rotation beds—such as the Roto Rest—promote postural drainage and peristalsis and help prevent complications of immobility and ventilator—associated pneumonia.[1,2,3] Because these beds hold the patient motionless, they're especially helpful for patients with spinal cord injury, multiple trauma, stroke, multiple sclerosis, coma, severe burns, hypostatic pneumonia, atelectasis, or other unilateral lung involvement causing poor ventilation and perfusion.

Rotation beds turn in an arc up to 90 degrees and can be set to pause on either side for up to 30 minutes. They can accommodate cervical traction devices and tongs. Arm and leg hatches on the bed fold down to allow for range-of-motion (ROM) exercises. Other bed features include a fan, access for X-rays, and supports and clips for chest tubes, catheters, and drains. Racks beneath the bed hold X-ray plates in place for chest and spinal films. (See *Understanding the Roto Rest bed.*)

Rotation beds are contraindicated for pregnant patients and patients who have severe claustrophobia, an open chest, an unstable pelvis, or an unstable cervical fracture without neurologic deficit and the complications of immobility. Patient transfer and positioning on the bed should be performed by at least two people to ensure the patient's safety.

The instructions given below apply to the Roto Rest bed.

Equipment

Rotation bed with appropriate accessories ▪ pillowcases or linen-saver pads ▪ flat sheet or padding ▪ gloves.

Preparation of equipment

When using the Roto Rest bed, carefully inspect the bed and run it through a complete cycle in both automatic and manual modes *to ensure that it's working properly.* Check the tightness of the set screws at the head of the bed if applicable for that model.

To prepare the bed for the patient, remove the counterbalance weights from the keel and place them in the base frame's storage area. Release the connecting arm by pulling down on the cam handle and depressing the lower side of the footboard. Next, lock the table in the horizontal position, and place all side supports in the extreme lateral position by loosening the cam handles on the underside of the table. Slide the supports off the bed. Note that all supports and packs are labeled "right" or "left" on the bottom *to facilitate reassembly.*

Remove the knee packs by depressing the snap button and rotating and pulling the packs from the tube. Then remove the abductor packs by depressing and sliding them toward the head of the bed. Next, loosen the foot and knee assemblies by lifting the cam handle at its base, and slide them to the foot of the bed. Finally, loosen the shoulder clamp assembly and knobs; swing the shoulder clamps to the vertical position and retighten them.

If applicable for the bed model, remove the cervical, thoracic, and perineal packs. Cover them with pillowcases or linen-saver pads, smooth all wrinkles, and replace the packs. Cover the upper half of the bed, which is a solid unit, with padding or a sheet. Install new disposable foam cushions for the patient's head, shoulders, and feet.

Implementation

▪ Perform hand hygiene and put on clean gloves, if necessary.[4,5,6]
▪ Confirm the patient's identity using at least two patient identifiers according to your facility's policy.[7]
▪ If possible, show the patient the bed before use. Explain and demonstrate its operation and reassure the patient that the bed will hold him securely. Answer all questions *to decrease anxiety and increase cooperation.*
▪ Before positioning the patient on the bed, make sure it's turned off. Then, place and lock the bed in horizontal position, out of gear. Latch all hatches and lock the wheels.
▪ Obtain assistance and transfer the patient. Move him gently to the center of the bed *to prevent contact with the pillar posts and to ensure proper balance during bed operation.* Smooth the pillowcase or linen-saver pad beneath his hips. Then place any tubes through the appropriate notches in the hatches and ensure that any traction weights hang freely.
▪ Insert the thoracic side supports in their posts. Adjust the patient's longitudinal position to allow a 1″ (2.5 cm) space between the axillae and the supports *to avoid pressure on the axillary blood vessels and the brachial plexus.* Push the supports against his chest

and lock the cam arms securely *to provide support and ensure patient safety.*
▪ Place the disposable supports under the patient's legs *to remove pressure from his heels and prevent pressure ulcers.*
▪ Install and adjust the foot supports so that the patient's feet lie in the normal anatomic position, *helping to prevent footdrop.* The foot supports should be in position for only 2 hours every shift *to prevent excessive pressure on the soles and toes.*
▪ Place the abductor packs in the appropriate supports, allowing a 6″ (15 cm) space between the packs and the patient's groin. Tighten the knobs on the bed's underside at the base of the support tubes.
▪ Install the leg side supports snugly against the patient's hips, and tighten the cam arms. Position the knee assemblies slightly above his knees and tighten the cam arms. Then place your hand on the patient's knee and move the knee pack until it rests lightly on the top of your hand. Repeat for the other knee.
▪ Loosen the retaining rings on the crossbar, and slide the head and shoulder assembly laterally. *The retaining rings maintain correct lateral position of the shoulder clamp assembly and head support pack.*
▪ Carefully lower the head and shoulder assembly into place and slide it to touch the patient's head.
▪ Place your hand on the patient's shoulder, and move the shoulder pack until it touches your hand. Tighten it in place. Repeat for the other shoulder. *The 1″ clearance between the shoulders and the packs prevents excess pressure, which can lead to pressure ulcers.*
▪ Place the head pack close to, but not touching, the patient's ears (or tongs).
▪ Tighten the head and shoulder assembly securely *so it won't lift off the bed.* Position the restraining rings next to the shoulder assembly bracket and tighten them.
▪ Place the patient's arms on the disposable supports. Install the side arm supports and secure the safety straps, placing one across the shoulder assembly and the other over the thoracic supports. If necessary, cover the patient with a flat sheet.

Balancing the bed

▪ Place one hand on the footboard *to prevent the bed from turning rapidly if it's unbalanced.* Then remove the locking pin. If the bed rotates to one side, reposition the patient in its center; if it tilts to the right, gently turn it slightly to the left and slide the packs on the right side toward the patient; if it tilts to the left, reverse the process. If a large imbalance exists, you may have to adjust the packs on both sides.
▪ After the patient is centered, gently turn the bed into position.
▪ Measure the space between the patient's chest, hip, and thighs and the inside of the packs. If the space appears too tight, slide both packs outward. *Excessively loose packs cause the patient to slide from side to side during turning, possibly resulting in unnecessary movement at fracture sites, skin irritation from shearing force, and bed imbalance. Overly tight packs can place pressure on the patient during turning.*
▪ After adjusting the packs, check the bed; balance it and make any necessary adjustments.

Initiating automatic bed rotation

■ Ensure that all packs are securely in place. Then hold the footboard firmly and remove the locking pin *to start the bed's motor.* The bed will continue to rotate until the pin is reinserted.

■ Raise the connecting arm cam handle until the connecting assembly snaps into place, locking the bed into automatic rotation.

■ Remain with the patient for at least three complete turns from side to side *to evaluate his comfort and safety.* Observe his response and offer him emotional support.

■ Perform hand hygiene.[4,5,6]

■ Document the procedure.[8]

Special considerations

■ If the patient goes into cardiac arrest while on the bed, perform cardiopulmonary resuscitation after taking the bed out of gear, locking it in horizontal position, removing the side arm support and the thoracic pack, lifting the shoulder assembly, and dropping the arm pack. Doing all these steps takes only 5 to 10 seconds. You won't need a cardiac board *because of the bed's firm surface.*

■ If the electricity fails, lock the bed in horizontal or lateral position and rotate it manually every 30 minutes *to prevent pressure ulcers.* If cervical traction causes the patient to slide upward, place the bed in reverse Trendelenburg's position; if extremity traction causes the patient to migrate toward the foot of the bed, use Trendelenburg's position.

■ Lock the bed in the extreme lateral position for access to the back of the head, thorax, and buttocks through the appropriate hatches.

■ Clean the mattress and nondisposable packs during patient care, and rinse them thoroughly *to remove all soap residue.*

■ When replacing the packs and hatches, take care not to pinch the patient's skin between the packs, *which can cause pain and tissue necrosis.*

■ Expect increased drainage from any pressure ulcers for the first few days the patient is on the bed *because the motion helps debride necrotic tissue and improves local circulation.*

■ Perform or schedule daily ROM exercises, as ordered, *because the bed allows full access to all extremities without disturbing spinal alignment.* Drop the arm hatch for shoulder rotation, remove the thoracic packs for shoulder abduction, and drop the leg hatch and remove leg and knee packs for hip rotation and full leg motion.

■ For female patients, tape an indwelling urinary catheter to the thigh before bringing it through the perineal hatch. For the male patient with spinal cord lesions, tape the catheter to the abdomen and then to the thigh *to facilitate gravity drainage.* Hang the drainage bag on the clips provided, and make sure it doesn't become caught between the bed frames during rotation.

■ If the patient has a tracheal or endotracheal tube and is on mechanical ventilation, attach the tube support bracket between the cervical pack and the arm packs. Tape the connecting T tubing to the support and run it beside the patient's head and off the center of the table *to help prevent reflux of condensation.*

■ For a patient with pulmonary congestion or pneumonia, suction secretions more often during the first 12 to 24 hours on the bed *because the motion will increase drainage.*

Documentation

Document the preparation of the bed and the transfer of the patient into the bed. Record changes in the patient's condition and his response to therapy in your progress notes. Note turning times and ongoing care on the flowchart.

REFERENCES

1 Staudinger, A., et al. (2009). Continuous lateral rotation therapy to prevent ventilator-associated pneumonia. *Critical Care Medicine, 38*(2), 486–490.

2 Swadener-Culpepper, L., et al. (2008). The impact of continuous lateral rotation therapy in overall clinical and financial outcomes of critically ill patients. *Critical Care Nursing Quarterly, 31*(3), 270–279.

3 Goldhill, D.R., et al. (2007). Rotational bed therapy to prevent and treat respiratory complications: A review and meta-analysis. *American Journal of Critical Care, 16*(1), 50–61; quiz 62.

4 The Joint Commission. (2012). Standard NPSG.07.01.01. *Comprehensive accreditation manual for hospitals: The official handbook.* Oakbrook Terrace, IL: The Joint Commission. (Level I)

5 Centers for Disease Control and Prevention. (October 2002). Guideline for hand hygiene in health-care settings. *Morbidity and Mortality Weekly Report, 51*(RR-16), 1–45. (Level I)

6 World Health Organization. (2009). *WHO guidelines on hand hygiene in health care: First global patient safety challenge. Clean care is safer care.* Geneva, Switzerland: World Health Organization. (Level I)

7 The Joint Commission. (2012). Standard NPSG.01.01.01. *Comprehensive accreditation manual for hospitals: The official handbook.* Oakbrook Terrace, IL: The Joint Commission. (Level I)

8 The Joint Commission. (2012). Standard RC.01.03.01. *Comprehensive accreditation manual for hospitals: The official handbook.* Oakbrook Terrace, IL: The Joint Commission. (Level I)

ADDITIONAL REFERENCES

Chandy, D., et al. (2007). Impact of kinetic beds on the incidence of atelectasis in mechanically ventilated patients. *American Journal of Therapeutics, 14*(3), 25–61.

Fleegler, B, et al. (2009). Continuous lateral rotation therapy for acute hypoxemic respiratory failure: The effect of timing. *Dimensions of Critical Care Nursing, 28*(6), 283–287.

Johnson, K.L., et al. (2009). Physiological rationale and current evidence for therapeutic positioning of critically ill Patients. *AACN Advances in Critical Care, 20*(3), 241–242.

Swadener-Culpepper, L., et al. (2010). Continuous lateral rotation therapy. *Critical Care Nurse, 30*(2), S5–S7.

S

Seizure management

Seizures are paroxysmal events associated with abnormal electrical discharges of neurons in the brain. Partial seizures are usually unilateral, involving a localized or focal area of the brain. Generalized seizures involve the entire brain. (See *Differentiating among seizure types,* page 642.) When a patient has a generalized seizure, nursing care aims to protect him from injury and prevent serious complications. Appropriate care also includes observation of seizure characteristics to help determine the area of the brain involved.

Patients considered at risk for seizures are those with a history of seizures and those with conditions that predispose them to seizures. These conditions include metabolic abnormalities, such as hypocalcemia and pyridoxine deficiency; brain tumors or other space-occupying lesions; infections, such as meningitis, encephalitis, and brain abscess; traumatic injury, especially if the dura mater was penetrated; ingestion of toxins, such as mercury, lead, or carbon monoxide; genetic abnormalities, such as tuberous sclerosis and phenylketonuria; perinatal injuries; and stroke. Patients at risk for seizures need precautionary measures to help prevent injury if a seizure occurs. (See *Precautions for generalized seizures,* page 643.)

Equipment

Oral airway ▪ suction equipment ▪ side rail pads ▪ seizure activity record ▪ IV catheter insertion equipment ▪ normal saline solution ▪ oxygen ▪ endotracheal intubation equipment.

Implementation

▪ If you are with a patient when he experiences an aura, help him into bed, raise the side rails, and adjust the bed flat. If he's away from his room, lower him to the floor and place a pillow, blanket, or other soft material under his head *to keep it from hitting the floor.*
▪ Provide privacy, if possible.
▪ Stay with the patient during the seizure, and be ready to intervene if complications such as airway obstruction develop.[1] If necessary, have another staff member obtain the appropriate equipment and notify the doctor of the obstruction.

NURSING ALERT *Depending on your facility's policy, if the patient is in the beginning of the tonic phase of the seizure, you may insert an oral airway so his tongue doesn't block his airway. If an oral airway isn't available, don't try to hold the patient's mouth open or place your hands inside because you may be bitten. After the patient's jaw becomes rigid, don't force an airway into place because you may break his teeth or cause another injury. Turn the patient on his side to allow secretions to drain and the tongue to fall forward. Never force any objects into the patient's mouth unless his airway is compromised.*

▪ Move hard or sharp objects out of the patient's way and loosen his clothing.

Understanding status epilepticus

Status epilepticus is defined as recurrent seizures without complete recovery of consciousness between attacks. If the patient has virtually continuous seizure activity for more than 30 minutes, with or without impaired consciousness, it may also be classified as status epilepticus.[1] The most serious and life-threatening type is a *generalized tonic-clonic status epilepticus*.[1]

Status epilepticus, always an emergency, is accompanied by respiratory distress. It can result from abrupt withdrawal of anticonvulsant medications, hypoxic or metabolic encephalopathy, acute head trauma, or septicemia secondary to encephalitis or meningitis.

Emergency treatment of status epilepticus usually consists of diazepam, phenytoin, or phenobarbital; dextrose 50% IV (when seizures are secondary to hypoglycemia); and thiamine IV (in the presence of chronic alcoholism or withdrawal).

▪ Don't forcibly restrain the patient or restrict his movements during the seizure *because the force of the patient's movements against restraints could cause muscle strain or even joint dislocation.*
▪ Continually assess the patient during the seizure. Observe the earliest signs and symptom, such as head or eye deviation, as well as how the seizure progresses, what form it takes, and how long it lasts. *Your description may help determine the seizure's type and cause.*[1]
▪ If this is the patient's first seizure, notify the doctor immediately. If the patient has had seizures before, notify the doctor only if the seizure activity is prolonged or if the patient fails to regain consciousness. (See *Understanding status epilepticus.*)
▪ If ordered, establish an IV catheter and infuse normal saline solution at a keep-vein-open rate.
▪ If the seizure is prolonged and the patient becomes hypoxemic, administer oxygen as ordered. Some patients may require endotracheal intubation.
▪ For a patient known to be diabetic, administer 50 mL of dextrose 50% in water by IV push as ordered. For a patient known to be an alcoholic, a 100-mg bolus of thiamine may be ordered to stop the seizure.
▪ After the seizure, turn the patient on his side and apply suction if necessary *to facilitate drainage of secretions and maintain a patent airway.* Insert an oral airway if needed.
▪ Check for injuries.
▪ Reorient and reassure the patient as necessary.
▪ Place side rail pads on the bed in case the patient experiences another seizure.
▪ After the seizure, monitor vital signs and mental status every 15 to 20 minutes for 2 hours or according to your facility policy.

Differentiating among seizure types

The hallmark of epilepsy is recurring seizures, which can be classified as partial or generalized. Some patients may be affected by more than one type of seizure.

Partial seizures (focal, local seizures)

Arising from a localized area in the brain, partial seizures cause specific symptoms. Categories of partial seizures include simple partial seizures (consciousness is intact), complex partial seizures (some loss of consciousness occurs), and partial seizures in which seizure activity may be spread to the entire brain, thereby causing a generalized seizure.[1]

Simple partial seizures

A simple partial seizure doesn't alter consciousness but, depending on the focal point in the brain, can cause various types of signs and symptoms, including:
- motor (jerking of the thumb or the cheek)
- somatosensory (visual, vestibular, gustatory, olfactory, or auditory hallucinations or sensations)
- autonomic (such as tachycardia, sweating, and pupillary dilation)
- psychic (such as feelings of déjà-vu or a dreamy state).

Complex partial seizures

Consciousness becomes impaired with a complex partial seizure.[1] This type of seizure begins as a simple partial seizure in which consciousness isn't impaired and evolves to an impairment of consciousness. The same signs and symptoms that present during a simple partial seizure are still seen as the seizure develops into a complex partial seizure.

Partial seizures evolving to generalized tonic-clonic seizures

A partial seizure can be either a simple or complex partial seizure that progresses to a generalized seizure. An aura may precede the progression. Loss of consciousness occurs immediately or within 1 to 2 minutes of the start of the progression.

Generalized seizures (convulsive or nonconvulsive)

As the term suggests, generalized seizures cause a general electrical abnormality within the brain. They include several distinct types.

Absence (petit mal) seizures

An absence seizure occurs commonly in children, but it may also affect adults. It usually begins with a brief change in the level of consciousness, indicated by blinking or rolling of the eyes, or a blank stare, and slight mouth movements.[1] Typically, the seizure lasts 1 to 10 seconds. The impairment is so brief that the patient (or parent) is sometimes unaware of it. If not properly treated, these seizures can recur as often as 100 times per day and may result in learning difficulties.

Myoclonic seizures

A myoclonic seizure is marked by abrupt muscle contractions of the body extremities.[1] They may occur in a rhythmic manner and may be accompanied by brief loss of consciousness.

Generalized tonic-clonic (grand mal) seizures

Typically, a generalized tonic-clonic seizure begins with a loud cry, precipitated by air rushing from the lungs through the vocal cords. The patient falls to the ground, losing consciousness. The body stiffens (tonic phase) and then alternates between episodes of muscle spasm and relaxation (clonic phase). Tongue biting, incontinence, labored breathing, apnea, and subsequent cyanosis may also occur. The seizure stops in 2 to 5 minutes, when abnormal electrical conduction of the neurons is completed. The patient then regains consciousness but is somewhat confused and may have difficulty talking. If he can talk, he may complain of drowsiness, fatigue, headache, muscle soreness, and arm or leg weakness. He may fall into a deep sleep after the seizure.

Atonic seizures (drop attacks)

Characterized by a general loss of postural tone and a temporary loss of consciousness, an atonic seizure occurs in young children. It's sometimes called a "drop attack" because it causes the child to fall.[1]

- Ask the patient about his aura and activities preceding the seizure. The type of aura (auditory, visual, olfactory, gustatory, or somatic) helps pinpoint the site in the brain where the seizure originated.
- Perform hand hygiene.[2,3,4]
- Document the event.[5]

Special considerations

- Because a seizure commonly indicates an underlying disorder such as meningitis or a metabolic or electrolyte imbalance, a complete diagnostic workup will be ordered if the cause of the seizure isn't evident.

- When a patient with a known seizure history is hospitalized, maintain IV access or an intermittent infusion device so there's IV access available to administer seizure medication, if needed.

Complications

The patient who experiences a seizure may experience an injury, respiratory difficulty, and decreased mental capability. Common injuries include scrapes and bruises suffered when the patient hits objects during the seizure and traumatic injury to the tongue caused by biting. If you suspect a serious injury, such as a fracture or deep laceration, notify the doctor and arrange for appropriate evaluation and treatment.

Changes in respiratory function may include aspiration, airway obstruction, and hypoxemia. After the seizure, complete a respiratory assessment and notify the doctor if you suspect a problem. Expect most patients to experience a postictal period of decreased mental status lasting 30 minutes to 24 hours. Reassure the patient that this doesn't indicate incipient brain damage.

Documentation

Document that the patient requires seizure precautions, and record all precautions taken.

Record the date and the time the seizure began as well as its duration and any precipitating factors. Identify any sensation that may be considered an aura. If the seizure was preceded by an aura, have the patient describe what he experienced.

Record any involuntary behavior that occurred at the onset, such as lip smacking, chewing movements, or hand and eye movements. Describe where the behavior began and the parts of the body involved. Note any progression or pattern to the activity. Document whether the patient's eyes deviated to one side and if the pupils changed in size, shape, equality, or reaction to light. Note if the patient's teeth were clenched or open. Record any incontinence, vomiting, or salivation that occurred during the seizure.

Note the patient's response to the seizure. Was the patient aware of what happened? Did he fall into a deep sleep following the seizure? Was he upset or ashamed? Also note any medications given, any complications experienced during the seizure, and any interventions performed. Finally, note the patient's postseizure mental status.

REFERENCES

1 American Association of Neuroscience Nurses. (2009). "AANN Clinical Practice Guideline Series: Care of the Patient with Seizures" (2nd ed.) [Online]. Accessed December 2011 via the Web at http://www.aann.org/pdf/cpg/aannseizures.pdf (Level I)
2 The Joint Commission. (2012). Standard NPSG.07.01.01. *Comprehensive accreditation manual for hospitals: The official handbook.* Oakbrook Terrace, IL: The Joint Commission. (Level I)
3 Centers for Disease Control and Prevention. (October 2002). Guideline for hand hygiene in health-care settings. *Morbidity and Mortality Weekly Report, 51*(RR-16), 1–45. (Level I)
4 World Health Organization. (2009). *WHO guidelines on hand hygiene in health care: First global patient safety challenge. Clean care is safer care.* Geneva, Switzerland: World Health Organization. (Level I)
5 The Joint Commission. (2012). Standard RC.01.03.01. *Comprehensive accreditation manual for hospitals: The official handbook.* Oakbrook Terrace, IL: The Joint Commission. (Level I)

ADDITIONAL REFERENCES

Fagley, M.U. (2007). Taking charge of seizure activity. *Nursing, 37*(9), 42–48.
Glauser, T.A., et al. (2008). Core elements of epilepsy diagnosis and management: Expert consensus from the Leadership in Epilepsy, Advocacy, and Development (LEAD) Faculty. *Current Medical Research and Opinion, 24*(12), 3463–3477.
Harden, C.L. (2008). Issues for mature women with epilepsy. *International Review of Neurobiology, 83*, 385–395.
Lynn-McHale Wiegand, D. (Ed.). (2011). *AACN procedure manual for critical care* (6th ed.). Philadelphia, PA: Saunders.

Nettina, S.M. (2010). *Lippincott manual of nursing practice* (9th ed.). Philadelphia, PA: Lippincott Williams & Wilkins.
Seneviratne, U. (2009). Management of the first seizure: An evidence based approach. *Postgraduate Medical Journal, 85*(1010), 667–673.
Sperling, M.R., et al. (2008). Self-perception of seizure precipitants and their relation to anxiety level, depression, and health locus of control in epilepsy. *Seizure, 17*(4), 302–307.
Thapar, A., et al. (2009). Stress, anxiety, depression, and epilepsy: Investigating the relationship between psychological factors and seizures. *Epilepsy and Behavior, 14*(1), 134–140.

Precautions for generalized seizures

By taking appropriate precautions, you can help protect a patient from injury, aspiration, and airway obstruction should he have a seizure. Plan your precautions using information obtained from the patient's history. What kind of seizure has the patient had before? Is he aware of exacerbating factors? Sleep deprivation, missed doses of anticonvulsants, even upper respiratory tract infections can increase seizure frequency in some people who have had seizures. Was his previous seizure an acute episode or did it result from a chronic condition?

Gather the equipment

Based on answers provided in the patient's history, you can tailor your precautions to his needs. Start by gathering the appropriate equipment, including a hospital bed with full-length side rails, commercial side rail pads or six bath blankets (four for a crib), adhesive tape, an oral airway, and oral or nasal suction equipment.

Bedside preparations

Now carry out the precautions you think appropriate for the patient. Remember that a patient with preexisting seizures who's being admitted for a change in medication, treatment of an infection, or detoxification may have an increased risk for seizures.

■ Explain the reasons for the precautions to the patient.

■ To protect the patient's limbs, head, and feet from injury if he has a seizure while in bed, cover the side rails, headboard, and footboard with side rail pads or bath blankets. If you use blankets, keep them in place with adhesive tape. Be sure to keep the side rails raised while the patient is in bed to prevent falls. Keep the bed in a low position to minimize any injuries that may occur if the patient climbs over the rails.

■ Place an airway at the patient's bedside or tape it to the wall above the bed, according to your facility's protocol. Keep suction equipment nearby in case you need to establish a patent airway. Explain to the patient how the airway will be used.

■ If the patient has frequent or prolonged seizures, prepare an IV heparin lock to facilitate administration of emergency medications.

Teaching the female patient self-catheterization

Instruct the female patient to hold the catheter in her dominant hand as if it were a pencil or a dart, about ½″ (1 cm) from its tip. Keeping the vaginal folds separated, she should slowly insert the lubricated catheter about 2″ to 4″ (5 to 10 cm) into the urethra. Once the catheter is inserted, tell her to press down with her abdominal muscles *to empty the bladder,* allowing all urine to drain through the catheter and into the toilet or drainage container.

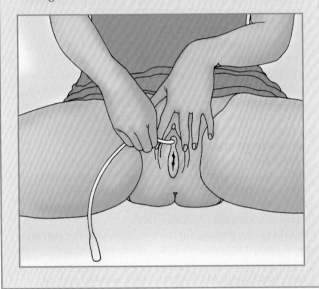

SELF-CATHETERIZATION

Self-catheterization is performed by many patients who have some form of impaired or absent bladder function. The two major advantages of self-catheterization are that the patient maintains independence and regains bladder control. Self-catheterization also allows normal sexual intimacy without the fear of incontinence, decreases the chance of urinary reflux, reduces the use of aids and appliances and, in many cases, allows the patient to return to work.

Self-catheterization requires thorough and careful teaching by the nurse. At home, the patient will use clean technique for self-catheterization.[1,2] In the health care facility, the nurse and patient can use either clean or sterile technique.[2] Studies have shown that clean intermittent catheterization doesn't increase the risk for urinary tract infections.[2]

Equipment

Rubber catheter ■ washcloth ■ soap and water ■ small packet of water-soluble lubricant ■ Optional: drainage container, paper towels, rubber or plastic sheets, gooseneck lamp, catheterization record, mirror.

Implementation

■ Confirm the patient's identity using at least two patient identifiers according to your facility's policy.[3]
■ Perform hand hygiene.[4,5,6]
■ Tell the patient to begin by trying to urinate into the toilet or, if a toilet isn't available or he needs to measure urine quantity, into a drainage container.
■ Have the patient perform hand hygiene.[4,5,6]
■ Demonstrate how the patient should perform the catheterization, explaining each step clearly and carefully. Position a gooseneck lamp nearby if room lighting is inadequate *to make the urinary meatus clearly visible.* Arrange the patient's clothing so that it's out of the way.

Teaching the male patient

■ Tell the patient to wash and rinse the end of his penis thoroughly with soap and water, pulling back the foreskin, if appropriate. He should keep the foreskin pulled back during the procedure.
■ Show him how to squeeze lubricant onto a paper towel and have him roll the first 6″ to 8″ (15 to 20 cm) of the catheter in the lubricant. *Tell him that copious lubricant will make the procedure more comfortable for him.* Then show him how to insert the catheter. (See *Teaching the male patient self-catheterization.*)
■ When the urine stops draining, tell him to remove the catheter slowly and, if necessary, pull the foreskin forward again. Have him get dressed.

Teaching the female patient

■ Demonstrate and explain to the patient that she should separate the vaginal folds as widely as possible with the fingers of her nondominant hand *to obtain a full view of the urinary meatus.* She may need to use a mirror to visualize the meatus. Ask if she's right- or left-handed and, if necessary, tell her which is her nondominant hand.
■ While holding her labia open with the nondominant hand, she should use the dominant hand to wash the perineal area thoroughly with a soapy washcloth, using downward strokes.[2] Tell her to rinse the area with the washcloth, using downward strokes as well.
■ Show her how to squeeze some lubricant onto the first 2″ to 4″ (5 to 10 cm) of the catheter and then how to insert the catheter. (See *Teaching the female patient self-catheterization.*)
■ When the urine stops draining, tell her to remove the catheter slowly and get dressed.

Completing the procedure

■ Tell the patient to dispose of equipment appropriately.
■ Perform hand hygiene and have the patient perform hand hygiene.[4,5,6]
■ Document the procedure.[7]

Special considerations

■ Instruct the patient to keep a supply of catheters at home and to use a new catheter each time.
■ Impress upon the patient that the timing of catheterization is critical *to prevent overdistention of the bladder, which can lead to*

infection. Self-catheterization is usually performed every 4 to 6 hours around the clock (or more often at first).[2]

■ Stress the importance of regulating fluid intake, as ordered, *to prevent incontinence while maintaining adequate hydration.* However, explain that incontinent episodes may occur occasionally. For managing incontinence, the doctor or a home health care nurse can help develop a plan such as more frequent catheterizations. After an incontinent episode, tell the patient to wash with soap and water, pat himself dry with a towel, and expose the skin to the air for as long as possible. Bedding and furniture can be protected by covering them with rubber or plastic sheets and then covering the rubber or plastic with fabric.

■ Stress the importance of taking medications, as ordered, *to increase urine retention and help prevent incontinence.*

■ Tell the patient that if he can't pass the catheter, and he can feel that his bladder is full, he should contact his doctor immediately.[2]

Complications

Overdistention of the bladder can lead to urinary tract infections and urine leakage. Improper hand hygiene or equipment cleaning can also cause a urinary tract infection. Incorrect catheter insertion can injure the urethral or bladder mucosa.

Documentation

Record the date and times of catheterization, character of the urine (color, odor, clarity, and presence of particles or blood), the amount of urine (increase, decrease, or no change), and any problems encountered during the procedure. Note whether the patient has difficulty performing a return demonstration.

REFERENCES

1 Gould, C.V., et al. (2009). "Guideline for Prevention of Catheter-associated Urinary Tract Infections, 2009" [Online]. Accessed November 2011 via the Web at http://www.cdc.gov/hicpac/cauti/001_cauti.html (Level I)

2 Society of Urologic Nurses and Associates. (2006). "Clinical Practice Guidelines: Adult Clean Intermittent Catheterization" [Online]. Accessed November 2011 via the Web at http://www.suna.org/resources/adultCICGuide.pdf (Level I)

3 The Joint Commission. (2012). Standard NPSG.01.01.01. *Comprehensive accreditation manual for hospitals: The official handbook.* Oakbrook Terrace, IL: The Joint Commission. (Level I)

4 Centers for Disease Control and Prevention. (October 2002). Guideline for hand hygiene in health-care settings. *Morbidity and Mortality Weekly Report, 51*(RR-16), 1–45. (Level I)

5 World Health Organization. (2009). *WHO guidelines on hand hygiene in health care: First global patient safety challenge. Clean care is safer care.* Geneva, Switzerland: World Health Organization. (Level I)

6 The Joint Commission. (2012). Standard NPSG.07.01.01. *Comprehensive accreditation manual for hospitals: The official handbook.* Oakbrook Terrace, IL: The Joint Commission. (Level I)

7 The Joint Commission. (2012). Standard RC.01.03.01. *Comprehensive accreditation manual for hospitals: The official handbook.* Oakbrook Terrace, IL: The Joint Commission. (Level I)

Teaching the male patient self-catheterization

Teach the patient to hold his penis in his nondominant hand, at a right angle to his body. He should hold the catheter in his dominant hand as if it were a pencil or a dart and slowly insert it 6″ to 8″ (15 to 20 cm) into the urethra—until urine begins flowing.[2] Then he should gently advance the catheter about 1″ (2.5 cm) farther, allowing all urine to drain into the toilet or drainage container.

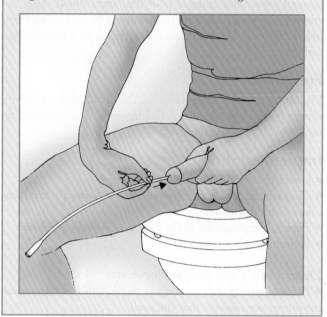

ADDITIONAL REFERENCES

Kessler, T.M., et al. (2009). Clean intermittent self-catheterization: A burden for the patient? *Neurology and Urodynamics, 28*(1), 18–21.

Nettina, S.M. (2010). *Lippincott manual of nursing practice* (9th ed.). Philadelphia, PA: Lippincott Williams & Wilkins.

Taylor, C., et al. (2011). *Fundamentals of nursing: The art and science of nursing care* (7th ed.). Philadelphia, PA: Lippincott Williams & Wilkins.

van Achterberg, T., et al. (2008). Adherence to clean intermittent self-catheterization procedures: Determinants explored. *Journal of Clinical Nursing, 17*(3), 394–402.

SEQUENTIAL COMPRESSION THERAPY

Safe, effective, and noninvasive, sequential compression therapy helps prevent deep vein thrombosis (DVT) in surgical patients. This therapy massages the legs in a wavelike, milking motion that promotes blood flow and deters thrombosis.

Typically, sequential compression therapy complements other preventive measures, such as antiembolism stockings and anticoagulant medications. Although patients at low risk for DVT may require only antiembolism stockings, those at moderate to high risk may require both antiembolism stockings and sequential compression therapy. These preventive measures are continued for as long as the patient remains at risk.

Both antiembolism stockings and sequential compression sleeves are commonly used preoperatively and postoperatively because blood clots tend to form during surgery. About 20% of blood clots form in the femoral vein. Sequential compression therapy counteracts blood stasis and coagulation changes, two of the three major factors that promote DVT. It reduces stasis by increasing peak blood flow velocity, helping to empty the femoral vein's valve cusps of pooled or static blood. Also, the compressions cause an anticlotting effect by increasing fibrinolytic activity, which stimulates the release of a plasminogen activator.

Equipment

Measuring tape and sizing chart for the brand of sleeves you're using ■ pair of compression sleeves in correct size ■ connecting tubing ■ compression controller.

Implementation

- Check the doctor's order.
- Confirm the patient's identity using at least two patient identifiers according to your facility's policy.[1]
- Explain the procedure to the patient *to increase cooperation.*
- Perform hand hygiene.[2,3,4]

Determining the proper sleeve size

- Before applying the compression sleeve, you must determine the proper size of sleeve that you need.
- Measure the circumference of the upper thigh while the patient rests in bed. Do this by placing the measuring tape under the thigh at the gluteal furrow (as shown below).

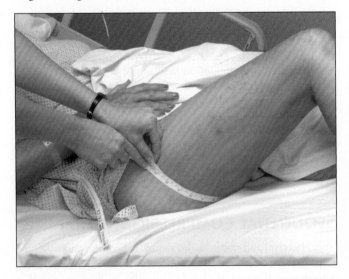

- Hold the tape snugly, but not tightly, around the patient's leg. Note the exact circumference.

- Find the patient's thigh measurement on the sizing chart, and locate the corresponding size of the compression sleeve.
- Remove the compression sleeves from the package and unfold them.
- Lay the unfolded sleeves on a flat surface with the cotton lining facing up (as shown below).

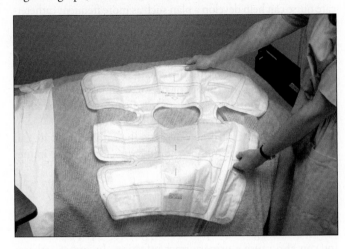

- Notice the markings on the lining denoting the ankle and the area behind the knee at the popliteal pulse point. Use these markings to position the sleeve at the appropriate landmarks.

Applying the sleeves

- Place the patient's leg on the sleeve lining. Position the back of the knee over the popliteal opening.
- Make sure that the back of the ankle is over the ankle marking.
- Starting at the side opposite the clear plastic tubing, wrap the sleeve snugly around the patient's leg.
- Fasten the sleeve securely with the Velcro fasteners. For the best fit, first secure the ankle and calf sections, and then the thigh.
- The sleeve should fit snugly but not tightly. Check the fit by inserting two fingers between the sleeve and the patient's leg at the knee opening. Loosen or tighten the sleeve by readjusting the Velcro fastener.
- Using the same procedure, apply the second sleeve (as shown below).

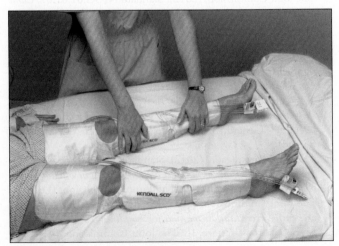

Operating the system

- Connect each sleeve to the tubing leading to the controller. Both sleeves must be connected to the compression controller for the system to operate. Line up the blue arrows on the sleeve connector with the arrows on the tubing connectors, and push the ends together firmly. Listen for a click, signaling a firm connection. Make sure that the tubing is not kinked.
- Plug the compression controller into the proper wall outlet. Turn on the power.
- The controller automatically sets the compression sleeve pressure at 45 mm Hg, which is the midpoint of the normal range (35 to 55 mm Hg).
- Observe to see how well the patient tolerates the therapy and the controller as the system completes its first cycle.
- Check the "audible alarm" key. The green light should be lit, indicating that the alarm is working.
- The compression sleeves should function continuously (24 hours daily) until the patient is fully ambulatory. Check the sleeves at least once each shift *to ensure proper fit and inflation.*[5,6,7,8]
- Remove the sleeves and assess and document skin integrity every 8 hours *to avoid skin breakdown,* especially in patients with decreased sensation or who are unresponsive.
- Perform hand hygiene.[2,3,4]
- Document the procedure.[9]

Removing the sleeves

- You may remove the sleeves when the patient is walking, bathing, or leaving the room for tests or other procedures. Reapply them immediately after any of these activities.[6,7,8] To disconnect the sleeves from the tubing, depress the latches on each side of the connectors and pull the connectors apart.
- Store the tubing and compression controller according to facility protocol. This equipment isn't disposable.

Special considerations

- The compression controller also has a mechanism to help cool the patient.
- If you're applying only one sleeve—for example, if the patient has a cast—leave the unused sleeve folded in the plastic bag. Cut a small hole in the bag's sealed bottom edge, and pull the sleeve connector (the part that holds the connecting tubing) through the hole. Then you can join both sleeves to the compression controller.
- If a malfunction triggers the instrument's alarm, you'll hear beeping. The system shuts off whenever the alarm is activated.
- To respond to the alarm, remove the operator's card from the slot on the top of the compression controller.
- Follow the instructions printed on the card next to the matching code.
- Assess the extremities for peripheral pulses, edema, changes in sensation, and movement at least once each shift.
- Don't use this therapy in a patient with acute DVT (or DVT diagnosed within the last 6 months); severe arteriosclerosis or any other ischemic vascular disease; massive edema of the legs resulting from pulmonary edema or heart failure; or any local condition that the compression sleeves would aggravate, such as dermatitis, vein ligation, gangrene, or recent skin grafting. A patient with a pronounced leg deformity also would be unlikely to benefit from the compression sleeves.

Complications

The most common complication of compression therapy is skin irritation.

Documentation

Document the procedure, the patient's response to and understanding of the procedure, and the status of the alarm and cooling settings.

REFERENCES

1 The Joint Commission. (2012). Standard NPSG.01.01.01. *Comprehensive accreditation manual for hospitals: The official handbook.* Oakbrook Terrace, IL: The Joint Commission. (Level I)
2 Centers for Disease Control and Prevention. (October 2002). Guideline for hand hygiene in health-care settings. *Morbidity and Mortality Weekly Report, 51*(RR-16), 1–45. (Level I)
3 World Health Organization. (2009). *WHO guidelines on hand hygiene in health care: First global patient safety challenge. Clean care is safer care.* Geneva, Switzerland: World Health Organization. (Level I)
4 The Joint Commission. (2012). Standard NPSG.07.01.01. *Comprehensive accreditation manual for hospitals: The official handbook.* Oakbrook Terrace, IL: The Joint Commission. (Level I)
5 Conner, R., et al. (Eds.). (2011). *Perioperative standards and recommended practices.* Denver, CO: AORN. (Level I)
6 ACOG Committee on Practice Bulletins. (2001, reaffirmed 2008). ACOG practice bulletin 19. Thromboembolism in pregnancy. *International Journal of Gynecology and Obstetrics, 75*(2), 203–212.
7 American Association of Critical-Care Nurses. (2005). "AACN Practice Alert: Deep Vein Thrombosis Prevention" [Online]. Accessed December 2011 via the Web at http://classic.aacn.org/AACN/practiceAlert.nsf/Files/DVT%20PA/$file/DVT%20Prevention%2012-2005.pdf (Level I)
8 Hirsch, J., et al. (2008). American College of Chest Physicians evidence-based clinical practice guidelines (8th ed.). *Chest, 133*(6), 71s–109s. (Level I)
9 The Joint Commission. (2012). Standard RC.01.03.01. *Comprehensive accreditation manual for hospitals: The official handbook.* Oakbrook Terrace, IL: The Joint Commission. (Level I)

ADDITIONAL REFERENCES

Craven, R.F., & Hirnle, C.J. (2012). *Fundamentals of nursing: Human health and function* (7th ed.). Philadelphia, PA: Lippincott Williams & Wilkins.
Nettina, S.M. (2010). *Lippincott manual of nursing practice* (9th ed.). Philadelphia, PA: Lippincott Williams & Wilkins.
Snow, V., et al. (2007). Management of venous thromboembolism: A clinical practice guideline from the American College of Physicians and the American Academy of Family Physicians. *Annals of Internal Medicine, 146*(3), 204–210.
Stewart, D., et al. (2006). A prospective study of nurse and patient education on compliance with sequential compression devices. *Annals of Surgery, 72*(10), 921–923.

Taylor, C., et al. (2011). *Fundamentals of nursing: The art and science of nursing care* (7th ed.). Philadelphia, PA: Lippincott Williams & Wilkins.

SEXUAL ASSAULT EXAMINATION

Each facility or agency has a specific protocol for specimen collection in cases involving sexual assault. Specimens can be collected from various sources, including blood, hair, nails, tissues, and such body fluids as urine, semen, saliva, and vaginal secretions. In addition, evidence can be obtained from the results of diagnostic tests, such as computed tomography and radiography. Regardless of the protocol or specimen source, accurate and precise specimen collection is essential in conjunction with thorough, objective documentation because in many cases this information will be used as evidence in legal proceedings.

Many institutions have a Sexual Assault Nurse Examiner (SANE) available to care for patients who are victims of sexual assault. SANEs are skilled rape crisis professionals who can evaluate the victim and collect specimens. They may also be called upon at a later date to testify in legal proceedings.

If you're responsible for collecting specimens in a sexual assault, follow these important guidelines:
■ Know your facility's policy and procedures for specimen collection in sexual assault cases.
■ When obtaining specimens, be sure to collect them from the victim and, if possible, from the suspect.
■ Inform local law enforcement about the suspected assault.[1,2]
■ Check with local law enforcement agencies about additional specimens that may be needed; for example, such trace evidence as soot, grass, gravel, glass, or other debris.
■ Wear gloves and change them frequently; use disposable equipment and instruments if possible.[3]
■ Avoid coughing, sneezing, or talking over specimens or touching your face, nose, or mouth when collecting specimens.
■ Include the victim's clothing as part of the collection procedure.
■ Place all items collected in a paper bag.[3]

NURSING ALERT *Never allow a specimen or item considered as evidence to be left unattended.*

■ Document each item or specimen collected; have another person witness each collection and document it.
■ Label each specimen in the presence of the patient to prevent mislabeling.[4]
■ Obtain photographs of all injuries for documentation.[3]
■ Include written documentation of the victim's physical and psychological condition on first encounter, throughout specimen collection, and afterward.

Equipment

Nonlubricated gloves ■ Wood's lamp ■ examination paper ■ clean paper bags (one for each article of clothing) ■ swabs for collecting specimens ■ comb ■ EDTA tube ■ supplies for venipuncture (See "Venipuncture," page 781) ■ camera for photographs ■ Optional: tetanus shot, antibiotics, human immunodeficiency virus (HIV) prophylaxis.

When possible, obtain a special Sexual Assault Evidence Collection Kit, which contains the necessary items for specimen collection based on the evidence required by the local crime laboratory. The kit also contains a form that the examiner must complete, sign, and date. Keep in mind that when collecting specimens of moist secretions, you'll typically use a one-swab technique; for dry secretions, use a two-swab technique.

Implementation
■ Perform hand hygiene.[5,6,7]
■ Ensure patient privacy throughout the collection procedure.[3]
■ Confirm the patient's identity using at least two patient identifiers according to your facility's policy.[8]
■ Assess the patient's ability to undergo the specimen collection procedure.
■ Explain the procedures that the patient will undergo, including what specimens will be collected and from where; provide emotional support throughout.[3]
■ Ask the patient if he or she would like someone, such as a family member, friend, or other person, to stay during the specimen collection.
■ Put on nonlubricated gloves.
■ Ask the patient to stand on a clean piece of examination paper if he or she can stand; if the patient can't stand, then have the patient remain on the examination table or bed.
■ Have the patient remove each article of clothing, one at a time, and place each article in a separate, clean paper bag.[3]
■ If the clothing is wet, allow it to dry first before placing the item into the paper bag.

NURSING ALERT *Never use plastic bags to collect clothing. Plastic promotes bacterial growth and can destroy deoxyribonucleic acid (DNA).*[3]

■ Fold the examination paper onto itself and place it into a clean paper bag.
■ Fold over, seal, label, and initial each bag.
■ Before obtaining specimens, inspect the genital area using a Wood's lamp. *This device uses long wave ultraviolet light to scan the area for secretions and aids in identifying areas of trauma.*

Vaginal or cervical secretion collection
■ Swab the vaginal area thoroughly with four swabs; swab the cervical area with two swabs, making sure to keep the vaginal swabs separate from the cervical swabs.
■ Run the vaginal swabs over a slide (supplied in the kit) and allow the slide and swabs to air-dry; do the same for the cervical swabs.
■ Place the vaginal swabs in the swab container and close it; then place the slide in the cardboard sleeve, close it, and tape it shut. Repeat this procedure for the cervical swabs.
■ Place the swab container and cardboard sleeve into the envelope, and seal it securely.
■ Complete the information as provided on the front of the envelope; if you've obtained both vaginal and cervical swabs, use a separate envelope for each.

Anal secretion collection
■ Moisten a single swab with sterile water.

■ Gently insert the swab about 1¼" (3 cm) into the patient's rectum.
■ Rotate the swab gently and then remove it.
■ Allow the swab to air-dry, and then place it in an envelope.
■ Seal and label the envelope appropriately.

Penile secretion collection
■ Moisten a single swab with sterile water.
■ Swab the entire external surface of the penis.
■ Repeat this at least one more time (so that at least two swabs are obtained).
■ Allow the swab to air-dry and then place it in an envelope.
■ Seal and label the envelope appropriately.

Pubic hair collection
■ Use the comb provided in the kit and comb through the pubic hair.
■ Collect approximately 20 to 30 pubic hairs and place them in the envelope.
■ Alternatively, obtain 20 to 30 plucked hairs from the patient; allow the patient the option of plucking his or her own pubic hair.
■ Place the hair in the envelope, and seal and label it appropriately.

Blood samples
■ After performing a venipuncture, obtain at least 5 mL of blood in an EDTA tube.
■ Write the patient's name and date on the label of the tube.
■ Remove the DNA stain card from the kit and label it with the patient's name.
■ Using the blood collected in this tube, withdraw 1 mL of blood and apply blood to each of the four circles on the card, completely filling each circle if possible.
■ Let the card air-dry and then place the card in the envelope.
■ Seal and label the envelope appropriately.
■ Place the blood tube into the tube holder supplied in the kit and seal the holder with the tape supplied in the kit (it may be referred to as evidence tape).
■ Place the tube and holder in the zippered bag provided.
■ Collect additional blood samples to test for pregnancy; sexually transmitted infections, such as gonorrhea, chlamydia, and syphilis; or toxicology as appropriate, and send them to the laboratory immediately.

Urine specimens
■ Obtain a random urine specimen from the patient. Remind the patient not to use cleaning wipes *to avoid destroying possible evidence.*

Specimen storage and transport
■ Refrigerate blood samples obtained.
■ Place all other specimens in the specimen kit and keep the kit at room temperature.
■ Remove and discard your gloves and perform hand hygiene.[5,6,7]
■ Give all the specimens to the police when they arrive.
■ Carefully document the handoff *to ensure proper chain of custody.*[3]

■ Document the procedure.[9]

Special considerations
■ Follow the directions in the kit precisely *to ensure that the chain of evidence is followed.*
■ Provide follow-up counseling and support to the patient.
■ If necessary, administer ordered medications, such as tetanus, antibiotics, or HIV prophylaxis.
■ Make sure that the patient has a support person to accompany him or her home.
■ Arrange a referral to a local support group or follow-up with a trained counselor.

Documentation
Document all specimens collected, including the type, location, time collected, patient's name and identification number, and any other relevant information. Include photographs as appropriate, including all relevant information about each photograph.

REFERENCES

1 The Joint Commission. (2012). Standard PC.01.02.09. *Comprehensive accreditation manual for hospitals: The official handbook.* Oakbrook Terrace, IL: The Joint Commission. (Level I)
2 The Joint Commission. (2012). Standard RI.01.06.03. *Comprehensive accreditation manual for hospitals: The official handbook.* Oakbrook Terrace, IL: The Joint Commission. (Level I)
3 U.S. Department of Justice, Office on Violence Against Women. (2004). "A National Protocol for Sexual Assault Medical Forensic Examinations" [Online]. Accessed December 2011 via the Web at http://www.ncjrs.gov/pdffiles1/ovw/206554.pdf
4 The Joint Commission. (2012). Standard NPSG.03.04.01. *Comprehensive accreditation manual for hospitals: The official handbook.* Oakbrook Terrace, IL: The Joint Commission. (Level I)
5 Centers for Disease Control and Prevention. (October 2002). Guideline for hand hygiene in health-care settings. *Morbidity and Mortality Weekly Report, 51*(RR-16), 1–45. (Level I)
6 World Health Organization. (2009). *WHO guidelines on hand hygiene in health care: First global patient safety challenge. Clean care is safer care.* Geneva, Switzerland: World Health Organization. (Level I)
7 The Joint Commission. (2012). Standard NPSG.07.01.01. *Comprehensive accreditation manual for hospitals: The official handbook.* Oakbrook Terrace, IL: The Joint Commission. (Level I)
8 The Joint Commission. (2012). Standard NPSG.01.01.01. *Comprehensive accreditation manual for hospitals: The official handbook.* Oakbrook Terrace, IL: The Joint Commission. (Level I)
9 The Joint Commission. (2012). Standard RC.01.03.01. *Comprehensive accreditation manual for hospitals: The official handbook.* Oakbrook Terrace, IL: The Joint Commission. (Level I)

ADDITIONAL REFERENCES

Anderson, S., et al. (2006). Genital findings of women after consensual and nonconsensual intercourse. *Journal of Forensic Nursing, 2*(2), 59–65.
Eckert, L.O., et al. (2004). Factors impacting injury documentation after sexual assault: Role of examiner experience and gender. *American Journal of Obstetrics and Gynecology, 190*(6), 1739–1743; discussion 1744–1746.

Ingemann-Hansen, O., et al. (2008). Characteristics of victims and assaults of sexual violence—Improving inquiries and prevention. *Journal of Forensic and Legal Medicine, 16*(4), 182–188.

Morgan, J.A. (2008). Comparison of cervical os versus vaginal evidentiary findings during sexual assault exam. *Journal of Emergency Nursing, 34*(2), 102–105.

Nettina, S.M. (2010). *Lippincott manual of nursing practice* (9th ed.). Philadelphia, PA: Lippincott Williams & Wilkins.

SHARP DEBRIDEMENT

Debridement involves removing necrotic tissue or contaminated foreign debris from a wound. As necrotic tissue develops, it becomes a barrier to wound healing and a medium for bacterial growth. Removing this tissue decreases the risk of infection, accelerates wound healing, and prevents further complications associated with tissue destruction. Surgical debridement is recommended for large or deep wounds. However, when surgical debridement isn't appropriate for the patient's condition, sharp, chemical (or enzymatic), mechanical, autolytic, or biosurgical debridement may be used.[1]

Sharp debridement involves using a scalpel, scissors, or other sharp instrument to excise a wound's necrotic material up to the viable tissue.[1] It's the most rapid form of debridement, and it may be combined with other forms of debridement as needed. Specially trained nurses may perform sharp debridement.[2]

Sharp debridement must be used cautiously in patients with compromised immune systems, compromised vascular supply to the limb, or sepsis.[2] Relative contraindications for sharp debridement include anticoagulant therapy and bleeding disorders.[2]

Equipment

Pain medication as ordered and as needed ▪ two pairs of sterile gloves ▪ two gowns or aprons ▪ mask ▪ cap ▪ sterile scissors or scalpel ▪ sterile forceps ▪ sterile solutions and medications to clean the wound (as ordered) ▪ knife ▪ dressing material ▪ Optional: sterile 4″ × 4″ gauze pads ▪ camera.

Implementation

▪ Confirm the patient's identity using at least two patient identifiers according to your facility's policy.[3]
▪ Explain the procedure to the patient *to allay his fears and promote cooperation.* Teach him distraction and relaxation techniques, if possible, *to minimize his discomfort.*
▪ Provide privacy.
▪ Theoretically, sharp debridement doesn't remove healthy tissue, so the patient shouldn't experience much pain. However, if the patient is awake and able to experience pain, administer an analgesic at an appropriate time before debridement begins based on the onset and peak of the medication prescribed, or give an IV analgesic immediately before the procedure.[1,2]
▪ Keep the patient warm. Expose only the area to be debrided *to prevent chilling and fluid and electrolyte loss.*
▪ If the wound to be debrided is on a lower extremity, perform a neurovascular assessment before beginning the procedure *to obtain baseline information.*[1,2]

▪ Perform hand hygiene and put on a cap, a mask, a gown or an apron, and sterile gloves.[4,5,6]
▪ Remove the dressings and clean the wound.
▪ Measure the wound *to determine how wound healing is progressing.* If applicable, photograph the wound for additional documentation.[2]
▪ Remove your gown or apron and dirty gloves, perform hand hygiene,[4,5,6] and change to another gown or apron and sterile gloves.
▪ Lift the necrotic tissue with forceps. Use the scalpel or scissors to cut the tissue. Keep the scalpel or scissors parallel to or angled away from the wound bed.
▪ Replace the dressing over the wound.
▪ Dispose of all equipment in the proper receptacle.
▪ Remove and discard your personal protective equipment.
▪ Perform hand hygiene.[4,5,6]
▪ Document the procedure.[7]

Special considerations

▪ *Because debridement removes dead tissue,* bleeding should be minimal. If bleeding occurs, apply gentle pressure on the wound with sterile 4″ × 4″ gauze pads. Then apply the hemostatic agent. If bleeding persists, notify the doctor, and maintain pressure on the wound until he arrives. Excessive bleeding or spurting vessels may require ligation.

Complications

Infection may develop despite the use of sterile technique and equipment. Bleeding, the most common complication, may occur if debridement exposes an eroded blood vessel or if you inadvertently cut a vessel. Fluid and electrolyte imbalances may result from exudate lost during the procedure.

Documentation

Record the date and time of wound debridement, the area debrided, and solutions and medications used. Describe the wound's condition, noting signs of infection or skin breakdown. Record the patient's tolerance of and reaction to the procedure. Note indications for additional therapy. Record the administration of preprocedure pain medication.

REFERENCES

1 Institute for Clinical Systems Improvement. (2010). "Health Care Protocol: Pressure Ulcer Prevention and Treatment Protocol" (2nd ed.) [Online]. Accessed December 2011 via the Web at http://www.icsi.org/pressure_ulcer_treatment_protocol__review_and_comment_/pressure_ulcer_treatment__protocol__.html

2 National Pressure Ulcer Advisory Panel and European Pressure Ulcer Advisory Panel. (2009). *Pressure ulcer prevention and treatment: Clinical practice guidelines.* Washington, DC: National Pressure Ulcer Advisory Panel.

3 The Joint Commission. (2012). Standard NPSG.01.01.01. *Comprehensive accreditation manual for hospitals: The official handbook.* Oakbrook Terrace, IL: The Joint Commission. (Level I)

4 Centers for Disease Control and Prevention. (October 2002). Guideline for hand hygiene in health-care settings. *Morbidity and Mortality Weekly Report, 51*(RR-16), 1–45. (Level I)

5   World Health Organization. (2009). *WHO guidelines on hand hygiene in health care: First global patient safety challenge. Clean care is safer care.* Geneva, Switzerland: World Health Organization. (Level I)

6   The Joint Commission. (2012). Standard NPSG.07.01.01. *Comprehensive accreditation manual for hospitals: The official handbook.* Oakbrook Terrace, IL: The Joint Commission. (Level I)

7   The Joint Commission. (2012). Standard RC.01.03.01. *Comprehensive accreditation manual for hospitals: The official handbook.* Oakbrook Terrace, IL: The Joint Commission. (Level I)

ADDITIONAL REFERENCES

Anderson, I. (2006). Debridement methods in wound care. *Nursing Standard, 20*(24), 65–66, 68, 70 passim.

Baranoski, S., & Ayello, E.A. (2008). *Wound care essentials: Practice principles* (2nd ed.). Philadelphia, PA: Lippincott Williams & Williams.

Fleck, C., & Chakravarthy, D. (2010). Newer debridement methods for wound bed preparation. *Advances in Skin and Wound Care, 23*(7), 313–315.

Keast, D.H., et al. (2007). Best practice recommendations for the prevention and treatment of pressure ulcers: Update 2006. *Advances in Skin and Wound Care, 20*(8), 447–460.

Wound, Ostomy and Continence Nurses Society. (2005). *Guideline for management of wounds in patients with lower-extremity venous disease.* Glenview, IL: WOCN.

Wound, Ostomy and Continence Nurses Society. (2005). "WOCN Position Statement: Clean versus Sterile: Management of Chronic Wounds" [Online]. Accessed February 2012 via the Web at http://www.wocn.org/resource/resmgr/docs/clvst.pdf

SHAVING

Performed with a safety or electric razor, shaving is part of the male patient's usual daily care. Besides reducing bacterial growth on the face, shaving promotes patient comfort by removing whiskers that can itch and irritate the skin and produce an unkempt appearance. Because nicks and cuts occur more frequently with a safety razor, a patient with a clotting disorder or on anticoagulant therapy should be shaved with an electric razor. Shaving may be contraindicated in the patient with a facial skin disorder or wound.

Equipment

For a safety razor

Shaving kit containing a razor and soap container ▪ gloves ▪ soap or shaving cream ▪ bath towel ▪ washcloth ▪ basin ▪ Optional: aftershave lotion, talcum powder.

For an electric razor

Electric razor ▪ bath towel ▪ gloves ▪ Optional: preshave and aftershave lotions, mirror, grounded three-pronged plug.

Preparation of equipment

With a safety razor, make sure the blade is sharp, clean, even, and rust-free. If necessary, insert a new blade securely into the razor. A razor may be used more than once, but only for the same patient. If the patient is bedridden, gather the equipment on the bedside stand or overbed table; if he's ambulatory, gather it at the sink.

When the patient is ready to shave, fill the basin or sink with warm water.

If you're using an electric razor, check its cord for fraying or other damage that could create an electrical hazard. If the razor isn't double-insulated or battery operated, use a grounded three-pronged plug. Examine the razor head for sharp edges and dirt. Read the manufacturer's instructions, if available. Gather the equipment at the bedside.

Implementation

▪ Perform hand hygiene.[1,2,3]
▪ Confirm the patient's identity using at least two patient identifiers according to your facility's policy.[4]
▪ Tell the patient that you're going to shave him, and provide privacy. Ask him to assist you as much as possible *to promote his independence.*
▪ Unless contraindicated, place the conscious patient in high Fowler's or semi-Fowler's position. If the patient is unconscious, elevate his head *to prevent soap and water from running behind it.*
▪ Direct bright light onto the patient's face, but not into his eyes.
▪ Put on gloves.

Using a safety razor

▪ Drape a bath towel around the patient's shoulders, and tuck it under his chin *to protect the bed from moisture and to catch falling whiskers.*
▪ Fill the basin with warm water. Using the washcloth, wet the patient's entire beard with warm water. Let the warm cloth soak the beard for at least 1 minute *to soften whiskers.*
▪ Apply shaving cream to the beard. Or, if you're using soap, rub it to form a lather.
▪ Gently stretch the patient's skin taut with one hand and shave with the other, holding the razor firmly. Ask the patient to puff his cheeks or turn his head, as necessary, to shave hard-to-reach areas.
▪ Begin at the sideburns and work toward the chin using short, firm, downward strokes in the direction of hair growth (as shown below). *This method reduces skin irritation and helps prevent nicks and cuts.*

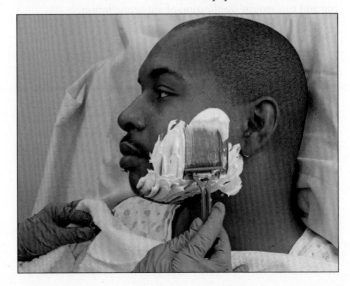

- Rinse the razor often *to remove whiskers*. Apply more warm water or shaving cream to the face, as needed, *to maintain adequate lather.*
- Shave across the chin and up the neck and throat. Use short, gentle strokes for the neck and the area around the nose and mouth *to avoid skin irritation.*
- Change the water, and rinse any remaining lather and whiskers from the patient's face. Then dry his face with a bath towel and, if the patient desires, apply aftershave lotion or talcum powder.
- Rinse the razor and basin, and then return the razor to its storage area or dispose of it in a sharps container.

Using an electric razor

- Plug in the razor and apply preshave lotion, if available, *to remove skin oils.* If the razor head is adjustable, select the appropriate setting.
- Using a circular motion and pressing the razor firmly against the skin, shave each area of the patient's face until smooth.
- If the patient desires, apply talcum powder or aftershave lotion.
- Clean the razor head, and return the razor to its storage area.

Completing the procedure

- Remove and discard your gloves and perform hand hygiene.[1,2,3]
- Document the procedure.[5]

Special considerations

- If the patient is conscious, find out his usual shaving routine. Although shaving in the direction of hair growth is most common, the patient may prefer the opposite direction.
- Don't interchange patients' shaving equipment *to prevent cross-contamination.*
- Shaving may be contraindicated if the patient is on anticoagulant therapy (for example, tissue plasminogen activator or heparin). Check your facility's policy.
- A safety inspection by medical maintenance may need to be performed before using an electric razor brought from home.

Complications

Cuts and abrasions are the most common complications of shaving and can require application of antiseptic lotion.

Documentation

If applicable, record nicks or cuts resulting from shaving.

REFERENCES

1 The Joint Commission. (2012). Standard NPSG.07.01.01. *Comprehensive accreditation manual for hospitals: The official handbook.* Oakbrook Terrace, IL: The Joint Commission. (Level I)
2 Centers for Disease Control and Prevention. (October 2002). Guideline for hand hygiene in health-care settings. *Morbidity and Mortality Weekly Report, 51*(RR-16), 1–45. (Level I)
3 World Health Organization. (2009). *WHO guidelines on hand hygiene in health care: First global patient safety challenge. Clean care is safer care.* Geneva, Switzerland: World Health Organization. (Level I)
4 The Joint Commission. (2012). Standard NPSG.01.01.01. *Comprehensive accreditation manual for hospitals: The official handbook.* Oakbrook Terrace, IL: The Joint Commission. (Level I)
5 The Joint Commission. (2012). Standard RC.01.03.01. *Comprehensive accreditation manual for hospitals: The official handbook.* Oakbrook Terrace, IL: The Joint Commission. (Level I)

ADDITIONAL REFERENCE

Craven, R.F., & Hirnle, C.J. (2012). *Fundamentals of nursing: Human health and function* (7th ed.). Philadelphia, PA: Lippincott Williams & Wilkins.

SITZ BATH

A sitz bath involves immersion of the pelvic area in warm or hot water. It is used to relieve discomfort, especially after perineal or rectal surgery or childbirth. The bath promotes wound healing by cleaning the perineum and anus, increasing circulation, and reducing inflammation. It also helps relax local muscles.

To be performed correctly, the sitz bath requires frequent checks of water temperature to ensure therapeutic effects as well as correct draping of the patient during the bath and prompt dressing after it to prevent vasoconstriction.

Equipment

Sitz tub, portable sitz bath, or regular bathtub ■ bath mat ■ rubber mat ■ bath (utility) thermometer ■ two bath blankets ■ towels ■ patient gown ■ gloves, if the patient has an open lesion or has been incontinent ■ Optional: rubber ring, footstool, overbed table, IV pole (to hold irrigation bag), wheelchair or cart, dressings.

A disposable sitz bath kit is available for single-patient use. It includes a plastic basin that fits over a commode and an irrigation bag with tubing and clamp.

Preparation of equipment

Make sure the sitz tub, portable sitz bath, or regular bathtub is clean and disinfected. Or obtain a disposable sitz bath kit from the central supply department.

Position the bath mat next to the bathtub, sitz tub, or commode. If you're using a tub, place the rubber mat on its surface *to prevent falls.* Place the rubber ring on the bottom of the tub *to serve as a seat for the patient,* and cover the ring with a towel *for comfort. Keeping the patient elevated improves water flow over the wound site and avoids unnecessary pressure on tender tissues.*

If you're using a commercial kit, open the package and familiarize yourself with the equipment.

Fill the sitz tub or bathtub one-third to one-half full *so that the water will reach the seated patient's umbilicus.* Use warm water (94° to 98° F [34.4° to 36.7° C]) for relaxation or wound cleaning and healing and hot water (110° to 115° F [43.3° to 46.1° C]) for heat application. Run the water slightly warmer than desired *because it will cool while the patient prepares for the bath.* Measure the water temperature using the bath thermometer.

If you're using a commercial kit, fill the basin to the specified line with water at the prescribed temperature. Place the basin under the commode seat, clamp the irrigation tubing to block water flow, and fill the irrigation bag with water of the same temperature as that in the basin. To create flow pressure, hang the bag above the patient's head on a hook, towel rack, or IV pole.

Implementation

- Check the doctor's order.
- Confirm the patient's identity using at least two patient identifiers according to your facility's policy.[1]
- Explain the procedure to the patient.
- Perform hand hygiene and put on gloves as needed.[2,3,4]
- Assess the patient's condition.
- Have the patient void.
- Assist the patient to the bath area, provide privacy, and make sure the area is warm and free of drafts. Help the patient undress, as needed.
- Remove and dispose of any soiled dressings. If a dressing adheres to a wound, allow it to soak off in the tub.
- Assist the patient into the tub or onto the commode, as needed. Instruct him to use the safety rail for balance. Explain that the sensation may be unpleasant initially *because the wound area is already tender.* Assure him that this discomfort will soon be relieved by the warm water.
- For any apparatus except a regular bathtub, if the patient's feet don't reach the floor and the weight of his legs presses against the edge of the equipment, place a small stool under the patient's feet *to decrease pressure on local blood vessels.* Also place a folded towel against the patient's lower back *to prevent discomfort and promote correct body alignment.*
- Drape the patient's shoulders and knees with bath blankets *to avoid chills that cause vasoconstriction.*
- If you're using the sitz bath kit, open the clamp on the irrigation tubing *to allow a stream of water to flow continuously over the wound site.* Refill the bag with water of the correct temperature as needed, and encourage the patient to regulate the flow himself. Place the patient's overbed table in front of him *to provide support and comfort.*
- If you're using a tub, check the water temperature frequently with the bath thermometer. If the temperature drops significantly, add warm water. For maximum safety, first help the patient stand up slowly *to prevent dizziness and loss of balance.* Then with the patient holding the safety rail *for support,* run warm water into the tub. Check water temperature. When the water reaches the correct temperature, help the patient sit down again to resume the bath.
- If necessary, stay with the patient during the bath. If you must leave, show him how to use the call bell, and ensure his privacy.
- Check the patient's color and general condition frequently. If he complains of feeling weak, faint, or nauseated or shows signs of cardiovascular distress, discontinue the bath, check the patient's pulse and blood pressure, and assist him back to bed. Use a wheelchair or cart to transport the patient to his room if necessary. Notify the doctor.
- When the prescribed bath time has elapsed—usually 15 to 20 minutes—tell the patient to use the safety rail *for balance,* and help him to a standing position slowly *to prevent dizziness and to allow him to regain his equilibrium.*
- If necessary, help the patient dry himself. Put on clean gloves and re-dress the wound as needed, provide a clean gown,

and help the patient dress and return to bed or back to his room.
- Dispose of soiled materials properly.
- Empty, clean, and disinfect the sitz tub, bathtub, or portable sitz bath. Return the commercial kit to the patient's bedside for later use.
- Remove and discard your gloves and perform hand hygiene.[2,3,4]
- Document the procedure.[5]

Special considerations

- Use a regular bathtub only if a special sitz tub, portable sitz bath, or commercial sitz bath kit is unavailable. *Because the application of heat to the extremities causes vasodilation and draws blood away from the perineal area,* a regular bathtub is less effective for local treatment than a sitz device.
- If the patient will be sitting in a bathtub with his extremities immersed in the hot water, check his pulse before, during, and after the bath *to help detect vasodilation that could make him feel faint when he stands up.*
- Tell the patient never to touch an open wound *because of the risk of infection.*

Complications

Weakness or faintness can result from heat or the exertion of changing position. Irregular or accelerated pulse may indicate cardiovascular distress.

Documentation

Record the date, time, duration, and temperature of the bath; wound condition before and after treatment, including color, odor, and amount of drainage; any complications; and the patient's response to treatment.

REFERENCES

1 The Joint Commission. (2012). Standard NPSG.01.01.01. *Comprehensive accreditation manual for hospitals: The official handbook.* Oakbrook Terrace, IL: The Joint Commission. (Level I)
2 Centers for Disease Control and Prevention. (October 2002). Guideline for hand hygiene in health-care settings. *Morbidity and Mortality Weekly Report, 51*(RR-16), 1–45. (Level I)
3 World Health Organization. (2009). *WHO guidelines on hand hygiene in health care: First global patient safety challenge. Clean care is safer care.* Geneva, Switzerland: World Health Organization. (Level I)
4 The Joint Commission. (2012). Standard NPSG.07.01.01. *Comprehensive accreditation manual for hospitals: The official handbook.* Oakbrook Terrace, IL: The Joint Commission. (Level I)
5 The Joint Commission. (2012). Standard RC.01.03.01. *Comprehensive accreditation manual for hospitals: The official handbook.* Oakbrook Terrace, IL: The Joint Commission. (Level I)

ADDITIONAL REFERENCES

Albers, L.L., & Borders, N. (2007). Minimizing genital tract trauma and related pain following spontaneous vaginal birth. *Journal of Midwifery and Women's Health, 52*(3), 246–253.

Craven, R.F., & Hirnle, C.J. (2012). *Fundamentals of nursing: Human health and function* (7th ed.). Philadelphia, PA: Lippincott Williams & Wilkins.

Taylor, C., et al. (2011). *Fundamentals of nursing: The art and science of nursing care* (7th ed.). Philadelphia, PA: Lippincott Williams & Wilkins.

SKIN BIOPSY

Skin biopsy is a diagnostic test in which a small piece of tissue is removed, under local anesthesia, from a lesion that's suspected of being malignant or from another dermatosis.

One of three techniques may be used: shave biopsy, punch biopsy, or excisional biopsy. *Shave biopsy* cuts the lesion above the skin line, which allows further biopsy of the site. *Punch biopsy* removes an oval or round core from the center of the lesion. *Excisional biopsy* removes the entire lesion and is indicated for rapidly expanding lesions, malignant or dysplastic tissue, ensuring clear margins of skin surrounding a lesion (when necessary), examining the border of a lesion surrounding normal skin, and sclerotic, bullous, or atrophic lesions.

Lesions suspected of being malignant usually have changed color, size, or appearance or have failed to heal properly. (See *The ABCDEs of malignant melanoma.*) Fully developed lesions should be selected for biopsy whenever possible because they provide more diagnostic information than lesions that are either resolving or in an early stage of development. For example, if the skin shows blisters, the biopsy should include the most mature ones.

Normal skin consists of squamous epithelium (epidermis) and fibrous connective tissue (dermis). Benign growths include cysts, seborrheic keratoses, warts, pigmented nevi (moles), keloids, dermatofibromas, and neurofibromas. Malignant tumors include dysplastic nevi, basal cell carcinoma, squamous cell carcinoma, and malignant melanoma.

Equipment

Gloves ▪ sterile gloves ▪ #15 scalpel for shave or excisional biopsy ▪ skin preparation product ▪ punch for punch biopsy ▪ local anesthetic ▪ specimen bottle containing 10% formaldehyde solution ▪ 3-0, 4-0, or 5-0 sutures for punch or excisional biopsy ▪ adhesive bandage ▪ forceps ▪ scissors ▪ adhesive strips.

Implementation

- Verify the doctor's order.
- Perform hand hygiene.[1,2,3]
- Confirm the patient's identity using at least two patient identifiers according to your facility's policy.[4]
- Explain to the patient that the biopsy provides a skin specimen for microscopic study. Describe the procedure and tell him who will perform it. Answer any questions he may have *to ease anxiety and ensure cooperation.*
- Inform the patient that he need not restrict food or fluids.
- Tell him that he'll receive a local anesthetic for pain.
- Inform him that the biopsy will take about 15 minutes and that the test results are usually available within 7 days, depending on the facility.
- Confirm that an informed consent has been obtained and is documented on the chart.[5]

- Check the patient's history for hypersensitivity to the local anesthetic.
- Perform hand hygiene and put on gloves.[1,2,3]
- Label all medications, medication containers, and other solutions on and off the sterile field.[6]
- Position the patient comfortably, and prepare the biopsy site before the local anesthetic is administered.
- For a *shave biopsy,* the growth is cut off at the skin line with a #15 scalpel. The tissue is placed immediately in a properly labeled specimen bottle containing 10% formaldehyde solution. Apply pressure to the biopsy area *to stop the bleeding.* Apply an adhesive bandage.
- For a *punch biopsy,* the skin surrounding the lesion is pulled taut, and the punch is firmly introduced into the lesion and rotated to obtain a tissue specimen. The plug is lifted with forceps or a needle and is severed as deeply into the fat layer as possible. The specimen is placed in a properly labeled specimen bottle containing 10% formaldehyde solution or in a sterile container if indicated. The method of closing the wound depends on the size of the punch and varies from using only an adhesive bandage to using two sutures.
- For an *excisional biopsy,* a #15 scalpel is used to excise the lesion; the incision is made as wide and as deep as necessary. The tissue specimen is removed and placed immediately in a properly labeled specimen bottle containing 10% formaldehyde solution. Apply pressure to the site *to stop the bleeding.* The size of the sutures required to close the wound vary from 3-0 to 5-0, depending on the location of the biopsy. If the incision is large, a skin graft may be required. If the incision is small, adhesive strips may be applied.
- Check the biopsy site for bleeding.
- Label the specimen container in the presence of the patient and send it to the laboratory immediately.[6]
- Remove and discard your gloves and perform hand hygiene.[1,2,3]
- If the patient experiences pain, administer analgesics as prescribed following safe medication administration practices.[7]
- Document the procedure.[8]

Special considerations

- Shave biopsies aren't recommended for suspected melanomas.

Patient teaching

Advise the patient going home with sutures to keep the area clean and as dry as possible for 24 hours. Tell him that facial sutures will be removed in 3 to 5 days and trunk sutures in 7 to 14 days. Instruct the patient with adhesive strips to leave them in place for 14 to 21 days or until they fall off. Instruct the patient to report signs of infection—including redness, swelling, pain, discharge from the wound, or skin that's warm or hot—to his doctor as soon as possible.

Complications

Possible complications may include bleeding and infection of the surrounding tissue.

Documentation

Document the time and location where the specimen was obtained, the appearance of the specimen and site, and whether bleeding occurred at the biopsy site. Document patient teaching.

The ABCDEs of malignant melanoma

Use the mnemonic ABCDE to remember the warning signs of malignant melanoma.

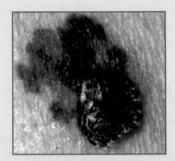

Asymmetry: One half of a mole or birthmark doesn't match the other.

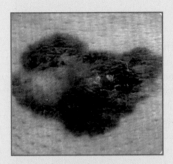

Diameter: The mole's diameter is greater than ¼″ (0.6 cm) or increases in size, especially over a short period of time.

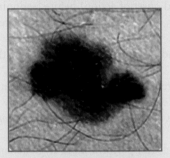

Border: The mole's edges are irregular, ragged, notched, or blurred.

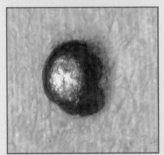

Elevation: The mole is elevated, or raised from the skin.

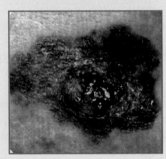

Color: The pigmentation isn't uniform; the mole may have varying degrees of brown, black, or occasionally red.

REFERENCES

1 Centers for Disease Control and Prevention. (October 2002). Guideline for hand hygiene in health-care settings. *Morbidity and Mortality Weekly Report, 51*(RR-16), 1–45. (Level I)

2 World Health Organization. (2009). *WHO guidelines on hand hygiene in health care: First global patient safety challenge. Clean care is safer care.* Geneva, Switzerland: World Health Organization. (Level I)

3 The Joint Commission. (2012). Standard NPSG.07.01.01. *Comprehensive accreditation manual for hospitals: The official handbook.* Oakbrook Terrace, IL: The Joint Commission. (Level I)

4 The Joint Commission. (2012). Standard NPSG.01.01.01. *Comprehensive accreditation manual for hospitals: The official handbook.* Oakbrook Terrace, IL: The Joint Commission. (Level I)

5 The Joint Commission. (2012). Standard RI.01.03.01. *Comprehensive accreditation manual for hospitals: The official handbook.* Oakbrook Terrace, IL: The Joint Commission. (Level I)

6 The Joint Commission. (2012). Standard NPSG.03.04.01. *Comprehensive accreditation manual for hospitals: The official handbook.* Oakbrook Terrace, IL: The Joint Commission. (Level I)

7 The Joint Commission. (2012). Standard MM.06.01.01. *Comprehensive accreditation manual for hospitals: The official handbook.* Oakbrook Terrace, IL: The Joint Commission. (Level I)

8 The Joint Commission. (2012). Standard RC.01.03.01. *Comprehensive accreditation manual for hospitals: The official handbook.* Oakbrook Terrace, IL: The Joint Commission. (Level I)

SKIN GRAFT CARE

A skin graft consists of healthy skin taken either from the patient (autograft) or a donor (allograft) and applied to a part of the patient's body, where the graft resurfaces an area damaged by burns, traumatic injury, or surgery. Although caring for an autograft or an allograft is essentially the same, an autograft requires care for two sites: the graft site and the donor site.

Understanding types of grafts

A burn patient may receive one or more of the graft types described below.

Split-thickness
A split-thickness graft is used most commonly for covering open burns. This graft includes the epidermis and part of the dermis. It may be applied as a sheet (usually on the face or neck *to preserve the cosmetic result*) or as a mesh. A mesh graft has tiny slits cut in it, which allow the graft to expand up to nine times its original size. Mesh grafts prevent fluids from collecting under the graft and typically are used over extensive full-thickness burns.

Full-thickness
A full-thickness graft includes the epidermis and the entire dermis. Consequently, the graft contains hair follicles, sweat glands, and sebaceous glands, which typically aren't included in split-thickness grafts. Full-thickness grafts usually are used for small burns that cause deep wounds.

Pedicle-flap
A pedicle-flap graft includes not only skin and subcutaneous tissue, but also subcutaneous blood vessels *to ensure a continued blood supply to the graft.* Pedicle-flap grafts may be used during reconstructive surgery *to cover previous defects.*

The graft itself may be one of several types: split-thickness, full-thickness, or pedicle-flap. (See *Understanding types of grafts.*) Successful grafting depends on various factors, including clean wound granulation with adequate vascularization, complete contact of the graft with the wound bed, sterile technique to prevent infection, adequate graft immobilization, and skilled care.

The size and depth of the patient's burns determine whether the burns will require grafting. Grafting usually occurs at the completion of wound debridement. The goal is to cover all wounds with an autograft or allograft within 2 weeks. With enzymatic debridement, grafting may be performed 5 to 7 days after debridement is complete; with surgical debridement, grafting can occur the same day as the surgery.

Depending on your facility's policy, a doctor or a specially trained nurse may change graft dressings. The dressings usually stay in place for 3 to 5 days after surgery *to avoid disturbing the graft site.* Meanwhile, the donor graft site needs diligent care. (See *How to care for a donor graft site.*)

Equipment
Ordered analgesic ▪ gloves ▪ sterile gloves ▪ sterile gown ▪ cap ▪ mask ▪ sterile forceps ▪ sterile scissors ▪ sterile scalpel ▪ sterile 4″ × 4″ gauze pads ▪ Xeroflo gauze ▪ elastic gauze dressing ▪ warm normal saline solution ▪ moisturizing cream ▪ topical medication (such as micronized silver sulfadiazine cream) ▪ Optional: sterile, cotton-tipped applicators.

Preparation of equipment
Verify the doctor's order. Gather the equipment on the dressing cart. Perform hand hygiene and prepare a sterile field.[1,2,3] Label all medications, medication containers, and solutions on and off the sterile field.[4]

Implementation
▪ Confirm the patient's identity using at least two patient identifiers according to your facility's policy.[5]
▪ Explain the procedure to the patient and provide privacy.
▪ Following safe medication administration practices,[6] administer an analgesic, as ordered, at an appropriate time (depending on the medication's peak and onset of action) before beginning the procedure. Alternatively, give an IV analgesic immediately before the procedure.
▪ Perform hand hygiene and put on the sterile gown and the clean mask, cap, and gloves.[1,2,3]
▪ Gently lift off all outer dressings. Soak the middle dressings with warm saline solution. Remove these carefully and slowly *to avoid disturbing the graft site.* Leave the Xeroflo intact *to avoid dislodging the graft.*
▪ Remove and discard the gloves, perform hand hygiene, and put on the sterile gloves.[1,2,3]
▪ Assess the condition of the graft. If you see purulent drainage, notify the doctor.
▪ Remove the Xeroflo with sterile forceps, and clean the area gently. If necessary, soak the Xeroflo with warm saline solution *to ease removal.*
▪ Inspect an allograft for signs of rejection, such as infection and delayed healing. Inspect a sheet graft frequently for blebs. If ordered, evacuate them carefully with a sterile scalpel. (See *Evacuating fluid from a sheet graft,* page 658.)
▪ Apply topical medication if ordered following safe medication administration practices.[6]
▪ Place fresh Xeroflo over the site *to promote wound healing and prevent infection.* Use sterile scissors to cut the appropriate size. Cover the Xeroflo with 4″ × 4″ gauze and elastic gauze dressing.
▪ Assess the donor site.
▪ Clean any completely healed areas, and apply prescribed moisturizing cream to them *to keep the skin pliable and to retard scarring.*
▪ Discard equipment and supplies according to your facility's policy.
▪ Remove and discard your personal protective equipment and perform hand hygiene.[1,2,3]
▪ Document the procedure.[7]

Special considerations
▪ *To avoid dislodging the graft,* hydrotherapy is usually discontinued by the doctor, as ordered, for 3 to 4 days after grafting. Avoid using a blood pressure cuff over the graft. Don't tug or pull dressings during dressing changes. Keep the patient from lying on the graft.

How to care for a donor graft site

Autografts are usually taken from another area of the patient's body with a dermatome, an instrument that cuts uniform, split-thickness skin portions—typically, about 0.013 to 0.05 cm thick. Autografting makes the donor site a partial-thickness wound, which may bleed, drain, and cause pain.

The donor site needs scrupulous care *to prevent infection, which could convert the site to a full-thickness wound.* Depending on the graft's thickness, tissue may be obtained from the donor site again in as few as 10 days.

Usually, Xeroflo grease gauze is applied to the donor site postoperatively. The outer gauze dressing can be taken off on the first postoperative day; the Xeroflo will protect the new epithelial proliferation. In addition to Xeroflo, the donor site may be dressed in scarlet red, an antibiotic-impregnated gauze, or a synthetic skin substitute.

Care for the donor site as you care for the autograft, using dressing changes at the initial stages to prevent infection and promote healing. Follow the guidelines below.

Dressing the wound
- Perform hand hygiene and put on sterile gloves.[1,2,3]
- Remove the outer gauze dressings within 24 hours. Inspect the Xeroflo for signs of infection; then leave it open to the air *to speed drying and healing.*
- Leave small amounts of fluid accumulation alone. Using sterile technique, aspirate larger amounts through the dressing with a small-gauge needle and syringe.
- Don't apply any creams to the donor site until it's dry.
- When dry, a thin layer of cream, according to the doctor's preference, may be applied on a daily basis to keep the skin tissue pliable.
- As the donor site heals, the Xeroflo starts to lift up at the edges. Excess Xeroflo may be trimmed away with scissors.

- If the graft dislodges, apply sterile skin compresses *to keep the area moist until the surgeon reapplies the graft.* If the graft affects an arm or a leg, elevate the affected extremity *to reduce postoperative edema.* Check for bleeding and signs of neurovascular impairment—increasing pain, numbness or tingling, coolness, and pallor.
- The patient is generally allowed to shower after the 5th postoperative day at the discretion of the doctor.

Patient teaching

Teach the patient about graft and donor site care. Teach the patient how to apply moisturizing cream to healed areas. Stress the importance of using a sunscreen with a sun protection containing titanium dioxide or oxybenzone factor of 20 or higher on all grafted areas *to avoid sunburn and discoloration.*

Complications

Graft failure may result from traumatic injury, hematoma or seroma formation, infection, an inadequate graft bed, rejection, or compromised nutritional status.

Documentation

Record the time and date of all dressing changes. Document all medications used, and note the patient's response to the medications. Describe the condition of the graft, and note any signs of infection or rejection. Record any additional treatment, and note the patient's reaction to the graft. Document any patient teaching provided.

REFERENCES

1 Centers for Disease Control and Prevention. (October 2002). Guideline for hand hygiene in health-care settings. *Morbidity and Mortality Weekly Report, 51*(RR-16), 1–45. (Level I)

2 World Health Organization. (2009). *WHO guidelines on hand hygiene in health care: First global patient safety challenge. Clean care is safer care.* Geneva, Switzerland: World Health Organization. (Level I)

3 The Joint Commission. (2012). Standard NPSG.07.01.01. *Comprehensive accreditation manual for hospitals: The official handbook.* Oakbrook Terrace, IL: The Joint Commission. (Level I)

4 The Joint Commission. (2012). Standard NPSG.03.04.01. *Comprehensive accreditation manual for hospitals: The official handbook.* Oakbrook Terrace, IL: The Joint Commission. (Level I)

5 The Joint Commission. (2012). Standard NPSG.01.01.01. *Comprehensive accreditation manual for hospitals: The official handbook.* Oakbrook Terrace, IL: The Joint Commission. (Level I)

6 The Joint Commission. (2012). Standard MM.06.01.01. *Comprehensive accreditation manual for hospitals: The official handbook.* Oakbrook Terrace, IL: The Joint Commission. (Level I)

7 The Joint Commission. (2012). Standard RC.01.03.01. *Comprehensive accreditation manual for hospitals: The official handbook.* Oakbrook Terrace, IL: The Joint Commission. (Level I)

ADDITIONAL REFERENCES

Joanna Briggs Institute. (2002). "Split Thickness Skin Graft Donor Sites: Post Harvest Management" [Online]. Accessed December 2011 via the Web at http://connect.jbiconnectplus.org/ViewSourceFile.aspx?0=4325

Siegel, J.D., et al. "2007 Guideline for Isolation Precautions: Preventing Transmission of Infectious Agents in Healthcare Settings" [Online]. Accessed December 2011 via the Web at http://www.cdc.gov/hicpac/2007ip/2007isolationprecautions.html

Terrill, P.J., et al. (2007). Split-thickness skin graft donor sites: A comparative study of two absorbent dressings. *Journal of Wound Care, 16*(10), 433–438.

Evacuating fluid from a sheet graft

When small pockets of fluid (called *blebs*) accumulate beneath a sheet graft, you'll need to evacuate the fluid using a sterile scalpel and cotton-tipped applicators. First, carefully perforate the center of the bleb with the scalpel.

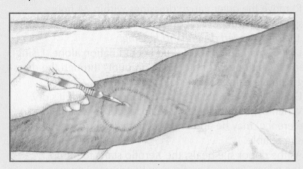

Gently express the fluid with the cotton-tipped applicators.

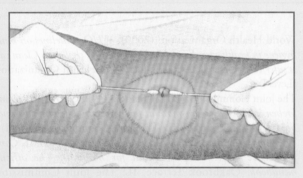

Never express fluid by rolling the bleb to the edge of the graft. This disturbs healing in other areas.

SKIN STAPLE AND CLIP REMOVAL

Skin staples or clips may be used instead of standard sutures to close lacerations or surgical wounds. Because they can secure a wound more quickly than sutures, they may substitute for surface sutures where cosmetic results aren't a prime consideration, such as in abdominal closure. When properly placed, staples and clips distribute tension evenly along the suture line with minimal tissue trauma and compression, promoting healing and minimizing scarring. Because staples and clips are made from surgical stainless steel, tissue reaction to them is minimal. Doctors typically remove skin staples and clips, but some facilities permit qualified nurses to perform this procedure.

Skin staples and clips are contraindicated when the wound's location requires cosmetically superior results or when the incision site makes it impossible to maintain at least a 5-mm distance between the staple and the underlying bone, vessels, or internal organs.

Equipment

Waterproof trash bag ■ adjustable light ■ gloves (if needed) ■ sterile gloves ■ sterile gauze pads ■ sterile staple or clip extractor ■ antiseptic cleaning agent ■ sterile cotton-tipped applicators ■ Optional: butterfly or regular adhesive strips, compound benzoin tincture or other skin protectant.

Prepackaged, sterile, disposable staple or clip extractors are available.

Preparation of equipment

Gather all equipment in the patient's room. Check the expiration date on each sterile package and inspect for tears. Open the waterproof trash bag, and place it near the patient's bed. Position the bag *to avoid reaching across the sterile field or the wound when disposing of soiled articles.* Form a cuff by turning down the top of the bag *to provide a wide opening, thus preventing contamination of instruments or gloves by touching the bag's edge.*

Implementation

■ If your facility allows you to remove skin staples and clips, check the doctor's order *to confirm the exact timing and details for this procedure.*
■ Confirm the patient's identity using at least two patient identifiers according to your facility's policy.[1]
■ Check for patient allergies, especially to adhesive tape and topical solutions or medications.
■ Explain the procedure to the patient. Tell him that he may feel a slight pulling or tickling sensation, but little discomfort, during staple removal. Reassure him that, *because his incision is healing properly,* removing the supporting staples or clips won't weaken the incision line.
■ Provide privacy, and place the patient in a comfortable position that doesn't place undue tension on the incision. *Because some patients experience nausea or dizziness during the procedure,* have the patient recline if possible. Adjust the light to shine directly on the incision.
■ Perform hand hygiene.[2,3,4]
■ If the patient's wound has a dressing, put on gloves and carefully remove it.
■ Discard the dressing and the gloves in the waterproof trash bag.
■ Perform hand hygiene.[2,3,4]
■ Assess the patient's incision. Notify the doctor of gaping, drainage, inflammation, and other signs of infection.
■ Establish a sterile work area with all the equipment and supplies you'll need for removing staples or clips and for cleaning and dressing the incision. Open the package containing the sterile staple or clip extractor, maintaining asepsis.
■ Perform hand hygiene and put on sterile gloves.[2,3,4]
■ Wipe the incision gently with sterile gauze pads soaked in an antiseptic cleaning agent or with sterile cotton-tipped applicators *to remove surface encrustations.*
■ Pick up the sterile staple or clip extractor. Then, starting at one end of the incision, remove the staple or clip. (See *Removing a staple.*) Hold the extractor over the trash bag, and release the handle to discard the staple or clip.
■ Repeat the procedure for each staple or clip until all are removed.

Removing a staple

Position the extractor's lower jaws beneath the span of the first staple (as shown below). Next, squeeze the handles until they're completely closed; then lift the staple away from the skin. The extractor changes the shape of the staple and pulls the prongs out of the intradermal tissue.

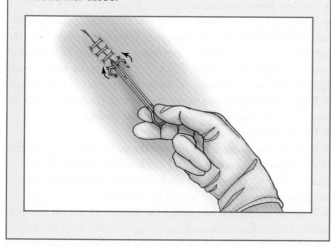

- Apply a sterile gauze dressing, if needed, *to prevent infection and irritation from clothing.*
- Make sure the patient is comfortable. According to the doctor's preference, inform the patient that he may shower in 1 or 2 days if the incision is dry and healing well.
- Properly dispose of solutions and the trash bag. Clean or dispose of soiled equipment and supplies according to facility policy.
- Remove and discard your gloves. Perform hand hygiene.[2,3,4]
- Document the procedure.[5]

Special considerations

- Carefully check the doctor's order for the time and extent of staple or clip removal. The doctor may want you to remove only alternate staples or clips initially and to leave the others in place for an additional day or two *to support the incision.*
- When removing a staple or clip, place the extractor's jaws carefully between the patient's skin and the staple or clip *to avoid patient discomfort.* If extraction is difficult, notify the doctor; *staples or clips placed too deeply within the skin or left in place too long may resist removal.*
- If the wound dehisces after staples or clips are removed, apply butterfly or regular adhesive strips to approximate and support the edges, and call the doctor immediately to repair the wound. (See *Types of adhesive skin closures.*)
- You may also apply butterfly or regular adhesive strips after removing staples or clips even if the wound is healing normally *to give added support to the incision and prevent lateral tension from forming a wide scar.* Use a small amount of compound benzoin tincture or other skin protectant *to ensure adherence.* Leave the strips in place for 3 to 5 days.

Types of adhesive skin closures

Regular adhesive strips are used as a primary means of keeping a wound closed after suture removal. They're made of thin strips of sterile, nonwoven, porous fabric tape.

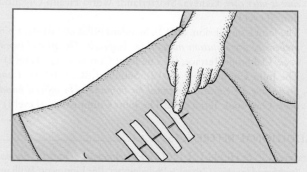

Butterfly adhesive strips consist of sterile, waterproof adhesive strips. A narrow, nonadhesive "bridge" connects the two expanded adhesive portions. These strips are used to close small wounds and to assist healing after suture removal.

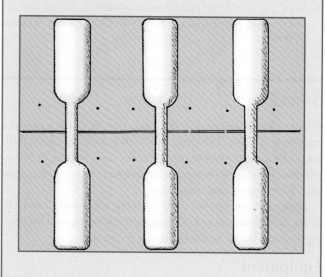

Patient teaching

If the patient is being discharged, teach him how to remove the dressing and care for the wound. Instruct him to call the doctor immediately if he observes wound discharge or any other abnormal change. Tell him the redness surrounding the incision should gradually disappear, and that after a few weeks only a thin line should show.

Documentation

Record the date and time of staple or clip removal, the number of staples or clips removed, appearance of the incision, dressings or adhesive strips applied, signs of wound complications, the patient's tolerance of the procedure, and any patient teaching provided.

REFERENCES

1 The Joint Commission. (2012). Standard NPSG.01.01.01. *Comprehensive accreditation manual for hospitals: The official handbook.* Oakbrook Terrace, IL: The Joint Commission. (Level I)

2 Centers for Disease Control and Prevention. (October 2002). Guideline for hand hygiene in health-care settings. *Morbidity and Mortality Weekly Report, 51*(RR-16), 1–45. (Level I)

3 World Health Organization. (2009). *WHO guidelines on hand hygiene in health care: First global patient safety challenge. Clean care is safer care.* Geneva, Switzerland: World Health Organization. (Level I)

4 The Joint Commission. (2012). Standard NPSG.07.01.01. *Comprehensive accreditation manual for hospitals: The official handbook.* Oakbrook Terrace, IL: The Joint Commission. (Level I)

5 The Joint Commission. (2012). Standard RC.01.03.01. *Comprehensive accreditation manual for hospitals: The official handbook.* Oakbrook Terrace, IL: The Joint Commission. (Level I)

ADDITIONAL REFERENCES

Craven, R.F., & Hirnle, C.J. (2012). *Fundamentals of nursing: Human health and function* (7th ed.). Philadelphia, PA: Lippincott Williams & Wilkins.

Dhillon, H., & Randhawa, V. (2009). The D stitch: An efficient method to facilitate suture removal. *Orthopedics, 32*(1), 29.

Nettina, S.M. (2010). *Lippincott manual of nursing practice* (9th ed.). Philadelphia, PA: Lippincott Williams & Wilkins.

Taylor, C., et al. (2011). *Fundamentals of nursing: The art and science of nursing care* (7th ed.). Philadelphia, PA: Lippincott Williams & Wilkins.

SOAKS

A soak involves immersion of a body part in warm water or a medicated solution. This treatment helps to soften exudates, facilitate debridement, enhance suppuration, clean wounds or burns, rehydrate wounds, apply medication to infected areas, and increase local blood supply and circulation.

Most soaks are applied with clean tap water and clean technique. Sterile solution and sterile equipment are required for treating wounds, burns, and other breaks in the skin.

Equipment

Basin, or arm or foot tub ■ bath (utility) thermometer ■ warm tap water or prescribed solution ■ cup ■ pitcher ■ linen-saver pad ■ overbed table ■ footstool ■ pillows ■ towels ■ gauze pads and other dressing materials ■ gloves ■ sterile gloves.

Preparation of equipment

Clean and disinfect the basin or tub. Run warm tap water into a pitcher or heat the prescribed solution, as applicable. Measure the water or solution temperature with a bath thermometer. If the temperature isn't within the prescribed range (usually 105° to 110° F [40.6° to 43.3° C]), add hot or cold water or reheat or cool the solution, as needed.

If you're preparing the soak outside the patient's room, heat the liquid slightly above the correct temperature *to allow for cooling during transport.* If the solution for a medicated soak isn't premixed, prepare the solution and heat it.

Implementation

■ Check the doctor's order and check for a history of an allergy to the medicated solution, as appropriate.

■ Confirm the patient's identity using at least two patient identifiers according to your facility's policy.[1]

■ Provide privacy. Explain the procedure to the patient.

■ Perform hand hygiene and put on gloves.[2,3,4]

■ If the soak basin or tub will be placed in bed, make sure the bed is flat beneath it *to prevent spills.* For an arm soak, have the patient sit erect. For a leg or foot soak, ask him to lie down and bend the appropriate knee. For a foot soak in the sitting position, let him sit on the edge of the bed or transfer him to a chair.

■ Place a linen-saver pad under the treatment site and, if necessary, cover the pad with a towel *to absorb spillage.*

■ Expose the treatment site.

■ Remove any dressing; dispose of the soiled dressing properly. If the dressing is encrusted and stuck to the wound, leave it in place and proceed with the soak. Remove the dressing several minutes later when it has begun to soak free.

■ Position the soak basin under the treatment site on the bed, overbed table, footstool, or floor, as appropriate. Pour the heated liquid into the soak basin or tub. Then lower the arm or leg into the basin gradually *to allow adjustment to the temperature change.* Make sure the soak solution covers the treatment site.

■ Support other body parts with pillows or towels as needed *to prevent discomfort and muscle strain.* Make the patient comfortable and ensure proper body alignment.

■ Check the temperature of the soak solution with the bath thermometer every 5 minutes. If the temperature drops below the prescribed range, remove some of the cooled solution with a cup. Then lift the patient's arm or leg from the basin *to avoid burns,* and add hot water or solution to the basin. Mix the liquid thoroughly and then check its temperature. If the temperature is within the prescribed range, lower the patient's affected part back into the basin.

■ Observe the patient for signs of tissue intolerance: extreme redness at the treatment site, excessive drainage, bleeding, or maceration. If such signs develop or the patient complains of pain, discontinue the treatment and notify the doctor.

■ After 15 to 20 minutes, or as ordered, lift the patient's arm or leg from the basin and remove the basin.

■ Dry the arm or leg thoroughly with a towel. If the patient has a wound, dry the skin around it without touching the wound.

■ While the skin is hydrated from the soak, use gauze pads to remove loose scales or crusts.

■ Observe the treatment area for general appearance, degree of swelling, debridement, suppuration, and healing.

■ Perform hand hygiene and put on sterile gloves and redress the wound, if appropriate.[2,3,4]

■ Remove the towel and linen-saver pad, and make the patient comfortable in bed.

■ Discard the soak solution, dispose of soiled materials properly, and clean and disinfect the basin.

- Remove and discard your gloves. Perform hand hygiene.[2,3,4]
- If the treatment is to be repeated, store the equipment in the patient's room, out of his reach; otherwise, return it to the central supply department.
- Document the procedure.[5]

Special considerations

- To treat large areas, particularly burns, a soak may be administered in a whirlpool or Hubbard tank.

Documentation

Record the date, time, and duration of the soak; treatment site; solution used and its temperature; skin and wound appearance before, during, and after treatment; and the patient's tolerance of treatment.

REFERENCES

1 The Joint Commission. (2012). Standard NPSG.01.01.01. *Comprehensive accreditation manual for hospitals: The official handbook.* Oakbrook Terrace, IL: The Joint Commission. (Level I)
2 Centers for Disease Control and Prevention. (October 2002). Guideline for hand hygiene in health-care settings. *Morbidity and Mortality Weekly Report, 51*(RR-16), 1–45. (Level I)
3 World Health Organization. (2009). *WHO guidelines on hand hygiene in health care: First global patient safety challenge. Clean care is safer care.* Geneva, Switzerland: World Health Organization. (Level I)
4 The Joint Commission. (2012). Standard NPSG.07.01.01. *Comprehensive accreditation manual for hospitals: The official handbook.* Oakbrook Terrace, IL: The Joint Commission. (Level I)
5 The Joint Commission. (2012). Standard RC.01.03.01. *Comprehensive accreditation manual for hospitals: The official handbook.* Oakbrook Terrace, IL: The Joint Commission. (Level I)

ADDITIONAL REFERENCES

Craven, R.F., & Hirnle, C.J. (2012). *Fundamentals of nursing: Human health and function* (7th ed.). Philadelphia, PA: Lippincott Williams & Wilkins.
Taylor, C., et al. (2011). *Fundamentals of nursing: The art and science of nursing care* (7th ed.). Philadelphia, PA: Lippincott Williams & Wilkins.

SPIRITUAL CARE

Religious beliefs can profoundly influence a patient's recovery rate, attitude toward treatment, and overall response to hospitalization. In certain religious groups, beliefs can preclude diagnostic tests and therapeutic treatments, require dietary restrictions, or prohibit organ donation and artificial prolongation of life. (See *Beliefs and practices of selected religions,* pages 662 and 663.)

Because of this, effective patient care requires recognition of and respect for the patient's religious beliefs. Recognizing his beliefs and need for spiritual care may require close attention to his nonverbal cues or to seemingly casual remarks that express his spiritual concerns. Respecting his beliefs may require setting aside your own beliefs to help the patient follow his. Providing spiritual care may require contacting an appropriate member of the clergy in the facility or community, gathering equipment needed to help the patient perform rites and administer sacraments, and preparing him for a pastoral visit.

Equipment

Clean towels (one or two) ▪ container of water (for emergency baptism), if appropriate ▪ other supplies specific to the patient's religious affiliation.

Some facilities, particularly those with a religious affiliation, provide baptismal trays. The clergy member may bring holy water, holy oil, or other religious articles to minister to the patient.

Preparation of equipment

For baptism, cover a small table with a clean towel. Fold a second towel and place it on the table, along with the teaspoon or medicine cup. For communion and anointing, cover the bedside stand with a clean towel.

Implementation

- Check the patient's admission record *to determine his religious affiliation.* Remember that some patients may claim no religious beliefs. However, even an agnostic may wish to speak with a clergy member, so watch and listen carefully for subtle expressions of this desire.
- Perform hand hygiene.[1]
- Evaluate the patient's behavior for signs of loneliness, anxiety, or fear—*emotions that may signal his need for spiritual counsel.* Also consider whether the patient is facing a health crisis, which may occur with chronic illness and before childbirth, surgery, or impending death. Remember that a patient may feel acutely distressed because of his inability to participate in religious observances. Help such a patient verbalize his beliefs *to relieve stress.* Listen to him and let him express his concerns, but carefully refrain from imposing your beliefs on him *to avoid conflict and further stress.*
- If the patient requests, arrange a visit by an appropriate member of the clergy. Consult this clergy member if you need more information about the patient's beliefs.
- If your patient faces the possibility of abortion, amputation, transfusion, or other medical procedures with important religious implications, try to discover his spiritual attitude. Also, try to determine your patient's attitude toward the importance of laying on of hands, confession, communion, observance of holy days (such as the Sabbath), and restrictions in diet or physical appearance. *Helping the patient continue his normal religious practices during hospitalization can help reduce stress.*
- If the patient is pregnant, find out her beliefs concerning infant baptism and circumcision, and comply with them after delivery.
- If a Jewish woman delivers a male infant prematurely or by cesarean birth, ask her whether she plans to observe the rite of circumcision, or a bris, a significant ceremony performed on the 8th day after birth. (*Because a patient who delivers a healthy, full-term*

Beliefs and practices of selected religions

A patient's religious beliefs can affect his attitudes toward illness and traditional medicine. By trying to accommodate the patient's religious beliefs and practices in your plan of care, you can increase his willingness to learn and comply with treatment regimens. Because religious beliefs may vary within particular sects, individual practices may differ from those described here.

Adventist
Birth and death rituals
None (baptism of adults only)
Dietary restrictions
Alcohol, coffee, tea, opioids, and stimulants prohibited; in many groups, meat as well
Practices in health crisis
Communion and baptism performed; some members believe in divine healing, anointing with oil, and prayer; some regard Saturday as the Sabbath

Baptist
Birth and death rituals
At birth, none (baptism of believers only); before death, counseling by clergy member and prayer
Dietary restrictions
Alcohol prohibited; in some groups, coffee and tea as well
Practices in health crisis
Some believe in healing by laying on of hands; resistance to medical therapy occasionally approved

Christian Scientist
Birth and death rituals
At birth, none; before death, counseling by a Christian Science practitioner
Dietary restrictions
Alcohol, coffee, and tobacco prohibited
Practices in health crisis
Many members refuse all treatment, including drugs, biopsies, physical examination, and blood transfusions and permit vaccination only when required by law; alteration of thoughts believed to cure illness; hypnotism and psychotherapy prohibited (Christian Scientist nurses and nursing homes honor these beliefs)

Church of Christ
Birth and death rituals
None (baptism at age 8 or older)
Dietary restrictions
Alcohol discouraged
Practices in health crisis
Communion, anointing with oil, laying on of hands, and counseling performed by a minister

Eastern Orthodox
Birth and death rituals
At birth, baptism and confirmation; before death, last rites; for members of the Russian Orthodox Church, arms are crossed after death, fingers set in cross, and unembalmed body clothed in natural fiber

Dietary restrictions
For members of the Russian Orthodox Church and usually the Greek Orthodox Church, no meat or dairy products on Wednesday or Friday or during Lent
Practices in health crisis
Anointing of the sick; for members of the Russian Orthodox Church, cross necklace is replaced immediately after surgery and shaving of male patients is prohibited except in preparation for surgery; for members of the Greek Orthodox Church, communion and Sacrament of Holy Unction

Episcopalian
Birth and death rituals
At birth, baptism; before death, occasional last rites
Dietary restrictions
For some members, abstention from meat on Friday, fasting before communion (which may be daily)
Practices in health crisis
Communion, prayer, and counseling performed by a minister

Jehovah's Witnesses
Birth and death rituals
None
Dietary restrictions
Abstention from foods to which blood has been added
Practices in health crisis
Typically, no blood transfusions permitted; a court order may be required for emergency transfusion

Judaism
Birth and death rituals
Ritual circumcision on 8th day after birth; burial of dead fetus; ritual washing of dead; burial (including organs and other body tissues) occurs as soon as possible; no autopsy or embalming
Dietary restrictions
For Orthodox and Conservative Jews, kosher dietary laws (for example, pork and shellfish prohibited); for Reform Jews, usually no restrictions
Practices in health crisis
Donation or transplantation of organs requires rabbinical consultation; for Orthodox and Conservative Jews, medical procedures may be prohibited on the Sabbath—from sundown Friday to sundown Saturday—and special holidays

Lutheran
Birth and death rituals
Baptism usually performed 6 to 8 weeks after birth
Dietary restrictions
None

Beliefs and practices of selected religions *(continued)*

Lutheran *(continued)*
Practices in health crisis
Communion, prayer, and counseling performed by a minister

Mormon
Birth and death rituals
At birth, none (baptism at age 8 or older); before death, baptism and Gospel preaching
Dietary restrictions
Alcohol, tobacco, tea, and coffee prohibited; meat intake limited
Practices in health crisis
Belief in divine healing through the laying on of hands; communion on Sunday; some members may refuse medical treatment; many wear a special undergarment

Muslim
Birth and death rituals
If spontaneous abortion occurs before 130 days, fetus treated as discarded tissue; after 130 days, as a human being; before death, confession of sins with family present; after death, only relatives or friends may touch the body
Dietary restrictions
Pork prohibited; daylight fasting during 9th month of Islamic calendar
Practices in health crisis
Faith healing for the patient's morale only; conservative members may reject medical therapy

Orthodox Presbyterian
Birth and death rituals
Infant baptism; scripture reading and prayer before death
Dietary restrictions
None
Practices in health crisis
Communion, prayer, and counseling performed by a minister

Pentecostal Assembly of God, Foursquare Church
Birth and death rituals
None (baptism only after age of accountability)
Dietary restrictions
Abstention from alcohol, tobacco, meat slaughtered by strangling, any food to which blood has been added, and sometimes pork
Practices in health crisis
Divine healing through prayer, anointing with oil, laying on of hands

Roman Catholic
Birth and death rituals
Infant baptism, including baptism of aborted fetus without sign of clinical death (tissue necrosis); before death, anointing of the sick
Dietary restrictions
Fasting or abstention from meat on Ash Wednesday and on Fridays during Lent; this practice usually waived for the hospitalized
Practices in health crisis
Burial of major amputated limb (sometimes) in consecrated ground; donation or transplantation of organs allowed if the benefit to recipient outweighs the donor's potential harm; Sacrament of the Sick also performed when patients are ill, not just before death, and sometimes performed shortly after admission

United Methodist
Birth and death rituals
None (baptism of children and adults only)
Dietary restrictions
None
Practices in health crisis
Communion before surgery or similar crisis; donation of body parts encouraged

---

baby vaginally is usually discharged quickly, this ceremony is normally performed outside the facility.) For a bris, ensure privacy and, if requested, sterilize the instruments.

■ If the patient requests communion, prepare him for it before the clergy member arrives. First, place him in Fowler's or semi-Fowler's position if his condition permits. Otherwise, allow him to remain supine. Tuck a clean towel under his chin and straighten the bed linens.

■ If a terminally ill patient requests the Sacrament of the Sick (last rites) or special treatment of his body after death, call an appropriate clergy member. For the Roman Catholic patient, call a Roman Catholic priest to administer the sacrament, even if the patient is unresponsive or comatose. *To prepare the patient for this sacrament,* uncover his arms and fold back the top linens to expose his feet. After the clergy member anoints the patient's forehead, eyes, nose, mouth, hands, and feet, straighten and retuck the bed linens.

■ Perform hand hygiene.[1,2,3]
■ Document the procedure.[4]

Special considerations
■ Handle the patient's religious articles carefully *to avoid damage or loss.*
■ Become familiar with religious resources in your facility. Some facilities employ one or more clergy members who counsel patients and staff members and link patients to other pastoral resources.
■ If the patient tries to convert you to his personal beliefs, tell him that you respect his beliefs but are content with your own. Likewise, avoid attempts to convert the patient to your personal beliefs.

Documentation
If baptism was performed, complete a baptismal form and attach it to the patient's record; send a copy of the form to the

EQUIPMENT

Rigid splint

A rigid splint can be used to immobilize a fracture or dislocation in an extremity, as shown on right. Ideally, two people should apply a rigid splint to an extremity.

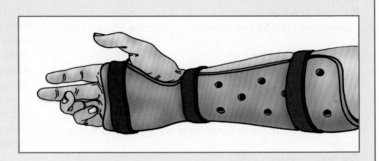

appropriate clergy member. Record the rites of circumcision and last rites in your notes. Also, record last rites in red on the Kardex so it won't be repeated unnecessarily.

REFERENCES

1 The Joint Commission. (2012). Standard NPSG.07.01.01. *Comprehensive accreditation manual for hospitals: The official handbook.* Oakbrook Terrace, IL: The Joint Commission. (Level I)
2 Centers for Disease Control and Prevention. (October 2002). Guideline for hand hygiene in health-care settings. *Morbidity and Mortality Weekly Report, 51*(RR-16), 1–45. (Level I)
3 World Health Organization. (2009). *WHO guidelines on hand hygiene in health care: First global patient safety challenge. Clean care is safer care.* Geneva, Switzerland: World Health Organization. (Level I)
4 The Joint Commission. (2012). Standard RC.01.03.01. *Comprehensive accreditation manual for hospitals: The official handbook.* Oakbrook Terrace, IL: The Joint Commission. (Level I)

ADDITIONAL REFERENCES

McBrien, B. (2010). Emergency nurses' provision of spiritual care: A literature review. *British Journal of Nursing, 19*(12), 768–773.
Robinson, S. (2008). *Spirituality, ethics and care.* Philadelphia, PA: Jessica Kingsley Publishers.
Sartori, P. (2010). Spirituality. 2: Exploring how to address patients' spiritual needs in practice. *Nursing Times, 106*(29), 23–25.

SPLINT APPLICATION

By immobilizing the site of an injury, a splint alleviates pain and allows the injury to heal in proper alignment. It also minimizes possible complications, such as excessive bleeding into tissues and restricted blood flow caused by bone pressing against vessels. In cases of multiple serious injuries, a splint allows caretakers to move the patient without risking further damage to bones, muscles, nerves, blood vessels, and skin.

A splint can be applied to immobilize a simple or compound fracture, a dislocation, or a subluxation. (See *Rigid splint.*)

During an emergency, any injury suspected of being a fracture, dislocation, or subluxation should be splinted. No contraindications exist for rigid splints.

Equipment

Rigid splint ▪ bindings ▪ padding ▪ sandbags or rolled towels or clothing ▪ Optional: rolled gauze, cloth strips, sterile compress, ice bag.

An inflatable semirigid splint, called an *air splint,* sometimes can be used to secure an injured extremity. (See *Using an air splint.*) Velcro straps, 2″ roller gauze, or 2″ cloth strips can be used as bindings. However, avoid using twine or rope, if possible, *because they can restrict circulation.*

Implementation

▪ Confirm the patient's identity using at least two patient identifiers according to your facility's policy.[1]
▪ Obtain a complete history of the injury, if possible.
▪ Provide emotional support to the patient. Explain all procedures to him *to allay his fears.*
▪ Perform hand hygiene, and follow standard precautions.[2,3,4]
▪ Begin a thorough head-to-toe assessment, inspecting for obvious deformities, swelling, or bleeding.
▪ Ask the patient if he can move his extremities.
▪ Inspect and palpate the injured area for evidence of fracture or dislocation.
▪ If necessary, remove or cut away the patient's clothing and remove jewelry.
▪ Check the neurovascular integrity distal to the injury site.
▪ If possible, align the injured extremity in its normal anatomic position.
▪ Don't attempt to straighten a dislocation *to avoid damaging misplaced vessels and nerves.*
▪ Apply a sterile compress to any open wound. Don't attempt reduction of a contaminated bone end *because this may cause additional laceration of soft tissues, vessels, and nerves as well gross contamination of deep tissues.*
▪ Choose a splint that will immobilize the joints above and below the fracture.
▪ Pad the splint, as needed, *to protect bony prominences.*

EQUIPMENT

Using an air splint

In an emergency, an air splint can be applied to immobilize a fracture or control bleeding, especially from a forearm or lower leg. This compact, comfortable splint is made of double-walled plastic and provides gentle, diffuse pressure over an injured area. The appropriate splint is chosen, wrapped around the affected extremity, secured with Velcro or other strips, and then inflated. The fit should be snug enough to immobilize the extremity without impairing circulation.

An air splint (shown on right) may actually control bleeding better than a local pressure bandage. It's clear plastic construction simplifies inspection of the affected site for bleeding, pallor, or cyanosis. An air splint also allows the patient to be moved without further damage to the injured limb.

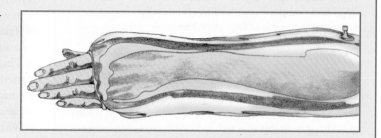

■ Support the injured extremity above and below the fracture site while applying firm, gentle traction.
■ Have an assistant place the splint under, beside, or on top of the extremity.
■ Have the assistant apply the bindings to secure the splint, being careful not to compromise the circulation.
■ Assess the neurovascular status of the extremity. If it's impaired by the bindings, release and reapply them.
■ Monitor the patient's vital signs frequently *to detect signs of shock.* Fractured bones may cause significant bleeding into surrounding tissues.
■ Monitor the patient's neurovascular status by assessing skin color, temperature of the extremities, level of pain, presence of paresthesia, and pulses as well as the patient's ability to move his extremities. Numbness or paralysis distal to an injury indicates nerve injury. (See *Assessing neurovascular status,* page 666.)
■ Apply ice to the injury.
■ Perform hand hygiene.[2,3,4]
■ Document the procedure.[5]

Special considerations

■ At an accident scene, always examine the patient completely for other injuries. Avoid unnecessary movement or manipulation of the patient, *which might cause additional pain or injury.*
■ Always consider the possibility of a cervical spine injury in an unconscious patient. If possible, apply the splint before repositioning the patient.
■ If the patient requires a rigid splint and one isn't available, another body part can be used as a splint. To splint a leg in this manner, pad the inner aspect and secure it to the other leg with rolled gauze or cloth strips.
■ Arrange transport of the patient to a hospital as soon as possible.
■ Under a doctor's direct supervision, apply gentle traction, and carefully remove a splint if there's evidence of improper application or vascular impairment.

Complications

Multiple transfers and repeated manipulation of fractures may cause fat embolism. This complication usually occurs within 24 to 72 hours of an injury or manipulation. Signs and symptoms of fat embolism include dyspnea, agitation, hypoxia, changes in mental status, and a petechial rash.

Documentation

Record the cause and circumstances surrounding the injury. Document the patient's subjective complaints, noting whether his symptoms are localized. Record the neurovascular assessment before and after applying the splint. Note the type of wound and the type and amount of any drainage. Note the time when the splint was applied. Be sure to note if the bone end slips into surrounding tissue or if transportation causes any change in the degree of dislocation.

REFERENCES

1 The Joint Commission. (2012). Standard NPSG.01.01.01. *Comprehensive accreditation manual for hospitals: The official handbook.* Oakbrook Terrace, IL: The Joint Commission. (Level I)
2 The Joint Commission. (2012). Standard NPSG.07.01.01. *Comprehensive accreditation manual for hospitals: The official handbook.* Oakbrook Terrace, IL: The Joint Commission. (Level I)
3 Centers for Disease Control and Prevention. (October 2002). Guideline for hand hygiene in health-care settings. *Morbidity and Mortality Weekly Report, 51*(RR-16), 1–45. (Level I)
4 World Health Organization. (2009). *WHO guidelines on hand hygiene in health care: First global patient safety challenge. Clean care is safer care.* Geneva, Switzerland: World Health Organization. (Level I)
5 The Joint Commission. (2012). Standard RC.01.03.01. *Comprehensive accreditation manual for hospitals: The official handbook.* Oakbrook Terrace, IL: The Joint Commission. (Level I)

ADDITIONAL REFERENCE

Proehl, J.A. (2008). *Emergency nursing procedures* (4th ed.). Philadelphia, PA: Saunders.

Assessing neurovascular status

When assessing an injured extremity, include these steps and compare your findings bilaterally.
- Inspect the color of fingers or toes.
- *To detect edema,* note the size of the digits.
- Simultaneously touch the digits of the affected and unaffected extremities and compare temperature.
- Check capillary refill by pressing on the distal tip of one digit until it's white. Then release the pressure and note how soon the normal color returns. It should return quickly in both the affected and unaffected extremities.
- Check sensation by touching the fingers or toes and asking the patient how they feel. Note reports of any numbness or tingling.
- *To check proprioception,* tell the patient to close his eyes; then move one digit and ask him which position it's in.
- *To test movement,* tell the patient to wiggle his toes or move his fingers.
- Palpate the distal pulses *to assess vascular patency.*

Record your findings for the affected and the unaffected extremities, using standard terminology to avoid ambiguity. Warmth, free movement, rapid capillary refill, and normal color, sensation, and proprioception indicate sound neurovascular status.

SPONGE BATH

A sponge bath with tepid water reduces fever by dilating superficial blood vessels, thus releasing heat and lowering body temperature. A tepid-water sponge bath may lower systemic temperature when routine fever treatments fail, particularly for infants and children, whose temperatures tend to rise very high, very quickly.

Equipment

Basin of tepid water, about 80° to 93° F (26.7° to 33.9° C) ▪ bath (utility) thermometer ▪ bath blanket ▪ linen-saver pad ▪ washcloths ▪ patient thermometer ▪ hot-water bottle and cover ▪ ice bag and cover ▪ towel ▪ clean patient gown ▪ gloves, if the patient has open lesions or has been incontinent ▪ antipyretics as ordered.

Preparation of equipment

Prepare a hot-water bottle and an ice bag. Then place the bath thermometer in a basin, and run water over it until the temperature reaches the high end of the tepid range (93° F) *because the water will cool during the bath.* Immerse the washcloths in the tepid solution until saturated.

Implementation

- Confirm the patient's identity using at least two patient identifiers according to your facility's policy.[1]
- Check the medication record for recent administration of an antipyretic *because this type of drug can affect the patient's response to the bath.*

- Explain the procedure to the patient, provide privacy, and make sure the room is warm and free from drafts.
- Perform hand hygiene and put on gloves, if necessary.[2,3,4]
- Place a linen-saver pad under the patient *to catch any spills* and a bath blanket over him *for privacy.* Then remove his gown. Also remove the top bed linen *to avoid wetting it.*
- Take the patient's temperature, pulse, and respirations *to serve as a baseline.*
- Place the hot-water bottle with protective covering on the patient's feet *to reduce the sensation of chilliness.* Place the covered ice bag on his head *to prevent headache and nasal congestion that occur as the rest of the body cools.*
- Wring out each washcloth before sponging the patient *so the water doesn't drip and cause discomfort.*
- Place moist washcloths over the major superficial blood vessels in the axillae, groin, and popliteal areas *to accelerate cooling.* Change the washcloths as they warm.
- Bathe each extremity separately for about 5 minutes; then sponge the chest and abdomen for 5 minutes. Turn the patient, and bathe his back and buttocks for 5 to 10 minutes. Keep the patient covered except for the body part you're sponging.
- Pat each area dry after sponging but avoid rubbing with the towel *because rubbing increases cell metabolism and produces heat.*
- Add warm water to the basin as necessary *to maintain the desired water temperature.*
- Check the patient's temperature, pulse, and respirations every 10 minutes. Notify the doctor if the patient's temperature doesn't fall within 30 minutes.
- Observe the patient for chills, shivering, pallor, mottling, cyanosis of the lips or nail beds, and changes in vital signs—especially a rapid, weak, or irregular pulse—*because such signs may indicate an emergency.* If any of these signs occur, discontinue the bath, cover the patient lightly, and notify the doctor.
- If no adverse effects occur, bathe the patient for at least 30 minutes or until the patient's temperature reaches 1° to 2° F (0.6° to 1° C) above the desired level *because his temperature will continue to fall naturally.* Continue to monitor his temperature until it stabilizes.
- After the bath, make sure the patient is dry and comfortable. Dress him in a fresh gown and cover him lightly.
- Dispose of liquids and soiled materials properly. If the treatment will be repeated, clean and store the equipment in the patient's room.
- Check the patient's temperature, pulse, and respirations 30 minutes after the bath *to determine the treatment's effectiveness.*
- Perform hand hygiene.[2,3,4]
- Document the procedure.[5]

Special considerations

- If ordered, administer an antipyretic 15 to 20 minutes before the sponge bath *to achieve more rapid fever reduction.* Consider covering the patient's trunk with a wet towel for 15 minutes *to speed cooling.* Resaturate the towel as necessary.
- Refrain from bathing the breasts of a postpartum patient *because they could become overly dry or fissures could develop on the nipples.*
- Take a rectal temperature, unless contraindicated, *for accuracy.* Axillary temperatures are unreliable *because the cool compresses*

applied to these areas alter the readings. However, taking a tympanic temperature gives the temperature reading more quickly.

Complications

Accelerated temperature reduction can provoke seizure activity.

Documentation

Record the date, time, and duration of the bath; the temperature of the water; the patient's temperature, pulse, and respirations before, during, and after the procedure; any complications and interventions; and the patient's tolerance to the treatment.

REFERENCES

1 The Joint Commission. (2012). Standard NPSG.01.01.01. *Comprehensive accreditation manual for hospitals: The official handbook.* Oakbrook Terrace, IL: The Joint Commission. (Level I)
2 Centers for Disease Control and Prevention. (October 2002). Guideline for hand hygiene in health-care settings. *Morbidity and Mortality Weekly Report, 51*(RR-16), 1–45. (Level I)
3 World Health Organization. (2009). *WHO guidelines on hand hygiene in health care: First global patient safety challenge. Clean care is safer care.* Geneva, Switzerland: World Health Organization. (Level I)
4 The Joint Commission. (2012). Standard NPSG.07.01.01. *Comprehensive accreditation manual for hospitals: The official handbook.* Oakbrook Terrace, IL: The Joint Commission. (Level I)
5 The Joint Commission. (2012). Standard RC.01.03.01. *Comprehensive accreditation manual for hospitals: The official handbook.* Oakbrook Terrace, IL: The Joint Commission. (Level I)

ADDITIONAL REFERENCES

Nettina, S.M. (2010). *Lippincott manual of nursing practice* (9th ed.). Philadelphia, PA: Lippincott Williams & Wilkins.
Taylor, C., et al. (2011). *Fundamentals of nursing: The art and science of nursing care* (7th ed.). Philadelphia, PA: Lippincott Williams & Wilkins.

SPUTUM COLLECTION

Secreted by mucous membranes lining the bronchioles, bronchi, and trachea, sputum helps protect the respiratory tract from infection. When expelled from the respiratory tract, sputum carries saliva, nasal and sinus secretions, dead cells, and normal oral bacteria from the respiratory tract. Sputum specimens may be cultured for identification of respiratory pathogens.

The usual method of sputum specimen collection, expectoration, may require ultrasonic nebulization, hydration, chest percussion, and postural drainage to help mobilize the secretions.

Tracheal suctioning is contraindicated within 1 hour of eating and in patients with esophageal varices, nausea, facial or basilar skull fractures, laryngospasm, or bronchospasm. It should be performed cautiously in patients with heart disease because it may precipitate arrhythmias.

Equipment

For expectoration

Sterile specimen container with tight-fitting cap ▪ gloves ▪ specimen label ▪ laboratory request form and laboratory biohazard transport bag ▪ facial tissues ▪ emesis basin ▪ mask ▪ goggles or face shield ▪ supplies for oral hygiene ▪ Optional: aerosol (10% sodium chloride, propylene glycol, acetylcysteine, or sterile or distilled water), as ordered.

For tracheal suctioning

#12 to #14 French sterile suction catheter ▪ water-soluble lubricant ▪ laboratory request form and laboratory biohazard transport bag ▪ specimen label ▪ sterile gloves ▪ mask ▪ goggles ▪ sterile in-line specimen trap (Lukens trap) ▪ normal saline solution ▪ portable suction machine, if wall unit is unavailable ▪ oxygen therapy equipment.

Commercial suction kits have all equipment except the suction apparatus and an in-line specimen container.

Implementation

▪ Verify the doctor's order.
▪ Gather the appropriate equipment.
▪ Perform hand hygiene.[1,2,3]
▪ Confirm the patient's identity using at least two patient identifiers according to your facility's policy.[4]
▪ Explain the need to collect a specimen of sputum (not saliva), and the procedure *to promote cooperation.* If possible, collect the specimen early in the morning, before breakfast, *because secretions have accumulated overnight, aiding in the collection process.*
▪ Have all supplies within reach.
▪ Instruct the patient to sit in a chair or at the edge of the bed. If he can't sit up, place him in high Fowler's position.
▪ Perform hand hygiene and put on a mask, eye protection, and gloves.[1,2,3]
▪ Perform nebulizer treatment, chest percussion, and postural drainage *to assist specimen production,* as needed.

Sputum collection by expectoration

▪ Ask the patient to rinse his mouth with water *to reduce specimen contamination.* (Avoid mouthwash or toothpaste *because they may affect the mobility of organisms in the sputum sample.*) Then tell him to cough deeply and expectorate directly into the specimen container. Instruct the patient not to touch the inside of the cup. Ask him to produce at least 15 mL of sputum, if possible.
▪ Cap the container and, if necessary, clean its exterior.

NURSING ALERT *If the patient has asthma or chronic bronchitis, watch for aggravated bronchospasms with the use of more than a 10% concentration of sodium chloride or acetylcysteine in an aerosol.*

Sputum collection by tracheal suctioning

▪ Explain the suctioning procedure to him and tell him that he may cough, gag, or feel short of breath during the procedure.
▪ Check the suction equipment *to make sure it's functioning properly.* Then place the patient in high Fowler's or semi-Fowler's position.
▪ Administer oxygen to the patient before beginning the procedure.
▪ Perform hand hygiene.[1,2,3]
▪ Put on a mask and eye protection, as appropriate.

EQUIPMENT

Attaching a specimen trap to a suction catheter

Wearing gloves, push the suction tubing onto the male adapter of the in-line trap.

Insert the suction catheter into the rubber tubing of the trap.

After suctioning, disconnect the in-line trap from the suction tubing and catheter. To seal the container, connect the rubber tubing to the male adapter of the trap.

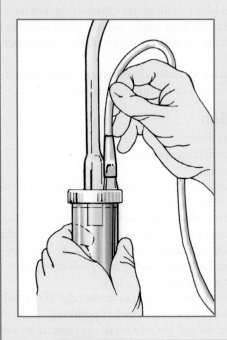

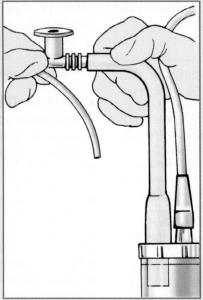

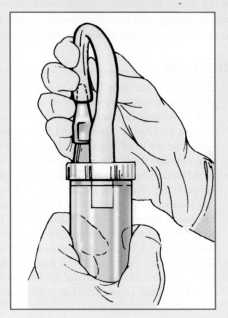

■ Put on sterile gloves. Consider the suction catheter hand sterile and the other hand clean *to prevent cross-contamination.*[5,6]

■ Connect the suction tubing to the male adapter of the in-line specimen trap. Attach the sterile suction catheter to the rubber tubing of the trap. (See *Attaching a specimen trap to a suction catheter.*)

■ Tell the patient to tilt his head back slightly. Then lubricate the catheter with normal saline solution, and gently pass it through the patient's nostril without suction.[6]

■ When the catheter reaches the larynx, the patient will cough. As he does, quickly advance the catheter into the trachea. Tell him to take several deep breaths through his mouth *to ease insertion.*

■ To obtain the specimen, apply suction for 5 to 10 seconds, but never for longer than 15 seconds *because prolonged suction can cause hypoxia.* If the procedure must be repeated, let the patient rest for four to six breaths. When collection is completed, discontinue the suction, gently remove the catheter, and administer oxygen.[7]

■ Detach the catheter from the in-line trap, gather it up in your dominant hand, and pull the glove cuff inside out and down around the used catheter to enclose it for disposal.

■ Detach the trap from the tubing connected to the suction machine. Seal the trap tightly by connecting the rubber tubing to the male adapter of the trap.

Completing the procedure

■ Remove and discard your gloves, and perform hand hygiene.[1,2,3]

■ Label the container in the presence of the patient *to prevent mislabeling.*[7]

■ Include on the laboratory request form whether the patient was febrile or taking antibiotics and whether sputum was induced *because such specimens commonly appear watery and may resemble saliva.*

■ Send the specimen to the laboratory immediately in a laboratory biohazard transport bag. *A delay in transport of the sample to the laboratory could damage the specimen and alter the accuracy of the results.*[8]

■ Offer the patient oral hygiene.

■ Perform hand hygiene.[1,2,3]

■ Document the procedure.[9]

Special considerations

■ Before sending the specimen to the laboratory, examine it *to make sure it's actually sputum, not saliva; saliva will produce inaccurate test results.*

■ *Because expectorated sputum is contaminated by normal mouth flora,* tracheal suctioning provides a more reliable specimen for diagnosis.

■ If you can't obtain a sputum specimen through tracheal suctioning, perform chest percussion *to loosen and mobilize secretions,* and position the patient for optimal drainage. After 20 to 30 minutes, repeat the tracheal suctioning procedure.

■ If the patient is suspected of having tuberculosis, don't use more than 20% propylene glycol with water when inducing a sputum specimen *because a higher concentration inhibits growth of the pathogen and causes erroneous test results.* If propylene glycol isn't available, use 10% to 20% acetylcysteine with water or sodium chloride.

■ As many as three consecutive morning specimens may be required if the suspected organism is *Mycobacterium tuberculosis.*

■ If tuberculosis is suspected, place the patient on airborne precautions in an airborne infection isolation room *to reduce the risk for transmission.*[10,11]

Complications

Patients with cardiac disease may develop arrhythmias during the procedure as a result of coughing.

Documentation

In your notes, record the collection method used, time and date of collection, how the patient tolerated the procedure, color and consistency of the specimen, and its proper disposition.

REFERENCES

1 Centers for Disease Control and Prevention. (October 2002). Guideline for hand hygiene in health-care settings. *Morbidity and Mortality Weekly Report, 51*(RR-16), 1–45. (Level I)

2 World Health Organization. (2009). *WHO guidelines on hand hygiene in health care: First global patient safety challenge. Clean care is safer care.* Geneva, Switzerland: World Health Organization. (Level I)

3 The Joint Commission. (2012). Standard NPSG.07.01.01. *Comprehensive accreditation manual for hospitals: The official handbook.* Oakbrook Terrace, IL: The Joint Commission. (Level I)

4 The Joint Commission. (2012). Standard NPSG.01.01.01. *Comprehensive accreditation manual for hospitals: The official handbook.* Oakbrook Terrace, IL: The Joint Commission. (Level I)

5 American Association for Respiratory Care. (1999). AARC clinical practice guideline: Suctioning of the patient in the home. *Respiratory Care, 44*(1), 99–104.

6 Centers for Disease Control and Prevention. (2004). Guidelines for preventing health-care–associated pneumonia, 2003. *Morbidity and Mortality Weekly Report, 53*(RR-03), 1–36. (Level I)

7 The Joint Commission. (2012). Standard NPSG.03.04.01. *Comprehensive accreditation manual for hospitals: The official handbook.* Oakbrook Terrace, IL: The Joint Commission. (Level I)

8 Occupational Safety and Health Administration. "Bloodborne Pathogens, Standard Number 1910.1030" [Online]. Accessed December 2011 via the Web at http://www.osha.gov/pls/oshaweb/owadisp.show_document?p_table=STANDARDS&p_id=10051 (Level I)

9 The Joint Commission. (2012). Standard RC.01.03.01. *Comprehensive accreditation manual for hospitals: The official handbook.* Oakbrook Terrace, IL: The Joint Commission. (Level I)

10 Siegel, J.D., et al. "2007 Guideline for Isolation Precautions: Preventing Transmission of Infectious Agents in Healthcare Settings" [Online]. Accessed December 2011 via the Web at http://www.cdc.gov/hicpac/2007ip/2007isolationprecautions.html (Level I)

11 Centers for Disease Control and Prevention. (December 2005). Guidelines for preventing the transmission of *Mycobacterium tuberculosis* in health care settings. *Morbidity and Mortality Weekly Report, 54*(RR-17), 1–141. (Level I)

ADDITIONAL REFERENCES

Craven, R.F., & Hirnle, C.J. (2012). *Fundamentals of nursing: Human health and function* (7th ed.). Philadelphia, PA: Lippincott Williams & Wilkins.

Fischbach, F., & Dunning, M.B. (2009). *A manual of laboratory and diagnostic tests* (8th ed.). Philadelphia, PA: Lippincott Williams & Wilkins.

Nettina, S.M. (2010). *Lippincott manual of nursing practice* (9th ed.). Philadelphia, PA: Lippincott Williams & Wilkins.

STANDARD PRECAUTIONS

Standard precautions were developed by the Centers for Disease Control and Prevention (CDC) to protect against the transmission of infection. CDC officials recommend that health care workers assume that all patients are potentially infected or colonized (carry the organism but not showing signs or symptoms of infection) with an organism that could be transmitted in the health care setting, regardless of their diagnosis.

One part of standard precautions includes wearing gloves for situations involving known or anticipated contact with blood, body fluids, tissue, mucous membrane, and nonintact skin.[1] If the task or procedure being performed may result in splashing or splattering of blood or body fluids to the face, a mask and goggles or face shield should be worn. If the task or procedure being performed may result in splashing or splattering of blood or body fluids to the body, a fluid-resistant gown or apron should be worn.[1,2] Additional protective clothing such as shoe covers may be appropriate to protect the feet in situations that may expose the health care worker to large amounts of blood or body fluids (or both), such as when caring for a trauma patient in the operating room or emergency department.

Standard precautions should be combined with transmission-based precautions for patients with confirmed or suspected infection with highly transmissible pathogens. (See *Transmission-based, precautions*, page 670 as well as "Airborne precautions," page 10; "Contact precautions," page 196; and "Droplet precautions," page 233.)

Equipment

Gloves ■ masks ■ goggles, glasses, or face shields ■ gowns ■ resuscitation bag ■ hospital-grade disinfectant ■ bags for specimens.

Implementation

■ Wash your hands immediately if they become contaminated with blood or body fluids, excretions, secretions, or drainage; perform hand hygiene before and after patient care and before and after putting on and discarding gloves. *Hand hygiene removes microorganisms from your skin.* If your hands aren't visibly soiled, an alcohol-based hand rub can be used for routine decontamination.[1]

Transmission-based precautions[1]

Depending on the patient's condition, these precautions may be necessary in addition to standard precautions.

PRECAUTION TYPE	INDICATIONS	NURSING ACTIONS
Airborne	When a patient is suspected of having or known to have an infection that's spread by the airborne route	■ Place the patient in an airborne infection isolation room with monitored negative pressure, if available. ■ Make sure that all people who enter the room wear a respirator mask.
Contact	To prevent the spread of epidemiologically important infectious organisms through direct or indirect contact with the patient or his environment	■ Place the patient in a single-patient room, if possible. ■ Wear a gown and gloves for all interactions with the patient or the patient's environment. ■ Follow your facility's infection-control plan to determine when to initiate contact precautions.[3]
Droplet	To prevent the spread of infectious organisms through close respiratory or mucous membrane contact with respiratory secretions from an infected individual	■ Place the patient in a single-patient room, if possible. ■ Put on a mask before entering the patient's room when coming within 3' (1 m) of the patient.

■ Wear gloves if you will or could come in contact with blood, specimens, tissue, body fluids, secretions or excretions, mucous membrane, broken skin, or contaminated surfaces or objects.

■ Change your gloves and perform hand hygiene when moving from a contaminated to a clean site during patient care, and in between patient contacts *to avoid cross-contamination.*[1]

■ Wear a fluid-resistant gown, face shield, or goggles and a mask during procedures likely to generate splash or splatter of blood or body fluids, such as surgery, endoscopic procedures, dialysis, assisting with intubation or manipulation of arterial lines, or any other procedure with potential for splashing or splattering of body fluids.[1,2]

■ Wear a mask during lumbar puncture procedures, such as a myelogram and spinal or epidural anesthesia. The health care worker performing the procedure should wear a face shield.[1]

■ Follow safe injection practices; whenever possible, use single-dose vials instead of multidose vials. Use a sterile, single-use disposable needle and syringe for each injection.[1]

■ Handle used needles and other sharp instruments carefully. Don't bend, break, reinsert them into their original sheaths, remove needles from syringes, or unnecessarily handle them. Activate any safety mechanisms immediately after use. Discard the instruments intact immediately after use into a puncture-resistant disposal box. Use tools to pick up broken glass or other sharp objects. *These measures reduce the risk of accidental injury or infection.* Use a needleless IV system whenever possible.[1,2]

■ Immediately notify your employee health provider (or the provider's designee) of all needle-stick or other sharp object injuries, mucosal splashes, or contamination of open wounds or nonintact skin with blood or body fluids *to allow investigation of the incident and appropriate care and documentation.* Complete all follow-up screening and care as recommended by your employee health provider.[2]

■ Properly label all specimens collected from patients in the presence of the patient and place them in laboratory biohazard transport bags at the collection site. Attach requisition slips to the outside of the bags.[2]

■ Place all items that have come in direct contact with the patient's secretions, excretions, blood, drainage, or body fluids—such as nondisposable utensils or instruments—in a single impervious bag or container before removal from the room. Place linens and trash in single bags of sufficient thickness to contain the contents.[1]

■ While wearing the appropriate personal protective equipment, promptly clean all blood and body fluid spills. Blot the spill with an absorbent material (such as a paper towel) first, and then clean the area with detergent and water. Notify the environmental services department of the spill *so they can properly clean the area.*

■ If you have an exudative lesion, avoid all direct patient contact until the condition has resolved and you've been cleared by the employee health provider.[3]

■ Properly clean and disinfect or sterilize reusable equipment with hospital-grade disinfectant before using it for another patient.[1,4,5,6]

■ If you have dermatitis or other conditions resulting in broken skin on your hands, avoid situations where you may have contact with blood and body fluids (even though gloves could be worn) until the condition has resolved and you've been cleared by the employee health care provider.

■ Teach patients, family members, and visitors about respiratory hygiene and cough etiquette. Provide a mask for anyone who presents with signs or symptoms of respiratory infection. Tell people to cover their mouths and noses with a tissue when coughing or sneezing, dispose of the tissue promptly, and then perform hand hygiene.[1]

Special considerations

■ Keep mouthpieces, resuscitation bags, and other ventilation devices nearby *to eliminate the need for emergency mouth-to-mouth resuscitation, thus reducing the risk of exposure to body fluids.*
■ Disposable food trays and dishes aren't necessary for standard precautions.[1]

NURSING ALERT Because you may not always know which organisms may be present in every clinical situation, *you must use standard precautions for every contact with blood, body fluids, secretions, excretions, drainage, mucous membranes, and nonintact skin. Use your judgment in individual cases about whether to implement additional isolation precautions, such as airborne, droplet, or contact precautions or a combination of them. Also, if your work requires you to be exposed to blood, you should receive the hepatitis B virus vaccine series.*

Complications

Failure to follow standard precautions may lead to exposure to blood-borne pathogens or other infectious agents and to all the complications they may cause.

Documentation

Record any special needs for isolation precautions on the nursing care plan and as otherwise indicated by your facility.

REFERENCES

1 Siegel, J.D., et al. "2007 Guideline for Isolation Precautions: Preventing Transmission of Infectious Agents in Healthcare Settings" [Online]. Accessed December 2011 via the Web at http://www.cdc.gov/hicpac/2007ip/2007isolationprecautions.html (Level I)
2 Occupational Safety & Health Administration. (2001). 29 CFR part 1920. Occupational exposure to bloodborne pathogens: Needlesticks and other sharps injuries: Final rule. *Federal Register, 66*(12), 5318–5325.
3 The Joint Commission. (2012). Standard IC.02.01.01. *Comprehensive accreditation manual for hospitals: The official handbook.* Oakbrook Terrace, IL: The Joint Commission. (Level I)
4 The Joint Commission. (2012). Standard IC.02.03.01. *Comprehensive accreditation manual for hospitals: The official handbook.* Oakbrook Terrace, IL: The Joint Commission. (Level I)
5 Rutala, W.A., et al. (2008). "Guideline for Disinfection and Sterilization in Healthcare Facilities, 2008" [Online]. Accessed October 2011 via the Web at http://www.cdc.gov/ncidod/dhqp/pdf/guidelines/Disinfection_Nov_2008.pdf (Level I)
6 The Joint Commission. (2012). Standard IC.02.02.01. *Comprehensive accreditation manual for hospitals: The official handbook.* Oakbrook Terrace, IL: The Joint Commission. (Level I)

STERILE TECHNIQUE, BASIC

Sterile technique is used to prevent contamination with microbes, preventing infection. It's used in conjunction with other procedures and isn't a procedure in itself. Sterile technique should be followed any time the patient's skin is intentionally perforated, during procedures that involve entry into a sterile body cavity, or when coming into contact with nonintact skin resulting from trauma or surgery. Procedures requiring sterile technique include inserting a urinary catheter, inserting an IV catheter, dispensing and administering IV drugs, and changing surgical dressings. A patient with a compromised immune system (such as a burn patient or a patient who has just had an organ transplant or is receiving chemotherapy or radiation therapy) also requires sterile technique, even for some procedures that would normally require only clean technique.

Equipment

Sterile gloves ■ personal protective equipment ■ sterile supplies, as required by the procedure to be performed ■ Optional: sterile bowl, sterile normal saline solution, sterile drape.

Many procedures have commercially prepared kits that provide all of the necessary components.

Preparation of equipment

Gather all the equipment in the patient's room. Check each package carefully and discard any that has a hole or tear or is wet.[1] Note the expiration date and discard any package that's beyond that date.[1] Make sure that the sterilization tape has turned the appropriate color. (See your facility's policy; color depends on the product used and sterilization method.) Prepare a clean surface to set up the equipment for the sterile procedure.

Implementation

■ Verify the doctor's order.
■ Perform hand hygiene.[2,3,4]
■ Confirm the patient's identity using at least two patient identifiers according to your facility's policy.[5]
■ Explain the procedure to the patient and family *to relieve anxiety and ensure understanding and cooperation.*
■ Remove rings and perform hand hygiene.[2,3,4]
■ Follow standard precautions by putting on the necessary personal protective equipment for the procedure. (See "Standard precautions," page 669.)

Opening sterile kits

■ Remove the plastic outer wrapper from the procedure kit, if one is present.
■ Place the inner wrapped kit on a clean, dry flat surface *because any moisture on the table could be absorbed through the wrapper and contaminate the sterile supplies.*
■ Position the kit so that the tip of the triangle-pointed wrapper is toward you *so you don't have to reach over the sterile contents after the other flaps are opened.*
■ Grasp the outer portion of this outermost flap *to avoid contaminating the sterile field.*[1]

■ Open the flap away from your body, keeping your arm outstretched to the side (as shown below) *so it doesn't cross over the sterile field.*[1]

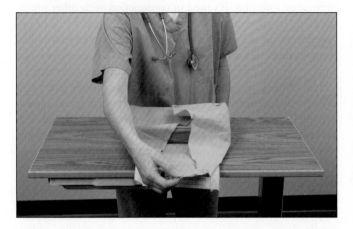

■ Grasp the outer surface of the first side flap with your hand on the same side as the flap to avoid crossing over the sterile field (as shown below).[1] Open the flap fully *to avoid allowing the wrapper to spring back into place.*

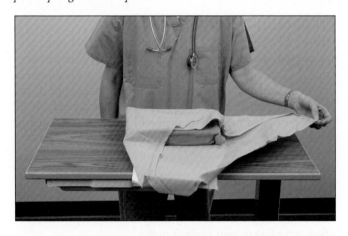

■ Grasp the outer surface of the second side flap and open it with your hand on the same side (as shown below).

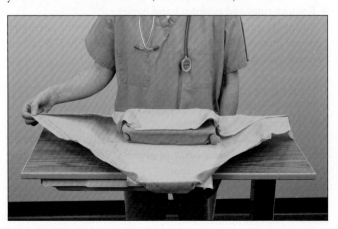

■ Grasp the outer surface of the innermost flap and open it toward your body (as shown below).[1]

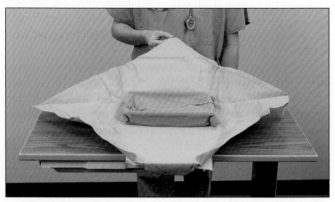

Opening wrapped sterile items

■ Grasp the sterile item wrapped in paper or linen in the nondominant hand.
■ Break the sterilization tape.
■ Use your dominant hand to grasp the outer surface of the top outermost flap *to avoid touching a sterile surface.*
■ Open the flap away from your body.
■ Grasp the outer surface of the first side flap and open it fully to the side.
■ Repeat with the other side flap.
■ Secure all flaps in your nondominant hand *to avoid dangling and contaminating the sterile field.*
■ Grasp the outer surface of the inner flap and open it toward you.
■ Place the item on the sterile field, ensuring that only sterile surfaces touch other sterile surfaces *to avoid contamination.*[1]
■ Make sure the item is at least 1″ (2.5 cm) from the edge of the sterile field *because any closer to the edge is considered unsterile.*

Opening peel-pack containers or pouches

■ Grasp the unsealed corner of the wrapper and pull it toward you.
■ If the item is light, it can be dropped onto the sterile field. Heavy items should be given to a scrubbed person or opened on a separate surface.[1]
■ Open a peel-pack pouch (such as gloves and syringes) by grasping each side of the unsealed edge with the thumb side of each hand parallel to the seal and pulling apart gently.
■ Hold the sides back so the wrap covers your hands and exposes the sterile item.
■ Don't allow the item to slide across the package side when dropping the item onto the sterile field.

Pouring sterile solutions

■ Open the wrapped package containing the sterile bowl as described above *to avoid contaminating the sterile field.* Label the bowl with the name of the solution to be poured into it.[6]
■ Place the bowl on the edge of the sterile field but inside of the 1″ safety margin *so that solution can be poured without reaching across the sterile field.*

- Unwrap the seal on the sterile solution bottle.
- Unscrew the cap without touching the edges of the bottle.
- Pour the solution into the bowl without reaching over the sterile field *to reduce the risk of touching sterile surfaces.*[1]
- Pour slowly *to avoid splashing onto the drape and contaminating the sterile field.*
- Discard any unused solution. *The edge of the container is considered contaminated after the contents have been poured.*

Opening and putting on sterile gloving

- Open the package containing the sterile gloves. Some commercially prepared kits (such as the kit for inserting an indwelling urinary catheter) include a pair of sterile gloves. If gloves are included they will be the uppermost item in the pack. Touch only the outer side of the glove wrapper.
- Grasp the paper glove wrapper and place it on a clean, dry, flat surface.
- Open the inner package, touching only the outer edges of the wrapper (as shown below).

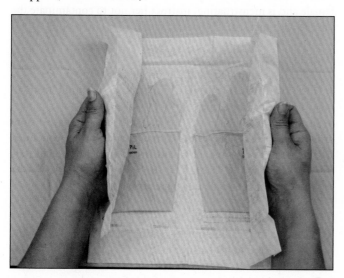

- Use the thumb and fingers of your nondominant hand to grasp the folded inner surface portion of the glove for the dominant hand, touching only the inner portion of the glove (as shown below) *to avoid contaminating the outer portion of the glove.*

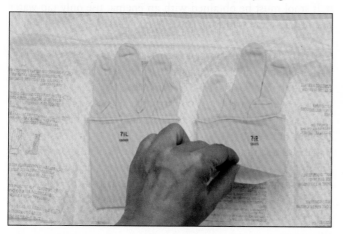

- Lift up the glove and insert your dominant hand into the glove, palm side up (as shown below).

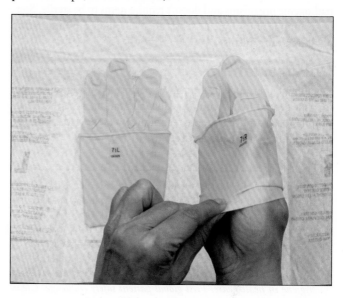

- Pull down the cuff by touching only the inner surface of the glove. Gently stretch the glove over your hand. Make sure the outside of the glove doesn't touch the nonsterile surface.[7]
- Insert the four fingers of your dominant gloved hand into the sterile outer cuff of the other glove, keeping your thumb pulled back out of the way (as shown below).

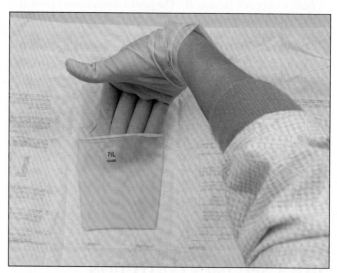

- Lift up the glove and insert the nondominant hand into the glove. Allow the cuff to come uncuffed as you finish putting it on, but don't touch the skin of the arm with your gloved hand.
- Adjust the fingers of the gloves after both your hands are gloved.
- Keep your hands above waist level *to decrease the potential for contamination.*[7]

Special considerations

- Be sure to open supplies away from the already setup sterile field *to avoid contaminating the field.* Hold the opened additional supplies above the sterile field and drop them onto the field.[1]

■ Medical asepsis, also called *clean technique,* isn't the same as sterile technique. Medical asepsis is focused on the absence of pathogenic organisms and doesn't require items to be sterile. Sterile technique and surgical asepsis are focused on the elimination of all microorganisms.

Documentation

Document the procedure that was performed using guidelines for that procedure. Within this documentation, note the sterile supplies used and that sterile technique was followed. Note the date and time of the procedure.

REFERENCES

1 Recommended practices for maintaining a sterile field. (2011). In R. Conner, et al. (Eds.). *Perioperative standards and recommended practices.* Denver, CO: AORN.
2 Centers for Disease Control and Prevention. (October 2002). Guideline for hand hygiene in health-care settings. *Morbidity and Mortality Weekly Report, 51*(RR-16), 1–45. (Level I)
3 World Health Organization. (2009). *WHO guidelines on hand hygiene in health care: First global patient safety challenge. Clean care is safer care.* Geneva, Switzerland: World Health Organization. (Level I)
4 The Joint Commission. (2012). Standard NPSG.07.01.01. *Comprehensive accreditation manual for hospitals: The official handbook.* Oakbrook Terrace, IL: The Joint Commission. (Level I)
5 The Joint Commission. (2012). Standard NPSG.01.01.01. *Comprehensive accreditation manual for hospitals: The official handbook.* Oakbrook Terrace, IL: The Joint Commission. (Level I)
6 The Joint Commission. (2012). Standard NPSG.03.04.01. *Comprehensive accreditation manual for hospitals: The official handbook.* Oakbrook Terrace, IL: The Joint Commission. (Level I)
7 Timby, B. (2009). *Fundamental nursing skills and concepts* (9th ed.). Philadelphia, PA: Lippincott Williams & Wilkins.

ADDITIONAL REFERENCES

Craven, R.F., & Hirnle, C.J. (2012). *Fundamentals of nursing: Human health and function* (7th ed.). Philadelphia, PA: Lippincott Williams & Wilkins.
The Joint Commission. (2012). Standard PC.01.02.07. *Comprehensive accreditation manual for hospitals: The official handbook.* Oakbrook Terrace, IL: The Joint Commission.

STOOL SPECIMEN COLLECTION

Stool is collected to determine the presence of blood, ova and parasites, pathogens, or such substances as ingested drugs. Gross examination of stool characteristics, including color, consistency, and odor, can reveal such conditions as GI bleeding and steatorrhea.

Stool specimens may be collected over a specific time period, such as 48, 72, or 96 hours. Typically, timed specimens are used to test for fat, porphyrins, urobilinogen, nitrogen, and electrolytes. Because stool specimens can't be obtained on demand, proper collection requires careful instructions to the patient to ensure an uncontaminated specimen.

Equipment

Sample container with lid ■ gloves ■ two tongue blades ■ paper towel or paper bag ■ bedpan or portable commode ■ laboratory request form and laboratory biohazard transport bag ■ specimen label ■ patient care reminder ■ enema equipment. (See "Enema Administration," page 272.)

Implementation

■ Verify the doctor's order for the stool collection.
■ Confirm the patient's identity using at least two patient identifiers according to your facility's policy.[1]
■ Explain the procedure to the patient and his family, if possible, *to ensure their cooperation and prevent inadvertent disposal of timed stool samples.*
■ Tell the patient to notify you when he has the urge to defecate. Have him defecate into a clean, dry bedpan or commode. Instruct him not to contaminate the sample with urine or toilet tissue *because urine inhibits fecal bacterial growth and toilet tissue contains bismuth, which interferes with test results.* If the patient is female and is menstruating, instruct her not to contaminate the sample with menstrual blood.

Random stool collection

■ Perform hand hygiene and put on gloves.[2,3,4]
■ If the patient is incontinent, collect a stool sample from an incontinence pad or diaper.
■ Using a tongue blade, transfer the most representative stool sample from the bedpan to the container, and cap the container.
■ If the patient passes blood, mucus, or pus with the stool, include this with the sample.
■ Wrap the tongue blade in a paper towel and discard it.

Timed stool collection

■ Place a patient-care reminder stating "save all stool" over the patient's bed and in his bathroom.
■ Tell the patient to notify you when he has the urge to defecate.
■ Begin timing with the passage of this first stool.
■ After performing hand hygiene put on gloves,[2,3,4] collect the first specimen, and include this in the total specimen.
■ Continue to collect stools passed, remembering to transfer all stool to the specimen container.
■ If stool must be obtained with an enema, use only tap water or normal saline solution.

Completing the procedure

■ Remove and discard your gloves, and perform hand hygiene thoroughly *to prevent cross-contamination.*[2,3,4]
■ Make sure the patient is comfortable after the procedure and that he has the opportunity to thoroughly clean his hands and perianal area.
■ Label the sample in the presence of the patient *to prevent mislabeling.*[5] The label should include the patient's name and identification number, type of sample, time and date of collection, and your name or initials in accordance with your facility's policy.[6]
■ Document the procedure.[7]

Special considerations

- Be sure to collect all stool passed during the specified time period.
- Never place a stool sample in a refrigerator that contains food or medication *to prevent contamination.*
- Notify the doctor if the stool sample looks unusual.
- If the patient is to collect a sample at home, instruct him to collect it in a clean container with a tight-fitting lid, to wrap the container in a brown paper bag, and to keep it in the refrigerator (separate from food items) until it can be transported.

Documentation

Record the time period for the specimen collection and time of transport to the laboratory. Note stool color, odor, consistency, and unusual characteristics; also note whether the patient had difficulty passing the stool.

REFERENCES

1 The Joint Commission. (2012). Standard NPSG.01.01.01. *Comprehensive accreditation manual for hospitals: The official handbook.* Oakbrook Terrace, IL: The Joint Commission. (Level I)
2 Centers for Disease Control and Prevention. (October 2002). Guideline for hand hygiene in health-care settings. *Morbidity and Mortality Weekly Report, 51*(RR-16), 1–45. (Level I)
3 World Health Organization. (2009). *WHO guidelines on hand hygiene in health care: First global patient safety challenge. Clean care is safer care.* Geneva, Switzerland: World Health Organization. (Level I)
4 The Joint Commission. (2012). Standard NPSG.07.01.01. *Comprehensive accreditation manual for hospitals: The official handbook.* Oakbrook Terrace, IL: The Joint Commission. (Level I)
5 The Joint Commission. (2012). Standard NPSG.03.04.01. *Comprehensive accreditation manual for hospitals: The official handbook.* Oakbrook Terrace, IL: The Joint Commission. (Level I)
6 Occupational Safety and Health Administration. "Bloodborne Pathogens, Standard Number 1910.1030" [Online]. Accessed December 2011 via the Web at http://www.osha.gov/pls/oshaweb/owadisp.show_document?p_table=STANDARDS&p_id=10051 (Level I)
7 The Joint Commission. (2012). Standard RC.01.03.01. *Comprehensive accreditation manual for hospitals: The official handbook.* Oakbrook Terrace, IL: The Joint Commission. (Level I)

ADDITIONAL REFERENCES

Craven, R.F., & Hirnle, C.J. (2012). *Fundamentals of nursing: Human health and function* (7th ed.). Philadelphia, PA: Lippincott Williams & Wilkins.
Fischbach, F., & Dunning, M.B. (2009). *A manual of laboratory and diagnostic tests* (8th ed.). Philadelphia, PA: Lippincott Williams & Wilkins.
Nettina, S.M. (2010). *Lippincott manual of nursing practice* (9th ed.). Philadelphia, PA: Lippincott Williams & Wilkins.

ST-SEGMENT MONITORING

A sensitive indicator of myocardial damage, the ST segment is normally flat or isoelectric. A depressed ST segment may result from cardiac glycosides, myocardial ischemia, or a subendocardial infarction. An elevated ST segment suggests myocardial infarction.

Continuous ST-segment monitoring is helpful for patients with acute coronary syndromes and for those who have received thrombolytic therapy or have undergone coronary angioplasty or cardiac surgery.[1] ST-segment monitoring allows early detection of reocclusion. It's also useful for patients who have had previous episodes of cardiac ischemia without chest pain, for those who have difficulty distinguishing cardiac pain from pain associated with other sources, and for those who have difficulty communicating. It gives the doctor the ability to identify and reverse ischemia by starting early interventions.[2]

Because ischemia typically occurs in only one portion of the heart muscle, not all electrocardiogram (ECG) leads detect it. Select the most appropriate lead by examining ECG tracings obtained during an ischemic episode. The leads showing ischemia are the same leads to use for ST-segment monitoring.

ST-segment monitoring isn't useful for patients with left or right bundle-branch block or ventricular paced rhythm or for those who are very restless.[2]

Equipment

ECG electrodes ▪ gauze pads ▪ ECG monitor cable ▪ leadwires ▪ alcohol pad ▪ cardiac monitor programmed for ST-segment monitoring.

Preparation of equipment

Plug the cardiac monitor into an electrical outlet and turn it on *to warm up while you prepare the equipment and the patient.*

Implementation

- Confirm the patient's identity using at least two patient identifiers according to your facility's policy.[3]
- Bring the equipment to the patient's bedside and explain the procedure to the patient. Provide privacy.
- Perform hand hygiene.[4,5,6]
- If the patient isn't already on a monitor, turn on the device and attach the cable.
- Select the sites for electrode placement and prepare the patient's skin for attachment as you would for continuous cardiac monitoring or a 12-lead ECG. Attach the leadwires to the electrodes and position the electrodes appropriately on the patient's skin.
- Activate ST-segment monitoring by pressing the "monitoring procedures" key and then the ST key. Activate individual ST parameters by pressing the "on/off parameter" key.
- Select the appropriate ECG for each ST channel to be monitored by pressing the "parameters" key and then the key labeled "ECG." If monitoring only one lead, choose the lead most likely to show arrhythmias and ST-segment changes.[2,7] Lead III is sensitive to inferior ischemia, and V_3 is sensitive to anterior or posterior ischemia.

Changes in the ST Segment

Closely monitoring the ST segment on a patient's electrocardiogram can help you detect ischemia or injury before the infarction develops.

ST-segment depression

An ST segment is considered depressed when it is 0.5 mm or more below the baseline. A depressed ST segment may indicate myocardial ischemia or digoxin toxicity.

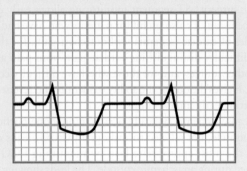

ST-segment elevation

An ST segment is considered elevated when it is 1 mm or more above the baseline. An elevated ST segment may indicate myocardial injury.

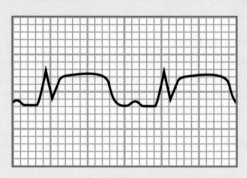

NURSING ALERT *Always give precedence to the lead that shows arrhythmias.*

■ Identify the ECG complex landmarks, as prompted by the monitor.

■ Adjust the ST point to 60 msec after the J point (as shown below).[2,7]

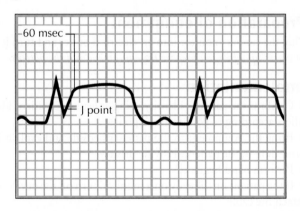

60 msec

J point

■ Set the alarm limits for each ST-segment parameter by manipulating the high and low limit keys.

■ Press the key labeled "standard display" to return to the display screen.

■ Assess the waveform shown on the monitor.

■ Evaluate for ST-segment depression or elevation. (See *Changes in the ST segment.*)

■ Document the procedure.[8]

Special considerations

■ Abrade the patient's skin gently *to ensure electrode adhesion and promote electrical conductivity.*

■ Verify limit parameters for the patient with the doctor. Commonly, when a limit is surpassed for more than 1 minute, visual and audible alarms are activated.

■ If you note ischemia, obtain a 12-lead ECG and assess the patient for signs and symptoms of acute ischemia, such as arrhythmias, angina, and hemodynamic changes.

Documentation

Document the leads being monitored and the ST-segment measurement points in the patient's medical record.

REFERENCES

1 Yan, A.T., et al. (2007). Long-term prognostic value and therapeutic implications of continuous ST-segment monitoring in acute coronary syndrome. *American Heart Journal, 153*(4), 500–506. (Level IV)

2 Drew, B.J., et al. (2005). AHA scientific statement: Practice standards for electrocardiographic monitoring in hospital settings. *Journal of Cardiovascular Nursing, 20*(2), 76–106. (Level I)

3 The Joint Commission. (2012). Standard NPSG.01.01.01. *Comprehensive accreditation manual for hospitals: The official handbook.* Oakbrook Terrace, IL: The Joint Commission. (Level I)

4 Centers for Disease Control and Prevention. (October 2002). Guideline for hand hygiene in health-care settings. *Morbidity and Mortality Weekly Report, 51*(RR-16), 1–45. (Level I)

5 World Health Organization. (2009). *WHO guidelines on hand hygiene in health care: First global patient safety challenge. Clean care is safer care.* Geneva, Switzerland: World Health Organization. (Level I)

6   The Joint Commission. (2012). Standard NPSG.07.01.01. *Comprehensive accreditation manual for hospitals: The official handbook.* Oakbrook Terrace, IL: The Joint Commission. (Level I)

7   American Association of Critical-Care Nurses. (2009). "AACN Practice Alert: ST Segment Monitoring" [Online]. Accessed April 2011 via the Web at http://www.aacn.org/WD/Practice/Docs/PracticeAlerts/ST_Segment_Monitoring_05-2009.pdf. (Level I)

8   The Joint Commission. (2012). Standard RC.01.03.01. *Comprehensive accreditation manual for hospitals: The official handbook.* Oakbrook Terrace, IL: The Joint Commission. (Level I)

ADDITIONAL REFERENCES

Flanders, S.A. (2006). Continuous ST-segment monitoring: Raising the bar. *Critical Care Nursing Clinics of North America, 18*(2), 169–177.

Flanders, S.A. (2007). ST-segment monitoring: Putting standards into practice. *AACN Advanced Critical Care, 18*(3), 275–284.

Foussas, S.G., et al. (2009). "Serial Snapshot Electrocardiograms and Continuous 12-lead ST-Segment Electrocardiographic Monitoring for the Prediction of Intravenous Thrombolysis Outcome in Patients with ST-Segment Elevation Myocardial Infarction" [Online]. Accessed April 2011 via the Web at http://www.internationaljournalofcardiology.com/article/S0167-5273(08)01585-4/fulltext

Landesberg, G., et al. (2005). Myocardial ischemia, cardiac troponin, and long-term survival of high-cardiac risk critically ill intensive care patients. *Critical Care Medicine, 33*(6), 1281–1287.

ST-segment monitoring. (2008). *Critical Care Nurse, 28*(4), 70–72.

STUMP AND PROSTHESIS CARE

Patient care immediately after limb amputation includes monitoring drainage from the stump, managing pain, reducing edema, positioning the affected limb, assisting with exercises prescribed by a physical therapist, and wrapping and conditioning the stump. Postoperative care of the stump varies slightly, depending on the amputation site (arm or leg) and the type of dressing applied to the stump (elastic bandage or plaster cast).

After limb amputation and stump healing, patient care includes routine daily care, such as proper hygiene and continued muscle-strengthening exercises. As the patient recovers from the physical and psychological trauma of amputation, he will need to learn correct procedures for routine daily care of the stump and any prosthesis he might have. A plastic prosthesis—the most common type—typically must be cleaned, lubricated, and checked for proper fit.

Equipment

For postoperative stump care

Gloves ▪ pressure dressing ▪ abdominal (ABD) pad ▪ suction equipment, if ordered ▪ overhead trapeze ▪ 1″ adhesive tape or bandage clips ▪ trochanter roll (for a leg) ▪ elastic stump shrinker or 4″ elastic bandage ▪ Optional: tourniquet (as a last resort to control bleeding).

For ongoing stump or prosthetic care

Mild soap or alcohol pads ▪ stump socks or athletic tube socks ▪ two washcloths ▪ two towels ▪ appropriate lubricating oil.

Implementation

▪ Confirm the patient's identity using at least two patient identifiers according to your facility's policy.[1]
▪ Explain the procedure to the patient.
▪ Perform hand hygiene and put on gloves.[2,3,4]
▪ Perform routine postoperative care. Frequently assess respiratory status and level of consciousness, monitor vital signs and IV infusions, check tube patency, and provide for the patient's comfort, pain management, and safety.

Monitoring stump drainage

▪ *Because gravity causes fluid to accumulate at the stump,* frequently check the amount of blood and drainage on the dressing. Notify the doctor if accumulations of drainage or blood increase rapidly. If excessive bleeding occurs, notify the doctor immediately and apply a pressure dressing or compress the appropriate pressure points. If this doesn't control bleeding, use a tourniquet only as a last resort.
▪ Tape the ABD pad over the moist part of the dressing as necessary. *Doing so provides a dry area to help prevent bacterial infection.*

Positioning the extremity

▪ Elevate the extremity for the first 24 hours *to reduce swelling and promote venous return.*
▪ *To prevent contractures,* position an arm with the elbow extended and the shoulder abducted.
▪ *To correctly position a leg,* elevate the foot of the bed slightly and place a trochanter roll against the hip *to prevent external rotation.*
NURSING ALERT *Don't place a pillow under the thigh to flex the hip* because this positioning can cause hip flexion contracture. *For the same reason, tell the patient to avoid prolonged sitting.*
▪ After a below-the-knee amputation, maintain knee extension *to prevent hamstring muscle contractures.*
▪ After any leg amputation, place the patient on a firm surface in the prone position for at least 2 hours a day, with his legs close together and without pillows under his stomach, hips, knees, or stump, unless this position is contraindicated. *This position helps prevent hip flexion, contractures, and abduction; it also stretches the flexor muscles.*

Assisting with prescribed exercises

▪ After arm amputation, encourage the patient to exercise the remaining arm *to prevent muscle contractures.* Help the patient perform isometric and range-of-motion (ROM) exercises for both shoulders, as prescribed by the physical therapist, *because use of a prosthesis requires both shoulders.*
▪ After leg amputation, stand behind the patient and, if necessary, support him with your hands at his waist during balancing exercises.
▪ Instruct the patient to exercise the affected and unaffected limbs *to maintain muscle tone and increase muscle strength.* The patient with a leg amputation may perform push-ups, as ordered (in the sitting position, arms at his sides), or pull-ups on the overhead trapeze *to strengthen his arms, shoulders, and back in preparation for using crutches.*

Wrapping a stump

Proper stump care helps protect the limb, reduces swelling, and prepares the limb for a prosthesis. As you perform the procedure, teach it to the patient.

Start by obtaining two 4″ elastic bandages. Center the end of the first 4″ bandage at the top of the patient's thigh. Unroll the bandage downward over the stump and to the back of the leg (as shown below).

Make three figure-eight turns to adequately cover the ends of the stump. As you wrap, be sure to include the roll of flesh in the groin area. Use enough pressure to ensure that the stump narrows toward the end so that it fits comfortably into the prosthesis.

Use the second 4″ bandage to anchor the first bandage around the waist. For a below-the-knee amputation, use the knee to anchor the bandage in place. Secure the bandage with clips or adhesive tape. Check the stump bandage regularly, and rewrap it if it bunches at the end.

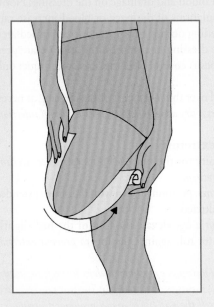
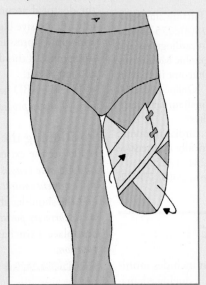
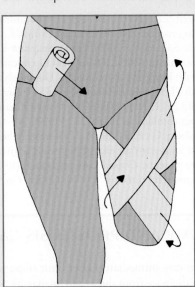

Wrapping and conditioning the stump

■ Apply an elastic stump shrinker *to prevent edema and shape the limb in preparation for the prosthesis.* Wrap the stump so that it narrows toward the distal end *to help ensure comfort when the patient wears the prosthesis.*

■ If an elastic stump shrinker isn't available, you can wrap the stump in a 4″ elastic bandage. To do this, stretch the bandage to about two-thirds its maximum length as you wrap it diagonally around the stump, with the greatest pressure distally. (Depending on the size of the leg, you may need to use two 4″ bandages.) Secure the bandage with clips, safety pins, or adhesive tape. Make sure the bandage covers all portions of the stump smoothly *because wrinkles or exposed areas encourage skin breakdown.* (See *Wrapping a stump.*)

■ If the patient experiences throbbing after the stump is wrapped, the bandage may be too tight; remove the bandage immediately and reapply it less tightly. *Throbbing indicates impaired circulation.*

■ Check the bandage regularly. Rewrap it when it begins to bunch up at the end (usually about every 12 hours for a moderately active patient) or as necessary.

■ After removing the bandage to rewrap it, massage the stump gently, always pushing toward the suture line rather than away from it. *Massage stimulates circulation and prevents scar tissue from adhering to the bone.*

■ When healing begins, instruct the patient to push the stump against a pillow. Then have him progress gradually to pushing against harder surfaces, such as a padded chair, then a hard chair. *These conditioning exercises will help the patient adjust to experiencing pressure and sensation in the stump.*

Caring for the healed stump

■ *To shape the stump,* have the patient wear an elastic bandage 24 hours a day except while bathing.

■ Bathe the stump but never shave it *to prevent infection.* If possible, bathe the stump at the end of the day *because the warm water may cause swelling, making reapplication of the prosthesis difficult.* Don't soak the stump for long periods of time.

■ Don't apply lotion to the stump; *lotion may clog follicles, which increases the risk of infection.*

■ Rub the stump with alcohol daily *to toughen the skin, reducing the risk of skin breakdown.* (Avoid using powders or lotions *because they can soften or irritate the skin.*) *Because alcohol may cause severe irritation in some patients,* instruct the patient to watch for and report this sign.

■ Inspect the stump for redness, swelling, irritation, and calluses. Report any of these to the doctor. Tell the patient to avoid putting weight on the stump. (The skin should be firm but not taut over the bony end of the limb.)

■ Continue muscle-strengthening exercises *so that the patient can build the strength he'll need to control the prosthesis.*

■ Change and wash the patient's elastic bandages every day *to avoid exposing the skin to excessive perspiration, which can be irritating.* Wash the elastic bandages in warm water and gentle nondetergent soap; lay them flat on a towel to dry. *Machine washing or drying may shrink the elastic bandages.*

■ Remove and discard your gloves and perform hand hygiene.[2,3,4]

■ Document the procedure.[5]

Caring for the plastic prosthesis

■ Wipe the plastic socket of the prosthesis with a damp cloth and mild soap or alcohol *to prevent bacterial accumulation.*

■ Wipe the insert (if the prosthesis has one) with a dry cloth.

■ Dry the prosthesis thoroughly; if possible, allow it to dry overnight.

■ Maintain and lubricate the prosthesis, as instructed by the manufacturer.

■ Check for malfunctions and adjust or repair the prosthesis as necessary *to prevent further damage.*

■ Check the condition of the shoe on a foot prosthesis frequently, and change it as necessary.

Applying the prosthesis

■ Perform hand hygiene.[2,3,4]

■ Apply a stump sock. Keep the seams away from bony prominences.

■ If the prosthesis has an insert, remove it from the socket, place it over the stump, and insert the stump into the prosthesis.

■ If it has no insert, slide the prosthesis over the stump. Secure the prosthesis onto the stump according to the manufacturer's directions.

■ Perform hand hygiene.[2,3,4]

■ Document the procedure.[5]

Special considerations

■ For a below-the-knee amputation, you may substitute an athletic tube sock for a stump sock by cutting off the elastic band.

Patient teaching

Emphasize to the patient that proper care of his stump can speed healing. Tell him to inspect his stump carefully every day, using a mirror, and to continue proper daily stump care. Instruct him to call the doctor if the incision appears to be opening, looks red or swollen, feels warm, is painful to touch, or is seeping drainage.

Make sure the patient knows the signs and symptoms that indicate problems in the stump. Explain that a 10-lb (4.5-kg) change in body weight will alter his stump size and require a new prosthesis socket *to ensure a correct fit.*

Tell the patient to massage the stump toward the suture line *to mobilize the scar and prevent its adherence to bone.* Advise him to avoid exposing the skin around the stump to excessive per-spiration, which can be irritating. Tell him to change his elastic bandages or stump socks daily to avoid this irritation.

Tell the patient that he may experience twitching, spasms, or phantom limb sensations (such as pain, warmth, cold, or itching) as his stump muscles adjust to amputation. Tell the patient that phantom pain usually peaks about 1 month after amputation, but a second peak may occur about 1 year after amputation.[6] Measures such as imagery, biofeedback, and distraction may help relieve phantom limb pain or other sensations. Advise him that he can decrease these symptoms with heat, massage, or gentle pressure. If his stump is sensitive to touch, tell him to rub it with a dry washcloth for 4 minutes three times a day.

Inform the patient that exercise of the remaining muscles in an amputated limb must begin the day after surgery. A physical therapist will direct these exercises. For example, arm exercises progress from isometrics to assisted ROM to active ROM. Leg exercises include rising from a chair, balancing on one leg, and ROM exercises of the knees and hips.

Stress the importance of performing prescribed exercises *to help minimize complications, maintain muscle strength and tone, prevent contractures, and promote independence.* Also stress the importance of positioning *to prevent contractures and edema.*

Complications

The most common postoperative complications include hemorrhage, stump infection, contractures, and a swollen or flabby stump. Complications that may develop at any time after an amputation include hematoma formation; skin breakdown or irritation from lack of ventilation; bone erosion or osteomyelitis; a sebaceous cyst or boil from tight socks; psychological problems, such as denial, depression, or withdrawal; and phantom limb pain caused by stimulation of nerves that once carried sensations from the distal part of the extremity.

Documentation

Record the date, time, and specific procedures of all postoperative care, including the amount and type of drainage, condition of the dressing, need for dressing reinforcement, and appearance of the suture line, surrounding tissue, and pain assessment. Also note any signs of skin irritation or infection, any complications and the nursing action taken, the patient's tolerance of exercises, and his psychological reaction to the amputation.

During routine daily care, document the date, time, type of care given, and condition of the skin and suture line, noting any signs of irritation, such as redness or tenderness. Also record the patient's progress in caring for the stump or prosthesis.

REFERENCES

1 The Joint Commission. (2012). Standard NPSG.01.01.01. *Comprehensive accreditation manual for hospitals: The official handbook.* Oakbrook Terrace, IL: The Joint Commission. (Level I)

2 Centers for Disease Control and Prevention. (October 2002). Guideline for hand hygiene in health-care settings. *Morbidity and Mortality Weekly Report, 51*(RR-16), 1–45. (Level I)

3 World Health Organization. (2009). *WHO guidelines on hand hygiene in health care: First global patient safety challenge. Clean care is safer care.* Geneva, Switzerland: World Health Organization. (Level I)

4 The Joint Commission. (2012). Standard NPSG.07.01.01. *Comprehensive accreditation manual for hospitals: The official handbook.* Oakbrook Terrace, IL: The Joint Commission. (Level I)

5 The Joint Commission. (2012). Standard RC.01.03.01. *Comprehensive accreditation manual for hospitals: The official handbook.* Oakbrook Terrace, IL: The Joint Commission. (Level I)

6 Schley, M.T., et al. (2008). Painful and nonpainful phantom and stump sensations in acute traumatic amputees. *Journal of Trauma, 65*(4), 858–864.

ADDITIONAL REFERENCES

Bevan, H. (2006). Save that stump: A multidisciplinary approach to changing stump dressing care on a vascular unit. *Journal of Vascular Nursing, 24*(3), 95.

Harker, J. (2006). "Wound Healing Complications Associated with Lower Limb Amputation" [Online]. Accessed December 2011 via the Web at http://www.worldwidewounds.com/2006/september/Harker/Wound-Healing-Complications-Limb-Amputation.html

Kelly, M., & Dowling, M. (2008). Patient rehabilitation following lower limb amputation, *Nurse Standard, 22*(49), 35–40.

Liu, F., et al. (2010). The lived experience of persons with lower extremity amputation. *Journal of Clinical Nursing, 19*(15–16), 2152–2161.

SUBCUTANEOUS INJECTION

When injected into the adipose (fatty) tissue beneath the skin, a drug moves into the bloodstream more rapidly than if given by mouth. Subcutaneous injection allows slower, more sustained drug administration than IM injection; it also causes minimal tissue trauma and carries little risk of striking large blood vessels and nerves.

Absorbed mainly through the capillaries, drugs recommended for subcutaneous injection include nonirritating aqueous solutions and suspensions contained in 0.5 to 2 mL of fluid. Heparin and insulin, for example, are usually administered subcutaneously. (Some diabetic patients may benefit from an insulin infusion pump.)

Drugs and solutions for subcutaneous injection are injected through a relatively short needle. The most common subcutaneous injection sites are the outer aspect of the upper arm, anterior thigh, loose tissue of the lower abdomen, upper hips, buttocks, and upper back. (See *Locating subcutaneous injection sites.*) Injection is contraindicated in sites that are inflamed, edematous, scarred, or covered by a mole, birthmark, or other lesion. It may also be contraindicated in patients with impaired coagulation mechanisms.

Equipment

Prescribed medication ▪ patient's medication administration record ▪ 25G to 27G ⅝″ to ½″ needle ▪ gloves ▪ 1- to 3-mL syringe ▪ alcohol pads ▪ filter needle ▪ Optional: antiseptic cleaning agent, insulin syringe. (See *Types of insulin infusion pumps,* page 682.)

Preparation of equipment

Verify the order on the patient's medication record by checking it against the doctor's order.[1] Also note whether the patient has any allergies, especially before the first dose.

Avoid distractions and interruptions when preparing and administering medication *to prevent medication errors.*[2]

Inspect the medication *to make sure it isn't abnormally discolored or cloudy and doesn't contain precipitates* (unless the manufacturer's instructions allow it).[1]

Perform hand hygiene.[3,4,5] Choose equipment appropriate to the prescribed medication and injection site.

Check the medication label against the patient's medication record. Read the label again as you draw up the medication for injection.

For single-dose ampules

Wrap an alcohol pad around the ampule's neck and snap off the top, directing the force away from your body. Attach a filter needle to the syringe and withdraw the medication, keeping the needle's bevel tip below the level of the solution. Tap the syringe *to clear air from it.* Cover the needle with the needle sheath.

Before discarding the ampule, check the medication label against the patient's medication record.[1]

Discard the filter needle and the ampule. Attach the appropriate needle to the syringe.

For single-dose or multidose vials

Reconstitute powdered drugs according to instructions. Make sure all crystals have dissolved in the solution. Warm the vial by rolling it between your palms *to help the drug dissolve faster.*

Clean the vial's rubber stopper with an alcohol pad. Pull the syringe plunger back until the volume of air in the syringe equals the volume of drug to be withdrawn from the vial.

Without inverting the vial, insert the needle into the vial. Inject the air, invert the vial, and keep the needle's bevel tip below the level of the solution as you withdraw the prescribed amount of medication. Cover the needle with the needle sheath. Tap the syringe *to clear any air from it.*

Check the medication label against the patient's medication record before discarding the single-dose vial or returning the multidose vial to the shelf.

Implementation

▪ Confirm the patient's identity using at least two patient identifiers according to your facility's policy.[6]

▪ If your facility uses a bar code scanning system, scan your identification badge, the patient's identification bracelet, and the medication's bar code, or follow the procedure for your facility's bar code system.

▪ Explain the procedure to the patient and provide privacy.

▪ Select an appropriate injection site. Rotate sites according to a schedule for repeated injections, using different areas of the body unless contraindicated. (Heparin, for example, should be injected only in the abdomen if possible.)

▪ Perform hand hygiene and put on gloves.[3,4,5]

■ Position the patient and expose the injection site.

■ Clean the injection site with an alcohol pad, beginning at the center of the site and moving outward in a circular motion. Allow the skin to dry before injecting the drug *to avoid a stinging sensation from introducing alcohol into subcutaneous tissues.*

■ Loosen the protective needle sheath.

■ With your nondominant hand, grasp the skin around the injection site firmly to elevate the subcutaneous tissue, forming a 1″ (2.5-cm) fat fold.

■ Holding the syringe in your dominant hand, insert the loosened needle sheath between the fourth and fifth fingers of your other hand while still pinching the skin around the injection site. Pull back the syringe with your dominant hand by grasping the syringe like a pencil *to uncover the needle.* Don't touch the needle.

■ Position the needle with its bevel up.

■ Tell the patient he'll feel a needle prick.

■ Insert the needle quickly in one motion at a 45- or 90-degree angle. (See *Technique for subcutaneous injections,* page 683.) Release the patient's skin *to avoid injecting the drug into compressed tissue and irritating nerve fibers.*

■ Pull back the plunger slightly *to check for blood return.* If none appears, begin injecting the drug slowly. If blood appears upon aspiration, withdraw the needle, prepare another syringe, and repeat the procedure.

NURSING ALERT *Don't aspirate for blood return when giving insulin or heparin.* It isn't necessary with insulin and may cause a hematoma with heparin.

■ After injection, remove the needle gently but quickly at the same angle used for insertion and, if present, activate the safety mechanism *to prevent accidental needle-stick injury.*[7]

■ Cover the site with an alcohol pad, and massage the site gently (unless contraindicated, as with heparin or insulin) *to distribute the drug and facilitate absorption.*

■ Remove the alcohol pad, and check the injection site for bleeding and bruising.

■ Dispose of injection equipment and gloves according to your facility's policy. *To avoid a needle-stick injury,* don't resheath the needle.[7]

■ Remove and discard your gloves and perform hand hygiene.[3,4,5]

■ Document the procedure.[8]

Special considerations

■ Aspiration for blood isn't recommended for the administration of immunizations and vaccines.[9]

■ If the medication isn't going to be administered immediately to the patient without a break in the process, clearly label the medication according to your facility's policy to prevent a medication error.[10]

■ When using prefilled syringes, adjust the angle and depth of insertion according to needle length.

For insulin injections

■ *To establish more consistent blood insulin levels,* rotate insulin injection sites within anatomic regions. Preferred insulin injection sites are the arms, abdomen, thighs, and buttocks.

Locating subcutaneous injection sites

Subcutaneous injection sites (as indicated by the shaded areas) include the fat pads on the abdomen, upper hips, upper back, and lateral upper arms and thighs. For subcutaneous injections administered repeatedly, such as insulin, rotate sites. Choose one injection site in one area, move to a corresponding injection site in the next area, and so on. When returning to an area, choose a new site in that area.

Preferred injection sites for insulin are the arms, abdomen, thighs, and buttocks. The preferred injection site for heparin is the lower abdominal fat pad, just below the umbilicus.

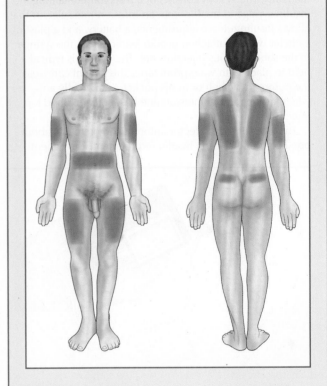

■ Make sure the type of insulin, unit dosage, and syringe are correct.

■ When combining insulins in a syringe, make sure they're compatible. Regular insulin can be mixed with all other types. Insulin zinc suspension (semilente insulin) can't be mixed with NPH insulin. Follow your facility's policy regarding which insulin to draw up first.

■ Before drawing up insulin suspension, gently roll and invert the bottle. Don't shake the bottle *because shaking can cause foam or bubbles to develop in the syringe.*

■ Insulin may be administered through an inserted insulin pump. However, before administering the drug, make sure the patient doesn't already have a pump in place.

EQUIPMENT

Types of insulin infusion pumps

A subcutaneous insulin infusion pump provides continuous, long-term insulin therapy for patients with type 1 diabetes mellitus. Complications include infection at the injection site, catheter clogging, and insulin loss from loose reservoir-catheter connections. Insulin pumps work on either an open-loop or a closed-loop system.

Open-loop system

The open-loop pump (shown below) is used most commonly. It infuses insulin but can't respond to changes in the patient's serum glucose levels. These portable, self-contained, programmable insulin pumps are small and unobtrusive.

The pump delivers insulin in small (basal) doses every few minutes and large (bolus) doses that the patient sets manually. The system consists of a reservoir containing the insulin syringe, a small pump, an infusion-rate selector that allows insulin release adjustments, a battery, and a plastic catheter with an attached needle leading from the syringe to the subcutaneous injection site. The needle is typically held in place with waterproof tape. The patient can wear the pump on his belt or in his pocket—practically anywhere as long as the infusion line has a clear path to the injection site.

The infusion-rate selector automatically releases about one-half the total daily insulin requirement. The patient

releases the remainder in bolus doses before meals and snacks. He must change the syringe daily and the needle, catheter, and injection site every other day.

Closed-loop system

The self-contained closed-loop system detects and responds to changing serum glucose levels. The typical closed-loop system includes a glucose sensor, a programmable computer, a power supply, a pump, and an insulin reservoir. The computer triggers continuous insulin delivery in appropriate amounts from the reservoir.

Nonneedle catheter system

In the nonneedle delivery system, a tiny plastic catheter is inserted into the skin over a needle using a special insertion device (shown below). The needle is then withdrawn, leaving the catheter in place. This catheter can be placed in the abdomen, thigh, or flank and should be changed every 2 to 3 days.

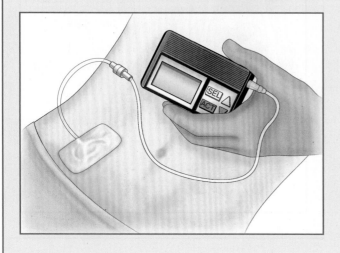

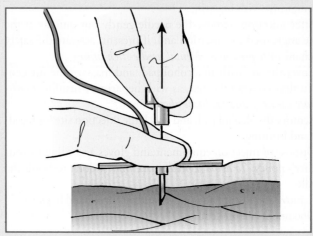

For heparin injections

■ The preferred site for a heparin injection is the lower abdominal fat pad, 2″ (5 cm) beneath the umbilicus, between the right and left iliac crests. *Injecting heparin into this area, which isn't involved in muscle activity, reduces the risk of local capillary bleeding.* Always rotate the sites from one side to the other.

■ Inject the drug slowly into the fat pad. Leave the needle in place for 10 seconds after injection, and then withdraw it.[11]

■ Don't administer any injections within 2″ of a scar, a bruise, or the umbilicus.

■ Don't aspirate to check for blood return *because this can cause bleeding into the tissues at the site.*

■ Don't rub or massage the site after the injection. *Rubbing can cause localized minute hemorrhages or bruises.*

■ If the patient bruises easily, apply ice to the site for the first 5 minutes after the injection *to minimize local hemorrhage,* and then apply pressure.

Complications

Concentrated or irritating solutions may cause sterile abscesses to form. Repeated injections in the same site can cause lipodystrophy. A natural immune response, lipodystrophy can be minimized by rotating injection sites.

Documentation

Record the time and date of the injection, medication and dose administered, injection site and route, and patient's response.

REFERENCES

1 The Joint Commission. (2012). Standard MM.06.01.01. *Comprehensive accreditation manual for hospitals: The official handbook.* Oakbrook Terrace, IL: The Joint Commission. (Level I)

2 Westbrook, J., et al. (2010). Association of interruptions with an increased risk and severity of medication administration errors. *Archives of Internal Medicine, 170*(8), 683–690.

3 Centers for Disease Control and Prevention. (October 2002). Guideline for hand hygiene in health-care settings. *Morbidity and Mortality Weekly Report, 51*(RR-16), 1–45. (Level I)

4 World Health Organization. (2009). *WHO guidelines on hand hygiene in health care: First global patient safety challenge. Clean care is safer care.* Geneva, Switzerland: World Health Organization. (Level I)

5 The Joint Commission. (2012). Standard NPSG.07.01.01. *Comprehensive accreditation manual for hospitals: The official handbook.* Oakbrook Terrace, IL: The Joint Commission. (Level I)

6 The Joint Commission. (2012). Standard NPSG.01.01.01. *Comprehensive accreditation manual for hospitals: The official handbook.* Oakbrook Terrace, IL: The Joint Commission. (Level I)

7 Occupational Safety and Health Administration. "Bloodborne Pathogens, Standard Number 1910.1030" [Online]. Accessed December 2011 via the Web at http://www.osha.gov/pls/oshaweb/owadisp.show_document?p_table=STANDARDS&p_id=10051

8 The Joint Commission. (2012). Standard RC.01.03.01. *Comprehensive accreditation manual for hospitals: The official handbook.* Oakbrook Terrace, IL: The Joint Commission. (Level I)

9 Petousis-Harris, H. (2008). Vaccine injection technique and reactogenicity—Evidence for practice. *Vaccine, 26*(50), 6299–6304.

10 The Joint Commission. (2012). Standard NPSG.03.04.01. *Comprehensive accreditation manual for hospitals: The official handbook.* Oakbrook Terrace, IL: The Joint Commission. (Level I)

11 Zaybak, A., & Khorshid, L. (2008). A study on the effect of the duration of subcutaneous heparin injection on bruising and pain. *Journal of Clinical Nursing, 17*(3), 378–385. (Level VI)

ADDITIONAL REFERENCES

Gittens, G., & Bunnell, T. (2009). Skin disinfection and its efficacy before administering injections. *Nursing Standard, 23*(39), 42–44.

Hunter, J. (2008). Subcutaneous injection technique. *Nursing Standard, 22*(21), 41–44.

Lynn, P. (2011). *Taylor's clinical nursing skills* (3rd ed.). Philadelphia, PA: Lippincott Williams & Wilkins.

Nettina, S.M. (2010). *Lippincott manual of nursing practice* (9th ed.). Philadelphia, PA: Lippincott Williams & Wilkins.

Taylor, C., et al. (2011). *Fundamentals of nursing: The art and science of nursing care* (7th ed.). Philadelphia, PA: Lippincott Williams & Wilkins.

Technique for subcutaneous injections

Before giving the injection, elevate the subcutaneous tissue at the site by grasping it firmly.

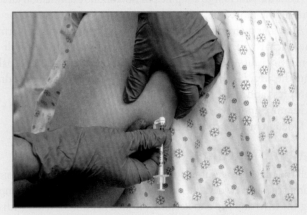

Insert the needle at a 45- or 90-degree angle to the skin surface, depending on needle length and the amount of subcutaneous tissue at the site. Some medications, such as heparin, should always be injected at a 90-degree angle.

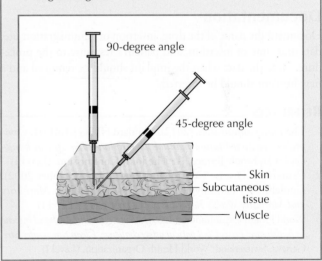

SUBDERMAL DRUG IMPLANTS

A method of drug delivery, subdermal implants come in the form of flexible capsules or rods, which are placed under the skin. This method is most commonly used to inject various hormones so they can be absorbed into the bloodstream.

Equipment

Sterile surgical drapes ▪ sterile gloves ▪ antiseptic solution ▪ local anesthetic ▪ implants ▪ needles ▪ 5-ml syringe ▪ #11 scalpel ▪ #10 trocar ▪ forceps ▪ sutures ▪ sterile gauze ▪ tape ▪ gloves.

Implementation

- Confirm the patient's identity using at least two patient identifiers according to your facility's policy.[1]
- Explain the procedure, including its benefits and risks, and show a set of implants to the patient.
- Perform hand hygiene and put on gloves.[2,3,4]
- Assist the patient into a supine position on the examination table. During the procedure, stay and provide support, as necessary.
- After anesthetizing the upper portion of the nondominant arm, the doctor will use a trocar to insert each capsule through a 2-mm incision. After insertion, he'll remove the trocar and palpate the area. He'll then close the incision and cover it with a dry compress and sterile gauze.
- Remove and discard your gloves. Perform hand hygiene.[2,3,4]
- Document the procedure.[5]

Patient teaching

Tell the patient to resume normal activities but to protect the site during the first few days after implantation. Recommend not bumping the insertion site and keeping the area dry and covered with a gauze bandage for 3 days. Tell the patient to report signs of bleeding or infection at the insertion site. Instruct the patient to notify the doctor immediately if one of the implants falls out before the skin heals. If it's a contraceptive implant, the patient should use alternative means of contraception until the drug is replaced.

Documentation

Document the name of the drug, insertion or administration site, date and time of insertion, and patient's response to the procedure. Note the date when the implant should be removed and a new implant should be inserted.

REFERENCES

1 The Joint Commission. (2012). Standard NPSG.01.01.01. *Comprehensive accreditation manual for hospitals: The official handbook.* Oakbrook Terrace, IL: The Joint Commission. (Level I)
2 Centers for Disease Control and Prevention. (October 2002). Guideline for hand hygiene in health-care settings. *Morbidity and Mortality Weekly Report, 51*(RR-16), 1–45. (Level I)
3 World Health Organization. (2009). *WHO guidelines on hand hygiene in health care: First global patient safety challenge. Clean care is safer care.* Geneva, Switzerland: World Health Organization. (Level I)
4 The Joint Commission. (2012). Standard NPSG.07.01.01. *Comprehensive accreditation manual for hospitals: The official handbook.* Oakbrook Terrace, IL: The Joint Commission. (Level I)
5 The Joint Commission. (2012). Standard RC.01.03.01. *Comprehensive accreditation manual for hospitals: The official handbook.* Oakbrook Terrace, IL: The Joint Commission. (Level I)

SURGICAL DRAIN REMOVAL

Surgical drains are important adjuncts to postoperative care because they promote wound healing by providing an exit site for fluid that accumulates in or near the wound bed. Drains should be removed when drainage becomes minimal or when they malfunction. Drains commonly inserted during surgery include the Hemovac, bulb suction, and Penrose.

Equipment

Sterile 4″ × 4″ gauze pads ▪ tape ▪ gloves ▪ gown ▪ face shield ▪ Optional: suture removal kit, ordered pain medications.

Implementation

- Verify the doctor's order.
- Review the patient's medical record to determine the type of drain to be removed, its location, and the method used to secure it *to ensure proper removal.*
- Perform hand hygiene.[1,2,3]
- Confirm the patient's identity using at least two patient identifiers according to your facility's policy.[4]
- Explain the procedure to the patient *to allay his fear and anxiety.*
- Perform a comprehensive pain assessment, using techniques appropriate for the patient's age, condition, and ability to understand.[5]
- Administer pain medications, as ordered, following safe medication administration practices.[6]
- Perform hand hygiene. Put on a gown, gloves, and a face shield, if necessary, *to protect yourself from splashing.*[7]
- Position the patient in a comfortable position that provides you with adequate access to the surgical site.
- If the drain contains suction from its initial closure, release the suction from the drain.
- Remove the drain dressing *to gain access to the exit site.*
- Open the suture removal kit and cut any sutures, if present.
- Place a 4″ × 4″ sterile gauze pad close to the exit site *to absorb any remaining drainage while the drain is removed.*[8]
- Have the patient breathe deeply and smoothly. While the patient is breathing as instructed, remove the drain in a quick, even motion, and then discard it in the appropriate receptacle. If you feel resistance, stop the procedure and notify the doctor.[8]
- Assess the exit site for signs of infection, such as redness, swelling, a foul odor, or purulent drainage.
- Remove and discard your gloves. Perform hand hygiene, and put on new gloves.[1,2,3]
- Place a sterile 4″ × 4″ gauze dressing over the drain exit site and secure it with tape. Label the dressing with the date, time, and your initials.[8]
- Discard used materials in an appropriate receptacle according to your facility's policy.
- Perform a follow-up pain assessment and notify the doctor if the patient's pain isn't adequately controlled.[5]
- Remove your gloves and other personal protective equipment and perform hand hygiene.[1,2,3]
- Document the procedure.[9]

Special considerations

- Drainage from the exit site should be minimal and cease within 24 hours of drain removal. If drainage continues, notify the doctor because fluid may be accumulating beneath the skin and require evacuation.[9]

Complications

Fluid accumulating under the skin may result in impaired wound healing. Infection may also be a complication of drain removal.

Documentation

Document the date and time of drain removal, the type of drain removed, the condition of the exit site, and the presence of drainage. Document your pain assessments and any medications given. Document the patient's tolerance of the procedure, patient teaching performed, and the patient's understanding of the teaching.

REFERENCES

1 Centers for Disease Control and Prevention. (October 2002). Guideline for hand hygiene in health-care settings. *Morbidity and Mortality Weekly Report, 51*(RR-16), 1–45. (Level I)
2 World Health Organization. (2009). *WHO guidelines on hand hygiene in health care: First global patient safety challenge. Clean care is safer care.* Geneva, Switzerland: World Health Organization. (Level I)
3 The Joint Commission. (2012). Standard NPSG.07.01.01. *Comprehensive accreditation manual for hospitals: The official handbook.* Oakbrook Terrace, IL: The Joint Commission. (Level I)
4 The Joint Commission. (2012). Standard NPSG.01.01.01. *Comprehensive accreditation manual for hospitals: The official handbook.* Oakbrook Terrace, IL: The Joint Commission. (Level I)
5 The Joint Commission. (2012). Standard PC.01.02.07. *Comprehensive accreditation manual for hospitals: The official handbook.* Oakbrook Terrace, IL: The Joint Commission. (Level I)
6 The Joint Commission. (2012). Standard MM.06.01.01. *Comprehensive accreditation manual for hospitals: The official handbook.* Oakbrook Terrace, IL: The Joint Commission. (Level I)
7 The Joint Commission. (2012). Standard NPSG.07.05.01. *Comprehensive accreditation manual for hospitals: The official handbook.* Oakbrook Terrace, IL: The Joint Commission. (Level I)
8 Lynn-McHale Wiegand, D. (Ed.). (2011). *AACN procedure manual for critical care* (6th ed.). Philadelphia, PA: Saunders.
9 The Joint Commission. (2012). Standard RC.01.03.01. *Comprehensive accreditation manual for hospitals: The official handbook.* Oakbrook Terrace, IL: The Joint Commission. (Level I)

SURGICAL WOUND MANAGEMENT

When caring for a surgical wound, you carry out procedures that help prevent infection by stopping pathogens from entering the wound. Besides promoting patient comfort, such procedures protect the skin surface from maceration and excoriation caused by contact with irritating drainage. They also allow you to measure wound drainage to monitor fluid balance.

Dressing is the primary method used to manage a draining surgical wound. Lightly seeping wounds with drains and wounds with minimal purulent drainage can typically be managed with packing and gauze dressings. Some wounds, such as those that become chronic, may require an occlusive dressing. If your patient has a surgical wound, monitor him closely and choose the appropriate dressing.

Dressing a wound calls for sterile technique and sterile supplies to prevent contamination. You may use the color of the wound to help determine which type of dressing to apply. (See *Tailoring wound care to wound color.*)

Tailoring wound care to wound color

Promote healing in any wound by keeping it moist, clean, and free of debris. For open wounds, use wound color to guide the specific management approach and to assess how well the wound is healing.

Red wounds

Red, the color of healthy granulation tissue, indicates normal healing. When a wound begins to heal, a layer of pale pink granulation tissue covers the wound bed. As this layer thickens, it becomes beefy red. Cover a red wound, keep it moist and clean, and protect it from trauma. Use a transparent dressing, hydrocolloid dressing, or gauze dressing moistened with sterile normal saline solution or impregnated with petroleum jelly or an antibiotic.

Yellow wounds

Yellow is the color of exudate produced by microorganisms in an open wound. When a wound heals without complications, the immune system removes microorganisms. However, if there are too many microorganisms to remove, exudate accumulates and becomes visible. Exudate usually appears whitish yellow, creamy yellow, yellowish green, or beige. Dry exudate appears darker.

If your patient has a yellow wound, clean it and remove exudate, using irrigation; then cover it with a moist dressing. Use absorptive products or a moist gauze dressing with or without an antibiotic. You may also use hydrotherapy with whirlpool or high-pressure irrigation.

Black wounds

Black, the least healthy color, signals necrosis. Dead, avascular tissue slows healing and provides a site for microorganisms to proliferate.

A black wound should be debrided. After removing dead tissue, apply a dressing to keep the wound moist and guard against external contamination. As ordered, use enzyme products, surgical debridement, hydrotherapy with whirlpool or irrigation, or a moist gauze dressing.

Multicolored wounds

You may note two or even all three colors in a wound. In this case, classify the wound according to the least healthy color present. For example, if your patient's wound is both red and yellow, classify it as a yellow wound.

Change the dressing frequently enough to keep the skin dry. Always follow standard precautions set by the Centers for Disease Control and Prevention.

Equipment

Waterproof trash bag ■ gloves ■ sterile gloves ■ gown and face shield or goggles, if indicated ■ sterile 4″ × 4″ gauze pads ■ large absorbent dressings, if indicated ■ sterile cotton-tipped applicators ■ sterile dressing set ■ povidone-iodine swabs ■ topical medication, if ordered ■ adhesive or other tape ■ soap and water ■ Optional: forceps; skin protectant; nonadherent pads; collodion spray or acetone-free adhesive remover; sterile normal saline solution; graduated container; prescribed irrigant and piston-style syringe; sterile scissors; Montgomery straps, fishnet tube elasticized dressing support, or T-binder.

Preparation of equipment

Identify the patient's allergies, especially to adhesive tape, povidone-iodine or other topical solutions, or medications. Gather all equipment in the patient's room. Check the expiration date on each sterile package, and inspect for tears.

Open the waterproof trash bag, and place it near the patient's bed. Position the bag to avoid reaching across the sterile field or the wound when disposing of soiled articles. Form a cuff by turning down the top of the trash bag *to provide a wide opening and to prevent contamination of instruments or gloves by touching the bag's edge.*

Implementation

■ Check the doctor's order for specific wound care and medication instructions.[1]
■ Note the location of surgical drains *to avoid dislodging them during the procedure.*
■ Confirm the patient's identity using at least two patient identifiers according to your facility's policy.[2]
■ Explain the procedure to the patient *to allay his fears and ensure his cooperation.*

Removing the old dressing

■ Provide privacy and position the patient, as necessary. *To avoid chilling him,* expose only the wound site.
■ Perform hand hygiene. Put on a gown and a face shield, if necessary. Then put on gloves.[3,4,5]
■ Assess the patient's condition.
■ Loosen the soiled dressing by holding the patient's skin and pulling the tape or dressing toward the wound. *This protects the newly formed tissue and prevents stress on the incision.*
■ Moisten the tape with acetone-free adhesive remover, if necessary, *to make the tape removal less painful (particularly if the skin is hairy).* Don't apply solvents to the incision *because they could contaminate the wound.*
■ Slowly remove the soiled dressing. If the gauze adheres to the wound, loosen the gauze by moistening it with sterile normal saline solution.
■ Observe the dressing for the amount, type, color, and odor of drainage.
■ Discard the dressing and gloves in the waterproof trash bag.

Caring for the wound

■ Perform hand hygiene.[3,4,5]
■ Establish a sterile field with all the equipment and supplies you'll need for suture-line care and the dressing change, including a sterile dressing set and povidone-iodine swabs. If the doctor has ordered ointment, squeeze the needed amount onto the sterile field. If you're using an antiseptic from an unsterile bottle, pour the antiseptic cleaning agent into a sterile container *so you won't contaminate your gloves.* Then put on sterile gloves.
■ Saturate the sterile gauze pads with the prescribed cleaning agent. Avoid using cotton balls *because they may shed fibers in the wound, causing irritation, infection, or adhesion.*
■ If ordered, obtain a wound culture; then proceed to clean the wound.
■ If ordered, irrigate the wound, using the specified solution and a piston-style syringe. (See "Wound irrigation," page 795.)
■ Pick up the moistened gauze pad or swab, and squeeze out the excess solution.
■ For an open wound, clean the wound in a full or half circle beginning in the center and working outwards (as shown below). Use a new swab or pad for each circle. Clean to at least 1″ (2.5 cm) beyond the end of the new dressing or 2″ (5 cm) beyond the wound margins if you aren't applying a dressing.

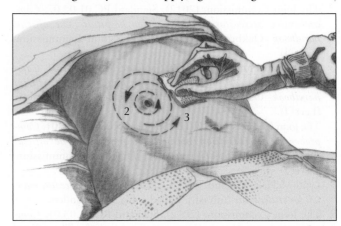

■ For a linear incision, work from the top of the incision, wipe once to the bottom, and then discard the gauze pad. With a second moistened pad, wipe from top to bottom in a vertical path next to the incision (as shown below).

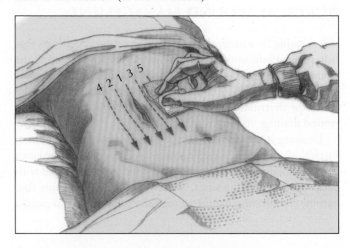

■ Continue to work outward from the incision in lines running parallel to it. Always wipe from the clean area toward the less clean area (usually from top to bottom). Use each gauze pad or swab for only one stroke *to avoid tracking wound exudate and normal body flora from surrounding skin to the clean areas.* Remember that the suture line is cleaner than the adjacent skin and the top of the suture line is usually cleaner than the bottom *because more drainage collects at the bottom of the wound.*

■ Use sterile, cotton-tipped applicators for efficient cleaning of tight-fitting wire sutures, deep and narrow wounds, and wounds with pockets. *Because the cotton on the swab is tightly wrapped,* it's less likely than a cotton ball to leave fibers in the wound. Remember to wipe only once with each applicator.

■ If the patient has a surgical drain, clean the patient's drain surface last. *Because moisture promotes bacterial growth,* the drain is the most contaminated area. Clean the skin around the drain by wiping in half or full circles from the drain site outward.

■ Clean all areas of the wound *to wash away debris, pus, blood, and necrotic material.* Try not to disturb sutures or irritate the incision. Clean to at least 1″ (2.5 cm) beyond the end of the new dressing.

■ Check to make sure the edges of the incision are lined up properly, and check for signs of infection (heat, redness, swelling, induration, and odor), dehiscence, and evisceration. If you observe such signs or if the patient reports pain at the wound site, notify the doctor.

■ Wash the skin surrounding the wound with soap and water, and pat dry using a sterile 4″ × 4″ gauze pad. Avoid oil-based soap *because it may interfere with tape adherence.* Apply any prescribed topical medication.

■ Apply a skin protectant, if needed.

■ If ordered, pack the wound with gauze pads or strips folded to fit, using a sterile forceps. Avoid using cotton-lined gauze pads *because cotton fibers can adhere to the wound surface and cause complications.* Pack the wound, using the wet-to-damp method. Soaking the packing material in solution and wringing it out so that it's slightly moist provides a moist wound environment that absorbs debris and drainage without disrupting new tissue when the packing is removed. Don't pack the wound tightly; doing so will exert pressure and may damage the wound.

Applying a fresh gauze dressing

■ Gently place sterile 4″ × 4″ gauze pads at the center of the wound, and move progressively outward to the edges of the wound site. Extend the gauze at least 1″ (2.5 cm) beyond the incision in each direction, and cover the wound evenly with enough sterile dressings (usually two or three layers) to absorb all drainage until the next dressing change. Use large absorbent dressings to form outer layers, if needed, *to provide greater absorbency.*

■ Secure the dressing's edges to the patient's skin with strips of tape to maintain the sterility of the wound site (as shown in next column top).

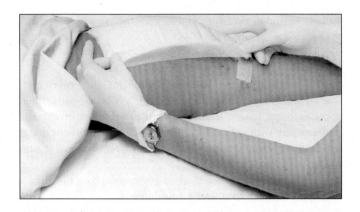

■ Alternatively, secure the dressing with a T-binder or Montgomery straps (as shown below) *to prevent skin excoriation,* which may occur with repeated tape removal necessitated by frequent dressing changes.

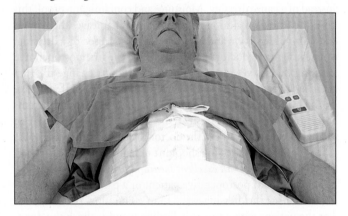

■ If the wound is on a limb, secure the dressing with a fishnet tube elasticized dressing support.

Dressing a wound with a drain

■ Use commercially precut sterile gauze dressings, or prepare a drain dressing by using sterile scissors to cut a slit in a sterile 4″ × 4″ gauze pad. Fold the pad in half; then cut inward from the center of the folded edge. Don't use a cotton-lined gauze pad *because cutting the gauze opens the lining and releases cotton fibers into the wound.* Prepare a second pad in the same way.

■ Gently press one drain dressing close to the skin around the drain so that the tubing fits into the slit. Press the second drain dressing around the drain from the opposite direction so that the two dressings encircle the drain.

■ Layer as many uncut sterile 4″ × 4″ gauze pads or large absorbent dressings around the tubing as needed *to absorb expected drainage.* Tape the dressing in place, or use a T-binder or Montgomery straps.

Completing the procedure

■ Make sure the patient is comfortable.

■ Properly dispose of the solutions and trash bag, and clean or discard soiled equipment and supplies according to your facility's policy. If your patient's wound has purulent drainage, don't return unopened sterile supplies to the sterile supply cabinet *because this could cause cross-contamination of other equipment.*

- Remove and discard your gloves. Perform hand hygiene.[3,4,5]
- Document the procedure.[6]

Special considerations

- If the patient has two wounds in the same area, cover each wound separately with layers of sterile 4″ × 4″ gauze pads. Then cover each site with a large absorbent dressing secured to the patient's skin with tape. Don't use a single large absorbent dressing to cover both sites *because drainage quickly saturates a pad, promoting cross-contamination.*
- If a wound drains more than an estimated 1½ oz (44 mL) a day, apply a pouch to collect excess drainage.
- When packing a wound, don't pack it too tightly *because this compresses adjacent capillaries and may prevent the wound edges from contracting.* Avoid overlapping damp packing onto surrounding skin *because it macerates the intact tissue.*
- If ordered, use a collodion spray or similar topical protectant instead of a gauze dressing. Moisture- and contaminant-proof, this covering dries in a clear, impermeable film that leaves the wound visible for observation and avoids the friction caused by a dressing.
- Because many doctors prefer to change the first postoperative dressing themselves to check the incision, don't change the first dressing unless you have specific instructions to do so. If you have no such order and drainage comes through the dressings, reinforce the dressing with fresh sterile gauze. Request an order to change the dressing, or ask the doctor to change it as soon as possible. A reinforced dressing shouldn't remain in place longer than 24 hours *because it's an excellent medium for bacterial growth.*
- For the recent postoperative patient or a patient with complications, check the dressing every 15 to 30 minutes, or as ordered. For the patient with a properly healing wound, check the dressing at least once every 8 hours.
- If the dressing becomes wet from the outside (for example, from spilled drinking water), replace it as soon as possible *to prevent wound contamination.*

Patient teaching

If your patient will need wound care after discharge, provide appropriate teaching. If he'll be caring for the wound himself, stress the importance of using sterile technique, and teach him how to examine the wound for signs of infection and other complications. Also show him how to change dressings, and give him written instructions for all procedures to be performed at home.

Complications

A major complication of a dressing change is an allergic reaction to an antiseptic cleaning agent, a prescribed topical medication, or adhesive tape. This reaction may lead to skin redness, rash, excoriation, or infection.

NURSING ALERT *Take care when removing adhesive tape to prevent skin tears, especially in elderly patients.*

Documentation

Document the date, time, and type of wound management procedure; amount of soiled dressing and packing removed; wound appearance (size, condition of margins, and presence of necrotic tissue) and odor (if present); type, color, consistency, and amount of drainage (for each wound); presence and location of drains; additional procedures, such as irrigation, packing, or application of a topical medication; type and amount of new dressing applied; the patient's tolerance of the procedure; and any patient teaching provided.

Document special or detailed wound care instructions and pain management steps on the care plan. Record the color and amount of drainage on the intake and output sheet.

REFERENCES

1 The Joint Commission. (2012). Standard MM.04.01.01. *Comprehensive accreditation manual for hospitals: The official handbook.* Oakbrook Terrace, IL: The Joint Commission. (Level I)
2 The Joint Commission. (2012). Standard NPSG.01.01.01. *Comprehensive accreditation manual for hospitals: The official handbook.* Oakbrook Terrace, IL: The Joint Commission. (Level I)
3 Centers for Disease Control and Prevention. (October 2002). Guideline for hand hygiene in health-care settings. *Morbidity and Mortality Weekly Report, 51*(RR-16), 1–45. (Level I)
4 World Health Organization. (2009). *WHO guidelines on hand hygiene in health care: First global patient safety challenge. Clean care is safer care.* Geneva, Switzerland: World Health Organization. (Level I)
5 The Joint Commission. (2012). Standard NPSG.07.01.01. *Comprehensive accreditation manual for hospitals: The official handbook.* Oakbrook Terrace, IL: The Joint Commission. (Level I)
6 The Joint Commission. (2012). Standard RC.01.03.01. *Comprehensive accreditation manual for hospitals: The official handbook.* Oakbrook Terrace, IL: The Joint Commission. (Level I)

ADDITIONAL REFERENCES

Baranoski, S., & Ayello, E.A. (2008). *Wound care essentials: Practice principles* (2nd ed.). Philadelphia, PA: Lippincott Williams & Williams.
Craven, R.F., & Hirnle, C.J. (2012). *Fundamentals of nursing: Human health and function* (7th ed.). Philadelphia, PA: Lippincott Williams & Wilkins.
Hess, C.T. (2008). *Clinical guide to skin & wound care* (6th ed.). Philadelphia, PA: Lippincott Williams & Wilkins.
Taylor, C., et al. (2011). *Fundamentals of nursing: The art and science of nursing care* (7th ed.). Philadelphia, PA: Lippincott Williams & Wilkins.
Vuolo, J. (2006). Assessment and management of surgical wounds in clinical practice. *Nursing Standard, 20*(52), 46–56.

SUTURE REMOVAL

The goal of this procedure is to remove skin sutures from a healed wound without damaging newly formed tissue. The timing of suture removal depends on the shape, size, and location of the sutured incision; the absence of inflammation, drainage, and infection; and the patient's general condition. For a sufficiently healed wound, sutures are typically removed 7 to 10 days after insertion.

Techniques for removal depend on the method of suturing, but all require sterile technique to prevent contamination. Although sutures usually are removed by a doctor, in many facilities, a nurse may remove them on the doctor's order.

Equipment

Waterproof trash bag ▪ adjustable light ▪ clean gloves, if the wound is dressed ▪ sterile gloves ▪ sterile forceps or sterile hemostat ▪ normal saline solution ▪ sterile gauze pads ▪ antiseptic cleaning agent ▪ sterile curve-tipped suture scissors ▪ povidone-iodine sponges ▪ Optional: butterfly or regular adhesive strips, compound benzoin tincture or other skin protectant.

Prepackaged, sterile suture-removal trays are available.

Preparation of equipment

Gather all equipment in the patient's room. Check the expiration date on each sterile package and inspect for tears. Open the waterproof trash bag, and place it near the patient's bed. Position the bag properly *to avoid reaching across the sterile field or the suture line when disposing of soiled articles.* Form a cuff on the bag by turning down the top *to provide a wide opening and prevent contamination of instruments or gloves by touching the bag's edge.*

Implementation

▪ If your facility allows you to remove sutures, check the doctor's order *to confirm the details of this procedure.*
▪ Confirm the patient's identity using at least two patient identifiers according to your facility's policy.[1]
▪ Check for patient allergies, especially to adhesive tape and povidone-iodine or other topical solutions or medications.
▪ Tell the patient that you're going to remove the stitches from his wound. Assure him that this procedure typically is painless, but that he may feel a pulling sensation as the stitches come out. Reassure him that because his wound is healing properly, removing the stitches won't weaken the incision.
▪ Provide privacy, and position the patient so he's comfortable without placing undue tension on the suture line. *Because some patients experience nausea or dizziness during the procedure,* have the patient recline if possible. Adjust the light to have it shine directly on the suture line.
▪ Perform hand hygiene. If the patient's wound has a dressing, put on clean gloves and carefully remove the dressing.[2,3,4]
▪ Discard the dressing and the gloves in the waterproof trash bag.
▪ Observe the patient's wound for possible gaping, drainage, inflammation, signs of infection, and embedded sutures. Notify the doctor if the wound has failed to heal properly. The absence of a healing ridge under the suture line 5 to 7 days after the incision indicates that the line needs continued support and protection during the healing process.
▪ Establish a sterile work area with all the equipment and supplies you'll need for suture removal and wound care.
▪ Perform hand hygiene and put on sterile gloves and open the sterile suture removal tray if you're using one.[2,3,4]
▪ Using sterile technique, clean the suture line *to decrease the number of microorganisms present and reduce the risk of infection.* The cleaning process should also moisten the sutures sufficiently *to ease removal.* Soften them further, if needed, with normal saline solution.
▪ Proceed according to the type of suture you're removing. (See *Methods for removing sutures,* pages 690 and 691.) *Because the visible part of a suture is exposed to skin bacteria and considered contaminated,* be sure to cut sutures at the skin surface on one side

of the visible part of the suture. Remove the suture by lifting and pulling the visible end off the skin *to avoid drawing this contaminated portion back through subcutaneous tissue.*
▪ If ordered, remove every other suture *to maintain some support for the incision.* Then go back and remove the remaining sutures.
▪ After removing sutures, wipe the incision gently with gauze pads soaked in an antiseptic cleaning agent or with a povidone-iodine sponge. Apply a light sterile gauze dressing, if needed, *to prevent infection and irritation from clothing.* Then discard your gloves.
▪ Make sure the patient is comfortable. According to the doctor's preference, inform the patient that he may shower in 1 or 2 days if the incision is dry and heals well.
▪ Properly dispose of the solutions and trash bag, and clean or dispose of soiled equipment and supplies according to your facility's policy.
▪ Perform hand hygiene.[2,3,4]
▪ Document the procedure.[5]

Special considerations

▪ Check the doctor's order for the time of suture removal. You'll typically remove sutures on the head and neck 3 to 5 days after insertion; on the chest and abdomen, 5 to 7 days after insertion; and on the lower extremities, 7 to 10 days after insertion.
▪ If the patient has interrupted sutures or an incompletely healed suture line, remove only those sutures specified by the doctor. He may want to leave some sutures in place for an additional day or two *to support the suture line.*
▪ If the patient has both retention and regular sutures in place, check the doctor's order for the sequence in which they are to be removed. *Because retention sutures link underlying fat and muscle tissue and give added support to the obese or slow-healing patient,* they usually remain in place for 14 to 21 days.
▪ Be particularly careful to clean the suture line before attempting to remove mattress sutures *to decrease the risk of infection when the visible, contaminated part of the stitch is too small to cut twice for sterile removal and must be pulled through the tissue.* After you have removed mattress sutures this way, monitor the suture line carefully *for subsequent infection.*
▪ If the wound dehisces during suture removal, apply butterfly or regular adhesive strips to support and approximate the edges and call the doctor immediately to repair the wound.
▪ Apply butterfly or regular adhesive strips after any suture removal, if desired, *to give added support to the incision line and prevent lateral tension on the wound from forming a wide scar.* Use a small amount of compound benzoin tincture or other skin protectant *to ensure adherence.* Leave the strips in place for 3 to 5 days, as ordered.

Patient teaching

If the patient is being discharged, teach him how to remove the dressing and care for the wound. Instruct him to call the doctor immediately if he observes wound discharge or any other abnormal change. Tell him that the redness surrounding the incision should gradually disappear and only a thin line should show after a few weeks.

Methods for removing sutures

Removal techniques depend in large part on the type of sutures to be removed. The illustrations here show removal steps for four common suture types. Keep in mind that for all suture types, it's important to grasp and cut sutures in the correct place to avoid pulling the exposed (thus contaminated) suture material through subcutaneous tissue.

Cutting the suture

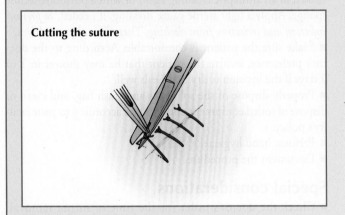

Grasping the suture

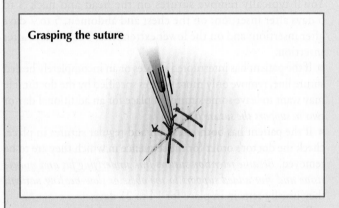

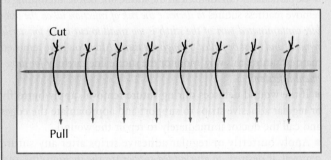

Cut

Pull

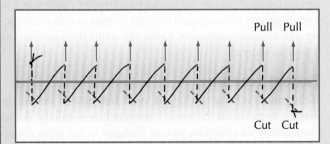

Pull Pull

Cut Cut

Plain interrupted sutures

Using sterile forceps, grasp the knot of the first suture and raise it off the skin. *Doing so exposes a small portion of the suture that was below skin level.* Place the rounded tips of sterile curved-tip suture scissors against the skin, and cut through the exposed portion of the suture.

Then, still holding the knot with the forceps, pull the cut suture up and out of the skin in a smooth continuous motion to *avoid causing the patient pain.*

Discard the suture. Repeat the process for every other suture, initially; if the wound doesn't gape, you can then remove the remaining sutures as ordered.

Plain continuous sutures

Cut the first suture on the side opposite the knot. Next, cut the same side of the next suture in line. Then lift the first suture out in the direction of the knot. Proceed along the suture line, grasping each suture where you grasped the knot on the first one.

Methods for removing sutures (continued)

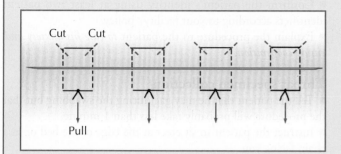

Cut   Cut

Pull

Mattress interrupted sutures

If possible, remove the small, visible portion of the suture opposite the knot by cutting it at each visible end and lifting the small piece away from the skin *to prevent pulling it through and contaminating subcutaneous tissue*. Then remove the rest of the suture by pulling it out in the direction of the knot. If the visible portion is too small to cut twice, cut it once and pull the entire suture out in the opposite direction. Repeat these steps for the remaining sutures, and monitor the incision carefully for infection.

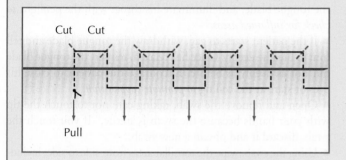

Cut   Cut

Pull

Mattress continuous sutures

Follow the procedure for removing mattress interrupted sutures, first removing the small visible portion of the suture, if possible, *to prevent pulling it through and contaminating subcutaneous tissue*. Then extract the rest of the suture in the direction of the knot.

Documentation

Record the date and time of suture removal, type and number of sutures, appearance of the suture line, signs of wound complications, dressings or adhesive strips applied, the patient's tolerance of the procedure, and any patient teaching provided.

REFERENCES

1 The Joint Commission. (2012). *Standard NPSG.01.01.01. Comprehensive accreditation manual for hospitals: The official handbook.* Oakbrook Terrace, IL: The Joint Commission. (Level I)

2 Centers for Disease Control and Prevention. (October 2002). Guideline for hand hygiene in health-care settings. *Morbidity and Mortality Weekly Report, 51*(RR-16), 1–45. (Level I)

3 World Health Organization. (2009). *WHO guidelines on hand hygiene in health care: First global patient safety challenge. Clean care is safer care.* Geneva, Switzerland: World Health Organization. (Level I)

4 The Joint Commission. (2012). *Standard NPSG.07.01.01. Comprehensive accreditation manual for hospitals: The official handbook.* Oakbrook Terrace, IL: The Joint Commission. (Level I)

5 The Joint Commission. (2012). *Standard RC.01.03.01. Comprehensive accreditation manual for hospitals: The official handbook.* Oakbrook Terrace, IL: The Joint Commission. (Level I)

ADDITIONAL REFERENCES

Craven, R.F., & Hirnle, C.J. (2012). *Fundamentals of nursing: Human health and function* (7th ed.). Philadelphia, PA: Lippincott Williams & Wilkins.

Taylor, C., et al. (2011). *Fundamentals of nursing: The art and science of nursing care* (7th ed.). Philadelphia, PA: Lippincott Williams & Wilkins.

SWAB SPECIMEN COLLECTION

Correct collection and handling of swab specimens helps laboratory staff members identify pathogens accurately with a minimum of contamination from normal bacterial flora.

Collection methods vary depending on the type of specimen being collected. For instance, collection of throat, nasopharyngeal, wound, external ear, and eye specimens usually involves sampling inflamed tissues and exudates, typically using sterile swabs of cotton or other absorbent material; wound exudate may also be aspirated into a syringe. Collection of fluid from the middle ear is performed by a doctor using a needle and syringe.

Because the normal bacterial flora in stool include several potentially pathogenic organisms, bacteriologic examinations are valuable for identifying pathogens that cause overt GI disease—such as typhoid and dysentery—and carrier states. A sensitivity test may follow isolation of the pathogen. Identifying the organism is vital to treat the patient, to prevent possible fatal complications (especially in a debilitated patient), and to prevent the spread of a severe infectious disease.

Equipment

Gloves ▪ penlight ▪ sterile swab (cotton wool or synthetic fiber) ▪ sterile culture tube with transport medium or commercial collection kit ▪ specimen label ▪ laboratory request form ▪ laboratory

Obtaining a nasopharyngeal specimen

When the swab passes into the nasopharynx, gently but quickly rotate it to collect a specimen. Then remove the swab, taking care not to injure the nasal mucous membrane.

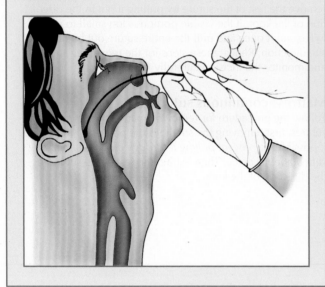

biohazard transport bag ■ Optional: mask and other personal protective equipment.

Additional equipment for throat and nasopharyngeal specimen collection
Tongue blade.

Additional equipment for wound specimen collection
Two pairs of sterile gloves ■ chlorhexidine swabs ■ sterile normal saline solution ■ sterile 10-mL syringe ■ sterile 21G needle ■ anaerobic culture tube ■ supplies to apply new dressing ■ Optional: rubber stopper for needle.

Additional equipment for middle ear specimen collection
Normal saline solution ■ 2″ × 2″ gauze pads ■ sterile 10-mL syringe and sterile 22G 1″ needle.

Additional equipment for eye specimen collection
Sterile normal saline solution ■ two 2″ × 2″ gauze pads ■ sterile wire culture loop (for corneal scraping).

Additional equipment for rectal specimen collection
Soap and water ■ washcloth ■ normal saline solution.

Implementation
■ Verify the doctor's order.
■ Perform hand hygiene and put on gloves.[1,2,3]
■ Confirm the patient's identity using at least two patient identifiers according to your facility's policy.[4]
■ Explain the procedure to the patient *to ease his anxiety and ensure cooperation.*

Throat specimen collection
■ Tell the patient that he may gag during the swabbing but that the procedure will probably take less than 1 minute.
■ Instruct the patient to sit erect at the edge of the bed or in a chair, facing you.
■ Ask the patient to tilt back his head. Depress his tongue with the tongue blade, and illuminate his throat with the penlight *to check for inflamed areas.*[5]
■ If the patient starts to gag, withdraw the tongue blade and tell him to breathe deeply. Once he's relaxed, reinsert the tongue blade but not as deeply as before. Encourage the patient to close his eyes or stare at the ceiling *to promote cooperation.*
■ Open and remove the swab, taking care not to touch the tip with your hands because the swab is sterile.[6] If you touch the swab, discard it and obtain a new swab.
■ Using the swab, wipe the tonsillar areas from side to side, including any inflamed or purulent sites. Make sure you don't touch the tongue, cheeks, saliva, or teeth with the swab *to avoid contaminating it with oral bacteria.*[5]
■ Move the swab into the posterior pharynx and wipe the area using a gentle side-to-side sweeping motion.
■ Withdraw the swab and immediately place it in the culture tube.[5] If you're using a commercial kit, crush the ampule of culture medium at the bottom of the tube, and then push the swab into the medium *to keep the swab moist.*

Nasopharyngeal specimen collection
■ Tell the patient that he may gag or feel the urge to sneeze during the swabbing but that the procedure takes less than 1 minute.
■ Have the patient sit erect at the edge of the bed or in a chair, facing you.
■ Put on a mask, and other personal protective equipment as necessary.[1,2,3]
■ Ask the patient to blow his nose *to clear his nasal passages.* Then check his nostrils for patency with a penlight.
■ Tell the patient to occlude one nostril first and then the other as he exhales. Listen for the more patent nostril *because you'll insert the swab through it.*
■ While it's still in the package, bend the sterile swab in a curve; then open the package without contaminating the swab.
■ Ask the patient to cough *to bring organisms to the nasopharynx for a better specimen.*
■ Ask the patient to tilt his head back, and gently pass the swab through the more patent nostril about 3″ to 4″ (7.5 to 10 cm) into the nasopharynx, keeping the swab near the septum and floor of the nose. Rotate the swab quickly and remove it. (See *Obtaining a nasopharyngeal specimen.*)

- Alternatively, depress the patient's tongue with a tongue blade, and pass the bent swab up behind the uvula. Rotate the swab and withdraw it.
- Remove the cap from the culture tube, insert the swab, and break off the contaminated end. Then close the tube tightly.

Wound specimen collection
- Carefully remove the dressing to expose the wound. Dispose of the soiled dressings properly.
- Discard your gloves and perform hand hygiene.[1,2,3]
- Prepare a sterile field and put on sterile gloves.
- Clean the area around the wound with a chlorhexidine swab *to reduce the risk of contaminating the specimen with skin bacteria.* Then allow the area to dry.[6]
- Clean the wound with sterile normal saline solution.
- For an aerobic culture of a deep wound, use a sterile swab to collect as much exudate as possible, or insert the swab deeply into the wound and gently rotate it. Remove the swab from the wound and immediately place it in the aerobic culture tube. Send the tube to the laboratory immediately with a completed laboratory request form. Never collect exudate from the skin and then insert the same swab into the wound; *this could contaminate the wound with skin bacteria.*
- For an anaerobic culture of a deep wound, insert the sterile swab deeply into the wound, rotate it gently, remove it, and immediately place it in the anaerobic culture tube. (See *Anaerobic specimen collection.*) Or insert a sterile 10-mL syringe, without a needle, into the wound and aspirate 1 to 5 mL of exudate into the syringe. Then attach the 21G needle to the syringe, expel all air from the syringe, and immediately inject the aspirate into the anaerobic culture tube.

External ear specimen collection
- Gently clean excess debris from the patient's ear with normal saline solution and gauze pads.
- Insert the sterile swab into the ear canal, and rotate it gently along the walls of the canal *to avoid damaging the eardrum.*
- Withdraw the swab, being careful not to touch other surfaces *to avoid contaminating the specimen.*
- Place the swab in the sterile culture tube with transport medium.

Middle ear specimen collection
- Clean the outer ear with normal saline solution and gauze pads.
- The doctor punctures the eardrum with a needle and aspirates fluid into the syringe.
- The doctor places the fluid in the sterile specimen container.

Eye specimen collection
- Gently clean excess debris from the outside of the patient's eye with sterile normal saline solution and gauze pads, wiping from the inner to the outer canthus.
- Retract the lower eyelid *to expose the conjunctival sac.* Gently rub the sterile swab over the conjunctiva, being careful not to touch other surfaces. Move from the inner canthus to the outer canthus. Hold the swab parallel to the eye, rather than pointed directly at it *to prevent corneal irritation or trauma due to sudden*

Anaerobic specimen collection

Some anaerobes die when exposed to oxygen. To facilitate anaerobic collection and culturing, tubes filled with carbon dioxide (CO_2) or nitrogen are used for oxygen-free transport.

The anaerobic specimen collector shown here consists of a rubber-stopper tube filled with CO_2, a small inner tube, and a swab attached to a plastic plunger. The drawing below left shows the tube before specimen collection. The small inner tube containing the swab is held in place by the rubber stopper.

After specimen collection (below right), the swab is quickly replaced in the inner tube, and the plunger is depressed. This procedure separates the inner tube from the stopper, forcing it into the larger tube and exposing the specimen to the CO_2-rich environment.

The tube should be kept upright.

Before

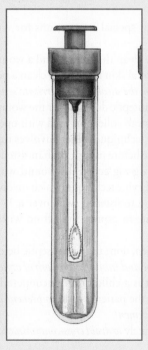

After

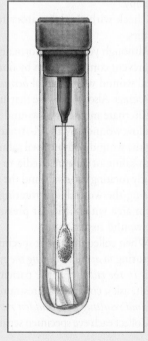

movement. (If a corneal scraping is required, this procedure is performed by a doctor, using a wire culture loop.)
- Immediately place the swab or wire loop in the culture tube with transport medium.

Rectal swab specimen collection
- Clean the area around the patient's anus using a washcloth and soap and water *to minimize contamination of the specimen.*
- Insert the swab, moistened with normal saline solution or sterile broth medium, through the anus and advance it about 1½″ (4 cm).[7] While withdrawing the swab, gently rotate it against the walls of the lower rectum *to sample a large area of the rectal mucosa.*

- Place the swab in a culture tube with transport medium.

Completing the procedure

- Remove and discard your gloves, and perform hand hygiene.[1,2,3]
- Label the specimen in the presence of the patient *to prevent mislabeling.*[7]
- On the laboratory request form, indicate whether any organism is strongly suspected, especially *Corynebacterium diphtheriae* (requires two swabs and special growth medium), *Bordetella pertussis* (requires a nasopharyngeal culture and special growth medium), and *Neisseria meningitidis* (requires enriched selective media).
- Place the specimen in a laboratory biohazard transport bag and send it to the laboratory immediately *to prevent growth or deterioration of microbes.*[8]
- Remove and discard your gloves and perform hand hygiene.[1,2,3]
- Document the procedure.[9]

Special considerations

- Note recent antibiotic therapy on the laboratory request form.
- If possible, obtain a specimen before starting antimicrobial therapy.
- Check with the laboratory for special instructions for viral studies.
- Although you would normally clean the area around a wound to prevent contamination by normal skin flora, don't clean a perineal wound with alcohol *because the alcohol could irritate sensitive tissues.* Also, make sure that antiseptic doesn't enter the wound.
- Alternate methods of wound swab collection used with open, shallow wounds are the Z-stroke technique, which involves rinsing the wound with normal saline before using a swab moistened with saline or culture media to zig-zag across the wound while gently rotating the swab, and the Levine technique, which involves rinsing the wound and rotating a moistened swab over a 1- to 2-cm area with sufficient pressure to express fluid from within the wound tissue.
- When collecting an eye specimen, don't use an antiseptic before culturing *to avoid irritating the eye and inhibiting growth of organisms in the culture.* If the patient is a child or an uncooperative adult, ask a coworker to restrain the patient's head *to prevent eye trauma resulting from sudden movement.*
- Collect each eye specimen separately *to avoid cross-contamination.*

Complications

If the patient has epiglottiditis or diphtheria, laryngospasm may occur after collecting a throat culture. Keep resuscitation equipment nearby.

Documentation

Record the time, date, and site of specimen collection and recent or current antibiotic therapy. Also note whether the specimen has an unusual appearance or odor. Document patient teaching.

REFERENCES

1 Centers for Disease Control and Prevention. (October 2002). Guideline for hand hygiene in health-care settings. *Morbidity and Mortality Weekly Report, 51*(RR-16), 1–45. (Level I)

2 World Health Organization. (2009). *WHO guidelines on hand hygiene in health care: First global patient safety challenge. Clean care is safer care.* Geneva, Switzerland: World Health Organization. (Level I)

3 The Joint Commission. (2012). Standard NPSG.07.01.01. *Comprehensive accreditation manual for hospitals: The official handbook.* Oakbrook Terrace, IL: The Joint Commission. (Level I)

4 The Joint Commission. (2012). Standard NPSG.01.01.01. *Comprehensive accreditation manual for hospitals: The official handbook.* Oakbrook Terrace, IL: The Joint Commission. (Level I)

5 Kotloff, K., & Van Beneden, C. (2008). "Standardization of Epidemiologic Protocols for Surveillance of Acute Diseases Caused by *Streptococcus pyogenes*: Pharyngitis, Impetigo, and Invasive Diseases" [Online]. Accessed January 2012 via the Web at http://www. niaid.nih.gov/topics/strepThroat/Documents/acute-groupastrep.pdf

6 Carrico, R. (Ed.). (2009). *APIC text of infection control and epidemiology* (3rd ed.). Washington, D.C.: Association for Professionals in Infection Control and Epidemiology, Inc.

7 The Joint Commission. (2012). Standard NPSG.03.04.01. *Comprehensive accreditation manual for hospitals: The official handbook.* Oakbrook Terrace, IL: The Joint Commission. (Level I)

8 Occupational Safety and Health Administration. "Bloodborne Pathogens, Standard Number 1910.1030"[Online]. Accessed December 2011 via the Web at http://www.osha.gov/pls/oshaweb/owadisp.show_document?p_table=STANDARDS&p_id=10051 (Level I)

9 The Joint Commission. (2012). Standard RC.01.03.01. *Comprehensive accreditation manual for hospitals: The official handbook.* Oakbrook Terrace, IL: The Joint Commission. (Level I)

ADDITIONAL REFERENCES

Baranoski, S., & Ayello, E.A. (2008). *Wound care essentials: Practice principles* (2nd ed.). Philadelphia, PA: Lippincott Williams & Williams.

Bonham, P.A. (2009). Swab cultures for diagnosing wound infections: A literature review and clinical guideline. *Journal of Wound, Ostomy and Continence Nursing, 36*(4), 389–395.

Centers for Disease Control and Prevention. (2004, January 8). "Public Health Guidance for Community-Level Preparedness and Response to Severe Acute Respiratory Syndrome (SARS), Version 2, Supplement F: Laboratory Guidance" [Online]. Accessed January 2012 via the Web at http://www.cdc.gov/sars/guidance/F-lab/index.html

Craven, R.F., & Hirnle, C.J. (2012). *Fundamentals of nursing: Human health and function* (7th ed.). Philadelphia, PA: Lippincott Williams & Wilkins.

Fischbach, F., & Dunning, M.B. (2009). *A manual of laboratory and diagnostic tests* (8th ed.). Philadelphia, PA: Lippincott Williams & Wilkins.

Nettina, S.M. (2010). *Lippincott manual of nursing practice* (9th ed.). Philadelphia, PA: Lippincott Williams & Wilkins.

Siegel, J.D., et al. "2007 Guideline for Isolation Precautions: Preventing Transmission of Infectious Agents in Healthcare Settings" [Online]. Accessed December 2011 via the Web at http://www.cdc.gov/hicpac/2007ip/2007isolationprecautions.html

SYNCHRONIZED CARDIOVERSION

Used to treat tachyarrhythmias, synchronized cardioversion delivers an electrical charge to the myocardium at the peak of the R wave. This charge causes immediate depolarization, interrupting reentry circuits and allowing the sinoatrial node to resume control. Synchronizing the electrical charge with the R wave ensures that the current won't be delivered on the vulnerable T wave, which would disrupt repolarization and possibly lead to ventricular fibrillation.

Synchronized cardioversion is the treatment of choice for arrhythmias that don't respond to vagal maneuvers or drug therapy, such as unstable supraventricular tachycardia resulting from reentry, unstable atrial flutter, unstable atrial fibrillation, and unstable monomorphic ventricular tachycardia with a pulse.[1] It may be performed as an elective or urgent procedure, depending on how well the patient tolerates the arrhythmia.[1] If a patient is hemodynamically unstable, for instance, he may require urgent cardioversion. When preparing for synchronized cardioversion with any patient, keep in mind that a patient's condition can deteriorate quickly, requiring immediate defibrillation.

Synchronized cardioversion should be performed according to the 2010 American Heart Association (AHA) guidelines and should follow an assessment of the patient's cardiac and metabolic status.[1] Assessment should include electrolyte levels, particularly potassium levels, which should be in the normal range; creatinine levels to determine renal function, which helps guide the dosage of adjunctive medications; and serum digoxin levels, which should be in the nontoxic range. If the patient has chronic lung disease, arterial blood gas (ABG) analysis may also be helpful.

When possible, the patient should be in optimal functional status at the time of the procedure. The doctor should discuss the procedure with the patient beforehand and obtain written informed consent. A general anesthetic or sedative agent as well as cardiopulmonary resuscitation equipment should be available during the procedure.

The AHA recommends immediate synchronized cardioversion for treatment of symptomatic (unstable) tachycardia. Signs and symptoms of unstable tachycardia include altered mental status, shock or hypotension, and ongoing chest pain.[1] If the patient is stable, he'll need a 12-lead electrocardiogram (ECG) to further classify the tachycardia.

Equipment

Gloves ■ cardioverter-defibrillator ■ self-adhesive cardioversion-defibrillation pads or anterior, posterior, or transverse paddles and conductive gel pads ■ ECG monitor with recorder ■ sedative ■ oxygen therapy equipment ■ airway ■ handheld resuscitation bag ■ emergency pacing equipment ■ emergency cardiac medications ■ automatic blood pressure cuff ■ pulse oximeter ■ IV catheter insertion equipment.

Implementation

■ Gather the appropriate equipment.
■ Have resuscitation equipment at the patient's bedside.
■ Perform hand hygiene and put on gloves.[2,3,4,5]

■ Confirm the patient's identity using at least two patient identifiers according to your facility's policy.[6]
■ Confirm that an informed consent has been obtained and that it's documented in the medical record.[7,8]
■ Check the patient's recent serum potassium and magnesium levels and ABG results. Also check recent digoxin levels. If the patient takes digoxin, withhold the dose on the day of the procedure, if ordered. *Although patients on digoxin therapy may undergo cardioversion, they tend to require lower energy levels to convert their cardiac rhythm.*
■ Maintain nothing-by-mouth status for 6 to 12 hours before the procedure, if possible.
■ Perform a preprocedure verification to make sure that all relevant documentation, related information, and equipment are available and correctly identified with the patient's identifiers.[9]
■ Obtain a 12-lead ECG *to serve as a baseline.*
■ Check to see if the doctor has ordered the administration of any cardiac drugs before the procedure. Also verify that the patient has a patent IV catheter in place in case drug administration becomes necessary; if he doesn't, insert one. (See "IV catheter insertion and removal," page 421.) Connect the patient to the monitor, a pulse oximeter, and an automatic blood pressure cuff.
■ Consider administering oxygen for 5 to 10 minutes before cardioversion *to promote myocardial oxygenation.* If the patient wears dentures, evaluate whether they support his airway or may cause an airway obstruction, in which case, you'll need to remove them.
■ Place the patient in the supine position and assess his vital signs, level of consciousness (LOC), cardiac rhythm, and peripheral pulses.
■ Conduct a time-out before starting the procedure, if time allows, to perform a final assessment that the correct patient and procedure are identified and that all relevant information and necessary equipment are available.[10]
■ A specially trained health care provider will administer moderate sedation or anesthesia.
■ Carefully monitor the patient's heart rate, blood pressure, and respiratory rate.
■ Press the power button to turn on the defibrillator. Next, push the sync button *to synchronize the machine with the patient's QRS complexes.* Make sure the sync button flashes with each of the patient's QRS complexes. You should also see a bright green flag flash on the monitor.
■ Advanced cardiac life support protocols call for an initial shock of 50 to 100 joules for a patient with unstable supraventricular tachycardia, 120 to 200 joules for a patient with atrial fibrillation, 50 to 100 joules for a patient with atrial flutter, and 100 joules for a patient who has monomorphic ventricular tachycardia with a pulse. If there's no response with the first shock, the health care provider should increase the joules in a step-wise manner.[1]
■ Turn the energy select dial to the ordered amount of energy.
■ Apply the self-adhesive cardioversion-defibrillation pads or remove the paddles from the machine, and prepare them as you would if you were defibrillating the patient. Place the self-adhesive pads or paddles and the conductive gel pads in the same positions as you would to defibrillate.
■ Make sure everyone stands away from the bed; then push the discharge buttons. Hold the paddles in place and wait for the

energy to be discharged; the machine has to synchronize the discharge with the QRS complex.

■ Assess the waveform on the monitor. If the arrhythmia fails to convert, repeat the procedure two or three more times at 3-minute intervals. Gradually increase the energy level with each additional countershock.[1]

■ After the cardioversion, frequently assess the patient's LOC and respiratory status, including airway patency, respiratory rate and depth, and the need for supplemental oxygen. *Because the patient will be heavily sedated,* he may require airway support.

■ Record a postcardioversion 12-lead ECG, and monitor the patient's ECG rhythm for 2 hours.

■ Inspect the patient's chest for electrical burns.

■ Discard used supplies, remove and discard your gloves, and perform hand hygiene.[2,3,4]

■ Document the procedure.[11]

Special considerations

■ If the patient is connected to a bedside or telemetry monitor, disconnect the unit before cardioversion. *The electrical current it generates could damage the equipment.*

■ Be aware that improper synchronization may result if the patient's ECG tracing contains artifact-like spikes, such as peaked T waves or bundle-branch heart blocks when the R′ wave may be taller than the R wave.

■ Although the electrical shock of cardioversion won't usually damage an implanted pacemaker, avoid placing the paddles directly over the pacemaker.

■ Remove any patches with metallic backing such as nitroglycerin patches. *This backing may cause arcing during cardioversion or burns.*

■ Remove all metal objects from the patient *because they may conduct electricity and cause a burn.*[12]

■ Reset the synchronization mode after each cardioversion *because many defibrillators automatically default back to the unsynchronized mode.*

■ Make sure the patient is in a dry environment and his chest is dry *because, if the rescuer or the patient comes in contact with water, the rescuer can receive a shock or the patient may receive a skin burn.*[12]

Complications

Common complications following cardioversion include transient, harmless arrhythmias, such as atrial, ventricular, and junctional premature beats. Serious ventricular arrhythmias such as ventricular fibrillation may also occur. However, this type of arrhythmia is more likely to result from high amounts of electrical energy, digoxin toxicity, severe heart disease, electrolyte imbalance, or improper synchronization with the R wave.

Documentation

Document the procedure, including the voltage delivered with each attempt, rhythm strips before and after the procedure, medications administered, and the patient's tolerance of the procedure. Note any emergency interventions required and the patient's response to these interventions. Record the patient's vital signs and your assessment findings. Document any patient teaching and the patient's understanding of your teaching.

REFERENCES

1 American Heart Association. (2010). 2010 American Heart Association guidelines for cardiopulmonary resuscitation and emergency cardiovascular care. *Circulation, 122*(Suppl. 3), S706–S719. (Level I)

2 Centers for Disease Control and Prevention. (October 2002). Guideline for hand hygiene in health-care settings. *Morbidity and Mortality Weekly Report, 51*(RR-16), 1–45. (Level I)

3 World Health Organization. (2009). *WHO guidelines on hand hygiene in health care: First global patient safety challenge. Clean care is safer care.* Geneva, Switzerland: World Health Organization. (Level I)

4 The Joint Commission. (2012). Standard NPSG.07.01.01. *Comprehensive accreditation manual for hospitals: The official handbook.* Oakbrook Terrace, IL: The Joint Commission. (Level I)

5 Siegel, J.D., et al. "2007 Guideline for Isolation Precautions: Preventing Transmission of Infectious Agents in Healthcare Settings" [Online]. Accessed December 2011 via the Web at http://www.cdc.gov/hicpac/2007ip/2007isolationprecautions.html

6 The Joint Commission. (2012). Standard NPSG.01.01.01. *Comprehensive accreditation manual for hospitals: The official handbook.* Oakbrook Terrace, IL: The Joint Commission. (Level I)

7 The Joint Commission. (2012). Standard RI.01.03.01. *Comprehensive accreditation manual for hospitals: The official handbook.* Oakbrook Terrace, IL: The Joint Commission. (Level I)

8 Centers for Medicare & Medicaid Services, Department of Health and Human Services. (2006). "Conditions of Participation: Patients' Rights," 42 CFR part 482.13 [Online]. Accessed November 2011 via the Web at https://www.cms.gov/CFCsAndCoPs/downloads/finalpatientrightsrule.pdf

9 The Joint Commission. (2012). Standard UP.01.01.01. *Comprehensive accreditation manual for hospitals: The official handbook.* Oakbrook Terrace, IL: The Joint Commission. (Level I)

10 The Joint Commission. (2012). Standard UP.01.03.01. *Comprehensive accreditation manual for hospitals: The official handbook.* Oakbrook Terrace, IL: The Joint Commission. (Level I)

11 The Joint Commission. (2012). Standard RC.01.03.01. *Comprehensive accreditation manual for hospitals: The official handbook.* Oakbrook Terrace, IL: The Joint Commission. (Level I)

12 Lynn-McHale Wiegand, D. (Ed.). (2011). *AACN procedure manual for critical care* (6th ed.). Philadelphia, PA: Saunders.

ADDITIONAL REFERENCES

American Association for Respiratory Care. (2004). AARC clinical practice guideline: Resuscitation and defibrillation in the health care setting—2004 revision & update. *Respiratory Care, 89*(9), 1085–1099.

Cakulev, I., et al. (2009). Cardioversion: Past, present, and future. *Circulation, 120*(16), 1623–1632.

Gibson, T. (2008). A practical guide to external direct current cardioversion. *Nursing Standard, 22*(37), 45–50.

Kim, S.K., et al. (2009). Clinical and serological predictors for the recurrence of atrial fibrillation after electrical cardioversion. *Europace, 11*(12), 1632–1638.

Nettina, S.M. (2010). *Lippincott manual of nursing practice* (9th ed.). Philadelphia, PA: Lippincott Williams & Wilkins.

Risius, T., et al. (2009). Comparison of antero-lateral versus antero-posterior electrode position for biphasic external cardioversion of atrial flutter. *American Journal of Cardiology, 104*(11), 1547–1550.

Sekhri, A., et al. (2009). Treatment of patients with supraventricular tachyarrhythmias in a medical intensive care unit. *Comprehensive Therapy, 35*(3–4), 188–191.

TEMPERATURE ASSESSMENT

Body temperature represents the balance between heat produced by metabolism, muscular activity, and other factors and heat lost through the skin, lungs, and body wastes. A stable temperature pattern promotes proper function of cells, tissues, and organs; a change in this pattern usually signals the onset of illness.

Temperature can be measured with an electronic digital, chemical-dot, or tympanic thermometer. Oral temperature in adults normally ranges from 97° to 99.5° F (36.1° to 37.5° C); rectal temperature, the most accurate reading, is usually 1° F (0.6° C) higher; axillary temperature, the least accurate, reads 1° to 2° F (0.6° to 1.1° C) lower; and tympanic temperature reads 0.5° to 1° (0.3° to 0.6°) higher.[1]

Temperature normally fluctuates with rest and activity. Lowest readings typically occur between 4 and 5 a.m.; the highest readings occur between 4 and 8 p.m. Other factors also influence temperature, including gender, age, emotional conditions, and environment. Keep the following principles in mind: Women normally have higher temperatures than men, especially during ovulation. Normal temperature is highest in neonates and lowest in the elderly. Heightened emotions raise temperature; depressed emotions lower it. A hot external environment can raise temperature; a cold environment lowers it.

Equipment

Electronic thermometer, chemical-dot thermometer, or tympanic thermometer ▪ facial tissue ▪ disposable thermometer sheath or probe cover (except for chemical thermometer) ▪ alcohol pad.

Preparation of equipment

If you use an electronic thermometer, make sure it's been recharged. (See *Types of thermometers,* page 698.)

Electronic thermometer

Insert the probe into a disposable probe cover (as shown below).

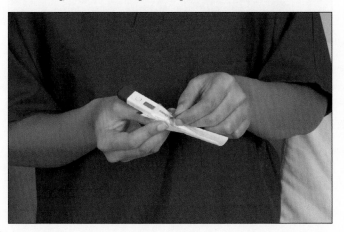

Chemical-dot thermometer

Remove the thermometer from its protective dispenser case by grasping the handle end with your thumb and forefinger, moving the handle up and down to break the seal, and pulling the handle straight out. Keep the thermometer sealed until use.

Implementation

▪ Perform hand hygiene.[2,3,4]
▪ Confirm the patient's identity using at least two patient identifiers according to your facility's policy.[5]
▪ Explain the procedure to the patient.
▪ If the patient has had hot or cold liquids, chewed gum, or smoked, wait 15 minutes before taking an oral temperature.[6]

Taking a tympanic temperature

▪ Make sure the lens under the probe is clean and shiny. Attach a disposable probe cover (as shown below).

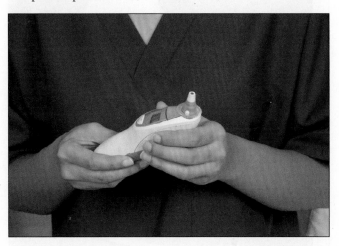

▪ Examine the patient's ear. It should be free from cerumen *to obtain an accurate reading.* If the patient has any visible lesions or drainage, don't perform a tympanic temperature.
▪ Stabilize the patient's head; then gently pull the ear up and back (as shown below).

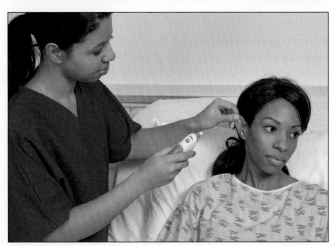

EQUIPMENT

Types of thermometers

You can take an oral, rectal, or axillary temperature with such instruments as a chemical-dot device or various electronic digital thermometers.

You'll use the oral route most for adults who are awake, alert, oriented, and cooperative. For infants, young children, and confused or unconscious patients, you may need to take the temperature rectally. The tympanic route may be used on almost all patients.

Chemical-dot thermometer

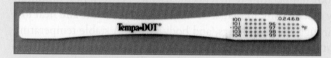

Tympanic thermometer

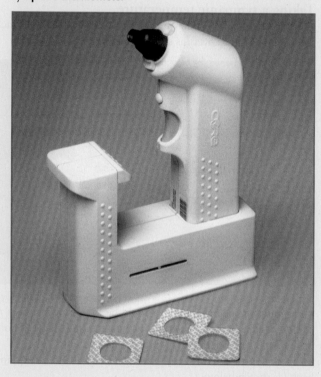

Institutional electronic digital thermometer

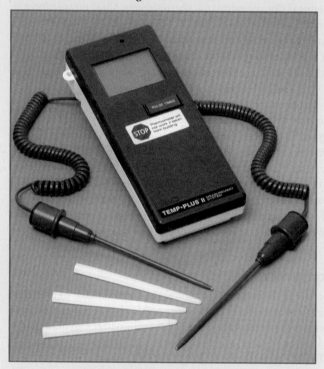

■ Insert the thermometer until the ear canal is sealed. The thermometer should be inserted toward the tympanic membrane in the same way that an otoscope is inserted. Then press the activation button and hold it for 1 second. The temperature will appear on the display.

Taking an oral temperature

■ Position the tip of the thermometer under the patient's tongue (as shown at right), as far back as possible on either side of the frenulum linguae. *Placing the tip in this area promotes contact with superficial blood vessels and contributes to an accurate reading.*

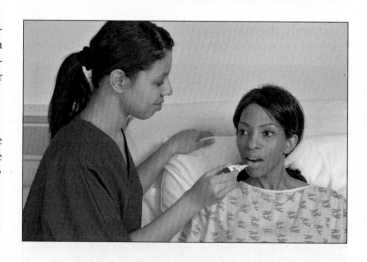

■ Instruct the patient to close her lips but to avoid biting down with her teeth.

■ Leave a chemical-dot thermometer in place for 45 seconds to register temperature; for an electronic thermometer, wait until the maximum temperature is displayed.

■ For an electronic thermometer, note the temperature; then remove and discard the probe cover. For the chemical-dot thermometer, read the temperature as the last dye dot that has changed color, or fired; then discard the thermometer and its dispenser case.

Taking an axillary temperature

■ Position the patient with the axilla exposed.

■ Gently pat the axilla dry with a facial tissue *because moisture conducts heat.* Avoid harsh rubbing, *which generates heat.*

■ Ask the patient to reach across her chest and grasp her opposite shoulder, lifting her elbow.

■ Position the thermometer probe in the center of the axilla (as shown below).

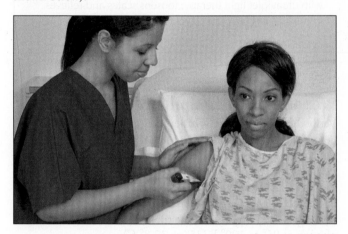

■ Tell her to keep grasping her shoulder and to lower her elbow and hold it against her chest. *This promotes skin contact with the thermometer probe.*

■ Remove an electronic thermometer when it displays the maximum temperature. Axillary temperature takes longer to register than oral or rectal temperature *because the thermometer isn't enclosed in a body cavity.*

Completing the procedure

■ Dispose of the probe cover or disposable thermometer.

■ Perform hand hygiene.[2,3,4]

■ Clean and disinfect the electronic model after use *to prevent cross-contaminaiton.*[7]

■ Return the electronic model to the charging base *so it is ready for the next use.*

■ Perform hand hygiene.[2,3,4]

■ Document the procedure.[8]

Special considerations

■ Make sure the probe cover doesn't have any wrinkles *because wrinkles can interfere with the reading.*

■ Oral measurement is contraindicated in patients who are unconscious, disoriented, or seizure-prone; in young children and infants; and in patients who must breathe through their mouths.

■ Use the same thermometer for repeated temperature taking *to avoid spurious variations caused by equipment differences.* Store chemical-dot thermometers in a cool area *because exposure to heat activates the dye dots.*

■ Don't avoid taking an oral temperature when the patient is receiving nasal oxygen; *oxygen administration raises oral temperature by only about 0.3° F (0.17° C).*

■ Make sure you document where the temperature was taken. Studies have shown that effective temperature measurement is based on consistency of the site used, not the actual site used.[9]

Documentation

Record the time, route, and temperature on the patient's chart.

REFERENCES

1 Jensen, B.N., et al. (2001). Accuray of digital tympanic, oral, axillary, and rectal thermometers compared with standard rectal mercury thermometers. *European Journal of Surgery, 166*(11), 848–851.

2 Centers for Disease Control and Prevention. (October 2002). Guideline for hand hygiene in health-care settings. *Morbidity and Mortality Weekly Report, 51*(RR-16), 1–45. (Level I)

3 World Health Organization. (2009). *WHO guidelines on hand hygiene in health care: First global patient safety challenge. Clean care is safer care.* Geneva, Switzerland: World Health Organization. (Level I)

4 The Joint Commission. (2012). Standard NPSG.07.01.01. *Comprehensive accreditation manual for hospitals: The official handbook.* Oakbrook Terrace, IL: The Joint Commission. (Level I)

5 The Joint Commission. (2012). Standard NPSG.01.01.01. *Comprehensive accreditation manual for hospitals: The official handbook.* Oakbrook Terrace, IL: The Joint Commission. (Level I)

6 Quatrara, B., et al. (2007). The effect of respiratory rate and ingestion of hot and cold beverages on the accuracy of oral temperature measurement by electronic thermometers. *Medsurg Nursing, 16*(2), 105–108. (Level II)

7 Rutala, W.A., et al. (2008). "Guideline for Disinfection and Sterilization in Healthcare Facilities, 2008" [Online]. Accessed January 2012 via the Web at http://www.cdc.gov/ncidod/dhqp/pdf/guidelines/Disinfection_Nov_2008.pdf (Level I)

8 The Joint Commission. (2012). Standard RC.01.03.01. *Comprehensive accreditation manual for hospitals: The official handbook.* Oakbrook Terrace, IL: The Joint Commission. (Level I)

9 Spitzer, O.P. (2008). Comparing tympanic temperatures in both ears to oral temperature in the critically ill adult. *Dimensions in Critical Care Nursing, 27*(1), 24–29. (Level VI)

ADDITIONAL REFERENCES

Craven, R.F., & Hirnle, C.J. (2012). *Fundamentals of nursing: Human health and function* (7th ed.). Philadelphia, PA: Lippincott Williams & Wilkins.

Davie, A., & Amoore, J. (2010). Best practice in measurement of body temperature. *Nursing Standard, 24*(42), 42–49.

Jensen, S. (2011). *Nursing health assessment: A best practice approach.* Philadelphia, PA: Lippincott Williams & Wilkins.

Comparing therapeutic baths

TYPE	AGENTS	PURPOSE
Antibacterial	■ Acetic acid ■ Potassium permanganate ■ Povidone-iodine	Used to treat infected eczema, dirty ulcerations, furunculosis, and pemphigus
Colloidal	■ Aveeno colloidal oatmeal ■ Aveeno colloidal oatmeal, oilated ■ Starch and baking soda ■ Soybean complex	Used to relieve pruritus and to soothe and coat irritated skin; indicated for any irritated or oozing condition, such as atopic eczema
Emollient	■ Bath oils ■ Chamomile ■ Mineral oil	Used to clean and hydrate the skin; indicated for any dry skin condition
Tar	■ Bath oils with tar ■ Coal tar concentrate	Used to treat scaly dermatoses, sometimes in combination with ultraviolet light therapy; loosens scales and relieves pruritus

THERAPEUTIC BATH

Also referred to as *balneotherapy,* the therapeutic bath combines water and additives to soothe and relax the patient, relieve fatigue and sore muscles and joints, clean the skin, relieve inflammation and pruritus, and soften and remove crusts, scales, debris, and old medications. Used primarily for their antipruritic and emollient actions, these baths coat irritated skin with a soothing, protective film. Because they constrict surface blood vessels, they also have an anti-inflammatory effect.

The addition of oatmeal powder, soluble cornstarch, or soybean complex to water creates a colloid bath, which has a soothing effect and is used to treat generalized itching. Oil baths are useful for lubricating dry skin and easing eczematous eruptions. Sodium bicarbonate added to water produces an alkaline bath that has a cooling effect and helps relieve pruritus. A medicated tar bath may be used to treat psoriasis. The film of tar left on the skin works in combination with ultraviolet light to inhibit the rapid cell turnover characteristic of psoriasis. (See *Comparing therapeutic baths.*)

A bedridden patient may benefit from a local soak with the therapeutic additive instead of a therapeutic tub bath.

Equipment

Bathtub ■ bath mat ■ rubber mat ■ bath (utility) thermometer ■ therapeutic additive ■ measuring device ■ colander or sieve for oatmeal powder ■ two washcloths ■ two towels ■ patient gown or loose-fitting cotton pajamas ■ lubricating cream or ointment, if ordered ■ gloves.

Preparation of equipment

Verify the doctor's order.[1] Gather the supplies and draw the bath before bringing the patient to the bath area *to prevent chilling him.* Make sure the tub is clean and disinfected *because a patient with skin breakdown is particularly vulnerable to infection.* Place the bath mat next to the tub and the rubber mat on the bottom of the tub *to prevent falls; the therapeutic additive may make the tub exceptionally slippery.* Fill the tub with 6″ to 8″ (15 to 20 cm) of water at 95° to 100° F (35° to 37.8° C).

The treatment's purpose and the type of additive used will determine the water temperature. Cool to lukewarm water is used for relieving pruritus and when adding tar or starch. Warm baths soothe, but water warmer than 100° F causes vasodilation, *which could aggravate pruritus.*

Measure the correct amount of therapeutic additive, according to the doctor's order or package instructions. As the tub is filling, thoroughly mix the additive in the water. Add most substances directly to the water, but place oatmeal powder in a sieve or colander under the tub faucet *to help it dissolve.* Begin with 2 tbs of oatmeal powder; then add more powder or water as needed to regulate the thickness of the oatmeal bath.

When giving a tar bath, wear a plastic apron or protective gown *because tar preparations stain clothing.*

Make sure that the bathroom is well ventilated. Some patients may experience allergic reactions or hypersensitivity to the additive in the water or to the smell of the additive. If a reaction occurs, limit the patient's time in the bath and notify the ordering doctor. If a skin reaction to the additive occurs, gently wash the additive from the skin and notify the ordering doctor.

Implementation

- Confirm the patient's identity using at least two patient identifiers according to your facility's policy.[2]
- Close the door *to provide privacy and eliminate drafts.*
- Explain the procedure to the patient and have him void.
- Escort the patient to the bath area.
- Perform hand hygiene.[3,4,5]
- Put on gloves.
- Check the water temperature. If necessary, help the patient undress and into the tub. Advise him to use the safety rails *to prevent falls.*
- Tell him that the bath may feel unpleasant at first *because his skin is irritated,* but assure him that the medication will soon coat and soothe his skin.
- Ask the patient to stretch out in the tub and submerge his body up to the chin. Support his head and neck, if needed. If he's capable, give him a washcloth to apply the bath solution gently to his face and other body areas not immersed if these areas require treatment.

NURSING ALERT *If the patient is taking a tar bath, tell him not to get the bath solution in his eyes* because tar is an eye irritant.

- Warn the patient against scrubbing his skin *to prevent further irritation.*
- Add warm water to the bath as needed *to maintain a comfortable temperature.*
- Remove and discard your gloves and perform hand hygiene.[3,4,5]
- Allow the patient to soak for 15 to 30 minutes. *Periods of soaking longer than this may cause skin softening and damage to the skin.* If you stay with him, pull the bath curtain *to give him some privacy and protect him from drafts.* If you must leave the room, show the patient how to use the call bell, and ensure his privacy.
- After the bath, assist the patient from the tub. Have him use the safety rails *to prevent falls.*
- Help the patient pat his skin dry with towels. Don't rub the skin *because rubbing removes some solutes and oils clinging to the skin and produces friction, worsening pruritus.*
- Put on new gloves.
- Apply lubricating cream or ointment, if ordered, *to help hold water in the newly hydrated skin.*
- Provide a fresh patient gown or loose-fitting cotton pajamas. *Tight clothing and scratchy or synthetic materials can aggravate skin conditions by causing friction and increasing perspiration.*
- Escort the patient to his room and make sure he's comfortable.
- Drain the bath water, clean and disinfect the tub, and dispose of soiled materials properly. *If you've given an oatmeal powder bath, drain and rinse the tub immediately or the powder will cake, making later removal difficult.*
- Remove and discard your gloves and perform hand hygiene.[3,4,5]
- Document the procedure.[6]

Special considerations

- *Because pruritus seems worse at night,* a therapeutic bath is best before bedtime, unless ordered otherwise, *to promote restful sleep. Because the patient with a skin disorder may be self-conscious,* maintain eye contact during conversation and avoid staring at his skin. Also avoid nonverbal expressions and gestures that show revulsion. If the patient wishes, allow him to talk about his condition and how it affects his self-esteem.
- Refrain from using soap during a therapeutic bath *because its drying effect counteracts the bath emollient.*
- *A patient with skin breakdown chills easily,* so protect him from drafts. But after the bath, avoid covering or dressing him too warmly *because perspiration aggravates pruritus.* Instruct the patient not to scratch his skin *to prevent excoriation and infection.*
- If the patient is confined to bed, you can place the therapeutic additive in a basin of water at 95° to 100° F (35° to 37.8° C) and apply it with a washcloth, using light, gentle strokes.

Patient teaching

Instruct the patient to bathe only as often as prescribed. *Excessive bathing can dry the skin.* Advise the patient to purchase commercial bath oil. *Salad or cooking oils may give clothes an unpleasant odor, and mineral oil mixes poorly with water.* Tell the patient to follow manufacturer's instructions for commercially prepared colloid preparations. Colloid for an oatmeal bath can be made at home by putting one-half cup of raw oatmeal into a blender and blending at medium-high speed until the material has the consistency of flour, then sifting it to remove unground pieces. Advise the patient to avoid wearing pajamas, underwear, or other clothing that isn't cotton and loose-fitting.

Documentation

Record the date, time, and duration of the bath. Note the water temperature, type and amount of additive, skin appearance before and after the bath, the patient's tolerance of the treatment, and the bath's effectiveness. Document patient teaching and the patient's understanding of your teaching.

REFERENCES

1 The Joint Commission. (2012). Standard MM.04.01.01. *Comprehensive accreditation manual for hospitals: The official handbook.* Oakbrook Terrace, IL: The Joint Commission. (Level I)
2 The Joint Commission. (2012). Standard NPSG.01.01.01. *Comprehensive accreditation manual for hospitals: The official handbook.* Oakbrook Terrace, IL: The Joint Commission. (Level I)
3 Centers for Disease Control and Prevention. (October 2002). Guideline for hand hygiene in health-care settings. *Morbidity and Mortality Weekly Report, 51*(RR-16), 1–45. (Level I)
4 World Health Organization. (2009). *WHO guidelines on hand hygiene in health care: First global patient safety challenge. Clean care is safer care.* Geneva, Switzerland: World Health Organization. (Level I)
5 The Joint Commission. (2012). Standard NPSG.07.01.01. *Comprehensive accreditation manual for hospitals: The official handbook.* Oakbrook Terrace, IL: The Joint Commission. (Level I)
6 The Joint Commission. (2012). Standard RC.01.03.01. *Comprehensive accreditation manual for hospitals: The official handbook.* Oakbrook Terrace, IL: The Joint Commission. (Level I)

ADDITIONAL REFERENCES

Falagas, M.E., et al. (2009). The therapeutic effect of balneotherapy: Evaluation of the evidence from randomised controlled trials. *International Journal of Clinical Practice, 63*(7), 1068–1084.

Hoffman, L., et al. (2008). Benefits of an emollient body wash for patients with chronic winter dry skin. *Dermatologic Therapy, 21*(5), 416–421.

Kesiktas, N., et al. (2011). The efficacy of balneotherapy and physical modalities on the pulmonary system of patients with fibromyalgia. *Journal of Back and Musculoskeletal Rehabilitation, 24*(1), 57–65.

Verhagen, A., et al. (2008). Balneotherapy for osteoarthritis. A Cochrane review. *Journal of Rheumatology, 35*(6), 1118–1123.

THORACENTESIS, ASSISTING

Thoracentesis involves aspiration of fluid or air from the pleural space. It relieves pulmonary compression and respiratory distress by removing accumulated air or fluid that results from injury or such conditions as tuberculosis, cancer, and heart failure. It also provides a specimen of pleural fluid or tissue for analysis and allows instillation of chemotherapeutic agents or other medications into the pleural space.

Thoracentesis is contraindicated in patients with bleeding disorders and should be used cautiously in patients who don't cooperate well, who have uncontrolled coughing, whose pleural fluid location is uncertain, who have only one functional lung, or who are on positive end-expiratory pressure mechanical ventilation.

Equipment

Most facilities use a prepackaged thoracentesis tray that typically includes the following:
Sterile gloves ▪ sterile drapes ▪ 1% or 2% lidocaine ▪ 5-mL syringe with 21G and 25G needles for anesthetic injection ▪ 17G thoracentesis needle for aspiration or Teflon over-the-needle catheters ▪ 50-mL syringe ▪ three-way stopcock and tubing ▪ sterile specimen containers ▪ sterile hemostat ▪ sterile 4″ × 4″ gauze pads ▪ antiseptic cleaning swabs.

You'll also need the following:
Sterile marker ▪ sterile labels ▪ adhesive tape ▪ sphygmomanometer or electronic vital signs monitor ▪ gown ▪ face shield ▪ gloves ▪ stethoscope ▪ laboratory request slips ▪ drainage bottles ▪ clippers ▪ biopsy needle ▪ prescribed sedative with 3-mL syringe and 21G needle ▪ drainage bottles if the doctor expects a large amount of drainage.

Preparation of equipment

Gather all equipment at the patient's bedside or in the treatment area. Check the expiration date on each sterile package, and inspect for tears. Prepare the necessary laboratory request form. List current antibiotic therapy on the laboratory forms *because this factor will be considered in analyzing the specimens.*

Implementation

▪ Perform hand hygiene.[1,2,3]
▪ Confirm the patient's identity using at least two patient identifiers according to your facility's policy.[4]
▪ Confirm that an informed consent has been obtained and that it is documented in the medical record.[5]

▪ Note any drug allergies, especially to the local anesthetic.
▪ Have the patient's chest X-rays available.
▪ Conduct a preprocedure verification *to make sure that all relevant documentation, related information, and equipment are available and correctly identified to the patient's identifiers.*[6]
▪ Explain the procedure to the patient. Inform him that he may feel some discomfort and a sensation of pressure during the needle insertion.
▪ Provide privacy and emotional support.
▪ Verify that the doctor has marked the procedure site with his initials or with another unambiguous mark set by your facility's policy before the procedure is performed. Confirm that the correct procedure has been identified for the correct patient at the correct site.[6]
▪ Administer the prescribed sedative or analgesia as ordered, following safe medication administration practices.[7]
▪ Obtain baseline vital signs, and assess respiratory function. Auscultate the patient's breath sounds.
▪ Position the patient. Make sure he's firmly supported and comfortable. (See *Positioning for thoracentesis.*)
▪ Remind the patient not to cough, breathe deeply, or move suddenly during the procedure *to avoid puncture of the visceral pleura or lung.* If the patient coughs, the doctor will briefly halt the procedure and withdraw the needle slightly *to prevent puncture.*
▪ Expose the patient's entire chest or back as appropriate.
▪ Clip hair from the aspiration site if needed.
▪ Perform hand hygiene; put on gloves, a gown, and a face shield; and follow standard precautions.[1,2,3]
▪ Using sterile technique, open the thoracentesis tray. Label all medications, medication containers, and other solutions on and off the sterile field.[8]
▪ Conduct a time-out immediately before starting the procedure *to perform a final assessment that the correct patient, site, positioning, and procedure are identified and that, as applicable, all relevant information and necessary equipment are available during and after the procedure.*[9,10]
▪ Assist the doctor as necessary in disinfecting the site and allowing it to dry.
▪ If an ampule of local anesthetic isn't included in the sterile tray and a multidose vial of local anesthetic is to be used, assist the doctor by disinfecting the rubber stopper with an alcohol pad and holding the inverted vial while the doctor withdraws the anesthetic solution.
▪ After draping the patient and injecting the local anesthetic, the doctor attaches a three-way stopcock with tubing to the aspirating needle and turns the stopcock *to prevent air from entering the pleural space through the needle.*
▪ Attach the other end of the tubing to the drainage bottle.
▪ The doctor then inserts the needle into the pleural space and attaches a 50-mL syringe to the needle's stopcock. A hemostat may be used *to hold the needle in place and prevent a pleural tear or lung puncture.* As an alternative, the doctor may introduce a Teflon catheter into the needle, remove the needle, and attach a stopcock and syringe or drainage tubing to the catheter *to reduce the risk of pleural puncture by the needle.*

■ Support the patient verbally throughout the procedure, and keep him informed of each step. Assess him for signs of anxiety, and provide reassurance as necessary.

■ Monitor vital signs regularly during the procedure. Continually observe the patient for signs of distress such as pallor, vertigo, faintness, weak and rapid pulse, decreased blood pressure, dyspnea, tachypnea, diaphoresis, chest pain, blood-tinged mucus, and excessive coughing. Alert the doctor if such signs develop *because they may indicate complications such as hypovolemic shock or tension pneumothorax.*

■ Assist the doctor as necessary in specimen collection, fluid drainage, and dressing the site.

■ After the doctor withdraws the needle or catheter, apply pressure to the puncture site using a sterile 4″ × 4″ gauze pad. Then apply a new sterile gauze pad and secure it with an occlusive dressing.

■ Place the patient in a comfortable position, obtain his vital signs, and assess his respiratory status.

■ Label the specimens properly in the presence of the patient *to prevent mislabeling* and send them to the laboratory.[8]

■ Discard disposable equipment in the appropriate receptacle.[11] Clean nondisposable items, and return them for sterilization.

■ Check the patient's vital signs and the dressing for drainage every 15 minutes for 1 hour. Then continue to assess the patient's vital signs and respiratory status as ordered or according to facility policy.

■ A chest X-ray may be ordered after the procedure.

■ Remove and discard your personal protective equipment and perform hand hygiene.[1,2,3]

■ Document the procedure.[12]

Special considerations

■ To prevent pulmonary edema and hypovolemic shock after thoracentesis, fluid is removed slowly, and no more than 1,000 mL of fluid is removed during the first 30 minutes.[13] *Removing the fluid increases the negative intrapleural pressure, which can lead to edema if the lung doesn't reexpand to fill the space.*

■ Some coughing is common as the lung reexpands.

■ Pleuritic or shoulder pain may indicate pleural irritation by the needle point.

■ The doctor may decide to place a small bore or "pig-tail" chest tube for continued drainage of a large effusion.

Complications

Pneumothorax (possibly leading to mediastinal shift and requiring chest tube insertion) can occur if the needle punctures the lung and air enters the pleural cavity. Hemoptysis may also occur if the lung is punctured. Pyogenic infection can result from contamination during the procedure. Hemothorax may occur if the thoracentesis needle punctures one of the intercostal vessels. Other potential difficulties include pain, cough, anxiety, dry taps, and subcutaneous hematoma and vasovagal syncope.

Documentation

Record the date and time of thoracentesis and the name of the doctor performing the procedure. Include the location of the

Positioning for thoracentesis

The choice of the position may vary. Usually, the patient sits upright and leans forward. If the patient is sitting on the edge of the bed, support his legs and have him lean forward and rest his head and arms on a pillow on the overbed table (as shown). If the patient can't sit, turn him on the unaffected side with the arm of the affected side raised comfortably above his head. The head of the bed may be elevated 30 to 45 degrees unless contraindicated. Recumbent thoracentesis may be performed with ultrasound guidance. *Proper positioning stretches the chest or back and allows easier access to the intercostal spaces.*

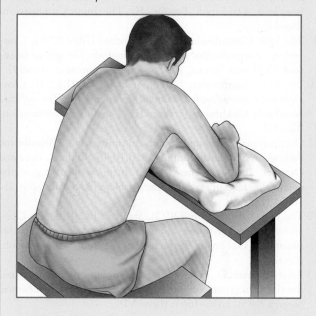

puncture site; volume and description (color, viscosity, and odor) of the fluid withdrawn; whether specimens were sent to the laboratory; vital signs and respiratory assessments before, during, and after the procedure; any postprocedure tests such as chest X-ray; any complications and nursing actions taken; and the patient's reaction to the procedure. If later signs and symptoms of pneumothorax, subcutaneous emphysema, or infection occur, notify the doctor immediately and document your observations and interventions on the chart.

REFERENCES

1 Centers for Disease Control and Prevention. (October 2002). Guideline for hand hygiene in health-care settings. *Morbidity and Mortality Weekly Report, 51*(RR-16), 1–45. (Level I)

2 World Health Organization. (2009). *WHO guidelines on hand hygiene in health care: First global patient safety challenge. Clean care is safer care.* Geneva, Switzerland: World Health Organization. (Level I)

3 The Joint Commission. (2012). Standard NPSG.07.01.01. *Comprehensive accreditation manual for hospitals: The official handbook.* Oakbrook Terrace, IL: The Joint Commission. (Level I)

4 The Joint Commission. (2012). Standard NPSG.01.01.01. *Comprehensive accreditation manual for hospitals: The official handbook.* Oakbrook Terrace, IL: The Joint Commission. (Level I)

5 The Joint Commission. (2012). Standard RI.01.03.01. *Comprehensive accreditation manual for hospitals: The official handbook.* Oakbrook Terrace, IL: The Joint Commission. (Level I)

6 The Joint Commission. (2012). Standard UP.01.01.01. *Comprehensive accreditation manual for hospitals: The official handbook.* Oakbrook Terrace, IL: The Joint Commission. (Level I)

7 The Joint Commission. (2012). Standard MM.06.01.01. *Comprehensive accreditation manual for hospitals: The official handbook.* Oakbrook Terrace, IL: The Joint Commission. (Level I)

8 The Joint Commission. (2012). Standard NPSG.03.04.01. *Comprehensive accreditation manual for hospitals: The official handbook.* Oakbrook Terrace, IL: The Joint Commission. (Level I)

9 The Joint Commission. (2012). Standard UP.01.02.01. *Comprehensive accreditation manual for hospitals: The official handbook.* Oakbrook Terrace, IL: The Joint Commission. (Level I)

10 The Joint Commission. (2012). Standard UP.01.03.01. *Comprehensive accreditation manual for hospitals: The official handbook.* Oakbrook Terrace, IL: The Joint Commission. (Level I)

11 Occupational Safety and Health Administration. "Bloodborne Pathogens, Standard Number 1910.1030" [Online]. Accessed October 2011 via the Web at http://www.osha.gov/pls/oshaweb/owadisp.show_document?p_table=STANDARDS&p_id=10051 (Level I)

12 The Joint Commission. (2012). Standard RC.01.03.01. *Comprehensive accreditation manual for hospitals: The official handbook.* Oakbrook Terrace, IL: The Joint Commission. (Level I)

13 Feller-Kopman, D., et al. (2007). Large-volume thoracentesis and the risk of reexpansion pulmonary edema. *Annals of Thoracic Surgery, 84*(5), 1656–1661. (Level VI)

ADDITIONAL REFERENCES

Centers for Medicare & Medicaid Services, Department of Health and Human Services. (2006). "Conditions of Participation: Patients' Rights," 42 CFR part 482.13 [Online]. Accessed November 2011 via the Web at https://www.cms.gov/CFCsAndCoPs/downloads/finalpatientrightsrule.pdf

Gordon, C.E., et al. (2010). Pneumothorax following thoracentesis: A systematic review and meta-analysis. *Archives of Internal Medicine, 170*(4), 332–339.

Liu, Y. et al. (2010). Ultrasound-guided pigtail catheters for drainage of various pleural diseases. *The American Journal of Emergency Medicine 28*(8), 915–921.

Lynn-McHale Wiegand, D. (Ed.). (2011). *AACN procedure manual for critical care* (6th ed.). Philadelphia, PA: Saunders.

Nettina, S.M. (2010). *Lippincott manual of nursing practice* (9th ed.). Philadelphia, PA: Lippincott Williams & Wilkins.

Peterson, W.G., & Zimmerman, R. (2000). Limited utility of chest radiography after thoracentesis. *Chest, 117*(4), 1038–1042.

Siegel, J.D., et al. "2007 Guideline for Isolation Precautions: Preventing Transmission of Infectious Agents in Healthcare Settings" [Online]. Accessed December 2011 via the Web at http://www.cdc.gov/hicpac/2007ip/2007isolationprecautions.html

THORACIC ELECTRICAL BIOIMPEDANCE MONITORING

A noninvasive alternative for tracking hemodynamic status, thoracic electrical bioimpedance monitoring, also known as *impedance cardiography,* provides information about a patient's cardiac index, preload, afterload, contractility, cardiac output, and blood flow. In this procedure, electrodes are placed on the patient's thorax. The electrodes have two purposes: to send harmless low-level electricity through the patient's body and to detect return electrical signals. These signals, which are interruptions in the electrical flow, come from changes in the volume and velocity of blood as it flows through the aorta. The bioimpedance monitor interprets the signals as a waveform. Cardiac output is then computed from this waveform and the electrocardiogram (ECG).

Thoracic electrical bioimpedance monitoring eliminates the risk of infection, bleeding, pneumothorax, emboli, and arrhythmias associated with traditional invasive monitoring. The accuracy of results obtained by this method proves comparable to that obtained by thermodilution; the bioimpedance monitor also automatically updates information every second to tenth heartbeat.[1]

Equipment

Thoracic electrical bioimpedance unit ∎ color-coded leadwires ∎ connecting cable ∎ four sets of thoracic electrical bioimpedance electrodes ∎ three ECG electrodes ∎ sterile 3″ × 3″ or 4″ × 4″ gauze pads ∎ tape measure ∎ gloves.

Implementation

∎ Perform hand hygiene and put on gloves.[2,3,4]
∎ Confirm the patient's identity using at least two patient identifiers according to your facility's policy.[5]
∎ Explain the procedure to the patient.
∎ Plug the thoracic electrical bioimpedance unit into a power supply.
∎ Press the power button. The initial display screen will appear.
∎ Enter information as prompted by the unit.
∎ Assist the patient onto his back with the head of the bed elevated no more than 30 degrees.
∎ Provide privacy and expose the patient's chest.
∎ Wet some sterile 4″ × 4″ or 3″ × 3″ gauze pads with warm water and clean the skin on each side of his neck from the base of the neck to 2″ (5 cm) above the base. Also clean the skin on both sides of the chest at the midaxillary line directly across the xiphoid process. *To ensure that you've cleaned a large enough area for electrode placement,* clean at least two fingerbreadths above and below the site.
∎ Place one electrode set vertically on the side of the neck in line with the ear. Make sure that the bottom of the electrode set isn't lower than the junction of the shoulder at the base of the neck.
∎ Place the second set of electrodes on the opposite side of the neck in line with the ear and about 180 degrees from the first set.
∎ Place the remaining two sets of electrodes on either side of the patient's chest. *To determine the correct location,* draw a line with your finger from the xiphoid process to the midaxillary line on one side of the chest. This is the site for the first chest electrode.

Make sure that the top portion of the electrode is at the level of the xiphoid process.
- Attach the ECG leadwires and try different lead selections until you obtain a consistent QRS signal. Don't remove the patient from the primary monitor. *The regular system must be maintained to ensure monitoring at the central station and to keep the alarms intact.*
- Attach the leadwires of the bioimpedance harness to the thoracic electrical bioimpedance electrodes and the ECG electrodes.
- Measure the distance between the bottom of an electrode set on one side of the patient's neck and the top of an electrode set on the same side of his chest. This distance, the thorax length, is the numeric value required by the monitor's computer to calculate accurate stroke volume. Enter this value on the patient data screen. Return to the waveform screen.
- Monitor the results provided by the unit.
- Remove and discard your gloves and perform hand hygiene.[2,3,4]
- Document the procedure.[6]

Special considerations
- Baseline bioimpedance values may be reduced in patients who have conditions characterized by increased fluid in the chest, such as pulmonary edema and pleural effusion.
- Bioimpedance values may be lower than thermodilution values in patients with tachycardia and other arrhythmias.

Documentation
Note the waveforms and values on the monitor and document the values by pressing "print" on the waveform screen to print a strip containing all the values monitored. Place the strip in the patient's chart.

REFERENCES

1 Gujjar, A.R., et al. (2008). Non-invasive cardiac output by transthoracic electrical bioimpedence in post-cardiac surgery patients: Comparison with thermodilution method. *Journal of Clinical Monitoring and Computing, 22*(3), 175–180. (Level VI)
2 Centers for Disease Control and Prevention. (October 2002). Guideline for hand hygiene in health-care settings. *Morbidity and Mortality Weekly Report, 51*(RR-16), 1–45. (Level I)
3 World Health Organization. (2009). *WHO guidelines on hand hygiene in health care: First global patient safety challenge. Clean care is safer care.* Geneva, Switzerland: World Health Organization. (Level I)
4 The Joint Commission. (2012). Standard NPSG.07.01.01. *Comprehensive accreditation manual for hospitals: The official handbook.* Oakbrook Terrace, IL: The Joint Commission. (Level I)
5 The Joint Commission. (2012). Standard NPSG.01.01.01. *Comprehensive accreditation manual for hospitals: The official handbook.* Oakbrook Terrace, IL: The Joint Commission. (Level I)
6 The Joint Commission. (2012). Standard RC.01.03.01. *Comprehensive accreditation manual for hospitals: The official handbook.* Oakbrook Terrace, IL: The Joint Commission. (Level I)

ADDITIONAL REFERENCES

Albert, N.M. (2006). Bioimpedance cardiography measurements of cardiac output and other cardiovascular parameters. *Critical Care Clinics of North America, 18*(2), 195–202.

Packer, M., et al. (2006). Utility of impedance cardiography for the identification of short-term risk of clinical decompensation in stable patients with chronic heart failure. *Journal of the American College of Cardiology, 47*(11), 2245–2252.
Parry, M.J., & McFetridge-Durdle, J. (2006). Ambulatory impedance cardiography: A systemic review. *Nursing Research, 55*(4), 283–291.
Sathyaprabha, T.N., et al. (2008). Noninvasive cardiac output measurement by transthoracic electrical bioimpedence: Influence of age and gender. *Journal of Clinical Monitoring and Computing, 22*(6), 401–408.

TILT TABLE

The tilt table, a padded table or bed-length board that can be raised gradually from a horizontal to a vertical position, can help prevent the complications of prolonged bed rest. Used for a patient with a spinal cord injury, brain damage, orthostatic hypotension, or other condition that prevents free standing, the tilt table increases tolerance for the upright position, conditions the cardiovascular system, stretches muscles, and helps prevent contractures, bone demineralization, and urinary calculus formation.[1,2] Tilting a patient with a tilt table is performed once or twice per day, usually in a separate room, depending on the patient's tolerance. In patients with orthostatic hypotension and postural orthostatic tachycardia, the tilt table is used as part of a diagnostic test meant to produce signs and symptoms characteristic of the disease.

Equipment
Tilt table with footboard and safety straps ■ sphygmomanometer and stethoscope or electronic vital signs monitor ■ antiembolism stockings or elastic bandages ■ Optional: abdominal binder, wooden block, stretcher.

Implementation
- Confirm the doctor's order.
- Perform hand hygiene.[3,4,5]
- Confirm the patient's identity using at least two patient identifiers according to your facility's policy.[6]
- Explain the use and benefits of the tilt table to the patient.
- Apply antiembolism stockings *to restrict vessel walls and help prevent blood pooling and edema.* If necessary, apply an abdominal binder *to avoid pooling of blood in the splanchnic region, which contributes to insufficient cerebral circulation and orthostatic hypotension.*
- Make sure the tilt table is locked in the horizontal position.
- Summon assistance and transfer the patient to the table, placing him in the supine position with feet flat against the footboard.
- If the patient can't bear weight on one leg, place a wooden block between the footboard and the weight-bearing foot, permitting the leg that can't bear weight to dangle freely.
- Fasten the safety straps.
- Take the patient's blood pressure and pulse rate.
- Tilt the table slowly in 15- to 30-degree increments, evaluating the patient constantly. Take his blood pressure every 3 to 5 minutes *because movement from the supine to the upright position*

decreases systolic pressure. Be alert for signs and symptoms of insufficient cerebral circulation: dizziness, nausea, pallor, diaphoresis, tachycardia, or a change in mental status. If the patient experiences any of these signs or symptoms, or hypotension or seizures, return the table immediately to the horizontal position.

NURSING ALERT *Never leave the patient unattended on the tilt table* because marked physiologic changes, such as hypotension or severe headache, can occur suddenly.

- If the patient tolerates the position shift, continue to tilt the table until reaching the desired angle, usually between 45 degrees and 80 degrees. A 60-degree tilt gives the patient the physiologic effects and sensations of standing upright.

- The patient may remain tilted for 5 to 45 minutes or until he becomes symptomatic. Signs and symptoms may include nausea, lightheadedness, diaphoresis, tachycardia, low blood pressure, and anxiety.

- Gradually return the patient to the horizontal position, and check his vital signs.

- Obtain assistance and transfer the patient onto a stretcher for transport back to his room.

- Perform hand hygiene.[3,4,5]

- Document the procedure.[7,8]

Special considerations

- If the tilt table is being used for diagnostic purposes, a cardiologist will be present and the patient should be on continuous electrocardiograph monitoring.

- Let the patient's response determine the angle of tilt and duration of elevation, but avoid prolonged upright positioning (greater than 45 minutes) *because it may lead to venous stasis.*

- In some instances, the patient may need to fast for up to 4 hours before the test.

Complications

Use of a tilt table can lead to sudden hypotension, severe headache, and other dramatic physiologic changes.

Documentation

Record the angle and duration of elevation; changes in the patient's pulse rate, blood pressure, and physical and mental status; and his response to treatment.[8,9]

REFERENCES

1 Chang, A.T., et al. (2004). Standing with the assistance of a tilt table improves minute ventilation in chronic critically ill patients. *Archives of Physical Medicine and Rehabilitation, 85*(12), 1972–1976.

2 Kinay, O., et al. (2004). Tilt training for recurrent neurocardiogenic syncope: Effectiveness, patient compliance, and scheduling the frequency of training sessions. *Japanese Heart Journal, 45*(5), 833–843.

3 Centers for Disease Control and Prevention. (October 2002). Guideline for hand hygiene in health-care settings. *Morbidity and Mortality Weekly Report, 51*(RR-16), 1–45. (Level I)

4 World Health Organization. (2009). *WHO guidelines on hand hygiene in health care: First global patient safety challenge. Clean care is safer care.* Geneva, Switzerland: World Health Organization. (Level I)

5 The Joint Commission. (2012). Standard NPSG.07.01.01. *Comprehensive accreditation manual for hospitals: The official handbook.* Oakbrook Terrace, IL: The Joint Commission. (Level I)

6 The Joint Commission. (2012). Standard NPSG.01.01.01. *Comprehensive accreditation manual for hospitals: The official handbook.* Oakbrook Terrace, IL: The Joint Commission. (Level I)

7 The Joint Commission. (2012). Standard RC.01.03.01. *Comprehensive accreditation manual for hospitals: The official handbook.* Oakbrook Terrace, IL: The Joint Commission. (Level I)

8 The Joint Commission. (2012). Standard RC.02.01.01. *Comprehensive accreditation manual for hospitals: The official handbook.* Oakbrook Terrace, IL: The Joint Commission. (Level I)

ADDITIONAL REFERENCE

Parry, S.W., et al. (2009). The Newcastle protocols 2008: An update on head-up tilt table testing and the management of vasovagal syncope and related disorders. *Heart, 95*(5), 416–420.

TOPICAL SKIN DRUG APPLICATION

Topical drugs are applied directly to the skin surface. They include lotions, pastes, ointments, creams, powders, shampoos, and aerosol sprays. Topical medications are absorbed through the epidermal layer into the dermis. The extent of absorption depends on the vascularity of the region.

Nitroglycerin, fentanyl, nicotine, and certain supplemental hormone replacements are used for systemic effects. Most other topical medications are used for local effects. Ointments have a fatty base, which is an ideal vehicle for such drugs as antimicrobials and antiseptics. Typically, topical medications should be applied two or three times a day to achieve their therapeutic effect.

Equipment

Patient's medication record and chart ▪ prescribed medication ▪ gloves ▪ sterile 4″ × 4″ gauze pads ▪ transparent semipermeable dressing ▪ adhesive tape ▪ solvent (such as cottonseed oil) ▪ Optional: sterile gloves.

Implementation

- Verify the doctor's order.[1]

- Avoid distractions and interruptions when preparing and administering the medication *to prevent medication errors.*[1]

- Compare the medication label to the order and verify that the medication is correct.[1]

- Check the expiration date on the medication; don't give the medication if it has expired.

- Check the patient's medical record for an allergy to the prescribed medication. If the patient has an allergy, don't administer the medication; notify the doctor.[1]

- Perform hand hygiene and put on gloves.[2,3,4]

- Confirm the patient's identity using at least two patient identifiers according to your facility's policy.[5]

- If your facility uses a bar code scanning system, scan your identification badge, the patient's identification bracelet, and the medication's bar code.
- Provide privacy.
- Explain the procedure thoroughly to the patient *because he may have to apply the medication by himself after discharge.*
- Help the patient assume a comfortable position that provides access to the area to be treated.
- Expose the area to be treated. Make sure the skin or mucous membrane is intact (unless the medication has been ordered to treat a skin lesion, such as an ulcer). *Applying medication to broken or abraded skin may cause unwanted systemic absorption and result in further irritation.*
- If necessary, clean the skin of debris, including crusts, epidermal scales, and old medication. You may have to change your gloves if they become soiled.

Applying paste, cream, or ointment

- Open the container. Place the lid or cap upside down *to prevent contamination of the inside surface.*
- Using your gloved hands, apply the medication to the affected area with long, smooth strokes that follow the direction of hair growth (as shown below). *This technique avoids forcing medication into hair follicles, which can cause irritation and lead to folliculitis.* Avoid excessive pressure when applying the medication *because it could abrade the skin.*

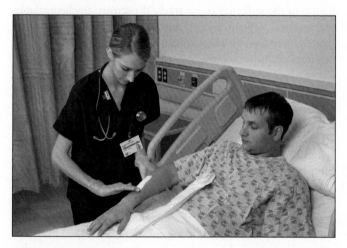

Removing ointment

- Perform hand hygiene and put on gloves. Then rub solvent on them and apply it liberally to the treated area in the direction of hair growth. Alternatively, saturate a sterile gauze pad with the solvent and use this pad to gently remove the ointment. Remove excess oil by gently wiping the area with a sterile gauze pad. Don't rub too hard to remove the medication *because you could irritate the skin.*

Applying other topical medications

- To apply shampoos, follow package directions. (See *Using medicated shampoos.*)
- To apply aerosol sprays, shake the container, if indicated, *to completely mix the medication.* Hold the container 6″ to 12″

Using medicated shampoos

Medicated shampoos include keratolytic and cytostatic agents, coal tar preparations, and lindane (gamma benzene hexachloride) solutions. They can be used to treat such conditions as dandruff, psoriasis, and head lice. However, they're contraindicated in patients with broken or abraded skin.

Because application instructions may vary among brands, check the label on the shampoo before starting the procedure *to ensure use of the correct amount.* Keep the shampoo away from the patient's eyes. If any shampoo should accidentally get in his eyes, irrigate promptly with water. Selenium sulfide, used in cytostatic agents, is extremely toxic if ingested.

To apply a medicated shampoo, follow these steps:
- Perform hand hygiene and put on gloves.[2,3,4]
- Prepare the patient for shampoo treatment.
- Shake the bottle of shampoo well *to mix the solution evenly.*
- Wet the patient's hair thoroughly and wring out excess water.
- Apply the proper amount of shampoo, as directed on the label.
- Work the shampoo into a lather, adding water as necessary. Part the hair and work the shampoo into the scalp, taking care not to use your fingernails.
- Leave the shampoo on the scalp and hair for as long as instructed (usually 5 to 10 minutes). Then rinse the hair thoroughly.
- Towel-dry the patient's hair.
- After the hair is dry, comb or brush it. Use a fine-tooth comb to remove nits if necessary.

(15 to 30 cm) from the skin, or follow the manufacturer's recommendation. Spray a thin film of medication evenly over the treatment area.
- To apply powders, dry the skin surface, making sure to spread skin folds where moisture collects. Then apply a thin layer of powder over the treatment area.
- *To protect applied medications and prevent them from soiling the patient's clothes,* tape an appropriate amount of sterile gauze pad or a transparent semipermeable dressing over the treated area. With certain medications (such as topical steroids), semipermeable dressings may be contraindicated. Check medication information and cautions.

PEDIATRIC ALERT *In children, topical medications (such as steroids) should be covered only loosely with a diaper. Do not use plastic pants.*
- Assess the patient's skin for signs of irritation, allergic reaction, or breakdown.
- Remove and discard your gloves and perform hand hygiene.[2,3,4]
- Document the procedure.[6,7]

Special considerations

- Never apply medication without first removing previous applications *to prevent skin irritation from an accumulation of medication.*
- Be sure to wear gloves *to prevent absorption by your own skin.* If the patient has an infectious skin condition, use sterile gloves and dispose of old dressings according to your facility's policy.
- Don't apply ointments to mucous membranes as liberally as you would to skin *because mucous membranes are usually moist and absorb ointment more quickly than skin does.* Also, don't apply too much ointment to any skin area *because it might cause irritation and discomfort, stain clothing and bedding, and make removal difficult.*
- Never apply ointment to the eyelids or ear canal unless ordered. *The ointment may congeal and occlude the tear duct or ear canal.*
- Inspect the treated area frequently for adverse effects, such as signs of an allergic reaction.
- When applying an aerosol spray or powder, make sure to prevent direct inhalation of the medication by the patient.

Complications

Skin irritation, a rash, or an allergic reaction may occur.

Documentation

Document the name of the medication, the dose, and the date and time it was administered in the patient's medication administration record. Include the route and site used. Document the appearance and integrity of the skin before administration. Record the presence or absence of adverse effects and whether the doctor was notified of adverse effects. Document the patient's response to and tolerance of therapy. Include teaching information given to the patient.

REFERENCES

1 The Joint Commission. (2012). Standard MM.06.01.01. *Comprehensive accreditation manual for hospitals: The official handbook.* Oakbrook Terrace, IL: The Joint Commission. (Level I)
2 Centers for Disease Control and Prevention. (October 2002). Guideline for hand hygiene in health-care settings. *Morbidity and Mortality Weekly Report, 51*(RR-16), 1–45. (Level I)
3 World Health Organization. (2009). *WHO guidelines on hand hygiene in health care: First global patient safety challenge. Clean care is safer care.* Geneva, Switzerland: World Health Organization. (Level I)
4 The Joint Commission. (2012). Standard NPSG.07.01.01. *Comprehensive accreditation manual for hospitals: The official handbook.* Oakbrook Terrace, IL: The Joint Commission. (Level I)
5 The Joint Commission. (2012). Standard NPSG.01.01.01. *Comprehensive accreditation manual for hospitals: The official handbook.* Oakbrook Terrace, IL: The Joint Commission. (Level I)
6 The Joint Commission. (2012). Standard RC.01.03.01. *Comprehensive accreditation manual for hospitals: The official handbook.* Oakbrook Terrace, IL: The Joint Commission. (Level I)
7 The Joint Commission. (2012). Standard RC.02.01.01. *Comprehensive accreditation manual for hospitals: The official handbook.* Oakbrook Terrace, IL: The Joint Commission. (Level I)

ADDITIONAL REFERENCES

Dunning, G. (2007). Emollients: Application of topical treatments to the skin. *British Journal of Nursing, 16*(21), 1342–1345.
Nettina, S.M. (2010). *Lippincott manual of nursing practice* (9th ed.). Philadelphia, PA: Lippincott Williams & Wilkins.
Taylor, C., et al. (2011). *Fundamentals of nursing: The art and science of nursing care* (7th ed.). Philadelphia, PA: Lippincott Williams & Wilkins.

TRACHEAL CUFF–PRESSURE MEASUREMENT

An endotracheal (ET) or tracheostomy cuff provides a closed system for mechanical ventilation, allowing a desired tidal volume to be delivered to the patient's lungs. To function properly, the cuff must exert enough pressure on the tracheal wall to seal the airway without compromising the blood supply to the tracheal mucosa.

The ideal pressure (known as *minimal occlusive volume*) is the lowest amount needed to seal the airway. Many authorities recommend maintaining a cuff pressure lower than venous perfusion pressure—usually about 20 to 30 mm Hg.[1] When cuff pressure is too low, oropharyngeal secretions can leak around the cuff, increasing the risk for ventilator-associated pneumonia. Overinflation of the cuff may cause tracheal necrosis, tracheomalacia, and tracheal stenosis.[1] Actual cuff pressure will vary with each patient, however. To keep pressure within safe limits, measure minimal occlusive volume at least once each shift or according to your facility's policy. Cuff pressure can be measured by a respiratory therapist or by the nurse.

Equipment

10-mL syringe ■ three-way stopcock ■ cuff pressure manometer ■ stethoscope ■ suction equipment ■ gloves ■ hospital-grade disinfectant.

Preparation of equipment

Assemble all equipment at the patient's bedside. If measuring with a blood pressure manometer, attach the syringe to one stopcock port; then attach the tubing from the manometer to another port of the stopcock. Turn off the stopcock port where you'll be connecting the pilot balloon cuff *so that air can't escape from the cuff.* Use the syringe to instill air into the manometer tubing until the pressure reading reaches 10 mm Hg. *Doing so prevents sudden cuff deflation when you open the stopcock to the cuff and the manometer.*

Implementation

- Verify the doctor's order.
- Perform hand hygiene and put on gloves.[2,3,4,5]
- Confirm the patient's identity using at least two patient identifiers according to your facility's policy.[6]
- Explain the procedure to the patient.

■ Hyperoxygenate the patient, if necessary. *Hyperoxygenation is recommended in critically ill patients who require full ventilator support; however, its benefit is unclear in patients who don't require full support.*[1] Then suction the ET or tracheostomy tube and the patient's oropharynx *to remove accumulated secretions above the cuff.*[7]

■ Attach the cuff pressure manometer to the pilot balloon port.

■ Place the diaphragm of the stethoscope over the trachea and listen for an air leak (as shown below). Keep in mind that a smooth, hollow sound indicates a sealed airway; a loud, gurgling sound indicates an air leak.

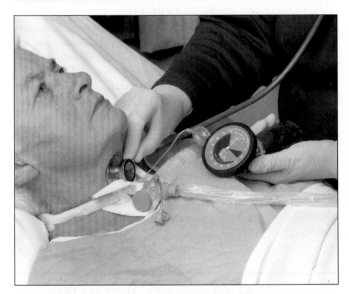

■ If you don't hear an air leak, press the red button under the dial of the cuff pressure manometer to slowly release air from the balloon on the tracheal tube (as shown below). Auscultate for an air leak.

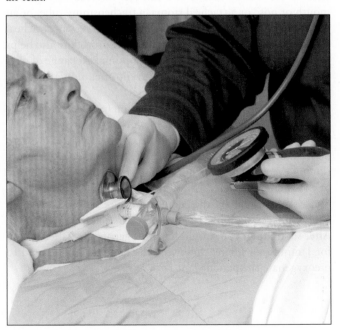

■ As soon as you hear an air leak, release the red button and gently squeeze the handle of the cuff pressure manometer to inflate the cuff (as shown below). Continue to add air to the cuff until you no longer hear an air leak.

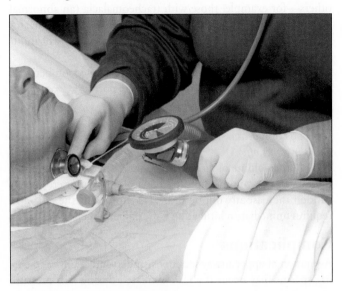

■ When the air leak ceases, read the dial on the cuff pressure manometer (as shown below). This number is the minimal pressure required to effectively occlude the trachea around the tracheal tube. In many cases, this pressure will fall within the green area (20 to 25 mm Hg) on the manometer dial.[7]

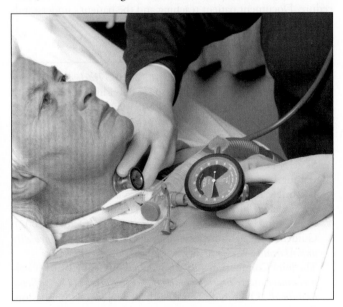

■ Disconnect the cuff pressure manometer from the pilot balloon port.

■ Remove your gloves and perform hand hygiene.[2,3,4,5]

■ Document the procedure and the cuff pressure.[8,9]

Special considerations

■ Measure cuff pressure at least every 8 hours *to avoid over-inflation.*[10]

■ Keep in mind that some patients require less pressure, whereas others—for example, those with tracheomalacia (an abnormal softening of the tracheal tissue)—require more pressure. Maintaining the cuff pressure at the lowest possible level will minimize cuff-related problems.

■ When measuring cuff pressure, keep the connection between the measuring device and the pilot balloon port tight *to avoid an air leak that could compromise cuff pressure.*

■ If you're using a stopcock, don't leave the manometer in the "off" position *because air will leak from the cuff if the syringe accidentally comes off.*

■ Note the volume of air needed to inflate the cuff. A gradual increase in this volume indicates tracheal dilation or erosion. A sudden increase in volume indicates rupture of the cuff and requires immediate reintubation if the patient is being ventilated.

Complications

Aspiration of upper airway secretions, underventilation, or coughing spasms may occur if a leak is created during cuff pressure measurement.

Documentation

Record the date and time of the procedure, cuff pressure, total amount of air in the cuff after the procedure, any complications and nursing actions taken, and the patient's tolerance of the procedure. Document patient teaching and the patient's understanding of your teaching.

REFERENCES

1 Morris, L.L., & Afifi, M.S. (Eds.). (2010). *Tracheostomies: The complete guide.* New York, NY: Sprier Publishing Company.
2 World Health Organization. (2009). *WHO guidelines on hand hygiene in health care: First global patient safety challenge. Clean care is safer care.* Geneva, Switzerland: World Health Organization. (Level I)
3 Siegel, J.D., et al. "2007 Guideline for Isolation Precautions: Preventing Transmission of Infectious Agents in Healthcare Settings" [Online]. Accessed December 2011 via the Web at http://www.cdc.gov/hicpac/2007ip/2007isolationprecautions.html
4 Centers for Disease Control and Prevention. (October 2002). Guideline for hand hygiene in health-care settings. *Morbidity and Mortality Weekly Report, 51*(RR-16), 1–45. (Level I)
5 The Joint Commission. (2012). Standard NPSG.07.01.01. *Comprehensive accreditation manual for hospitals: The official handbook.* Oakbrook Terrace, IL: The Joint Commission. (Level I)
6 The Joint Commission. (2012). Standard NPSG.01.01.01. *Comprehensive accreditation manual for hospitals: The official handbook.* Oakbrook Terrace, IL: The Joint Commission. (Level I)
7 Lynn-McHale Wiegand, D. (Ed.). (2011). *AACN procedure manual for critical care* (6th ed.). Philadelphia, PA: Saunders.
8 The Joint Commission. (2012). Standard RC.01.03.01. *Comprehensive accreditation manual for hospitals: The official handbook.* Oakbrook Terrace, IL: The Joint Commission. (Level I)
9 The Joint Commission. (2012). Standard RC.02.01.01. *Comprehensive accreditation manual for hospitals: The official handbook.* Oakbrook Terrace, IL: The Joint Commission. (Level I)
10 Vyas, D., et al. (2002). Measurement of tracheal tube cuff pressure in critical care. *Anaesthesia, 57*(3), 275–307. (Level VI)

ADDITIONAL REFERENCES

Centers for Disease Control and Prevention. (2004). Guidelines for preventing health-care–associated pneumonia, 2003. *Morbidity and Mortality Weekly Report, 53*(RR-03), 1–36.
Galinski, M., et al. (2006). Intracuff pressure of endotracheal tubes in the management of airway emergencies: The need for pressure monitoring. *Annals of Emergency Medicine, 47*(6), 545–547.
Nseir, S., et al. (2009). Variations in endotracheal cuff pressure in intubated critically ill patients: Prevalence and risk factors. *European Journal of Anesthesiology, 26*(3), 229–234.
Svenson, J.E., et al. (2007). Endotracheal intracuff pressures in the ED and prehospital setting: Is there a problem? *American Journal of Emergency Medicine, 25*(1), 53–56.
Young, P.J., & Wyncoll, D.L. (2007). Continuous cuff pressure control and the prevention of ventilator-associated pneumonia. *Critical Care Medicine, 35*(10), 2470–2471; author reply 2471.
Young, P.J., et al. (2006). A low-volume, low-pressure tracheal tube cuff reduces pulmonary aspiration. *Critical Care Medicine, 34*(3), 632–639.

TRACHEAL SUCTIONING, INTUBATED PATIENT

Tracheal suction involves the removal of secretions from the trachea or bronchi by means of a catheter inserted through the mouth or nose or a tracheal stoma, a tracheostomy tube, or an endotracheal (ET) tube. Besides removing secretions, tracheal suctioning stimulates the cough reflex. The procedure also helps maintain a patent airway to promote optimal exchange of oxygen and carbon dioxide and to prevent pneumonia that can result from pooling secretions.[1,2]

According to the American Association for Respiratory Care (AARC) guidelines, before you suction a patient, you should hyperoxygenate him with 100% oxygen for at least 30 to 60 seconds, using sterile technique.[1,3] The duration of each suctioning event—which includes the placement and withdrawal of the suction catheter—should take no longer than 15 seconds.[3] You should set the suction pressure as low as possible while still keeping it high enough to clear secretions effectively. After suctioning, you should hyperoxygenate the patient again for 1 minute or longer, following the same technique used to preoxygenate the patient.[3]

Equipment

Oxygen source (wall or portable unit, handheld resuscitation bag with a mask, 15-mm adapter, or a positive end-expiratory pressure valve, if indicated) ■ wall or portable suction apparatus ■ collection container ■ connecting tube ■ suction catheter kit or a sterile suction catheter, one sterile glove, one clean glove, goggles, and a disposable sterile solution container ■ 1-L bottle of sterile water or normal saline solution ■ syringe for deflating cuff of ET or tracheostomy tube ■ waterproof trash bag ■ personal protective equipment ■ Optional: sterile towel.

Preparation of equipment

Choose a suction catheter of appropriate size. The diameter should be no larger than one-half the inside diameter of the tracheostomy or ET tube *to minimize hypoxia during suctioning.* (A #12 or #14 French catheter may be used for an 8-mm or larger tube.)[3,4,5] Place the suction apparatus on the patient's overbed table or bedside stand. Position the table or stand on your preferred side of the bed *to facilitate suctioning.*

Attach the collection container to the suction unit and the connecting tube to the collection container. Label and date the normal saline solution or sterile water. Open the waterproof trash bag.

Implementation

■ Before suctioning, determine whether your facility requires a doctor's order and obtain one, if necessary.
■ Perform hand hygiene.[1,6,7,8,9] Put on personal protective equipment as appropriate.[3,9]
■ Confirm the patient's identity using at least two patient identifiers according to your facility's policy.[10]
■ Assess the patient's vital signs, breath sounds, and general appearance *to establish a baseline for comparison after suctioning.* Review the patient's arterial blood gas values and oxygen saturation levels if they're available. Attach the patient to a pulse oximeter *to assess oxygen saturation before and after the procedure.*[3] Evaluate the patient's ability to cough and deep-breathe *to help move secretions up the tracheobronchial tree.*[3]
■ Explain the procedure to the patient even if he's unresponsive. Tell him that suctioning usually causes transient coughing or gagging but that coughing helps remove secretions. If the patient has been suctioned previously, summarize the reasons for suctioning. Continue to reassure the patient throughout the procedure *to minimize anxiety, promote relaxation, and decrease oxygen demand.*
■ Unless contraindicated, place the patient in semi-Fowler's or high Fowler's position *to promote lung expansion and productive coughing.*
■ Remove the top from the normal saline solution or water bottle.
■ Open the package containing the sterile solution container.
■ Using strict sterile technique, open the suction catheter kit, and put on the gloves. If using individual supplies, open the suction catheter and the gloves, placing first the nonsterile glove on your nondominant hand and then the sterile glove on your dominant hand.[1,3]

■ Using your nondominant (nonsterile) hand, pour the normal saline solution or sterile water into the solution container.
■ Place a sterile towel over the patient's chest, if desired, *to provide an additional sterile area.*
■ Using your dominant (sterile) hand, remove the catheter from its wrapper. Keep it coiled *so it can't touch a nonsterile object.* Using your other hand to manipulate the connecting tubing, attach the catheter to the tubing (as shown below).[3]

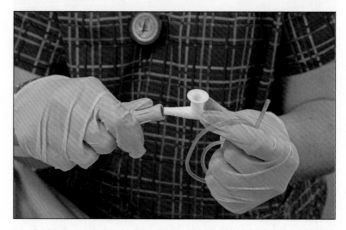

■ Using your nondominant hand, set the suction pressure according to facility policy. Pressure should be set as low as possible but high enough to clear secretions; less than 150 mm Hg is recommended for adults.[3,11] *Higher pressures don't enhance secretion removal and may cause traumatic injury.* Occlude the suction port *to assess suction pressure.*
■ Dip the catheter tip in the saline solution or sterile water (as shown below) *to lubricate the outside of the catheter and reduce tissue trauma during insertion.*

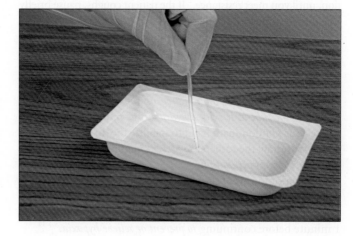

■ With the catheter tip in the sterile saline or water, occlude the control valve with the thumb of your nondominant hand (as shown below). Suction a small amount of solution through the catheter *to lubricate the inside of the catheter, which facilitates passage of secretions through it.*

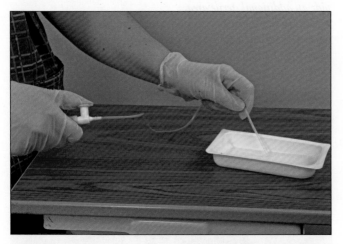

■ If the patient is being mechanically ventilated, hyperoxygenate him for at least 30 seconds.[2,3,11] First, adjust the fraction of inspired oxygen (FiO_2) and tidal volume according to your facility's policy and the patient's needs. Next, either use the sigh mode or manually deliver three to six breaths with a manual resuscitation bag. If you have an assistant for the procedure, the assistant can manage the patient's oxygen needs while you perform the suctioning.

■ Using your nonsterile hand, disconnect the patient from the ventilator. (If you're using a closed system, see *Closed tracheal suctioning.*)

■ Using your sterile hand, gently insert the suction catheter into the artificial airway. Advance the catheter, without applying suction, until you meet resistance.[2] If the patient coughs, pause briefly and then resume advancement.

■ After inserting the catheter, apply suction intermittently by removing and replacing the thumb of your nondominant hand over the control valve. Simultaneously use your dominant hand to withdraw the catheter as you roll it between your thumb and forefinger. *This rotating motion prevents the catheter from pulling tissue into the tube as it exits, avoiding tissue trauma.*

■ Use your nondominant hand to stabilize the tip of the ET tube as you withdraw the catheter *to prevent mucous membrane irritation or accidental extubation.*

■ The suctioning event should take no longer than 15 seconds.[3]

■ Resume oxygen delivery by reconnecting the source of oxygen or ventilation and hyperoxygenating the patient's lungs for at least 1 minute before continuing *to prevent or relieve hypoxia.*[2,3,11]

■ Observe the patient, and allow him to rest for a few minutes before the next suctioning. The timing of each suctioning and the length of each rest period depend on the patient's tolerance of the procedure and the absence of complications. *To enhance secretion removal,* encourage the patient to cough between suctioning attempts. Don't attempt more than two suctioning passes.

■ Observe the secretions. If they're thick, clear the catheter periodically by dipping the tip in the saline solution and applying suction. Normally, sputum is watery and tends to be sticky. Tenacious or thick sputum usually indicates dehydration. Watch for color variations. White or translucent color is normal, yellow or green secretions may indicate infection, brown usually indicates old blood, and red indicates fresh blood. When sputum contains blood, note whether it's streaked or well mixed. Also, note how often blood appears. If the patient's heart rate and rhythm are being monitored, observe for arrhythmias. If they occur, stop suctioning and ventilate the patient.

■ After suctioning, hyperoxygenate the patient for 1 minute using the same technique described earlier.[2,3,11]

■ Readjust the FiO_2 and, for ventilated patients, the tidal volume to the ordered settings.

■ After suctioning the lower airway, assess the patient's need for upper airway suctioning. If the cuff of the ET or tracheostomy tube is inflated, suction the upper airway before deflating the cuff with a syringe[1,2] (See "Oronasopharyngeal suction," page 533.) Always change the catheter and sterile glove before resuctioning the lower airway *to avoid introducing microorganisms into the lower airway.*[1]

■ Clear the connecting tubing by aspirating the remaining saline solution or water.

■ Remove and discard your gloves and catheter in the waterproof trash bag.

■ Discard suction equipment and supplies in the appropriate receptacle and replace according to your facility's policy.

■ Maintain the head of the patient's bed at 30 to 45 degrees, if the patient's condition allows, *to prevent ventilator-associated pneumonia.*[12,13,14]

■ Auscultate the patient's lungs bilaterally and take vital signs, if indicated, *to assess the procedure's effectiveness.*

■ Perform hand hygiene.[1,6,7,8,9]

■ Document the procedure.[15,16]

Special considerations

■ Shallow suctioning is recommended *to prevent trauma to the trachea* instead of deep suctioning *because deep suctioning may be associated with more adverse events.*

■ Studies show that instillation of normal saline solution into the trachea before suctioning may stimulate the patient's cough but doesn't liquefy his secretions. Keeping the patient adequately hydrated and using bronchial hygiene techniques seem to have a greater effect on mobilizing secretions. Instilling normal saline solution may also decrease arterial and mixed venous oxygenation and contribute to lower airway contamination, increasing the risk of ventilator-associated pneumonia.[3,11,17]

■ Don't allow the collection container on the suction machine to become more than three-quarters full *to keep from damaging the machine.*

■ Patients who can't mobilize secretions effectively may need to perform tracheal suctioning after discharge.

Closed tracheal suctioning

The closed tracheal suction system can ease removal of secretions and reduce patient complications. Consisting of a sterile suction catheter in a clear plastic sleeve, the system permits the patient to remain connected to the ventilator during suctioning. *Because the catheter remains in a protective sleeve,* the system also reduces the risk of infection, even when the same catheter is used many times.[1,2] The caregiver doesn't need to touch the catheter and the ventilator circuit remains closed.

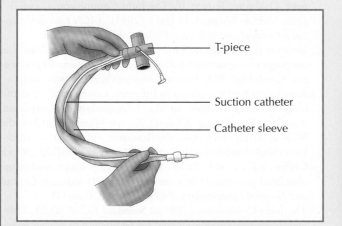

T-piece

Suction catheter

Catheter sleeve

Closed tracheal suctioning allows the tidal volume, oxygen concentration, and positive end-expiratory pressure delivered by the ventilator to be maintained while the patient is being suctioned, reducing the risk of suction-induced hypoxemia. In patients receiving intermittent mandatory mechanical ventilation, the system may reduce arterial desaturation and eliminate the need for preoxygenation.

Because suction catheters are considered contaminated after a single use, researchers studied whether closed tracheal suctioning increased the rate of health care–associated pneumonia in mechanically ventilated patients. They found that patients receiving closed tracheal suctioning had lower—not higher—rates of health care–associated pneumonia than those receiving open suctioning. Moreover, researchers found that changing closed tracheal suction catheters as needed was just as effective in preventing ventilator-associated pneumonia as daily catheter changes.[3]

On the negative side, closed tracheal suctioning has been found to produce increased negative airway pressure when certain ventilatory modes are used, increasing the risk of atelectasis and hypoxemia.

Implementation

To perform the procedure, gather the closed suction system, consisting of a control valve, a T-piece to connect the artificial airway to the ventilator breathing circuit, and a catheter sleeve that encloses the catheter and has connections at each end for the control valve and the T-piece. Then follow these steps:

■ Perform hand hygiene.[1,6,7,8,9]
■ Remove the closed suction system from its wrapping. Attach the control valve to the connecting tubing.

■ Depress the thumb suction control valve, and keep it depressed while setting the suction pressure to the desired level.
■ Connect the T-piece to the ventilator breathing circuit; make sure that the irrigation port is closed. Then connect the T-piece to the patient's endotracheal or tracheostomy tube.
■ Hyperoxygenate the patient for 30 to 60 seconds using the ventilator.[2,3,11]
■ Perform hand hygiene and put on clean gloves.[1,6,7,8,9] Steadying the T-piece, use the thumb and index finger of the other hand to advance the catheter through the tube and into the patient's tracheobronchial tree (as shown). You may need to gently retract the catheter sleeve as you advance the catheter.

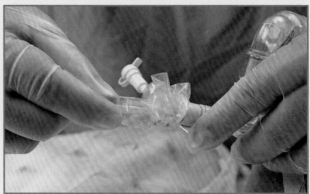

■ While continuing to hold the T-piece and control valve, apply intermittent suction and withdraw the catheter until it reaches its fully extended length in the sleeve (as shown). Repeat the procedure only if necessary.

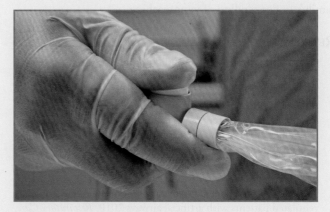

■ After you've finished suctioning, flush the catheter by maintaining suction while slowly introducing normal saline solution or sterile water into the irrigation port.
■ Place the thumb control valve in the "off" position.
■ Dispose of and replace the suction equipment and supplies according to your facility's policy.
■ Remove and discard your gloves and perform hand hygiene.[1,6,7,8,9]

Patient teaching

Teach the patient and his family about measures to prevent ventilator-associated pneumonia, and involve them in maintaining the head of the bed at 30 to 45 degrees.

Complications

Because oxygen is removed along with secretions, the patient may experience hypoxemia and dyspnea. Anxiety may alter respiratory patterns. Cardiac arrhythmias can result from hypoxia and stimulation of the vagus nerve in the tracheobronchial tree. Tracheal or bronchial trauma can result from traumatic or prolonged suctioning.

Patients with compromised cardiovascular or pulmonary status are at risk for hypoxemia, arrhythmias, hypertension, or hypotension. Patients with a history of nasopharyngeal bleeding, those who are taking anticoagulants, those who have undergone a tracheostomy recently, and those who have a blood dyscrasia are at increased risk for bleeding as a result of suctioning. Use caution when suctioning patients who have increased intracranial pressure because suction may further increase pressure.

If the patient experiences laryngospasm or bronchospasm (rare complications) during suctioning, disconnect the suction catheter from the connecting tubing and allow the catheter to act as an airway. Discuss with the patient's doctor the use of bronchodilators or lidocaine to reduce the risk of this complication.

Documentation

Record the date and time of the procedure; the technique used; the reason for suctioning; the amount, color, consistency, and odor (if any) of the secretions; any complications and nursing actions taken; and pertinent data regarding the patient's subjective response to the procedure. Document patient and family teaching. If the patient will be performing the procedure at home, document return demonstration and the patient's and family's understanding of your teaching.

REFERENCES

1 Centers for Disease Control and Prevention. (2004). Guidelines for preventing health-care–associated pneumonia, 2003. *Morbidity and Mortality Weekly Report, 53*(RR-03), 1–36. (Level I)
2 American Association of Critical-Care Nurses. (2008). "AACN Practice Alert: Ventilator Associated Pneumonia" [Online]. Accessed December 2011 via the Web at http://www.aacn.org/WD/Practice/DOCS/Ventilator_Associated_Pneumonia_1-2008.pdf (Level I)
3 American Association for Respiratory Care. (2010). AARC clinical practice guideline: Endotracheal suctioning of mechanically ventilated patients with artificial airways 2010. *Respiratory Care, 55*(6), 758–764. (Level I)
4 Morris, L.L., & Afifi, M.S. (Eds.). (2010). *Tracheostomies: The complete guide.* New York, NY: Sprier Publishing Company.
5 Vanner, R., & Bick, E. (2008). Tracheal pressures during open suctioning. *Anesthesia, 63*(3), 313–315. (Level VI)
6 Centers for Disease Control and Prevention. (October 2002). Guideline for hand hygiene in health-care settings. *Morbidity and Mortality Weekly Report, 51*(RR-16), 1–45. (Level I)
7 World Health Organization. (2009). *WHO guidelines on hand hygiene in health care: First global patient safety challenge. Clean care is safer care.* Geneva, Switzerland: World Health Organization. (Level I)
8 Siegel, J.D., et al. "2007 Guideline for Isolation Precautions: Preventing Transmission of Infectious Agents in Healthcare Settings" [Online]. Accessed December 2011 via the Web at http://www.cdc.gov/hicpac/2007ip/2007isolationprecautions.html
9 The Joint Commission. (2012). Standard NPSG.07.01.01. *Comprehensive accreditation manual for hospitals: The official handbook.* Oakbrook Terrace, IL: The Joint Commission. (Level I)
10 The Joint Commission. (2012). Standard NPSG.01.01.01. *Comprehensive accreditation manual for hospitals: The official handbook.* Oakbrook Terrace, IL: The Joint Commission. (Level I)
11 Lynn-McHale Wiegand, D. (Ed.). (2011). *AACN procedure manual for critical care* (6th ed.). Philadelphia, PA: Saunders.
12 Institute for Healthcare Improvement. (2010). *5 million lives campaign getting started kit: Prevent ventilator-associated pneumonia.* Cambridge, MA: Institute for Healthcare Improvement.
13 Association for Professional in Infection Control and Epidemiology. (2009). "Guide to the Elimination of Ventilator-Associated Pneumonia" [Online]. Accessed January 2012 via the Web at http://www.apic.org/Resource_/EliminationGuideForm/18e326ad-b484-471c-9c35-6822a53ee4a2/File/VAP_09.pdf
14 Coffin, S.E., et al. (2008). Strategies to prevent ventilator-associated pneumonia in acute care hospitals. *Infection Control and Hospital Epidemiology, 29*(1), S31–S40. (Level I)
15 The Joint Commission. (2012). Standard RC.01.03.01. *Comprehensive accreditation manual for hospitals: The official handbook.* Oakbrook Terrace, IL: The Joint Commission. (Level I)
16 The Joint Commission. (2012). Standard RC.02.01.01. *Comprehensive accreditation manual for hospitals: The official handbook.* Oakbrook Terrace, IL: The Joint Commission. (Level I)
17 Rauen, C.A., et al. (2008). Seven evidence-based practice habits: Putting some sacred cows out to pasture. *Critical Care Nurse, 28*(2), 98–124.

ADDITIONAL REFERENCES

Lorente, L., et al. (2006). Tracheal suction by closed system without daily change versus open system. *Intensive Care Medicine, 32*(4), 538–544.
Muscedere, J., et al. (2008). Comprehensive evidence-based clinical practice guidelines for ventilator-associated pneumonia: Prevention. *Journal of Critical Care, 23*(1), 126–137.
Niel-Weise, B.S., et al. (2007). Policies for endotracheal suctioning of patients receiving mechanical ventilation: A systematic review of randomized controlled trials. *Infection Control and Hospital Epidemiology, 28*(5), 531–536.
Pedersen, C.M., et al. (2009). Endotracheal suctioning of the adult intubated patient—What is the evidence? *Intensive and Critical Care Nursing, 25*(1), 21–30.
Subirana, M., et al. (2007). Closed tracheal suction systems versus open tracheal suction systems for mechanically ventilated adult patients. *Cochrane Database of Systematic Reviews* (4), CD004581.
Taylor, C., et al. (2011). *Fundamentals of nursing: The art and science of nursing care* (7th ed.). Philadelphia, PA: Lippincott Williams & Wilkins.

TRACHEOSTOMY AND VENTILATOR SPEAKING VALVE

Patients with a conventional tracheostomy tube can't speak because the cuffed tracheostomy tube that directs air into the lungs on inspiration expels air through the tracheostomy tube rather than the vocal cords, mouth, and nose. Providing a means of communication for such patients is crucial for their physical and emotional well-being. Nonverbal means of communicating, such as writing, lip-reading, alphabet boards, and gestures, can be frustrating for the patient and family members as well as for health care facility personnel. Until recently, the only alternatives were cuffed tracheostomy speaking tubes and the use of an artificial larynx.

The Passy-Muir Tracheostomy and Ventilator Speaking Valve (PMV) allows the ventilator-dependent patient to speak. The PMV is a positive-closure, one-way speaking valve developed by David Muir (a ventilator-dependent patient). It opens upon inspiration to allow the patient to inspire through the tracheostomy tube and then closes after inspiration, redirecting the exhaled air around the tube, through the vocal cords, and out of the mouth.

Other speaking valves, such as the Montgomery Ventrach, the Shiley Phonate, and a variety of others, have since been developed. Some have a closed valve like the PMV, whereas others have valves containing an alternate design.[1]

Ideally, the tracheostomy should be cuffless; however, if you're using a cuffed tube, the tracheostomy cuff must be *completely* deflated to enable the patient to exhale and to function safely.[1] For maximum airflow around the tube, the tube should be no larger than two-thirds the size of the tracheal lumen.

The PMV 005 is most commonly used by nonventilated tracheostomy patients, but it can be used by ventilator patients with rubber, nondisposable ventilator tubing. The PMV 007 fits easily into the ventilator tubing used by mechanically ventilated tracheostomy patients.[1] Both valves fit the 15-mm hub of adult, pediatric, and neonatal tracheostomy tubes and can be used by patients either on or off the ventilator.

Two other PMV valves are available: the PMV 2000 and the PMV 2001. Both of these valves are low-profile and low-resistance, feature the positive-closure design, and can be used on or off the ventilator. The PMV 2000 is clear in color and is used more readily in the home care setting because it's less noticeable. The PMV 2001 is a bright purple color and is used more often in health care facility settings because the color is more noticeable. These valves also include safety ties that prevent valve loss if the patient inadvertently coughs the PMV out of the tracheostomy tube.

A PMV oxygen adapter is now available for use with the PMV 2000 series speaking valves. This adapter allows improved mobility and comfort for patients who require a tracheostomy tube, speaking valve, and low-flow supplemental oxygen.

Short- and long-term adult, pediatric, and infant tracheostomy and ventilator-dependent patients may benefit from the use of a PMV.

PMV use is contraindicated in patients with severe tracheal or laryngeal stenosis, laryngectomy, or excessive oral secretions and in patients who are unconscious or at risk for aspiration.[1,2]

PMV use requires a multidisciplinary team approach. A doctor's order is required for placement of the PMV and sometimes for cuff deflation. The nurse and the respiratory therapist monitor and assess the patient while he's using the PMV. The respiratory therapist makes ventilator adjustments for the ventilator-dependent tracheostomy patient. A speech-language pathologist should assess the patient's cognitive, language, and oral motor function and may also evaluate swallowing status and risk for aspiration. The patient must also be involved in the decision to use the PMV.

An initial trial assesses the patient's tolerance. During this trial period, the nurse should make sure the patient understands how the PMV functions and what to expect during the trial. If he's anxious, especially during cuff deflation, he may be unwilling to use the valve, so he'll need emotional support. The patient shouldn't be left unsupervised with the valve in place until tolerance is determined.[1]

If the patient can't tolerate the PMV initially, the team should troubleshoot to determine the cause. The problem can usually be easily remedied (for example, by repositioning the patient, downsizing the tracheostomy tube, changing to a cuffless tube, or correcting an airway obstruction). Some patients will only be able to wear the PMV for a few minutes at a time, building up time gradually, as tolerated.

If repeated trials fail, the speech-language pathologist should assess the patient for other communication options.

Equipment

Appropriate size PMV ▪ gloves ▪ suction equipment ▪ 10-mL luer-lock syringe ▪ PMV instruction booklet.
Note: The PMV 005 is for the more ambulatory tracheostomy patient and can be used with flexible rubber tubing. The PMV 007 is more convenient to use with disposable ventilator tubing. Its color, which is different from the ventilator tubing, makes it easier to identify when it's in position in the ventilator circuitry.

Implementation

▪ Gather the appropriate equipment.
▪ Perform hand hygiene and put on gloves.[3,4,5,6]
▪ Confirm the patient's identity using at least two patient identifiers according to your facility's policy.[7]
▪ Explain the procedure to the patient, and make sure that he's comfortable with the procedure before beginning. Provide him with written instructions included in the PMV booklet. Allay any fear and anxiety he might feel before proceeding. If this is the patient's first wearing experience, coordinate the trial with the respiratory therapist and speech-language pathologist.
▪ Elevate the head of the patient's bed about 45 degrees.
▪ Assess the patient's vital signs, breath sounds, level of consciousness, work of breathing, and tracheal and oral secretions.[2]
▪ Perform tracheal and oral suctioning *to clear the airway of pooled secretions that could leak past the cuff after the cuff is deflated, increasing the patient's risk for pneumonia.*[2]

■ Deflate the cuff slowly *so the patient can become accustomed to using his upper airways again.* Do this by attaching a 10-mL syringe to the tracheostomy tube's pilot balloon and removing the air until air can no longer be extracted and a vacuum is created (as shown below).

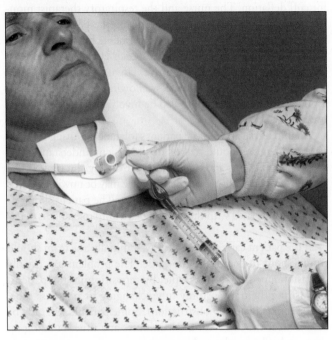

■ Suction the trachea and oral cavity as needed. The tracheostomy cuff *must* be completely deflated before the PMV is placed.

NURSING ALERT Never *place the PMV on the tracheostomy tube before deflating the cuff* because the patient won't be able to breathe.

■ Hold the PMV between your fingers. For a patient who isn't ventilator-dependent, attach the PMV to the hub of the existing tracheostomy hub with a quarter-turn twist (as shown below).

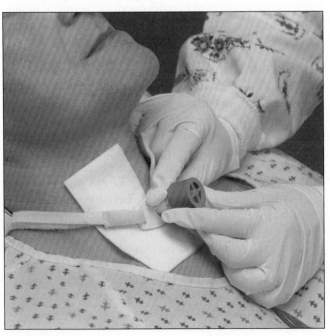

■ The PMV 007 is more convenient to use on patients who are ventilator-dependent *because it's tapered to fit into disposable ventilator tubing.* Insert the PMV into the end of the wide-mouth, short-flex tubing (as shown below).

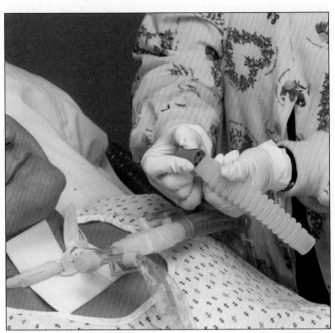

■ Connect the other end of the short-flex tubing to the ventilator tubing. Then attach the PMV (connected to the short-flex tubing) and the ventilator tubing to the closed-suction system (as shown below).

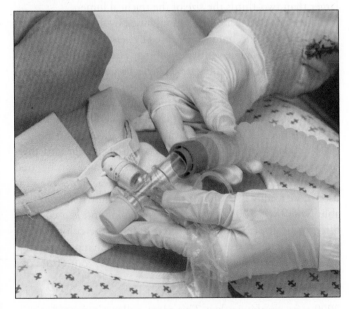

■ The PMV can also be attached between the swivel adapter and the short-flex tubing and ventilator tubing.

■ After the PMV is in place, encourage the patient to relax and concentrate on exhaling through his mouth and nose as he becomes accustomed to using his upper airways. Then have him slowly

count aloud to 10, or ask him to speak as he becomes comfortable breathing with the PMV in place. The speech-language pathologist can facilitate voice production and speech.
■ Evaluate the patient's response during PMV use. Obtain blood pressure, heart rate, and respiratory status.

NURSING ALERT *Remove the PMV at once if the patient shows signs and symptoms of distress, such as a significant change in blood pressure or heart rate, increased respiratory rate, dyspnea, diaphoresis, anxiety, uncontrollable coughing, or arterial oxygen saturation less than 90%. Reassess the patient before trying the valve again.*[2]

■ Post cuff-deflation warning signs in the room. Also, label the tracheostomy pilot balloon *to remind health care providers to reinflate the pilot balloon after removing the PMV.*[2]
■ Gently twist the PMV to remove it. Only when it's removed and the original setup is in place should you return the ventilator settings to their original levels and reinflate the pilot balloon cuff. Always remember to reinflate the tracheostomy cuff *after* removing the PMV.
■ Remove and discard your gloves and perform hand hygiene.[3,4,6]
■ Document the procedure.[8,9]

Special considerations

■ Remove the PMV before administering medicated nebulizer treatments. If the PMV is inadvertently used during a nebulizer treatment, remove it immediately and rinse it thoroughly *to remove the medication residue.*[2]
■ If the patient's tracheostomy tube has a disposable inner cannula with a grasp ring, it may be necessary to remove the inner cannula if the grasp ring extends beyond the tracheostomy tube hub.[2]
■ A PMV may be used 48 to 72 hours after the tracheotomy is performed in patients who aren't ventilator-dependent if tracheal edema and secretions from the surgical procedure have decreased.[2]
■ If tracheal swelling or bronchospasm occur as a result of tracheostomy tube change, PMV use may need to be delayed for 48 to 72 hours after the procedure.[2]

Documentation

Document the type of PMV used and the time the device was placed. Note the patient's response to the procedure, including how long the PMV has been in place, respiratory and hemodynamic status, secretion management, and ability to vocalize. Document patient teaching and the patient's understanding of your teaching.

REFERENCES

1 Morris, L.L., & Afifi, M.S. (Eds.). (2010). *Tracheostomies: The complete guide.* New York, NY: Sprier Publishing Company.
2 Passy-Muir, Inc. (2008). *Passy-Muir tracheostomy & ventilator swallowing and speaking valves instruction booklet.* Irvine, CA: Passy-Muir, Inc.
3 World Health Organization. (2009). *WHO guidelines on hand hygiene in health care: First global patient safety challenge. Clean care is safer care.* Geneva, Switzerland: World Health Organization. (Level I)

4 Siegel, J.D., et al. "2007 Guideline for Isolation Precautions: Preventing Transmission of Infectious Agents in Healthcare Settings" [Online]. Accessed December 2011 via the Web at http://www.cdc.gov/hicpac/2007ip/2007isolationprecautions.html
5 Centers for Disease Control and Prevention. (October 2002). Guideline for hand hygiene in health-care settings. *Morbidity and Mortality Weekly Report, 51*(RR-16), 1–45. (Level I)
6 The Joint Commission. (2012). Standard NPSG.07.01.01. *Comprehensive accreditation manual for hospitals: The official handbook.* Oakbrook Terrace, IL: The Joint Commission. (Level I)
7 The Joint Commission. (2012). Standard NPSG.01.01.01. *Comprehensive accreditation manual for hospitals: The official handbook.* Oakbrook Terrace, IL: The Joint Commission. (Level I)
8 The Joint Commission. (2012). Standard RC.01.03.01. *Comprehensive accreditation manual for hospitals: The official handbook.* Oakbrook Terrace, IL: The Joint Commission. (Level I)
9 The Joint Commission. (2012). Standard RC.02.01.01. *Comprehensive accreditation manual for hospitals: The official handbook.* Oakbrook Terrace, IL: The Joint Commission. (Level I)

ADDITIONAL REFERENCES

Hess, D.R. (2005). Facilitating speech in the patient with a tracheostomy. *Respiratory Care, 50*(4), 519–525.
Nettina, S.M. (2010). *Lippincott manual of nursing practice* (9th ed.). Philadelphia, PA: Lippincott Williams & Wilkins.
Nomori, H. (2004). Tracheostomy tube enabling speech during mechanical ventilation. *Chest, 125*(3), 1046–1051.

TRACHEOSTOMY CARE

Whether a tracheotomy is performed in an emergency situation or after careful preparation, as a permanent measure or as temporary therapy, tracheostomy care has identical goals: to ensure airway patency by keeping the tube free of mucus buildup, to maintain mucous membrane and skin integrity, to prevent infection, and to provide psychological support.

The patient may have one of three types of tracheostomy tube—uncuffed, cuffed, or fenestrated. Tube selection depends on the patient's condition and the doctor's preference.

An *uncuffed tube,* which may be plastic or metal, allows air to flow freely around the tracheostomy tube and through the larynx, reducing the risk of tracheal damage. A *cuffed tube,* made of plastic, is disposable. The cuff and the tube won't separate accidentally inside the trachea because the cuff is bonded to the tube. Also, it doesn't require periodic deflating to lower pressure because cuff pressure is low and evenly distributed against the tracheal wall. Although cuffed tubes may cost more than other tubes, they reduce the risk of tracheal damage. A plastic *fenestrated tube* permits speech through the upper airway when the external opening is capped and the cuff is deflated. It also allows easy removal of the inner cannula for cleaning. However, a fenestrated tube may become occluded. (See *Types of tracheostomy tubes,* page 718.)

Whichever tube is used, tracheostomy care should be performed using sterile technique until the stoma has healed to prevent infection. For recently performed tracheotomies, use sterile gloves for all manipulations at the tracheostomy site. When the

EQUIPMENT

Types of tracheostomy tubes

Cuffed and uncuffed tracheostomy tubes each have advantages and disadvantages. Cuffed tubes help seal the area between the tube and trachea, decreasing the patient's risk of aspiration; however, if the cuff pressure isn't regularly monitored, it may erode the trachea. Also, if the cuff is inflated, the patient can't talk and needs an alternate means of communication.

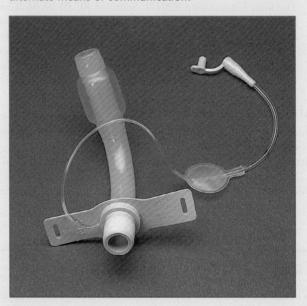

Uncuffed tubes allow the patient to eat and talk, but this type of tube can't be used in a patient who is receiving mechanical ventilation *because oxygen may escape from around the tube.*

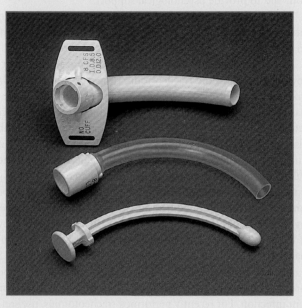

stoma has healed, clean gloves may be substituted for sterile ones. Changing tracheostomy ties helps prevent infection and the skin underneath the ties from becoming excoriated and wet. Tracheostomy ties should be changed at least once each day, or as needed.

Equipment

For cuff inflation and deflation
10-mL syringe ▪ gloves ▪ stethoscope ▪ handheld resuscitation bag.

For tracheostomy ties change
30" (76-cm) length of tracheostomy twill tape or commercially prepared tracheostomy ties ▪ bandage scissors ▪ clean or sterile gloves ▪ hemostat.

For tracheostomy tube cannula and stoma care
Disposable inner cannula ▪ waterproof trash bag ▪ two sterile solution containers ▪ normal saline solution or sterile water ▪ sterile cotton-tipped applicators ▪ sterile 4" × 4" gauze pads ▪ sterile gloves ▪ prepackaged sterile tracheostomy dressing (or 4" × 4" gauze pad) ▪ equipment and supplies for suctioning and for mouth care ▪ materials, as needed, for cuff procedures and for changing tracheostomy ties ▪ personal protective equipment ▪ tracheostomy cleaning brush or sterile pipe cleaner ▪ Optional: water-soluble lubricant or topical antibiotic cream, third sterile solution container.

Keep supplies in full view in the patient's room at all times for easy access in case of emergency. Consider taping an emergency sterile tracheostomy tube in a sterile wrapper above the head of the bed for access in an emergency.

Preparation of equipment
Perform hand hygiene[1,2,3,4] and gather all equipment and supplies in the patient's room.

For tracheostomy tube cannula and stoma care
Check the expiration date on each sterile package and inspect the package for tears. Open the waterproof trash bag and place it next to you *so that you can avoid reaching across the sterile field or the patient's stoma when discarding soiled items.* Establish a sterile field near the patient's bed (usually on the overbed table), and place equipment and supplies on it. Pour normal saline solution or sterile water into one of the sterile solution containers; then pour normal saline solution or sterile water into the second sterile container for rinsing. For inner-cannula care, you may use a third sterile solution container to hold the gauze pads and cotton-tipped applicators saturated with normal saline solution. Hydrogen peroxide is no longer recommended for cleaning inner cannulas or tracheostomy sites.[5] If you'll be replacing the disposable inner cannula, open the package containing the new inner cannula while maintaining sterile technique.[5] Obtain or prepare new tracheostomy ties, if indicated.

Implementation

- Confirm the patient's identity using at least two patient identifiers according to your facility's policy.[6]
- Explain the procedure to him, provide privacy and reassure him.
- Perform hand hygiene and put on gloves.[1,2,3,4]
- Assess the patient's condition.
- Help the patient into semi-Fowler's position, if possible, or place him in a supine position with the head of the bed elevated as tolerated *to prevent aspiration of secretions.*
- Hyperoxygenate the patient for at least 1 minute and then perform deep oropharyngeal suctioning *to remove accumulated secretions from above the cuff and prevent pooled secretions from descending into the trachea after cuff deflation; these secretions have been implicated in the development of ventilator-associated pneumonia.*[7,8,9,10]

For cuff inflation and deflation

- Read the cuff manufacturer's instructions *because cuff types and procedures vary widely.*
- Remove the ventilation device or humidified oxygen.
- Insert a 10-mL syringe into the cuff pilot balloon. Ventilate the patient with a handheld resuscitation bag and slowly withdraw air from the cuff until a small leak is heard during inspiration. Leave the syringe attached to the tubing for later reinflation of the cuff.[5] *Slow deflation allows positive lung pressure to push secretions upward from the bronchi. Cuff deflation may also stimulate the patient's cough reflex, producing additional secretions.*
- Reinflate the cuff using the minimal-leak technique or the minimal occlusive volume technique *to help gauge the proper inflation point.*
- If you're inflating the cuff using cuff pressure measurement, be careful not to exceed 25 mm Hg. If pressure exceeds 25 mm Hg, notify the doctor *because you may need to change to a larger size tube, use higher inflation pressures, or permit a larger air leak.*
- After you've inflated the cuff, remove the syringe.
- Reattach the ventilation device or humidified oxygen.
- Check for minimal leaks at the cuff seal. You shouldn't feel air coming from the patient's mouth, nose, or tracheostomy site, and a conscious patient shouldn't be able to speak.
- Observe the patient for adequate ventilation.
- Be alert for air leaks from the cuff itself. Suspect a leak if injection of air fails to inflate the cuff or increase cuff pressure, if you're unable to inject the amount of air you withdrew, if the patient can speak, if ventilation fails to maintain adequate respiratory movement with pressures or volumes previously considered adequate, or if air escapes during the ventilator's inspiratory cycle.
- Note the exact amount of air used to inflate the cuff *to detect tracheomalacia if more air is consistently needed.*

For ties change

- Obtain assistance from another nurse or a respiratory therapist *because of the risk of accidental tube expulsion during this procedure.* Patient movement or coughing can dislodge the tube.
- Discard your gloves, perform hand hygiene, and put on a new pair of sterile or clean gloves.[1,2,3,4]

- If you aren't using commercially packaged tracheostomy ties, prepare new ties from a 30″ (76-cm) length of tracheostomy twill tape by folding one end back 1″ (2.5 cm) on itself. Then, with the bandage scissors, cut a ½″ (1.3-cm) slit down the center of the tape from the folded edge.
- Prepare the other end of the tape the same way.
- Hold both ends together and, using scissors, cut the resulting circle of tape so that one piece is approximately 10″ (25 cm) long and the other is about 20″ (51 cm) long.
- After your assistant puts on clean or sterile gloves, instruct her to hold the tracheostomy tube in place *to prevent its expulsion during replacement of the ties.* If you must perform the procedure without assistance, fasten the clean ties in place before removing the old ties *to prevent tube expulsion.*
- With the assistant's gloved fingers holding the tracheostomy tube in place, cut the soiled tracheostomy ties with the bandage scissors or untie them and discard the ties. Be careful not to cut the tube of the pilot balloon.
- Thread the slit end of one new tie a short distance through the eye of one tracheostomy tube flange from the underside; use the hemostat, if needed, to pull the tie through. Then thread the other end of the tie completely through the slit end, and pull it taut so it loops firmly through the flange. *This technique avoids knots that can cause throat discomfort, tissue irritation, pressure, and necrosis of the patient's throat.*
- Fasten the second tie to the opposite flange in the same manner.
- Instruct the patient to flex his neck while you bring the ties around to the side, and tie them together with a square knot. *Flexion produces the same neck circumference as coughing and helps prevent an overly tight tie.* Instruct your assistant to place one finger under the tapes as you tie them *to ensure that they're tight enough to avoid slippage but loose enough to prevent choking or jugular vein constriction. Placing the closure on the side allows easy access and prevents pressure necrosis at the back of the neck when the patient is recumbent.*
- After securing the ties, cut off the excess tape with the scissors and instruct your assistant to release the tracheostomy tube.
- Check tracheostomy-tie tension often on patients with traumatic injury, radical neck dissection, or cardiac failure *because neck diameter can increase from swelling and cause constriction;* also check neonatal or restless patients frequently *because ties can loosen and cause tube dislodgment.*
- Provide oral care, as needed, *because the oral cavity can become dry and malodorous or develop sores from encrusted secretions.*
- Observe soiled dressings and any suctioned secretions for amount, color, consistency, and odor.

For tracheostomy tube cannula and stoma care

- Discard gloves, perform hand hygiene, and put on sterile gloves.[1,2,3,4]
- With your nondominant hand, remove any humidification or ventilation device.

■ Using sterile technique, suction the tracheostomy tube *to clear the airway of any secretions that may hinder oxygenation.* Determine the volume of secretions and assess them for color, consistency, and odor.

■ With your nondominant hand, reconnect the patient to the humidifier or ventilator, if necessary.

■ Remove the patient's tracheostomy dressing; inspect it for drainage and then discard it.[5]

■ Remove and discard your gloves and perform hand hygiene.[2,3,4]

Cleaning a nondisposable inner cannula

■ Perform hand hygiene and put on sterile gloves.[2,3,4,5]

■ Using your nondominant hand, disconnect the ventilator or humidification device, and unlock the tracheostomy tube's inner cannula by rotating it counterclockwise (as shown below).[5]

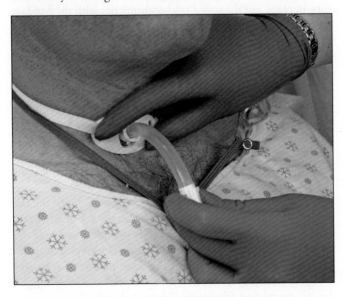

■ Place the ventilator oxygen device or humidification device over or near the outer cannula *to maintain oxygen supply.*

■ Working quickly, use your dominant hand to scrub the cannula with the sterile nylon brush (as shown below).[5] If the brush doesn't slide easily into the cannula, use a sterile pipe cleaner.

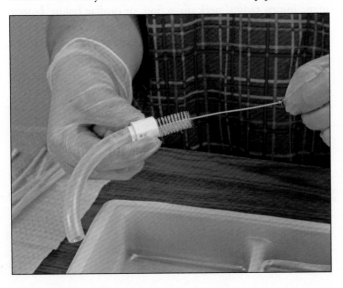

■ Immerse the cannula in the container of normal saline solution or sterile water, and agitate it for about 10 seconds (as shown below) *to rinse it thoroughly.*

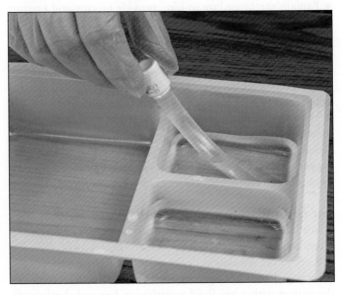

■ Inspect the cannula for cleanliness. Repeat the cleaning process, if necessary. If it's clean, tap it gently against the inside edge of the sterile container *to remove excess liquid and prevent aspiration.* Don't dry the outer surface *because a thin film of moisture acts as a lubricant during insertion.*

■ Reinsert the inner cannula into the patient's tracheostomy tube (as shown below). Lock it in place and then gently pull on it *to make sure it's positioned securely.* Reconnect the mechanical ventilator or humidification device.[5]

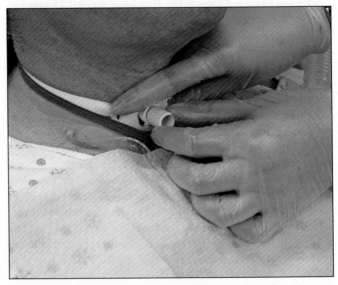

■ If the patient can't tolerate being disconnected from the ventilator for the time it takes to clean the inner cannula, replace the existing inner cannula with a clean one and reattach the mechanical ventilator. Then clean the cannula just removed from the patient, and store it in a sterile container for the next time.[5]

Caring for a disposable inner cannula
- Perform hand hygiene and put on sterile gloves.[1,2,3,4]
- Using your dominant hand, remove the patient's inner cannula.[5] After evaluating the secretions in the cannula, discard it properly.
- Pick up the new inner cannula, touching only the outer locking portion. Insert the cannula into the tracheostomy and, following the manufacturer's instructions, lock it securely.[5]
- Replace any humidification or ventilation device.[5]

Cleaning the stoma and outer cannula
- Perform hand hygiene and put on sterile gloves.[1,2,3,4]
- With your dominant hand, moisten a sterile gauze pad with the normal saline solution or sterile water. Squeeze out the excess liquid *to prevent accidental aspiration.* Then wipe the patient's neck under the tracheostomy tube flanges and twill tapes.
- Assess the stoma site for redness, swelling, and drainage, *which may indicate infection.*[5]
- Use a cotton-tipped applicator and a gauze pad to clean the stoma site and the tube's flanges. Wipe only once with each applicator or gauze pad and then discard it *to prevent contamination of a clean area with a soiled applicator or pad.*[5]
- Rinse debris with one or more sterile 4″ × 4″ gauze pads dampened in normal saline solution or sterile water.
- Dry the area thoroughly with additional sterile gauze pads; then apply a new sterile tracheostomy dressing.[5,10]

Completing cannula care
- Provide oral care routinely according to your facility's policy (usually every 2 to 4 hours) *because the oral cavity can become dry and malodorous or develop sores from encrusted secretions.* Brush the patient's teeth, gums, and tongue at least twice a day using a soft toothbrush.[7] Perform oral care daily using chlorhexidine solution as prescribed *to prevent ventilator-associated pneumonia.*[13]
- Make sure the head of the patient's bed is elevated 30 to 45 degrees *to prevent ventilator-associated pneumonia.*[13,14,15]

Completing the procedure
- Make sure the patient is comfortable and can easily reach the call bell and communication aids.
- Properly clean or dispose of all equipment, supplies, and trash according to your facility's policy.
- Remove and discard your gloves and any other personal protective equipment and perform hand hygiene.[1,2,3,4]
- Replenish any used supplies, and make sure all necessary emergency supplies are at the bedside.
- Document the procedure.[11,12]

Special considerations
- Keep appropriate equipment at the patient's bedside for immediate use in an emergency. (See "Tracheotomy, assisting," page 722.)
- Consult the doctor about first-aid measures you can use for your tracheostomy patient should an emergency occur. Follow your facility's policy for what to do if a tracheostomy tube is expelled or if the outer cannula becomes blocked. If the patient's breathing is obstructed—for example, when the tube is blocked with mucus that can't be removed by suctioning or by withdrawing the inner cannula—call the appropriate code, and provide manual resuscitation with a handheld resuscitation bag or reconnect the patient to the ventilator. Don't remove the tracheostomy tube entirely *because removal may allow the airway to close completely.* Use extreme caution when attempting to reinsert an expelled tracheostomy tube *because of the risk of tracheal trauma, perforation, compression, and asphyxiation.* Reassure the patient until the doctor arrives.
- Refrain from changing tracheostomy ties unnecessarily during the immediate postoperative period before the stoma track is well formed (usually 4 days) *to avoid accidental dislodgement and expulsion of the tube.* Unless secretions or drainage is a problem, ties can be changed once a day.
- Refrain from changing a single-cannula tracheostomy tube or the outer cannula of a double-cannula tube. *Because of the risk of tracheal complications,* the doctor usually changes the cannula; the frequency of change depends on the patient's condition.
- If the patient's neck or stoma is excoriated or infected, apply a water-soluble lubricant or topical antibiotic cream as ordered. Remember not to use a powder or an oil-based substance on or around a stoma *because aspiration can cause infection and abscess.*
- If the outer cannula of a cuffed tracheostomy tube is accidentally removed or coughed out, never use hydrogen peroxide to clean it. *Using hydrogen peroxide may affect the integrity of the cuff.* Replace it with a new tracheostomy tube.
- Replace all equipment, including solutions, regularly according to your facility's policy *to reduce the risk of health care–acquired infections.*

Patient teaching
If the patient is being discharged with a tracheostomy, start self-care teaching as soon as he's receptive. Teach the patient how to change and clean the tube. If he's being discharged with suction equipment, make sure he and his family feel knowledgeable and comfortable about using this equipment.

Teach the patient and his family about measures to prevent ventilator-associated pneumonia, including maintaining the head of the bed at 30 to 45 degrees, and encourage them to alert staff members when the bed doesn't appear to be positioned correctly.[13]

Complications
Secretions that collect under dressings can encourage skin excoriation and infection. Hardened mucus or a slipped cuff can occlude the cannula opening and obstruct the airway. Tube displacement can stimulate the cough reflex if the tip rests on the carina, or it can cause blood vessel erosion and hemorrhage. Just the presence of the tube or excessive cuff pressure can produce tracheal erosion and necrosis.

Complications associated with changing tracheostomy ties include dislodgement of the tube and tissue necrosis caused by ties that are placed too tightly.

Documentation

Record the date and time of the procedure; the type of procedure; the amount, consistency, color, and odor of secretions; stoma and skin condition; the patient's respiratory status; changing of the tracheostomy tube by the doctor; the duration of any cuff deflation; the amount of any cuff inflation; and cuff pressure readings and specific body position. Note complications and nursing actions taken, patient or family teaching and their comprehension of the teaching and progress, and the patient's tolerance of the treatment.

REFERENCES

1 Siegel, J.D., et al. "2007 Guideline for Isolation Precautions: Preventing Transmission of Infectious Agents in Healthcare Settings" [Online]. Accessed December 2011 via the Web at http://www.cdc.gov/hicpac/2007ip/2007isolationprecautions.html

2 World Health Organization. (2009). *WHO guidelines on hand hygiene in health care: First global patient safety challenge. Clean care is safer care.* Geneva, Switzerland: World Health Organization. (Level I)

3 Centers for Disease Control and Prevention. (October 2002). Guideline for hand hygiene in health-care settings. *Morbidity and Mortality Weekly Report, 51*(RR-16), 1–45. (Level I)

4 The Joint Commission. (2012). Standard NPSG.07.01.01. *Comprehensive accreditation manual for hospitals: The official handbook.* Oakbrook Terrace, IL: The Joint Commission. (Level I)

5 Lynn-McHale Wiegand, D. (Ed.). (2011). *AACN procedure manual for critical care* (6th ed.). Philadelphia, PA: Saunders.

6 The Joint Commission. (2012). Standard NPSG.01.01.01. *Comprehensive accreditation manual for hospitals: The official handbook.* Oakbrook Terrace, IL: The Joint Commission. (Level I)

7 American Association of Critical Care Nurses. (2008). "AACN Practice Alert: Ventilator Associated Pneumonia" [Online]. Accessed December 2011 via the Web http://www.aacn.org/WD/Practice/DOCS/Ventilator_Associated_Pneumonia_1-2008.pdf (Level I)

8 Centers for Disease Control and Prevention. (2004). Guidelines for preventing health-care–associated pneumonia, 2003. *Morbidity and Mortality Weekly Report, 53*(RR-03), 1–36. (Level I)

9 American Association for Respiratory Care. (2010). AARC clinical practice guideline: Endotracheal suctioning of mechanically ventilated patients with artificial airways 2010. *Respiratory Care, 55*(6), 758–764. (Level I)

10 Morris, L.L., & Afifi, M.S. (Eds.). (2010). *Tracheostomies: The complete guide.* New York, NY: Sprier Publishing Company.

11 The Joint Commission. (2012). Standard RC.01.03.01. *Comprehensive accreditation manual for hospitals: The official handbook.* Oakbrook Terrace, IL: The Joint Commission. (Level I)

12 The Joint Commission. (2012). Standard RC.02.01.01. *Comprehensive accreditation manual for hospitals: The official handbook.* Oakbrook Terrace, IL: The Joint Commission. (Level I)

13 Institute for Healthcare Improvement. (2010). *5 million lives campaign getting started kit: Prevent ventilator-associated pneumonia.* Cambridge, MA: Institute for Healthcare Improvement.

14 Association for Professional in Infection Control and Epidemiology. (2009). "Guide to the Elimination of Ventilator-Associated Pneumonia" [Online]. Accessed January 2012 via the Web at http://www.apic.org/Resource_/EliminationGuideForm/18e326ad-b484-471c-9c35-6822a53ee4a2/File/VAP_09.pdf

15 Coffin, S.E. et al. (2008). Strategies to prevent ventilator-associated pneumonia in acute care hospitals. *Infection Control and Hospital Epidemiology, 29*(1), S31–S40.

ADDITIONAL REFERENCES

Björling, G., et al. (2007). Tracheostomy inner cannula care: A randomized crossover study of two decontamination procedures. *American Journal of Infection Control, 35*(9), 600–605.

Frace, M.A. (2010). Tracheostomy care on the medical-surgical unit. *Medsurg Nursing, 19*(1), 58–61.

Garrubba, M., et al. (2009). Multidisciplinary care for tracheostomy patients: A systematic review. *Critical Care Medicine, 13*(6), R177.

Nettina, S.M. (2010). *Lippincott manual of nursing practice* (9th ed.). Philadelphia, PA: Lippincott Williams & Wilkins.

Taylor, C., et al. (2011). *Fundamentals of nursing: The art and science of nursing care* (7th ed.). Philadelphia, PA: Lippincott Williams & Wilkins.

Vyas, D., et al. (2002). Measurement of tracheal tube cuff pressure in critical care. *Anaesthesia, 57*(3), 275–277.

Webber-Jones, J. (2010). Obstructed tracheostomy tubes: Clearing the air. *Nursing, 40*(1), 49–50.

TRACHEOTOMY, ASSISTING

A tracheotomy involves the surgical creation of an external opening—called a *tracheostomy*—into the trachea and insertion of an indwelling tube to maintain the airway's patency. If all other attempts to establish an airway have failed, a doctor may perform a tracheotomy at a patient's bedside. This procedure may be necessary when an airway obstruction results from laryngeal edema, foreign-body obstruction, or a tumor. An emergency tracheotomy also may be performed when endotracheal intubation is contraindicated.

Use of a cuffed tracheostomy tube provides and maintains a patent airway, prevents the unconscious or paralyzed patient from aspirating food or secretions, allows removal of tracheobronchial secretions from the patient unable to cough, replaces an endotracheal tube, and permits the use of positive-pressure ventilation.

When laryngectomy accompanies a tracheostomy, a laryngectomy tube—a shorter version of a tracheostomy tube—may be inserted by the doctor. In addition, the patient's trachea is sutured to the skin surface. Consequently, with a laryngectomy, accidental tube expulsion doesn't precipitate immediate closure of the tracheal opening. When healing occurs, the patient has a permanent neck stoma through which respiration takes place.

Although tracheostomy tubes come in plastic and metal, plastic tubes are much more commonly used because they have a universal adapter for respiratory support equipment, such as a mechanical ventilator, and a cuff to allow positive-pressure ventilation.

Equipment

Tracheostomy tube of the proper size with obturator ■ sterile tracheotomy tray (typically contains tracheal dilator, vein retractor, hemostats, and clamps) ■ sutures and needles ■ 4″ × 4″ gauze pads ■ gloves ■ sterile drapes, gloves, mask, and gown ■ sterile bowls ■ stethoscope ■ dressing ■ pillow ■ tracheostomy ties ■ suction apparatus and tubing ■ alcohol pad ■ antiseptic cleaning solution ■ sterile water ■ 5-mL syringe with 22G needle ■ local anesthetic (such as lidocaine with epinephrine) ■ oxygen therapy device ■ oxygen source ■ syringe for cuff inflation.

Many facilities use prepackaged sterile tracheotomy trays.

Preparation of equipment

Have one person stay with the patient while another obtains the necessary equipment. Perform hand hygiene.[1,2,3,4] Then, maintaining sterile technique, open the tray.[1,2,3] Take the tracheostomy tube from its container and place it on the sterile field. If necessary, set up the suction equipment and make sure it works. When the doctor opens the sterile bowls, pour in the antiseptic cleaning solution.

Implementation

■ Perform hand hygiene and put on gloves.[1,2,3,4]
■ Confirm the patient's identity using at least two patient identifiers according to your facility's policy.[5]
■ Explain the procedure to the patient even if he's unresponsive.
■ If possible, make sure that an informed consent has been obtained and is documented in the medical record.[6]
■ Conduct a preprocedure verification process *to make sure that all relevant documentation, related information, and equipment are available and correctly identified to the patient's identifiers.*[7]
■ Assess the patient's condition and provide privacy. Maintain ventilation until the tracheotomy is performed.
■ Make sure the patient has patent IV access; insert an IV catheter if necessary.[8]
■ Sedate the patient, as ordered, for the procedure following safe medication administration practices *to decrease pain and anxiety.*[9]
■ Monitor the patient's cardiac rhythm, oxygen saturation, blood pressure, and capnography throughout the procedure.[8]
■ Conduct a time-out immediately before starting the procedure *to perform a final assessment that the correct patient, site, positioning, and procedure are identified and that, as applicable, all relevant information and necessary equipment are available during and after the procedure.*[10]
■ Before the doctor begins, place a shoulder roll under the patient's shoulders and neck to extend his neck. If the patient is in respiratory distress and optimal neck extensions isn't tolerated, place the patient in semi-Fowler's position.[8]
■ Disinfect the top of the local anesthetic vial with an alcohol pad. Invert the vial so that the doctor can withdraw the anesthetic using the 22G needle attached to the 5-mL syringe.
■ The doctor will put on sterile gloves, gown, and mask.[4]
■ Assist with the procedure as needed. (See *Assisting with a tracheotomy,* page 724.)
■ When the tube is in position, attach it to the appropriate oxygen therapy device, which is connected to an oxygen source.
■ Inject air into the distal cuff port *to inflate the cuff.*
■ Auscultate the patient's lungs using a stethoscope.
■ The doctor will suture the corners of the incision.

■ Remove and discard your gloves. Perform hand hygiene and put on sterile gloves.[1,2,3,4]
■ Apply the sterile tracheostomy dressing under the tracheostomy tube flange. Place the tracheostomy ties through the openings of the tube flanges, and tie them on the side of the patient's neck. *Doing so allows easy access and prevents pressure necrosis at the back of the neck.*
■ Clean or dispose of the used equipment according to facility policy. Replenish all supplies as needed.
■ Remove and discard your gloves and perform hand hygiene.[1,2,3,4]
■ Assess the patient's vital signs and respiratory status every 15 minutes for 1 hour, then every 30 minutes for 2 hours, then every 2 hours until his condition is stable, or according to facility policy.
■ Make sure that a chest X-ray is ordered *to confirm tube placement.*
■ Document the procedure.[11,12]

Special considerations

■ Monitor the patient carefully for signs of infection. Ideally, the tracheotomy should be performed using sterile technique as described. But in an emergency, this may not be possible.
■ Make sure the following equipment is always at the patient's bedside: suctioning equipment *because the patient may need his airway cleared at any time;* the sterile obturator used to insert the tracheostomy tube *in case the tube is expelled;* a sterile tracheostomy tube and obturator (the same size as the one used) *in case the tube must be replaced quickly;* a spare, sterile inner cannula *that can be used if the cannula is expelled;* a sterile tracheostomy tube and obturator one size smaller than the one used, *which may be needed if the tube is expelled and the trachea begins to close;* and a sterile tracheal dilator or sterile hemostats *to maintain an open airway before inserting a new tracheostomy tube.*
■ Review emergency first-aid measures, and always follow your facility's policy concerning an expelled or blocked tracheostomy tube. When a blocked tube can't be cleared by suctioning or withdrawing the inner cannula, policy may require you to stay with the patient while someone else calls the doctor or the appropriate code. You should continue trying to ventilate the patient with whatever method works such as a handheld resuscitation bag. Don't remove the tracheostomy tube entirely; *doing so may close the airway completely.*
■ Use extreme caution if you try to reinsert an expelled tracheostomy tube *to avoid tracheal trauma, perforation, compression, and asphyxiation.*

Complications

A tracheotomy can cause an airway obstruction (from improper tube placement), hemorrhage, edema, a perforated esophagus, subcutaneous or mediastinal emphysema, aspiration of secretions, tracheal necrosis (from cuff pressure), infection, or lacerations of arteries, veins, or nerves.

Documentation

Record the reason for the procedure, the date and time it took place, and the patient's respiratory status before and after the

Assisting with a tracheotomy

After preparing the skin with an antiseptic and allowing it to dry, the doctor will make a horizontal or vertical incision into the skin. (A vertical incision helps avoid arteries, veins, and nerves on the lateral borders of the trachea.) Then he'll dissect subcutaneous fat and muscle and move the muscle aside with vein retractors *to locate the tracheal rings.* He'll make an incision between the second and third tracheal rings, using hemostats *to control bleeding.*

Next, he'll inject a local anesthetic into the tracheal lumen *to suppress the cough reflex* and create a stoma in the trachea. When this is done, carefully apply suction to remove blood and secretions that may obstruct the airway or be aspirated into the lungs. The doctor will then insert the tracheostomy tube and obturator into the stoma (as shown). After inserting the tube, he'll remove the obturator.

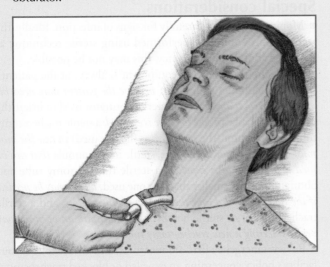

Apply a sterile tracheostomy dressing, and anchor the tube with tracheostomy ties (as shown). Check for air movement through the tube and auscultate the lungs *to ensure proper placement.*

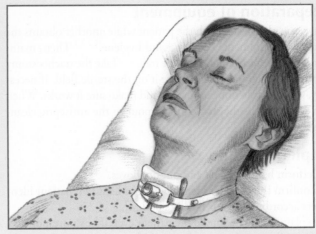

An alternative approach

In another approach, the doctor inserts the tracheostomy tube percutaneously at the bedside. Using either a series of dilators or a pair of forceps, he creates a stoma for tube insertion. Unlike the surgical technique, this method dilates rather than cuts the tissue structures.

After the skin is prepared and anesthetized, the doctor makes a 1-cm midline incision. When the stoma reaches the desired size, the doctor inserts the tracheostomy tube. After the tube is in place, inflate the cuff, secure the tube, and check the patient's breath sounds. Then obtain a portable chest X-ray.

procedure. Note the type and size of tube used. Include any complications that occurred during the procedure, the amount of cuff pressure, and the respiratory therapy initiated after the procedure. Also note the patient's response to respiratory therapy.

References

1 Centers for Disease Control and Prevention. (October 2002). Guideline for hand hygiene in health-care settings. *Morbidity and Mortality Weekly Report, 51*(RR-16), 1–45. (Level I)

2 World Health Organization. (2009). *WHO guidelines on hand hygiene in health care: First global patient safety challenge. Clean care is safer care.* Geneva, Switzerland: World Health Organization. (Level I)

3 Siegel, J.D., et al. "2007 Guideline for Isolation Precautions: Preventing Transmission of Infectious Agents in Healthcare Settings" [Online]. Accessed December 2011 via the Web at http://www.cdc.gov/hicpac/2007ip/2007isolationprecautions.html

4 The Joint Commission. (2012). Standard NPSG.07.01.01. *Comprehensive accreditation manual for hospitals: The official handbook.* Oakbrook Terrace, IL: The Joint Commission. (Level I)

5 The Joint Commission. (2012). Standard NPSG.01.01.01. *Comprehensive accreditation manual for hospitals: The official handbook.* Oakbrook Terrace, IL: The Joint Commission. (Level I)

6 The Joint Commission. (2012). Standard RI.01.03.01. *Comprehensive accreditation manual for hospitals: The official handbook.* Oakbrook Terrace, IL: The Joint Commission. (Level I)

7 The Joint Commission. (2012). Standard UP.01.01.01. *Comprehensive accreditation manual for hospitals: The official handbook.* Oakbrook Terrace, IL: The Joint Commission. (Level I)

8 Morris, L.L., & Afifi, M.S. (Eds.). (2010). *Tracheostomies: The complete guide.* New York, NY: Sprier Publishing Company.

9 The Joint Commission. (2012). Standard MM.06.01.01. *Comprehensive accreditation manual for hospitals: The official handbook.* Oakbrook Terrace, IL: The Joint Commission. (Level I)

10 The Joint Commission. (2012). Standard UP.01.03.01. *Comprehensive accreditation manual for hospitals: The official handbook.* Oakbrook Terrace, IL: The Joint Commission. (Level I)

11 The Joint Commission. (2012). Standard RC.01.03.01. *Comprehensive accreditation manual for hospitals: The official handbook.* Oakbrook Terrace, IL: The Joint Commission. (Level I)

12 The Joint Commission. (2012). Standard RC.02.01.01. *Comprehensive accreditation manual for hospitals: The official handbook.* Oakbrook Terrace, IL: The Joint Commission. (Level I)

ADDITIONAL REFERENCES

Barbetti, J.K., et al. (2009). Prospective observational study of postoperative complications after percutaneous dilatational or surgical tracheostomy in critically ill patients, *Critical Care Resuscitation, 11*(4), 244–249.

Engels, P.T., et al. (2009). Tracheostomy: From insertion to decannulation. *Canadian Journal of Surgery, 52*(5), 427–433.

Garrubba, M., et al. (2009). Multidisciplinary care for tracheostomy patients: A systematic review. *Critical Care Medicine* 13(6): R177.

Lynn-McHale Wiegand, D. (Ed.). (2011). *AACN procedure manual for critical care* (6th ed.). Philadelphia, PA: Saunders.

Nettina, S.M. (2010). *Lippincott manual of nursing practice* (9th ed.). Philadelphia, PA: Lippincott Williams & Wilkins.

U.S. Food and Drug Administration. (2009). "Look. Check. Connect.: Safe Medical Device Connections Save Lives" [Online]. Accessed December 2011 via the Web at http://www.fda.gov/downloads/MedicalDevices/Safety/AlertsandNotices/UCM134873.pdf

TRANSABDOMINAL TUBE FEEDING AND CARE

To access the stomach, duodenum, or jejunum, the doctor may place a tube through the patient's abdominal wall. This procedure may be done surgically or percutaneously.

A gastrostomy or jejunostomy tube is usually inserted during intra-abdominal surgery. The tube may be used for feeding during the immediate postoperative period or it may provide long-term enteral access, depending on the type of surgery. Typically, the doctor will suture the tube in place to prevent gastric contents from leaking.

In contrast, a percutaneous endoscopic gastrostomy (PEG) or percutaneous endoscopic jejunostomy (PEJ) tube can be inserted endoscopically without the need for laparotomy or general anesthesia. Typically, the insertion is done in the endoscopy suite or at the patient's bedside. Ultrasound can be used to confirm placement. A PEG or PEJ tube may be used for nutrition, drainage, and decompression. Contraindications to endoscopic placement include obstruction (such as an esophageal stricture or duodenal blockage), previous gastric surgery, morbid obesity, and ascites. These conditions would necessitate surgical placement.

With PEJ tube placement, feedings may begin after 24 hours (or when peristalsis resumes). A PEG tube can be used for feedings within 2 hours of placement in adults and 6 hours in infants and children.[1]

After a time, the tube may need to be replaced and the doctor may recommend a gastrostomy button—a skin-level feeding tube. Tubes not intended for use as enteral feeding devices, such as urinary or GI drainage tubes, shouldn't be used because these tubes don't have an external anchoring device. Use of these tubes

may lead to misconnection or tube migration, which may cause obstruction of the gastric pylorus or small bowel.[1]

Nursing care for patients receiving transabdominal feedings includes providing skin care at the tube exit site, maintaining the feeding tube, administering feeding formula, monitoring the patient's response to feeding, adjusting the feeding schedule, and preparing the patient for self-care after discharge.

Equipment

For continuous or intermittent feeding
Feeding formula ■ large-bulb or catheter-tip syringe ■ 120 mL of water ■ 4" × 4" gauze pads ■ gravity-drip administration bags ■ mouthwash, toothpaste, or mild salt solution ■ gloves ■ Optional: enteral infusion pump, sterile water.

For site care
4" × 4" gauze pads ■ soap ■ cotton-tipped applicators ■ skin protectant ■ normal saline solution ■ hypoallergenic tape ■ gloves.

Preparation of equipment
Always check the expiration date on commercially prepared feeding formulas. If the formula has been prepared by the dietitian or pharmacist, check the preparation time and date. Discard any opened formula within 24 hours of preparation if not used.[1]

For continuous feedings
Commercially prepared administration sets and enteral pumps allow continuous formula administration. Set up the equipment according to the manufacturer's guidelines. Fill the feeding bag and purge air form the administration tubing. If a prefilled container is available, attach it to the administration set and then purge air from the tubing. Make sure that the feeding bag or container is clearly labeled with a statement such as "WARNING! For Enteral Use Only—Not for IV Use" *to prevent administration errors.*[1]

To avoid contamination, hang only a 4-hour supply of reconstituted formula at a time. Sterile, decanted formula can hang for 8 hours. Closed-system formulas can hang for 24 to 48 hours according to the manufacturer's guidelines.[1]

For intermittent feedings
Prepare the gavage set and administration equipment. Make sure the formula is room temperature. *Cold formula may cause cramping.*

Implementation
■ Verify the doctor's order for continuous or intermittent transabdominal tube feeding.
■ Review the patient's medical record to make sure that catheter placement was confirmed before beginning the feeding.
■ Perform hand hygiene and put on gloves.[2,3,4,5]
■ Confirm the patient's identity using at least two patient identifiers according to your facility's policy.[6]
■ Provide privacy.
■ Explain the procedure to the patient. Tell him that feedings usually start at a slow rate (for continuous feeding) or slow

volume (for intermittent feedings) and increase, as tolerated. If the patient is receiving continuous feedings, explain that after he tolerates this type of feeding, he may progress to intermittent feedings as ordered.

■ Assess the patient to determine his risk for aspiration.[1]

■ Assess for bowel sounds before feeding, *which indicate adequate GI motility,* and monitor for abdominal distention

■ Check the external length of the catheter *to determine whether the catheter has migrated.*[1] If you suspect catheter migration, don't administer the feeding, and notify the doctor.

■ Have the patient sit, or elevate the head of the bed at least 30 degrees (45 degrees is preferred) unless contraindicated by the patient's condition. If the patient can't tolerate an elevation of this type, use reverse Trendelenburg's position unless contraindicated.[1]

For continuous feeding

■ Trace the administration tubing from the patient to its point of origin and then connect it to the feeding tube *to make sure that you're connecting it to the proper port.*[1,7]

■ Route the tubing in a unique direction; for example, route the tube feeding administration set toward the patient's feet and the IV tubing toward the patient's head *to prevent misconnections.*[1,7]

■ If your tube-feeding equipment isn't color-coded, label the tubing and connectors so staff members can easily identify that they are for enteral use only, not for IV use.[1,7]

■ Set the drip rate on the pump and push "start."

■ Monitor the gravity drip rate or pump infusion rate frequently *to ensure accurate delivery of formula.*

■ Monitor the patient's fluid and electrolyte status *to anticipate and detect fluid and electrolyte imbalances.*

For intermittent feeding

■ Begin intermittent feeding with a low volume (200 mL) daily. According to the patient's tolerance, increase the volume each feeding as needed to reach the desired calorie intake.

■ Before starting the feeding, trace the feeding tubing from the patient to its point of origin and then attach the syringe to the feeding tube. Aspirate gastric contents to measure gastric residual volume. If the contents measure more than half of the previous feeding volume, hold the tube feeding.[1]

■ Flush the tube with 30 mL of water *to establish patency.*[1]

■ Trace the administration tubing from its point of origin and connect it to the transabdominal tube *to make sure you're connecting the tubing to the proper port.* Allow gravity to help the formula flow over 30 to 45 minutes. *Faster infusions may cause bloating, cramps, or diarrhea.*

■ When the feeding is complete, flush the feeding tube with 30 mL of water *to maintain patency and provide hydration.*[1]

■ Cap the tube *to prevent leakage.*

■ Rinse the feeding administration set thoroughly with hot water *to avoid contaminating subsequent feedings.* Allow it to dry between feedings.

For site care

■ Gently remove the dressing by hand. Never cut away the dressing over the catheter *because you might cut the tube or the sutures holding the tube in place.*

■ Remove and discard your gloves, perform hand hygiene, and put on a new pair of gloves.[2,3,4,5]

■ Until healing occurs, clean the skin immediately around the tube's exit site daily (and as needed) using a cotton-tipped applicator moistened with normal saline solution. Next, using a 4″ × 4″ gauze pad soaked in normal saline solution, clean the adjacent skin and pat it dry using another gauze pad. When healed, wash the skin around the exit site daily with soap and water. Rinse the area with water and pat dry. Apply skin protectant, if necessary, *to prevent skin maceration.*

■ Secure a gastrostomy or jejunostomy tube to the skin with hypoallergenic tape *to prevent peristaltic migration of the tube and tension on the suture anchoring the tube in place.*

■ Coil the tube, if necessary, and tape it to the abdomen *to prevent pulling and contamination of the tube.* (See *Caring for a PEG or PEJ site.*)

Completing the procedure

■ Remove and discard your gloves and perform hand hygiene.[2,3,4,5]

■ Document the procedure.[8,9]

Special considerations

■ If the patient vomits or complains of nausea, feels too full, or regurgitates, stop the feeding immediately and assess his condition.[1] Flush the feeding tube and attempt to restart the feeding in 1 hour (measure residual gastric contents first). You may have to decrease the volume or rate of feedings. If the patient develops dumping syndrome, which includes nausea, vomiting, cramps, pallor, and diarrhea, the feedings may have been given too quickly.

■ Provide oral hygiene frequently. Brush all surfaces of the teeth, gums, and tongue at least twice daily using mouthwash, toothpaste, or a mild salt solution.

■ Control diarrhea resulting from dumping syndrome by diluting the feeding formula, decreasing the infusion rate, or adding antidiarrheals to the formula. Assess whether diarrhea may result from milk intolerance.

■ Don't mix medications together when administering them through the enteral feeding tube *because of the risk for physical and chemical incompatibilities.*[1]

■ Liquid dosage forms of medication should be administered when available; only immediate-release solid dosage forms may be substituted. Grind tablets to a fine powder and mix them with sterile water; open hard gelatin capsules and mix the powder with sterile water before administration.[1]

For continuous feeding

■ Replace administration sets for open-system enteral feedings at least every 24 hours; for closed-systems, follow the manufacturer's instructions.[1]

■ Flush the feeding tube with 30 mL of water every 4 hours during continuous feedings and after residual volume measurements *to maintain tube patency and to provide hydration.* Use sterile or

Caring for a PEG or PEJ site

The exit site of a percutaneous endoscopic gastrostomy (PEG) or percutaneous endoscopic jejunostomy (PEJ) tube requires routine observation and care. Follow these care guidelines:

■ Change the dressing daily while the tube is in place. After removing the dressing, carefully slide the tube's outer bumper away from the skin (as shown below) about ½″ (1 cm).

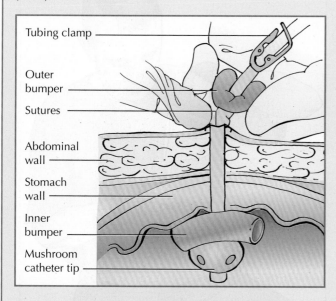

■ Examine the skin around the tube. Look for redness and other signs of infection or erosion.
■ Gently depress the skin surrounding the tube and inspect for drainage (as shown in next column). Expect minimal wound drainage initially after implantation, which should subside in about 1 week.

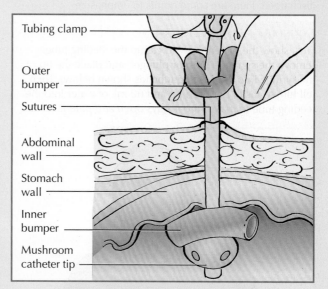

■ Inspect the tube for wear and tear. (A tube that wears out will need replacement.)
■ Clean the site with the prescribed cleaning solution.
■ Apply antibacterial ointment over the exit site according to your facility's guidelines.
■ Rotate the outer bumper 90 degrees (*to avoid repeating the same tension on the same skin area*), and slide the outer bumper back over the exit site.
■ If leakage appears at the PEG site, or if the patient risks dislodging the tube, apply a sterile gauze dressing over the site. Don't put sterile gauze underneath the outer bumper. *Loosening the anchor this way allows the feeding tube free play, which could lead to wound abscess.*
■ Write the date and time of the dressing change on the tape.

---

purified water for patients who have a compromised immune system.[1]
■ Check gastric residual volume every 4 hours during the first 48 hours for gastrically fed patients; after the enteral feeding goal rate is achieved, check gastric residual volume every 6 to 8 hours unless the patient is critically ill; then continue to monitor every 4 hours or according to facility policy.[1]
■ If gastric residual volume is 250 mL or greater after a second residual check, notify the doctor; a promotility agent may be needed. Hold the feeding if gastric residual volume is greater than 500 mL; reassess the patient's tolerance by assessing his GI status and glycemic control. Minimize the use of sedation, if possible, and administer a promotility agent as prescribed.[1]
■ Before administering medication, stop the feeding and flush the tube with at least 15 mL of water. Administer the medica-

tion and then flush the tube again with at least 15 mL of water, taking into consideration the patient's fluid status. Repeat with each subsequent medication. Restart the feeding within 30 minutes when withholding the feeding is necessary to prevent interference with drug bioavailability *to prevent compromising the patient's nutritional status.*[1]

Patient teaching

Teach the patient and his family members or other caregivers all aspects of transabdominal tube feedings, including tube maintenance and site care. Specify signs and symptoms to report to the doctor, define emergency situations, and review actions to take.

When the tube needs replacement, advise the patient that the doctor may insert a replacement gastrostomy button after

Teaching the patient about syringe feeding

If the patient plans to feed himself by syringe when he returns home, you'll need to teach him how to do this before he's discharged. Here are some points to emphasize.

Initial instructions

First, show the patient how to clamp the feeding tube, remove the syringe's bulb or plunger, and place the tip of the syringe into the feeding tube (as shown below). Then tell him to instill between 30 and 60 mL of water into the feeding tube *to make sure it stays open and patent.*

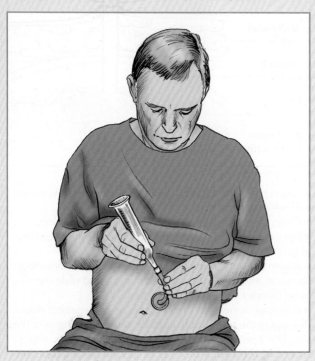

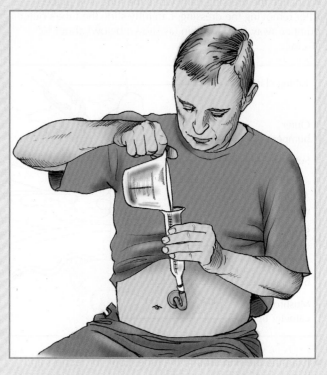

Next, tell him to pour the feeding solution into the syringe and begin the feeding (as shown at top of next column). As the solution flows into the stomach, show him how to tilt the syringe *to allow air bubbles to escape.* Describe the discomfort that air bubbles may cause.

Tips for free flow

When about one-fourth of the feeding solution remains, direct the patient to refill the syringe. Caution him to avoid letting the syringe empty completely. *Doing so may result in abdominal cramping and gas.*

Show the patient how to increase and decrease the solution's flow rate by raising or lowering the syringe. Explain that he may need to dilute a thick solution *to promote free flow.*

Finishing up

Inform the patient that the feeding infusion process should take at least 15 minutes. If the process takes less than 15 minutes, dumping syndrome may result.

Show the patient the steps needed to finish the feeding, including how to flush the tube with water, clamp the tube, and clean the equipment for later use. If he's using disposable gear, urge him to discard it properly. Review instructions for storing unused feeding solution as appropriate.

removing the initial feeding tube. The procedure may be done in the doctor's office or your facility's endoscopy suite.

As the patient's tolerance of intermittent tube feeding improves, he may wish to try syringe feedings rather than intermittent feedings. If appropriate, teach him how to feed himself by the syringe method. (See *Teaching the patient about syringe feeding.*)

Complications

Common complications related to transabdominal tubes include GI or other systemic problems, mechanical malfunction, and metabolic disturbances. Cramping, nausea, vomiting, bloating, and diarrhea may be related to medication; rapid infusion rate; formula contamination, osmolarity, or temperature (too cold or too warm); fat malabsorption; or intestinal atrophy from malnutrition. Constipation may result from inadequate hydration or insufficient exercise.

Systemic problems may be caused by pulmonary aspiration, infection at the tube exit site, or contaminated formula.

Typical mechanical problems include tube dislodgment, obstruction, or impairment. For example, a PEG or PEJ tube may migrate if the external bumper loosens. Occlusion may result from incompletely crushed and liquefied medication particles or inadequate tube flushing. The tube may also rupture or crack from age, drying, or frequent manipulation.

Other complications include vitamin and mineral deficiencies, impaired glucose tolerance, and fluid and electrolyte imbalances, which may follow bouts of diarrhea or constipation.

Documentation

On the intake and output record, note the date, time, and amount of each feeding and the water volume instilled. Maintain total volumes for nutrients and water separately to allow calculation of nutrient intake. In your notes, document the type of formula, the infusion method and rate, the patient's tolerance of the procedure and formula, and the amount of residual gastric contents. Also record complications and abdominal assessment findings. Note patient-teaching topics covered and the patient's progress in self-care. Note the date and time site care was performed. Record the appearance of the site, including any signs of infection, such as redness, swelling, and drainage.

REFERENCES

1 Bankhead, R. et al. (2009). Enteral nutrition practice recommendations. *The American Society for Parenteral and Enteral Nutrition, 2*(33), 122–167. (Level I)

2 Siegel, J.D., et al. "2007 Guideline for Isolation Precautions: Preventing Transmission of Infectious Agents in Healthcare Settings" [Online]. Accessed December 2011 via the Web at http://www.cdc.gov/hicpac/2007ip/2007isolationprecautions.html

3 Centers for Disease Control and Prevention. (October 2002). Guideline for hand hygiene in health-care settings. *Morbidity and Mortality Weekly Report, 51*(RR-16), 1–45. (Level I)

4 World Health Organization. (2009). *WHO guidelines on hand hygiene in health care: First global patient safety challenge. Clean care is safer care.* Geneva, Switzerland: World Health Organization. (Level I)

5 The Joint Commission. (2012). Standard NPSG.07.01.01. *Comprehensive accreditation manual for hospitals: The official handbook.* Oakbrook Terrace, IL: The Joint Commission. (Level I)

6 The Joint Commission. (2012). Standard NPSG.01.01.01. *Comprehensive accreditation manual for hospitals: The official handbook.* Oakbrook Terrace, IL: The Joint Commission. (Level I)

7 U.S. Food and Drug Administration. (2009). "Look. Check. Connect.: Safe Medical Device Connections Save Lives" [Online]. Accessed December 2011 via the Web at http://www.fda.gov/downloads/MedicalDevices/Safety/AlertsandNotices/UCM134873.pdf

8 The Joint Commission. (2012). Standard RC.01.03.01. *Comprehensive accreditation manual for hospitals: The official handbook.* Oakbrook Terrace, IL: The Joint Commission. (Level I)

9 The Joint Commission. (2012). Standard RC.02.01.01. *Comprehensive accreditation manual for hospitals: The official handbook.* Oakbrook Terrace, IL: The Joint Commission. (Level I)

ADDITIONAL REFERENCES

Baskin, W.N. (2006). Acute complications associated with bedside placement of feeding tubes. *Nutrition in Clinical Practice, 21*(1), 40–55.

Lynn-McHale Wiegand, D. (Ed.). (2011). *AACN procedure manual for critical care* (6th ed.). Philadelphia, PA: Saunders.

Nettina, S.M. (2010). *Lippincott manual of nursing practice* (9th ed.). Philadelphia, PA: Lippincott Williams & Wilkins.

Taylor, C., et al. (2011). *Fundamentals of nursing: The art and science of nursing care* (7th ed.). Philadelphia, PA: Lippincott Williams & Wilkins.

TRANSCRANIAL DOPPLER MONITORING

Transcranial Doppler ultrasonography is a noninvasive method of monitoring blood flow in the intracranial vessels, specifically the circle of Willis. This procedure is used on the intensive care unit to monitor patients who have experienced cerebrovascular disorders, such as stroke, head trauma, or subarachnoid hemorrhage. It can help detect intracranial stenosis, vasospasm, and arteriovenous malformations as well as assess collateral pathways. Because it has the advantage of monitoring a continuous waveform, it can be used in intraoperative monitoring of cerebral circulation.

Transcranial Doppler ultrasonography is also used to monitor the effect of intracranial pressure changes on the cerebral circulation, to monitor patient response to various medications, and to evaluate carbon dioxide reactivity, which may be impaired or lost from arterial obstruction or trauma. In addition, it has been used to confirm brain death.

The transcranial Doppler unit transmits pulses of high-frequency ultrasound, which are then reflected back to the transducer by the red blood cells moving in the vessel being monitored. This information is then processed by the instrument into an audible signal and a velocity waveform, which is displayed on the monitor. The displayed waveform is actually a moving graph of blood flow velocities with *time* displayed along the horizontal axis, *velocity* displayed along the vertical axis, and *amplitude* represented by various colors or intensities within the waveform. The heart's contractions speed up the movement of blood cells during systole and slow it down during diastole, resulting in a waveform that varies in velocity over the cardiac cycle.

The major benefits of transcranial Doppler monitoring are that it provides instantaneous, real-time information about cerebral blood flow and that it's noninvasive and painless for the patient. Also, the unit itself is portable and easy to use. The major disadvantage is that it relies on the ability of the ultrasound waves to penetrate thin areas of the cranium; this is difficult if the patient has thickening of the temporal bone, which increases with age.

The transcranial Doppler unit should always be used with its power set at the lowest level needed to provide an adequate waveform. This procedure requires specialized training to ensure accurate vessel identification and correct interpretation of the signals.

Equipment

Transcranial Doppler unit ■ transducer with an attachment system ■ terry cloth headband ■ ultrasonic coupling gel ■ marker.

Implementation

- Verify the doctor's order.
- Perform hand hygiene.[1,2,3]
- Confirm the patient's identity using at least two patient identifiers according to your facility's policy.[4]
- Explain the procedure to the patient, and answer any questions he has about the procedure as thoroughly as possible.
- Place the patient in the proper position, usually the supine position.
- Turn the Doppler unit on and observe as it performs a self-test.
- Enter information as prompted by the Doppler unit. Depending on the unit you're using, you may need to enter the patient's name, identification number, diagnosis, or the doctor's name.
- Indicate the vessel that you wish to monitor, usually the right or left middle cerebral artery. You'll also need to set the approximate depth of the vessel within the skull (50 mm to 56 mm for the middle cerebral artery).
- Increase the power level to 100% to initially locate the signal. You can later decrease the level as needed, depending on the thickness of the patient's skull.
- Examine the temporal region of the patient's head, and mentally identify the three windows of the transtemporal access route: posterior, middle, and anterior (as shown below).

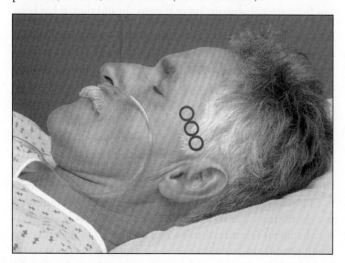

- Apply a generous amount of ultrasonic gel at the level of the temporal bone between the tragus of the ear and the end of the eyebrow, over the area of the three windows.

- Place the transducer on the posterior window. Angle the transducer slightly in an anterior direction, and slowly move it in a narrow circle. This movement is commonly called the *flashlighting* technique. As you hold the transducer at an angle and perform flashlighting, also begin to very slowly move the transducer forward across the temporal area. As you do this, listen for the audible signal with the highest pitch. This sound corresponds to the highest velocity signal, which corresponds to the signal of the vessel you are assessing. You can also use headphones *to let you better evaluate the audible signal and provide patient privacy.*
- After you've located the highest-pitched signal, use a marker to draw a circle around the transducer head on the patient's temple (as shown below). Note the angle of the transducer *so that you can duplicate it after the transducer attachment system is in place.*

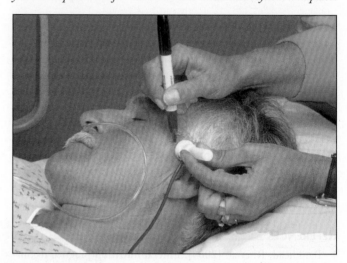

- Next, place the transducer system on the patient. To do this, first place the plate of the transducer attachment system over the patient's temporal area; match the circular opening in the plate exactly with the circle drawn on the patient's head. Then, holding the plate in place, encircle the patient's head with the straps attached to the system. Finally, tighten the straps so that the transducer attachment system will stay in place on the patient's head.
- Fill the circular opening in the plate with the ultrasonic gel.
- Place the transducer in the gel-filled opening in the attachment system plate. Using the plastic screws provided, loosely secure the two plates together *to hold the transducer in place but allow it to rotate for the best angle.*
- Adjust the position and angle of the transducer until you again hear the highest-pitched audible signal. When you hear this signal, look at the waveform on the monitor screen. You should see a clear waveform with a bright white line (called an *envelope*) at the upper edge of the waveform. The envelope exactly follows the contours of the waveform itself.
- If the envelope doesn't follow the waveform's contours, adjust the gain setting. If the signal is wrapping around the screen, increase the scale to drop the baseline.

Comparing velocity waveforms

A normal transcranial Doppler signal is usually characterized by mean velocities that fall within the normal reported values. Additional information can be gathered by evaluating the shape of the velocity waveform.

Effect of significant proximal vessel obstruction

A delayed systolic upstroke can be seen in a waveform when significant proximal vessel obstruction is present.

Normal

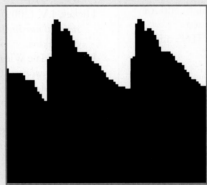

Proximal vessel obstruction

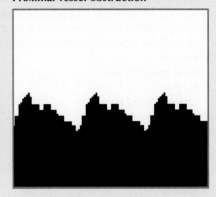

Effect of increased cerebrovascular resistance

Changes in cerebrovascular resistance, such as those that occur with increased intracranial pressure, cause a decrease in diastolic flow.

Normal

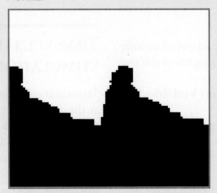

Increased resistance

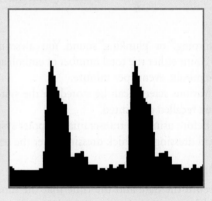

■ When you've determined that you have the strongest, highest-pitched signal and the best waveform, lock the transducer in place by tightening the plastic screws (as shown below). The tightened plates will hold the transducer at the angle you've chosen. Disconnect the transducer handle.

■ Place a wide terry cloth headband over the transducer attachment system, and secure it around the patient's head *to provide additional stability for the transducer.*

■ Look at the monitor screen. You should be able to see a waveform and read the numeric values of the peak, mean velocities, and pulsatility index (PI+) above the displayed waveform. The shape of the waveform reveals more information. (See *Comparing velocity waveforms.*)

■ Perform hand hygiene.[1,2,3]

■ Document the procedure.[5,6]

Special considerations

■ Velocity changes in the transcranial Doppler signal correlate with changes in cerebral blood flow. The parameter that most clearly reflects this change is the mean velocity. To determine this, first establish a baseline for the mean velocity. Then, as the patient's velocity increases or decreases, the value (%) will change negatively or positively from the baseline.

■ Emboli appear as high-intensity transients occurring randomly during the cardiac cycle. Emboli make a distinctive "clicking,"

Current uses of TENS

Transcutaneous electrical nerve stimulation (TENS) must be prescribed by a doctor and is most successful if it's administered and taught to the patient by a therapist skilled in its use. TENS has been used for temporary relief of acute pain, such as postoperative pain, and for ongoing relief of chronic pain, such as sciatica.

Among the types of pain that respond to TENS are:

- arthritis
- bone fracture pain
- bursitis
- cancer-related pain
- musculoskeletal pain
- myofascial pain
- neuralgias and neuropathies
- phantom limb pain
- postoperative incision pain
- sciatica
- whiplash.

"chirping," or "plunking" sound. You can set up an emboli counter to count either the total number of emboli aggregates or the rate of embolic events per minute.

- Various screens can be stored on the system's hard drive and then recalled or printed.
- Before using the transcranial Doppler system, remove turban head dressings or thick dressings over the test site.

Documentation

Record the date and the time that the monitoring began and which artery is being monitored. Document any patient teaching as well as the patient's tolerance of the procedure.

REFERENCES

1 World Health Organization. (2009). *WHO guidelines on hand hygiene in health care: First global patient safety challenge. Clean care is safer care.* Geneva, Switzerland: World Health Organization. (Level I)
2 Centers for Disease Control and Prevention. (October 2002). Guideline for hand hygiene in health-care settings. *Morbidity and Mortality Weekly Report, 51*(RR-16), 1–45. (Level I)
3 The Joint Commission. (2012). Standard NPSG.07.01.01. *Comprehensive accreditation manual for hospitals: The official handbook.* Oakbrook Terrace, IL: The Joint Commission. (Level I)
4 The Joint Commission. (2012). Standard NPSG.01.01.01. *Comprehensive accreditation manual for hospitals: The official handbook.* Oakbrook Terrace, IL: The Joint Commission. (Level I)
5 The Joint Commission. (2012). Standard RC.01.03.01. *Comprehensive accreditation manual for hospitals: The official handbook.* Oakbrook Terrace, IL: The Joint Commission. (Level I)
6 The Joint Commission. (2012). Standard RC.02.01.01. *Comprehensive accreditation manual for hospitals: The official handbook.* Oakbrook Terrace, IL: The Joint Commission. (Level I)

ADDITIONAL REFERENCES

Carrera, E., et al. (2009). Transcranial Doppler for predicting delayed cerebral ischemia after subarachnoid hemorrhage. *Neurosurgery, 65*(2), 316–323; discussion 323–324.
Hickey, J.V. (2009). *The clinical practice of neurological and neurosurgical nursing* (6th ed.). Philadelphia, PA: Lippincott Williams & Wilkins.
Lynn-McHale Wiegand, D. (Ed.). (2011). *AACN procedure manual for critical care* (6th ed.). Philadelphia, PA: Saunders.
Rubiera, M., et al. (2010). Diagnostic criteria and yield of real-time transcranial Doppler monitoring of intra-arterial reperfusion procedures. *Stroke, 41*(4), 695–699.
Saqqur, M., et al. (2007). Role of transcranial Doppler in neurocritical care. *Critical Care Medicine* 35(5 Suppl):S216–S223.
Tsivgoulis, G., et al. (2009). Advances in transcranial Doppler ultrasonography. *Current Neurology and Neuroscience Reports, 9*(1), 46–54.

TRANSCUTANEOUS ELECTRICAL NERVE STIMULATION

Transcutaneous electrical nerve stimulation (TENS) is defined as the application of electrical stimulation to the skin for pain relief. It's based on the gate-control theory of pain, which proposes that painful impulses pass through a "gate" in the brain. TENS is performed with a portable, battery-powered device that transmits painless electrical current to peripheral nerves or directly to a painful area over relatively large nerve fibers. This treatment effectively alters the patient's perception of pain by blocking painful stimuli traveling over smaller fibers.

Used for postoperative patients and those with chronic pain, TENS reduces the need for analgesic drugs and may allow the patient to resume normal activities. Typically, a course of TENS treatments lasts 3 to 5 days. Some conditions, such as phantom limb pain, may require continuous stimulation; other conditions, such as a painful arthritic joint, require shorter periods (3 to 4 hours). TENS has also been found to decrease knee pain associated with osteoarthritis. However, recent studies have shown TENS isn't helpful in patients with chronic lower back pain.[1] (See *Current uses of TENS.*)

TENS is contraindicated for patients with cardiac pacemakers because it can interfere with pacemaker function. The procedure is also contraindicated for pregnant patients because its effect on the fetus is unknown. It's also contraindicated in patients with dementia. TENS should be used cautiously in all patients with cardiac disorders. TENS electrodes shouldn't be placed on the head or neck of patients with vascular or seizure disorders.

EQUIPMENT

Positioning TENS electrodes

With transcutaneous electrical nerve stimulation (TENS), electrodes placed around peripheral nerves (or an incisional site) transmit mild electrical pulses to the brain. The current is thought to block pain impulses. The patient can influence the level and frequency of his pain relief by adjusting the controls on the device.

Typically, electrode placement varies even though patients may have similar complaints. Electrodes can be placed in several ways:

■ to cover the painful area or surround it, as with muscle tenderness or spasm or painful joints

■ to "capture" the painful area between electrodes, as with incisional pain.

With peripheral nerve injury, electrodes should be placed proximal to the injury (between the brain and the injury site) to avoid increasing pain. Placing electrodes in a hypersensitive area also increases pain. In an area lacking sensation, electrodes should be placed on adjacent dermatomes.

The illustrations show combinations of electrode placement (red squares) and areas of nerve stimulation (shaded pink) for lower back and leg pain.

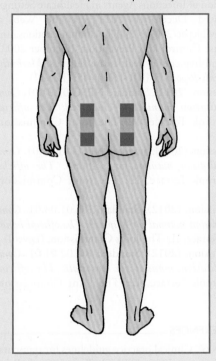
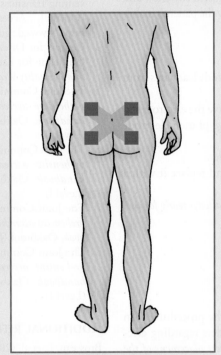
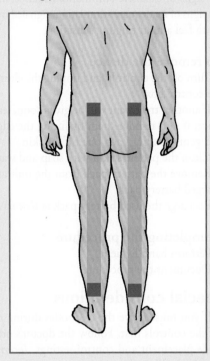

Equipment

TENS device ■ pregelled, self-stick electrodes ■ warm water and soap ■ leadwires ■ charged battery pack ■ battery recharger ■ Optional: alcohol pads, hypoallergenic tape.

Commercial TENS kits are available. They include the stimulator, leadwires, electrodes, spare battery pack, battery recharger, and sometimes the adhesive patch.

Preparation of equipment

Before beginning the procedure, always test the battery pack *to make sure it's fully charged.*

Implementation

■ Verify the doctor's order.
■ Perform hand hygiene and follow standard precautions, as appropriate.[2,3,4,5]

■ Confirm the patient's identity using at least two patient identifiers according to your facility's policy.[6]
■ Provide privacy.
■ If the patient has never seen a TENS unit, show him the device and explain the procedure.

Before TENS treatment

■ Using soap and water, thoroughly clean the skin where the electrode will be applied. Dry the skin before application. Use an alcohol pad, if necessary, to remove excess oil or lotion.
■ Apply the ordered number of electrodes on the proper skin area, leaving at least 2″ (5 cm) between them. (See *Positioning TENS electrodes.*) If necessary, secure them with the hypoallergenic tape. Tape all sides evenly *so that the electrodes are firmly attached to the skin.*

- Plug the pin connectors into the electrode sockets. *To protect the cords,* hold the connectors—not the cords themselves—during insertion.
- Turn the channel controls to the off position or as recommended in the operator's manual.
- Plug the leadwires into the jacks in the control box.
- Turn the amplitude and rate dials slowly as the manual directs. (The patient should feel a tingling sensation.) Then adjust the controls on this device to the prescribed settings or to settings that are most comfortable for the patient. Most patients select stimulation frequencies of 60 to 100 Hz.
- Attach the TENS control box to part of the patient's clothing, such as a belt, pocket, or bra.
- *To make sure the device is working effectively,* monitor the patient for signs of excessive stimulation, such as muscle twitches, and for signs of inadequate stimulation, signaled by the patient's inability to feel a mild tingling sensation.

To remove the device
- Turn off the controls, and unplug the electrode leadwires from the control box.
- If another treatment will be given soon, leave the electrodes in place; if not, remove them by lifting the edge of each electrode and gently pulling each one off the skin.
- Clean the patient's skin with soap and water.
- Remove the battery pack from the unit and replace it with a charged battery pack.
- Recharge the used battery pack *so that it's always ready for use.*

Completing the procedure
- Perform hand hygiene.[2,3,4,5]
- Document the procedure.[7,8]

Special considerations
- If you must move the electrodes during the procedure, turn off the controls first. Follow the doctor's orders regarding electrode placement and control settings. *Incorrect placement of the electrodes will result in inappropriate pain control.*
- Setting the controls too high can cause pain; setting them too low will fail to relieve pain.

NURSING ALERT *Never place the electrodes near the patient's eyes or over the nerves that innervate the carotid sinus or laryngeal or pharyngeal muscles* to avoid interference with critical nerve function.

- If TENS is used continuously for postoperative pain, remove the electrodes at least daily *to check for skin irritation, provide skin care, and rotate sites of electrode placement.*
- If appropriate, let the patient study the operator's manual. Teach him how to place the electrodes properly and how to take care of the TENS unit.

Documentation
On the patient's medical record and the nursing care plan, record the electrode sites and the control settings. Document the patient's tolerance for treatment. Also evaluate pain control, and record the location of pain and how the patient rates his pain using a pain scale. Document patient teaching and the patient's understanding of your teaching.

REFERENCES

1 Dubinsky, R.M., & Miyasaki, J. (2010). Assessment: Efficacy of transcutaneous electric nerve stimulation in the treatment of pain in neurologic disorders (An evidence-based review): Report of the Therapeutics and Technology Assessment Subcommittee of the American Academy of Neurology. *Neurology, 74*(2), 173–176. (Level I)
2 World Health Organization. (2009). *WHO guidelines on hand hygiene in health care: First global patient safety challenge. Clean care is safer care.* Geneva, Switzerland: World Health Organization. (Level I)
3 Siegel, J.D., et al. "2007 Guideline for Isolation Precautions: Preventing Transmission of Infectious Agents in Healthcare Settings" [Online]. Accessed December 2011 via the Web at http://www.cdc.gov/hicpac/2007ip/2007isolationprecautions.html
4 Centers for Disease Control and Prevention. (October 2002). Guideline for hand hygiene in health-care settings. *Morbidity and Mortality Weekly Report, 51*(RR-16), 1–45. (Level I)
5 The Joint Commission. (2012). Standard NPSG.07.01.01. *Comprehensive accreditation manual for hospitals: The official handbook.* Oakbrook Terrace, IL: The Joint Commission. (Level I)
6 The Joint Commission. (2012). Standard NPSG.01.01.01. *Comprehensive accreditation manual for hospitals: The official handbook.* Oakbrook Terrace, IL: The Joint Commission. (Level I)
7 The Joint Commission. (2012). Standard RC.01.03.01. *Comprehensive accreditation manual for hospitals: The official handbook.* Oakbrook Terrace, IL: The Joint Commission. (Level I)
8 The Joint Commission. (2012). Standard RC.02.01.01. *Comprehensive accreditation manual for hospitals: The official handbook.* Oakbrook Terrace, IL: The Joint Commission. (Level I)

ADDITIONAL REFERENCES

Brosseau, L. et al. (2006). Clinical practice guidelines for transcutaneous electrical nerve stimulation (TENS). *Topics in Stroke Rehabilitation, 13*(2), 61–63.
Desantana, J.M., et al. (2008). Effectiveness of transcutaneous electrical nerve stimulation for treatment of hyperalgesia and pain. *Current Rheumatology Reports, 10*(6), 492–499.
Hickey, J.V. (2009). *The clinical practice of neurological and neurosurgical nursing* (6th ed.). Philadelphia, PA: Lippincott Williams & Wilkins.

TRANSCUTANEOUS PACING

Transcutaneous pacing is a method of external electrical stimulation of the heart through a set of electrode pads. It isn't as efficient as transvenous pacing because the electrical stimulus (the pad) isn't in direct contact with the heart muscle.

In a life-threatening situation, when time is critical, a transcutaneous pacemaker is the best choice. (See *Indications for transcutaneous pacing.*)

The device works by sending an electrical impulse from the pulse generator to the patient's heart by way of two electrodes, which are placed on the front and back of the patient's chest. Transcutaneous pacing is quick and effective, but it's used only until the doctor can institute transvenous pacing.

Transcutaneous pacing is recommended by the 2010 American Heart Association guidelines for cardiopulmonary resuscitation and emergency cardiovascular care for symptomatic bradycardia when a pulse is present. It isn't recommended for cardiac arrest because research shows that it's ineffective in cardiac arrest.[1]

Equipment

Transcutaneous pacing generator ■ transcutaneous pacing electrodes ■ cardiac monitor ■ electrocardiogram (ECG) electrodes ■ ECG cables and monitor ■ washcloth ■ towel ■ nonemollient soap ■ Optional: clippers.

Implementation

■ Perform hand hygiene[2,3,4]
■ Confirm the patient's identity using at least two patient identifiers according to your facility's policy.[5]
■ If applicable, explain the procedure to the patient.
■ Assist the patient to a supine position and expose his torso.[6]
■ If necessary, clip the hair over the areas of electrode placement.[6] However, don't shave the area. *If you nick the skin, the current from the pulse generator could cause discomfort and the nicks could become irritated or infected after the electrodes are applied.*
■ Prepare the skin on the patient's chest and back by washing it with nonemollient soap and water; dry the skin thoroughly *to improve electrode adherence.*[6]
■ Attach monitoring electrodes to the patient in lead I, II, or III position. Do this even if the patient is already on telemetry monitoring *because you'll need to connect the electrodes to the pacemaker.* If you select the lead II position, adjust the LL (left leg) electrode placement to accommodate the anterior pacing electrode and the patient's anatomy.
■ Plug the patient cable into the ECG input connection on the front of the pacing generator. Set the selector switch to the "monitor on" position.
■ You should see the ECG waveform on the monitor. Adjust the R-wave beeper volume to a suitable level and activate the alarm by pressing the "alarm on" button. Set the alarm for 10 to 20 beats lower and 20 to 30 beats higher than the intrinsic rate.
■ Press the appropriate button for a printout of the waveform.
■ To apply the two pacing electrodes, pull off the protective strip from the posterior electrode (marked "back") and apply the electrode on the left side of the back, just below the scapula and to the left of the spine.[6]
■ The anterior pacing electrode (marked "front") has two protective strips—one covering the jellied area and one covering the outer rim. Expose the jellied area and apply it to the skin in the anterior position—to the left side of the precordium in the usual V_2 to V_5 position. Move this electrode around to get the best waveform. Then expose the electrode's outer rim and firmly press it to the skin. (See *Transcutaneous electrode placement,* page 736.)

Indications for transcutaneous pacing[1]

The American Heart Association recommends transcutaneous pacing for these class IIa indications:
■ Bradycardia with hemodynamic instability unresponsive to atropine while preparing for emergent transvenous pacing
■ High-degree block (Mobitz type II second-degree block or third-degree atrioventricular block)
■ Symptomatic bradycardia
■ Sinus arrest

■ Now you're ready to pace the heart. After making sure the energy output in milliamperes (mA) is on 0, connect the electrode cable to the monitor output cable.
■ Check the waveform, looking for a tall QRS complex in lead II.
■ Next, turn the selector switch to "pacer on." Tell the patient that he may feel a thumping or twitching sensation. Reassure him that you'll give him medication if he can't tolerate the discomfort.
■ Now set the rate dial to a rate that adequately maintains cardiac output. Look for pacer artifact or spikes, which will appear as you increase the rate. Some pacemakers have a default setting, such as 80 beats/minute, that can be adjusted as needed.[6]
■ Slowly increase the amount of energy delivered to the heart by adjusting the output mA dial. Do this until capture is achieved—you'll see a pacer spike followed by a widened QRS complex that resembles a premature ventricular contraction. This is the pacing threshold. *To ensure consistent capture,* increase output by 10%. Don't go any higher *because you could cause the patient needless discomfort.*
■ With full capture, the patient's heart rate should be approximately the same as the pacemaker rate set on the machine. The usual pacing threshold is between 40 and 80 mA. Be sure to check the patient's pulse; don't just rely on the monitor to determine heart rate.
■ Perform hand hygiene.[2,3,4]
■ Document the procedure.[7,8]

Special considerations

■ Take care to prevent microshock. This includes warning the patient not to use any electrical equipment that isn't grounded, such as telephones, electric shavers, televisions, or lamps.
■ Don't place the electrodes over a bony area *because bone conducts current poorly.* With female patients, place the anterior electrode under the patient's breast but not over her diaphragm.
■ After application of a transcutaneous pacemaker, assess the patient's vital signs, skin color, level of consciousness, and peripheral pulses *to determine the effectiveness of the paced rhythm.* Perform a 12-lead ECG *to serve as a baseline,* and then perform

Transcutaneous electrode placement

For a noninvasive temporary pacemaker, the two pacing electrodes are placed at heart level on the patient's chest and back (as shown). This type of pacemaker can be quickly applied in an emergency but is uncomfortable for the patient.

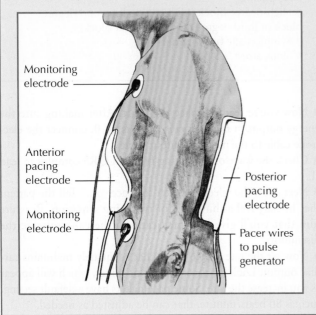

Monitoring electrode

Anterior pacing electrode

Monitoring electrode

Posterior pacing electrode

Pacer wires to pulse generator

REFERENCES

1 American Heart Association. (2010). 2010 American Heart Association guidelines for cardiopulmonary resuscitation and emergency cardiovascular care. *Circulation, 122*(Suppl. 3), S706–S767. (Level I)

2 Centers for Disease Control and Prevention. (October 2002). Guideline for hand hygiene in health-care settings. *Morbidity and Mortality Weekly Report, 51*(RR-16), 1–45. (Level I)

3 World Health Organization. (2009). *WHO guidelines on hand hygiene in health care: First global patient safety challenge. Clean care is safer care.* Geneva, Switzerland: World Health Organization. (Level I)

4 The Joint Commission. (2012). Standard NPSG.07.01.01. *Comprehensive accreditation manual for hospitals: The official handbook.* Oakbrook Terrace, IL: The Joint Commission. (Level I)

5 The Joint Commission. (2012). Standard NPSG.01.01.01. *Comprehensive accreditation manual for hospitals: The official handbook.* Oakbrook Terrace, IL: The Joint Commission. (Level I)

6 Lynn-McHale Wiegand, D. (Ed.). (2011). *AACN procedure manual for critical care* (6th ed.). Philadelphia, PA: Saunders.

7 The Joint Commission. (2012). Standard RC.01.03.01. *Comprehensive accreditation manual for hospitals: The official handbook.* Oakbrook Terrace, IL: The Joint Commission. (Level I)

8 The Joint Commission. (2012). Standard RC.02.01.01. *Comprehensive accreditation manual for hospitals: The official handbook.* Oakbrook Terrace, IL: The Joint Commission. (Level I)

ADDITIONAL REFERENCES

American Association for Respiratory Care. (2004). AARC clinical practice guideline: Resuscitation and defibrillation in the health care setting—2004 revision & update. *Respiratory Care, 89*(9), 1085–1099.

Gibson T. (2008). A practical guide to external cardiac pacing. *Nursing Standard, 22*(20), 45–48.

Woods, S., et al. (2010). *Cardiac nursing* (6th ed.). Philadelphia, PA: Lippincott Williams & Wilkins.

additional ECGs according to your facility's policy or with clinical changes. Also, if possible, obtain a rhythm strip before, during, and after pacemaker placement; any time that pacemaker settings are changed; and whenever the patient receives treatment because of a complication resulting from the pacemaker.

■ Continuously monitor the ECG reading, noting capture, sensing, rate, intrinsic beats, and competition of paced and intrinsic rhythms. If the pacemaker is sensing correctly, the sense indicator on the pulse generator should flash with each beat.

Complications

Complications associated with pacemaker therapy include microshock, equipment failure, and competitive or fatal arrhythmias. Transcutaneous pacemakers may also cause skin breakdown as well as muscle pain and twitching when the pacemaker fires.

Documentation

Record the reason for pacing, the date and time it started, the type of pacemaker, and the locations of the electrodes. Also record the pacemaker settings. Note the patient's response to the procedure, along with any complications and interventions taken. If possible, obtain rhythm strips before, during, and after pacemaker placement and whenever pacemaker settings are changed or when the patient receives treatment for a complication caused by the pacemaker.

TRANSDERMAL DRUG APPLICATION

Through a measured dose of ointment or an adhesive patch applied to the skin, transdermal drugs deliver constant, controlled medication directly into the bloodstream for a prolonged systemic effect.

Nitroglycerin, one of the more common transdermal ointments, dilates coronary vessels for up to 4 hours.

Medications available as transdermal patches include scopolamine, used to treat motion sickness; estradiol, used for postmenopausal hormone replacement; clonidine, used to treat hypertension; nicotine, used for smoking cessation; and fentanyl, an opioid analgesic used to control chronic pain. Transdermal scopolamine can relieve motion sickness for as long as 72 hours, transdermal estradiol lasts for up to 1 week, transdermal clonidine and nicotine last for 24 hours, and transdermal fentanyl can last for up to 72 hours.

Contraindications for transdermal drug application include skin allergies or skin reactions to the drug. Transdermal drugs

Applying nitroglycerin ointment

Unlike most topical medications, nitroglycerin ointment is used for its transdermal systemic effect. It's used to dilate the veins and arteries, improving cardiac perfusion in a patient with cardiac ischemia or angina pectoris.

To apply nitroglycerin ointment, start by taking the patient's baseline blood pressure *so that you can compare it with later readings.* Remove any previously applied nitroglycerin ointment. Gather your equipment. Nitroglycerin ointment, which is prescribed by the inch, comes with a rectangular piece of ruled paper to be used in applying the medication. Squeeze the prescribed amount of ointment onto the ruled paper (as shown below). Put on gloves, if desired, *to avoid contact with the medication.*

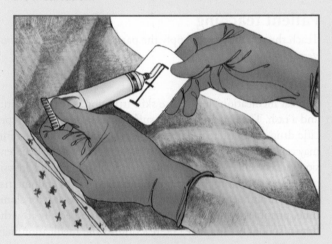

After measuring the correct amount of ointment, tape the paper—drug side down—directly to the skin (as shown below). (Some facilities require you to use the paper to apply the medication to the patient's skin, usually on the chest or arm. Spread a thin layer of the ointment over a 3″ [7.6-cm] area.) For increased absorption, the doctor may request that you cover the site with a transparent semipermeable dressing.

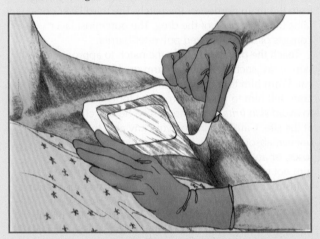

After 5 minutes, record the patient's blood pressure. If it has dropped significantly and he has a headache (from vasodilation of blood vessels in his head), notify the doctor immediately; he may reduce the dose. If the patient's blood pressure has dropped but he has no symptoms, instruct him to lie still until it returns to normal.

shouldn't be applied to broken or irritated skin, which would increase irritation, or to scarred or callused skin, which might impair absorption.

Equipment

Patient's medication administration record and medical record ■ gloves ■ prescribed medication ■ application strip or measuring paper (for nitroglycerin ointment) ■ adhesive tape ■ Optional: semipermeable dressing.

Implementation
■ Verify the doctor's order order.[1]
■ Avoid distractions and interruptions when preparing and administering the medication *to prevent medication errors.*[2]
■ Compare the medication label to the order and verify that the medication is correct.[3]
■ Check the expiration date on the medication; don't give the medication if it has expired.
■ Check the patient's medical record for an allergy to the prescribed medication. If an allergy is present, don't administer the medication; notify the doctor.

■ Perform hand hygiene and put on gloves.[4,5,6]
■ Confirm the patient's identity using at least two patient identifiers according to your facility's policy.[7]
■ If your facility uses a bar code scanning system, be sure to scan your identification badge, the patient's identification bracelet, and the medication's bar code.
■ Explain the procedure to the patient and provide privacy.
■ Remove any previously applied medication.

Applying transdermal ointment
■ Place the prescribed amount of ointment on the application strip or measuring paper, taking care not to get any on your skin. (See *Applying nitroglycerin ointment.*)
■ Apply the strip to any dry, hairless area of the body. Don't rub the ointment into the skin.
■ Tape the strip and ointment to the skin.
■ If desired, cover the application strip with the semipermeable dressing.

Applying a transdermal medication patch

If the patient will be receiving medication by transdermal patch, instruct him in its proper use. Explain to the patient that the patch consists of several layers. The layer closest to his skin contains a small amount of the drug and allows prompt introduction of the drug into the bloodstream. The next layer controls release of the drug from the main portion of the patch. The third layer contains the main dose of the drug. The outermost layer consists of an aluminized polyester barrier.

Teach the patient to apply the patch to appropriate skin areas, such as the upper arm or chest or behind the ear. Warn him to avoid touching the gel or surrounding tape. Tell him to use a different site for each application *to avoid skin irritation.* If necessary, he can clip the hair at the site. Caution him to avoid any area that may cause uneven absorption, such as skin folds, scars, and calluses, or any irritated or damaged skin areas. Also, tell him not to apply the patch below the elbow or knee.

Instruct the patient to wash his hands after application *to remove any medication that may have rubbed off.*

Warn the patient not to get the patch wet. Tell him to discard it if it leaks or falls off and then to clean the site and apply a new patch at a different site.

Instruct the patient to apply the patch at the same time at the prescribed interval *to ensure continuous drug delivery. Bedtime application is ideal because body movement is reduced during the night.* Finally, tell him to apply a new patch about 30 minutes before removing the old one.

Applying a transdermal patch
- Open the package and remove the patch.
- Without touching the adhesive surface, remove the clear plastic backing.
- Apply the patch to a dry, hairless area—behind the ear, for example, as with scopolamine.
- Write the date, the time, and your initials on the dressing

Completing the procedure
- Store the medication, as ordered.
- Instruct the patient to keep the area around the ointment as dry as possible.
- Remove and discard your gloves and perform hand hygiene immediately after applying the ointment or patch *to avoid absorbing the drug yourself.*[4,5,6]
- Document the procedure.[8,9]

Special considerations
- Reapply transdermal medications at the same time every day *to ensure a continuous effect,* but alternate the application sites *to avoid skin irritation.*
- Before reapplying nitroglycerin ointment, remove the plastic wrap, application strip, and any remaining ointment from the patient's skin at the previous site.
- Avoid shaving an area to apply the ointment. *Shaving removes the top layer of skin, which may cause the medication to absorb faster than with unshaved skin.* If necessary, use clippers to remove excess hair.
- When applying a scopolamine or fentanyl patch, instruct the patient not to drive or operate machinery until his response to the drug has been determined.
- Warn a patient using a clonidine patch to check with his doctor before taking an over-the-counter cough preparation *because such drugs may counteract clonidine's effects.*

Patient teaching
Teach the patient how to apply the patch. (See *Applying a transdermal medication patch.*)

Complications
Topical medications may cause skin irritation, such as pruritus and a rash. The patient may also suffer adverse effects of the specific drug administered. For example, transdermal nitroglycerin may cause headaches and, in elderly patients, orthostatic hypotension. Adverse effects of scopolamine include dry mouth and drowsiness (most common); for estradiol, increased risk of endometrial cancer, thromboembolic disease, and birth defects; and for clonidine, possible severe rebound hypertension, especially if withdrawn suddenly. Anaphylactic reaction to the medication may occur. Monitor for signs and symptoms of this complication.

Documentation
Document the name of the medication, the dose, and the date and time it was administered in the patient's medication administration record. Include the route and site used. Document the appearance and integrity of the skin before administration. Record the presence or absence of adverse effects and whether the doctor was notified of adverse effects. Document the patient's response to and tolerance of therapy. Include teaching information given to the patient.

REFERENCES

1 The Joint Commission. (2012). Standard MM.04.01.01. *Comprehensive accreditation manual for hospitals: The official handbook.* Oakbrook Terrace, IL: The Joint Commission. (Level I)
2 Westbrook, J. et al. (2010). Association of interruptions with an increased risk and severity of medication administration errors. *Archives of Internal Medicine, 170*(8), 683–690.
3 The Joint Commission. (2012). Standard MM.06.01.01. *Comprehensive accreditation manual for hospitals: The official handbook.* Oakbrook Terrace, IL: The Joint Commission. (Level I)

4 Centers for Disease Control and Prevention. (October 2002). Guideline for hand hygiene in health-care settings. *Morbidity and Mortality Weekly Report, 51*(RR-16), 1–45. (Level I)

5 World Health Organization. (2009). *WHO guidelines on hand hygiene in health care: First global patient safety challenge. Clean care is safer care.* Geneva, Switzerland: World Health Organization. (Level I)

6 The Joint Commission. (2012). Standard NPSG.07.01.01. *Comprehensive accreditation manual for hospitals: The official handbook.* Oakbrook Terrace, IL: The Joint Commission. (Level I)

7 The Joint Commission. (2012). Standard NPSG.01.01.01. *Comprehensive accreditation manual for hospitals: The official handbook.* Oakbrook Terrace, IL: The Joint Commission. (Level I)

8 The Joint Commission. (2012). Standard RC.01.03.01. *Comprehensive accreditation manual for hospitals: The official handbook.* Oakbrook Terrace, IL: The Joint Commission. (Level I)

9 The Joint Commission. (2012). Standard RC.02.01.01. *Comprehensive accreditation manual for hospitals: The official handbook.* Oakbrook Terrace, IL: The Joint Commission. (Level I)

ADDITIONAL REFERENCES

Nettina, S.M. (2010). *Lippincott manual of nursing practice* (9th ed.). Philadelphia, PA: Lippincott Williams & Wilkins.

Taylor, C., et al. (2011). *Fundamentals of nursing: The art and science of nursing care* (7th ed.). Philadelphia, PA: Lippincott Williams & Wilkins.

TRANSDUCER SYSTEM SETUP

The exact type of transducer system used depends on the patient's needs and the doctor's preference. Some systems monitor pressure continuously, whereas others monitor pressure intermittently. Single-pressure transducers monitor only one type of pressure—for example, pulmonary artery pressure (PAP). Multiple-pressure transducers can monitor two or more types of pressure, such as PAP and central venous pressure.

Equipment

Bag of flush solution (usually 500 mL of normal saline solution) ■ pressure infusion bag ■ medication-added label ■ preassembled disposable pressure tubing with flush device and disposable transducer ■ monitor and monitor cable ■ IV pole with transducer mount ■ leveling device ■ sterile, nonvented stopcock caps ■ sterile gauze package ■ Optional: 500 to 1,000 units of heparin to add to flush bag.

Implementation

To set up and zero a single-pressure transducer system, perform the following steps.

Setting up the system

■ Gather the appropriate equipment
■ Perform hand hygiene.[1,2,3]
■ Follow your facility's policy on adding heparin to the flush solution. If your patient has a history of bleeding or clotting problems, use heparin with caution. Add the ordered amount of heparin to the solution—usually 1 to 2 units of heparin per milliliter of solution—and then label the bag.[4]

■ Put the pressure module into the monitor, if necessary, and connect the transducer cable to the monitor.

■ Remove the preassembled pressure tubing from the package. If necessary, connect the pressure tubing to the transducer. Tighten all tubing connections.

■ Position all stopcocks so the flush solution flows through the entire system. Then roll the tubing's flow regulator to the "off" position.

■ Spike the flush solution bag with the tubing, invert the bag, open the roller clamp, and squeeze all the air through the drip chamber. Then compress the tubing's drip chamber, filling it no more than halfway with the flush solution.

■ Place the flush solution bag into the pressure infuser bag. To do this, hang the pressure infuser bag on the IV pole, and then position the flush solution bag inside the pressure infuser bag. Don't inflate the pressure bag *because priming the tubing under pressure can cause air bubbles to enter the system.*

■ Open the tubing's flow regulator, uncoil the tube if you haven't already done so, and remove the protective cap at the end of the pressure tubing. Squeeze the continuous flush device slowly to prime the entire system, including the stopcock ports, with the flush solution.

■ As the solution nears the disposable transducer, hold the transducer at a 45-degree angle (as shown below). *This forces the solution to flow upward to the transducer. In doing so, the solution forces any air out of the system.*

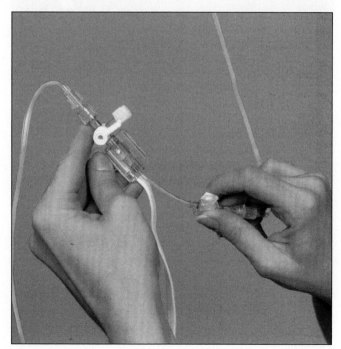

■ When the solution nears a stopcock, open the stopcock to air, allowing the solution to flow into the stopcock (as shown below). When the stopcock fills, close it to air and turn it open to the remainder of the tubing. Do this for each stopcock.

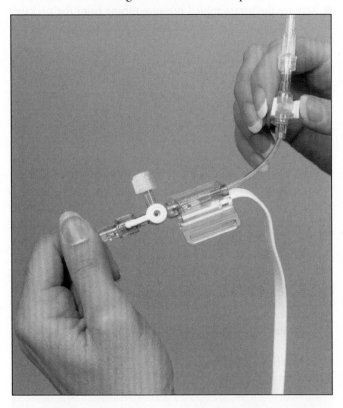

■ After removing the air from the stopcock, replace the vented cap with a sterile nonvented cap *to prevent air from entering the system.*

■ After you've completely primed the system, replace the protective cap at the end of the tubing.

■ Inflate the pressure infuser bag to 300 mm Hg. *This bag keeps the pressure in the arterial line higher than the patient's systolic pressure, preventing blood backflow into the tubing and ensuring a continuous flow rate.* When you inflate the pressure bag, make sure that the drip chamber doesn't completely fill with fluid. Afterward, flush the system again *to remove all air bubbles.*

■ If you're going to mount the transducer on an IV pole, insert the device into its holder.

Zeroing the system

■ Perform hand hygiene.[1,2,3]

■ Position the patient and the transducer on the same level each time you zero the transducer or record a pressure *to ensure accuracy.* Typically, the patient lies flat in bed, if he can tolerate that position.[5]

■ Use the leveling device to position the air-reference stopcock or the air-fluid interface of the transducer level with the phlebostatic axis (midway between the posterior chest and the sternum at the fourth intercostal space, midaxillary line).[6] Alternatively, you may level the air-reference stopcock or the air-fluid interface to the same position as the catheter tip.

■ After leveling the transducer, turn the stopcock next to the transducer off to the patient and open to air. Remove the cap to the stopcock port. Place the cap inside an opened sterile gauze package to prevent contamination.

■ Now zero the transducer. To do so, follow the manufacturer's directions for zeroing.

■ When you've finished zeroing, turn the stopcock on the transducer so that it's closed to air and open to the patient. This is the monitoring position. Replace the cap on the stopcock. You're then ready to attach the single-pressure transducer to the patient's catheter. Now you've assembled a single-pressure transducer system (as shown below).

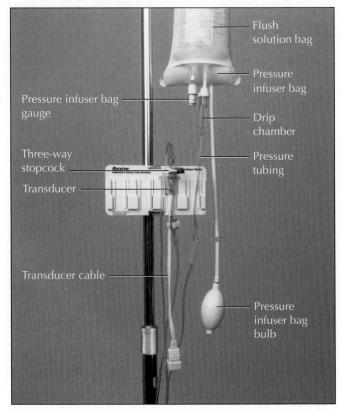

■ Perform hand hygiene.[1,2,3]

■ Document the procedure.[7]

Special considerations

■ You may use any of several methods to set up a multiple-pressure transducer system. But the easiest way is to add to the single-pressure system. You'll also need another bag of heparin flush solution in a second pressure infuser bag. Then you'll prime the tubing, mount the second transducer, and connect an additional cable to the monitor. Finally, you'll zero the second transducer.

■ Alternatively, your facility may use a Y-type tubing setup with two attached pressure transducers. This method requires only one bag of flush solution. To set up the system, proceed as you would for a single transducer, with this exception: First, prime one branch of the Y-type tubing and then the other. Next, attach two cables to the monitor in the modules for each pressure that you'll be measuring. Finally, zero each transducer.

- Minimize the number of manipulations and entries into the pressure monitoring system *to reduce the risk of infection.*[8]
- If the pressure monitoring system is accessed through a diaphragm instead of a stopcock, thoroughly disinfect the diaphragm with an antiseptic pad using friction before accessing the system.[8]
- Change the flush bag, tubing, and other components of the system every 96 hours, immediately when contamination is suspected or when the integrity of the product or system is compromised, or according to your facility's policy.[9]

Documentation

Document the patient's position for zeroing so that other health care team members can replicate the placement. Document the flush solution used and the date and time of tubing changes.

REFERENCES

1 Centers for Disease Control and Prevention. (October 2002). Guideline for hand hygiene in health-care settings. *Morbidity and Mortality Weekly Report, 51*(RR-16), 1–45. (Level I)
2 World Health Organization. (2009). *WHO guidelines on hand hygiene in health care: First global patient safety challenge. Clean care is safer care.* Geneva, Switzerland: World Health Organization. (Level I)
3 The Joint Commission. (2012). Standard NPSG.07.01.01. *Comprehensive accreditation manual for hospitals: The official handbook.* Oakbrook Terrace, IL: The Joint Commission. (Level I)
4 American Association of Critical Care Nurses. (1993). Evaluation of the effects of heparinized and nonheparinized flush solution on the patency of arterial pressure monitoring lines: The AACN Thunder Project. *American Journal of Critical Care, 2*(1), 3–15. (Level II)
5 Laulive, J.L. (1982). Pulmonary artery pressure and position changes in the critically ill adult. *Dimensions in Critical Care Nursing, 1*(1), 28–34. (Level VI)
6 Lynn-McHale Wiegand, D. (Ed.). (2011). *AACN procedure manual for critical care* (6th ed.). Philadelphia, PA: Saunders.
7 The Joint Commission. (2012). Standard RC.01.03.01. *Comprehensive accreditation manual for hospitals: The official handbook.* Oakbrook Terrace, IL: The Joint Commission. (Level I)
8 O'Grady, N.P., et al. (2011). "Guidelines for the Prevention of Intravascular Catheter-Related Infections" [Online]. Accessed December 2011 via the Web at http://www.cdc.gov/hicpac/pdf/guidelines/bsi-guidelines-2011.pdf (Level I)
9 Standard 43. Administration set change. Infusion nursing standards of practice. (2011). *Journal of Infusion Nursing, 34*(1S), S55–S57. (Level I)

TRANSFER WITHIN A FACILITY

Patient transfer requires thorough preparation and careful documentation. Preparation includes an explanation of the transfer to the patient and his family and discussion of the patient's condition and care plan with staff members on the receiving unit. Documentation of the patient's condition before and during transfer and adequate communication between the nursing staff from each unit ensures continuity of nursing care and provides legal protection for the transferring unit and its staff members.[1]

Equipment

Admission inventory of belongings ▪ patient's medical record and medication record ▪ medications ▪ bag or suitcase ▪ wheelchair or stretcher, as necessary.

Implementation

- If the patient is being transferred from or to an intensive care unit, your facility may require new care orders from the patient's doctor. If so, review the new orders with the nursing staff at the receiving unit.
- Perform hand hygiene.[2,3,4]
- Confirm the patient's identity using at least two patient identifiers according to your facility's policy.[5]
- Explain the transfer to the patient and his family.[6] If the patient is anxious about the transfer or his condition precludes patient teaching, explain the reason for the transfer to his family, especially if the transfer is the result of a serious change in the patient's condition.
- Assess the patient's physical condition to determine the means of transfer, such as a wheelchair or a stretcher.
- Using the admissions inventory of belongings as a checklist, collect the patient's property. Check the entire room, including the closet, bedside stand, overbed table, and bathroom.
- Gather the patient's medications from the cart and the refrigerator. If the patient is being transferred to another unit, take or send the medications to the receiving unit.
- Notify the business office and other appropriate departments of the transfer.
- Have a staff person notify the dietary department, the pharmacy, and the facility telephone operator about the transfer.
- Provide the nursing staff members on the receiving unit with a detailed report about the patient's condition and drug regimen and review the patient's nursing care plan with them *to ensure continuity of care.* Allow an opportunity for questioning.
- Take or send the patient's chart, accurate medication reconciliation list, laboratory request slips, Kardex, special equipment, and other required materials to the receiving unit.[7]
- Use a wheelchair to transport the ambulatory patient to the newly assigned room unless it's on the same unit as his present one, in which case he may be allowed to walk. Use a stretcher or bed to transport the bedridden patient.
- Introduce the patient to the nursing staff members at the receiving unit. Then take the patient to his room and, depending on his condition, place him in the bed or seat him in a chair.
- Introduce him to his new roommate, if appropriate, and tell him about any unfamiliar equipment such as the call bell.
- Perform hand hygiene[2,3,4]
- Document the procedure.[8]

Special considerations

- Before the patient is transferred, make sure none of these patient care measures have been omitted: suctioning of airway, administering prescribed medications, changing soiled dressing, bathing an incontinent patient, and emptying drainage collection devices.

Documentation

Record the time and date of transfer, the patient's condition during transfer, the name of the receiving unit, and the means of transportation. Include equipment accompanying the patient, such as IV lines and pumps, surgical drains, and oxygen therapy. Note the name and title of the person you gave your report to; also include the names of staff or family members accompanying the patient.

References

1 The Joint Commission. (2012). Standard PC.04.01.01. *Comprehensive accreditation manual for hospitals: The official handbook.* Oakbrook Terrace, IL: The Joint Commission. (Level I)
2 Centers for Disease Control and Prevention. (October 2002). Guideline for hand hygiene in health-care settings. *Morbidity and Mortality Weekly Report, 51*(RR-16), 1–45. (Level I)
3 World Health Organization. (2009). *WHO guidelines on hand hygiene in health care: First global patient safety challenge. Clean care is safer care.* Geneva, Switzerland: World Health Organization. (Level I)
4 The Joint Commission. (2012). Standard NPSG.07.01.01. *Comprehensive accreditation manual for hospitals: The official handbook.* Oakbrook Terrace, IL: The Joint Commission. (Level I)
5 The Joint Commission. (2012). Standard NPSG.01.01.01. *Comprehensive accreditation manual for hospitals: The official handbook.* Oakbrook Terrace, IL: The Joint Commission. (Level I)
6 The Joint Commission. (2012). Standard PC.04.01.05. *Comprehensive accreditation manual for hospitals: The official handbook.* Oakbrook Terrace, IL: The Joint Commission. (Level I)
7 The Joint Commission. (2012). Standard PC.04.02.01. *Comprehensive accreditation manual for hospitals: The official handbook.* Oakbrook Terrace, IL: The Joint Commission. (Level I)
8 The Joint Commission. (2012). Standard RC.01.03.01. *Comprehensive accreditation manual for hospitals: The official handbook.* Oakbrook Terrace, IL: The Joint Commission. (Level I)

Additional references

Chaboyer, W., et al. (2007). The effect of an ICU liaison nurse on patient's and family's anxiety prior to transfer to the ward: An intervention study. *Intensive and Critical Care Nurse, 23*(6), 362–369.
Committee on Patient Safety and Quality Improvement. (2012). "ACOG Committee Opinion Number 517: Communication Strategies for Patient Handoffs" [Online]. Accessed March 2012 via the Web at http://www.acog.org/Resources_And_Publications/Committee_Opinions/Committee_on_Patient_Safety_and_Quality_Improvement/Communication_Strategies_for_Patient_Handoffs

TRANSFUSION OF BLOOD AND BLOOD PRODUCTS

The transfusion of blood and blood products should be performed only as a last resort in patients with chronic anemia or acute bleeding. Prevention and early diagnosis of anemia or bleeding can help minimize the need for transfusion of blood and blood products. For a patient with chronic anemia, the use of iron and vitamin supplements is often sufficient to raise the hemoglobin level enough so a transfusion isn't required.

If the patient is experiencing acute bleeding, the first line of treatment should be IV fluids, such as crystalloids or colloids, to help increase the circulating volume. If the patient requires a blood transfusion, it's very important to make sure that the right patient is receiving the right blood or blood product. If a patient receives the wrong blood or blood product, it could cause a serious reaction and possibly death. Before administering blood or a blood product, you should be familiar with the different types of blood and blood products (See *Transfusing blood and selected blood products.*)

Equipment

Blood or blood component administration set as appropriate ▪ IV pole ▪ gloves ▪ blood or blood product ▪ 10-mL syringe ▪ 250 mL of normal saline solution ▪ IV catheter equipment, if necessary (should include 14G to 24G catheter).[3]

Straight line and Y-type blood administration sets (Y-type is most commonly used) contain a standard blood filter designed to eliminate blood clots and cellular debris that occur during blood storage. A standard blood filter will trap particles that are 170 microns or larger. There are times, however, when a specialized blood filter may be required. (See *Specialized blood filters,* page 745.)

Preparation of equipment

Avoid obtaining the blood or blood product until you're ready to begin the transfusion. The transfusion should begin within 30 minutes of obtaining the blood or blood product *to decrease the risk of bacterial growth.*[3] Prepare the equipment when you're ready to start the infusion.

NURSING ALERT *Never store blood in a non–blood bank refrigerator. Return the blood to the blood bank refrigerator if a delay of 30 minutes or more is anticipated.*[3,4]

Implementation

▪ Make sure that a written order is in the patient's medical record. Confirm that the order and the medical record are labeled with the patient's name and assigned identification number.[3,5]
▪ Verify that the patient or his legally authorized representative has signed an informed consent form before transfusion therapy is initiated and that the form is in the patient's medical record according to your facility's policy.[6,7] Some facilities don't require consent for blood components such as albumin; make sure you're familiar with your facility's policy.
▪ Ensure that the indication for the transfusion is documented in the patient's medical record.
▪ Gather the equipment.
▪ Confirm the patient's identity using at least two patient identifiers according to your facility's policy.[11]
▪ Explain the procedure to the patient.
▪ Perform hand hygiene and put on gloves[8,9,10,15]
▪ If the patient doesn't have an IV catheter in place, insert one. Use a catheter that's 24G or larger in diameter.[3] The selection of the catheter size depends on the location, size, and integrity of the patient's veins. A smaller catheter usually requires a slower rate of transfusion. (See "IV catheter insertion and removal," page 421.)

Transfusing blood and selected blood products

BLOOD COMPONENT	INDICATIONS	COMPATIBILITY	NURSING CONSIDERATIONS
Packed red blood cells (RBCs) Same RBC mass as whole blood but with 80% of the plasma removed	▪ To restore or maintain oxygen-carrying capacity ▪ To correct anemia and surgical blood loss ▪ To increase RBC mass ▪ For red cell exchange	▪ Group A receives A or O ▪ Group B receives B or O ▪ Group AB receives AB, A, B, or O ▪ Group O receives O ▪ Rh type must match[1]	▪ Use blood administration tubing to infuse within 4 hours. ▪ Use only with normal saline solution. ▪ Avoid administering packed RBCs for anemic conditions correctable by nutritional or drug therapy.
Leukocyte-poor RBCs Same as packed RBCs with about 70% of the leukocytes removed	▪ Same as packed RBCs ▪ To prevent febrile reactions from leukocyte antibodies ▪ To treat immunocompromised patients ▪ To restore RBCs to patients who have had two or more nonhemolytic febrile reactions	▪ Same as packed RBCs ▪ Rh type must match	▪ Use blood administration tubing. ▪ May require a 40-micron filter suitable for hard-spun, leukocyte-poor RBCs. ▪ Use only with normal saline solution. ▪ Cells expire 24 hours after washing.
Platelets Platelet sediment from RBCs or plasma platelets	▪ To treat bleeding caused by decreased circulating platelets or functionally abnormal platelets ▪ To improve platelet count preoperatively in a patient whose count is 50,000/μL or less[1]	▪ ABO compatibility identical; Rh-negative recipients should receive Rh-negative platelets[1]	▪ Use a blood filter or leukocyte-reduction filter. ▪ As prescribed, premedicate with antipyretics and antihistamines if the patient's history includes a platelet transfusion reaction or to reduce chills, fever, and allergic reactions. ▪ Complete transfusion within 20 minutes or at the fastest rate the patient can tolerate. ▪ Use single-donor platelets if the patient has a need for repeated transfusions. ▪ Platelets aren't used to treat autoimmune thrombocytopenia or thrombocytopenic purpura unless patient has a life-threatening hemorrhage.
Fresh frozen plasma (FFP) Uncoagulated plasma separated from RBCs and rich in coagulation factors V, VIII, and IX	▪ To correct a coagulation factor deficiency ▪ To replace a specific factor when that factor isn't available ▪ For warfarin reversal ▪ To treat thrombotic thrombocytopenic purpura	▪ ABO compatibility required ▪ Rh match not required	▪ Use a blood administration set. ▪ Complete the transfusion within 20 minutes or at the fastest rate the patient can tolerate. ▪ Keep in mind that large-volume transfusions of FFP may require correction for hypocalcemia because the citric acid in FFP binds calcium. ▪ Must be infused within 6 hours of being thawed.

(continued)

Transfusing blood and selected blood products *(continued)*

BLOOD COMPONENT	INDICATIONS	COMPATIBILITY	NURSING CONSIDERATIONS
Albumin 5% (buffered saline); albumin 25% (salt-poor) A small plasma protein prepared by fractionating pooled plasma	■ To replace volume lost because of shock from burns, trauma, surgery, or infections ■ To treat hypoproteinemia (with or without edema)	■ Not required	■ Use the administration set supplied by the manufacturer and set the rate based on the patient's condition and response. ■ Keep in mind that albumin is contraindicated in severe anemia. ■ Administer cautiously in cardiac and pulmonary disease *because heart failure may result from circulatory overload.*
Factor VIII concentrate (antihemophilic factor) Cold insoluble portion of plasma recovered from FFP	■ To treat a patient with hemophilia A ■ To treat a patient with von Willebrand's disease	■ ABO compatibility not required	■ Administer by IV injection using a filter needle, or use the administration set supplied by the manufacturer.
Cryoprecipitate Insoluble plasma portion of FFP containing fibrinogen, factor VIIIc, factor VIIvWF, factor XIII, and fibronectin	■ To treat factor VIII deficiency and fibrinogen disorders ■ To treat significant factor XIII deficiency	■ ABO compatibility required[1,2] ■ Rh match not required[1,2]	■ Administer with a blood administration set. ■ Add normal saline solution to each bag of cryoprecipitate, as necessary, *to facilitate infusion.* ■ Keep in mind that cryoprecipitate must be administered within 6 hours of thawing. ■ Before administration, check laboratory studies to confirm a deficiency of one of the specific clotting factors present in cryoprecipitate. ■ Be aware that patients with hemophilia A or von Willebrand's disease should only be treated with cryoprecipitate when appropriate factor VIII concentrates aren't available.

If an existing IV catheter is in place, verify it's an appropriate size and that it's patent by using a 10-mL syringe to aspirate for blood return.[12] Central venous access devices also may be used for transfusion therapy.

■ Record the patient's baseline vital signs.

■ Obtain the blood or blood product from the blood bank. Check the expiration date on the blood bag, and observe for abnormal color, red blood cell (RBC) clumping, gas bubbles, and extraneous material.[2,3] Return outdated or abnormal blood to the blood bank.

■ Use a two-person verification process to match the blood or blood component to the doctor's order and to match the patient to the blood component.[3] One of the individuals conducting the verification must be the qualified person, usually a registered nurse, who will administer the blood or blood component to the patient. The second individual conducting the verification must be qualified to participate in the process as determined by your facility's policy.[13]

■ Compare the name and identification number on the patient's wristband with those on the blood bag label. Check the blood bag identification number, ABO blood group, and Rh compatibility. Also, compare the patient's blood bank identification number with the number on the blood bag.[2]

■ When using a Y-type set, close all the clamps on the set. Insert the spike of the line you're using for the normal saline solution into the bag of saline solution. Next, open the port on the blood bag, and insert the spike of the line you're using to administer the blood or blood product into the port. Hang the bag of normal saline solution and blood or blood product on the IV pole, open the clamp on the line of saline solution, and squeeze the drip chamber until it's half full. Then remove the adapter cover at the tip of the blood administration set, open the main flow clamp, prime the tubing with saline solution, and then close the clamp.

■ If necessary, when administering packed RBCs with a Y-type set, you can add saline solution to the bag to dilute the cells by closing the clamp between the patient and the drip chamber and opening the clamp from the blood. Then lower the blood bag below the saline container and let 30 to 50 mL of saline solution flow into the packed cells. Finally, close the clamp to the blood bag, rehang the bag, rotate it gently *to mix the cells and saline solution,* and close the clamp to the saline container.

■ Thoroughly disinfect the port of the venous access device with a disinfectant pad using friction.

■ Trace the blood administration set tubing from the patient to its point of origin, and then attach it to the venous access device, open the clamp, and flush it with normal saline solution.[12] Then close the clamp to the saline solution and open the clamp between the blood bag and the patient.

NURSING ALERT *When administering blood, never mix or administer simultaneously any other IV solution except normal saline solution,[3] which is isotonic and calcium-free. Calcium will bind with the citrate anticoagulant in the blood bag and promote clotting in the tubing. Excess glucose causes hemolysis and shortens RBC survival. Also, a blood administration set shouldn't be piggybacked into a main line that has been used for any solution other than normal saline solution.*

■ Monitor the patient closely and adjust the flow rate to no greater than 2 mL/minute for the first 15 minutes of the transfusion *to observe for a possible transfusion reaction.*[2] If such signs develop, record vital signs and stop the transfusion. Infuse saline solution at a keep-vein-open rate, and notify the doctor immediately. Report the transfusion reaction according to your facility's policy. (See "Transfusion reaction management," page 747.) If no signs of a reaction appear within 15 minutes, you'll need to adjust the flow clamp to the ordered infusion rate. The rate of infusion should be as rapid as the patient's circulatory system can tolerate. It's undesirable for blood products to remain at room temperature for more than 4 hours.[3,5] If the infusion rate must be so slow that the entire unit can't be infused within 4 hours, it may be appropriate for the blood bank to divide the unit and keep one portion refrigerated until it can be safely administered.

■ Remove and discard your gloves and perform hand hygiene.[8,9,10,14,15]

■ Recheck the patient's vital signs, including temperature, every 15 minutes for the first 30 minutes after beginning the infusion, and then according to facility policy.[2,5]

■ Perform hand hygiene and put on gloves[8,9,10,15]

■ After completing the transfusion, flush the administration set and IV catheter with the normal saline solution.

■ Using sterile technique, remove and discard the used infusion equipment. If additional units are being given, repeat the procedure. Otherwise, as indicated, reconnect the original IV fluid, saline lock the site, or discontinue the IV infusion.

■ Discard the blood bag, tubing and filter in the appropriate hazardous waste container.

■ Remove and discard your gloves and perform hand hygiene.[8,9,10,14,15]

■ Record the patient's vital signs.

■ Document the procedure.[16,17]

Special considerations

■ If necessary, using sterile technique, change the blood or blood component administration set after each unit is infused or after 4 hours. Change it immediately if contamination is suspected or the integrity of the product or system has been compromised.[18]

■ Change the filter whenever you change the tubing unless otherwise indicated by a manufacturer's labeled use and directions.[19]

■ Use a blood warmer, as ordered, in special situations, such as when transfusing multiple units of refrigerated blood to a patient with a large volume of blood loss, performing exchange transfusions, or transfusing to a patient with cold agglutinin disease. Always follow the manufacturer's instructions.[5,20]

■ For rapid blood replacement, you may need to use a pressure bag or a positive pressure electronic infusion device. Always follow the manufacturer's instructions for use. Pressure bags should be equipped with a pressure gauge and exert uniform pressure. Be aware that excessive pressure may develop, leading to broken blood vessels and extravasation, with hematoma and hemolysis of the infusing RBCs.

Documenting blood transfusions

After matching the patient's name, medical record number, blood group (or type) and Rh factor (the patient's and the donor's), the crossmatch data, and the blood bank identification number with the label on the blood bag, you'll need to clearly document that you did so. The blood or blood component must be identified and documented properly by two health care professionals as well.

On the transfusion record, document:
- the date and time the transfusion was started and completed
- the name of the health care professional who verified the information
- the type and gauge of the catheter
- the total amount of the transfusion
- the patient's vital signs before and after the transfusion
- any infusion device used
- the flow rate and if any blood warming unit used.

If the patient receives his own blood, document in the intake and output records:
- the amount of autologous blood retrieved
- the amount reinfused in the intake and output records
- laboratory data during and after the autotransfusion
- the patient's pretransfusion and posttransfusion vital signs.

Pay particular attention to:
- the patient's coagulation profile
- hemoglobin and hematocrit values and arterial blood gas and calcium levels
- the patient's tolerance of the procedure, especially fluid status.

- If the transfusion stops, take the following steps as needed: Check that the IV container is at least 3' (1 m) above the level of the IV site. Make sure that the flow clamp is open and that the blood completely covers the filter. If it doesn't, squeeze the drip chamber until it does. Gently rock the bag back and forth, agitating any blood cells that may have settled. Untape the dressing over the IV site to check catheter placement. Reposition the catheter if necessary. Flush the line with saline solution, aspirate for blood return, and restart the transfusion. When using a Y-type set, close the flow clamp to the patient and lower the blood bag. Next, open the saline clamp and allow some saline solution to flow into the blood bag. Rehang the blood bag, open the flow clamp to the patient, and reset the flow rate.
- If a hematoma develops at the IV site, immediately stop the infusion. Remove the IV cannula. Notify the doctor and expect to place ice on the site intermittently for 8 hours and then apply warm compresses. Follow your facility's policy.
- If the blood bag empties before the next one arrives, administer normal saline solution slowly. If you're using a Y-type set, close the blood-line clamp, open the saline clamp, and let the saline run slowly until the new blood arrives. Decrease the flow rate or clamp the line before attaching the new unit of blood.

- Keep in mind that blood products must be infused within 4 hours of removal from the blood bank refrigerator.[2,3] If any blood product remains after 4 hours, discontinue the infusion and discard the remaining product in the hazardous waste container in the patient's room *to prevent accidental exposure.*
- Monitor the patient's intake and output and lung status and watch for edema *to prevent fluid overload.*
- Be aware that whole blood is rarely used. It may be used on rare occasions to restore blood volume from hemorrhage or in an exchange transfusion.
- If the patient is a Jehovah's Witness, special written permission from him is required for a transfusion.

Complications

Despite improvements in crossmatching precautions, transfusion reactions can still occur during a transfusion or within 96 hours after a transfusion. Transfusion reactions typically stem from a major antigen-antibody reaction. The nurse must closely monitor for signs and symptoms, especially if the patient can't report the symptoms. A transfusion reaction requires prompt nursing action *to prevent further complications and, possibly, death.*

Unlike a transfusion reaction, an infectious disease transmitted during a transfusion may go undetected until days, weeks, or even months later, when it produces signs and symptoms. Measures to prevent disease transmission include laboratory testing of blood products and careful screening of potential donors, neither of which is guaranteed.

Hepatitis C accounts for most posttransfusion hepatitis cases. The tests that detect hepatitis B and hepatitis C can produce false-negative results and may allow some hepatitis cases to go undetected.

When testing for antibodies to human immunodeficiency virus (HIV), keep in mind that antibodies don't appear until 6 to 12 weeks after exposure. The American Association of Blood Banks estimates the risk of acquiring HIV from a single blood transfusion is between 1 in 40,000 to 1 in 153,000.

Many blood banks screen blood for cytomegalovirus (CMV). Blood with CMV is especially dangerous for an immunosuppressed, seronegative patient. Blood banks also test blood for syphilis, but refrigerating blood virtually eliminates the risk of transfusion-related syphilis.

Circulatory overload and hemolytic, allergic, febrile, and pyogenic reactions can result from any transfusion. Coagulation disturbances, citrate intoxication, hyperkalemia, acid-base imbalance, loss of 2,3-diphosphoglycerate, ammonia intoxication, and hypothermia can result from massive transfusion.

Documentation

Record the date and time of the transfusion, that informed consent was obtained, the indications for the transfusion, the type and amount of transfusion product, the amount of normal saline solution, the patient's vital signs, your check of all identification data, and the patient's response. Document any transfusion reaction and treatment provided. Note any patient teaching and the patient's understanding of your teaching. (See *Documenting blood transfusions.*)

REFERENCES

1 American Red Cross. (2007). *Practice guidelines for blood transfusion: A compilation from recent peer-reviewed literature* (2nd ed.) [Online]. Accessed December 2011 via the Web at http://www.red-crossblood.org/sites/arc/files/pdf/practiceguidelinesforblood-trans.pdf (Level I)

2 American Association of Blood Banks, America's Blood Banks, and the American Red Cross. (2002). *Circular of information for use of human blood and blood components (WNV language inserted, April 2006)*. Bethesda, MD: American Association of Blood Banks. (Level I)

3 Standard 66. Transfusion therapy. Infusion nursing standards of practice (2011). *Journal of Infusion Nursing, 34*(1S), S93–94. (Level I)

4 Occupational Safety and Health Administration. "Bloodborne Pathogens, Standard Number 1910.1030" [Online]. Accessed October 2011 via the Web at http://www.osha.gov/pls/oshaweb/owadisp.show_document?p_table=STANDARDS&p_id=10051 (Level I)

5 American Association of Blood Banks. (2009). *Standards for blood banks and transfusion services* (26th ed.). Bethesda, MD: American Association of Blood Banks. (Level I)

6 Centers for Medicare & Medicaid Services, Department of Health and Human Services. (2006). "Conditions of Participation: Patients' Rights," 42 CFR part 482.13 [Online]. Accessed November 2011 via the Web at https://www.cms.gov/CFCsAnd-CoPs/downloads/finalpatientrightsrule.pdf

7 Standard 12. Informed consent. Infusion nursing standards of practice (2011). *Journal of Infusion Nursing, 34*(1S), S17–18. (Level I)

8 The Joint Commission. (2012). Standard NPSG.07.01.01. *Comprehensive accreditation manual for hospitals: The official handbook.* Oakbrook Terrace, IL: The Joint Commission. (Level I)

9 Centers for Disease Control and Prevention. (October 2002). Guideline for hand hygiene in health-care settings. *Morbidity and Mortality Weekly Report, 51*(RR-16), 1–45. (Level I)

10 World Health Organization. (2009). *WHO guidelines on hand hygiene in health care: First global patient safety challenge. Clean care is safer care.* Geneva, Switzerland: World Health Organization. (Level I)

11 The Joint Commission. (2012). Standard NPSG.01.01.01. *Comprehensive accreditation manual for hospitals: The official handbook.* Oakbrook Terrace, IL: The Joint Commission. (Level I)

12 Standard 61. Parenteral medication and solution administration. Infusion nursing standards of practice (2011). *Journal of Infusion Nursing, 34*(1S), S86–87. (Level I)

13 The Joint Commission. (2012). Standard NPSG.01.03.01. *Comprehensive accreditation manual for hospitals: The official handbook.* Oakbrook Terrace, IL: The Joint Commission. (Level I)

14 O'Grady, N.P., et al. (2011). "Guidelines for the Prevention of Intravascular Catheter-Related Infections" [Online]. Accessed December 2011 via the Web at http://www.cdc.gov/hicpac/pdf/guidelines/bsi-guidelines-2011.pdf

15 Standard 19. Hand hygiene. Infusion nursing standards of practice (2011). *Journal of Infusion Nursing, 34*(1S), S26–S27. (Level I)

16 The Joint Commission. (2012). Standard RC.01.03.01. *Comprehensive accreditation manual for hospitals: The official handbook.* Oakbrook Terrace, IL: The Joint Commission. (Level I)

17 The Joint Commission. (2012). Standard RC.02.01.01. *Comprehensive accreditation manual for hospitals: The official handbook.* Oakbrook Terrace, IL: The Joint Commission. (Level I)

18 Standard 43. Administration set change. Infusion nursing standards of practice (2011). *Journal of Infusion Nursing, 34*(1S), S55–S56. (Level I)

19 Standard 28. Filters. Infusion nursing standards of practice (2011). *Journal of Infusion Nursing, 34*(1S), S33–S34. (Level I)

20 Standard 34. Blood and fluid warmers. Infusion nursing standards of practice (2011). *Journal of Infusion Nursing, 34*(1S), S35. (Level I)

ADDITIONAL REFERENCES

Alexander, M., et al. (Eds.). (2010). *Infusion nursing: An evidence-based approach* (3rd ed.). Philadelphia, PA: Elsevier.

Infusion Nurses Society. (2011). *Policies and procedures for infusion nursing* (4th ed.). Boston, MA: Infusion Nurses Society.

Nettina, S.M. (2010). *Lippincott manual of nursing practice* (9th ed.). Philadelphia, PA: Lippincott Williams & Wilkins.

Roback, J., et al. (2008). *Technical manual* (16th ed.). Bethesda, MD: American Association of Blood Banks.

Siegel, J.D., et al. "2007 Guideline for Isolation Precautions: Preventing Transmission of Infectious Agents in Healthcare Settings" [Online]. Accessed December 2011 via the Web at http://www.cdc.gov/hicpac/2007ip/2007isolationprecautions.html

TRANSFUSION REACTION MANAGEMENT

A transfusion reaction typically stems from a major antigen-antibody reaction and can result from a single or massive transfusion of blood or blood products. It's estimated that 1% to 2% of all patients who receive a transfusion of blood or blood products experience a transfusion reaction.[1] Although many reactions occur during transfusion or within 96 hours afterward, infectious diseases transmitted during a transfusion may go undetected until days, weeks, or months later, when signs and symptoms appear.

A transfusion reaction requires immediate recognition and prompt nursing action to prevent further complications and, possibly, death—particularly if the patient is unconscious or so heavily sedated that he can't report the common symptoms. (See *Guide to transfusion reactions*, pages 748 and 749.)

Equipment

Gloves ▪ normal saline solution ▪ IV administration set ▪ sterile urine specimen container ▪ supplies for blood collection (see "Venipuncture," page 781) ▪ transfusion reaction report form ▪ stethoscope ▪ blood pressure cuff ▪ pulse oximeter ▪ thermometer ▪ laboratory specimen labels ▪ laboratory request form ▪ laboratory biohazard transport bags ▪ Optional: oxygen, epinephrine, hypothermia blanket, leukocyte removal filter.

Implementation

▪ Perform hand hygiene.[2,3,4]
▪ Confirm the patient's identity using at least two patient identifiers according to your facility's policy.[5]
▪ As soon as you suspect an adverse reaction, stop the transfusion and notify the doctor and the blood bank.[6,7]
▪ Prepare a normal saline infusion using a new macrodrip IV administration set.

(Text continues on page 750.)

Guide to transfusion reactions

Any patient receiving a transfusion of blood or blood products is at risk for a transfusion reaction. A transfusion reaction may be immediate, occurring during the transfusion or within several hours of the completion of the transfusion, or delayed. The chart below describes immediate and delayed reactions.

REACTION	CAUSES	SIGNS AND SYMPTOMS	PREVENTION	NURSING INTERVENTIONS
IMMEDIATE REACTIONS				
Acute hemolytic	Administration of incompatible blood	Chest pain, dyspnea, facial flushing, fever, chills, hypotension, flank pain, bloody oozing at the infusion or surgical incision site, nausea, tachycardia	■ Carefully check the patient's identity against the blood or blood product. ■ Monitor the patient at the start of the transfusion of each unit. ■ Correctly label all blood samples and blood request forms.	■ Monitor the patient carefully for the first 15 minutes of any transfusion. ■ Administer IV fluids, oxygen, epinephrine, and a vasopressor as ordered. ■ Observe patient for signs of coagulopathy.
Bacterial contamination	Contamination of blood product	Chills, fever, vomiting, abdominal cramping, diarrhea, shock	■ Use careful technique when collecting or administering blood. ■ Change the blood tubing and filter at least every 4 hours.[6] ■ Transfuse blood or blood product within 30 minutes of receiving.[6] ■ Complete transfusion of blood within 4 hours.[1,6]	■ Provide broad-spectrum antibiotics, as prescribed. ■ Monitor the patient for fever for several hours after completion of the transfusion. ■ Obtain blood cultures from a site other than the IV infusion site.[13,17] ■ Keep all blood bags and tubing and send them to the blood bank.
Febrile non-hemolytic	Bacterial lipopolysaccharides; antileukocyte recipient antibodies directed against donor white blood cells	Fever within 2 hours of transfusion, chills, rigors, headache, palpitation, cough, tachycardia	■ Premedicate the patient with antipyretics. ■ Limit the number of transfusions the patient receives, if possible.	■ Relieve symptoms with an antipyretic. ■ If the patient requires further transfusions, consider using a leukocyte removal filter.[13,17]
Transfusion-related acute lung injury (TRALI)	Granulocyte antibodies in the donor or recipient cause complement and histamine release	Severe respiratory distress within 6 hours of transfusion, fever, chills, cyanosis, hypotension[13,17]	■ No prevention is known.	■ Provide oxygen as needed. ■ Monitor pulse oximetry. ■ Prepare for intubation and ventilatory support and hemodynamic monitoring.
Allergic reaction	Allergen in donor blood	Urticaria, fever, nausea, vomiting, anaphylaxis (facial swelling, laryngeal edema, respiratory distress) in extreme cases	■ Administer antihistamines if the patient has a history of allergic reaction.[13,17]	■ Administer antihistamine, corticosteroid, or epinephrine as ordered. ■ Prepare for intubation and respiratory support if patient develops anaphylaxis.

Guide to transfusion reactions (continued)

REACTION	CAUSES	SIGNS AND SYMPTOMS	PREVENTION	NURSING INTERVENTIONS
IMMEDIATE REACTIONS (continued)				
Transfusion-associated circulatory overload (TACO)	Rapid infusion of blood; excessive volume of transfusion	Chest tightness, chills, dyspnea, tachypnea, hypoxemia, hypertension, jugular vein distention; occurs within 2 to 6 hours after transfusion	■ Infuse at the slowest rate needed while keeping total transfusion time in mind. ■ Ask the blood bank to divide the unit into smaller aliquots.	■ Monitor intake and output, breath sounds, and blood pressure. ■ Administer diuretics as needed. ■ Keep in mind that elderly patients and those with history of cardiac disease at higher risk.
Hypocalcemia	Rapid infusion of citrate-treated blood (citrate binds to calcium)	Arrhythmias, hypotension, muscle cramps, nausea and vomiting, seizures, prolonged Q-T interval	■ Monitor ionized calcium levels in patients receiving large amounts of transfused blood.	■ Administer calcium gluconate IV, as ordered. ■ Monitor the ECG for arrhythmias or prolonged QT interval. ■ Monitor patients with an elevated potassium level closely; they're at higher risk for hypocalcemia.
DELAYED REACTIONS				
Delayed hemolytic	Production of antibodies by red blood cells to antigens on transfused red blood cells	Fever, anemia, jaundice; occurs 5 to 10 days after transfusion	■ No prevention is known.	■ Recheck the patient's blood group. ■ Administer antipyretics for fever.
Infection transmission	Transmission of infectious agent in the blood	Depends on infection transmitted	■ Careful screening of blood helps prevent this reaction.	■ Treatment is based on individual infection transmitted.
Posttransfusion purpura	Destruction of autologous and allogenic platelets	Thrombocytopenia, bleeding; occurs 7 to 10 days after transfusion	■ Limit transfusion in patients with a history of sensitization from either pregnancy or previous transfusion.[13]	■ Administer high doses of IV immune globulin, as ordered.[17]
Graft-versus-host disease	T-lymphocytes in blood or blood product react against patient's tissue antigens	Fever, skin rash and desquamation, diarrhea, pancytopenia; occurs 10 to 12 days after transfusion; usually fatal	■ Transfuse irradiated blood components to immunocompromised patients.	■ Provide supportive care to the patient and family.

- Perform hand hygiene[2,3,4,8,9] and put on gloves.[10,11]
- Trace the tubing on the administration set from the patient to its point of origin and then disconnect it from the IV catheter.[12] Replace the blood administration set with the normal saline solution set *to prevent the infusion of any additional blood remaining in the blood administration tubing.* Start the normal saline infusion at a keep-vein-open rate *to maintain venous access.*[1] Increase the infusion rate, as ordered, if rapid fluid replacement is necessary. Don't discard the blood bag or blood administration set unless it's indicated by your facility's policy.[1]
- Monitor the patient's vital signs and oxygenation level every 15 minutes or as indicated by the severity and type of reaction.
- Compare the labels on all blood containers with corresponding patient identification forms *to verify that the transfusion was the correct blood or blood product and that it was being administered to the correct patient.*
- Notify the blood bank of a possible transfusion reaction and collect blood samples, according to your facility's policy, from a site opposite the transfusion site. (See "Venipuncture," page 781.)
- If bacterial contamination is suspected, obtain blood cultures.[13] (See "Blood culture sample collection," page 74.)
- Label all samples in the presence of the patient *to prevent mislabeling.*
- Place all the samples, all transfusion containers (even if empty), and the administration set in a laboratory biohazard transport bag and immediately send the bag to the blood bank or follow your facility's policy. Also complete and send the appropriate documentation, usually a transfusion reaction form. The blood bank will test these materials *to further evaluate the reaction.*[14]
- Discard used supplies in the appropriate container, remove and discard your gloves, and perform hand hygiene.[2,3,4,8,9]
- Collect the first posttransfusion urine specimen, place it in the urine specimen container, and label it in the presence of the patient *to prevent mislabeling.*
- Mark the collection slip "Possible transfusion reaction," place the specimen in a laboratory transport bag, and send it to the laboratory immediately. *The laboratory tests this urine specimen for the presence of hemoglobin, which indicates a hemolytic reaction.*
- Closely monitor intake and output. Note evidence of oliguria or anuria *because hemoglobin deposition in the renal tubules can cause renal damage.* Be prepared to administer fluid to maintain a urine output of at least 100 mL/hour *to prevent acute tubular necrosis.*
- If prescribed, administer oxygen, epinephrine, or other drugs following safe medication administration practices and apply a hypothermia blanket *to reduce fever.*
- As ordered, obtain specimens for laboratory tests, such as blood urea nitrogen and creatinine, *to monitor renal function* and coagulation studies (prothrombin time, fibrinogen levels, and partial thromboplastin time) *to identify extensive red blood cell destruction and possible disseminated intravascular coagulation.* Monitor results and report abnormalities to the doctor.
- Make the patient as comfortable as possible and provide reassurance as necessary.
- Perform hand hygiene.[2,3,4]
- Document your actions.[15,16]

Special considerations

- Treat all transfusion reactions as serious until proven otherwise. If the doctor anticipates a transfusion reaction, such as one that may occur in a leukemia patient, he may order prophylactic treatment with antihistamines or antipyretics to precede blood administration.
- Be aware that transfusion-related acute lung injury (TRALI) is the leading cause of transfusion-related mortality. Monitor the patient closely for signs and symptoms of TRALI.
- Be alert for signs and symptoms of shock or cardiovascular collapse. Be prepared to intervene with emergency medications and rapid fluid administration. Follow advanced cardiac life support protocols if respiratory or cardiac arrest occurs.
- *To avoid a possible febrile reaction,* the doctor may order the blood washed to remove as many leukocytes as possible, or a leukocyte removal filter may be used during the transfusion.
- All fatalities from a blood or blood product transfusion must be reported to the Food and Drug Administration within 24 hours.

Documentation

Record the time and date of the transfusion reaction, the type and amount of infused blood or blood products, the clinical signs of the transfusion reaction in order of occurrence, the patient's vital signs and oxygenation levels, any specimens sent to the laboratory for analysis, nursing interventions performed, any treatment given, and the patient's response to treatment and interventions. Note any unexpected outcomes and interventions performed in response to them. If required by policy, complete the transfusion reaction form. Document patient teaching.

REFERENCES

1 World Health Organization. (2002). *The clinical use of blood handbook.* Geneva, Switzerland: World Health Organization.
2 Centers for Disease Control and Prevention. (October 2002). Guideline for hand hygiene in health-care settings. *Morbidity and Mortality Weekly Report, 51*(RR-16), 1–45. (Level I)
3 World Health Organization. (2009). *WHO guidelines on hand hygiene in health care: First global patient safety challenge. Clean care is safer care.* Geneva, Switzerland: World Health Organization. (Level I)
4 The Joint Commission. (2012). Standard NPSG.07.01.01. *Comprehensive accreditation manual for hospitals: The official handbook.* Oakbrook Terrace, IL: The Joint Commission. (Level I)
5 The Joint Commission. (2012). Standard NPSG.01.01.01. *Comprehensive accreditation manual for hospitals: The official handbook.* Oakbrook Terrace, IL: The Joint Commission. (Level I)
6 Standard 66. Transfusion therapy. Infusion nursing standards of practice (2011). *Journal of Infusion Nursing, 34*(1S), S93–S94. (Level I)
7 Centers for Medicare & Medicaid Services, Department of Health and Human Services. (2006). "Conditions of Participation: Patients' Rights," 42 CFR part 482.13 [Online]. Accessed November 2011 via the Web at https://www.cms.gov/CFCsAndCoPs/downloads/finalpatientrightsrule.pdf
8 Standard 19. Hand hygiene. Infusion nursing standards of practice (2011). *Journal of Infusion Nursing, 34*(1S), S26–S27. (Level I)

9 O'Grady, N. P., et al. (2011). "Guidelines for the Prevention of Intravascular Catheter-Related Infections" [Online]. Accessed December 2011 via the Web at http://www.cdc.gov/hicpac/pdf/guidelines/bsi-guidelines-2011.pdf (Level I)

10 Siegel, J.D., et al. "2007 Guideline for Isolation Precautions: Preventing Transmission of Infectious Agents in Healthcare Settings" [Online]. Accessed December 2011 via the Web at http://www.cdc.gov/hicpac/2007ip/2007isolationprecautions.html

11 Standard 18. Infection prevention. Infusion nursing standards of practice (2011). *Journal of Infusion Nursing, 34*(1S), S25–26. (Level I)

12 U.S. Food and Drug Administration. (2009). "Look. Check. Connect.: Safe Medical Device Connections Save Lives" [Online]. Accessed December 2011 via the Web at http://www.fda.gov/downloads/MedicalDevices/Safety/AlertsandNotices/UCM134873.pdf

13 American Red Cross. (2007). *Practice guidelines for blood transfusion: A compilation from recent peer-reviewed literature* (2nd ed.) [Online]. Accessed December 2011 via the Web at http://www.redcrossblood.org/sites/arc/files/pdf/practiceguidelinesforbloodtrans.pdf (Level V)

14 American Association of Blood Banks. (2009). *Standards for blood banks and transfusion services* (26th ed.). Bethesda, MD: American Association of Blood Banks. (Level V)

15 The Joint Commission. (2012). Standard RC.01.03.01. *Comprehensive accreditation manual for hospitals: The official handbook.* Oakbrook Terrace, IL: The Joint Commission. (Level I)

16 The Joint Commission. (2012). Standard RC.02.01.01. *Comprehensive accreditation manual for hospitals: The official handbook.* Oakbrook Terrace, IL: The Joint Commission. (Level I)

17 American Association of Blood Banks, America's Blood Banks, and the American Red Cross. (2002). *Circular of information for use of human blood and blood components (WNV language inserted, April 2006).* Bethesda, MD: American Association of Blood Banks. (Level V)

ADDITIONAL REFERENCES

Kopko, P. (2010). Transfusion-related acute lung injury. *Journal of Infusion Nursing, 33*(1), 32–37.

Ruffolo, D. (2009). Seeing red: Complications of blood transfusions. *Nursing2009 Critical Care, 4*(3), 28–34.

TRANSVENOUS PACING

Usually inserted in an emergency, a temporary pacemaker consists of an external, battery-powered pulse generator and a lead or electrode system. The purpose of a transvenous pacemaker is to maintain circulatory integrity by providing for standby pacing should sudden complete heart block ensue, to increase the heart rate during periods of symptomatic bradycardia and, occasionally, to control sustained supraventricular or ventricular tachycardia.

In addition to being more comfortable for the patient, a transvenous pacemaker is more reliable than a transcutaneous pacemaker. Transvenous pacing involves threading an electrode catheter through a vein into the patient's right atrium or right ventricle. Veins used for insertion include the subclavian, brachial, internal jugular, and femoral.[1] The femoral site should be used as a last resort because it's associated with an increased risk of infection. The electrode then attaches to an external pulse generator. As a result, the pulse generator can provide an electrical stimulus directly to the endocardium.

Indications for transvenous pacing include management of symptomatic bradycardia, tachyarrhythmias, and other conduction system disturbances; it may also help diagnose conduction abnormalities.

According to the 2010 American Heart Association Guidelines for Cardiopulmonary Resuscitation and Emergency Cardiovascular Care, pacing isn't recommended in cardiac arrest.[2]

Equipment

Temporary pacemaker generator with new battery ■ guide wire or introducer ■ electrode catheter ■ gloves ■ sterile gloves ■ sterile dressings ■ adhesive tape ■ antiseptic solution (preferably a chlorhexidine-based solution) ■ nonconducting tape or rubber surgical glove ■ pouch for external pulse generator ■ emergency cardiac drugs ■ intubation equipment ■ defibrillator ■ cardiac monitor with strip-chart recorder ■ equipment to start a peripheral IV line, if appropriate ■ IV fluids ■ sedative ■ bridging cable ■ percutaneous introducer tray or venous cutdown tray ■ sterile gowns ■ mask, head cover, and goggles or face shield ■ linen-saver pad ■ antimicrobial soap ■ alcohol pads ■ vial of 1% lidocaine ■ 5-mL syringe ■ fluoroscopy equipment, if necessary ■ fenestrated drape ■ sutures ■ dextrose 5% in water ■ Optional: elastic bandage or gauze strips, restraints, clippers.

Implementation

■ Gather the appropriate equipment.

■ Make sure that informed consent has been obtained and that it's documented in the patient's medical record.[3,4]

■ Conduct a preprocedure verification *to make sure that all relevant documentation, related information, and equipment are available and correctly identified to the patient's identifiers.*[5]

■ Perform hand hygiene and put on gloves.[6,7,8]

■ Confirm the patient's identity using at least two patient identifiers according to your facility's policy.[9]

■ If applicable, explain the procedure to the patient.

■ Check the patient's history for hypersensitivity to local anesthetics. Then attach the cardiac monitor to the patient and obtain a baseline assessment, including the patient's vital signs, skin color, level of consciousness (LOC), heart rate and rhythm, and emotional state. Next, if ordered, insert a peripheral IV catheter (see "IV catheter insertion and removal," page 421) and initiate the ordered IV infusion at the ordered rate.

■ Insert a new battery into the external pacemaker generator, and test it to make sure it has a strong charge. Connect the bridging cable to the generator, and align the positive and negative poles. *This cable allows slack between the electrode catheter and the generator, reducing the risk of accidental catheter displacement.*

■ Place the patient in the supine position. If necessary, clip the hair around the insertion site.

■ Remove and discard your gloves and perform hand hygiene.[6,7,8]

■ Open the supply tray while maintaining a sterile field. Label all medications, medication containers, and other solutions on and off the sterile field.[10]

■ If assisting with the insertion, put on a mask, head cover, goggles or face shield, sterile gown, and sterile gloves.[11,12]

■ Conduct a time-out immediately before starting the procedure *to perform a final assessment that the correct patient, site, positioning, and procedure are identified and that, as applicable, all relevant information and necessary equipment are available.*[13]

■ Assist as needed with cleaning the insertion site with antimicrobial soap and antiseptic solution. Allow the antiseptic solution to dry. If fluoroscopy is used during the placement of leadwires, put on a protective apron.

■ Following maximal barrier precautions, the doctor puts on a mask, a head cover, goggles or a face shield, a sterile gown, and sterile gloves, and then covers the patient from head to toe with a sterile drape, leaving a small opening for the insertion site.

■ After anesthetizing the insertion site, the doctor will puncture the brachial, femoral, subclavian, or jugular vein. Then he'll insert a guide wire or an introducer and advance the electrode catheter.

■ As the catheter advances, watch the cardiac monitor. When the electrode catheter reaches the right atrium, you'll notice large P waves and small QRS complexes. Then, as the catheter reaches the right ventricle, the P waves will become smaller while the QRS complexes enlarge. When the catheter touches the right ventricular endocardium, expect to see elevated ST segments, premature ventricular contractions, or both.

■ When the electrode catheter is in the right ventricle, it will send an impulse to the myocardium, causing depolarization. If the patient needs atrial pacing, either alone or with ventricular pacing, the doctor may place an electrode in the right atrium.

■ Meanwhile, continuously monitor the patient's cardiac status and treat any arrhythmias, as appropriate. Also assess the patient for jaw pain and earache; *these symptoms indicate that the electrode catheter has missed the superior vena cava and has moved into the neck instead.*

■ When the electrode catheter is in place, attach the catheter leads to the bridging cable, lining up the positive and negative poles.

■ Turn the pacemaker on and assist with determining the correct settings (mode, rate, and output).

■ The doctor will then secure the catheter to the insertion site, usually by suturing.

■ Assess and monitor the patient's response to pacing according to your facility's policy.

■ Apply a sterile dressing to the site. Label the dressing with the date and time of application.

■ Discard supplies in the appropriate receptacle.

■ Remove and discard all personal protective equipment and perform hand hygiene.[6,7,8,12]

■ Document the procedure.[14,15]

Special considerations

■ Positioning of the leadwire may be confirmed by ultrasound, fluoroscopy, or chest X-ray.[1]

■ You'll need to take care to prevent microshock. This includes warning the patient not to use any electrical equipment that isn't grounded, such as telephones, electric shavers, televisions, or lamps.

■ Other safety measures you'll want to take include placing a plastic cover supplied by the manufacturer over the pacemaker controls *to avoid an accidental setting change.* Also, insulate the pacemaker by covering all exposed metal parts, such as electrode connections and pacemaker terminals, with nonconducting tape, or place the pacing unit in a dry, rubber surgical glove. If the patient needs emergency defibrillation, make sure the pacemaker can withstand the procedure. If you're unsure, disconnect the pulse generator *to avoid damage.*

■ After insertion of any temporary pacemaker, assess the patient's vital signs, skin color, LOC, and peripheral pulses *to determine the effectiveness of the paced rhythm.* Perform a 12-lead electrocardiogram (ECG) *to serve as a baseline,* and then perform additional ECGs daily or with clinical changes. Also, if possible, obtain a rhythm strip before, during, and after pacemaker placement; any time that pacemaker settings change; and whenever the patient receives treatment because of a complication caused by the pacemaker.

■ Continuously monitor the ECG reading, noting capture, sensing, rate, intrinsic beats, and competition of paced and intrinsic rhythms.[16] If the pacemaker is sensing correctly, the sense indicator on the pulse generator should flash with each beat. (See *Handling pacemaker malfunctions.*)

Complications

Complications associated with pacemaker therapy include microshock, equipment failure, and competitive or fatal arrhythmias. Transvenous pacemakers may cause such complications as pneumothorax or hemothorax, cardiac perforation and tamponade, diaphragmatic stimulation, pulmonary embolism, thrombophlebitis, and infection. Also, if the doctor threads the electrode through the antecubital or femoral vein, venous spasm, thrombophlebitis, or lead displacement may result.

Documentation

Record the reason for pacing, the time it started, and the locations of the electrodes. Also note the date and time, the reason for a temporary pacemaker, and pacemaker settings. Note the patient's response to the procedure, along with any complications and interventions taken. If possible, obtain rhythm strips before, during, and after pacemaker placement and whenever pacemaker settings are changed or when the patient receives treatment for a complication caused by the pacemaker. As you monitor the patient, record his response to temporary pacing and note any changes in his condition.

TROUBLESHOOTING

Handling pacemaker malfunctions

Occasionally, a temporary pacemaker may fail to function appropriately. When this occurs, you need to take immediate action to correct the problem. Follow these guidelines when your patient's pacemaker fails to pace, capture, or sense intrinsic beats.

Failure to pace
This happens when the pacemaker either doesn't fire or fires too often. The pulse generator may not be working properly, or it may not be conducting the impulse to the patient.

Nursing interventions
■ If the pacing or sensing indicator flashes, check the connections to the cable and the position of the pacing electrode in the patient by X-ray. The cable may have come loose, or the electrode may have been dislodged, pulled out, or broken.
■ If the pulse generator is turned on but the indicators still aren't flashing, change the battery. If that doesn't help, use a different pulse generator.
■ Check the settings if the pacemaker is firing too rapidly. If they're correct, or if altering them (according to your facility's policy or the doctor's order) doesn't help, change the pulse generator.

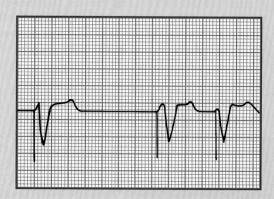

Failure to capture
Here, you see pacemaker spikes but the heart isn't responding. This may be caused by changes in the pacing threshold from ischemia, an electrolyte imbalance (high or low potassium or magnesium levels), acidosis, an adverse reaction to a medication, a perforated ventricle, fibrosis, or the electrode position.

Nursing interventions
■ If the patient's condition has changed, notify the doctor and ask him for new settings.
■ If pacemaker settings are altered by the patient or others, return them to their correct positions. Then make sure that the face of the pacemaker is covered with a plastic shield. Also, tell the patient or others not to touch the dials.

   If the heart isn't responding, try any or all of these suggestions: Carefully check all connections; increase the milliamperes slowly (according to your facility's policy or the doctor's order); turn the patient on his left side, then on his right (if turning him to the left

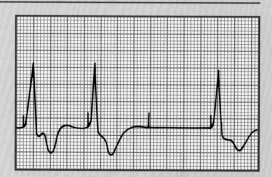

didn't help); reverse the cable in the pulse generator so the positive electrode wire is in the negative terminal and the negative electrode wire is in the positive terminal; or schedule an anteroposterior or lateral chest X-ray to determine the electrode position.

Failure to sense intrinsic beats
This could cause ventricular tachycardia or ventricular fibrillation if the pacemaker fires on the vulnerable T wave. This could result from the pacemaker sensing an external stimulus as a QRS complex, which could lead to asystole, or by the pacemaker not being sensitive enough, which means it could fire anywhere within the cardiac cycle.

Nursing interventions
■ If the pacing is undersensing, turn the sensitivity control completely to the right. If it's oversensing, turn it slightly to the left.
■ If the pacemaker isn't functioning correctly, change the battery or the pulse generator.
■ Remove items in the room causing electromechanical interference (razors, radios, cautery devices). Check the ground wires on the bed and other equipment for obvious damage. Unplug each piece and see if the interference stops. When you locate the cause, notify the staff engineer and ask him to check it.

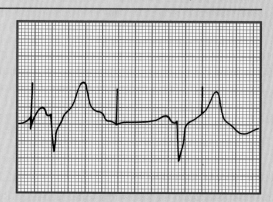

■ If the pacemaker is still firing on the T wave and all else has failed, turn off the pacemaker. Make sure that atropine is available in case the patient's heart rate drops and he becomes symptomatic. Be prepared to call a code and start cardiopulmonary resuscitation.

REFERENCES

1 Lynn-McHale Wiegand, D. (Ed.). (2011). *AACN procedure manual for critical care* (6th ed.). Philadelphia, PA: Saunders.

2 American Heart Association. (2010). 2010 American Heart Association guidelines for cardiopulmonary resuscitation and emergency cardiovascular care. *Circulation, 122*(Suppl. 3), S729–S767. (Level I)

3 Centers for Medicare & Medicaid Services, Department of Health and Human Services. (2006). "Conditions of Participation: Patients' Rights," 42 CFR part 482.13 [Online]. Accessed November 2011 via the Web at https://www.cms.gov/CFCsAndCoPs/downloads/finalpatientrightsrule.pdf

4 The Joint Commission. (2012). Standard RI.01.03.01. *Comprehensive accreditation manual for hospitals: The official handbook.* Oakbrook Terrace, IL: The Joint Commission. (Level I)

5 The Joint Commission. (2012). Standard UP.01.01.01. *Comprehensive accreditation manual for hospitals: The official handbook.* Oakbrook Terrace, IL: The Joint Commission. (Level I)

6 Centers for Disease Control and Prevention. (October 2002). Guideline for hand hygiene in health-care settings. *Morbidity and Mortality Weekly Report, 51*(RR-16), 1–45. (Level I).

7 The Joint Commission. (2012). Standard NPSG.07.01.01. *Comprehensive accreditation manual for hospitals: The official handbook.* Oakbrook Terrace, IL: The Joint Commission. (Level I)

8 World Health Organization. (2009). *WHO guidelines on hand hygiene in health care: First global patient safety challenge. Clean care is safer care.* Geneva, Switzerland: World Health Organization. (Level I)

9 The Joint Commission. (2012). Standard NPSG.01.01.01. *Comprehensive accreditation manual for hospitals: The official handbook.* Oakbrook Terrace, IL: The Joint Commission. (Level I)

10 The Joint Commission. (2012). Standard NPSG.03.04.01. *Comprehensive accreditation manual for hospitals: The official handbook.* Oakbrook Terrace, IL: The Joint Commission. (Level I)

11 The Joint Commission. (2012). Standard NPSG.07.05.01. *Comprehensive accreditation manual for hospitals: The official handbook.* Oakbrook Terrace, IL: The Joint Commission. (Level I)

12 Occupational Safety and Health Administration. "Bloodborne Pathogens, Standard Number 1910.1030" [Online]. Accessed October 2011 via the Web at http://www.osha.gov/pls/oshaweb/owadisp.show_document?p_table=STANDARDS&p_id=10051 (Level I)

13 The Joint Commission. (2012). Standard UP.01.03.01. *Comprehensive accreditation manual for hospitals: The official handbook.* Oakbrook Terrace, IL: The Joint Commission. (Level I)

14 The Joint Commission. (2012). Standard RC.01.03.01. *Comprehensive accreditation manual for hospitals: The official handbook.* Oakbrook Terrace, IL: The Joint Commission. (Level I)

15 The Joint Commission. (2012). Standard RC.02.01.01. *Comprehensive accreditation manual for hospitals: The official handbook.* Oakbrook Terrace, IL: The Joint Commission. (Level I)

16 Drew, B., et al. (2004). American Heart Association scientific statement: Practice standards for electrocardiographic monitoring in hospital settings. *Circulation,* 110, 2721–2746.

ADDITIONAL REFERENCES

American Association for Respiratory Care. (2004). AARC clinical practice guideline: Resuscitation and defibrillation in the health care setting—2004 revision & update. *Respiratory Care, 89*(9), 1085–1099.

Woods, S., et al. (2010). *Cardiac nursing* (6th ed.). Philadelphia, PA: Lippincott Williams & Wilkins.

TRAUMATIC WOUND MANAGEMENT

Traumatic wounds include abrasions, lacerations, puncture wounds, and amputations. A puncture wound occurs when a pointed object, such as a knife or glass fragment, penetrates the skin.

When caring for a patient with a traumatic wound, your first priority is to assess his circulation, airway, and breathing.[1] Once these are stabilized, you can turn your attention to the traumatic wound. Initial management concentrates on controlling bleeding, usually by applying firm, direct pressure and elevating any affected extremity. If bleeding continues, you may need to compress a pressure point. You'll next need to assess the condition of the wound; management and cleaning technique typically depend on the specific type of wound and degree of contamination.

Equipment

Sterile basin ▪ normal saline solution ▪ sterile 4″ × 4″ gauze pads ▪ sterile gloves ▪ clean gloves ▪ dry, sterile dressing, nonadherent pad, or petroleum gauze ▪ linen-saver pad ▪ Optional: goggles, mask, gown, scissors, 50-mL catheter-tip syringe, antibacterial ointment, porous tape, sutures and suture set, clippers, surgical scrub brush.

Preparation of equipment

Place a linen-saver pad under the area to be cleaned. Remove any clothing covering the wound. If necessary, clip hair around the wound with scissors *to promote cleaning and treatment.*

Gather needed equipment at the patient's bedside. Fill a sterile basin with normal saline solution. Make sure the treatment area has enough light *to allow close observation of the wound.* Depending on the nature and location of the wound, wear sterile or clean gloves *to avoid spreading infection.*

Implementation

▪ Check the patient's medical history for previous tetanus immunization and, if needed and ordered, arrange for immunization.
▪ Perform hand hygiene and put on gloves.[2,3,4]
▪ Confirm the patient's identity using at least two patient identifiers according to your facility's policy.[5]
▪ Explain the procedure to the patient.
▪ Perform a comprehensive pain assessment using techniques appropriate for the patient's age, condition, and ability to understand.[6]
▪ Administer pain medication as ordered, following safe medication administration practices.[7]
▪ Put on other personal protective equipment, such as a gown, mask, and goggles, if spraying or splashing of body fluids is possible.

For a traumatic puncture wound

▪ If the wound is minor, allow it to bleed for a few minutes before cleaning it *to help remove possible contaminates from the wound.*
▪ For a larger puncture wound, you may need to irrigate it before applying a dry dressing. The doctor may request a radiologic study *to rule out foreign matter remaining in the wound.*

- Stabilize any embedded foreign object until the doctor can remove it. After he removes the object and bleeding is stabilized, moisten a sterile 4″ × 4″ gauze pad with normal saline solution. Clean the wound gently, working outward from its center to about 2″ (5 cm) beyond its edges. Discard the soiled gauze pad and use a fresh one, as necessary. Continue until the wound appears clean.
- Remove and discard your gloves, perform hand hygiene, and put on new gloves.[2,3,4]
- Assist the doctor with suturing the wound using a suture kit, or apply sterile strips of porous tape.
- Apply the prescribed antibacterial ointment *to help prevent infection.*
- Apply a dry, sterile dressing over the wound *to absorb drainage and help prevent bacterial contamination.*

For a traumatic abrasion
- Flush the scraped skin with normal saline solution.
- Remove dirt or gravel with a sterile 4″ × 4″ gauze pad moistened with normal saline solution. Rub in the direction opposite that from which the dirt or gravel became embedded.
- If the wound is extremely dirty, you may use a surgical brush to scrub it.
- With a small wound, allow it to dry and form a scab. With a larger wound, you may need to cover it with a nonadherent pad or petroleum gauze and a light dressing. Apply antibacterial ointment, if ordered.

For a traumatic laceration
- Moisten a sterile 4″ × 4″ gauze pad with normal saline solution. Clean the wound gently, working outward from its center to about 2″ (5 cm) beyond its edges. Discard the soiled gauze pad and use a fresh one, as necessary. Continue until the wound appears clean.
- If the wound is dirty, you may irrigate it with a 50-mL catheter-tip syringe and normal saline solution.
- Remove and discard your gloves, perform hand hygiene, and put on a new pair of gloves.[2,3,4]
- Assist the doctor with suturing the wound using a suture kit, or apply sterile strips of porous tape.
- Apply the prescribed antibacterial ointment *to help prevent infection.*
- Apply a dry, sterile dressing over the wound *to absorb drainage and help prevent bacterial contamination.*

For a traumatic amputation
- Apply a dry, sterile dressing over the amputation site *to control hemorrhage.* Elevate the affected part, and immobilize it for surgery.
NURSING ALERT *If the patient is actively bleeding, the dressing must be dry or the bleeding may worsen.*
- Recover the amputated part if possible, and prepare it for transport to a facility where microvascular surgery is performed. (See *Caring for a severed body part,* page 756.)

Completing the procedure
- Reassess the patient's pain and respond appropriately.[6]

- Discard used supplies in the appropriate receptacle.
- Remove and discard your gloves and perform hand hygiene.[2,3,4]
- Document the procedure.[8,9]

Special considerations
- When irrigating a traumatic wound, avoid using more than 8 psi of pressure. *High-pressure irrigation can seriously interfere with healing, kill cells, and allow bacteria to infiltrate the tissue.*
- Avoid cleaning a traumatic wound with alcohol *because alcohol causes pain and tissue dehydration.* Also, avoid using antiseptics for wound cleaning *because they can impede healing.* In addition, never use a cotton ball or cotton-filled gauze pad to clean a wound *because cotton fibers left in the wound can cause contamination.*
- After a wound has been cleaned, the doctor may want to debride it *to remove dead tissue and reduce the risk of infection and scarring.* If this is necessary, pack the wound with gauze pads soaked in normal saline solution until debridement.
- Observe for signs and symptoms of infection, such as warm, red skin at the site or purulent discharge. *Be aware that infection of a traumatic wound can delay healing, increase scar formation, and trigger systemic infection, such as septicemia.*
- Observe all dressings. If edema is present, adjust the dressing *to avoid impairing circulation to the area.*
- Large abrasions, or "road rash" may require initial management in the operating room if the abrasion is greatly contaminated.
- An X-ray may be necessary to rule out the presence of a foreign body, especially when gravel or other materials are present in the blood.

Complications
Cleaning and care of traumatic wounds may temporarily increase the patient's pain. Excessive, vigorous cleaning may further disrupt tissue integrity.

Documentation
Document the date and time of the procedure, wound size and condition, medication administration, specific wound care measures, and patient teaching provided and the patient's understanding of your teaching.

REFERENCES

1 Berg, R.A., et al. (2010). Part 5: Adult basic life support: 2010 American Heart Association guidelines for cardiopulmonary resuscitation and emergency cardiovascular care. *Circulation, 122*(Suppl. 3), S685–S705. (Level I)
2 The Joint Commission. (2012). Standard NPSG.07.01.01. *Comprehensive accreditation manual for hospitals: The official handbook.* Oakbrook Terrace, IL: The Joint Commission. (Level I)
3 Centers for Disease Control and Prevention. (October 2002). Guideline for hand hygiene in health-care settings. *Morbidity and Mortality Weekly Report, 51*(RR-16), 1–45. (Level I)
4 World Health Organization. (2009). *WHO guidelines on hand hygiene in health care: First global patient safety challenge. Clean care is safer care.* Geneva, Switzerland: World Health Organization. (Level I)

Caring for a severed body part

After traumatic amputation, a surgeon may be able to reimplant the severed body part through microsurgery. The chance of successful reimplantation is much greater if the amputated part has received proper care.

If a patient arrives at the health care facility with a severed body part, first make sure that bleeding at the amputation site has been controlled. Then follow these guidelines for preserving the body part.

■ Perform hand hygeine.[2,3,4] Put on sterile gloves. Place several sterile gauze pads and an appropriate amount of sterile roller gauze in a sterile basin, and pour sterile normal saline or sterile lactated Ringer's solution over them. *Never* use any other solution, and don't try to scrub or debride the part.

■ Holding the body part in one gloved hand, carefully pat it dry with sterile gauze. Place saline-moistened gauze pads over the stump; then wrap the whole body part with saline-moistened roller gauze. Wrap the gauze with a sterile towel, if available. Then put this package in a watertight container or bag and seal it.

NURSING ALERT *Don't oversoak the gauze because the body part may become macerated.*

■ Fill another plastic bag with ice and water to make an ice-water slurry and place the part, still in its watertight container, inside. Seal the outer bag. (Always protect the part from direct contact with ice—and *never* use dry ice—*to prevent irreversible tissue damage, which would make the part unsuitable for reimplantation.*) Keep this bag ice-cold until the doctor is ready to do the reimplantation surgery.

■ Label the bag with the patient's name, identification number, identification of the amputated part, the health care facility's identification number, and the date and time when cooling began.

Note: The body part must be wrapped and cooled quickly. *Irreversible tissue damage occurs after only 6 hours at ambient temperature.* However, hypothermic management seldom preserves tissues for more than 24 hours.

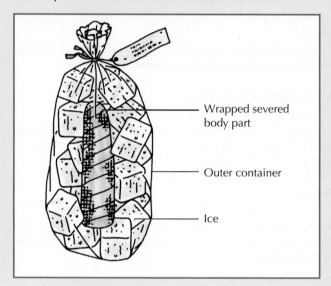

Wrapped severed body part

Outer container

Ice

5 The Joint Commission. (2012). Standard NPSG.01.01.01. *Comprehensive accreditation manual for hospitals: The official handbook.* Oakbrook Terrace, IL: The Joint Commission. (Level I)

6 The Joint Commission. (2012). Standard PC.01.02.07. *Comprehensive accreditation manual for hospitals: The official handbook.* Oakbrook Terrace, IL: The Joint Commission. (Level I)

7 The Joint Commission. (2012). Standard MM.06.01.01. *Comprehensive accreditation manual for hospitals: The official handbook.* Oakbrook Terrace, IL: The Joint Commission. (Level I)

8 The Joint Commission. (2012). Standard RC.01.03.01. *Comprehensive accreditation manual for hospitals: The official handbook.* Oakbrook Terrace, IL: The Joint Commission. (Level I)

9 The Joint Commission. (2012). Standard RC.02.01.01. *Comprehensive accreditation manual for hospitals: The official handbook.* Oakbrook Terrace, IL: The Joint Commission. (Level I)

ADDITIONAL REFERENCES

Ketz, A.K. (2008). Pain management in the traumatic amputee. *Critical Care Clinics of North America, 20*(1), 51–57.

Khan, M.N., & Naqvi, A.H. (2006). Antiseptics, iodine, povidone iodine and traumatic wound cleansing. *Journal of Tissue Viability, 16*(4), 6–10.

Laskowski-Jones, L. (2006). First aid for amputation. *Nursing, 36*(4), 50–52.

Laskowski-Jones, L. (2006). First aid for bleeding wounds. *Nursing, 36*(9), 50–51.

T-TUBE CARE

The T tube (or *biliary drainage tube*) may be placed in the common bile duct after cholecystectomy, choledochostomy, or liver transplant and during treatment for cholelithiasis to promote biliary drainage.

The surgeon inserts the short end (crossbar) of the T tube in the common bile duct and draws the long end through the incision. The tube then connects to a closed drainage system. (See *Understanding T-tube placement.*) Postoperatively, the tube remains in place between 7 and 14 days—potentially longer after liver transplant. T-tube dressings are changed routinely, as ordered, to prevent infection and skin excoriation from bile drainage. The T-tube drainage bag should be emptied every 12 hours unless there's significant drainage or a specific doctor's order. In preparation for removal, the tube may be clamped to assess the patient's tolerance to the return of bile flow and to aid in digestion.

Understanding T-tube placement

The T tube is placed in the common bile duct, anchored to the abdominal wall, and connected to a closed drainage system.

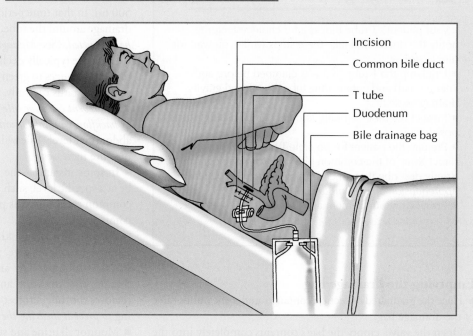

- Incision
- Common bile duct
- T tube
- Duodenum
- Bile drainage bag

Equipment

Clean gloves ▪ small plastic bag ▪ sterile gloves ▪ sterile 4″ × 4″ gauze pads ▪ transparent dressing ▪ normal saline solution ▪ sterile skin cleaning solution ▪ two sterile basins ▪ antiseptic pads ▪ sterile precut drain dressings ▪ hypoallergenic paper tape ▪ skin protectant, such as petroleum jelly, zinc oxide, or aluminum-based gel ▪ clamp or rubber band ▪ clean gauze ▪ graduated collection container.

Implementation

- ▪ Verify the doctor's order and check the patient's medical recorder for a history of allergies.
- ▪ Gather all necessary equipment at the bedside. Label all solution containers and a reusable collection container with the patient's name and date.
- ▪ Perform hand hygiene and put on gloves.[1,2,3,4]
- ▪ Confirm the patient's identity using at least two patient identifiers according to your facility's policy.[5]
- ▪ Provide privacy, and explain the procedure to the patient *to decrease anxiety and ensure cooperation.*

Changing the dressing

- ▪ Raise the bed to a comfortable working height, and position the patient *to allow clear access to the dressing.*
- ▪ Without dislodging the T tube, carefully remove the old dressing *to avoid skin tears.*
- ▪ Dispose of the dressing in a small plastic bag, using standard precautions. Remove and discard your gloves.

- ▪ Perform hand hygiene[1,2,3,4] and create a sterile field. Put on sterile gloves and follow strict sterile technique *to prevent contamination of the incision.*
- ▪ Inspect the incision and tube site for signs and symptoms of infection, such as redness, edema, warmth, tenderness, induration, or skin excoriation. Assess for wound dehiscence or evisceration, if applicable.
- ▪ Use sterile cleaning solution, as prescribed, to clean and remove dried matter or drainage from around the tube. Always start at the tube site and gently wipe outward in a continuous circular motion *to prevent recontamination of the incision.*
- ▪ Use normal saline solution to rinse the area. Dry the area with a sterile 4″ × 4″ gauze pad.
- ▪ Using an antiseptic pad, wipe the incision site in a circular motion. Allow the area to dry thoroughly.
- ▪ Lightly apply a skin protectant, such as petroleum jelly, zinc oxide, or aluminum-based gel, *to protect the skin from injury caused by bile drainage.*
- ▪ Apply sterile precut drain dressings, one from either side of the T tube, *to absorb drainage.*
- ▪ Apply a sterile 4″ × 4″ gauze pad or transparent dressing over the T tube and the drain dressings. Don't kink the tubing, *which may block the drainage.* Secure the dressings with the hypoallergenic paper tape.
- ▪ Return the patient's bed to the lowest position *for patient safety.*
- ▪ Dispose of used equipment and materials appropriately.

TROUBLESHOOTING

Managing T-tube obstruction

If your patient's T tube blocks after cholecystectomy, notify the doctor and take these steps while you wait for him to arrive:

- Unclamp the T tube (if it was clamped before and after a meal) and connect the tube to a closed gravity-drainage system.
- Inspect the tube carefully *to detect any kinks or obstructions.*
- Prepare the patient for possible T-tube irrigation or direct X-ray of the common bile duct (cholangiography). Briefly describe these measures *to reduce the patient's apprehension and promote cooperation.*
- Provide encouragement and support.

Emptying the drainage bag

- Place the graduated collection container under the outlet valve of the drainage bag.
- Open the valve, empty the bag's contents completely into the container, and close the outlet valve, without contaminating the valve, tubing, or clamp, if used.
- Wipe the end of the valve with a clean gauze pad *to remove residual drainage that may remain after closing.*
- Carefully measure and record the character, color, and amount of drainage.
- *To ensure patient comfort and safety,* check bile drainage amounts regularly. Be alert for such signs and symptoms of obstructed bile flow as chills, fever, tachycardia, nausea, right-upper-quadrant fullness and pain, jaundice, dark foamy urine, and clay-colored stools. Report them immediately.
- Discard the fluid appropriately and rinse or discard the container according to your facility's policy.

Clamping the tube

- Occlude the tube lightly with a clamp, or fold the tubing back on itself and wrap a rubber band around the kink. *Clamping the tube 1 hour before and after meals diverts bile back to the duodenum to aid digestion.*
- Monitor the patient's response to clamping the T tube.
- Unclamp the tube at the specified time.
- *To ensure patient comfort and safety,* check bile drainage amounts regularly. Be alert for such signs and symptoms of obstructed bile flow as chills, fever, tachycardia, nausea, right-upper-quadrant fullness and pain, jaundice, dark foamy urine, and clay-colored stools. Report them immediately.

Completing the procedure

- Remove and discard your gloves, and perform hand hygiene.[1,2,3,4]
- Document the procedure[6,7]

Special considerations

- The T tube usually drains 300 to 500 mL of blood-tinged bile in the first 24 hours after surgery. Report drainage that exceeds 500 mL in that time period; if it's 50 mL or less, and there's bile drainage around the tube, notify the doctor *because the tube may be obstructed.* (See *Managing T-tube obstruction.*)
- Drainage typically declines to 200 mL or less after 4 days, and the color changes to green-brown. Monitor fluid, electrolyte, and acid-base status carefully.
- *To prevent excessive bile loss (over 500 mL in the first 24 hours) or backflow contamination,* secure the T-tube drainage system at abdominal level. Bile will flow into the bag only when biliary pressure increases.
- In some instances, the doctor may order the drainage bag to be at a specific level, such as above the insertion point. The most common reason for this positioning is to test the patency of the common bile duct.
- Provide meticulous skin care and frequent dressing changes. Observe for bile leakage, *which may indicate obstruction.*
- Assess tube patency and site condition hourly for the first 8 hours after insertion and then every 4 hours until the doctor removes the tube. Protect the skin edges, and avoid excessive taping *to prevent shearing the skin.*
- Monitor all urine and stool for color changes. Assess for icteric skin and sclera, *which may signal jaundice.*

Patient teaching

Inform the patient that loose bowel movements commonly occur in the first few weeks after surgery. Teach him how to care for the tube at home, including meticulous skin care and dressing changes, and tell him the signs and symptoms of T-tube and biliary obstruction that he should report to the doctor. Caution him that bile stains clothing. Instruct the patient to keep the bag lower than the insertion site *to promote drainage.*

Complications

Obstructed bile flow, skin excoriation or breakdown, tube dislodgment, drainage reflux, and infection are the most common complications related to a biliary T tube.

Documentation

Record the appearance of the dressing and surrounding skin. Record the color, character, and volume of bile collected. Keep a precise record of the patient's temperature, and the amount and frequency of urination and bowel movements. Document any patient teaching provided.

REFERENCES

1 Centers for Disease Control and Prevention. (October 2002). Guideline for hand hygiene in health-care settings. *Morbidity and Mortality Weekly Report, 51*(RR-16), 1–45. (Level I)

2 Siegel, J. D., et al. "2007 Guideline for Isolation Precautions: Preventing Transmission of Infectious Agents in Healthcare Settings" [Online]. Accessed December 2011 via the Web at http://www.cdc.gov/hicpac/2007ip/2007isolationprecautions.html

3 The Joint Commission. (2012). Standard NPSG.07.01.01. *Comprehensive accreditation manual for hospitals: The official handbook.* Oakbrook Terrace, IL: The Joint Commission. (Level I)

4 World Health Organization. (2009). *WHO guidelines on hand hygiene in health care: First global patient safety challenge. Clean care is safer care.* Geneva, Switzerland: World Health Organization. (Level I)

5 The Joint Commission. (2012). Standard NPSG.01.01.01. *Comprehensive accreditation manual for hospitals: The official handbook.* Oakbrook Terrace, IL: The Joint Commission. (Level I)

6 The Joint Commission. (2012). Standard RC.01.03.01. *Comprehensive accreditation manual for hospitals: The official handbook.* Oakbrook Terrace, IL: The Joint Commission. (Level I)

7 The Joint Commission. (2012). Standard RC.02.01.01. *Comprehensive accreditation manual for hospitals: The official handbook.* Oakbrook Terrace, IL: The Joint Commission. (Level I)

ADDITIONAL REFERENCES

Hess, C.T. (2008). *Clinical guide to skin and wound care* (6th ed.). Philadelphia, PA: Lippincott Williams & Wilkins.
Taylor, C., et al. (2011). *Fundamentals of nursing: The art and science of nursing care* (7th ed.). Philadelphia, PA: Lippincott Williams & Wilkins.

TUB BATHS AND SHOWERS

Tub baths and showers provide personal hygiene, stimulate circulation, and reduce tension for the patient. They also allow you to observe skin conditions and assess joint mobility and muscle strength. If not precluded by the patient's condition or safety considerations, privacy during bathing promotes the patient's sense of well-being by allowing him to assume responsibility for his own care.

Patients who are recovering from recent surgery, who are emotionally unstable, or who have casted extremities or dressings in place usually require the doctor's permission for a tub bath or shower.

Equipment

One or two washcloths ■ bath towels ■ bath blanket ■ skin cleaner (such as soap or a hypoallergenic equivalent) ■ nonskid bath mat, if tub lacks nonskid strips ■ nonskid shower chair for shower ■ towel mat ■ bath (utility) thermometer ■ occupied sign ■ clean clothing or hospital gown ■ hospital-grade disinfectant ■ Optional: chair, shower cap, clear plastic bag and tape, bath oil, shampoo or mild castile soap.

Preparation of equipment

Prepare the bathing area before the patient arrives. Close any doors or windows and adjust the room temperature *to avoid chilling the patient.* Check that the bathtub or shower is clean. Then gather bathing articles and observe appropriate safety measures.

For a bath

Position a chair next to the tub *to help the patient get in and out of the tub and to provide a seat if he becomes weak.* Place a bath blanket over the chair *to cover the patient if he becomes chilled.* Fill the tub halfway with water, and test the temperature with a bath thermometer. The temperature should range from 100° to 110° F (38° to 43° C). If you don't have a bath thermometer, test the temperature by immersing your elbow in the water; it should feel comfortable to the touch. Besides the obvious risk of scalding the patient, excessively hot water can cause cutaneous vasodilation, *which alters blood flow to the brain and may lead to dizziness or fainting.* Place a rubber mat in the tub and place a towel mat on the floor in front of the tub *to prevent slipping.*

For a shower

Place a nonskid chair in the shower *to provide support.* The chair also allows the patient to sit down while washing his legs and feet, *reducing the risk of falling.*

Cover the floor of the shower with a nonskid mat unless it already has nonskid strips. Next, place a towel mat next to the bathing area. Remove electrical appliances, such as hair dryers and heaters, from the patient's reach *to prevent electrical accidents.* Adjust water flow and temperature just before the patient gets into the shower. Place a rubber mat in the tub and place a towel mat on the floor in front of the tub *to prevent slipping.*

Implementation

■ Perform hand hygiene and follow standard precautions.[1,2,3]
■ Confirm the patient's identity using at least two patient identifiers according to your facility's policy.[4]
■ Explain the procedure to the patient.
■ Escort the patient to the bathing area, and help him undress as necessary. Offer him a shower cap if he wants to keep his hair dry. Otherwise, provide shampoo or mild castile soap.
■ Help the patient into the tub or shower. Provide washcloths and skin cleaner. If he has dry skin, add bath oil to the water. Wait until after he gets into the tub before adding bath oil *because oil makes the tub slick and increases the risk of falling.*
■ Taking care to respect his privacy, help the patient bathe, as needed; he may appreciate help washing his back. If you can safely leave the patient alone, place the call bell within easy reach and show him how to use it.
■ Tell the patient to leave the door unlocked *for his own safety,* but assure him that you'll post an "occupied" sign on the door. Stay nearby in case of emergency, and check on the patient every 5 to 10 minutes.
■ When the patient finishes bathing, drain the tub or turn off the shower.
■ Assist the patient onto the bath mat *to prevent him from falling.* Then help him to dry off and put on a clean gown or other clothing, as appropriate.
■ Escort the patient to his room or to his bed.
■ Dry the floor of the bathing area well *to prevent slipping.*
■ Ensure that the tub or shower is cleaned and disinfected.[5]
■ Dispose of soiled towels and return the patient's personal belongings to his bedside.

- Perform hand hygiene.[1,2,3]
- Document the procedure.[6,7]

Special considerations

■ If you're giving a tub bath to a patient with a cast or dressing on an arm or leg, wrap the extremity in a clear plastic bag. Secure the bag with tape, being careful not to constrict circulation. Instruct the patient to dangle the arm or leg over the edge of the tub, and keep it out of the water.

■ Encourage the patient to use safety devices, bars, and rails when bathing.

■ *Because bathing in warm water causes vasodilation,* the patient may feel faint. If so, open the drain or turn off the shower. Cover the patient's shoulders and back with a bath towel, and instruct him to lean forward in the tub and to lower his head. Alternatively, assist him out of the shower onto a chair, lower his head, and summon help. If you have an ampule of aromatic spirits of ammonia readily available, break it open and wave it under the patient's nostrils. Never leave the patient unattended to obtain an ampule. When the patient recovers, escort him to bed and monitor his vital signs.

Documentation

Describe the patient's skin condition and record any discoloration or redness in your notes. Document the patient's tolerance of the procedure.

REFERENCES

1 The Joint Commission. (2012). Standard NPSG.07.01.01. *Comprehensive accreditation manual for hospitals: The official handbook.* Oakbrook Terrace, IL: The Joint Commission. (Level I)

2 Centers for Disease Control and Prevention. (October 2002). Guideline for hand hygiene in health-care settings. *Morbidity and Mortality Weekly Report, 51*(RR-16), 1–45. (Level I)

3 World Health Organization. (2009). *WHO guidelines on hand hygiene in health care: First global patient safety challenge. Clean care is safer care.* Geneva, Switzerland: World Health Organization. (Level I)

4 The Joint Commission. (2012). Standard NPSG.01.01.01. *Comprehensive accreditation manual for hospitals: The official handbook.* Oakbrook Terrace, IL: The Joint Commission. (Level I)

5 Rutala, W.A., et al. (2008). "Guideline for Disinfection and Sterilization in Healthcare Facilities, 2008" [Online]. Accessed January 2012 via the Web at http://www.cdc.gov/ncidod/dhqp/pdf/guidelines/Disinfection_Nov_2008.pdf (Level I)

6 The Joint Commission. (2012). Standard RC.01.03.01. *Comprehensive accreditation manual for hospitals: The official handbook.* Oakbrook Terrace, IL: The Joint Commission. (Level I)

7 The Joint Commission. (2012). Standard RC.02.01.01. *Comprehensive accreditation manual for hospitals: The official handbook.* Oakbrook Terrace, IL: The Joint Commission. (Level I)

ADDITIONAL REFERENCES

Burkhart, C.G. (2008). Clinical assessment by atopic dermatitis patients of response to reduced soap bathing: Pilot study. *International Journal of Dermatology, 47*(11), 1216–1217.

Carr, D., & Benoit, R. (2009). The role of interventional patient hygiene in improving clinical and economic outcomes. *Advances in Skin and Wound Care, 22*(2), 74–78.

Craven, R.F., & Hirnle, C.J. (2012). *Fundamentals of nursing: Human health and function* (7th ed.). Philadelphia, PA: Lippincott Williams & Wilkins.

Hoffman, L., et al. (2008). Benefits of an emollient body wash for patients with chronic winter dry skin. *Dermatologic Therapy, 21*(5), 416–421.

TUBE FEEDINGS

Tube feedings involve delivery of a liquid feeding formula directly to the stomach (known as *gastric gavage*). Tube feedings typically are indicated for a patient who can't eat normally because of dysphagia or oral or esophageal obstruction or injury. They also may be given to an unconscious or intubated patient or to a patient recovering from GI tract surgery who can't ingest food orally.

Duodenal or jejunal feedings decrease the risk of aspiration because the formula bypasses the pylorus. Jejunal feedings result in reduced pancreatic stimulation; as a result, the patient may require an elemental diet.

Enteral feedings should be started postoperatively in surgical patients without waiting for flatus or a bowel movement; current literature indicates within 24 to 48 hours.

Patients usually receive tube feedings on an intermittent schedule. However, for duodenal or jejunal feedings, most patients seem to better tolerate a continuous slow drip.

Liquid nutrient solutions come in various formulas for administration through a nasogastric tube, small-bore feeding tube, gastrostomy or jejunostomy tube, percutaneous endoscopic gastrostomy tube, or gastrostomy feeding button. Tube feeding is contraindicated in patients who have no bowel sounds or a suspected bowel obstruction, upper GI bleeding, or intractable vomiting and diarrhea.

Equipment

Feeding formula ■ gloves ■ graduated container ■ sterile water ■ gavage bag with tubing and flow regulator clamp or enteral administration set containing a gavage container, drip chamber, roller clamp or flow regulator, tube connector, and Y-connector (if needed) ■ towel or linen-saver pad ■ 60-mL syringe ■ pH test strip ■ Optional: infusion controller, tubing set (for continuous administration), adapter to connect gavage tubing to feeding tube, carbon dioxide (CO_2) detector designed for gastric tube placement.

A bulb syringe or large catheter-tip syringe may be substituted for a gavage bag after the patient demonstrates tolerance for a gravity-drip infusion. The doctor may order an infusion pump *to ensure accurate delivery of the prescribed formula.*

Preparation of equipment

Be sure to refrigerate formulas prepared in the dietary department or pharmacy. Refrigerate commercial formulas only after opening them. Check the formula against the doctor's orders. Check the date on all formula containers, discarding expired commercial formula. Use powdered formula within 24 hours of mixing.[1] Always shake the container well to mix the solution thoroughly.

Allow the formula to warm to room temperature before administration. *Cold formula can increase the chance of diarrhea.* Never warm it over direct heat or in a microwave *because heat may curdle the formula or change its chemical composition. Also, hot formula may injure the patient.*

Perform hand hygiene and put on gloves.[2,3,4,5] Pour 60 mL of water into the graduated container. After closing the flow clamp on the administration set, pour the appropriate amount of formula into the gavage bag. Hang no more than a 4-hour supply at one time *to prevent bacterial growth.*

If using a sterile, decanted tube-feeding formula, attach the administration set directly to the container. Sterile, decanted formula should have a hang time of 8 hours.

Open the flow clamp on the administration set *to remove air from the lines; doing so keeps air from entering the patient's stomach and causing distention and discomfort.*

Implementation

■ Perform hand hygiene and put on gloves.[2,3,4,5]
■ Provide privacy.
■ Confirm the patient's identity using at least two patient identifiers according to your facility's policy.[6]
■ Inform the patient that he'll receive nourishment through the tube, and explain the procedure to him. If possible, give him a schedule of subsequent feedings.
■ Cover his chest with a towel or linen-saver pad to protect him and the bed linens from spills.
■ Assess the patient's abdomen for bowel sounds and distention.[1]
■ To limit the risk for aspiration and reflux, raise the head of the patient's bed 30 to 45 degrees during feeding and for 1 hour after feeding.[2,8] Use intermittent or continuous feeding regimens rather than the rapid bolus method.

For gastric feeding

■ Check placement of the feeding tube *to be sure it hasn't slipped out since the last feeding.*[1,7]
■ Observe for a change in the external length of the tube by determining whether the mark placed at the tube's exit site has moved.
■ *To check tube patency and position,* remove the cap or plug from the feeding tube, and use the syringe to inject 5 to 10 mL of air through the tube *to clear the tube.* Then, aspirate gastric contents

(as shown below) *to be sure the tube is in the stomach.* Look at the appearance of the aspirate and check its pH.[7] Alternatively, use a CO_2 detector designed for gastric tube placement.

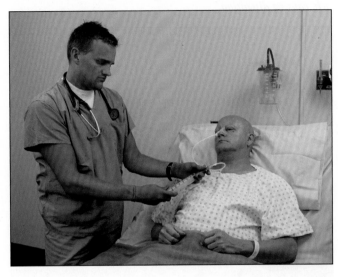

■ *To assess gastric emptying,* aspirate and measure residual gastric volume. Reinstill any aspirate obtained. Hold feedings if residual volume is greater than 500 mL.[1]
■ Flush the feeding tube with 30 mL of water; use sterile water in immunocompromised or critically ill patients, especially when the safety of tap water can't be reasonably assumed.[1]
■ Connect the gavage bag tubing to the feeding tube. Depending on the type of tube used, you may need to use an adapter to connect the two (as shown below).

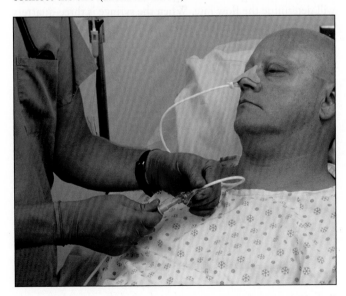

■ Trace the tubing from the patient to its point of origin *to make sure you've connected it to the proper port.*[9]

■ If you're using a bulb or catheter-tip syringe, remove the bulb or plunger (as shown below) and attach the syringe to the pinched-off feeding tube *to prevent excess air from entering the patient's stomach, causing distention.*

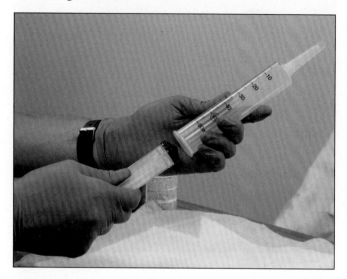

■ If you're using an infusion controller, thread the tube from the formula container through the controller according to the manufacturer's instructions. Purge the tubing of air and attach it to the feeding tube.

■ Open the regulator clamp on the gavage bag tubing, and adjust the flow rate appropriately. When using a bulb syringe, fill the syringe with formula and release the feeding tube *to allow formula to flow through it.* The height at which you hold the syringe will determine the flow rate. When the syringe is three-quarters empty, pour more formula into it (as shown below).

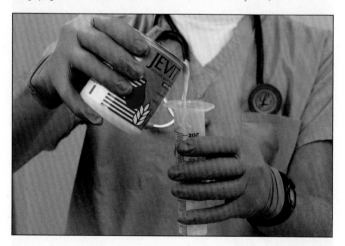

■ *To prevent air from entering the tube and the patient's stomach,* never allow the syringe to empty completely. If you're using an infusion controller, set the flow rate according to the manufacturer's instructions. Always administer a tube feeding slowly—typically 200 to 350 mL over 30 to 45 minutes, depending on the patient's tolerance and the doctor's order—*to prevent sudden stomach distention, which can cause nausea, vomiting, cramps, or diarrhea.*

■ After administering the appropriate amount of formula, add 30 mL of water to the gavage bag or bulb syringe (as shown below) or manually flush the feeding tube using a barrel syringe.[1] *Flushing maintains the tube's patency by removing excess formula, which could occlude the tube.*

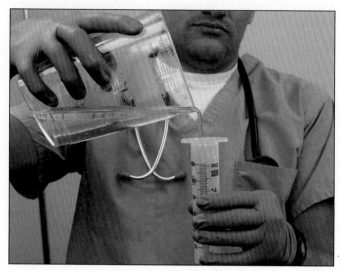

■ If you're administering a continuous feeding, flush the feeding tube with 30 mL of water every 4 hours. Flush the feeding tube with 30 mL of sterile water before and after medication administration *to help prevent tube occlusion.*

■ Measure gastric residual volume every 4 hours for the first 48 hours. After the enteral feeding goal rate is achieved and a small-bore feeding tube is inserted, measure gastric residual volume every 6 to 8 hours if the patient isn't critically ill; continue monitoring every 4 hours in a critically ill patient.[1]

■ To discontinue gastric feeding (depending on the equipment you're using), close the regulator clamp on the gavage bag tubing, disconnect the syringe from the feeding tube, or turn off the infusion controller.

■ Cover the end of the feeding tube with its plug or cap *to prevent leakage and contamination of the tube.*

■ Leave the patient in semi-Fowler's or high Fowler's position for at least 1 hour.[1,7]

■ Rinse all reusable equipment with warm water. Dry it and store it in a convenient place for the next feeding. Change equipment every 24 hours or according to your facility's policy.

■ Make sure that all equipment and products are labeled with the date and time that they were first used or opened.

■ Assess the patient for any discomfort and adverse reactions. Provide appropriate comfort measures as needed.

For duodenal or jejunal feeding

■ If you're using a nasoduodenal tube, measure its external length *to check tube placement.* Remember that you may not get any residual when you aspirate the tube.

■ Flush the feeding tube with 30 mL of water; use sterile water in immunocompromised or critically ill patients, especially when the safety of tap water can't be reasonably assumed.

■ Connect the administration set to the feeding tube, trace the tube from the patient to its point of origin *to make sure it's connected to the proper port,*[8] open the flow clamp, and regulate the flow to the desired rate. To regulate the rate using an enteral infusion pump, follow the manufacturer's instructions for setting up the equipment. Most patients receive small amounts initially, with volumes increasing gradually once tolerance is established.

■ Flush the tube every 4 hours with 30 mL of water *to maintain patency and provide hydration.* A needle catheter jejunostomy tube may require flushing every 2 hours *to prevent formula buildup inside the tube.* A Y-connector may also be useful for frequent flushing. Attach the continuous feeding to the main port and use the side port for flushes.

Completing the procedure
■ Remove and discard your gloves and perform hand hygiene.[2,3,4,5]
■ Document the procedure.[9,10]

Special considerations
■ If the feeding solution doesn't initially flow through a bulb syringe, attach the bulb and squeeze it gently to start the flow. Then remove the bulb. Never use the bulb to force the formula through the tube.

■ If the patient becomes nauseated or vomits, stop the feeding immediately and notify the doctor. The patient may vomit if his stomach becomes distended from overfeeding or delayed gastric emptying.

■ *To reduce oropharyngeal discomfort from the tube,* allow the patient to brush his teeth or care for his dentures regularly, and encourage frequent gargling. If the patient is unconscious, administer oral care with sponge swabs every 4 hours. Use petroleum jelly on dry, cracked lips. (*Note:* Dry mucous membranes may indicate dehydration, which requires increased fluid intake.) Clean the patient's nostrils with cotton-tipped applicators, apply lubricant along the mucosa, and assess the skin for signs of breakdown.

■ During continuous feedings, assess the patient frequently for abdominal distention.[1]

■ If the patient develops diarrhea, notify the doctor and administer small, frequent, less-concentrated feedings, or administer bolus feedings over a longer time. Also, make sure the formula isn't cold and that proper storage and sanitation practices have been followed. *The loose stools associated with tube feedings make extra perineal and skin care necessary.* The doctor may change to a formula with more fiber to help eliminate liquid stools. Studies have shown that banana flakes are also effective at controlling diarrhea in patients receiving tube feedings.

■ If the patient becomes constipated, the doctor may increase the fruit, vegetable, or sugar content of the formula. Assess the patient's hydration status *because dehydration may produce constipation.* Increase fluid intake, as necessary. If the condition persists, administer an appropriate drug or enema, as ordered.

■ Drugs can be administered through the feeding tube. Flush the tubing with at least 15 mL of sterile water before administration.[1] Except for enteric-coated drugs or sustained-release medications, crush tablets or open and dilute capsules in sterile water

before administering them. Be sure to flush the tubing afterward *to ensure full instillation of medication.* Avoid mixing medications together *because of the risk for physical and chemical incompatabilities.*[1] Keep in mind that some drugs may change the osmolarity of the feeding formula and cause diarrhea. Many drugs can be ordered through the pharmacy in a suspension, decreasing the risk of clogged tubes from large drug particles.

■ Small-bore feeding tubes may kink, making instillation impossible. If you suspect this problem, try changing the patient's position, or withdraw the tube a few inches and restart. Never use a guide wire to reposition the tube.

■ Constantly monitor the flow rate of a blended or high-residue formula *to determine if the formula is clogging the tubing as it settles. To prevent such clogging,* squeeze the bag frequently to agitate the solution.

■ Collect laboratory specimens as ordered by the doctor. *Glycosuria, hyperglycemia, and diuresis can indicate an excessive carbohydrate level, leading to hyperosmotic dehydration, which may be fatal.* Monitor urine and blood glucose levels *to assess glucose tolerance.* (A patient with a serum glucose level of less than 200 mg/dL and without glycosuria is considered stable.) Also monitor serum levels of electrolytes, blood urea nitrogen, and glucose as well as serum osmolality and other pertinent findings *to determine the patient's response to therapy and to assess his hydration status.*[1]

■ Until the patient acquires a tolerance for the formula, you may need to dilute it to half or three-quarters strength to start and increase it gradually, as ordered by the doctor.

■ Patients under stress or who are receiving steroids may experience a pseudodiabetic state. Assess such patients frequently *to determine the need for insulin.*

For gastric feeding
■ Check gastric residual volume (GVR) every 4 hours during the first 48 hours for gastrically fed patients. After the enteral feeding goal rate is achieved, gastric residual monitoring may be decreased to every 6 to 8 hours in noncritically ill patients. However, measurements every 4 hours are prudent in critically ill patients.[1]

■ If the GRV is greater than 250 mL after a second gastric residual check, a promotility agent should be considered in adult patients. A GRV greater than 500 mL should result in holding the feeding and reassessing the patient tolerance's using an established algorithm, including physical assessment, GI assessment, evaluation of glycemic control, minimization of sedation, and consideration of promotility agent use, if not already prescribed.[1]

For duodenal or jejunal feeding
■ During continuous feedings, assess the patient frequently for abdominal distention.[1] Flush the tubing by adding 30 mL of water to the gavage bag or bulb syringe. *Doing so maintains the tube's patency by removing excess formula, which could occlude the tube.*

■ Check the flow rate hourly *to ensure correct infusion.*

■ For duodenal or jejunal feeding, most patients tolerate a continuous drip better than bolus feedings. *Bolus feedings can cause*

Managing tube feeding problems

COMPLICATIONS	NURSING INTERVENTIONS
Aspiration of gastric secretions	■ Always keep the head of the bed elevated to a minimum of 30 degrees, preferably to 45 degrees. ■ Discontinue feeding immediately. ■ Perform tracheal suction of aspirated contents if possible. ■ Notify the doctor. *He may order prophylactic antibiotics and chest physiotherapy.* ■ Check tube placement before feeding *to prevent complications.*
Tube obstruction	■ Flush the tube with warm water. If necessary, replace the tube. ■ Flush the tube with 50 mL of water after each feeding *to remove excess sticky formula, which could occlude the tube.*
Oral, nasal, or pharyngeal irritation or necrosis	■ Provide frequent oral hygiene using mouthwash. Use petroleum jelly on cracked lips. ■ Change the tube's position. If necessary, replace the tube.
Vomiting, bloating, diarrhea, or cramps	■ Reduce the flow rate. ■ Administer metoclopramide, as ordered, *to increase GI motility.* ■ Warm the formula to prevent GI distress. ■ For at least 1 hour after feeding, position the patient in semi-Fowler's or high Fowler's position *to facilitate gastric emptying.* ■ Notify the doctor. *He may want to reduce the amount of formula being given during each feeding.*
Constipation	■ Provide additional fluids if the patient can tolerate them. ■ Administer a bulk-forming laxative as ordered. ■ Increase fruit, vegetable, or sugar content of the feeding.
Electrolyte imbalance	■ Monitor electrolyte levels. ■ Monitor intake and output ■ Notify the doctor. *He may want to adjust the formula content to correct the deficiency.*
Hyperglycemia	■ Monitor blood glucose levels. ■ Notify the doctor of elevated levels. ■ Administer insulin if ordered. ■ The doctor may adjust the sugar content of the formula.

such complications as hyperglycemia, glycosuria, and diarrhea. Jejunal feedings should never be bolused *to reduce the risk of bowel rupture.*

Patient teaching

Patient education for home tube feeding includes instructions on an infusion control device to maintain accuracy, use of the syringe or bag and tubing, care of the tube and insertion site, and formula mixing. Formula may be mixed in an electric blender according to package directions. Formula not used within 24 hours must be discarded. If the formula must hang for more than 4 hours, advise the patient to use a gavage or pump administration set with an ice pouch *to decrease the incidence of bacterial growth.* Tell him to use a new bag daily.

Teach family members signs and symptoms to report to the doctor or home care nurse as well as measures to take in an emergency.

Complications

Erosion of esophageal, tracheal, nasal, and oropharyngeal mucosa can result if tubes are left in place for a long time. (See *Managing tube feeding problems.*)

Using the gastric route, frequent or large-volume feedings can cause bloating and retention. Dehydration, diarrhea, and vomiting can cause metabolic disturbances. Glycosuria, cramping, and abdominal distention usually indicate intolerance.

Clogging of the feeding tube is common when using the duodenal or jejunal route. The patient may experience metabolic, fluid, and electrolyte abnormalities, including hyperglycemia, glycosuria, hyperosmolar dehydration, coma, edema, hypernatremia, and essential fatty acid deficiency.

The patient may also experience dumping syndrome, in which a large amount of hyperosmotic solution in the duodenum causes excessive diffusion of fluid through the semipermeable membrane and results in diarrhea. In a patient with low serum albumin levels, these signs and symptoms may result from low oncotic pressure in the duodenal mucosa.

Documentation

On the intake and output sheet, record the date, volume of formula, and volume of water. In your notes, document abdominal assessment findings (including tube exit site, if appropriate), amount of residual gastric contents, tube patency, and verification of tube placement. Also note the amount, type, and time of feeding and the patient's tolerance of the feeding, including nausea, vomiting, cramping, diarrhea, and distention.

Note the result of blood and urine tests, hydration status, and any drugs given through the tube. Include the date and time of administration set changes, oral and nasal hygiene performed, and results of specimen collections.

REFERENCES

1 Bankhead, R. et al. (2009). Enteral nutrition practice recommendations. *The American Society for Parenteral and Enteral Nutrition, 2*(33), 122–167. (Level I)
2 Centers for Disease Control and Prevention. (October 2002). Guideline for hand hygiene in health-care settings. *Morbidity and Mortality Weekly Report, 51*(RR-16), 1–45. (Level I)
3 The Joint Commission. (2012). Standard NPSG.07.01.01. *Comprehensive accreditation manual for hospitals: The official handbook.* Oakbrook Terrace, IL: The Joint Commission. (Level I)
4 World Health Organization. (2009). *WHO guidelines on hand hygiene in health care: First global patient safety challenge. Clean care is safer care.* Geneva, Switzerland: World Health Organization. (Level I)
5 Siegel, J.D., et al. "2007 Guideline for Isolation Precautions: Preventing Transmission of Infectious Agents in Healthcare Settings" [Online]. Accessed December 2011 via the Web at http://www.cdc.gov/hicpac/2007ip/2007isolationprecautions.html
6 The Joint Commission. (2012). Standard NPSG.01.01.01. *Comprehensive accreditation manual for hospitals: The official handbook.* Oakbrook Terrace, IL: The Joint Commission. (Level I)
7 American Association of Critical-Care Nurses. (2009). "AACN Practice Alert: Verification of Feeding Tube Placement" [Online]. Accessed December 2011 via the Web at http://www.aacn.org/WD/Practice/Docs/PracticeAlerts/Verification_of_Feeding_Tube_Placement_05-2005.pdf (Level I)
8 U.S. Food and Drug Administration. (2009). "Look. Check. Connect.: Safe Medical Device Connections Save Lives" [Online]. Accessed December 2011 via the Web at http://www.fda.gov/downloads/MedicalDevices/Safety/AlertsandNotices/UCM134873.pdf
9 The Joint Commission. (2012). Standard RC.01.03.01. *Comprehensive accreditation manual for hospitals: The official handbook.* Oakbrook Terrace, IL: The Joint Commission. (Level I)
10 The Joint Commission. (2012). Standard RC.02.01.01. *Comprehensive accreditation manual for hospitals: The official handbook.* Oakbrook Terrace, IL: The Joint Commission. (Level I)

ADDITIONAL REFERENCES

Hsu, C.W., et al. (2009). Duodenal versus gastric feeding in medical intensive care unit patients: A prospective, randomized, clinical study. *Critical Care Medicine, 37*(6), 1866–1872.
Lynn-McHale Wiegand, D. (Ed.). (2011). *AACN procedure manual for critical care* (6th ed.). Philadelphia, PA: Saunders.
Nettina, S.M. (2010). *Lippincott manual of nursing practice* (9th ed.). Philadelphia, PA: Lippincott Williams & Wilkins.
Taylor, C., et al. (2011). *Fundamentals of nursing: The art and science of nursing care* (7th ed.). Philadelphia, PA: Lippincott Williams & Wilkins.

ULTRAVIOLET LIGHT THERAPY

Ultraviolet (UV) light causes profound biological changes, including temporary suppression of epidermal basal cell division followed by a later increase in cell turnover, and UV light-induced immune suppression. As a result, such skin conditions as psoriasis, mycosis fungoides, atopic dermatitis, and uremic pruritus may respond to therapy that uses timed exposure to UV light rays.

Emitted by the sun, the UV spectrum is subdivided into three bands—A, B, and C—each of which affects the skin differently. Ultraviolet A (UVA) radiation (with a relatively long wavelength of 320 to 400 nm) rapidly darkens preformed melanin pigment, may augment ultraviolet B (UVB) in causing sunburn and skin aging, and may induce phototoxicity in the presence of some drugs. UVB radiation (with a wavelength of 280 to 320 nm) causes sunburn and erythema. Ultraviolet C (UVC) radiation (with a wavelength of 200 to 280 nm) normally is absorbed by the earth's ozone layer and doesn't reach the ground. However, UVC kills bacteria and is used in operating-room germicidal lamps.

The drug methoxsalen, a psoralen agent, creates artificial sensitivity to UVA by binding with the deoxyribonucleic acid in epidermal basal cells. When administered before UVA light treatment, it photosensitizes the skin to enhance UVA's therapeutic effect in a treatment called psoralen plus UVA (PUVA) therapy, or photochemotherapy. Other drugs used in combination with PUVA therapy include acitretin (Soriatane), an oral vitamin A derivative, and methotrexate.

Comparing skin types

SKIN TY	SUNBURN AND TANNING HISTORY
I	Always burns; never tans; sensitive ("Celtic" skin)
II	Burns easily; tans minimally
III	Burns moderately; tans gradually to light brown (average Caucasian skin)
IV	Burns minimally; always tans well to moderately brown (olive skin)
V	Rarely burns; tans profusely to dark (brown skin)
VI	Never burns; deeply pigmented; not sensitive (black skin)

Contraindications to PUVA and UVB therapy include a history of photosensitivity diseases, skin cancer, arsenic ingestion, or cataracts or cataract surgery; current use of photosensitivity-inducing drugs; and previous skin irradiation (which can induce skin cancer). Ultraviolet light therapy is also contraindicated in patients who have undergone previous ionizing chemotherapy and patients who are using photosensitizing or immunosuppressant drugs. PUVA is also contraindicated in pregnant women.

Equipment
For UVA radiation
Fluorescent black-light lamp ▪ high-intensity UVA fluorescent bulbs.

For UVB radiation
Fluorescent sunlamp or hot quartz lamp ▪ sunlamp bulbs.

For all UV treatments
Oral or topical phototherapeutic medications if necessary ▪ body-sized light chamber or smaller light box ▪ dark, polarized goggles ▪ sunscreen if necessary ▪ hospital gown ▪ towels.

Preparation of equipment
The patient can undergo UV light therapy in a health care facility, in a doctor's office, or at home. Typically set into a reflective cabinet, the light source consists of a bank of high-intensity fluorescent bulbs. (At home, the patient may use a small fluorescent sunlamp.)

Verify the doctor's orders to confirm the light treatment type and dose.[1] For PUVA, the initial dose is based on the patient's skin type and is increased according to the treatment protocol and as tolerated. (See *Comparing skin types*.)

Implementation
▪ Confirm the patient's identity using at least two patient identifiers according to your facility's policy.[1]
▪ Inform the patient that UV light treatments produce a mild sunburn that will help reduce or resolve skin lesions.
▪ Review the patient's health history for contraindications to UV light therapy. Also ask whether he's currently taking photosensitizing drugs, such as anticonvulsants, certain antihypertensives, phenothiazines, salicylates, sulfonamides, tetracyclines, tretinoin, and various cancer drugs.
▪ If the patient will have PUVA therapy, make sure he took methoxsalen (with food) 1½ hours before treatment.
▪ Perform hand hygiene.[2,3,4]
▪ To begin therapy, instruct the patient to disrobe and put on a hospital gown. Have him remove the gown or expose just the treatment area once he's in the phototherapy unit. Make sure that he wears goggles *to protect his eyes* and a sunscreen, towels, or the hospital gown *to protect vulnerable skin areas*. All male patients receiving PUVA must wear protection over the groin area.
▪ If the patient is having local UVB treatment, position him at the correct distance from the light source. For instance, for facial treatment with a sunlamp, position the patient's face about 12″ (30.5 cm) from the lamp. For body treatment, position the patient's body about 30″ (76 cm) from either the sunlamp or the hot quartz lamp.
▪ During therapy, make sure the patient wears goggles at all times. If you're observing him through light-chamber windows, you should wear goggles, too. If the patient must stand for the treatment, ask him to report any dizziness *to ensure his safety*.
▪ After delivering the prescribed UVB dose, help the patient out of the unit and instruct him to shield exposed areas of skin from sunlight for 8 hours after therapy.
▪ Perform hand hygiene.[2,3,4]
▪ Document the procedure.[5]

Special considerations
▪ Overexposure to UV light (sunburn) can result from prolonged treatment and an inadequate distance between the patient and light sources. It can also result from the use of photosensitizing drugs or from overly sensitive skin.
▪ To prevent eye damage, the patient undergoing UVB therapy should wear gray or green polarized lenses and the patient undergoing PUVA therapy should wear UV-opaque sunglasses for 24 hours after treatment *because methoxsalen can cause photosensitivity*.
▪ Tell the patient to look for marked erythema, blistering, peeling, or other signs of overexposure 4 to 6 hours after UVB therapy and 24 to 48 hours after UVA therapy. In either case, the erythema should disappear within another 24 hours. Tell him that mild dryness and desquamation will occur in 1 to 2 days. Teach him appropriate skin care measures. (See *Skin care guidelines*.) Advise him to notify the doctor if overexposure occurs. Typically, the doctor recommends stopping treatment for a few days and then starting over at a lower exposure level.

■ Before giving methoxsalen, check to ensure that baseline liver function studies have been done. Keep in mind that both drugs are hepatotoxic agents and are never given together. Liver function and blood lipid studies are required before treatment with acitretin and at regular intervals during treatment. Liver function studies and a complete blood count are required before and during methotrexate treatment.

■ If the doctor prescribes tar preparations with UVB treatment, watch for signs of sensitivity, such as erythema, pruritus, and eczematous reactions. If you apply carbonis detergens to the patient's skin before UV light therapy, be sure to remove it completely with mineral oil just before treatment begins *to let the light penetrate the skin.*

Complications

Erythema is the major adverse effect of UVB therapy. Minimal erythema without discomfort is acceptable, but treatments are suspended if marked edema, swelling, or blistering occurs.

Erythema, nausea, and pruritus are the three major short-term adverse effects of PUVA. Long-term adverse effects are similar to those caused by excessive exposure to sun—premature aging (neurosis, wrinkles, and mottled skin), lentigines, telangiectasia, increased risk of skin cancer, and ocular damage if eye protection isn't used. The patient can minimize effects by using emollients, sunscreens, and cover-ups.

Documentation

Record the date and time of initial and subsequent treatments, the UV wavelength used, and the name and dose of any oral or topical medications given. Record the exact duration of therapy, the distance between the light source and the skin, and the patient's tolerance. Note safety measures used such as eye protection. Also describe the patient's skin condition before and after treatment. Note improvements and adverse reactions, such as increased pruritus, oozing, and scaling.

REFERENCES

1 The Joint Commission. (2012). Standard NPSG.01.01.01. *Comprehensive accreditation manual for hospitals: The official handbook.* Oakbrook Terrace, IL: The Joint Commission. (Level I)
2 Centers for Disease Control and Prevention. (October 2002). Guideline for hand hygiene in health-care settings. *Morbidity and Mortality Weekly Report, 51*(RR-16), 1–45. (Level I)
3 World Health Organization. (2009). *WHO guidelines on hand hygiene in health care: First global patient safety challenge. Clean care is safer care.* Geneva, Switzerland: World Health Organization. (Level I)
4 The Joint Commission. (2012). Standard NPSG.07.01.01. *Comprehensive accreditation manual for hospitals: The official handbook.* Oakbrook Terrace, IL: The Joint Commission. (Level I)
5 The Joint Commission. (2012). Standard RC.01.03.01. *Comprehensive accreditation manual for hospitals: The official handbook.* Oakbrook Terrace, IL: The Joint Commission. (Level I)

ADDITIONAL REFERENCES

Bornstein, E. (2009). A review of current research in light-based technologies for treatment of podiatric infectious disease states. *Journal of the American Podiatric Medical Association, 99*(4), 348–352.
Menter, A., et al. (2010). Guidelines of care for the management of psoriasis and psoriatic arthritis: Section 5—Guidelines of care for the treatment of psoriasis with phototherapy and photochemotherapy. *Journal of the American Academy of Dermatologists, 62*(1), 114–135.
Rogers, C. (2006). Calcipotriol (Dovobet) ointment in combination with UVB therapy for psoriasis treatment. *Dermatology Nursing, 18*(3), 258–261.

UNNA'S BOOT APPLICATION

Named for dermatologist Paul Gerson Unna, this nonelastic paste bandage boot can be used to treat uninfected, nonnecrotic leg and foot ulcers that result from such conditions as venous insufficiency and stasis dermatitis. A commercially prepared Unna's boot is a gauze compression dressing that's impregnated with a preparation known as *Unna's paste* (gelatin, zinc oxide, calamine lotion, and glycerin). The dressing wraps around the affected foot and leg. The boot's effectiveness results from compression applied by the bandage to decrease edema, combined with moisture supplied by the paste.

Unna's boot is contraindicated in patients allergic to any ingredient used in the paste and in patients with arterial ulcers, weeping eczema, or cellulitis.

Equipment

Gauze sponge with ordered cleaning agent ■ normal saline solution ■ commercially prepared paste bandage impregnated with zinc oxide, glycerin, gelatin, and possibly calamine ■ bandage scissors ■ gloves ■ elastic bandage or self-adherent wrap to cover Unna's boot ■ Optional: extra gauze for excessive drainage.

Implementation

■ Verify the doctor's orders.[1]
■ Confirm the patient's identity using at least two patient identifiers according to your facility's policy.[2]
■ Explain the procedure to the patient and provide privacy.
■ Perform hand hygiene and put on gloves.[3,4,5]
■ Assess the ulcer and the surrounding skin. Evaluate ulcer size, drainage, and appearance.
■ Perform a neurovascular assessment of the affected foot *to ensure adequate circulation.* If you don't detect a pulse in the foot by palpation or Doppler, check with the ordering doctor before applying Unna's boot.
■ Place the patient in a supine position, elevating the leg on which you're going to place Unna's boot.
■ Open all the bandage wrappers. Make sure that you have enough supplies to cover the extremity.
■ Have the patient dorsiflex his foot 90 degrees.
■ Clean the affected area gently with the sponge and cleaning agent *to retard bacterial growth and to remove dirt and wound debris, which may create pressure points after you apply the bandage.* Rinse with normal saline solution.
■ Apply the prepared bandage in a spiral motion without tension, from just above the toes to 1″ (2.5 cm) below the knee. Be sure to cover the heel. The wrap should be snug but not tight. *To cover the area completely,* make sure each turn overlaps the previous one by one-half of the bandage width. (See *How to wrap Unna's boot.*)
■ Continue wrapping the patient's leg up to the knee, using firm, even pressure. Stop the dressing 1″ below the popliteal fossa *to prevent irritation when the knee is bent.* Mold the boot with your free hand as you apply the bandage *to make it smooth and even.*
■ Cover the boot with an elastic bandage *to provide external compression.*

■ Instruct the patient to remain in bed with his leg outstretched and elevated on a pillow until the paste dries (approximately 30 minutes). Observe the patient's foot for signs of impairment, such as cyanosis, loss of feeling, and swelling. *These signs indicate that the bandage is too tight and must be removed.*
■ Leave the boot on for 3 to 7 days or as ordered. Instruct the patient to walk on and handle the wrap carefully to avoid damaging it. Tell him the boot will stiffen but won't be as hard as a cast.
■ Change the boot weekly or as ordered *to assess the underlying skin and ulcer healing.* The boot should also be changed when the patient detects a loosening of the boot or anytime the wrap becomes saturated with drainage. Remove the boot by unwrapping the bandage from the knee back to the foot.
■ Remove and discard your gloves. Perform hand hygiene.[3,4,5]
■ Document the procedure.[6]

Special considerations

■ If the boot is applied over a swollen leg, it must be changed as the edema subsides—if necessary, more frequently than every 5 days.
■ Don't make reverse turns while wrapping the bandage. *This could create excessive pressure areas that may cause discomfort as the bandage hardens.*
■ For bathing, instruct the patient to cover the boot with a plastic bag sealed at the knee with an elastic bandage *to avoid wetting the boot. A wet boot softens and loses its effectiveness.* If the patient's safety is a concern, instruct him to take a sponge bath.
■ Other two- or four-layer wraps are available that follow the same principles as Unna's boot. Some products can be removed daily, such as compression stockings, which require measurement for accurate fit after any edema has subsided.

Complications

Contact dermatitis may result from hypersensitivity to Unna's paste.

Documentation

Record the date and time of application and the presence of a pulse in the affected foot. Specify which leg you bandaged. Describe the appearance of the patient's skin before and after boot application. Name the equipment used (a commercially prepared bandage or Unna's paste and lightweight gauze). Describe any allergic reaction.

REFERENCES

1 The Joint Commission. (2012). Standard MM.04.01.01. *Comprehensive accreditation manual for hospitals: The official handbook.* Oakbrook Terrace, IL: The Joint Commission. (Level I)
2 The Joint Commission. (2012). Standard NPSG.01.01.01. *Comprehensive accreditation manual for hospitals: The official handbook.* Oakbrook Terrace, IL: The Joint Commission. (Level I)
3 Centers for Disease Control and Prevention. (October 2002). Guideline for hand hygiene in health-care settings. *Morbidity and Mortality Weekly Report, 51*(RR-16), 1–45. (Level I)
4 World Health Organization. (2009). *WHO guidelines on hand hygiene in health care: First global patient safety challenge. Clean care is safer care.* Geneva, Switzerland: World Health Organization. (Level I)

5   The Joint Commission. (2012). Standard NPSG.07.01.01. *Comprehensive accreditation manual for hospitals: The official handbook.* Oakbrook Terrace, IL: The Joint Commission. (Level I)

6   The Joint Commission. (2012). Standard RC.01.03.01. *Comprehensive accreditation manual for hospitals: The official handbook.* Oakbrook Terrace, IL: The Joint Commission. (Level I)

ADDITIONAL REFERENCES

Grace, P. (Ed.). (2006). *Leg ulcer guidelines: A pocket guide for practice.* Dublin, Ireland: Smith & Nephew, Ltd.

Wound, Ostomy and Continence Nurses Society. (2005). *Guideline for management of wounds in patients with lower-extremity venous disease.* Glenview, IL: WOCN.

URINARY DIVERSION STOMA CARE

Urinary diversions provide an alternative route for urine flow when a disorder, such as an invasive bladder tumor, impedes normal drainage. A permanent urinary diversion is indicated in any condition that requires a total cystectomy. In conditions requiring temporary urinary drainage or diversion, a suprapubic or urethral catheter is usually inserted to divert the flow of urine temporarily. The catheter remains in place until the incision heals.

Urinary diversions may also be indicated for patients with neurogenic bladder, congenital anomaly, traumatic injury to the lower urinary tract, or severe chronic urinary tract infection.

Ileal conduit and continent urinary diversion are the two types of permanent urinary diversions with stomas. (See *Types of permanent urinary diversion*, page 770.) These procedures usually require the patient to wear a urine-collection appliance and to care for the stoma created during surgery. Evaluation by a wound ostomy continence nurse will facilitate site selection and postoperative stoma care.

Equipment

Soap and warm water ▪ gloves ▪ waste receptacle (such as an impervious or wax-coated bag) ▪ linen-saver pad ▪ hypoallergenic paper tape ▪ antiseptic swab ▪ urine collection container ▪ rubber catheter (usually #14 or #16 French) ▪ stoma measuring guide ▪ scissors ▪ urine-collection appliance (with or without antireflux valve) ▪ graduated cylinder ▪ cottonless gauze pads (some rolled, some flat) ▪ washcloth ▪ skin barrier in liquid, paste, wafer, or sheet form ▪ stoma covering (nonadherent gauze pad or panty liner) ▪ two pairs of gloves ▪ Optional: liquid skin sealant, adhesive remover pads, irrigating syringe, tampon, hair dryer, hair clipper, regular gauze pads, vinegar, deodorant tablets.

Commercially packaged stoma care kits are available. In place of soap and water, you can use adhesive remover pads, if available.

Some appliances come with a semipermeable skin barrier (impermeable to liquid but permeable to vapor and oxygen, which is essential for maintaining skin integrity). Wafer-type barriers may offer more protection against irritation than adhesive appliances. For example, a carbon-zinc barrier is economical and easy to apply. Its puttylike consistency allows it to be rolled between the palms to form a "washer" that can encircle the base of the

How to wrap Unna's boot

After cleaning and drying the patient's skin thoroughly, flex his knee. Then, starting with the foot positioned at a right angle to the leg, wrap the medicated gauze bandage firmly—not tightly—around the patient's foot. Wrap the bandage twice around the patient's toes without tension. Make sure the dressing covers the heel. Continue wrapping upward, overlapping the dressing 50% or more with each turn. Smooth the boot with your free hand as you go (as shown below).

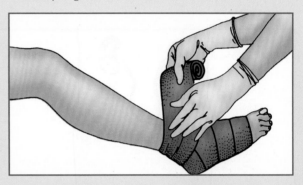

Stop wrapping about 1″ (2.5 cm) below the knee. If necessary, make a 2″ (5-cm) slit in the boot just below the knee *to relieve constriction that may develop as the dressing hardens.*

If drainage is excessive, you may wrap a roller gauze dressing over the Unna's boot. As the final layer, wrap an elastic bandage in a figure-eight pattern.

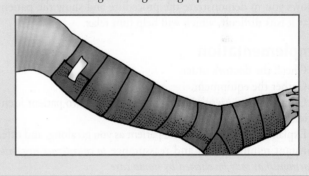

stoma. This barrier can withstand enzymes, acids, and other damaging discharge material. All semipermeable barriers are easily removed along with the adhesive, causing less damage to the skin.

Preparation of equipment

Gather all the equipment on the patient's overbed table. Tape the waste receptacle to the table *for ready access.* Provide privacy for the patient, perform hand hygiene[1,2,3] and follow standard precautions. Measure the diameter of the stoma with the measuring guide. Cut the opening of the appliance with the scissors—it shouldn't be more than ⅛″ to ⅙″ (0.3 to 0.4 cm) larger than the diameter of the stoma. Moisten the faceplate of the appliance with a small amount of water or liquid skin sealant *to prepare it*

Types of permanent urinary diversion

The steps involved in creating an ileal conduit or a continent urinary diversion are described below.

Ileal conduit

A segment of the ileum is excised, and the two ends of the ileum that result from excision of the segment are sutured closed. Then the ureters are dissected from the bladder and anastomosed to the ileal segment. One end of the ileal segment is closed with sutures; the opposite end is brought through the abdominal wall, forming a stoma.

Continent urinary diversion (Indiana pouch)

The surgeon introduces the ureters into a segment of ileum and cecum. Urine is drained periodically by inserting a catheter into the stoma.

Another type of continent urinary diversion (Kock pouch) is "hooked" back to the male urethra, making a stoma unnecessary.

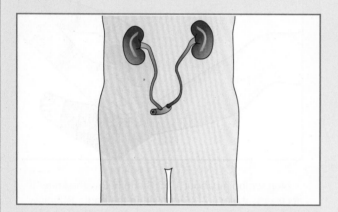

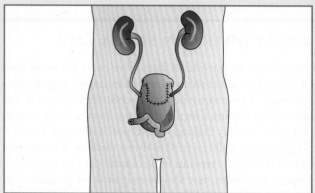

for adhesion. Performing these preliminary steps at the bedside allows you to demonstrate the procedure and show the patient that it isn't difficult, which will help him relax.

Implementation

- Check the doctor's order.
- Gather the equipment.
- Confirm the patient's identity using at least two patient identifiers according to your facility's policy.[4]
- Explain the procedure to the patient as you go along, and offer constant reinforcement and reassurance *to counteract negative reactions that may be elicited by stoma care.*
- Place the bed in low Fowler's position so the patient's abdomen is flat. *This position eliminates skin folds that could cause the appliance to slip or irritate the skin and allows the patient to observe or participate.*
- Perform hand hygiene again and put on gloves.[1,2,3]
- Place the linen-saver pad under the patient's side, near the stoma.
- Open the drain valve of the appliance being replaced *to empty the urine into the graduated cylinder.* Then, *to remove the appliance,* use a washcloth to apply soap and water or use an adhesive remover pad as you gently push the skin back from the pouch.
- If the appliance is disposable, discard it into the waste receptacle. If it's reusable, clean it with soap and lukewarm water and let it air-dry.

- *To prevent a constant flow of urine onto the skin while you're changing the appliance,* wick the urine with an absorbent, lint-free material. (See *Wicking urine from a stoma.*)
- Use water to carefully wash off any crystal deposits that may have formed around the stoma. If urine has stagnated and has a strong odor, use soap to wash it off. Be sure to rinse thoroughly *to remove any oily residue that could cause the appliance to slip.*
- Follow your facility's skin care protocol to treat any minor skin problems.
- Dry the peristomal area thoroughly with a gauze pad *because moisture will keep the appliance from sticking.* Use a hair dryer if you wish. Remove any hair from the area with clippers *to prevent hair follicles from becoming irritated when the pouch is removed, which can cause folliculitis.*
- Inspect the stoma *to see if it's healing properly and to detect complications.* Check the color and the appearance of the suture line, and examine any moisture or drainage. Inspect the peristomal skin for redness, irritation, and intactness.
- For a pouch with an attached skin barrier (one-piece system), measure the stoma with the measuring guide. Select an opening size that matches the stoma.
- For an adhesive-backed pouch with a separate skin barrier (two-piece), measure the stoma with the measuring guide and select the opening that matches the stoma. Trace the selected size opening onto the paper back of the skin barrier's adhesive side. Cut out the opening. (If the pouch has precut openings, which

can be handy for a round stoma, select an opening no more than ⅛" [0.3 cm] larger than the stoma. If the pouch comes without an opening, cut a hole ⅛" wider than the measured tracing.) Many pouching systems can be fit up to the stoma's edge without risk of trauma to the stoma. The cut-to-fit system works best for an irregularly shaped stoma.

■ If you're using a barrier paste, open the tube, squeeze out a small amount, and then discard it. Then squeeze a ribbon of paste directly onto the peristomal skin about ½" (1.3 cm) from the stoma, making a complete circle. Make several more concentric circles outward. Dip your fingers into lukewarm water, and smooth the paste until the skin is completely covered from the edge of the stoma to 3" to 4" (7.5 to 10 cm) outward. The paste should be ¼" to ½" (0.6 to 1.3 cm) thick.

■ Remove the material used for wicking urine, and place it in the waste receptacle.

■ Center the one-piece system over the stoma, adhesive side down, and gently press it to the skin. When using a two-piece system, apply the wafer; then gently press the pouch opening onto the ring until it snaps into place. When using a two-piece adhesive coupling device, line up the adhesive portion of the pouch to the "landing zone" of the wafer. Press together for adhesion. If the patient is still experiencing incisional discomfort, the pouches used in a two-piece system can be attached to the wafer before application.

■ Dispose of the used materials appropriately.

■ Encourage the patient to stay quietly in position for 5 minutes *to promote appliance adhesion.*

■ Remove and discard your gloves and perform hand hygiene.[1,2,3]

■ Document the procedure.[5]

Special considerations

■ The patient's attitude toward his urinary diversion stoma plays a big part in determining how well he'll adjust to it. *To encourage a positive attitude,* help him get used to the idea of caring for his stoma and the appliance as though they're natural extensions of himself. When teaching him to perform the procedure, give him written instructions and provide positive reinforcement after he completes each step. Suggest that he perform the procedure in the morning when urine flows most slowly.

■ Help the patient choose between disposable and reusable appliances by telling him the advantages and disadvantages of each. Emphasize the importance of correct placement and of a well-fitted appliance *to prevent seepage of urine onto the skin.* When positioned correctly, most appliances remain in place for at least 3 days and for as long as 5 days if no leakage occurs. After 5 days, the appliance should be changed. With the improved adhesives and pouches available, belts aren't always necessary.

■ Because urine flows constantly, it accumulates quickly, becoming even heavier than stools. *To prevent the weight of the urine from loosening the seal around the stoma and separating the* appliance *from the skin,* tell the patient to empty the appliance through the drain valve when it's one-third to one-half full.

■ Instruct the patient to connect his appliance to a urine-collection container before he goes to sleep. *The continuous flow*

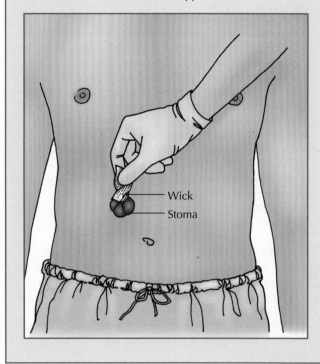

Wicking urine from a stoma

Use a piece of rolled, cottonless gauze or a tampon to wick urine from a stoma. Working by capillary action, wicking absorbs urine while you prepare the patient's skin to hold a urine-collection appliance.

Wick
Stoma

of urine into the container during the night prevents the urine from accumulating and stagnating in the appliance.

■ Teach the patient sanitary and dietary measures that can protect the peristomal skin and control the odor that commonly results from alkaline urine, infection, or poor hygiene. Reusable appliances should be washed with soap and lukewarm water and then air-dried thoroughly *to prevent brittleness.* Soaking the appliance in vinegar and water or placing deodorant tablets in it can further dissipate stubborn odors. Generous fluid intake also helps to reduce odors by diluting the urine.

■ Tell the patient that mucus may normally be present in the urine.

■ If the patient has a continent urinary diversion, make sure you know how to meet his special needs. (See *Caring for the patient with a continent urinary diversion,* page 772.)

■ Tell the patient about ostomy clubs and the American Cancer Society. Members of these organizations routinely visit health care facilities to explain ostomy care and the types of appliances available and to help patients learn to function normally with a stoma.

Patient teaching

The patient or a family member can learn to care for a urinary diversion stoma at home. However, the patient's emotional adjustment to the stoma must be given special consideration before he

Caring for the patient with a continent urinary diversion

In this procedure, an alternative to the traditional ileal conduit, a pouch created from the ascending colon and terminal ileum serves as a new bladder, which empties through a stoma. To drain urine continuously, several drains are inserted into this reconstructed bladder and left in place for 3 to 6 weeks until the new stoma heals. The patient will be discharged from the health care facility with the drains in place. He'll return to have them removed and to learn to catheterize his stoma.

First hospitalization care

■ Immediately after surgery, monitor intake and output from each drain. Be alert for decreased output, *which may indicate that urine flow is obstructed.*
■ Watch for common postoperative complications, such as infection or bleeding. Also watch for signs of urinary leakage, which include increased abdominal distention and urine appearing around the drains or midline incision.
■ Irrigate the drains as ordered.
■ Clean the area around the drains daily—first with an antiseptic swab and then with sterile water. Apply a dry, sterile dressing to the area. Use precut 4″ × 4″ drain dressings around the drains to absorb leakage.
■ To increase the patient's mobility and comfort, connect the drains to a leg bag.

Second hospitalization or outpatient care

■ After the patient's drains are removed, teach the patient how to catheterize the stoma. Begin by gathering the following equipment on a clean towel: rubber catheter (usually #14 or #16 French), water-soluble lubricant, washcloth, stoma covering (nonadherent gauze pad or panty liner), hypoallergenic adhesive tape, and an irrigating solution (optional).
■ Apply water-soluble lubricant to the catheter tip *to facilitate insertion.*
■ Remove and discard the stoma cover. Using the washcloth, clean the stoma and the area around it, starting at the stoma and working outward in a circular motion.

■ Hold the urine-collection container under the catheter; then slowly insert the catheter into the stoma. Urine should begin to flow into the container. If it doesn't, gently rotate the catheter or redirect its angle. If the catheter drains slowly, it may be plugged with mucus. Irrigate it with sterile saline solution or sterile water to clear it. When the flow stops, pinch the catheter closed and remove it.

Patient teaching

■ Teach the patient how to care for the drains and their insertion sites during the 3 to 6 weeks he'll be at home before their removal, and teach him how to attach them to a leg bag. Also teach him how to recognize the signs of infection and obstruction.
■ After the drains are removed, teach the patient how to empty the pouch, and establish a schedule. Initially, he should catheterize the stoma and empty the pouch every 2 to 3 hours. Later, he should catheterize every 4 hours while awake and also irrigate the pouch each morning and evening, if ordered. Instruct him to empty the pouch whenever he feels a sensation of fullness.
■ Tell the patient that the catheters are reusable, but only after they've been cleaned. He should clean the catheter thoroughly with warm, soapy water; rinse it thoroughly; and hang it to dry over a clean towel. He should store cleaned and dried catheters in plastic bags. Tell him he can reuse catheters for up to 1 month before discarding them. However, he should immediately discard any catheter that becomes discolored or cracked.

can be expected to maintain it properly. Arrange for a visiting nurse or an enterostomal therapist to assist the patient at home.

Complications

Because intestinal mucosa is delicate, an ill-fitting appliance can cause bleeding. Bleeding is especially likely with an ileal conduit, the most common urinary diversion stoma, *because a segment of the intestine forms the conduit.*

Peristomal skin may become reddened or excoriated from too-frequent changing or improper placement of the appliance, poor skin care, or allergic reaction to the appliance or adhesive. Constant leakage around the appliance can result from improper placement of the appliance or from poor skin turgor.

Documentation

Record the appearance and color of the stoma and whether it's inverted, flush with the skin, or protruding. If it protrudes, note by how much it protrudes above the skin. (The normal range is ½″ to ¾″ [1.3 to 2 cm].) Record the appearance and condition of the peristomal skin, noting any redness or irritation or complaints by the patient of itching or burning.

REFERENCES

1 Centers for Disease Control and Prevention. (October 2002). Guideline for hand hygiene in health-care settings. *Morbidity and Mortality Weekly Report, 51*(RR-16), 1–45. (Level I)
2 World Health Organization. (2009). *WHO guidelines on hand hygiene in health care: First global patient safety challenge. Clean care is safer care.* Geneva, Switzerland: World Health Organization. (Level I)
3 The Joint Commission. (2012). Standard NPSG.07.01.01. *Comprehensive accreditation manual for hospitals: The official handbook.* Oakbrook Terrace, IL: The Joint Commission. (Level I)

4 The Joint Commission. (2012). Standard NPSG.01.01.01. *Comprehensive accreditation manual for hospitals: The official handbook.* Oakbrook Terrace, IL: The Joint Commission. (Level I)

5 The Joint Commission. (2012). Standard RC.01.03.01. *Comprehensive accreditation manual for hospitals: The official handbook.* Oakbrook Terrace, IL: The Joint Commission. (Level I)

ADDITIONAL REFERENCES

Black, P. (2007). Peristomal skin care: An overview of available products. *British Journal of Nursing, 16*(17), 1048, 1050, 1052–1054 passim.

Burch, J. (2010). Caring for peristomal skin: What every nurse should know. *British Journal of Nursing, 19*(3), 166, 168, 170 passim.

Colwell, J.C., & Beitz, J. (2007). Survey of wound, ostomy and continence (WOC) nurse clinicians on stomal and peristomal complications: A content validation study. *Journal of Wound, Ostomy and Continence Nursing, 34*(1), 57–69.

Haugen, V., et al. (2006). Perioperative factors that affect long-term adjustment to an incontinent ostomy. *Journal of Wound, Ostomy and Continence Nursing, 33*(5), 525–535.

Richbourg, L. (2007). Difficulties experienced by the ostomate after hospital discharge. *Journal of Wound, Ostomy and Continence Nursing, 34*(1), 70–79.

Smeltzer, S.C., et al. (2010). *Brunner & Suddarth's textbook of medical-surgical nursing* (12th ed.). Philadelphia, PA: Lippincott Williams & Wilkins.

World Health Organization (WHO) Consensus Conference on Bladder Cancer. (2007). Urinary diversion. *Urology, 69*(1 Suppl.), 17–49.

URINE COLLECTION, 12- OR 24-HOUR TIMED

Because hormones, proteins, and electrolytes are excreted in small, variable amounts in urine, specimens for measuring these substances must typically be collected over an extended period to yield quantities of diagnostic value. A 24-hour specimen is used most commonly because it provides an average excretion rate for substances eliminated during this period. Timed specimens may also be collected for shorter periods, such as 12 hours, depending on the specific information needed.

Equipment

Large collection bottle with a cap or stopper, or a commercial plastic container ∎ preservative, if necessary ∎ gloves ∎ bedpan, urinal, or bedside commode if the patient doesn't have an indwelling catheter ∎ specimen collection hat ∎ graduated container, if intake and output are being measured ∎ ice-filled basin, if a refrigerator isn't available ∎ specimen label ∎ laboratory request form and laboratory biohazard transport container ∎ patient-care reminders.

Implementation

∎ Verify the doctor's order for specimen collection.
∎ Check with the laboratory to find out which preservatives may need to be added to the specimen or whether a dark collection bottle is required.

∎ Gather the equipment and check the expiration date on the preservative container.
∎ Perform hand hygiene.[1,2,3]
∎ Confirm the patient's identity using at least two patient identifiers according to your facility's policy.[4]
∎ Label the specimen container in the presence of the patient *to prevent mislabeling.*[5] The label should include the patient's name and identification number, the date, the start and end times of the collection, and your initials.
∎ Explain the procedure to the patient and his family, as necessary, *to enlist their cooperation and prevent accidental disposal of urine during the collection period.* Emphasize that failure to collect even one specimen during the collection period invalidates the test and requires that it begin again.
∎ Place the collection container at the bedside or in the bathroom. Place the container in an ice basin, as indicated. Replace the ice as needed. Explain that urine is to be kept and stored in the same collection container during the 12- or 24-hour period.
∎ Explain dietary or drug restrictions, and make sure the patient understands and is willing to comply with them.
∎ Place patient-care reminders over the patient's bed, in his bathroom, and on the urinal or indwelling catheter collection bag. Include the date and the collection interval.
∎ Instruct the patient to save all urine during the collection period, to notify you after each voiding, and to avoid contaminating the urine with stool or toilet tissue.
∎ If the patient is using the bathroom toilet, place a specimen collection hat in the toilet bowl to collect and measure urine.
∎ If possible, instruct the patient to drink two to four 8-oz (480 to 960 mL) glasses of water about 30 minutes before collection begins. After 30 minutes, tell him to void. Measure the amount of urine if output is being recorded. Note this time as the beginning time for the collection.
∎ Perform hand hygiene and put on gloves[1,2,3] to discard this specimen *so the patient starts the collection period with an empty bladder.*
∎ Remove and discard your gloves and perform hand hygiene.
∎ If an indwelling urinary catheter is in place, put on gloves, empty the drainage bag, measure the amount of urine if output is being recorded, and discard all the urine. Note this time as the beginning time for collection.
∎ Perform hand hygiene and put on gloves.[1,2,3]
∎ Measure the amount of urine if output is to be recorded, pour the first urine specimen to be saved into the collection bottle, and add the required preservative if not already present. Then refrigerate the bottle or keep it on ice until the next voiding, as appropriate.
∎ If possible, offer the patient a glass of water at least every hour during the collection period *to stimulate urine production.*
∎ After each voiding, perform hand hygiene and put on gloves[1,2,3] and add the specimen to the collection bottle.
∎ Collect all urine voided during the prescribed period. Just before the collection period ends, ask the patient to void again, if possible. Perform hand hygiene and put on gloves and add this last specimen to the collection bottle. Note the ending time on the specimen label.

■ If an indwelling urinary catheter is in place, perform hand hygiene and put on gloves each time and empty the drainage bag at regular intervals during the collection period. Measure the amount of urine if output is to be recorded, and place each specimen in the collection bottle. When collection time is complete, add the last specimen to the container and note the time on the specimen label as the ending time for collection.

■ Place the collection bottle in an approved laboratory biohazard transport container. Remove and discard your gloves and perform hand hygiene, then immediately send the container to the laboratory with a properly completed laboratory request form.[6]

■ Remove the patient-care reminder signs and inform the patient and family that the specimen collection period is complete.

■ Document the procedure.[7]

Special considerations

■ Keep the patient well hydrated before and during the test *to ensure adequate urine flow.*

■ Before collection of a timed specimen, make sure the laboratory will be open when the collection period ends *to help ensure prompt, accurate results.* Never store a specimen in a refrigerator that contains food or medication *to avoid contamination.*

■ If the patient has an indwelling catheter in place, put the collection bag in an ice-filled container at his bedside.

■ Instruct the patient to avoid exercise and ingestion of coffee, tea, or drugs (unless directed otherwise by the doctor) before the test to avoid altering test results.

■ If you accidentally discard a specimen during the collection period, you'll need to restart the collection. Emphasize the need to save all of the patient's urine during the collection period to everyone involved in his care as well as to his family and other visitors.

■ If the patient must continue collecting urine at home, provide written instructions for the appropriate method. Tell him that he can keep the collection bottle in a brown bag in his refrigerator at home, separate from other refrigerator contents.

■ There is only a 2-hour urine collection for pediatric patients.

Documentation

Record the date and intervals of specimen collection and when the collection bottle was sent to the laboratory.

REFERENCES

1 Centers for Disease Control and Prevention. (October 2002). Guideline for hand hygiene in health-care settings. *Morbidity and Mortality Weekly Report, 51*(RR-16), 1–45. (Level I)

2 World Health Organization. (2009). *WHO guidelines on hand hygiene in health care: First global patient safety challenge. Clean care is safer care.* Geneva, Switzerland: World Health Organization. (Level I)

3 The Joint Commission. (2012). Standard NPSG.07.01.01. *Comprehensive accreditation manual for hospitals: The official handbook.* Oakbrook Terrace, IL: The Joint Commission. (Level I)

4 The Joint Commission. (2012). Standard NPSG.01.01.01. *Comprehensive accreditation manual for hospitals: The official handbook.* Oakbrook Terrace, IL: The Joint Commission. (Level I)

5 The Joint Commission. (2012). Standard NPSG.03.04.01. *Comprehensive accreditation manual for hospitals: The official handbook.* Oakbrook Terrace, IL: The Joint Commission. (Level I)

6 Occupational Safety and Health Administration. "Bloodborne Pathogens, Standard Number 1910.1030" [Online]. Accessed December 2011 via the Web at http://www.osha.gov/pls/oshaweb/owadisp.show_document?p_table=STANDARDS&p_id=10051 (Level I)

7 The Joint Commission. (2012). Standard RC.01.03.01. *Comprehensive accreditation manual for hospitals: The official handbook.* Oakbrook Terrace, IL: The Joint Commission. (Level I)

ADDITIONAL REFERENCES

Craven, R.F., & Hirnle, C.J. (2012). *Fundamentals of nursing: Human health and function* (7th ed.). Philadelphia, PA: Lippincott Williams & Wilkins.

Fischbach, F., & Dunning, M.B. (2009). *A manual of laboratory and diagnostic tests* (8th ed.). Philadelphia, PA: Lippincott Williams & Wilkins.

Nettina, S.M. (2010). *Lippincott manual of nursing practice* (9th ed.). Philadelphia, PA: Lippincott Williams & Wilkins.

Tormo, C., et al. (2009). Strategies for improving the collection of 24-hour urine for analysis in clinical laboratory: Redesigned instructions, opinion surveys, and application of reference change value in micturition. *Archives of Pathology and Laboratory Medicine, 133*(12), 1954–1960.

URINE GLUCOSE AND KETONE TESTS

Reagent strip tests are used to monitor urine glucose and ketone levels and to screen for diabetes. Urine ketone tests monitor fat metabolism, help diagnose carbohydrate deprivation and diabetic ketoacidosis, and help distinguish between diabetic and nondiabetic coma. Urine glucose testing isn't as accurate as blood glucose testing, and should be used only when blood glucose testing isn't available. However, testing for ketones should be done when the patient is ill or glucose levels are elevated.[1]

Glucose oxidase tests (such as Diastix and Clinistix strips) produce color changes when patches of reagents implanted in handheld plastic strips react with glucose in the patient's urine. Urine ketone strip tests (such as Keto-Diastix and Ketostix) are similar. All test results are read by comparing color changes with a standardized reference chart.

Equipment

Specimen container ■ gloves ■ glucose or ketone test strips ■ reference color chart.

Wear gloves as barrier protection when performing all urine tests.

Implementation

■ Verify the doctor's order for testing.

■ Check the patient's history for medications that may interfere with test results.

- Perform hand hygiene.[2,3,4]
- Confirm the patient's identity using at least two patient identifiers according to your facility's policy.[5]
- Explain the test to the patient, and if he's a newly diagnosed diabetic, teach him to perform the test himself.
- Before each test, instruct the patient not to contaminate the urine specimen with stool or toilet tissue.
- Put on gloves before collecting a specimen for the test.
- Instruct the patient to void. Ask him to drink a glass of water, if possible, and collect a second-voided specimen after 30 to 45 minutes. (See "Urine specimen collection," page 776.)
- Test the urine specimen immediately after the patient voids.

Glucose oxidase strip tests
- If you're using a Clinistix strip, dip the reagent end of the strip into the urine for 2 seconds. Remove excess urine by tapping the strip against the container's rim, wait for exactly 10 seconds, and then compare its color with the color chart on the test strip container. Ignore color changes that occur after 10 seconds. Record the result.
- If you're using a Diastix strip, dip the reagent end of the strip into the urine for 2 seconds. Tap off excess urine, wait for exactly 30 seconds, and then compare the strip's color with the standardized color chart on the test strip container. Ignore color changes that occur after 30 seconds.
- Discard the specimen.
- Remove and discard your gloves.
- Perform hand hygiene.[2,3,4]
- Document the procedure and the test results.[6]

Ketone strip tests
- If you're using a Ketostix strip, dip the reagent end of the strip into the specimen and remove it immediately. Wait exactly 15 seconds, and then compare the color of the strip with the color chart on the test strip container. Ignore color changes that occur after 15 seconds.
- If you're using a Keto-Diastix strip, dip the reagent end of the strip into the specimen and remove it immediately. Tap off excess urine, and hold the strip horizontally *to prevent mixing of chemicals between the two reagent squares*. Wait exactly 15 seconds, and then compare the color of the ketone part of the strip with the color chart on the test strip container. After 30 seconds, compare the color of the glucose part of the strip with the color chart.
- Discard the specimen.
- Remove and discard your gloves.
- Perform hand hygiene.[2,3,4]
- Document the procedure and the test results.[6]

Special considerations
- Keep reagent strips in a cool, dry place at a temperature below 86° F (30° C), but don't refrigerate them.
- Keep the containers tightly closed. Don't use discolored or outdated strips.

Documentation
Record test results according to the information on the reagent containers, or use a flowchart designed to record this information. Indicate whether the doctor was notified of the test results. If you're teaching a patient how to perform the test, keep a record of his progress. Also, record any treatment given as a result of the testing.

REFERENCES
1 American Diabetes Association. (2009). Standards of medical care in diabetes—2010. *Diabetes Care, 32*(Suppl. 1), S13–S61. (Level VII)
2 Centers for Disease Control and Prevention. (October 2002). Guideline for hand hygiene in health-care settings. *Morbidity and Mortality Weekly Report, 51*(RR-16), 1–45. (Level I)
3 World Health Organization. (2009). *WHO guidelines on hand hygiene in health care: First global patient safety challenge. Clean care is safer care.* Geneva, Switzerland: World Health Organization. (Level I)
4 The Joint Commission. (2012). Standard NPSG.07.01.01. *Comprehensive accreditation manual for hospitals: The official handbook.* Oakbrook Terrace, IL: The Joint Commission. (Level I)
5 The Joint Commission. (2012). Standard NPSG.01.01.01. *Comprehensive accreditation manual for hospitals: The official handbook.* Oakbrook Terrace, IL: The Joint Commission. (Level I)
6 The Joint Commission. (2012). Standard RC.01.03.01. *Comprehensive accreditation manual for hospitals: The official handbook.* Oakbrook Terrace, IL: The Joint Commission. (Level I)

ADDITIONAL REFERENCES
Craven, R.F., & Hirnle, C.J. (2012). *Fundamentals of nursing: Human health and function* (7th ed.). Philadelphia, PA: Lippincott Williams & Wilkins.
Fischbach, F., & Dunning, M.B. (2009). *A manual of laboratory and diagnostic tests* (8th ed.). Philadelphia, PA: Lippincott Williams & Wilkins.
International Diabetes Federation. (2005). "Position Statement— Urine Glucose Monitoring: The Role of Urine Glucose Monitoring in Diabetes" [Online]. Accessed February 2012 via the Web at http://www.idf.org/position-statement-urine-glucose-monitoring (Level VII)
Taboulet, P., et al. (2007). Correlation between urine ketones (acetoacetate) and capillary blood ketones (3-beta-hydroxybutyrate) in hyperglycaemic patients. *Diabetes and Metabolism, 33*(2), 135–139.
Wei, O.Y., & Teece, S. (2006). Best evidence topic report. urine dipsticks in screening for diabetes mellitus. *Emergency Medicine Journal, 23*(2), 138.

URINE pH

The pH of urine—its alkalinity or acidity—reflects the kidneys' ability to maintain a normal hydrogen ion concentration in plasma and extracellular fluids. The normal hydrogen ion concentration in urine varies, ranging from pH 4.6 to 8.0, but it usually averages around pH 6.0.

The simplest procedure for testing the pH of urine consists of dipping a reagent strip (such as Combistix) into a fresh specimen of the patient's urine and comparing the resultant color change with a standardized color chart.

An alkaline pH (above 7.0), resulting from a diet low in meat but high in vegetables, dairy products, and citrus fruits, causes turbidity and the formation of phosphate, carbonate, and amorphous crystals. Alkaline urine may also result from urinary tract infection and from metabolic or respiratory alkalosis.

An acid pH (below 7.0), resulting from a high-protein diet, also causes turbidity as well as the formation of oxalate, cystine, amorphous urate, and uric acid crystals. Acid urine may also result from renal tuberculosis, phenylketonuria, alkaptonuria, pyrexia, diarrhea, starvation, renal failure, and all forms of acidosis. Low urine pH is also associated with insulin resistance and metabolic syndrome.[1]

Measuring urine pH can also help monitor some medications—such as methenamine, ammonium chloride, and some diuretics—that are active only at certain pH levels.

Equipment

Clean-catch kit ▪ urine specimen container ▪ gloves ▪ reagent strips that include pH indicators.

Implementation

- Perform hand hygiene.[2,3,4]
- Confirm the patient's identity using at least two patient identifiers according to your facility's policy.[5]
- Explain the procedure to the patient.
- Put on gloves.
- Provide the patient with a specimen container, and instruct him to collect a clean-catch midstream specimen. (See "Urine specimen collection.")
- Dip the reagent strip into the urine, remove it, and tap off the excess urine from the strip.
- Hold the strip horizontally *to avoid mixing reagents from adjacent test areas on the strip.* Then, compare the color on the strip with the standardized color chart on the strip package. This comparison can be made up to 60 seconds after immersing the strip.
- Discard the urine specimen. If you're monitoring the patient's intake and output, measure the amount of urine discarded.
- Remove and discard your gloves.
- Perform hand hygiene.[2,3,4]
- Document the procedure.[6]

Special considerations

- Use only a fresh urine specimen *because bacterial growth at room temperature changes urine pH.*
- Avoid letting a drop of urine run off the reagent strip onto adjacent reagent spots on the strip *because the other reagents can change the pH result.*
- Be aware that urine collected at night is usually more acidic than urine collected during the day.

Documentation

Record the test results, time of voiding, and amount voided.

REFERENCES

1 Maalouf, N.M., et al. (2007). Low urine pH: A novel feature of the metabolic syndrome. *Clinical Journal of the American Society of Nephrology, 2*(5), 883–888.
2 Centers for Disease Control and Prevention. (October 2002). Guideline for hand hygiene in health-care settings. *Morbidity and Mortality Weekly Report, 51*(RR-16), 1–45. (Level I)
3 World Health Organization. (2009). *WHO guidelines on hand hygiene in health care: First global patient safety challenge. Clean care is safer care.* Geneva, Switzerland: World Health Organization. (Level I)
4 The Joint Commission. (2012). Standard NPSG.07.01.01. *Comprehensive accreditation manual for hospitals: The official handbook.* Oakbrook Terrace, IL: The Joint Commission. (Level I)
5 The Joint Commission. (2012). Standard NPSG.01.01.01. *Comprehensive accreditation manual for hospitals: The official handbook.* Oakbrook Terrace, IL: The Joint Commission. (Level I)
6 The Joint Commission. (2012). Standard RC.01.03.01. *Comprehensive accreditation manual for hospitals: The official handbook.* Oakbrook Terrace, IL: The Joint Commission. (Level I)

ADDITIONAL REFERENCES

Craven, R.F., & Hirnle, C.J. (2012). *Fundamentals of nursing: Human health and function* (7th ed.). Philadelphia, PA: Lippincott Williams & Wilkins.
Fischbach, F., & Dunning, M.B. (2009). *A manual of laboratory and diagnostic tests* (8th ed.). Philadelphia, PA: Lippincott Williams & Wilkins.
Taboulet, P., et al. (2007). Correlation between urine ketones (acetoacetate) and capillary blood ketones (3-beta-hydroxybutyrate) in hyperglycaemic patients. *Diabetes and Metabolism, 33*(2), 135–139.

URINE SPECIMEN COLLECTION

A random urine specimen is usually collected as part of the physical examination or at various times during hospitalization. This specimen permits laboratory screening for urinary and systemic disorders; it's also used for drug screening. The clean-catch urine specimen, also called a *clean-catch midstream specimen method,* is commonly used in place of random specimen collection because it provides a virtually uncontaminated specimen without the need for catheterization. Obtaining a clean-catch midstream specimen also provides a specimen that more accurately indicates the constituents of the urine being produced by the body.

An indwelling urinary catheter specimen—obtained by aspiration with a syringe—requires sterile collection technique to prevent catheter contamination and urinary tract infection. This method is contraindicated after genitourinary surgery.

Equipment

For a random specimen

Bedpan, bedside commode, or urinal with cover, if necessary ▪ specimen collection hat (if using the bathroom toilet) ▪ gloves ▪ graduated container ▪ specimen container with lid ▪ specimen label ▪ laboratory request form and laboratory biohazard transport bag.

For a clean-catch midstream specimen

Basin ▪ soap and water ▪ towel and washcloth ▪ sterile gloves ▪ gloves ▪ commercial clean-catch kit, containing antiseptic towelettes and a sterile specimen container with lid and label ▪ laboratory request form and laboratory biohazard transport bag ▪ bedpan or bedside commode, if necessary ▪ Optional: graduated container, specimen collection hat (if using the bathroom toilet).

If a commercially prepared kit isn't used, you'll need gloves, three sterile 2″ × 2″ gauze pads or cotton balls, antiseptic solution, a sterile towel, a specimen label, and a sterile specimen container with lid.

For an indwelling catheter specimen

Gloves ▪ antiseptic pad ▪ 3-mL or 20-mL syringe (depending on volume of urine required for ordered tests) ▪ tube clamp ▪ sterile or nonsterile specimen container with lid (depending on ordered test) ▪ specimen label ▪ laboratory request form and laboratory biohazard transport bag ▪ Optional: 21G or 22G 1½″ blunt-tipped needle.

Implementation

- Verify the doctor's order.
- Perform hand hygiene.[1,2,3]
- Confirm the patient's identity using at least two patient identifiers according to your facility's policy.[4]
- Explain to the patient that you need a urine specimen for laboratory analysis.
- Explain the procedure to the patient and family *to promote cooperation, prevent accidental disposal of specimens, and ensure a virtually uncontaminated specimen.* If possible, provide illustrations *to emphasize the correct collection technique.*
- Assess the level of assistance required by the patient.
- Provide privacy. Allow an ambulatory patient to collect the specimen in the bathroom. Place a specimen collection hat in the bathroom toilet bowl if output is being recorded. For patients with limited activity, use a bedside commode or bedpan.

Collecting a random specimen

- Instruct the patient on bed rest to void into a clean bedpan or urinal; ask the ambulatory patient to void into either one or a specimen collection hat placed in the toilet in the bathroom.
- Put on gloves. Then pour at least 120 mL of urine into the specimen container, and cap the container securely.
- If the patient's urine output must be measured and recorded, pour the remaining urine into the graduated container. Otherwise, discard the remaining urine. If you inadvertently spill urine on the outside of the container, clean and dry it *to prevent cross-contamination.*
- Clean the graduated container and urinal, bedside commode, or bedpan, and return them to their proper storage area.

Collecting a clean-catch midstream specimen, female

- Tell the patient to remove all clothing from the waist down.
- Have the patient clean the periurethral area (labial folds, vulva, and urinary meatus) with soap and water. If the patient requires

assistance, put on gloves and assist the patient with cleaning the periurethral area. Then discard gloves and perform hand hygiene.[1,2,3]
- If appropriate, assist the patient onto a bedpan or bedside commode or walk her to the bathroom. Instruct her to sit far back on the toilet seat or bedside commode and spread her legs.
- Perform hand hygiene and, using sterile technique, prepare the commercial kit or create a sterile field. If assisting the patient, put on sterile gloves.[1,2,3]
- If not using a commercial kit, pour the antiseptic over the sterile 2″ × 2″ gauze pads or cotton balls.
- Open the sterile specimen container and place the cap with the sterile inside surface facing up. Avoid touching the inside, and also instruct the patient to avoid touching the inside of the container *to prevent contamination of the specimen.*
- Assist or have the patient spread her labial folds with the thumb and forefinger of her nondominant hand and wipe the area three times, each time with a fresh antiseptic wipe or the presoaked sterile 2″ × 2″ gauze pads or cotton balls. Tell her or assist her to wipe down one side with the first pad and discard it, to wipe the other side with the second pad and discard it and, lastly, to wipe down the center over the urinary meatus with the third pad and discard it. Stress the importance of cleaning from front to back *to avoid contaminating the genital area with fecal matter.*
- Tell the patient to straddle the bedpan or toilet to allow labial spreading and to keep her labia separated while voiding.
- Instruct the patient to begin voiding into the bedpan, bedside commode, or toilet. Without stopping the urine stream, the patient (or you, if assisting) should move the collection container into the stream, collecting 30 to 50 mL at the midstream portion of the voiding. Then have the patient finish voiding into the bedpan, bedside commode, or toilet.
- If you weren't assisting the patient, put on gloves.
- Take the sterile container from the patient, and cap it securely. Avoid touching the inside of the container or the lid. If the outside of the container is soiled, clean it and wipe it dry.
- Measure the remaining urine (from the first and last portions of the voiding) in a graduated container if intake and output are being recorded. Include the amount in the specimen container when recording the total amount voided.
- Tell the patient to wash her hands.[1,2,3]

Collecting a clean-catch midstream specimen, male

- Have the patient clean the periurethral area (tip of the penis) with soap and water. If the patient requires assistance, put on gloves and assist the patient with cleaning the periurethral area. Then discard gloves and perform hand hygiene.[1,2,3]
- If appropriate, assist the patient onto a bedpan, sit him on or stand him next to a bedside commode, or walk him to the bathroom. If the patient is able to stand and is using the bathroom toilet, instruct him to stand in front of the bowl as for urination. If the patient is unable to stand, tell him to sit far back on the toilet seat or bedside commode and spread his legs.
- Perform hand hygiene and, using sterile technique, prepare the commercial kit or create a sterile field. If assisting the patient, put on sterile gloves.[1,2,3]

■ If not using a commercial kit, pour the antiseptic over the sterile 2″ × 2″ gauze pads or cotton balls.

■ Open the sterile specimen container and place the cap with the sterile inside surface facing up. Avoid touching the inside, and also instruct the patient to avoid touching the inside of the container *to prevent contamination of the specimen.*

■ Assist or have the patient hold his penis with one hand. Use the other hand to clean the meatus and head of the penis with the antiseptic wipes or the presoaked sterile 2″ × 2″ gauze pads or cotton balls. Instruct the uncircumcised male patient to retract his foreskin *to effectively clean the meatus* and to keep it retracted during voiding.

■ Instruct the patient to begin voiding into the bedpan, bedside commode, or toilet. Without stopping the urine stream, the patient (or you, if assisting) should move the collection container into the stream, collecting 30 to 50 mL at the midstream portion of the voiding. Then have the patient finish voiding into the bedpan, bedside commode, or toilet.

■ If you weren't assisting the patient, put on gloves.

■ Take the sterile container from the patient, and cap it securely. Avoid touching the inside of the container or the lid. If the outside of the container is soiled, clean it and wipe it dry.

■ Measure the remaining urine (from the first and last portions of the voiding) in a graduated container if intake and output are being recorded. Include the amount in the specimen container when recording the total amount voided.

■ Tell the patient to wash his hands.[1,2,3]

Collecting an indwelling catheter specimen

■ About 30 minutes before collecting the specimen, clamp the drainage tube *to allow urine to accumulate.*

■ Perform hand hygiene and put on gloves, if necessary.[2,3,4]

■ If the drainage tube has a built-in sampling port, wipe the port with an antiseptic pad. If the sampling port is needleless, attach the syringe to the port. If the sampling port is not needleless, uncap the blunt-tipped needle on the syringe, and insert it into the sampling port at a 90-degree angle to the tubing. Aspirate the specimen into the syringe.

■ Slowly transfer the specimen to the appropriate container and secure the lid.

■ Unclamp the drainage tube after collecting the specimen *to prevent urine backflow, which may cause bladder distention and infection.*

Completing the procedure

■ Remove your gloves and discard them properly.

■ Perform hand hygiene.[1,2,3] Tell the patient to wash his hands also.

■ Label the container with the patient's name and identification number, collection time, and date while in the presence of the patient *to avoid mislabeling.*[4] If needed, complete the laboratory request form. If a urine culture has been ordered, note any current antibiotic therapy on the laboratory request form.[5]

■ Place the specimen in a laboratory biohazard transport bag and send the container and completed laboratory request form to the laboratory immediately or place it on ice *to prevent specimen deterioration and altered test results.*[5]

■ Document the procedure.[6]

Special considerations

■ If the specimen is to be collected by the patient at home, make sure the patient understands the procedure for collection; emphasize the need to avoid touching the inside of the container.

■ For a home specimen, instruct the patient to collect the specimen in the appropriate container with a tight-fitting lid and to keep it on ice or in the refrigerator (separate from food items) for up to 24 hours.

Documentation

Record the time of specimen collection and when the specimen was transported to the laboratory. Specify the test as well as the appearance, odor, color, and any unusual characteristics of the specimen. If necessary, record the urine volume on the intake and output record.

REFERENCES

1 Centers for Disease Control and Prevention. (October 2002). Guideline for hand hygiene in health-care settings. *Morbidity and Mortality Weekly Report, 51*(RR-16), 1–45. (Level I)

2 World Health Organization. (2009). *WHO guidelines on hand hygiene in health care: First global patient safety challenge. Clean care is safer care.* Geneva, Switzerland: World Health Organization. (Level I)

3 The Joint Commission. (2012). Standard NPSG.07.01.01. *Comprehensive accreditation manual for hospitals: The official handbook.* Oakbrook Terrace, IL: The Joint Commission. (Level I)

4 The Joint Commission. (2012). Standard NPSG.01.01.01. *Comprehensive accreditation manual for hospitals: The official handbook.* Oakbrook Terrace, IL: The Joint Commission. (Level I)

5 Occupational Safety and Health Administration. "Bloodborne Pathogens, Standard Number 1910.1030" [Online]. Accessed December 2011 via the Web at http://www.osha.gov/pls/oshaweb/owadisp.show_document?p_table=STANDARDS&p_id=10051 (Level I)

6 The Joint Commission. (2012). Standard RC.01.03.01. *Comprehensive accreditation manual for hospitals: The official handbook.* Oakbrook Terrace, IL: The Joint Commission. (Level I))

ADDITIONAL REFERENCES

Clinical Practice Guidelines Task Force; Society of Urologic Nurses and Associates. (2006). Care of the patient with an indwelling catheter. *Urologic Nursing, 26*(1), 80–81.

Craven, R.F., & Hirnle, C.J. (2012). *Fundamentals of nursing: Human health and function* (7th ed.). Philadelphia, PA: Lippincott Williams & Wilkins.

Fischbach, F., & Dunning, M.B. (2009). *A manual of laboratory and diagnostic tests* (8th ed.). Philadelphia, PA: Lippincott Williams & Wilkins.

Higgins, D. (2008). Specimen collection: Obtaining a midstream specimen of urine. *Nursing Times, 104*(17), 26–27.

Nettina, S. M. (2010). *Lippincott manual of nursing practice* (9th ed.). Philadelphia, PA: Lippincott Williams & Wilkins.

URINE STRAINING, FOR CALCULI

Renal calculi, or kidney stones, may develop anywhere in the urinary tract. They may be excreted with the urine or become lodged in the urinary tract, causing hematuria, urine retention, renal colic and, possibly, hydronephrosis.

Ranging in size from microscopic to several centimeters, calculi form in the kidneys when mineral salts—principally calcium oxalate or calcium phosphate—collect around a nucleus of bacterial cells, blood clots, or other particles. Other substances involved in calculus formation include uric acid, xanthine, and ammonia.

Renal calculi result from many causes, including hypercalcemia, which may occur with hyperparathyroidism, excessive dietary intake of calcium, prolonged immobility, abnormal urine pH levels, dehydration, hyperuricemia associated with gout, and some hereditary disorders. Most commonly, calculi form as a result of urine stasis stemming from dehydration (which concentrates urine), benign prostatic hyperplasia, neurologic disorders, or urethral strictures.

Testing for the presence of calculi requires careful straining of all of the patient's urine through a gauze pad or fine-mesh sieve and, at times, quantitative laboratory analysis of questionable specimens. Such testing typically continues until the patient passes the calculi or until surgery, as ordered.

Equipment

Fine-mesh sieve or 4″ × 4″ gauze pad ▪ graduated container ▪ rubber band, if needed ▪ specimen label ▪ tape ▪ urinal or bedpan ▪ gloves ▪ laboratory request form ▪ three patient-care reminders ▪ specimen container ▪ biohazard laboratory transport bag.

Implementation

- Gather all equipment.
- Perform hand hygiene.[1,2,3]
- Confirm the patient's identity using at least two patient identifiers according to your facility's policy.[4]
- Explain the procedure to the patient and his family, if possible, *to ensure cooperation and to stress the importance of straining all the patient's urine.*
- Post patient-care reminders stating "strain all urine" over the patient's bed, in his bathroom, and on the collection container.
- Tell the patient to notify you after each voiding.
- If a commercial strainer isn't available, unfold a 4″ × 4″ gauze pad, place it over the top of a graduated measuring container, and secure it with a rubber band.
- Leave the container in reach of the patient.
- After the patient voids, perform hand hygiene and put on gloves.[1,2,3]
- With the strainer secured over the mouth of the collection container, pour the specimen from the urinal or bedpan into the container. If the patient has an indwelling catheter in place, strain all urine from the collection bag before discarding it.
- Examine the strainer for calculi. If you detect calculi or if the filter looks questionable, notify the doctor and place the filtrate in a specimen container.
- Label the specimen in the presence of the patient *to prevent mislabeling.*[4]
- Send the specimen to the laboratory in a biohazard laboratory transport bag with a laboratory request form.
- If the strainer is intact, rinse it carefully and reuse it. If it has become damaged, discard it and replace it with a new strainer.
- Remove and discard your gloves and perform hand hygiene.[1,2,3]
- Document the procedure.[5]

Special considerations

- Save and send to the laboratory any small or suspicious-looking residue in the specimen container *because even tiny calculi can cause hematuria and pain.*
- Don't leave calculi in contact with urine or other fluids *because this contact may alter the results of the analysis.*
- Be aware that calculi may appear in various colors, each of which has diagnostic value.

Patient teaching

If the patient will be straining his urine at home, teach him how to use a strainer and the importance of straining all his urine for the prescribed period.

Documentation

Chart the time of the specimen collection and transport to the laboratory, if necessary. Describe any filtrate passed, and note any pain or hematuria that occurred during the voiding.

REFERENCES

1 World Health Organization. (2009). *WHO guidelines on hand hygiene in health care: First global patient safety challenge. Clean care is safer care.* Geneva, Switzerland: World Health Organization. (Level I)
2 Centers for Disease Control and Prevention. (October 2002). Guideline for hand hygiene in health-care settings. *Morbidity and Mortality Weekly Report, 51*(RR-16), 1–45. (Level I)
3 The Joint Commission. (2012). Standard NPSG.07.01.01. *Comprehensive accreditation manual for hospitals: The official handbook.* Oakbrook Terrace, IL: The Joint Commission. (Level I)
4 The Joint Commission. (2012). Standard NPSG.01.01.01. *Comprehensive accreditation manual for hospitals: The official handbook.* Oakbrook Terrace, IL: The Joint Commission. (Level I)
5 The Joint Commission. (2012). Standard RC.01.03.01. *Comprehensive accreditation manual for hospitals: The official handbook.* Oakbrook Terrace, IL: The Joint Commission. (Level I)

ADDITIONAL REFERENCES

Ciacci, C., et al. (2008). Urinary stone disease in adults with celiac disease: Prevalence, incidence and urinary determinants. *Journal of Urology, 180*(3), 974–979.
Craven, R.F., & Hirnle, C.J. (2012). *Fundamentals of nursing: Human health and function* (7th ed.). Philadelphia, PA: Lippincott Williams & Wilkins.
Taylor, C., et al. *Fundamentals of nursing: The art and science of nursing care* (7th ed.). Philadelphia: Lippincott Williams & Wilkins, 2011.

VAGINAL MEDICATION ADMINISTRATION

Vaginal medications include creams, gels, ointments, and suppositories. They can be inserted as a topical treatment for infection (particularly *Trichomonas vaginalis* and monilial vaginitis) or inflammation or be used as a contraceptive.

Vaginal medications usually come with a disposable applicator that enables placement of medication in the anterior and posterior fornices. Administration is most effective when the patient can remain lying down afterward to retain the medication.

Vaginal suppositories can also be inserted as a topical treatment for infection (particularly *Trichomonas vaginalis* and monilial vaginitis) or inflammation. Suppositories melt when they come into contact with the vaginal mucosa, and their medication diffuses topically (as effectively as creams, gels, and ointments).

Equipment

Patient's medication record and chart ▪ prescribed medication and applicator, if necessary ▪ water-soluble lubricant ▪ gloves ▪ small sanitary pad.

Implementation

▪ Verify the order on the patient's medication record by checking it against the doctor's order.[1,2]
▪ Check the medication label three times against the patient's medication record.[1]
▪ Confirm the patient's identity using at least two patient identifiers according to your facility's policy.[3]
▪ If your facility uses a bar code scanning system, scan your identification badge, the patient's identification bracelet, and the medication's bar code.
▪ Provide privacy and explain the procedure to the patient.
▪ Ask the patient to void.
▪ Ask the patient if she would rather insert the medication herself. If so, provide appropriate instructions. If not, proceed with the following steps.
▪ Perform hand hygiene.[4,5,6]
▪ Put on gloves.
▪ Help her into the lithotomy position.
▪ Expose only the perineum.
▪ Wash the vaginal orifice with warm water, wiping from front to back.

Administration of vaginal creams, gels, and ointments

▪ Insert the plunger into the applicator. Then attach the applicator to the tube of medication.
▪ Gently squeeze the tube to fill the applicator with the prescribed amount of medication. Detach the applicator from the tube, and lubricate the applicator.

▪ Expose the vagina by spreading the labia with your fingers.
▪ Insert the applicator as you would a small suppository, and administer the medication by depressing the plunger on the applicator. (See *How to insert a vaginal cream*).
▪ Wash the applicator with soap and warm water and store it, unless it's disposable. If the applicator can be used again, label it *so that it will be used only for the same patient.*

Administration of a vaginal suppository

▪ Remove the suppository from the wrapper and lubricate it with water-soluble lubricant.
▪ Expose the vagina by spreading the labia.
▪ With an applicator or the forefinger of your free hand, insert the suppository about 2″ (5 cm) into the vagina.

Completing the procedure

▪ Remove and discard your gloves. Perform hand hygiene.[4,5,6]
▪ *To prevent the medication from soiling the patient's clothing and bedding,* provide a sanitary pad.
▪ Help the patient return to a comfortable position, and advise her to remain in bed as much as possible for the next several hours.
▪ Document the procedure.[7]

Special considerations

▪ If possible, plan to insert vaginal medications at bedtime, *when the patient is recumbent.*

Patient teaching

If possible, teach the patient how to insert the vaginal medication *because she may have to administer it herself after discharge.* Give her a patient-teaching sheet if one is available. Instruct the patient not to wear a tampon after inserting vaginal medication *because it would absorb the medication and decrease its effectiveness.* Instruct the patient to avoid sexual intercourse during treatment.

Complications

Vaginal medications may cause local irritation.

Documentation

Record the medication administered as well as the time and date. Note any adverse effects and any other pertinent information.

REFERENCES

1 The Joint Commission. (2012). Standard MM.06.01.01. *Comprehensive accreditation manual for hospitals: The official handbook.* Oakbrook Terrace, IL: The Joint Commission. (Level I)
2 The Joint Commission. (2012). Standard MM.04.01.01. *Comprehensive accreditation manual for hospitals: The official handbook.* Oakbrook Terrace, IL: The Joint Commission. (Level I)
3 The Joint Commission. (2012). Standard NPSG.01.01.01. *Comprehensive accreditation manual for hospitals: The official handbook.* Oakbrook Terrace, IL: The Joint Commission. (Level I)
4 Centers for Disease Control and Prevention. (October 2002). Guideline for hand hygiene in health-care settings. *Morbidity and Mortality Weekly Report, 51*(RR-16), 1–45. (Level I)

5 World Health Organization. (2009). *WHO guidelines on hand hygiene in health care: First global patient safety challenge. Clean care is safer care.* Geneva, Switzerland: World Health Organization. (Level I)
6 The Joint Commission. (2012). Standard NPSG.07.01.01. *Comprehensive accreditation manual for hospitals: The official handbook.* Oakbrook Terrace, IL: The Joint Commission. (Level I)
7 The Joint Commission. (2012). Standard RC.01.03.01. *Comprehensive accreditation manual for hospitals: The official handbook.* Oakbrook Terrace, IL: The Joint Commission. (Level I)

Additional references

Nettina, S.M. (2010). *Lippincott manual of nursing practice* (9th ed.). Philadelphia, PA: Lippincott Williams & Wilkins.
Taylor, C., et al. (2011). *Fundamentals of nursing: The art and science of nursing care* (7th ed.). Philadelphia, PA: Lippincott Williams & Wilkins.

Venipuncture

Performed to obtain a venous blood sample, venipuncture involves piercing a vein with a needle and collecting blood in a syringe or evacuated tube. Typically, venipuncture is performed using the antecubital fossa. If necessary, however, it can be performed on a vein in the dorsal forearm, the dorsum of the hand or foot, or another accessible location. The inner wrist is not advised because of the high risk for damage to the underlying structures. Although laboratory personnel usually perform this procedure in the health care facility setting, the nurse may perform it.

Before performing venipuncture, assess the patient for possible risks of venipuncture, such as anticoagulant therapy, low platelet count, bleeding disorders, and other abnormalities that increase the risk of bleeding and hematoma formation.

Equipment

Tourniquet ▪ gloves ▪ syringe or evacuated tubes and needle holder ▪ alcohol pads ▪ 20G or 21G needle for the forearm or 25G needle for the wrist, hand, and ankle ▪ color-coded collection tubes containing appropriate additives (see *Guide to color-top collection tubes,* page 782) ▪ labels ▪ laboratory biohazard transport bag ▪ laboratory request form ▪ 2″ × 2″ gauze pads ▪ adhesive bandage.

Preparation of equipment

If you're using evacuated tubes, open the needle packet, attach the needle to its holder, and select the appropriate tubes. If you're using a syringe, attach the appropriate needle to it. Choose a syringe large enough to hold all the blood required for the test. Label all collection tubes clearly with the patient's name and identification number, the doctor's name, and the date and time of collection while at the patient's bedside.[1,2]

Implementation

▪ Verify the order.
▪ Perform hand hygiene and put on gloves.[3,4,5]

How to insert a vaginal cream

Fill the applicator with the prescribed amount of medication. Then lubricate the applicator, hold it by the cylinder, and insert it into the vagina. *To ensure the patient's comfort,* direct the applicator down initially, toward the spine, and then up and back, toward the cervix (as shown below).

Administer the medication by depressing the plunger. Remove the applicator while the plunger is still depressed.

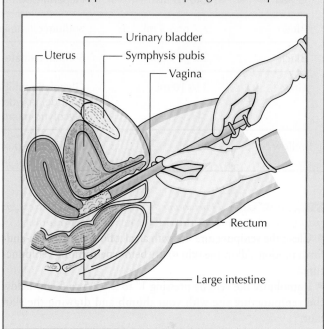

▪ Confirm the patient's identity using at least two patient identifiers according to your facility's policy.[6]
▪ Tell the patient that you're about to take a blood sample; then explain the procedure *to ease his anxiety and ensure his cooperation.* Ask him if he's ever felt faint, sweaty, or nauseated when having blood drawn.
▪ If the patient is on bed rest, ask him to lie supine, with his head slightly elevated and his arms at his sides. Ask the ambulatory patient to sit in a chair and support his arm securely on an armrest or table.
▪ Assess the patient's veins *to determine the best puncture site.* (See *Common venipuncture sites,* page 783.)
▪ Observe the skin for the vein's blue color, or palpate the vein for a firm rebound sensation.
▪ Tie a tourniquet 2″ (5 cm) proximal to the area chosen. *By impeding venous return to the heart while still allowing arterial flow, a tourniquet produces venous dilation.* If arterial perfusion remains adequate, you'll be able to feel the radial pulse.
NURSING ALERT *Don't leave the tourniquet in place for more than 1 minute* because of the risk for hemoconcentration.[7]
▪ If the tourniquet fails to dilate the vein, have the patient open and close his fist a few times. Then ask him to close his fist as you insert the needle and to open it again when the needle is in place.

EQUIPMENT

Guide to color-top collection tubes

TUBE COLOR	DRAW VOLUME	ADDITIVE	PURPOSE
Red	2 to 20 mL	None	Serum studies
Lavender	2 to 10 mL	EDTA	Whole-blood studies
Green	2 to 15 mL	Heparin (sodium, lithium, or ammonium)	Plasma studies
Blue	2.7 or 4.5 mL	Sodium citrate and citric acid	Coagulation studies on plasma
Black	2.7 or 4.5 mL	Sodium oxalate	Coagulation studies on plasma
Gray	3 to 10 mL	Glycolytic inhibitor, such as sodium fluoride, powdered oxalate, or glycolytic-microbial inhibitor	Glucose determinations on serum or plasma
Yellow	12 mL	Acid-citrate-dextrose	Whole-blood studies

NURSING ALERT *Don't allow the patient to open and close his fist vigorously* because of the risk for hemoconcentration.[7]

■ Clean the venipuncture site with an alcohol pad in a back-and-forth motion. Allow the skin to dry before performing venipuncture.

■ Immobilize the vein by pressing 1″ to 2″ (2.5 to 5 cm) below the venipuncture site with your thumb and drawing the skin taut.[7]

■ Position the needle holder or syringe with the needle bevel up and the shaft parallel to the path of the vein and at a 30-degree angle to the arm. Insert the needle into the vein. If you're using a syringe, venous blood will appear in the hub; withdraw the blood slowly, pulling the plunger of the syringe gently *to create steady suction* until you obtain the required sample. *Pulling the plunger too forcibly may collapse the vein.* If you're using a needle holder and an evacuated tube, grasp the holder securely to stabilize it in the vein, and push down on the collection tube until the needle punctures the rubber stopper. Blood will flow into the tube automatically.

■ Remove the tourniquet as soon as blood flows adequately *to prevent stasis and hemoconcentration, which can impair test results.* If the flow is sluggish, leave the tourniquet in place longer, but always remove it before withdrawing the needle.

■ Continue to fill the required tubes, removing one and inserting another. Gently rotate each tube as you remove it *to help mix the additive with the sample.*

■ After you've drawn the sample, place a gauze pad over the puncture site, and slowly and gently remove the needle from the vein. When using an evacuated tube, remove it from the needle holder *to release the vacuum* before withdrawing the needle from the vein. Activate the needle protector safety device, if necessary.

■ Apply gentle pressure to the puncture site for 2 or 3 minutes or until bleeding stops. *This prevents extravasation into the surrounding tissue, which can cause a hematoma.*[1]

■ After bleeding stops, apply an adhesive bandage.

■ If you've used a syringe, transfer the sample to a collection tube. Be careful to avoid foaming, *which can cause hemolysis.*

■ Finally, check the venipuncture site *to see if a hematoma has developed.* If it has, apply pressure until you are sure the bleeding has stopped; then you may apply warm soaks to the site *to help reabsorption.*

■ Place all tubes in a laboratory biohazard transport bag.

■ Discard syringes and needles in the appropriate containers.[8]

■ Remove and discard your gloves. Perform hand hygiene.[3,4,5]

■ Send the specimen tubes and the completed laboratory request form to the laboratory.

■ Document the procedure.[9]

Special considerations

■ Never draw a venous sample from an arm or leg that is already being used for IV therapy or blood administration *because this may affect test results.*[1]

■ Don't collect a venous sample from an infection site *because pathogens may be introduced into the vascular system.* Likewise, avoid drawing blood from edematous areas or sites of previous hematoma or vascular injury.

■ If the patient has large, distended, highly visible veins, perform venipuncture without a tourniquet *to minimize the risk for hematoma formation.* If the patient has a clotting disorder or is receiving anticoagulant therapy, maintain firm pressure on the venipuncture site for at least 5 minutes after withdrawing the needle *to prevent hematoma formation.*

■ Avoid using veins in the patient's legs for venipuncture, if possible, *because this increases the risk for thrombophlebitis.* Some

Common venipuncture sites

The illustrations below show the anatomic locations of veins commonly used for venipuncture. The most commonly used sites are on the forearm, followed by those on the hand.

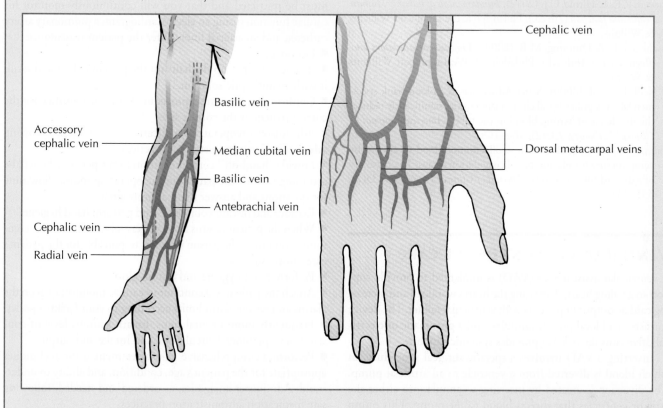

facilities require a doctor's order to collect blood from a leg or foot vein. Check the policy and procedure at your facility.

■ Don't use an arm on the side of a mastectomy *because reduced lymphatic drainage increases the risk for infection at the site.*

■ Never use an arm with an arteriovenous fistula *because of the increased risk for clotting and bleeding.*

Complications

A hematoma at the needle insertion site is the most common complication of venipuncture. Infection may result from poor technique.

Documentation

Record the date, time, and site of venipuncture; name of the test; the time the sample was sent to the laboratory; the amount of blood collected; and any adverse reactions to the procedure.

References

1 Clinical Laboratory and Standards Institute. (2007). "Procedures for the Collection of Diagnostic Blood Specimens by Venipuncture; Approved Standard—Sixth Edition" [Online]. Accessed December 2011 via the Web at http://www.clsi.org/source/orders/free/H3-a6.pdf

2 The Joint Commission. (2012). Standard NPSG.03.04.01. *Comprehensive accreditation manual for hospitals: The official handbook.* Oakbrook Terrace, IL: The Joint Commission. (Level I)

3 Centers for Disease Control and Prevention. (October 2002). Guideline for hand hygiene in health-care settings. *Morbidity and Mortality Weekly Report, 51*(RR-16), 1–45. (Level I)

4 World Health Organization. (2009). *WHO guidelines on hand hygiene in health care: First global patient safety challenge. Clean care is safer care.* Geneva, Switzerland: World Health Organization. (Level I)

5 The Joint Commission. (2012). Standard NPSG.07.01.01. *Comprehensive accreditation manual for hospitals: The official handbook.* Oakbrook Terrace, IL: The Joint Commission. (Level I)

6 The Joint Commission. (2012). Standard NPSG.01.01.01. *Comprehensive accreditation manual for hospitals: The official handbook.* Oakbrook Terrace, IL: The Joint Commission. (Level I)

7 Standard 57. Phlebotomy. Infusion nursing standards of practice. (2011). *Journal of Infusion Nursing, 34*(1S), S77–S79.

8 Occupational Safety and Health Administration. "Bloodborne Pathogens, Standard Number 1910.1030" [Online]. Accessed December 2011 via the Web at http://www.osha.gov/pls/oshaweb/owadisp.show_document?p_table=STANDARDS&p_id=10051 (Level I)

9 The Joint Commission. (2012). Standard RC.01.03.01. *Comprehensive accreditation manual for hospitals: The official handbook.* Oakbrook Terrace, IL: The Joint Commission. (Level I)

ADDITIONAL REFERENCES _____

Cengiz, M., et al. (2009). Influence of tourniquet application of venous blood sampling for serum chemistry, hematological parameters, leukocyte activation, and erythrocyte mechanical properties. *Clinical Chemistry and Laboratory Medicine, 47*(6), 769–776.

Craven, R.F., & Hirnle, C.J. (2012). *Fundamentals of nursing: Human health and function* (7th ed.). Philadelphia, PA: Lippincott Williams & Wilkins.

Fischbach, F., & Dunning, M.B. (2009). *A manual of laboratory and diagnostic tests* (8th ed.). Philadelphia, PA: Lippincott Williams & Wilkins.

O'Neill, E., et al. (2009). Strict Adherence to a blood bank specimen labeling policy by all clinical laboratories significantly reduces the incidence of 'wrong blood in the tube.' *American Journal of Clinical Pathology, 132*(2), 164–168.

Raijmakers, M. T., et al. (2010). Collection of blood specimens by venipuncture for plasma-based coagulation assays: The necessity of a discard tube. *American Journal of Clinical Pathology, 133*(2), 331–335.

VENTRICULAR ASSIST DEVICE CARE

A ventricular assist device (VAD) is implanted to provide support to a failing heart, decreasing the heart's workload and increasing cardiac output in patients with ventricular failure. The device consists of a blood pump, cannulas, and a pneumatic or electrical drive console. A VAD provides systemic support.

Inserting a VAD involves a specific surgical procedure, in which blood is diverted from a ventricle to an artificial pump. The diversion is created by inserting a cannula into either the atria or ventricles that directs blood to the pump. This pump then functions as the ventricle.

The typical VAD is implanted in the upper abdominal wall. An inflow cannula drains blood from the left atrium or ventricle into a pump (part of the VAD), which then pushes the blood into the aorta through the outflow cannula. (See *VAD: Help for the failing heart.*)

Candidates for a VAD include patients with massive myocardial infarction, irreversible cardiomyopathy, acute myocarditis, an inability to be weaned from cardiopulmonary bypass, valvular disease, bacterial endocarditis, heart transplant rejection, or cardiogenic shock that doesn't respond to maximal pharmacologic therapy. VADs are also commonly used as a bridge to cardiac transplantation in patients awaiting a heart transplant.

Equipment

VAD to be inserted in the operating room ▪ clippers ▪ antiseptic solution ▪ ordered analgesics ▪ thermometer ▪ heparin ▪ dressing supplies ▪ gloves.

Implementation

▪ Make sure that the doctor has obtained informed consent and that the consent form is in the patient's medical record.[1,2]
▪ Conduct a preprocedure verification *to make sure that all relevant documentation, related information, and equipment are available and correctly identified to the patient's identifiers.*[3]
▪ Perform hand hygiene.[4,5,6]

▪ Confirm the patient's identity using at least two patient identifiers according to your facility's policy.[7]
▪ Reinforce preoperative teaching and answer any questions *to reduce anxiety.*
▪ Before surgery, explain to the patient that food and fluid intake must be restricted and that you will continuously monitor his cardiac function (using an electrocardiogram, a pulmonary artery catheter, and an arterial line). Offer the patient reassurance.
▪ Put on gloves.
▪ If time permits, clip the hairs on the patient's chest and scrub it with an antiseptic solution.[8]
▪ Confirm that the correct procedure has been identified for the correct patient at the correct site.[3]
▪ Administer preoperative medications, as ordered, following safe medication administration practices.
▪ Provide "hand-off" communication to the person who will be assuming care for the patient in the operating room; allow time for questions and answer them appropriately.
▪ Remove and discard your gloves and perform hand hygiene.[4,5,6]
▪ When the patient returns from surgery, obtain "hand-off" communication from the person who was responsible for the patient's care during surgery.
▪ Perform hand hygiene and put on gloves.[4,5,6]
▪ Attach the patient to a continuous cardiac monitor; turn on the alarms and set the alarm limits according to your facility's policy.
▪ Frequently monitor vital signs, breath sounds, level of consciousness, peripheral circulation, and intake and output.
▪ Perform a comprehensive pain assessment using techniques appropriate for the patient's age, condition, and ability to understand. Administer analgesics, as ordered and needed, following safe medication administration practices.
▪ Initially, keep the patient immobile *to prevent accidental extubation, contamination, or disconnection of the VAD.* Log roll the patient side-to-side every 2 hours *to help prevent skin breakdown.* Perform active and passive range-of-motion (ROM) exercises with the patient.
▪ Monitor pulmonary artery pressures. If you've been trained to adjust the pump, maintain cardiac output at about 5 to 8 L/minute, central venous pressure at about 8 to 16 mm Hg, pulmonary capillary wedge pressure at about 10 to 20 mm Hg, mean arterial pressure at greater than 60 mm Hg, and left atrial pressure between 4 and 12 mm Hg.
▪ Monitor the patient for signs and symptoms of poor perfusion and ineffective pumping, including arrhythmias, hypotension, slow capillary refill, cool skin, oliguria or anuria, confusion, anxiety, and restlessness.
▪ Monitor the VAD's function and troubleshoot any problems. Follow the manufacturer's guidelines.

NURSING ALERT *Heparin is considered a "high-alert" medication because it can cause significant harm when used in error.*[9]

▪ Administer heparin, as prescribed, *to prevent thrombus formation and clotting in the pump head.* Before administering heparin, have another nurse perform an independent double-check according to your facility's policy *to verify the patient's identity as well as to make sure that the correct medication is being administered in the prescribed concentration, that the medication's indication corresponds with the patient's diagnosis, that the dosage calculations are correct*

EQUIPMENT

VAD: Help for the failing heart

A ventricular assist device (VAD) functions somewhat like an artificial heart. The major difference is that a VAD assists the heart, whereas an artificial heart replaces it. A VAD is designed to aid one or both ventricles. The pumping chambers themselves aren't usually implanted in the patient.

A permanent VAD is implanted in the patient's chest cavity, although it still provides only temporary support. The device receives power through the skin by a belt of electrical transformer coils (worn externally as a portable battery pack). It can also operate off an implanted, rechargeable battery for up to 1 hour at a time.

VADs are available as continuous flow (axial flow) or pulsatile pumps. A continuous flow pump fills continuously and returns blood to the aorta at a constant rate. A pulsatile pump may work in one of two ways: it may fill during systole and pump blood into the aorta during diastole or it may pump regardless of the patient's cardiac cycle.

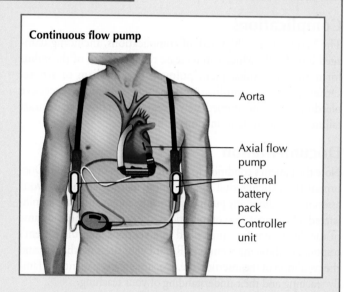

Continuous flow pump

- Aorta
- Axial flow pump
- External battery pack
- Controller unit

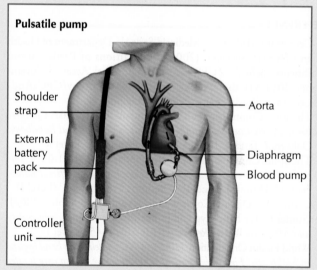

Pulsatile pump

- Shoulder strap
- External battery pack
- Controller unit
- Aorta
- Diaphragm
- Blood pump

---

and the dosing formula used to derive the final dose is correct, that the route of administration is safe and proper for the patient, that the pump settings are correct, and that the infusion line is attached to the correct port, if applicable.[10]

- After comparing the results of the independent double-check with the other nurse, administer the medication if there are no discrepancies. If discrepancies exist, rectify them before administering the medication.[10]
- Check for bleeding, especially at the operative sites. Monitor laboratory studies, as ordered, especially complete blood count and coagulation studies.
- Assess the patient's incisions and the cannula insertion sites for signs of infection and bleeding. Monitor the patient's white blood cell count and differential daily, and take rectal or core temperatures every 4 hours.

- Change the dressing over the cannula sites according to your facility's policy.
- Provide supportive care, including ROM exercises and oral and skin care.
- Remove and discard your gloves and perform hand hygiene.[4,5,6]
- Document the procedure.[11]

Special considerations

- If ventricular function fails to improve, the patient may need a transplant. If so, provide psychological support for the patient and his family as they go through the referral process. You may also initiate the transplant process by contacting the appropriate agency according to your facility's policy.

■ The psychological effects of the VAD can cause stress in the patient, his family, and his close friends. Provide emotional support and education for the patient and his family. If appropriate, refer them to other support personnel.

Complications

The VAD carries a high risk of complications, including damaged blood cells, which can increase the likelihood of thrombus formation and subsequent pulmonary embolism or stroke. Other possible complications include infection, excessive bleeding (especially immediately after implantation), acute heart failure and, rarely, malfunction of the device.

Documentation

Note the patient's condition following insertion of the VAD. Document the patient's vital signs, hemodynamic parameters, your assessment findings, any pump adjustments, and medications administered. Document any complications, the date and time, the name of the doctor notified, prescribed interventions, and the patient's response to those interventions. Record your dressing changes and the condition of the insertion site. Document any patient and family teaching and their understanding of your teaching.

REFERENCES

1 Centers for Medicare & Medicaid Services, Department of Health and Human Services. (2006). "Conditions of Participation: Patients' Rights," 42 CFR part 482.13 [Online]. Accessed November 2011 via the Web at https://www.cms.gov/CFCsAndCoPs/downloads/finalpatientrightsrule.pdf

2 The Joint Commission. (2012). Standard RI.01.03.01. *Comprehensive accreditation manual for hospitals: The official handbook.* Oakbrook Terrace, IL: The Joint Commission. (Level I)

3 The Joint Commission. (2012). Standard UP.01.01.01. *Comprehensive accreditation manual for hospitals: The official handbook.* Oakbrook Terrace, IL: The Joint Commission. (Level I)

4 Centers for Disease Control and Prevention. (October 2002). Guideline for hand hygiene in health-care settings. *Morbidity and Mortality Weekly Report, 51*(RR-16), 1–45. (Level I)

5 World Health Organization. (2009). *WHO guidelines on hand hygiene in health care: First global patient safety challenge. Clean care is safer care.* Geneva, Switzerland: World Health Organization. (Level I)

6 The Joint Commission. (2012). Standard NPSG.07.01.01. *Comprehensive accreditation manual for hospitals: The official handbook.* Oakbrook Terrace, IL: The Joint Commission. (Level I)

7 The Joint Commission. (2012). Standard NPSG.01.01.01. *Comprehensive accreditation manual for hospitals: The official handbook.* Oakbrook Terrace, IL: The Joint Commission. (Level I)

8 The Joint Commission. (2012). Standard NPSG.07.05.01. *Comprehensive accreditation manual for hospitals: The official handbook.* Oakbrook Terrace, IL: The Joint Commission. (Level I)

9 Institute of Safe Medication Practices. "ISMP's List of High-Alert Medications." [Online]. Accessed October 2011 via the Web at http://www.ismp.org/tools/highalertmedications.pdf

10 Institute for Safe Medication Practices. (2008). "Conducting an Independent Double-check." *ISMP Medication Safety Alert! Nurse Advise-ERR, 6*(12), 1 [Online]. Accessed October 2011 via the Web at http://www.ismp.org/newsletters/nursing/Issues/NurseAdviseERR200812.pdf

11 The Joint Commission. (2012). Standard RC.01.03.01. *Comprehensive accreditation manual for hospitals: The official handbook.* Oakbrook Terrace, IL: The Joint Commission. (Level I)

ADDITIONAL REFERENCES

Barnes, K. (2008). Complications in patients with ventricular assist devices. *Dimensions in Critical Care Nursing, 27*(6), 233–241; quiz 242–243.

El-Hamamsy, I., et al. (2009). Results following implantation of mechanical circulatory support systems: The Montreal Heart Institute experience. *Canadian Journal of Cardiology, 25*(2), 107–110.

Heilmann, C., et al. (2011). Supportive psychotherapy for patients with heart transplantation or ventricular assist devices. *European Journal of Cardio-thoracic Surgery, 39*(4), e44–e50.

Long, J.W. (2011). Improving outcomes with long-term 'destination' therapy using left ventricular assist devices. *Journal of Thoracic Cardiovascular Surgery, 135*(6), 1353–1360.

Lynn-McHale Wiegand, D. (Ed.). (2011). *AACN procedure manual for critical care* (6th ed.). Philadelphia, PA: Saunders.

Majeed, F., et al. (2009). Prospective observational study of antiplatelet and coagulation biomarkers as predictors of thromboembolic events after implantation of ventricular assist devices. *National Clinical Practice. Cardiovascular Medicine, 6*(2), 147–157.

Mountis, M.M., & Starling, R.C. (2009). Management of left ventricular assist devices after surgery: Bridge, destination, and recovery. *Current Opinions in Cardiology, 24*(3), 252–256.

Richards, N.M., & Stahl, M.A. (2007). Ventricular assist devices in the adult. *Critical Care Nursing Quarterly, 30*(2), 104–118.

Stahl, M., & Richards, N. (2009). Update on ventricular assist device technology. *AACN Advanced Critical Care, 20*(1), 26–34.

Woods, S., et al. (2010). *Cardiac nursing* (6th ed.). Philadelphia, PA: Lippincott Williams & Wilkins.

VENTRICULAR DRAIN INSERTION, ASSISTING

Cerebrospinal fluid (CSF) drainage aims to reduce CSF pressure to the desired level and then to maintain it at that level. Depending on the indication and the desired outcome, fluid can be withdrawn from the lateral ventricle (ventriculostomy) or the lumbar subarachnoid space via a catheter or a ventriculostomy tube in a sterile, closed-drainage collection system. Ventricular drainage is used to reduce increased intracranial pressure (ICP).

To place the ventricular drain, the doctor inserts a ventricular catheter through a burr hole in the patient's skull. This is typically done in the operating room, with the patient receiving a general anesthetic, but it can also be done in the emergency department or on the intensive care unit.

Equipment

Overbed table ■ sterile gloves, gown, mask, and cap ■ sterile cotton-tipped applicators ■ antiseptic solution ■ alcohol pads ■ sterile fenestrated drape ■ 3-mL syringe for local anesthetic ■ 25G ¾" needle for injecting anesthetic ■ local anesthetic (usually 1% lidocaine) ■ 18G or 20G sterile spinal needle or Tuohy needle ■ #5 French whistle-tip catheter or ventriculostomy tube ■ CSF drainage set (includes drainage tubing and sterile collection bag) ■ suture material ■ 4″ × 4″ dressings ■ paper tape ■ lamp or another light source ■ IV pole ■ sterile occlusive dressing ■ twist drill ■ Optional: pain medication, anti-infective agent (such as an antibiotic).

Some of the equipment may be available in a prepackaged ventriculostomy tray.

Preparation of equipment

If the procedure is done in the operating room, equipment is prepared there using sterile technique. If the procedure is to be performed at the bedside, perform hand hygiene and open all equipment using sterile technique. Check all packaging for breaks in seals and for expiration dates. Label all medications, medication containers, and other solutions, on and off the sterile field.[1]

Implementation

■ Confirm the patient's identity using at least two patient identifiers according to your facility's policy.[2]
■ Explain the procedure to the patient. Discuss activity restrictions that will need to be adhered to after the drain is placed.
■ The doctor should obtain consent from the patient or a responsible family member and should document this according to your facility's policy.[3]
■ Perform hand hygiene and follow standard precautions.[4,5,6]
■ Perform a baseline neurologic assessment, including vital signs, *to help detect alterations or signs of deterioration.*
■ Conduct a preprocedure verification process *to make sure that all relevant documentation, related information, and equipment are available and correctly identified to the patient's identifiers.*[7]
■ Place the patient in the supine position.
■ Place the equipment tray on the overbed table, and unwrap the tray.
■ Adjust the height of the bed *so that the doctor can perform the procedure comfortably.*
■ Illuminate the area of the catheter insertion site.
■ Conduct a time-out immediately before starting the procedure *to perform a final assessment to ensure that the correct patient, site, positioning, and procedure are identified and that, as applicable, all relevant information and necessary equipment are available during and after the procedure.*[8]
■ The doctor will clean the insertion site, administer a local anesthetic, and clip the hair from the area of the insertion site. He'll put on sterile gloves, mask, gown, and cap and will drape the insertion site.
■ To insert the drain, the doctor will request a ventriculostomy tray with a twist drill. After completing the ventriculostomy, he'll cover the insertion site with a sterile dressing.
■ After the doctor places the catheter, trace the tubing from the patient to the point of origin and then connect it to the external drainage system tubing. Secure connection points with tape or a connector.
■ Place the collection system, including drip chamber and collection bag, on an IV pole.
■ After the ventriculostomy is inserted, monitor vital signs, neurologic status, and ICP at least every hour or according to your facility's policy.

■ Make sure the collection system tubing is secured with tape or a luer-lock connector.
■ Maintain the drainage system at the level ordered by the doctor.
■ Monitor the patient for signs and symptoms of infection or of CSF leak.
■ Remove and discard your gloves. Perform hand hygiene.[4,5,6]
■ Document the procedure.[9]

Special considerations

■ Maintaining a continual hourly output of CSF is essential *to prevent overdrainage or underdrainage.* Overdrainage can occur if the drip chamber is placed too far below the catheter insertion site. Underdrainage may reflect kinked tubing, catheter displacement, or a drip chamber placed higher than the catheter insertion site.
■ Raising or lowering the head of the bed can affect the CSF flow rate. When changing the patient's position, reposition the drip chamber.
■ Patients may experience a chronic headache during continuous CSF drainage. Reassure the patient that this symptom isn't unusual; administer analgesics, as appropriate.
■ Assess for signs and symptoms of hemorrhage, which may include headache.
■ Make sure ICP waveforms are being monitored at all times.
■ Leaving the patient floor—for instance, to perform tests and procedures on the patient—is discouraged *to prevent dislodgement of the catheter.* Check your facility's policy for scheduling such tests and procedures at the patient's bedside.
■ Follow strict sterile technique when connecting tubing or flushing, when taking samples from the drainage system, and during dressing changes.

Patient teaching

Teach the patient and family members about the reason for the drain. Explain to the patient that his activity level must be restricted. The patient may not sit up, stand, or walk when the drain is open and must ask for assistance with movement. The system must be turned off when the patient is repositioned or transferred. Instruct the patient to avoid straining, coughing, and sneezing.

Complications

Signs of excessive CSF drainage include headache, tachycardia, diaphoresis, and nausea. Acute overdrainage may result in collapsed ventricles, tonsillar herniation, and medullary compression.

NURSING ALERT *If drainage accumulates too rapidly, clamp the system, notify the doctor immediately, and perform a complete neurologic assessment. This complication constitutes a potential neurosurgical emergency.*

Cessation of drainage may indicate clot formation. If you can't quickly identify the cause of the obstruction, notify the doctor. If drainage is blocked, the patient may develop signs of increased ICP.

Infection may cause meningitis. To prevent this complication, administer antibiotics, as ordered. Maintain a sterile closed system and a dry, sterile dressing over the site.

Documentation

Record the time and date of the insertion procedure and the patient's tolerance of the procedure. Record routine vital signs and neurologic assessment findings and ICP at least every 4 hours. Document the color, clarity, and amount of CSF at least every 8 hours or according to your facility's policy. Record hourly and 24-hour CSF output, and describe the condition of the dressing.

REFERENCES

1 The Joint Commission. (2012). Standard NPSG.03.04.01. *Comprehensive accreditation manual for hospitals: The official handbook.* Oakbrook Terrace, IL: The Joint Commission. (Level I)

2 The Joint Commission. (2012). Standard NPSG.01.01.01. *Comprehensive accreditation manual for hospitals: The official handbook.* Oakbrook Terrace, IL: The Joint Commission. (Level I)

3 The Joint Commission. (2012). Standard RI.01.03.01. *Comprehensive accreditation manual for hospitals: The official handbook.* Oakbrook Terrace, IL: The Joint Commission. (Level I)

4 Centers for Disease Control and Prevention. (October 2002). Guideline for hand hygiene in health-care settings. *Morbidity and Mortality Weekly Report, 51*(RR-16), 1–45. (Level I)

5 World Health Organization. (2009). *WHO guidelines on hand hygiene in health care: First global patient safety challenge. Clean care is safer care.* Geneva, Switzerland: World Health Organization. (Level I)

6 The Joint Commission. (2012). Standard NPSG.07.01.01. *Comprehensive accreditation manual for hospitals: The official handbook.* Oakbrook Terrace, IL: The Joint Commission. (Level I)

7 The Joint Commission. (2012). Standard UP.01.01.01. *Comprehensive accreditation manual for hospitals: The official handbook.* Oakbrook Terrace, IL: The Joint Commission. (Level I)

8 The Joint Commission. (2012). Standard UP.01.03.01. *Comprehensive accreditation manual for hospitals: The official handbook.* Oakbrook Terrace, IL: The Joint Commission. (Level I)

9 The Joint Commission. (2012). Standard RC.01.03.01. *Comprehensive accreditation manual for hospitals: The official handbook.* Oakbrook Terrace, IL: The Joint Commission. (Level I)

ADDITIONAL REFERENCE

Lynn-McHale Wiegand, D. (Ed.). (2011). *AACN procedure manual for critical care* (6th ed.). Philadelphia, PA: Saunders.

VOLUME-CONTROL SET PREPARATION

A volume-control set—an IV administration set with a graduated chamber—delivers precise amounts of fluid and shuts off when the fluid is exhausted, preventing air from entering the IV catheter. It may be used as a secondary line in adults for intermittent infusion of medication.

Equipment

Volume-control set ▪ IV pole ▪ IV solution ▪ antiseptic pads (alcohol, tincture of iodine, or chlorhexidine-based) ▪ medication in labeled syringe ▪ tape ▪ label.

Although various models of volume-control sets are available, each one consists of a graduated fluid chamber (120 to 250 mL) with a spike and a filtered air line on top and administration tubing underneath. Floating-valve sets have a valve at the bottom that closes when the chamber empties; membrane-filter sets have a rigid filter at the bottom that, when wet, prevents the passage of air.

Preparation of equipment

Ensure the sterility of all equipment and inspect it carefully *to ensure the absence of flaws.* Take the equipment to the patient's bedside.

Implementation

- Verify the doctor's order for IV fluid administration.[1]
- Perform hand hygiene.[2,3,4]
- Confirm the patient's identity using at least two patient identifiers according to your facility's policy.[5]
- Explain the procedure to the patient.
- If an IV catheter is already in place, assess the insertion site for signs of infiltration and infection.
- Remove the volume-control set from its box and close all the clamps.
- Remove the protective cap from the volume-control set spike, insert the spike into the IV solution container, and hang the container on the IV pole.
- Open the air vent clamp and close the upper slide clamp.
- Open the lower clamp on the IV tubing, slide it upward until it's slightly below the drip chamber, and close the clamp.
- Open the upper clamp until the fluid chamber fills with about 30 mL of solution. Then close the clamp.
- Gently squeeze the chamber.
- Release the drip chamber and let it fill about halfway with fluid.
- Open the lower clamp, prime the tubing, and close the clamp. To use the set as a primary line, insert the distal end of the tubing into the catheter or needle hub.
- To use the set as a secondary line, thoroughly disinfect the Y-port of the primary tubing with an antiseptic pad using friction, and attach the distal end of the tubing to the Y-port of the primary tubing, following the manufacturer's instructions.
- To add medication, thoroughly disinfect the injection port on the volume-control set with an antiseptic pad using friction, and inject the medication (as shown below). Make sure that you follow safe medication administration practices.[6]

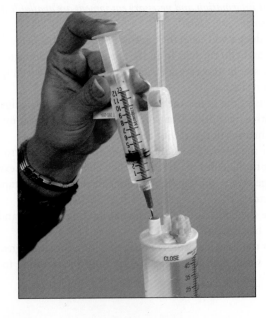

■ Place a label on the chamber, indicating the drug, dose, date, and your initials. Don't write directly on the chamber *because the plastic absorbs ink.*

■ Open the upper clamp (as shown below), fill the fluid chamber with the prescribed amount of solution and close the clamp. Gently rotate the chamber *to mix the medication.*

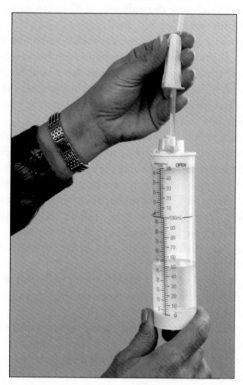

■ Turn off the primary solution (if present) or lower the drip rate *to maintain an open line.*

■ Trace the tubing from the patient to its point of origin to make sure that the set is connected to the proper port.[7,8]

■ Open the lower clamp on the volume-control set, and adjust the drip rate as ordered. After completion of the infusion, open the upper clamp and let 10 mL of IV solution flow into the chamber and through the tubing *to flush them.*

■ If you're using the volume-control set as a secondary IV line, close the lower clamp and reset the flow rate of the primary line. If you're using the set as a primary IV line, close the lower clamp, refill the chamber to the prescribed amount, and begin the infusion again.

■ Perform hand hygiene.[2,3,4]

■ Document the procedure.[9]

Special considerations

■ Always check compatibility of the medication and the IV solution. If you're using a membrane-filter set, avoid administering suspensions, lipid emulsions, blood, or blood components through it.

■ If you're using a floating-valve set, the diaphragm may stick after repeated use. If it does, close the air vent and upper clamp, invert the drip chamber, and squeeze it. If the diaphragm opens, reopen the clamp and continue to use the set.

■ If the drip chamber of a floating-valve diaphragm set overfills, immediately close the upper clamp and air vent, invert the chamber, and squeeze the excess fluid from the drip chamber back into the graduated fluid chamber.

Documentation

If you add a drug to the volume-control set, record the amount and type of medication, amount of fluid used to dilute it, and date and time of infusion. Document the patient's response to the medication, patient teaching, and the patient's understanding of your teaching.

REFERENCES

1 The Joint Commission. (2012). Standard MM.04.01.01. *Comprehensive accreditation manual for hospitals: The official handbook.* Oakbrook Terrace, IL: The Joint Commission. (Level I)

2 World Health Organization. (2009). *WHO guidelines on hand hygiene in health care: First global patient safety challenge. Clean care is safer care.* Geneva, Switzerland: World Health Organization. (Level I)

3 Centers for Disease Control and Prevention. (October 2002). Guideline for hand hygiene in health-care settings. *Morbidity and Mortality Weekly Report, 51*(RR–16), 1–45. (Level I)

4 The Joint Commission. (2012). Standard NPSG.07.01.01. *Comprehensive accreditation manual for hospitals: The official handbook.* Oakbrook Terrace, IL: The Joint Commission. (Level I)

5 The Joint Commission. (2012). Standard NPSG.01.01.01. *Comprehensive accreditation manual for hospitals: The official handbook.* Oakbrook Terrace, IL: The Joint Commission. (Level I)

6 Standard 26. Add-on devices: Infusion nursing standards of practice. (2011). *Journal of Infusion Nursing, 34*(1S), S31. (Level I)

7 Standard 61. Parenteral medication and solution administration: Infusion nursing standards of practice. (2011). *Journal of Infusion Nursing, 34*(1S),S86–87. (Level I)

8 U.S. Food and Drug Administration. (2009). "Look. Check. Connect.: Safe Medical Device Connections Save Lives" [Online]. Accessed December 2011 via the Web at http://www.fda.gov/downloads/MedicalDevices/Safety/AlertsandNotices/UCM134873.pdf

9 The Joint Commission. (2012). Standard RC.01.03.01. *Comprehensive accreditation manual for hospitals: The official handbook.* Oakbrook Terrace, IL: The Joint Commission. (Level I)

ADDITIONAL REFERENCES

O'Grady, N.P., et al. (2011). "Guidelines for the Prevention of Intravascular Catheter-Related Infections" [Online]. Accessed December 2011 via the Web at http://www.cdc.gov/hicpac/pdf/guidelines/bsi-guidelines-2011.pdf

Standard 19. Hand hygiene: Infusion nursing standards of practice. (2011). *Journal of Infusion Nursing, 34*(1S), S26–S27. (Level I)

Standard 43. Administration set change: Infusion nursing standards of practice. (2011). *Journal of Infusion Nursing, 34*(1S), S55. (Level I)

Taylor, C., et al. (2011). *Fundamentals of nursing: The art and science of nursing care* (7th ed.). Philadelphia, PA: Lippincott Williams & Wilkins.

WALKERS

A walker consists of a metal frame with handgrips and four legs that buttresses the patient on three sides. One side remains open. Because this device provides greater stability and security than other ambulatory aids, it's recommended for the patient with insufficient strength and balance to use crutches or a cane, or with weakness requiring frequent rest periods.

Attachments for standard walkers and modified walkers help meet special needs. For example, a walker may have a platform added to support an injured arm.

Equipment

Walker ▪ platform or wheel attachments, as necessary.

Various types of walkers are available. The standard walker is used by the patient with unilateral or bilateral weakness or an inability to bear weight on one leg. It requires arm strength and balance. Platform attachments may be added to a standard walker for the patient with arthritic arms or a casted arm, who can't bear weight directly on his hand, wrist, or forearm. With the doctor's approval, wheels may be placed on the front legs of the standard walker to allow the extremely weak or poorly coordinated patient to roll the device forward, instead of lifting it. However, wheels are applied infrequently *because they may be a safety hazard.*

The stair walker—used by the patient who must negotiate stairs without bilateral handrails—requires good arm strength and balance. Its extra set of handles extends toward the patient on the open side. The rolling walker—used by the patient with very weak legs—has four wheels and may have a seat. The reciprocal walker—used by the patient with very weak arms—allows one side to be advanced ahead of the other.

Preparation of equipment

Obtain the appropriate walker with the advice of a physical therapist, and adjust it to the patient's height: His elbows should be flexed at a 15- to 30-degree angle when standing comfortably within the walker with his hands on the grips. To adjust the walker, turn it upside down, and change the leg length by pushing in the button on each shaft and releasing it when the leg is in the correct position. Make sure the walker is level before the patient attempts to use it.

Implementation

▪ Perform hand hygiene.[1,2,3]
▪ Confirm the patient's identity using at least two patient identifiers according to your facility's policy.[4]
▪ Help the patient stand within the walker, and instruct him to hold the handgrips firmly and equally. Make sure that the patient is standing as upright as possible. Stand behind him, closer to the involved leg.

▪ If the patient has one-sided leg weakness, tell him to advance the walker 6″ to 8″ (15 to 20 cm) and to step forward with the involved leg and follow with the uninvolved leg, supporting himself on his arms. Encourage him to take equal strides. If he has equal strength in both legs, instruct him to advance the walker 6″ to 8″ and to step forward with either leg. If he can't use one leg, tell him to advance the walker 6″ to 8″ and to swing onto it, supporting his weight on his arms.
▪ If the patient is using a reciprocal walker, teach him the two-point gait. Instruct the patient to stand with his weight evenly distributed between his legs and the walker. Stand behind him, slightly to one side. Tell him to simultaneously advance the walker's right side and his left foot. Then have the patient advance the walker's left side and his right foot.
▪ If the patient is using a reciprocal walker, you may also teach him the four-point gait. Instruct the patient to evenly distribute his weight between his legs and the walker. Stand behind him and slightly to one side. Then have him move the right side of the walker forward. Then have the patient move his left foot forward. Next, instruct him to move the left side of the walker forward. Then have him move his right foot forward.
▪ Instruct the patient to step into the walker with each step, and not to walk behind it.
▪ If the patient is using a wheeled or stair walker, reinforce the physical therapist's instructions. Stress the need for caution when using a stair walker.
▪ Teach the patient how to safely move from a walker to a chair and back. (See *Teaching safe use of a walker.*)
▪ Observe the patient as he returns the demonstration, and assist the patient as necessary.
▪ Perform hand hygiene.[1,2,3]
▪ Document the procedure.[5]

Special considerations

▪ If the patient starts to fall, support his hips and shoulders *to help maintain an upright position if possible.* If unsuccessful, ease him slowly to the closest surface—bed, floor, or chair.
▪ If the patient will be using the walker on carpet, you can place cut tennis balls on the rubber tips *to help ease movement.*

Complications

An improperly fitted walker can lead to falls and injury.

Documentation

Record the type of walker and attachments used, the degree of guarding required, the distance walked, and the patient's tolerance of ambulation.

REFERENCES

1 Centers for Disease Control and Prevention. (October 2002). Guideline for hand hygiene in health-care settings. *Morbidity and Mortality Weekly Report, 51*(RR-16), 1–45. (Level I)
2 World Health Organization. (2009). *WHO guidelines on hand hygiene in health care: First global patient safety challenge. Clean care is safer care.* Geneva, Switzerland: World Health Organization. (Level I)

Teaching safe use of a walker

Sitting down

■ First, tell the patient to stand with the back of his stronger leg against the front of the chair, his weaker leg slightly off the floor, and the walker directly in front.

■ Tell him to grasp the armrests on the chair one arm at a time while supporting most of his weight on the stronger leg. (In the illustrations below, the patient has left leg weakness.)

■ Tell the patient to lower himself into the chair and slide backward. After he is seated, he should place the walker beside the chair.

Getting up

■ After bringing the walker to the front of his chair, tell the patient to slide forward in the chair. Placing the back of his stronger leg against the seat, he should then advance the weaker leg.

■ Next, with both hands on the armrests, the patient can push himself to a standing position. Supporting himself with the stronger leg and the opposite hand, the patient should grasp the walker's handgrip with his free hand.

■ Then have the patient grasp the free handgrip with his other hand.

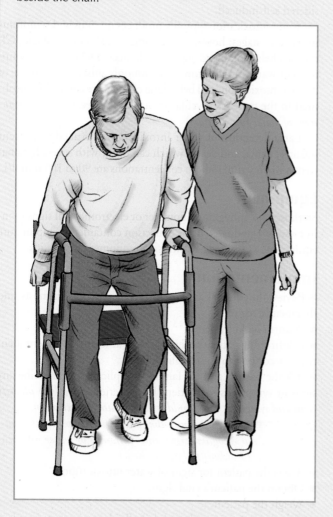

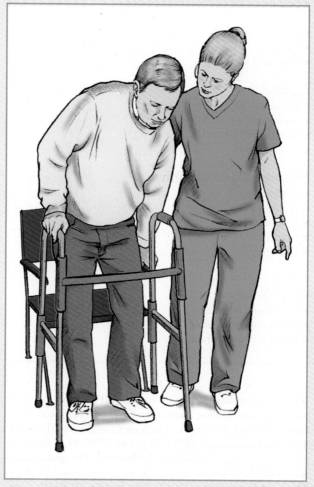

Signs and symptoms of water intoxication

These signs and symptoms of water intoxication may occur over time.

Neurologic
- Headache
- Vertigo
- Drowsiness
- Muscle cramps
- Blurred vision
- Weakness
- Tremors
- Lethargy
- Seizures

GI
- Nausea
- Repeated vomiting

Cardiac
- Hypotension
- Tachycardia
- Cardiac arrhythmias
- Heart failure

Behavioral and cognitive
- Restlessness
- Agitation
- Disorientation
- Confusion
- Delirium

Other
- Rapid breathing
- Decreased urination
- Sudden weight gain
- Metabolic abnormalities

3   The Joint Commission. (2012). Standard NPSG.07.01.01. *Comprehensive accreditation manual for hospitals: The official handbook.* Oakbrook Terrace, IL: The Joint Commission. (Level I))

4   The Joint Commission. (2012). Standard NPSG.01.01.01. *Comprehensive accreditation manual for hospitals: The official handbook.* Oakbrook Terrace, IL: The Joint Commission. (Level I)

5   The Joint Commission. (2012). Standard RC.01.03.01. *Comprehensive accreditation manual for hospitals: The official handbook.* Oakbrook Terrace, IL: The Joint Commission. (Level I)

ADDITIONAL REFERENCES

Craven, R.F., & Hirnle, C.J. (2012). *Fundamentals of nursing: Human health and function* (7th ed.). Philadelphia, PA: Lippincott Williams & Wilkins.

Nettina, S.M. (2010). *Lippincott manual of nursing practice* (9th ed.). Philadelphia, PA: Lippincott Williams & Wilkins.

WATER INTOXICATION ASSESSMENT

Water intoxication occurs when the body's water and sodium levels become imbalanced as a result of excessive water intake that's accompanied by inadequate sodium intake, resulting in severe hyponatremia. This imbalance allows more water to enter the cells, causing them to swell and place excess pressure on the body's organs, especially the brain.

In patients with chronic psychiatric disorders, water intoxication may result from compulsive water drinking, or *psychogenic polydipsia*. The cause of psychogenic polydipsia is unknown, but the condition may be related to the interaction of several factors, including delusions having to do with fluid intake, adverse effects of medications, and hyperactivity of hypothalamic thirst centers. Water intoxication resulting from psychogenic polydipsia is considered self-induced.

Water intoxication typically produces no signs and symptoms in its early stages; however, over time, it causes neurologic, GI, cardiac, behavioral, and cognitive changes. The signs and symptoms of water intoxication are commonly mistaken for those of alcohol intoxication, and behavioral changes are commonly attributed to the patient's psychiatric diagnosis. (See *Signs and symptoms of water intoxication.*)

Early detection of water intoxication is crucial to prevent seizures, coma, and death, which can occur with severe hyponatremia when serum sodium concentrations are 90 to 105 mmol/L.

Equipment

Stethoscope ▪ sphygmomanometer or electronic vital signs monitor ▪ scale ▪ graduated urine collection container ▪ venipuncture equipment ▪ Optional: IV infusion equipment and fluids.

Implementation

- Review the patient's medical history, psychiatric diagnosis, and therapeutic regimen.
- Perform hand hygiene.[1,2,3]
- Confirm the patient's identity using at least two patient identifiers according to your facility's policy.[4]
- Ask the patient and his family, if applicable, to describe any signs or symptoms the patient has experienced *to help identify signs and symptoms that would indicate water intoxication.*

NURSING ALERT *Be aware that patients with psychiatric disorders may not recognize signs and symptoms of water intoxication or may not admit to having them.*

- Assess the patient for signs of water intoxication.
- Obtain the patient's vital signs.
- Weigh the patient.
- Calculate an estimated total daily fluid requirement based on the patient's body weight *to assess for excess water intake.* (See *Calculating maintenance fluid requirements.*)
- Verify the doctor's treatment orders.
- Perform a venipuncture to obtain baseline and serial serum sodium levels, as ordered, and report results promptly. (See "Venipuncture," page 781.)
- Provide interventions as ordered, which may include IV administration of a hypertonic saline solution.

- Monitor the patient's water intake *to prevent self-induced water intoxication.*
- Measure the patient's urine output hourly or as ordered. Immediately report an output of less than 30 mL/hour.
- Monitor the patient, using one-to-one precautions as necessary, *to decrease excessive water intake.*
- Provide alternative activities *to redirect the patient from drinking excessive amounts of water while awake.*
- Continue to monitor the patient's mental status, behavior, level of consciousness, weight, vital signs, and serum sodium levels.
- Perform hand hygiene.[1,2,3]
- Document the procedure.[5]

Special considerations

- If the patient has severe water intoxication, the doctor may order IV furosemide *to promote diuresis.*

Patient teaching

Teach the patient and his family about the dangers related to excess water intake. Provide suggestions on ways for the family to redirect the patient during waking hours. If the patient demonstrates that he's willing to cooperate with restrictions, suggest alternative behaviors when he has the urge to drink excessively.

Provide the patient and his family with the patient's estimated total daily fluid requirement based on his body size *to ensure that the patient is adequately hydrated.* Review the signs and symptoms of water intoxication with the family, and instruct them to call the doctor or seek medical attention immediately if the patient exhibits them.

Complications

Untreated or undiagnosed water intoxication can lead to seizures, coma, and death. Too-rapid replacement of saline could lead to permanent brain damage.

Documentation

Record your assessment findings and the patient's vital signs, serum sodium levels, and weight in his medical record. Also record all signs and symptoms of water intoxication, any treatment given, and the patient's response to treatment. Document the patient's estimated total daily fluid requirement and the efforts made to maintain this amount. Document intake and output. Note any teaching provided to the patient and family members and their understanding of the information.

REFERENCES

1 Centers for Disease Control and Prevention. (October 2002). Guideline for hand hygiene in health-care settings. *Morbidity and Mortality Weekly Report, 51*(RR-16), 1–45. (Level I)
2 World Health Organization. (2009). *WHO guidelines on hand hygiene in health care: First global patient safety challenge. Clean care is safer care.* Geneva, Switzerland: World Health Organization. (Level I)

Calculating maintenance fluid requirements

The formula below helps you calculate the maintenance fluid requirements for your patient:

(1,500 mL for the first 20 kg) + (20 mL for each kg over 20)

For example, if you have a patient who weighs 75 kg, use the formula as follows:

1,500 mL + (20 mL × 55) = 1,500 + 1,100
= 2,600 mL of fluid per day.

---

3 The Joint Commission. (2012). Standard NPSG.07.01.01. *Comprehensive accreditation manual for hospitals: The official handbook.* Oakbrook Terrace, IL: The Joint Commission. (Level I)
4 The Joint Commission. (2012). Standard NPSG.01.01.01. *Comprehensive accreditation manual for hospitals: The official handbook.* Oakbrook Terrace, IL: The Joint Commission. (Level I)
5 The Joint Commission. (2012). Standard RC.01.03.01. *Comprehensive accreditation manual for hospitals: The official handbook.* Oakbrook Terrace, IL: The Joint Commission. (Level I)

ADDITIONAL REFERENCES

Dundas, B., et al. (2007). Psychogenic polydipsia review: Etiology, differential, and treatment. *Current Psychiatry Reports, 9*(3), 236–241.
Mohr, W.K. (2008). *Psychiatric-mental health nursing: Evidence-based concepts, skills, and practices* (7th ed.). Philadelphia, PA: Lippincott Williams & Wilkins.
Nettina, S.M. (2010). *Lippincott manual of nursing practice* (9th ed.). Philadelphia, PA: Lippincott Williams & Wilkins.

WOUND DEHISCENCE AND EVISCERATION MANAGEMENT

Although surgical wounds typically heal without incident, occasionally, the edges of a wound may fail to join or may separate even after they seem to be healing normally. This development, called *wound dehiscence,* may lead to an even more serious complication: evisceration, in which a portion of the viscera (usually a bowel loop) protrudes through the incision. Evisceration, in turn, can lead to peritonitis and septic shock. (See *Recognizing dehiscence and evisceration,* page 794.) Dehiscence and evisceration are most likely to occur 6 or 7 days after surgery. By then, sutures may have been removed and the patient can cough easily and breathe deeply—both of which strain the incision.

Several factors can contribute to these complications. Poor nutrition—whether from inadequate intake or a condition such as diabetes mellitus—may hinder wound healing. Chronic pulmonary or cardiac disease and metastatic cancer can also slow

Recognizing dehiscence and evisceration

In wound dehiscence, the layers of the surgical wound separate. With evisceration, the viscera (in this case, a bowel loop) protrude through the surgical incision.

Wound dehiscence

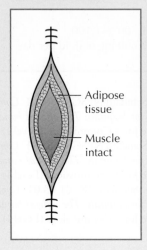

- Adipose tissue
- Muscle intact

Evisceration of bowel loop

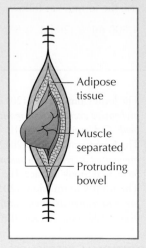

- Adipose tissue
- Muscle separated
- Protruding bowel

healing because the injured tissue doesn't get needed nutrients and oxygen. Localized wound infection may limit closure, delay healing, and weaken the incision. Stress on the incision from coughing or vomiting may cause abdominal distention or severe stretching.[1] A midline abdominal incision, for instance, poses a high risk of wound dehiscence.

Equipment

Sterile towels ▪ 1 L of sterile normal saline solution ▪ sterile irrigation set, including a basin, a solution container, and a 50-mL catheter-tip syringe ▪ several large abdominal dressings ▪ sterile, waterproof drape ▪ linen-saver pads ▪ gloves ▪ sterile gloves.

If the patient will return to the operating room, make sure you also gather an IV administration set and IV fluids, equipment for nasogastric (NG) intubation, prescribed sedative, and suction apparatus.

Implementation

- Perform hand hygiene and put on gloves.[2,3,4]
- Provide reassurance and support *to ease the patient's anxiety.* Tell him to stay in bed. If possible, stay with him while someone else notifies the doctor and collects the necessary equipment.
- Explain the procedure to the patient.
- Place a linen-saver pad under the patient *to keep the sheets dry when you moisten the exposed viscera.*
- Using sterile technique (see "Sterile technique, basic," page 671), unfold a sterile towel *to create a sterile field.* Open the

package containing the irrigation set, and place the basin, solution container, and 50-mL syringe on the sterile field.

- Open the bottle of sterile normal saline solution and pour about 400 mL into the solution container. Also pour about 200 mL into the sterile basin.
- Open several large abdominal dressings and place them on the sterile field.
- Remove and discard your gloves and perform hand hygiene.[2,3,4]
- Put on the sterile gloves and place one or two of the large abdominal dressings into the basin *to saturate them with saline solution.*[5]
- Place the moistened dressings over the exposed viscera.[5,6] Then place a sterile, waterproof drape over the dressings *to prevent the sheets from getting wet.*

Maintaining a moistened dressing

- To keep the dressing moist, perform hand hygiene and put on gloves[2,3,4] and then moisten the dressings every hour (or as ordered) by withdrawing saline solution from the container through the syringe and then gently squirting the solution on the dressings.
- When you moisten the dressings, inspect the color of the viscera. If it appears dusky or black, notify the doctor immediately. *With its blood supply interrupted, a protruding organ may become ischemic and necrotic.*
- Remove and discard your gloves and perform hand hygiene.[2,3,4]
- Keep the patient on absolute bed rest in low Fowler's position (no more than 20 degrees' elevation) with his knees flexed *to prevent injury and reduce stress on an abdominal incision.*[5,6]
- Don't allow the patient to have anything by mouth *to decrease the risk of aspiration during surgery.*
- Monitor the patient's pulse, respirations, blood pressure, and temperature frequently *to detect shock.*

Preparing the patient for surgery

- If necessary, prepare the patient to return to the operating room.
- Perform hand hygiene[2,3,4] and gather the appropriate equipment. Put on gloves and start an IV infusion, as ordered.
- Insert an NG tube and connect it to continuous or intermittent low suction, as ordered.
- Administer preoperative medications to the patient as ordered, following safe medication administration practices.[7]
- Continue to reassure the patient while you prepare him for surgery.
- Confirm that an informed consent has been obtained and documented in the medical record.[8]
- Provide hand-off communication to the person who will assume responsibility for care of the patient during surgery.

Completing the procedure

- Remove and discard your gloves and perform hand hygiene.[2,3,4]
- Document the procedure.[9]

Special considerations

- Depending on the circumstances, some of these procedures may not be performed at the bedside. For example, NG intubation may make the patient gag or vomit, causing further evisceration. For this reason, the doctor may choose to have the NG tube inserted in the operating room with the patient under anesthesia.
- The best treatment is prevention. If you're caring for a postoperative patient who's at risk for poor healing, make sure he gets an adequate supply of protein, vitamins, and calories. Monitor his dietary deficiencies, and discuss any problems with the doctor and the dietitian.
- When teaching the patient to cough and deep-breathe postoperatively, have him reinforce the dressing by holding a pillow or bath blanket tightly against his abdomen *to equalize the internal pressure that coughing places on the incision.*
- When changing wound dressings, always use sterile technique. Inspect the incision with each dressing change, and if you recognize the early signs of infection, start treatment before dehiscence or evisceration can occur. If local infection develops, clean the wound as ordered *to eliminate a buildup of purulent drainage.* Make sure bandages aren't so tight that they limit blood supply to the wound.

Complications

Infection, which can lead to peritonitis and possibly septic shock, is the most severe and most common complication of wound dehiscence and evisceration.

Documentation

Document when the dehiscence occurred, the patient's activity preceding the dehiscence, and your full assessments. Describe the appearance of the wound or eviscerated organ; the amount, color, consistency, and odor of any drainage; and any nursing interventions taken. Revise your care plan to reflect nursing interventions required to promote proper healing.

REFERENCES

1 Iqbal, A., et al. (2008). A study of intragastric and intravesicular pressure changes during rest, coughing, weight lifting, retching, and vomiting. *Surgical Endoscopy, 22*(12), 2571–2575. (Level VI)
2 Centers for Disease Control and Prevention. (October 2002). Guideline for hand hygiene in health-care settings. *Morbidity and Mortality Weekly Report, 51*(RR-16), 1–45. (Level I)
3 World Health Organization. (2009). *WHO guidelines on hand hygiene in health care: First global patient safety challenge. Clean care is safer care.* Geneva, Switzerland: World Health Organization. (Level I)
4 The Joint Commission. (2012). Standard NPSG.07.01.01. *Comprehensive accreditation manual for hospitals: The official handbook.* Oakbrook Terrace, IL: The Joint Commission. (Level I)
5 Taylor, C., et al. (2011). *Fundamentals of nursing: The art and science of nursing care* (7th ed.). Philadelphia, PA: Lippincott Williams & Wilkins.
6 Smeltzer, S.C., et al. (2010). *Brunner & Suddarth's textbook of medical-surgical nursing* (12th ed.). Philadelphia, PA: Lippincott Williams & Wilkins.
7 The Joint Commission. (2012). Standard MM.06.01.01. *Comprehensive accreditation manual for hospitals: The official handbook.* Oakbrook Terrace, IL: The Joint Commission. (Level I)
8 The Joint Commission. (2012). Standard RI.01.03.01. *Comprehensive accreditation manual for hospitals: The official handbook.* Oakbrook Terrace, IL: The Joint Commission. (Level I)
9 The Joint Commission. (2012). Standard RC.01.03.01. *Comprehensive accreditation manual for hospitals: The official handbook.* Oakbrook Terrace, IL: The Joint Commission. (Level I)

ADDITIONAL REFERENCE

Nettina, S.M. (2010). *Lippincott manual of nursing practice* (9th ed.). Philadelphia, PA: Lippincott Williams & Wilkins.

WOUND IRRIGATION

Irrigation cleans tissues and flushes cell debris and drainage from an open wound. Irrigation with a commercial wound cleaner helps the wound heal properly from the inside tissue layers outward to the skin surface; it also helps prevent premature surface healing over an abscess pocket or infected tract. After irrigation, open wounds usually are packed to absorb additional drainage.

Equipment

Waterproof trash bag ▪ linen-saver pad ▪ emesis basin ▪ gloves ▪ goggles, if indicated ▪ gown, if indicated ▪ prescribed irrigant such as sterile normal saline solution ▪ sterile water or normal saline solution ▪ sterile irrigating syringe ▪ sterile container ▪ sterile gauze ▪ sterile dressing ▪ commercial wound cleaner ▪ 35-mL piston syringe ▪ skin-protectant wipe ▪ gauze sponge.

Preparation of equipment

Assemble all equipment in the patient's room. Perform hand hygiene.[1,2,3] Check the expiration date on each sterile package and inspect for tears. Check the sterilization date and the date that each bottle of irrigating solution was opened; don't use any solution that's been open longer than 24 hours. Using sterile technique, dilute the prescribed irrigant to the correct proportions with sterile water or normal saline solution, if necessary. Let the solution stand until it reaches room temperature, or warm it to 90° to 95° F (32.2° to 35° C).[4]

Open the waterproof trash bag and place it near the patient's bed. Position the bag *to avoid reaching across the sterile field or the wound when disposing of soiled articles.* Form a cuff on the bag by turning down the top *to provide a wide opening, preventing contamination by touching the bag's edge.*

Implementation

- Verify the doctor's order.[5]
- Perform hand hygiene and put on gloves.[1,2,3]
- Confirm the patient's identity using at least two patient identifiers according to your facility's policy.[6]
- Assess the patient's condition.
- Identify the patient's allergies, especially to povidone-iodine or other topical solutions or medications.
- Explain the procedure to the patient, provide privacy, and position the patient correctly for the procedure.
- Place the linen-saver pad under the patient *to catch any spills and avoid linen changes.*
- Place the emesis basin below the wound *so that the irrigating solution flows from the wound into the basin and drains from the clean to the dirty end of the wound.*
- Perform hand hygiene. Put on gloves.[1,2,3]
- Remove the soiled dressing; then discard the dressing and gloves in the trash bag.
- Perform hand hygiene and put on gloves and a gown, if indicated.[1,2,3]
- Assess the wound and the surrounding tissue *to gauge the healing process or for the presence of infection.*
- Establish a clean field with all the equipment and supplies you'll need for irrigation and wound care. Pour the prescribed amount of irrigating solution into a container.
- Fill the syringe with the irrigating solution (as shown below).

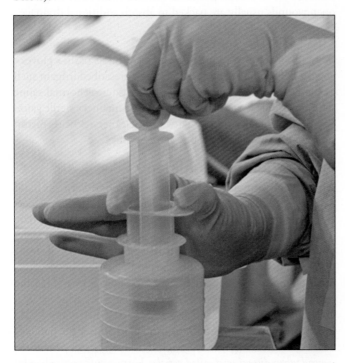

- Gently instill a slow, steady stream of irrigating solution into the wound until the syringe empties.

- Position the syringe so the solution flows from the clean to the dirty area of the wound (as shown below) *to prevent contamination of clean tissue by exudate.* Also make sure the solution reaches all areas of the wound.

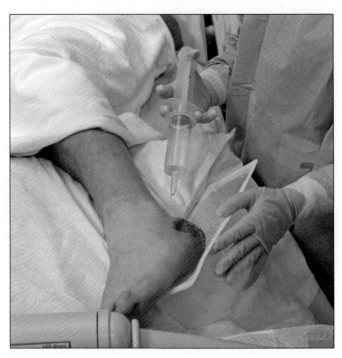

- Refill the syringe, and repeat the irrigation.
- Continue to irrigate the wound until you've administered the prescribed amount of solution or until the solution returns clear.[7] Note the amount of solution administered. Then discard the syringe in the waterproof trash bag.
- Keep the patient positioned *to allow further wound drainage into the basin.*
- Dry intact skin with a gauze sponge. Apply a skin-protectant wipe and allow it to dry well *to help prevent skin breakdown and infection.*
- Pack the wound, if ordered, and apply a sterile dressing.
- Dispose of used supplies in the appropriate receptacles.
- Remove and discard your gloves and gown. Perform hand hygiene.[1,2,3]
- Document the procedure.[8]

Special considerations

- Try to coordinate wound irrigation with the doctor's visit *so he can inspect the wound.*
- Use only the irrigant specified by the doctor *because others may be erosive or otherwise harmful.*
- If the procedure is likely to cause the patient pain, premedicate him before beginning irrigation, as ordered.
- Some facilities may use a splash guard for wound irrigation. This helps decrease the risk of contaminated fluid splashing onto the linens, surrounding areas, or you.

Patient teaching

If the wound must be irrigated at home, teach the patient or a family member how to perform it using strict sterile technique. Ask for a return demonstration of the proper technique. Provide written instructions. Arrange for home health supplies and nursing visits, as appropriate. Urge the patient to call the doctor if he detects signs of infection.

Complications

Wound irrigation increases the risk of infection and may cause excoriation and increased pain. Too much pressure causes trauma to the wound and directs bacteria back into the tissue.

Documentation

Record the date and time of irrigation, amount and type of irrigant, appearance of the wound, any sloughing tissue or exudate, amount of solution returned, skin care performed around the wound, dressings applied, and the patient's tolerance of the treatment.

REFERENCES

1 Centers for Disease Control and Prevention. (October 2002). Guideline for hand hygiene in health-care settings. *Morbidity and Mortality Weekly Report, 51*(RR-16), 1–45. (Level I)
2 World Health Organization. (2009). *WHO guidelines on hand hygiene in health care: First global patient safety challenge. Clean care is safer care.* Geneva, Switzerland: World Health Organization. (Level I)
3 The Joint Commission. (2012). Standard NPSG.07.01.01. *Comprehensive accreditation manual for hospitals: The official handbook.* Oakbrook Terrace, IL: The Joint Commission. (Level I)
4 Fernandez, R., & Griffiths, R. (2008). Water for wound cleansing. *Cochrane Database of Systematic Reviews* (1), CD003861. (Level I)
5 The Joint Commission. (2012). Standard MM.04.01.01. *Comprehensive accreditation manual for hospitals: The official handbook.* Oakbrook Terrace, IL: The Joint Commission. (Level I)
6 The Joint Commission. (2012). Standard NPSG.01.01.01. *Comprehensive accreditation manual for hospitals: The official handbook.* Oakbrook Terrace, IL: The Joint Commission. (Level I)
7 Fernandez, R., et al. (2006). "JBI Best Practice Technical Report: Effectiveness of Solutions, Techniques and Pressure in Wound Cleansing" [Online]. Accessed December 2011 via the Web at http://connect.jbiconnectplus.org/ViewSourceFile.aspx?0=4406 (Level I)
8 The Joint Commission. (2012). Standard RC.01.03.01. *Comprehensive accreditation manual for hospitals: The official handbook.* Oakbrook Terrace, IL: The Joint Commission. (Level I)

ADDITIONAL REFERENCES

Baranoski, S., & Ayello, E.A. (2012). *Wound care essentials: Practice principles* (3rd ed.). Philadelphia, PA: Lippincott Williams & Wilkins.
Craven, R.F., & Hirnle, C.J. (2012). *Fundamentals of nursing: Human health and function* (7th ed.). Philadelphia, PA: Lippincott Williams & Wilkins.
Hassinger, S.M., et al. (2005). High-pressure pulsatile lavage propagates bacteria into soft tissue. *Clinical Orthopaedics and Related Research, 439,* 27–31.

Joanna Briggs Institute. (2008). Solutions, techniques, and pressure in wound cleansing. *Nursing Standard, 22*(27), 35–39.
Moore, Z., & Cowman, S. (2008). A systematic review of wound cleansing for pressure ulcers. *Journal of Clinical Nursing, 17*(15), 1963–1972.
Nettina, S.M. (2010). *Lippincott manual of nursing practice* (9th ed.). Philadelphia, PA: Lippincott Williams & Wilkins.
Spear, M., et al. (2011). Wound cleansing: Solutions and techniques. *Plastic Surgical Nursing, 31,* 29–31.
Taylor, C., et al. (2011). *Fundamentals of nursing: The art and science of nursing care* (7th ed.). Philadelphia, PA: Lippincott Williams & Wilkins.

Z-TRACK INJECTION

The Z-track method of IM injection is the preferred method for administering IM injections because it prevents leakage, or tracking, of medication into the subcutaneous tissue. Lateral displacement of the skin during the injection helps to seal the drug in the muscle.

This procedure requires careful attention to technique because leakage into subcutaneous tissue can cause patient discomfort and may permanently stain some tissues.

Equipment

Patient's medication record and medical record ▪ two 20G 1¼" to 2" needles ▪ prescribed medication ▪ gloves ▪ 3- to 5-mL syringe ▪ two alcohol pads.

Preparation of equipment

Avoid distractions and interruptions when preparing and administering the medication to prevent medication errors.[1] Compare the medication label to the order and verify that the medication is correct.[1] Check the expiration date on the medication; don't give the medication if it has expired. Check the patient's medical record for an allergy to the prescribed medication. If an allergy is present, don't administer the medication; notify the doctor. Perform hand hygiene.[2,3,4]

Gather the appropriate equipment. Make sure the needle you're using is long enough to reach the muscle. As a rule of thumb, a 200-lb (91-kg) patient requires a 2" needle; a 100-lb (45-kg) patient, a 1¼" to 1½" needle.

Attach one needle to the syringe, and draw up the prescribed medication. Remove the first needle and attach the second *to prevent tracking the medication through the subcutaneous tissue as the needle is inserted.*

Implementation

▪ Verify the doctor's order.[1,5]
▪ Perform hand hygiene and put on gloves.[2,3,4]

Displacing the skin for Z-track injection

By blocking the needle pathway after injection, the Z-track technique allows IM injection while minimizing the risk of subcutaneous irritation and staining from such drugs as iron dextran. The illustrations below show how to perform a Z-track injection.

Before the procedure begins, the skin, subcutaneous fat, and muscle lie in their normal positions.

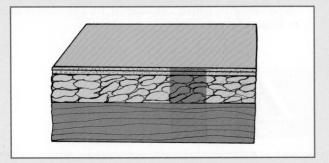

To begin, place your finger on the skin surface, and pull the skin and subcutaneous layers out of alignment with the underlying muscle. You should move the skin about ½″ (1 cm).

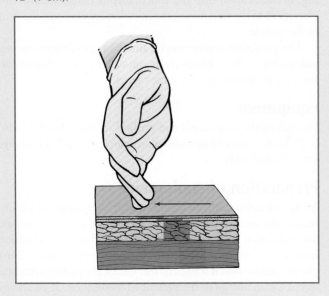

Insert the needle at a 90-degree angle at the site where you initially placed your finger. Inject the drug and withdraw the needle.

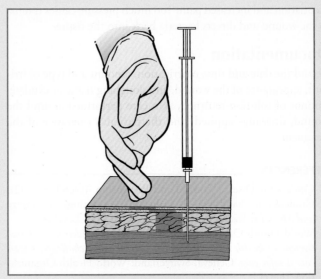

Finally, remove your finger from the skin surface, allowing the layers to return to their normal positions. The needle track is now broken at the junction of each tissue layer, trapping the drug in the muscle.

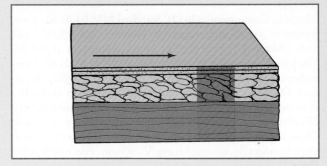

- Confirm the patient's identity using at least two patient identifiers according to your facility's policy.[6]
- If your facility uses a bar code scanning system, scan your identification badge, the patient's identification bracelet, and the medication's bar code.
- Explain the procedure to the patient and provide privacy.
- Expose the injection site.
- Clean the site with an alcohol pad.
- Displace the skin laterally by pulling it away from the injection site. (See *Displacing the skin for Z-track injection.*)

- Insert the needle into the muscle at a 90-degree angle.
- Aspirate for blood return if appropriate; if none appears, inject the drug slowly, followed by the air. *Injecting air after the drug helps clear the needle and prevents tracking the medication through subcutaneous tissues as the needle is withdrawn.*
- If blood appears, stop the injection, prepare a new syringe with medication, and inject it in another site.
- Wait 10 seconds before withdrawing the needle *to ensure dispersion of the medication.*

■ Withdraw the needle slowly. Then release the displaced skin and subcutaneous tissue *to seal the needle track*. Don't massage the injection site or allow the patient to wear a tight-fitting garment over the site *because it could force the medication into subcutaneous tissue*.
■ Encourage the patient to walk or to move about in bed *to facilitate absorption of the drug from the injection site*.
■ Discard the needles and syringe in an appropriate sharps container. Don't recap needles *to avoid needle-stick injuries*.
■ Remove and discard your gloves. Perform hand hygiene.[2,3,4]
■ Document the procedure.[7]

Special considerations

■ Never inject more than 5 mL of solution into a single site using the Z-track method. Alternate sites for repeat injections.
■ Always encourage the patient to relax the muscles you'll be injecting *because injections into tense muscle are more painful than usual and may bleed more readily*.
■ If the patient is on bed rest, encourage active range-of-motion (ROM) exercises or perform passive ROM exercises *to facilitate absorption from the injection site*.
■ IM injections can damage local muscle cells, causing elevated serum enzyme levels (for example, of creatine kinase) that can be confused with the elevated enzyme levels resulting from damage to cardiac muscle, as in myocardial infarction. If measuring enzyme levels is important, suggest that the doctor switch to IV administration and adjust dosages accordingly.

Complications

Discomfort and tissue irritation may result from drug leakage into subcutaneous tissue. Failure to rotate sites in patients who require repeated injections can interfere with the absorption of medication. Unabsorbed medications may build up in deposits. Such deposits can reduce the desired pharmacologic effect and may lead to abscess formation or tissue fibrosis.

Documentation

Record the medication, dosage, date, time, and site of injection on the patient's medication record. Include the patient's response to the injected drug.

REFERENCES

1 The Joint Commission. (2012). Standard MM.06.01.01. *Comprehensive accreditation manual for hospitals: The official handbook*. Oakbrook Terrace, IL: The Joint Commission. (Level I)
2 Centers for Disease Control and Prevention. (October 2002). Guideline for hand hygiene in health-care settings. *Morbidity and Mortality Weekly Report, 51*(RR-16), 1–45. (Level I)
3 World Health Organization. (2009). *WHO guidelines on hand hygiene in health care: First global patient safety challenge. Clean care is safer care.* Geneva, Switzerland: World Health Organization. (Level I)
4 The Joint Commission. (2012). Standard NPSG.07.01.01. *Comprehensive accreditation manual for hospitals: The official handbook*. Oakbrook Terrace, IL: The Joint Commission. (Level I)
5 The Joint Commission. (2012). Standard MM.04.01.01. *Comprehensive accreditation manual for hospitals: The official handbook*. Oakbrook Terrace, IL: The Joint Commission. (Level I)
6 The Joint Commission. (2012). Standard NPSG.01.01.01. *Comprehensive accreditation manual for hospitals: The official handbook*. Oakbrook Terrace, IL: The Joint Commission. (Level I)
7 The Joint Commission. (2012). Standard RC.01.03.01. *Comprehensive accreditation manual for hospitals: The official handbook*. Oakbrook Terrace, IL: The Joint Commission. (Level I)

ADDITIONAL REFERENCES

Gittens, G., & Bunnell, T. (2009). Skin disinfection and its efficacy before administering injections. *Nursing Standard, 23*(39), 42–44.
Hunt, C.W. (2008). Which site is best for an I.M. injection? *Nursing, 38*(11), 62.
Hunter, J. (2008). Intramuscular injection techniques. *Nursing Standard, 22*(24), 35–40.
Malkin, B. (2009). Are techniques used for intramuscular injection based on research evidence? *Nursing Times, 104*(50–51), 48–51.
Nettina, S.M. (2010). *Lippincott manual of nursing practice* (9th ed.). Philadelphia, PA: Lippincott Williams & Wilkins.
Westbrook, J. et al. (2010). Association of interruptions with an increased risk and severity of medication administration errors. *Archives of Internal Medicine, 170*(8), 683–690.

Index

---

i refers to an illustration; t refers to a table.

i refers to an illustration; t refers to a table.

i refers to an illustration; t refers to a table.

i refers to an illustration; t refers to a table.

---

i refers to an illustration; t refers to a table.

i refers to an illustration; t refers to a table.

i refers to an illustration; t refers to a table.

i refers to an illustration; t refers to a table.

i refers to an illustration; t refers to a table.

V

Vaginal medications, inserting, 780, 781i
Vaginal suppositories, administration of, 780
Valsalva's maneuver, teaching, 139
Vascular access device. *See* Implanted port.
Vascular access port. *See* Implanted port.
Vasopressin, 183t
Venipuncture, 781–783, 782t, 783i
  risks of, assessment for, 781
  sites for, 783i
Venous sheath removal, 27–29
Ventricular assist device (VAD), 784
  candidates for, 784–785
  caring for, 784–786
  for failing heart, 784, 784i
Ventricular drain insertion, 786–787
Venturi mask, 540i
Verapamil, 183t
Vest restraint, 631, 632
Visual pain rating scale, 545i
Vital signs
  electronic monitor, 79i
  recording of, on admission, 3
Volume-control sets, 788–789
Volumetric pumps, 438

W

Walkers, 790
  teaching safe use of, 790, 791i
Warming system, 350i
Washcloth mitt, making of, 49i

Water intoxication
  assessment of, 792–793
  signs and symptoms of, 792
Water mattress, 56, 57, 57i
Weight, measuring, 332–334
  guideline for determining healthy weights, 333
  scales for, 332i
Wheezing, 630
Winged infusion set, 422i
Wong-Baker FACES pain rating scale, 545i
World Health Organization (WHO), 325
  on hand hygiene, 325, 326i
Wound dehiscence and evisceration
  managing, 793–795
  recognizing, 794i
Wound irrigation, 795–797
Wound specimen collection, 693

X

Xylocaine. *See* Lidocaine.

Y

Yellow wounds, 685

Z

Z-track injection, 797–799
  displacing skin for, 798i